Laboratory Medicine

Test Selection and Interpretation

LABORATORY MEDICINE

Test Selection and Interpretation

Editors

Joan H. Howanitz, M.D.
Peter J. Howanitz, M.D.

Section Editors

P. Joanne Cornbleet, M.D., Ph.D.
Ron B. Schifman, M.D.
Lawrence D. Petz, M.D.

Churchill Livingstone
New York, Edinburgh, London, Melbourne, Tokyo

Library of Congress Cataloging-in-Publication Data

Laboratory medicine : test selection and interpretation / editors,
    Joan H. Howanitz, Peter J. Howanitz ; section editors, P. Joanne
    Cornbleet, Ron B. Schifman, Lawrence D. Petz.
           p.   cm.
       Includes bibliographical references and index.
       ISBN 0-443-08576-5
       1. Diagnosis, Laboratory.   I. Howanitz, Joan H. II. Howanitz,
    Peter J.
       [DNLM: 1. Diagnosis, Laboratory. 2. Diagnostic Tests, Routine.
    QY 4 L1233]
    RB37.L2752 1991
    616.07'5—dc20
    DNLM/DLC
    for Library of Congress   91-23261
                                                                   CIP

© Churchill Livingstone Inc. 1991

All rights reserved. No part of this publication may be reproduced, stored in a retrieval system, or transmitted in any form or by any means, electronic, mechanical, photocopying, recording, or otherwise, without prior permission of the publisher (Churchill Livingstone Inc., 650 Avenue of the Americas, New York, NY 10011).

Distributed in the United Kingdom by Churchill Livingstone, Robert Stevenson House, 1–3 Baxter's Place, Leith Walk, Edinburgh EH1 3AF, and by associated companies, branches, and representatives throughout the world.

Accurate indications, adverse reactions, and dosage schedules for drugs are provided in this book, but it is possible that they may change. The reader is urged to review the package information data of the manufacturers of the medications mentioned.

The Publishers have made every effort to trace the copyright holders for borrowed material. If they have inadvertently overlooked any, they will be pleased to make the necessary arrangements at the first opportunity.

Acquisitions Editor: *Beth Kaufman Barry*
Assistant Acquisitions Editor: *Nancy Terry*
Copy Editor: *Bridgett Dickinson*
Production Designer: *Patricia McFadden*
Production Supervisor: *Sharon Tuder*
Indexer: *Irving Conde Tullar*
Printed in the United States of America

First published in 1991   7 6 5 4 3 2 1

Contributors

Bruce Ackerman, Pharm.D.
Associate Professor, Department of Pharmacy Practice, College of Pharmacy, University of Arkansas for Medical Sciences; Consultant, Clinical Pharmacokinetic Monitoring Service, University of Arkansas Medical Center, Little Rock, Arkansas

John K. Ashton, M.D.
Clinical Professor, Department of Pathology, University of Medicine and Dentistry of New Jersey–Robert Wood Johnson Medical School, Piscataway, New Jersey; Director of Laboratories, Department of Pathology, Muhlenberg Regional Medical Center, Plainfield, New Jersey

Robert Astarita, M.D.
Clinical Professor, Department of Pathology, University of California, San Diego, School of Medicine; Chief, Anatomical Pathology, Veterans Affairs Medical Center, La Jolla, California

Leona W. Ayers, M.D.
Associate Professor, Department of Pathology, Ohio State University College of Medicine; Division Director, Departments of Clinical Microbiology and Hospital Epidemiology, Ohio State University Hospital, Columbus, Ohio

James Baker, M.D.
Clinical Professor, Department of Pathology, University of California, Irvine, School of Medicine, Irvine, California; Associate Pathologist, Department of Pathology, Memorial Hospital, Long Beach, California

Robert C. Barnes, M.D.
Clinical Assistant Professor, Infectious Diseases Section, Emory University School of Medicine; Chief, Chlamydia Section, Sexually Transmitted Diseases Laboratory Program, Centers for Disease Control, Atlanta, Georgia

John T. Brandt, M.D.
Associate Professor, Department of Pathology, Ohio State University College of Medicine; Associate Director of Clinical Laboratories, and Director of Laboratory Hematology, Department of Pathology, Ohio State University Hospitals, Columbus, Ohio

Joseph M. Campos, Ph.D.
Associate Professor, Departments of Pediatrics, Pathology, and Microbiology/Immunology, George Washington University School of Medicine and Health Sciences; Director, Microbiology Laboratory, Department of Laboratory Medicine, Children's National Medical Center, Washington, D.C.

P. Joanne Cornbleet, M.D., Ph.D.
Associate Professor, Department of Pathology, Stanford University School of Medicine, Stanford, California

Robert De Cresce, M.D.
Assistant Professor, Department of Clinical Pathology, University of Illinois College of Medicine; Acting Chief, Department of Pathology, Humana Hospital—Michael Reese, Chicago, Illinois

John H. Eckfeldt, M.D., Ph.D.
Associate Professor, Department of Laboratory Medicine and Pathology, University of Minnesota Medical School—Minneapolis; Director, Clinical Chemistry Section, University of Minnesota Hospital and Clinic, Minneapolis, Minnesota

Daniel J. Fink, M.D., M.P.H.
Associate Clinical Professor, Department of Pathology, Columbia University College of Physicians and Surgeons; Associate Director, Laboratory Information Services, Columbia Presbyterian Hospital, New York, New York

Thomas R. Fritsche, M.D., Ph.D.
Associate Professor, Departments of Laboratory Medicine and Microbiology, University of Washington School of Medicine; Associate Director, Clinical Microbiology Laboratory, University of Washington Medical Center, Seattle, Washington

Paul C. Fu, Ph.D.
Professor, Department of Pathology and Laboratory Medicine, University of California, Los Angeles, UCLA School of Medicine, Los Angeles, California; Director of Clinical Biochemistry and Toxicology, Department of Pathology, Harbor UCLA Medical Center, Torrance, California

Peter C. Fuchs, M.D., Ph.D.
Director of Microbiology, Department of Pathology, St. Vincent Hospital and Medical Center, Portland, Oregon

Wayne W. Grody, M.D., Ph.D.
Assistant Professor, Department of Pathology and Laboratory Medicine, University of California, Los Angeles, UCLA School of Medicine; Co-Director, Diagnostic Molecular Pathology Laboratory, UCLA Medical Center, Los Angeles, California

Gene L. Gulati, Ph.D., S.H.(A.S.C.P.)
Clinical Associate Professor, Department of Pathology, Jefferson Medical College of Thomas Jefferson University; Assistant Director of Hematology, Clinical Laboratories, Thomas Jefferson University Hospital, Philadelphia, Pennsylvania

James A. Harker, M.D.
Resident, Department of Pathology, University of Illinois College of Medicine; Resident, Department of Pathology, Humana Hospital—Michael Reese, Chicago, Illinois

Mary Jane Hicks, M.D.
Pathologist, Tucson Pathology Associates, Carondelet–St. Joseph's Hospital, Tucson, Arizona

Lee H. Hilborne, M.D., M.P.H.
Assistant Professor, Departments of Medicine and Pathology and Laboratory Medicine, University of California, Los Angeles, UCLA School of Medicine; Physician Advisor, Quality Management Services, UCLA Medical Center, Los Angeles, California

Joan H. Howanitz, M.D.
Professor and Vice Chair, Department of Pathology and Laboratory Medicine, University of California, Los Angeles, UCLA School of Medicine; Chief, Laboratory Service, West Los Angeles Veterans Administration Medical Center, Los Angeles, California

Peter J. Howanitz, M.D.
Professor, Department of Pathology and Laboratory Medicine, University of California, Los Angeles, UCLA School of Medicine; Director, Clinical Laboratories, UCLA Medical Center, Los Angeles, California

Bong Hak Hyun, M.D., D.Sc.
Clinical Professor, Department of Pathology and Cell Biology, Jefferson Medical College of Thomas Jefferson University; Director of Hematology, Clinical Laboratories, Thomas Jefferson University Hospital, Philadelphia, Pennsylvania

Henry D. Isenberg, Ph.D.
Professor, Department of Laboratory Medicine, Long Island Campus for Albert Einstein College of Medicine; Chief of Microbiology, Department of Clinical Pathology, Long Island Jewish Medical Center, New Hyde Park, New York

William Jones, M.S.
Adjunct Clinical Professor, Department of Pharmacy Practice, University of Arizona College of Pharmacy; Clinical Pharmacy Supervisor, Department of Pharmacy Service, Tucson Veterans Affairs Medical Center, Tucson, Arizona

Gerald Lancz, Ph.D.
Associate Professor, Department of Medical Microbiology and Immunology, University of South Florida College of Medicine, Tampa, Florida

Allen I. Lipsey, M.D., M.P.A.
Associate Professor of Clinical Pathology, Departments of Pathology and Pediatrics, University of Southern California School of Medicine; Director, Clinical Laboratories, Children's Hospital, Los Angeles, California

James H. McBride, Ph.D.
Assistant Professor, Department of Pathology and Laboratory Medicine, University of California, Los Angeles, UCLA School of Medicine; Assistant Head of Clinical Chemistry, UCLA Medical Center, Los Angeles, California

Robert M. Nakamura, M.D.
Adjunct Professor, Department of Pathology, University of California, San Diego, School of Medicine; Chairman, Department of Pathology, Scripps Clinic Research Foundation, La Jolla, California

Amin Nanji, M.D., F.R.C.P.C., M.R.C.Path.
Associate Professor, Department of Pathology, Harvard Medical School; Chief of Clinical Biochemistry, Department of Pathology, New England Deaconess Hospital, Boston, Massachusetts

Alex A. Pappas, M.D.
Associate Professor, Department of Pathology, College of Medicine, University of Arkansas for Medical Sciences; Director, Department of Clinical Laboratories, University of Arkansas for Medical Sciences, Little Rock, Arkansas

Lawrence D. Petz, M.D.
Professor, Department of Pathology and Laboratory Medicine, University of California, Los Angeles, UCLA School of Medicine; Director of Transfusion Medicine, UCLA Medical Center, Los Angeles, California

Ales Pindur, M.D.
Fellow of Clinical Microbiology, Department of Pathology, University of Arizona College of Medicine, Tucson, Arizona

Joseph Rindone, Pharm.D.
Adjunct Clinical Professor, Department of Pharmacy Practice, University of Arizona College of Medicine; Clinical Pharmacist, Department of Pharmacy, Tucson Veterans Affairs Medical Center, Tucson, Arizona

Denis O. Rodgerson, Ph.D.
Professor, Department of Pathology and Laboratory Medicine, University of California, Los Angeles, UCLA School of Medicine; Head of Clinical Chemistry, UCLA Medical Center, Los Angeles, California

Leonard Rossoff, M.D.
Assistant Professor, Department of Internal Medicine, Long Island Campus for Albert Einstein College of Medicine; Head of Critical Care, Pulmonary Division, Department of Medicine, Long Island Jewish Medical Center, New Hyde Park, New York

Michael A. Saubolle, Ph.D.
Director, Microbiology Sections, Department of Pathology, Good Samaritan Hospital and Medical Center, Phoenix, Arizona

Ron B. Schifman, M.D.
Associate Professor, Department of Pathology, University of Arizona College of Medicine; Director of Clinical Pathology, Department of Pathology, Tucson Veterans Affairs Medical Center, Tucson, Arizona

George P. Schmid, M.D.
Clinical Associate Professor of Medicine, Departments of Medicine and Microbiology Epidemiology, Morehouse School of Medicine; Chief, Clinical Research Branch, Division of Sexually Transmitted Diseases/HIV Prevention, Center for Prevention Services, Centers for Disease Control, Atlanta, Georgia

Elizabeth Sengupta, M.D.
Instructor, Department of Pathology, University of Chicago Division of the Biological Sciences Pritzker School of Medicine; Attending Pathologist, Department of Pathology, University of Chicago Hospitals and Clinics, Billings Hospital, Chicago, Illinois

Steven Specter, Ph.D.
Professor, Department of Medical Microbiology and Immunology, University of South Florida College of Medicine, Tampa, Florida

E. Howard Taylor, Ph.D.
Laboratory Director, Substance Abuse Division, National Reference Laboratory, Nashville, Tennessee

Ernest S. Tucker III, M.D.
Clinical Professor, Department of Pathology, University of California, School of Medicine, San Francisco; Chairman, Department of Pathology, Pacific Presbyterian Medical Center, San Francisco, California

Raymond Widen, Ph.D.
Assistant Professor, Department of Medical Microbiology and Immunology, University of South Florida College of Medicine; Director, Virology Laboratory, Tampa General Hospital, Tampa, Florida

Paul L. Wolf, M.D.
Clinical Professor, Department of Pathology and Laboratory Medicine, University of California, San Diego, School of Medicine; Director of Autopsy, Veterans Affairs Medical Center, La Jolla, California

Preface

Laboratory testing is an integral part of medicine, both in the diagnosis of disease as well as in the monitoring of patients during therapy. Selection of appropriate tests, however, is often problematic. Clinicians treating patients must know the effectiveness and limitations of various testing strategies. Laboratory technicians must know how to correlate and coordinate testing performed in all areas of the clinical laboratory.

Laboratory Medicine presents a rationale for the collection and processing of clinical specimens, for general methodology and analytic approaches, and for the interpretation of test results. Essentially, the book addresses two important questions facing physicians and laboratory technicians: What test(s) should be ordered and how should the results be interpreted?

For easy access to information, the book is organized around the clinician's order, namely the specific tests, rather than by disease entity. Tests are subdivided along traditional laboratory disciplines: chemistry, hematology, microbiology, immunology, and blood banking (transfusion medicine). In the chemistry, hematology, and immunology sections, organization is based on the clinician's order for a specific test. For microbiology, the format is based on the specimen collected, and in blood banking, the product requested.

Individual chapters within each of these sections cover laboratory methods as related to specific tests. Chapter 1 addresses general principles in conducting and interpreting tests and explains how information can be found in the standard chapter format. Each chapter is subdivided into groups of tests, with each test organized around a standard format. The specific sections in the test format are *test selection and background* (when and why the test is indicated and, where appropriate, background material relating to the test is included); *logistics* (patient preparation, specimen collection, and laboratory analysis); and *interpretation of results* (including reference ranges). For test groups for which the pattern of results is important, a separate section of pattern interpretation is included.

As laboratory testing often determines the course of diagnosis and treatment, it is a central facet of medical care. *Laboratory Medicine* was written to make the process of test selection and interpretation more accessible to all categories of laboratory workers, non-laboratory based clinicians, residents, and medical technology students. We believe that it will increase the effectiveness of laboratory testing for all involved, but particularly for the patients in our care.

Joan H. Howanitz, M.D.
Peter J. Howanitz, M.D.

Contents

Color Insert		xvii
1.	**Principles of Laboratory Medicine** Joan H. Howanitz and Peter J. Howanitz	1

Chemistry

2.	**Pulmonary and Cardiac Function** Daniel J. Fink and James A. Harker	11
3.	**Renal Function** Denis O. Rodgerson	41
4.	**Liver Function** Paul L. Wolf	67
5.	**Pancreatic and Gastrointestinal Function** Lee H. Hilborne and John H. Eckfeldt	85
6.	**Body Fluids** Amin Nanji	107
7.	**Carbohydrates** Peter J. Howanitz and Joan H. Howanitz	127
8.	**Amino Acids and Proteins** James H. McBride	143
9.	**Lipids, Lipoproteins, and Apolipoproteins** Paul C. Fu	173
10.	**Metals, Vitamins, and Nutritional Factors** Robert De Cresce and Elizabeth Sengupta	199

11.	**Hormones** Joan H. Howanitz and Peter J. Howanitz	237
12.	**Serum Tumor Markers** Peter J. Howanitz and Joan H. Howanitz	307
13.	**Therapeutic Drug Monitoring** Bruce Ackerman and Alex A. Pappas	333
14.	**Toxicology and Drugs of Abuse** Alex A. Pappas, E. Howard Taylor, and Bruce Ackerman	369
15.	**Pregnancy and Genetics** Wayne W. Grody, Peter J. Howanitz, and Allen I. Lipsey	399

Hematology

16.	**Hematopoiesis and Blood Cell Morphology** Bong Hak Hyun, Gene L. Gulati, and John K. Ashton	425
17.	**Erythrocyte Disorders** James Baker and P. Joanne Cornbleet	447
18.	**Hemostasis** John T. Brandt	499
19.	**White Blood Cell and Platelet Disorders** P. Joanne Cornbleet, Robert Astarita, and Paul L. Wolf	553

Microbiology/Immunology

20.	**Blood and Bone Marrow** Thomas R. Fritsche, Gerald Lancz, Ron B. Schifman, and Steven Specter	619
21.	**Eye, Ear, Nose, and Throat** Joseph M. Campos, Thomas R. Fritsche, Gerald Lancz, Ron B. Schifman, and Steven Specter	635
22.	**Lower Respiratory Tract Specimens** Henry D. Isenberg, Thomas R. Fritsche, Gerald Lancz, Steven Specter, Ron B. Schifman, and Leonard Rossoff	655
23.	**Skin, Wound, and Tissue Specimens** Leona W. Ayers, Thomas R. Fritsche, Gerald Lancz, Ales Pindur, and Steven Specter	675
24.	**Urine** Thomas R. Fritsche, Gerald Lancz, Ron B. Schifman, and Steven Specter	721

25.	**Genital Tract** George P. Schmid, Robert C. Barnes, and Thomas R. Fritsche	733
26.	**Gastrointestinal Tract** Joseph M. Campos, Thomas R. Fritsche, Gerald Lancz, and Steven Specter	747
27.	**Central Nervous System** Joseph M. Campos, Thomas R. Fritsche, Gerald Lancz, and Steven Specter	769
28.	**Antimicrobial Therapy** *Part I. In Vitro Susceptibility* Peter C. Fuchs *Part II. Therapeutic Monitoring of Antibiotics* Joseph Rindone and William Jones	787
29.	**Serodiagnosis of Infectious Disease** Thomas R. Fritsche, Gerald Lancz, Ron B. Schifman, Steven Specter, Michael A. Saubolle, and Raymond Widen	803
30.	**Diagnostic Immunology** *Part I. Humoral Immunology* Ernest S. Tucker III and Robert M. Nakamura *Part II. Cellular Immunology* Mary Jane Hicks	835

Blood Bank

31.	**Blood Bank and Transfusion Service** Lawrence D. Petz	865

Index

897

Color Plates

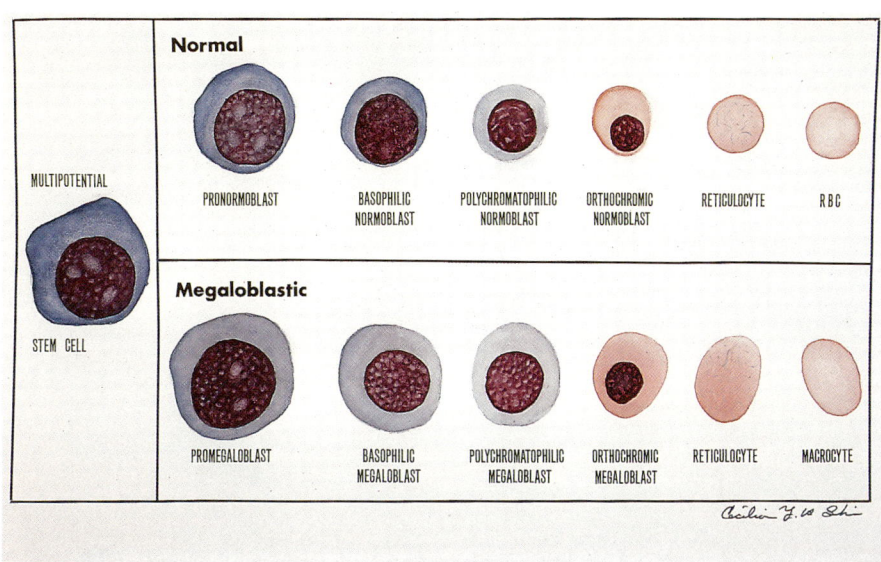

Plate 1

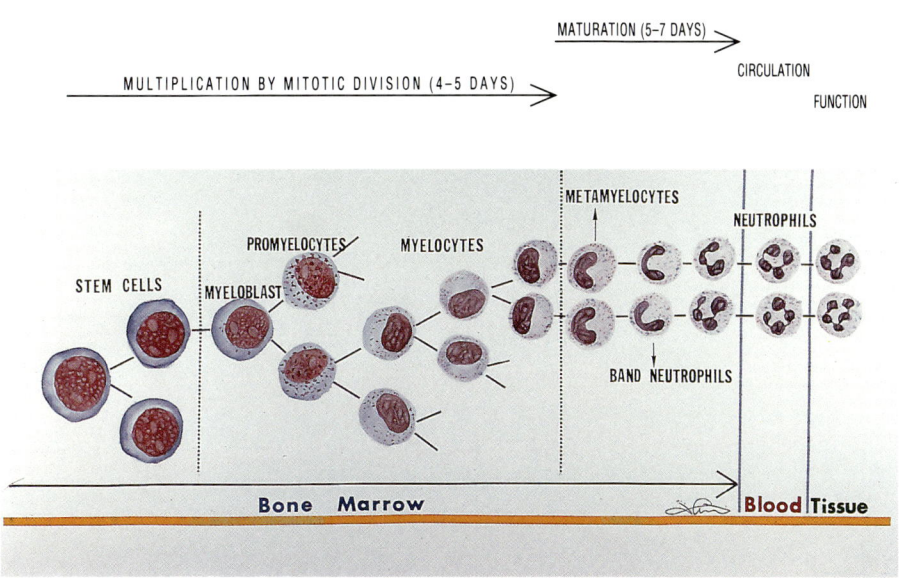

Plate 2

Plate 1. Maturation of the erythrocytic series. (From Hyun et al.,[13] with permission.)

Plate 2. Maturation of the granulocytic series. (From Hyun et al.,[13] with permission.)

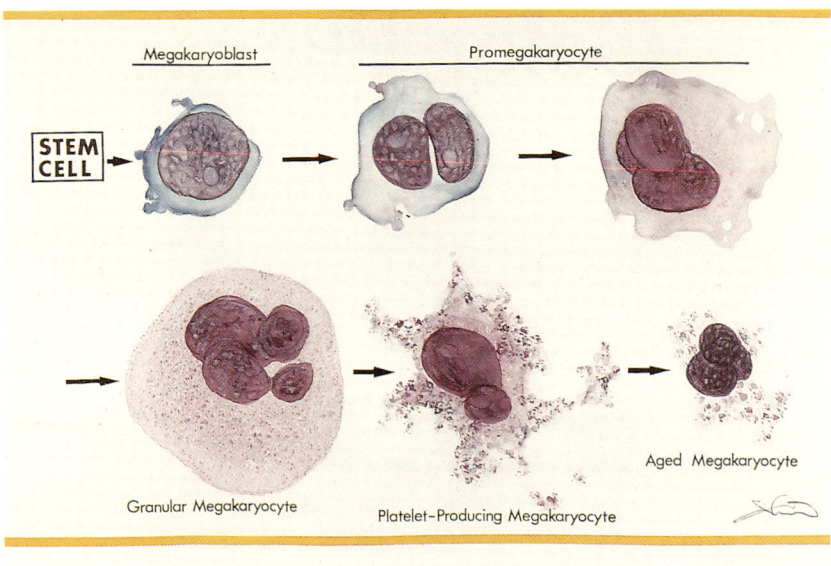

Plate 3

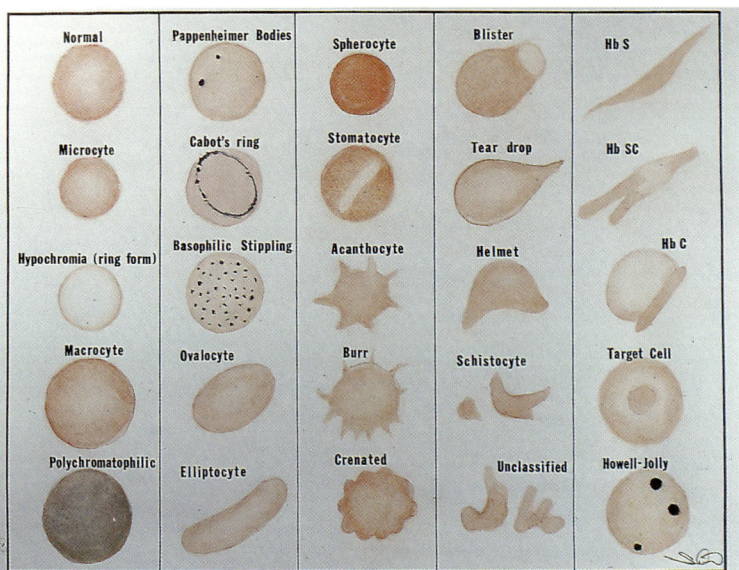

Plate 4

Plate 3. Maturation of the megakaryocytic series. (From Hyun et al.,[13] with permission.)

Plate 4. Red blood cell morphology. (From Hyun et al.,[13] with permission.)

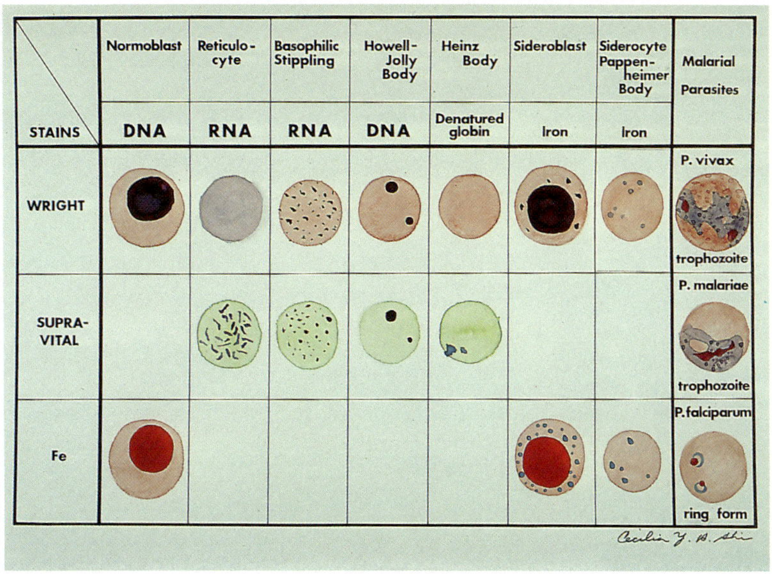

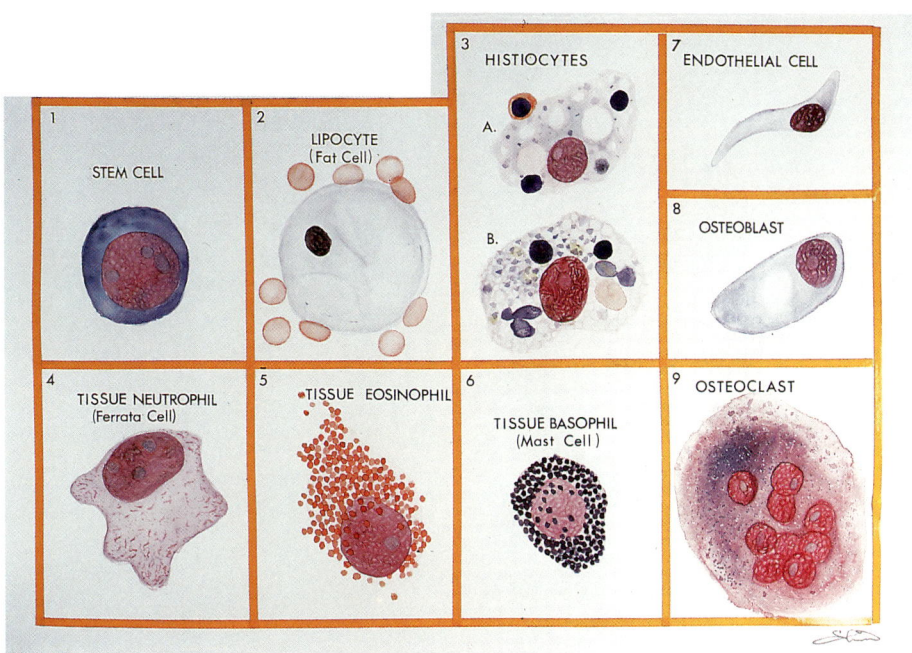

Plate 5. Red blood cell inclusions. (From Hyun et al.,[13] with permission.)

Plate 6. Cells occasionally found in the bone marrow film. (From Hyun et al.,[13] with permission.)

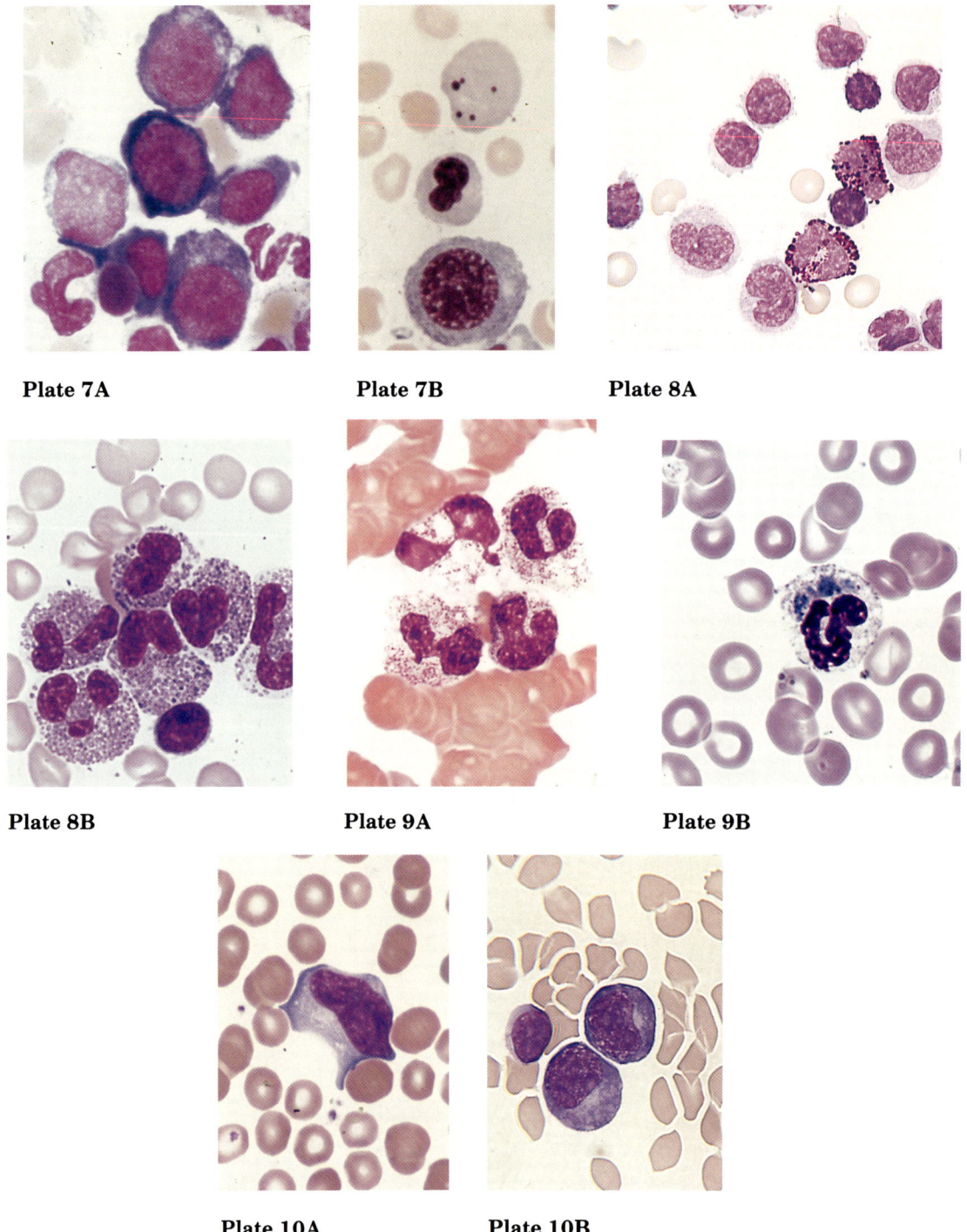

Plate 7. Pernicious anemia. **(A)** Numerous promegaloblasts. **(B)** Polychromatophilic megaloblast, orthochromic megaloblast with irregular nuclear shape, and large polychromatophilic red blood cell with many Howell-Jolly bodies. Bone marrow specimens. (Wright-Giemsa stain, 400×.)

Plate 8. Miscellaneous normal leukocytes. **(A)** Lymphocytes, monocytes, and basophils. Peripheral blood specimen. (Wright-Giemsa stain, 313×.) **(B)** Eosinophils. Peripheral blood specimen. (Wright-Giemsa stain, 400×.)

Plate 9. **(A)** Toxic granulation and vacuoles in neutrophils. Peripheral blood specimen. (Wright-Giesma stain, 400×.) **(B)** Döhle bodies in band neutrophil. Peripheral blood specimen. (Wright-Giemsa stain, 400×.)

Plate 10. **(A)** Reactive lymphocyte. Peripheral blood specimen. (Wright-Giemsa stain, 400×.) **(B)** Plasmacytoid reactive lymphocytes. Peripheral blood specimen. (Wright-Giemsa stain, 400×.)

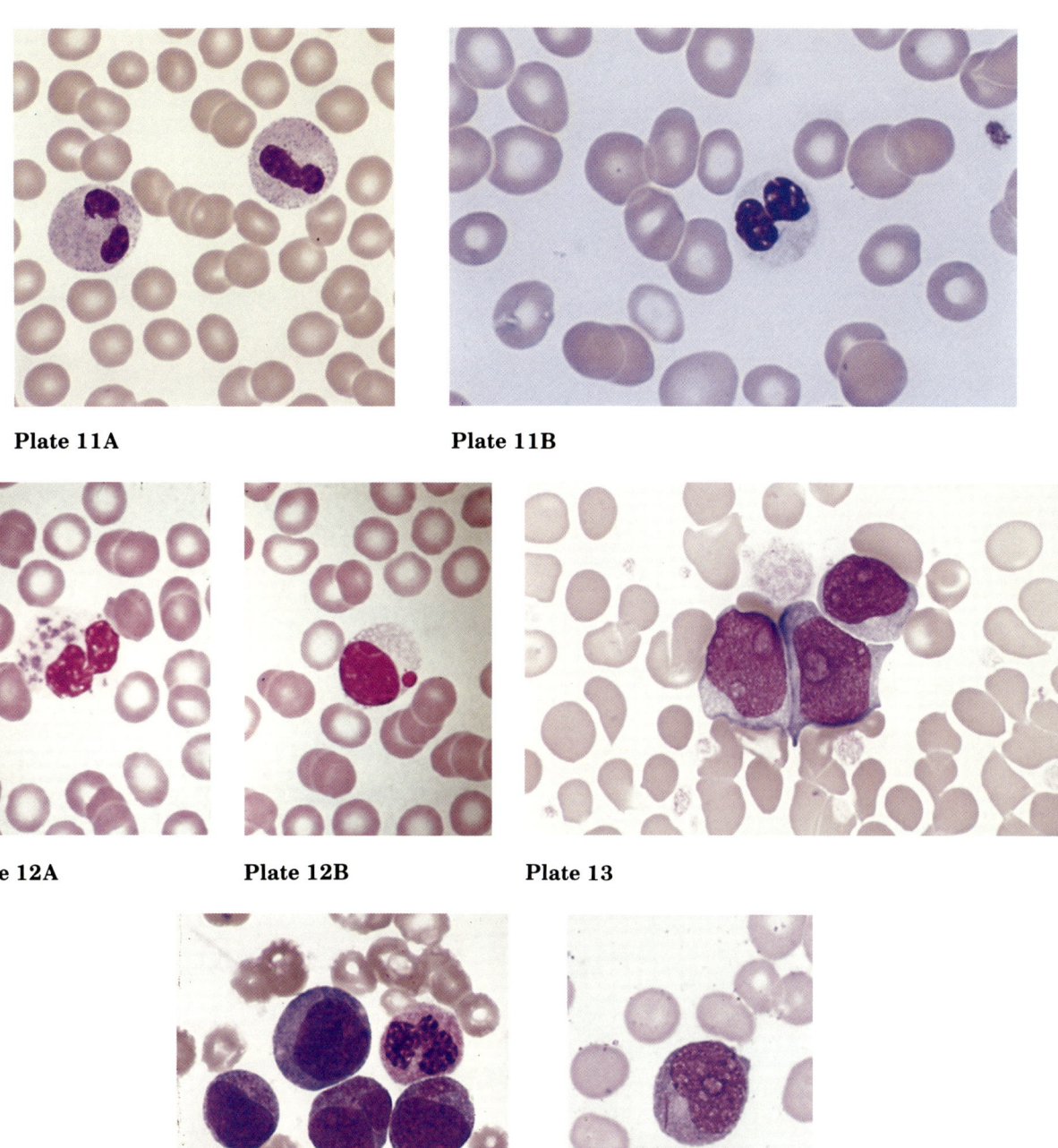

Plate 11. (A) Pelger-Huët anomaly, abnormal nuclear lobation. Peripheral blood specimen. (Wright-Giesma stain, 400×.) (B) Dysplastic neutrophil in myelodysplastic syndrome. Pseudo-Pelger-Huët nuclear change and agranular cytoplasm can be seen. Peripheral blood specimen. (Wright-Giemsa stain, 400×.)

Plate 12. Chédiak-Higashi disease. (A) Neutrophil with giant azurophilic granules. (B) Lymphocyte with large pink cytoplasmic granule. Peripheral blood specimen. (Wright-Giemsa stain, 400×.)

Plate 13. Acute myelocytic leukemia, M1. Myeloblasts. Peripheral blood specimen. (Wright-Giemsa stain, 400×.)

Plate 14. Acute myelocytic leukemia, M2. (A) Myeloblast, myelocytes, and a neutrophil with dysplastic (pelgeroid) nucleus. (B) Myeloblast with Auer body. Peripheral blood specimens. (Wright-Giemsa stain, 400×.)

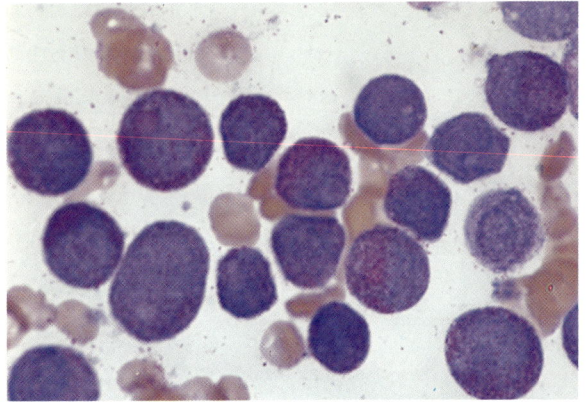
Plate 15

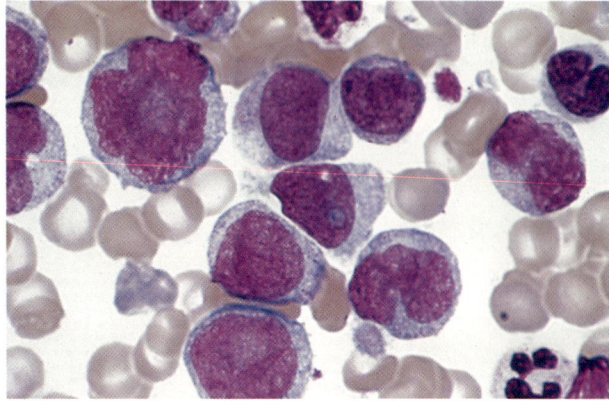
Plate 16

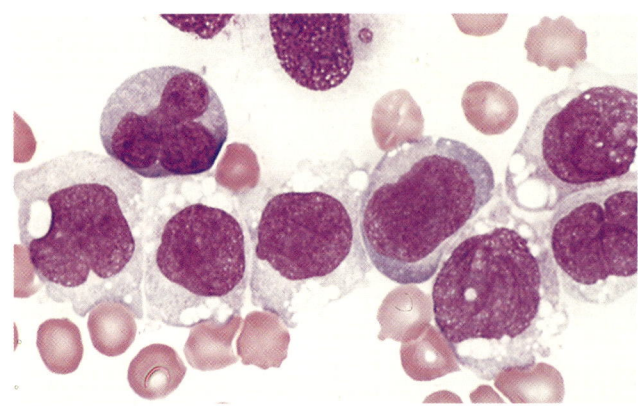
Plate 17

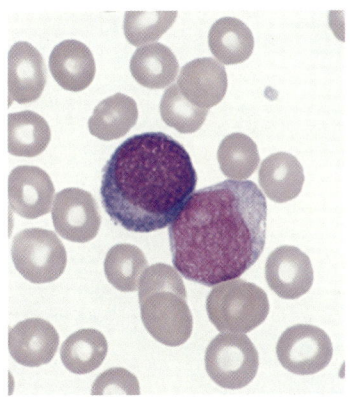
Plate 18A

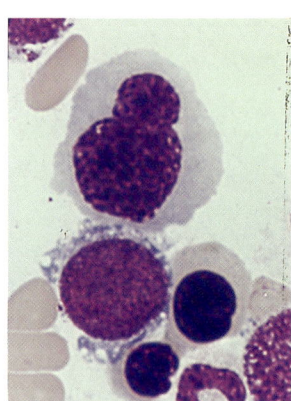
Plate 18B

Plate 15. Acute myelocytic leukemia, M3 (promyelocytic). Many hypergranular promyelocytes may be seen. Peripheral blood specimen. (Wright-Giemsa stain, 400×.)

Plate 16. Acute myelocytic leukemia, M4 (myelomonocytic). Myeloblasts with some monocytoid cells. Peripheral blood specimen. (Wright-Giemsa stain, 400×.)

Plate 17. Acute myelocytic leukemia, M5 (monocytic). Monoblasts with indented nuclei and large amount of cytoplasm. Peripheral blood specimen. (Wright-Giemsa stain, 400×.)

Plate 18. Acute myelocytic leukemia, M6 (erythroleukemia). **(A)** Myeloblast and pronormoblast. Peripheral blood specimen. (Wright-Giemsa stain, 400×.) **(B)** Leukemic erythroblasts. Bone marrow specimen. (Wright-Giemsa stain, 400×.)

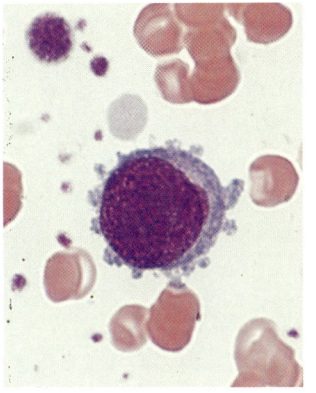
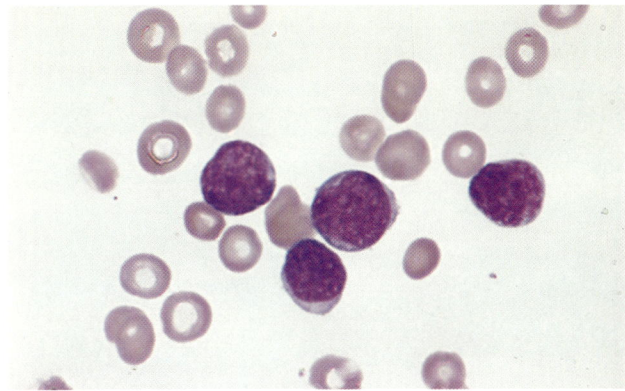

Plate 19   Plate 20

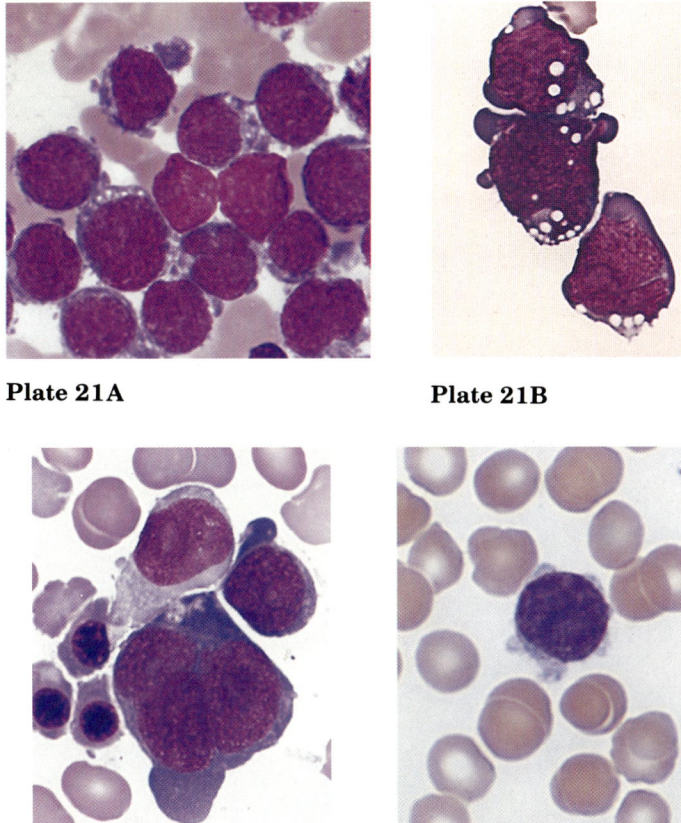

Plate 21A   Plate 21B

Plate 22A   Plate 22B

Plate 19. Acute myelocytic leukemia, M7 (megakaryocytic). Megakaryoblast. Peripheral blood specimen. (Wright-Giemsa stain, 400×.)

Plate 20. Acute lymphocytic leukemia, L1. Small lymphoblasts with sparse cytoplasm. Peripheral blood specimen. (Wright-Giemsa stain, 400×.)

Plate 21. Acute lymphocytic leukemia, L3 (Burkitt's leukemia/lymphoma). **(A)** Lymphoblsts. Bone marrow specimen. (Wright-Giemsa stain, 400×.) **(B)** Blasts in pleural fluid. (Wright-Giemsa stain, 400×.)

Plate 22. Myelodysplastic syndrome. **(A)** Multinucleate erythroblast, megaloblastoid polychromatophilic normoblasts, and two myeloblasts. Bone marrow specimen. **(B)** Micromegakaryocyte. Peripheral blood specimens. (Wright-Giemsa stain, 400×.)

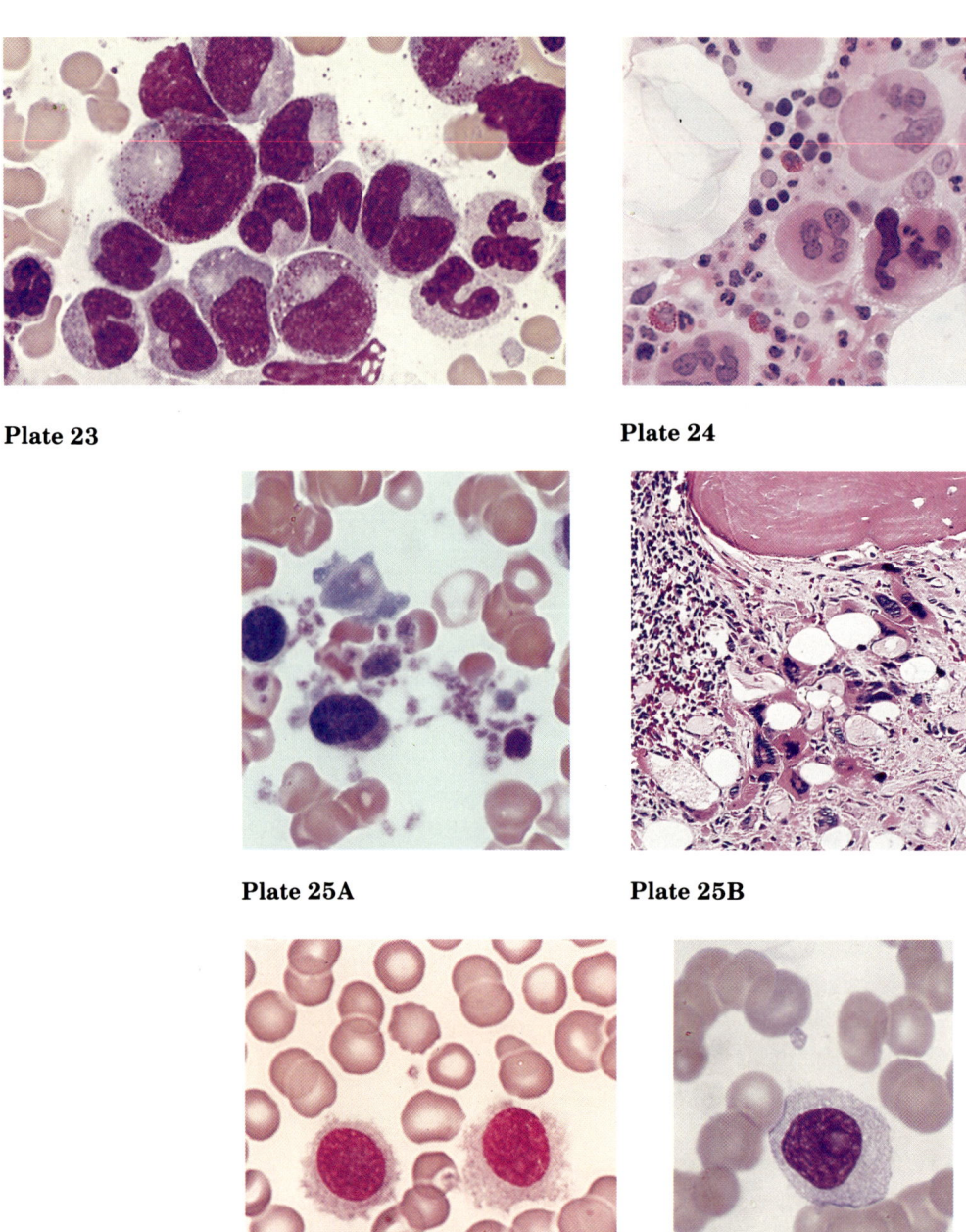

Plate 23. Chronic myelocytic leukemia. Neutrophilia with granulocytes in varying stages of development. Peripheral blood specimen. (Wright-Giemsa stain, 400×.)

Plate 24. Myeloproliferative disorder, idiopathic thrombocythemia type. Bone marrow specimen. (H&E stain, 160×.)

Plate 25. Myeloproliferative disorder, myelofibrosis with myeloid metaplasia. (A) Thrombocytosis with giant platelets and micromegakaryocytes. Peripheral blood specimen. (Wright-Giemsa stain, 400×.) (B) Marrow fibrosis and megakaryocytosis. Bone marrow specimen. (H&E stain, 160×.)

Plate 26. (A) Hairy cell leukemia (leukemic reticuloendotheliosis). Medium-sized lymphoid cells with hairy cytoplasm. (B) Prolymphocytic leukemia. Large prolymphocyte with abundant cytoplasm and prominent nucleolus. Peripheral blood specimens. (Wright-Giemsa stain, 400×.)

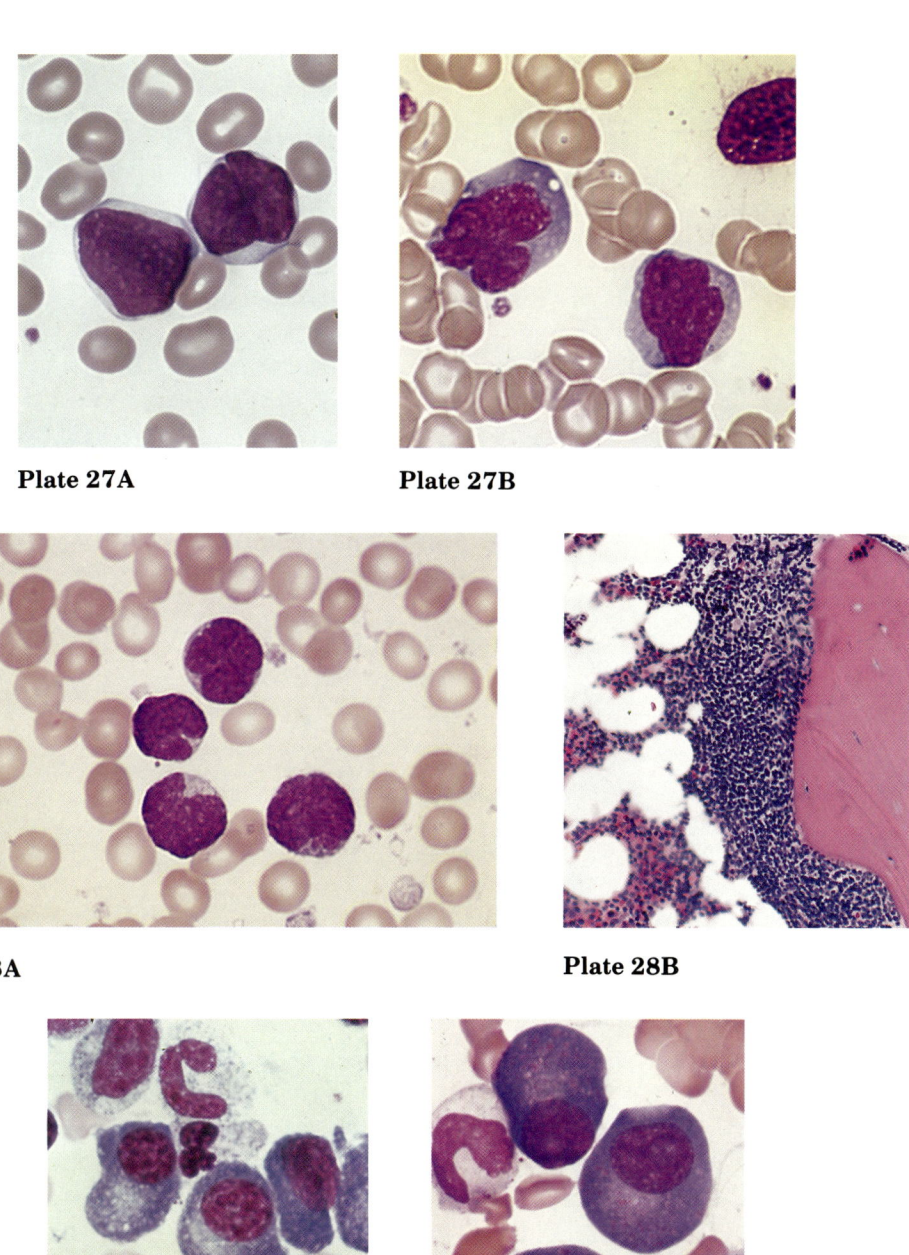

Plate 27. **(A)** Sézary syndrome, large cell type. Large convoluted nuclei with scanty cytoplasm. **(B)** Large cell lymphoma, leukemia phase. Large blastic cells with irregular-shaped nuclei and basophilic cytoplasm. Peripheral blood specimens. (Wright-Giemsa stain, 400×.)

Plate 28. **(A)** Follicular small cleaved cell lymphoma, leukemic phase. Small lymphs have very high nuclear to cytoplasmic (N/C) ratio with hypercondensed nuclear chromatin. Peripheral blood specimen. (Wright-Giemsa stain, 160×.) **(B)** Follicular small cleaved cell lymphoma. Paratrabecular lymphoid infiltrate. Bone marrow specimen. (H&E stain, 160×.)

Plate 29. **(A)** Reactive plasmacytosis in bone marrow. Mature plasma cells. **(B)** Multiple myeloma. Malignant plasma cells with nucleoli. Bone marrow specimens. (Wright-Giemsa stain, 400×.)

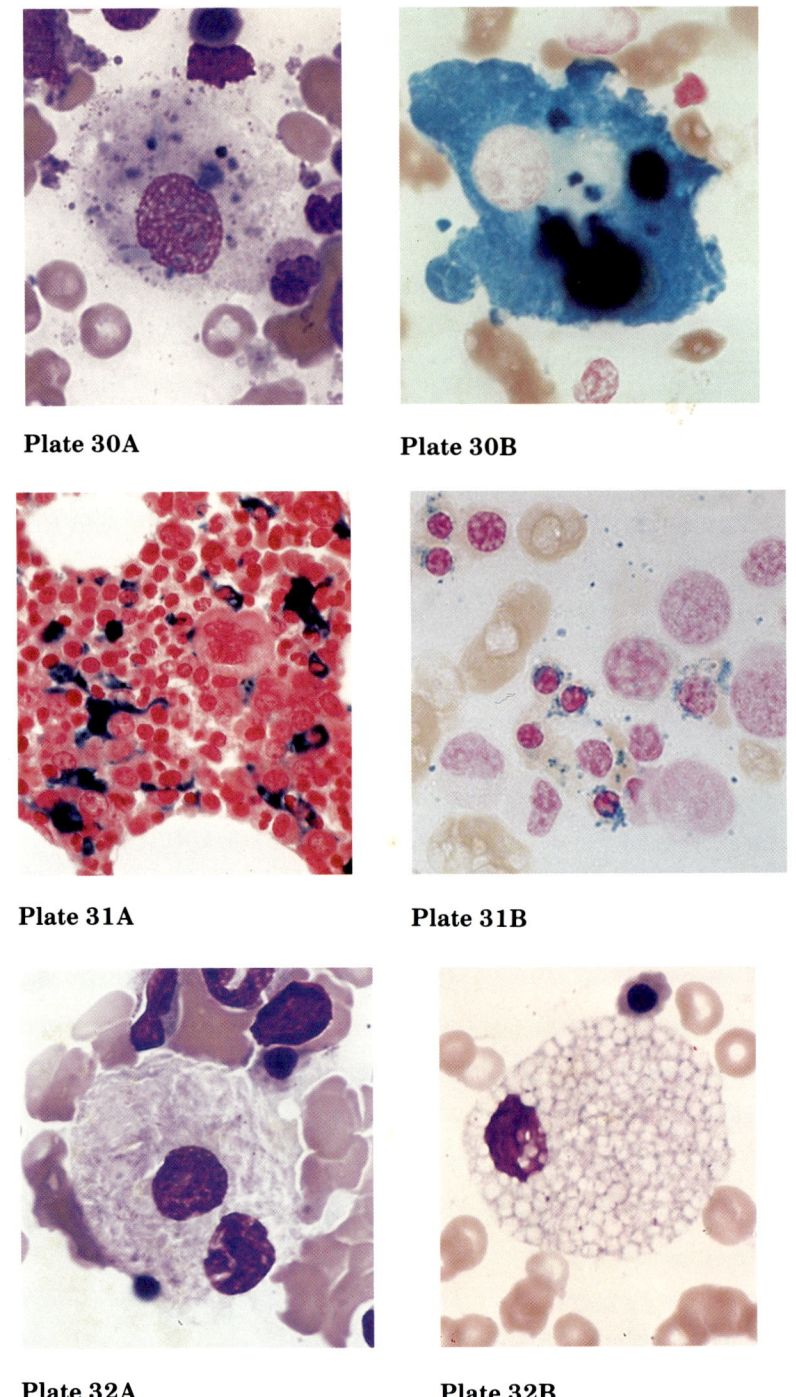

Plate 30. **(A)** Histiocyte (macrophage) containing hemosiderin particles. Bone marrow specimen. (Wright-Giemsa stain, 400×.) **(B)** Histiocyte with excess iron deposit. Bone marrow specimen. (Prussian blue stain, 400×.)

Plate 31. **(A)** Increased iron in macrophages in aspartate section. (Prussian blue stain, 160×.) **(B)** Myelodysplastic syndrome, refractory anemia with ringed sideroblasts. Bone marrow specimen. Prussian blue stain, 400×.)

Plate 32. **(A)** Gaucher's disease. A Gaucher cell (histiocyte) with reticular cytoplasm. **(B)** Niemann-Pick disease. Foamy histiocyte is characteristic but not specific. Bone marrow specimens. (Wright-Giemsa stain, 400×.)

1 Principles of Laboratory Medicine

Joan H. Howanitz
Peter J. Howanitz

INTRODUCTION

In the United States, we spend about $27 billion a year on laboratory tests.[1] Reasons for this heavy reliance on laboratory testing have been attributed to the physician's fear of litigation and lack of clinical skills. Another explanation for this phenomenon is that medicine, in aspiring to be a science, requires "hard" data. Therefore, laboratory results have become an important part of the database from which medical decisions are made. Laboratory personnel attempt to provide precise and accurate tests performed in a timely manner, but for optimum cost-effective patient care, clinicians must select appropriate tests or sets of tests and must properly interpret the results. Over-reliance on laboratory tests is expensive and dangerous. This introductory chapter addresses the general principles of laboratory medicine that are essential to understanding prudent test selection and correct interpretation of results.

LABORATORY TESTS

A laboratory test begins with proper test selection and proceeds through patient preparation, specimen acquisition and processing, laboratory analysis, reporting, and interpretation of results (Fig 1-1).

Test Selection

Laboratory tests usually are ordered for one of three main reasons: (1) diagnosis, (2) screening for disease, or (3) patient management, including determining prognosis and therapy.

Diagnosis

Because prognosis and treatment depend on accurate diagnosis, it is essential that the physician render the correct diagnosis. The approach to making a diagnosis has been compared with a process not unlike that described in the detective fiction of Sir Conan Doyle in its testing, refutation, and reformulation of hypotheses. Others conclude that most diagnosis is based on recognition, which is in turn based on knowledge and experience.[2-4] Whichever the case, the laboratory results provide clues or patterns but the physician must recognize discordant data to be protected from diagnostic error.

The clinician must grasp that in the real world, as a rule, perfect tests do not exist. That is, not all patients with a certain disease have a positive test for a given analyte (they have false negative results), and a test may be positive in some patients without disease (they have false positive results). Although the popular belief

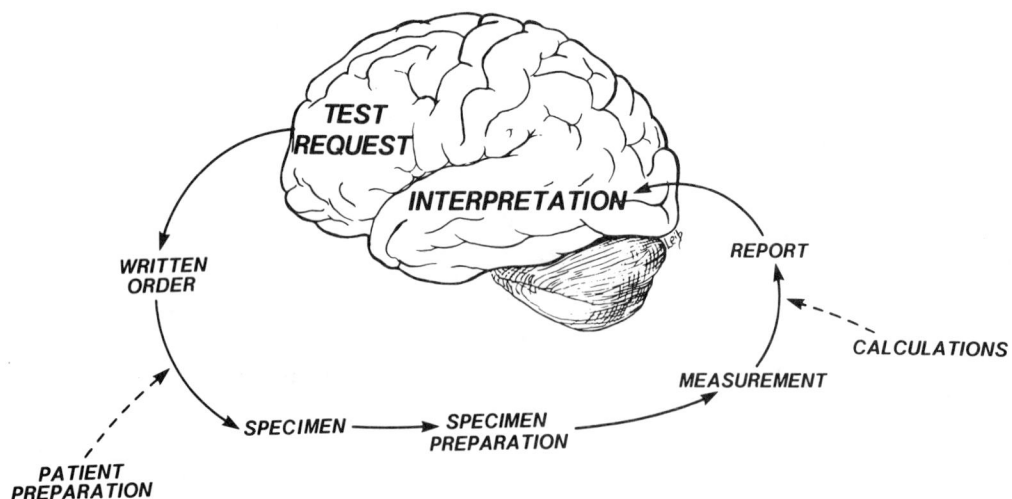

Fig. 1-1. Process of test selection and interpretation of results. (From Howanitz and Howanitz,[12] with permission.)

is that results of a test make or break a diagnosis, tests only affect the probability that a given disorder is present or absent. A test then is of value only to the extent it can alter or revise the probability estimate. Diagnostic sensitivity and diagnostic specificity of a test refer to its ability to classify individuals into true positives (a positive test and presence of disease) and true negatives (a negative test and absence of disease), respectively. These characteristics can be expressed by a binary (2 by 2 or four-fold) table (Fig. 1-2).

Diagnostic sensitivity is the proportion of patients with the disease who have a positive test, and it is given by the true positive ratio $[(a/a + b) \times 100]$. The true negative ratio $[(d/c + d) \times 100]$ expresses the specificity of the test, that is, the proportion of patients who will be correctly identified by the test as not having the disease. The post-test or posterior probability is the probability of the presence or absence of disease given the test results. Positive predictive value is the probability that a positive test result will occur in an individual with disease, whereas the negative predictive value is the probability that a negative test result will occur in an individual without disease. The positive predictive value is given by $(a/a + c) \times 100$ and the negative predictive value is given by $(d/b + d) \times 100$. The estimation of these probabilities depends on not only the diagnostic sensitivity and specificity of the test but also the likelihood of the disease before the test is ordered (pretest probability). With an uncommon disease, a positive test will identify a large number of healthy subjects (false positive findings) along with those individuals who have the disease. When the test is used for a large, generally healthy population, even a test with a diagnostic specificity and sensitivity of 95% will lead to a large number of false positive tests.

The number of false results depends on the prevalence of the disorder; for example, if the prevalence of the disorder in question is 5%, false positive results will equal true positive results. Because low disease prevalence gives rise to large numbers of false positive tests, low expectation of an abnormal result is a contraindication for ordering a diagnostic test.[5] In contrast, the predictive value of a negative test is adversely effected by high disease prevalence, but only slightly (Table 1-1). The diagnostic sensitivity and specificity of a test also influence how the test should be used when pursuing a clinical suspicion; a very sensitive test, when normal, serves to effectively rule out a suspected disorder, whereas a very specific test, when abnormal, serves to confirm the presence of disease.[6]

Although the influence of disease prevalence on test results is appreciated intellectually, the concept is often ignored in practice, with the attendant expense and confusion of an unexpected result. Ordering a diagnostic test is often the first misstep leading to clinical problems because it appears to hold minimal risks while promising to provide additional information. Ordering a test is not thought to cause any harm and by doing something, physicians diminish their own anxiety about patient problems.[7] An unexpected result, however, offers the opportunity for inappropriate care. A false positive or false negative result introduces a question that can only be resolved by further testing and examination. Once the cycle is triggered, even if inappropriately, it is virtually impossible to stop fur-

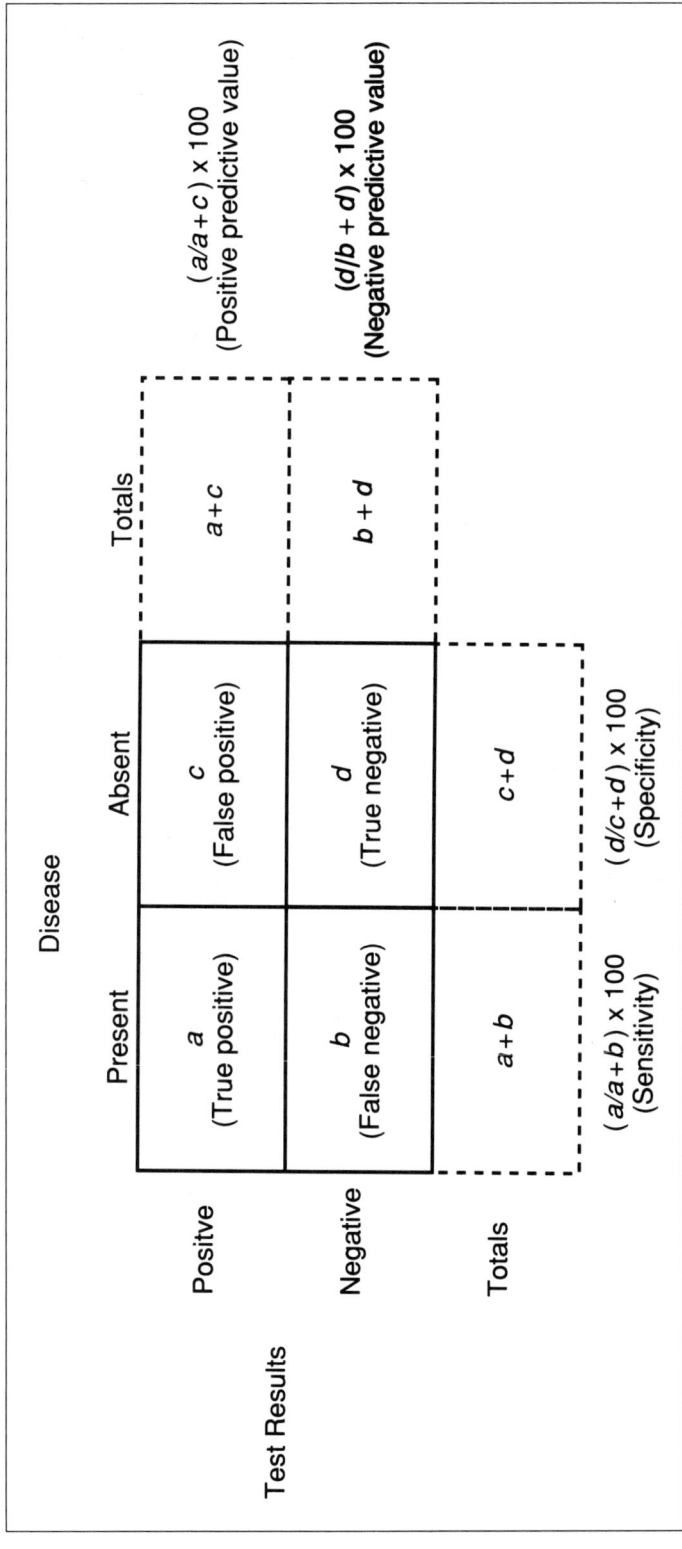

Fig. 1-2. Decision matrix. (See text for explanation.)

Table 1-1. The Relationship of Positive and Negative Predictive Value to Disease Prevalence[a]

Disease Prevalence (%)	Predictive Value	
	Positive (% of Time Positive Test Detects Disease)	Negative (% of Time Negative Test Predicts Nondisease)
1	6.1	99.9
2	27.9	99.9
5	50.0	99.7
50	95.0	95.0
75	98.3	83.7
100	100.0	—

[a] Test sensitivity and specificity = 95%.
(Modified from Vecchio,[29] with permission.)

ther testing. The phenomenon has been called the cascade effect, as well as colorfully described by a number of analogies. These include the "Tar-Baby effect" (the Tar-Baby distracts and entraps the inquisitive Brer Rabbit); lighting a candle in a fireworks factory (where it may be better "to curse the darkness than to light the wrong candle")[5]; and the "Ulysses syndrome," after the Homeric figure of the same name (because the patient embarks on a series of perilous, but pointless, diagnostic misadventures).[8] When faced with an unexpected result in an individual patient, the overall calculated reliability of a test does little to dissuade the physician from becoming embroiled in the cascade effect. This is true because the physician realizes failure to reconcile abnormal results can lead to diagnostic errors.

When a false result occurs, the physician is committed to proving that the result is spurious; this in turn leads to a situation that is costly, dangerous, and seemingly both unavoidable and unnecessary. Because pretest probability of disease effects its post-test probability, physicians should consider the incidence of the disorder in question before ordering a test. When a physician assesses a patient clinically and orders appropriate tests based on that assessment, he is increasing the incidence of the disorder in the population in question, thus improving the chance of getting the correct result. As far as diagnostic tests are concerned, more is not necessarily better.

Screening

Screening is an effort to detect the presence of disease in an unselected population of asymptomatic individuals. To make screening worthwhile, a number of clinical criteria must be met (Table 1-2). The incidence of the disease as well as the diagnostic sensitivity and specificity of the tests used must be sufficient to make the screening procedure practical. Because of the problem of false positive tests with biochemical screens, especially those that include large numbers of tests (Table 1-3), screening should be limited to subpopulations in which the incidence of a given disorder is relatively high. Moreover, screening is appropriate only when (1) the disorder in question is accompanied by significant mortality and morbidity if not treated, (2) effective therapy is available, and (3) treatment in the presymptomatic phase results in benefits greater than those obtained when treated in the early symptomatic

Table 1-2. Criteria for Evaluating the Usefulness of Diagnostic Screening Tests

Will the test detect disease that would otherwise remain undetected until later in time?
What are the risks, sensitivity, specificity, cost, and patient acceptability of the test?
How does the test's diagnostic value compare with unaided clinical judgment?
Will earlier disease detection have a favorable impact on patient status?
What is the risk, cost, efficiency, and effectiveness of therapy at an earlier stage of disease?
How will earlier diagnosis affect the patient's psychological well-being?
What are the costs of testing that result from diagnostic misclassification?
What are the induced costs and risks of further diagnostic evaluation?
What are the induced costs and risks of mistreatment?
What are the nonmedical consequences of diagnostic labeling?
Do the potential benefits of testing outweigh the costs and risks?
What is the current societal burden of suffering related to the target diseases?
What is the potential impact of testing on the individual person?

(From Cebul and Beck,[30] with permission.)

Table 1-3. Probability a Healthy Person Will Have All Test Results Within the Reference Range

Number of Tests Ordered	Probability (%)
1	95
6	74
12	54
20	36
100	0.6

phase. Currently, these constraints make screening ineffective or impractical for all but a few disorders. In addition, physicians often ignore laboratory data generated from screening programs. This response generally is believed to be a barrier to effective screening and to result in suboptimal patient care. Studies have shown, however, that when physicians ignore abnormal laboratory results they are in fact making clinical judgments based on the degree of abnormality, the likelihood further workup will affect therapy, and the risk associated with further diagnostic maneuvers.[9] They realize, especially when test results are continuously distributed, that overlapping values occur in patients with and without a given disease.

For convenience, multiple tests also have been used in what has been called the "panel" approach, usually targeting one specific organ. For example, the cardiac panel, consisting of serum creatine kinase and lactate dehydrogenase along with their isoenzymes, commonly is ordered for the laboratory confirmation of myocardial infarction. Because the panel approach to choosing tests potentially has some of the disadvantages of screening tests, it is important that panels only be ordered in well selected patients. Ordering panels is helpful in many diagnostic situations because a complete set of data is available to assess the pattern of results.

Patient Monitoring

Over one-half of all clinical laboratory tests are ordered for the purpose of monitoring.[10] Tests are used in patient management to monitor disease progression or resolution, to identify complications of treatment, to ensure therapeutic drug levels, and to assess prognosis. Additionally, tests are ordered to evaluate unexpected changes in patient status and to resolve unusual test or procedure results. Test precision is the most important characteristic in patient management because the physician usually assesses change in results. The optimal frequency of monitoring is not well established for most tests. Perhaps this is caused by the many factors that can influence test results, for example, change in disease progression or regression, normal physiologic variation, intercurrent disease, and influence of therapeutic measures.

Change between successive measurements depends on two basic components, analytic and biologic variation. Between assay precision of a measurement can be used to calculate whether or not a change in a result is significant above and beyond what can be explained on an analytic basis. Using the relationship between the largest expected range and the standard deviation (SD) of the measurement, variability due to technical factors can be estimated from the "between run" SD (see below). If two results differ by at least 2.8 SD, it is about 95% certain that a significant difference between the two results exists, that is, it is unlikely that the difference is caused by analytic variation alone. For patient monitoring, test sensitivity and specificity also are important parameters. For some clinical situations, a combination of tests is used to improve test performance. For example, carcinoembryonic antigen and cancer antigen 19-9 (CA 19-9) have been used together in following patients with malignancy of the gastrointestinal tract.

Patient Preparation and Specimen Acquisition

After a test is selected, the patient must be prepared and the appropriate specimen must be obtained at the proper time. The specimen must arrive in good condition at the test site where it is properly prepared for the test procedure. This step is a major source of laboratory interferences, which clinicians endure and which are known to laboratory personnel as preanalytic variation. There are myriad ways in which this step can be adversely affected (Table 1-4). For some tests, such as the glucose tolerance test, the patient's diet is important. Drugs can cause changes in the measured concentration of analyte by having a physiologic effect on the patient or by interfering with the analysis. The specimen must be obtained at the correct time and without introducing elements that increase or decrease the analyte in question. Stress during blood drawing and length of time the tourniquet is in place are two causes of change in analyte concentration. Considerable diurnal variation occurs not only with hormone measurements, such as cortisol, but with other analytes, for example, iron. The container in which the specimen is placed, the preservative or anticoagulant used, and the

Table 1-4. Important Considerations in Patient Preparation and in Specimen Collection, Transport, and Processing

Diet
Time since last meal
Smoking
Stress
Posture
Medications
Time of specimen collection
Collection container and preservative
Transport conditions
Storage prior to processing
Processing step (time, temperature, etc)
Storage following processing

conditions the container endures before and during preparation of the specimen for the test procedure all can affect results. Storage requirements vary with the analyte as well as the specimen and analytic method used. It is not always the case that interferences for a given analyte give rise to increased values (hyperlipemia results in low sodium as measured by indirect ion specific electrode) or that storage inadequacies yield low values (ammonia increases with improper storage). The method of analysis can influence the details of the precautions that must be taken at this step. For example, a patient may be receiving a drug that interferes with a given analyte's result when measured by fluorescence methods, but the drug may not interfere with immunoassays for that same analyte.

In order to provide insight on the important types of problems that can occur and the effects they have on data interpretation, major specimen handling and method problems are covered in the "logistics" segment for each analyte. More complete information is contained in a series of handbooks on patient preparation and specimen handling published by the College of American Pathologists, for example, the publication on therapeutic drug monitoring and toxicology.[11]

Laboratory Analysis

The clinician depends on the laboratory to provide precise, sensitive, and specific assays for the tests requested. Additionally, the laboratory's assay should be as free as possible from interferences and the results should be reported in a timely manner along with the appropriate reference range. For quantitative clinical laboratory analyses, there are well developed procedures for monitoring assay precision, which is the closeness with which replicate analyses can be made. Imprecision is quantitated using control sample results. With each analytic run, control samples at two or three levels are analyzed along with patient specimens, and control results are used to calculate assay variability. Data from these so-called internal controls are used to determine necessity of systems correction and whether patient results should be reported. Precision data can be used to estimate the amount of variability due to technical causes (see above); however, when clinicians have a question as to the spread of the results, they routinely repeat the test. This maneuver has several effects including substantiation of assay precision and verification specimen integrity (see below).

Dramatic differences in assay results occur between laboratories and, unfortunately, may not always be adequately reflected by differences in reference ranges. External quality control systems are used to assess assay comparability between laboratories. External quality control systems or survey programs refer to systems by which results from different laboratories are compared retrospectively. Because it is frequently impossible to determine true analyte concentration, accuracy comes to mean conformance with an assumed value determined by the state of the art in measuring an analyte. With external quality control programs, participants' results are compared with those of their peer group, often using the mean ± 2 SD from the mean as the evaluation criteria. Thus, a result determined by a very precise method may be close to a mean, but can be designated as unacceptable if the percent coefficient of variation (%, CV) for the peer group is small. In contrast, results obtained with a less precise method may be relatively far from the mean, but may receive "a better grade." This problem has led to introduction of other evaluation criteria.[12]

Both internal and external quality control systems have their limitations. Quality control systems are not effective in detecting blunders, such as mislabeled specimens, and no quality control system can compensate for the deficiencies of an unsound analytic procedure. Reliability of a laboratory result depends on an assay's precision and accuracy as well as on its sensitivity and specificity, plus freedom from mistakes. Additionally, preanalytic variation and other causes of interference must be carefully regulated and the reference interval carefully chosen. Assay specificity and sensitivity are controlled by the choice of analytic method. A series of guidelines for evaluating assay performance are available from the National Committee for Clinical Laboratory Standards (NCCLS).[13]

Laboratory methods have improved in sensitivity and specificity over time, but introduction of new methods and new treatments require ongoing vigilance of laboratory personnel and clinicians to prevent problems. Causes of interference with many types of assays occur with icteric, hemolyzed, or lipemic specimens. Other interferences are very specific depending on the particular method employed. For example, circulating antibodies to animal immunoglobulins have been reported to interfere with thyroid-stimulating hormone (TSH) assays. Circulating antibodies to mouse immunoglobulins may interfere with mouse monoclonal TSH antibodies, whereas circulating antibodies to rabbit immunoglobulins may interfere with polyclonal (rabbit) TSH antibodies.[14] A publication entitled *Drug Interference and Effects in Clinical Chemistry* provides an extensive list of interferences that affect various chemistry tests.[15] Because specificity problems are usually assay related and thus change rapidly as new assays are introduced, this aspect of laboratory medicine is not emphasized in this book.

Reports

Ideally, the reference range is included in the laboratory report along with some visual clues to highlight abnormal results. Graphic displays that summarize or reduce data can assist in the perception of abnormalities, but display needs vary depending on whether tests are used for diagnosis or screening.[16] In spite of efforts to convert to the International System (SI) of units, the reference range is reported in various units of measure in the United States. A number of arguments have been given for and against the use of SI units.[17] In this book conventional units are used with SI units given in parentheses.

Interpretation of Results

In interpreting results, the clinician compares patient results with the normal range or, in more recent parlance, the reference range or interval. Unfortunately, information regarding the reference range is too often the weakest link between the clinical laboratory and the clinician. The reference range depends on many factors (Table 1-5), including the method of analysis and the population used for its determination.[18] For

Table 1-5. Influences on References Ranges

Reference population and how it was chosen.
The environmental and physiologic conditions under which the specimens were obtained.
The techniques and timing of specimen collection, transport, preparation, and storage.
Analytic method including specificity, precision, and standardization.
Data collection and methods used to derive the reference range.

analytes that are influenced by such factors as age or gender, establishing separate reference ranges for these individual characteristics may help with interpretation of results.

Reference ranges are customarily defined as limits within 2 SD from the mean, thus about 2.5% of results from healthy individuals are either above or below the normal range. By convention, the limits are determined assuming the underlying distribution is gaussian even though this often is not the case. Assuming a gaussian distribution obviates using nonparametric statistics, which require large sample numbers and are sensitive to distortion by outliers. Outliers can occur by including specimens from individuals with unrecognized disease and by technical or clerical errors. Unfortunately, there appears to be limited understanding that a small percentage of healthy individuals will have test results that fall more than 2 SD from the mean and thus by convention are labeled "abnormal."[19] One way clinicians cope with this problem is to repeat the test. This maneuver assesses the possibility of laboratory error or problem with precision and also takes advantage of regression to the mean, that is, extreme values occurring simply on a physiologic or statistical basis are likely to become less extreme on repeat measurement. Thus, an abnormal test result from a healthy individual is likely to be within the reference range, or at least less abnormal, when measured a second time.[20]

Although the reference range theoretically encompasses approximately 95% of healthy individuals, the actual situation is more complicated. Many, if not most, analytes do not follow a gaussian distribution; the population used to determine the reference range may contain some individuals with disease, and the reference range may be inadequately adjusted for such parameters as age and gender. Moreover, there often is considerable overlap of values in healthy persons and individuals with disease in spite of the idea some clini-

8 • Laboratory Medicine

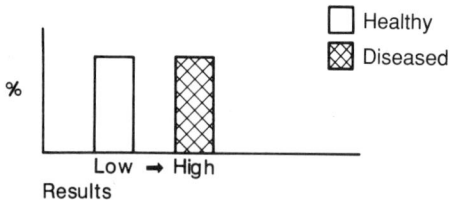

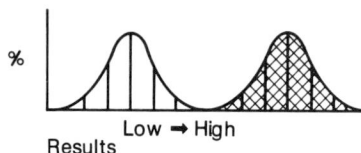

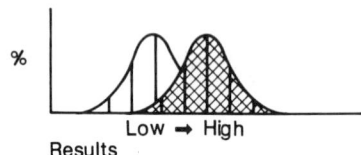

Fig. 1-3. Perceptions of test result distribution (result versus percent of population tested. (Modified from Cochrane,[21] with permission.)

cians have that the normal range is widely separated from a separate and distinct abnormal range (Fig. 1-3). Instead of bimodal distribution of normal and abnormal results, there exists in reality distributions that overlap and demonstrate various degrees of skewness (Fig. 1-4).[21]

Reference ranges, as indicated above are determined from results obtained from a group of healthy individuals. Although there may be little overlap of results from healthy individuals and those individuals with the specific disorder, there is often a patient group with intermediate values. For example, healthy men have lower serum prostatic acid phosphatase (PAP) results than men with benign prostatic hypertrophy. Thus, when applying the reference range for healthy men to a patient group with prostatic hypertrophy and carcinoma, PAP results give a higher false positive rate than if a range was determined with a population suspected of having prostatic carcinoma.

Because most clinical laboratory test results fall on a continuous scale (Fig. 1-5), the cutoff point at which a test is called positive or negative is arbitrary. The cutoff limit can be chosen to make the test very sensitive, but if this is done, the number of false positive results increases unavoidably (Fig. 1-6). If a different cutoff point is used to increase the specificity, sensitivity is compromised. The diagnostic specificity and sensitivity for a particular test depend on a number of test parameters including the clinical situation in which the test is used. In addition, selection of an appropriate cutoff depends on the probability of the disease in the population of interest and the clinical implications of a diagnostic error. For tests that have a continuous distribution, different cutoff points will yield different amounts of information.

The ratio of the true positive ratio to the false positive ratio is known as the likelihood ratio. Tests having a high likelihood ratio are better discriminators of disease than ones with low likelihood ratios, that is, they correctly identify a large portion of individuals with disease and do not include many individuals without disease. It should be kept in mind, however, that there

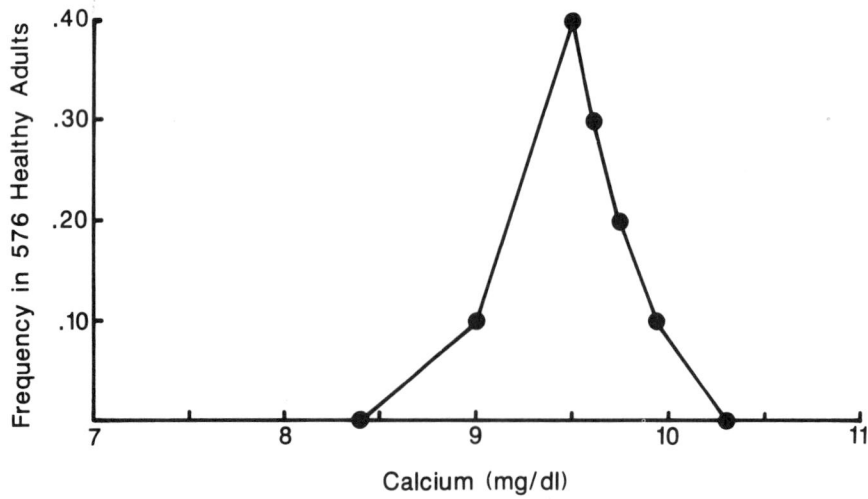

Fig. 1-4. Distribution of serum calcium in healthy adults. (Modified from Elveback et al.,[27] with permission.)

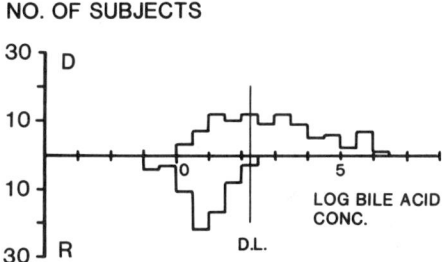

Fig. 1-5. Frequency histogram for log (bile acid concentrations in serum) in reference, R, and diseased, D, groups of subjects. *DL*, discrimination limit (0.975 fractile of the R-distribution). (From Linnet,[28] with permission.)

is not a single likelihood for a test, but rather a continuum of pairs of sensitivities and specificities that characterize the test's performance in a given clinical situation, including the time after disease onset. The test's performance in a given situation can be graphed on a relative (receiver) operating characteristic (ROC) curve (Fig. 1-7) by plotting the true positive ratio (sensitivity) as a function of false positive ratio (1 − specificity) at various cutoff levels.[22,23] Because the true positive ratios and false positive ratios depend on the incidence of the disorder in the population studied, there is a different ROC curve for each given clinical situation. Moreover, different cutoff values can be chosen depending on the consequences of a false negative or false positive test result. When risks of treatment appear small and benefits large, false positive interpretations appear less harmful, and thus liberal criteria often are chosen for a positive test. However, because positive criteria are liberally chosen, test sensitivity improves and false positive tests become more common. In contrast, as positive criteria are more conservatively chosen, test specificity improves, but false negative results become more common.[24]

Insight into diagnostic accuracy can be obtained from ROC curves and may be helpful in determining decision levels for specific diagnostic purposes. The diagnostic sensitivity and specificity are set according to assumptions made regarding the risk/benefit ratio of treatment. There is, however, no absolute measure of diagnostic accuracy. Sensitivity and specificity data are no more accurate than assumptions concerning who is sick and who is not, and the accuracy of these

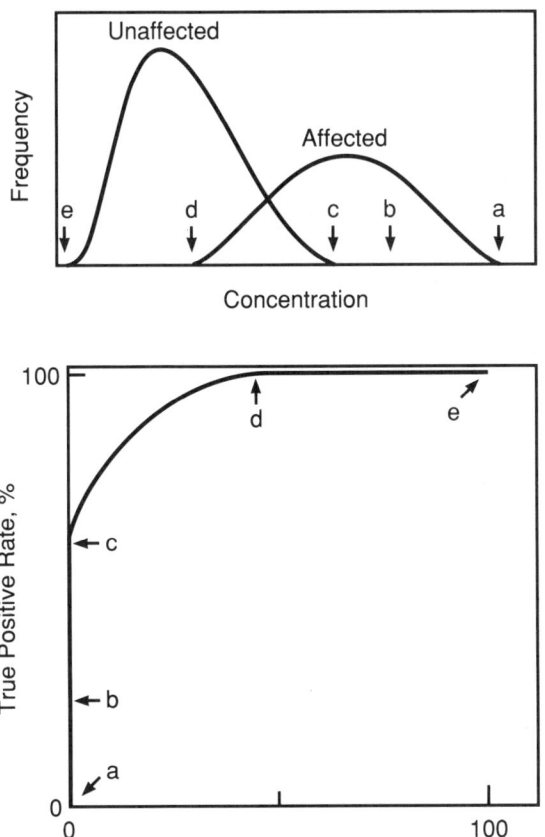

Fig. 1-6. (A) Hypothetical frequency distribution. (B) Receiver operating characteristic curve (ROC) (corresponding to data in Fig. A) generated by varying decision level and plotting resulting pairs of true and false positive rates. Points *a* through *e* on ROC curve correspond to decision levels in frequency distribution. Curve from *c* to *d* describes the test's accuracy in overlap region. (From Zweig,[22] with permission.)

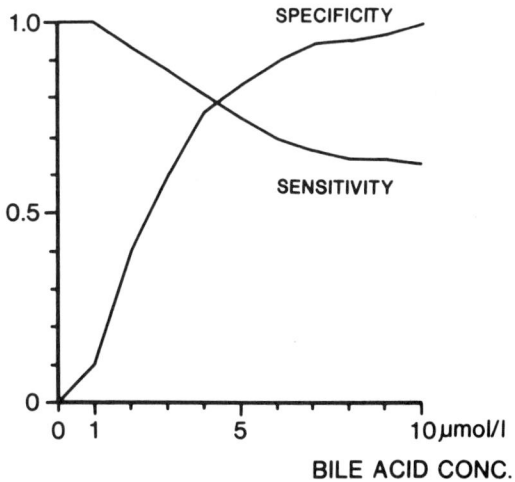

Fig. 1-7. Receiver operator curves. Specificity and sensitivity are seen as functions of the discrimination limit measured on the original bile acid concentration scale (μmol/L). (From Linnet,[28] with permission.)

assumptions is unmeasureable.[24] The greater the difference between the certainty of diagnosis before a test is performed and the certainty after it is performed, the more information the test will provide. Whenever it is known with reasonable certainty who is sick and who is not, a diagnostic test is not needed. The area under the ROC is proportional to reliability and therefore offers an opportunity to improve test interpretation, but ROC is difficult to calculate because of the reasons stated above.

CONCLUSIONS

The recognition of patterns and significant deviations in those patterns is as important in interpreting laboratory results as it is in other aspects of diagnosis and depends on experience as well as knowledge. Clinicians must recognize that the diagnostic implications of a given test result vary from patient to patient depending on other findings.[25] Unfortunately, diagnostic errors can occur because data inconsistent with preconceived conclusions are often ignored, whereas data suggesting preconceived ideas are exaggerated. Clinicians see what they expect dismissing the anomalous; thus they are both "blessed and cursed" with a suppressive mechanism. Clinicians are blessed if they can detect a significant pattern in spite of aberrant data, but cursed when significant but seemingly irrelevant data are not appreciated.[26]

REFERENCES

1. Tresnowski BR: Guidelines on diagnostic testing will lead to cost savings, better patient care. Press release. Blue Cross and Blue Shield Association. Chicago, IL, April 2, 1987.
2. McCormick JS: Diagnosis: The need for demystification. Lancet 1986;2:1434–1435.
3. Campbell EJM: The diagnosing mind. Lancet 1987;1:849–851.
4. Editorial: Diagnosis: Logic and psycho-logic. Lancet 1987;1:840–841.
5. Ober KP: Uncle Remus and the cascade effect in clinical medicine. Am J Med 1987;82:1009–1013.
6. Griner PF, Mayewski RJ, Mushlin AI, Greenland P: Principles of test selection and use. Ann Intern Med 1981;94:559–563.
7. Mold JW, Stein HF: The cascade effect in the clinical care of patient. N Engl J Med 1986;314:512–514.
8. Bensen ES: Initiatives toward effective decision making and laboratory use. Hum Pathol 1980;11:440–448.
9. Link K, Centor R, Buchsbaum D, Witherspoon J: Why physicians don't pursue abnormal laboratory tests: an investigation of hypercalcemia and the follow-up of abnormal testing results. Hum Pathol 984;15:75–78.
10. Beeler MF, Sappenfield R: Medical monitoring. What is it, how can it be improved? Am J Clin Pathol 1987;87:285–288.
11. Committee on Patient Preparation and Specimen Handling: Clinical Laboratory Handbook for Patient Preparation and Specimen Handling. Fascicle IV Therapeutic Drug Monitoring and Toxicology. College of American Pathologists, 1985.
12. Howanitz JH, Howanitz PJ: Introduction to quality assurance. pp. 1–19. In Howanitz PJ, Howanitz JH (eds): Laboratory Quality Assurance. New York, McGraw-Hill, 1987.
13. National Committee for Clinical Laboratory Standards. 771 East Lancaster Avenue, Villanova, PA 19085.
14. Zweig MH, Csako G, Benson CL et al: Interference by anti-immunoglobulin G antibodies in immunoradiometric assays of thyrotropin involving mouse monoclonal antibodies. Clin Chem 1987;33:840–844.
15. Drug Interference and Effects in Clinical Chemistry: Apoteksbolaget AB, Socialstyrelsen. Stockholm and Uppsala, 1984.
16. Politser PE: How to make laboratory information more informative. Clin Chem 1986;32:1510–1516.
17. Conn RB: Scientific medicine and Système International units. Arch Pathol Lab Med 1987;111:16–19.
18. Sunderman FW: Current concepts of "normal values", "reference values", and "discrimination values" in clinical chemistry. Clin Chem 1975;21:1873–1877.
19. Casscells W, Schoenberger A, Graboys TB: Interpretation by physicians of clinical laboratory results. N Engl J Med 1978;299:999–1001.
20. Cebul RD, Beck JR: Biochemical profiles: applications in ambulatory screening and preadmission testing of adults. Ann Intern Med 1987;106:403–413.
21. Cochrane AL: Effectiveness and Efficiency. Cardiff, Wales, Nuffield Provincial Hospitals Trust, 1972, pp. 33–44.
22. Zweig MH: Evaluation of the clinical accuracy of laboratory tests. Arch Pathol Lab Med 1988;112:383–386.
23. Swets JA: Measuring the accuracy of diagnostic systems. Science 1988;240:1285–1291.
24. Dix D: On the role of diagnostic tests in clinical decision analysis: A critical review. Clin Chem Enzymol Commission 1988;1:3–9.
25. Pauker SG, Kassirer JP: Decision analysis. N Engl J Med 1987;316:250–258.
26. Melman KL: Will the sighted physician see? Pharos 1984;Winter:2–6.
27. Elveback ER, Guillier CL, Keating FR: Health, normality and the ghost of Gauss. JAMA 1970;211:69–75.
28. Linnet K: A review on the methodology for assessing diagnostic tests. Clin Chem 1988;34:1379–1386.
29. Vecchio JJ: Predictive value of a single diagnostic test in unselected populations. N Engl J Med 1966;274:1171–1173.
30. Cebul RD, Beck JR: Biochemical profiles. Applications in ambulatory screening and preadmission testing of adults. pp. 278–304. In Sox HC (ed): Common Diagnostic Tests: Use and Interpretation. Philadelphia, American College of Physicians, 1987.

2 Pulmonary and Cardiac Function

Daniel J. Fink
James A. Harker

INTRODUCTION

Assays are performed for arterial blood gases to evaluate a patient's respiratory and/or acid-base system. The acid-base status affects respiratory rate, O_2 release from red blood cells (RBCs), and partial pressure of carbon dioxide (pCO_2). Likewise, the partial pressure of oxygen (pO_2) and the pCO_2 can affect the acid-base status.

Respiratory System

Arterial blood gases (ABG) also are used to evaluate respiratory function. The respiratory system can be divided into three functional components: ventilation, respiration, and O_2 delivery.

Ventilation is the mechanical movement of gases into and out of the lungs. Total ventilation is the sum of two components, alveolar ventilation and dead space ventilation. Dead space ventilation consists of several components, anatomic dead space (trachea and bronchi), alveolar dead space (alveoli that are ventilated but not perfused), and venous admixture (alveoli in which there is a mismatch between ventilation and perfusion). Roughly 30% of total ventilatory effort is used to ventilate dead space.[1]

Ventilation is not uniform throughout the lungs, but is greatest at the apex and lowest at the base. This is the opposite of perfusion, which is lowest at the apex and greatest at the base of the lungs because of the effect of gravity. Alveolar dead space is largest at the apex and venous admixture is largest at the base of the lungs.

Respiration, which is the exchange of gases in the lungs, depends on perfusion of the alveoli, alveolar gas content, and the status of the alveoli and the alveolar membranes. Inappropriate matching of ventilation to perfusion leads to increased dead space and decreased gas exchange. Both the overperfusion of poorly ventilated regions or underperfusion of well ventilated regions produce a mismatch. Most of the lung in healthy individuals has well matched ventilation and perfusion.

Alveolar air is rich in O_2 and low in CO_2 as compared with venous blood. Thus, when blood enters the alveolar capillary, the forces of diffusion cause O_2 to cross from the alveolus into the blood and CO_2 to cross from the blood into the alveolus. In healthy individuals, blood O_2 and CO_2 concentrations achieve equilibrium with the alveolar gas concentrations before leaving the alveolus. Carbon dioxide equilibrium is reached first because the permeability of CO_2 through the alveolar membrane is 10–20 times that of O_2.[2]

Pulmonary capillary O_2 concentration equals that of the alveolus, whereas the mixed arterial O_2 concentration is lower than that of alveolar gas owing to dead space and shunting of blood around the lungs. Blood passing through dead space is not oxygenated because of poor perfusion. Blood shunted around the lungs is not oxygenated because of the lack of exposure to alveolar air. The unoxygenated blood mixes with pulmonary blood, causing arterial blood to have a lower O_2 concentration than alveolar air. The difference in alveolar-arterial O_2 concentration in healthy individuals increases with age from about 3 mmHg in young people to more than 25 mmHg in older people.[3,4]

Respiration is enhanced by the related interactions of hemoglobin (Hgb) with O_2 and CO_2. In the lungs, the high affinity and rapid binding of O_2 by deoxyhemoglobin increase the rate of diffusion of O_2 into the RBC by maintaining an O_2 gradient. The oxyhemoglobin produced has a lower affinity for CO_2 than the deoxyhemoglobin leading to the release of CO_2 bound to hemoglobin. Because the oxyhemoglobin produced is also a stronger acid than deoxyhemoglobin, the hydrogen ion (H^+) is released and combines with intracellular HCO_3^- to produce CO_2. These reactions lead to an increase in RBC CO_2 and increased diffusion of CO_2 out of the RBC. The reverse of these reactions takes place in the tissue capillaries.

Damage to the alveolar membrane is the main cause of decreased gas exchange in adequately ventilated and perfused alveoli. Thickening, coating, or destruction of alveolar membranes leads to insufficient perfused alveolar surface area in contact with alveolar air and/or slowed diffusion such that equilibrium of gas exchange does not occur. This affects blood pO_2 before the pCO_2 because of the much higher permeability of the alveolar membrane to CO_2. The result of the failure to reach equilibrium is a widening of the alveolar-arterial O_2 difference and less O_2 transport.

Acid-Base System

Function

The function of the acid-base system is to maintain the blood and intracellular pH within a narrow range in the presence of normal, increased, or decreased rates of metabolic acid production and excretion.[5,6] The usual end point of metabolism is the production of an acid, primarily carbonic acid (H_2CO_3). Sulfuric, phosphoric, and small amounts of a variety of organic acids are also produced. The pH is regulated by the physiologic buffers, production of base (primarily bicarbonate), and control of acid excretion by the lungs and kidneys. The primary volatile acid, H_2CO_3, is excreted as CO_2 by the lungs and as H^+ and ammonium ion (NH_4^+) by the kidneys; "fixed" acids such as sulfuric, phosphoric, and the organic acids are excreted by the kidneys.

The equilibrium concentrations in solution of any acid (HB) and its conjugate base (B^-) are described by the equation:

$$HB \longleftrightarrow H^+ + B^-$$

At equilibrium:

$$K_a = \frac{[H^+][B^-]}{[HB]}$$

where K_a is the dissociation constant for the acid, [HB] is the concentration of undissociated acid, [H^+] is the concentration of hydrogen ion, and [B^-] is the concentration of the conjugate base. The higher the dissociation constant, the stronger the acid, that is, the higher the K_a, the higher the [H^+]. Buffers exert their effect by keeping [H^+] nearly constant despite the addition of an acid or base to the solution. If an acid is added to a buffered solution, the added H^+ combines with the conjugate base B^-, thus increasing the concentration of undissociated acid HB, but maintaining [H^+] nearly constant. Likewise, the addition of a base leads to increased dissociation of the acid HB providing additional H^+ to combine with the added base, also maintaining [H^+] nearly constant. It is their ability to maintain [H^+] within a narrow range in the face of changing metabolic and respiratory requirements that makes the physiologic buffers so important.

The buffering power (β) of an acid is defined as the amount of strong base that must be added to a solution in order to raise the pH by 1 pH unit or

$$\beta = \frac{\text{Amount of strong acid added}}{\text{resultant pH decrease}}$$
$$= \frac{\text{Amount of strong base added}}{\text{resultant pH increase}}$$

The higher the buffering power, the smaller the pH change when an acid or base is added. Buffers with a high buffering power will maintain a more stable pH than buffers with a low buffering power.

Open and Closed Buffering Systems

Another characteristic of buffers is the difference in the buffering capacity of an open versus a closed buffering system. In a closed buffer system, the amount of buffer acid plus conjugate base is constant. As H^+ is added, it combines with conjugate base to form the buffer acid HB and the concentration of conjugate base B^- decreases. As the concentration of conjugate base B^- decreases, the buffer solution loses its buffering ability and the pH decreases. In contrast, an open buffer system is one in which the amount of buffer acid plus conjugate base is not constant. Buffer acid (or base) is continually added from an external source, maintaining an available supply of buffer acid (or base). As the conjugate base is consumed by combining with the added acid, more conjugate base becomes available by dissociation of the added buffer acid. Thus, in an open system, there is always a ready supply of conjugate base and the pH remains nearly constant over wide ranges of input. The blood buffers constitute an open system because the concentration of HCO_3^- changes as CO_2 is produced by the tissues and removed by the lungs.

Physiologic Buffers

Bicarbonate, Hgb, protein, and phosphate are the physiologically important buffers. The pH is normally controlled by the bicarbonate and Hgb buffer systems with the protein and phosphate buffers accounting for less than 5% of the buffer capacity of blood. The bicarbonate buffer system is the buffer most closely linked to production and excretion of metabolic acids and serves as the intermediary buffer between both the blood and the lungs and the blood and the kidneys.

Table 2-1 summarizes the buffering power of the physiologic buffers in the blood for both open and closed systems. The bicarbonate buffer in blood is an open system because CO_2, transported as HCO_3^-, is produced by the tissues and removed by the lungs. Approximately 53% of the buffering capacity of blood is contained in the RBCs and 47% in the plasma.[7,8] Bicarbonate is the primary buffer in plasma providing about 90% of the plasma buffering capacity.[7,8] Hemoglobin is the predominant buffer inside RBCs providing about 72% of the RBC buffering capacity with the bicarbonate system providing most of the remainder.[7,8]

Application of the acid-base equilibrium equation to the bicarbonate buffer system gives:

$$K_a = \frac{[H^+][HCO_3^-]}{[H_2CO_3]}$$

which with rearrangement can be written as:

$$pH = pK_a + \log \frac{[HCO_3^-]}{[H_2CO_3]}$$

This is the Henderson-Hasselbalch equation where the pH is $-\log_{10}[H^+]$ and pK_a is $-\log_{10} K_a$.

The concentration of H_2CO_3 in the blood is also described by the equilibrium:

$$CO_2 + H_2O \longleftrightarrow H_2CO_3$$

with the equilibrium equation:

$$K_h = \frac{[H_2CO_3]}{[H_2O][CO_2]}$$

Table 2-1. The Buffering Capacity of the Physiologic Buffers in Blood When Viewed as an Open System and as a Closed System[a]

	In Vivo, $pCO_2 = 40$ mmHg (5.3 kPa); Hematocrit = 45%		In Vitro, Closed System Constant Total $CO_2 + H_2CO_3 + HCO_3^- = 25.2$ mEq/L (25.2 mmol/L)	
	β^b	%	β^b	%
Plasma pH 7.4 CO_2—H_2CO_3—HCO_3^- (25.2 mM)	30.4	42	1.4	4
Proteins (7 g/dL plasma [70 g/L])	3.9	5	3.9	12
Red blood cells Intracellular CO_2—H_2CO_3—HCO_3^-	10.4	15	0.5	2
Hemoglobin (15 g/dL [150 g/L] whole blood)	27.0	38	27.0	82
Total	71.7	100	32.8	100

[a] Note that the relative importance of the buffers and their buffering capacity is very different between an open and a closed system. In vivo, the physiologic buffers constitute an open system.
[b] Buffer value, β, mEq of H^+ or OH^-/(liter of whole blood × pH unit).
(Modified from Seldin and Gerhard,[8] with permission.)

or, with rearrangement:

$$[H_2CO_3] = K_h \times [CO_2] \times [H_2O]$$

This equation shows that $[H_2CO_3]$ is proportional to $[CO_2]$, the concentration of dissolved CO_2. At physiologic pH, almost no H_2CO_3 is found in the blood. If this equation is combined with the Henderson-Hasselbalch equation, $[H_2CO_3]$ can be eliminated and the equation becomes:

$$pH = pK_a' + \log \frac{[HCO_3^-]}{[CO_2]}$$

where K_a' is the combined equilibrium constants divided by $[H_2O]$, which is taken to be constant. From the application of Henry's law, the concentration of dissolved CO_2 in a fluid is related to the pCO_2 of a gas in contact with the fluid by the equation:

$$[CO_2] = \alpha \times pCO_2$$

where α is the solubility coefficient for CO_2. Conversely, a fluid with a known concentration of dissolved CO_2 has a partial pressure associated with it that corresponds to the pCO_2 required in a gas in contact with the fluid to achieve the observed concentration of dissolved CO_2. Substituting this relationship into the above gives the modified Henderson-Hasselbalch equation:

$$pH = pK' + \log \frac{[HCO_3^-]}{\alpha \times pCO_2},$$

where pK' in plasma at 37°C is 6.1 and the solubility coefficient α for CO_2 in plasma at 37°C is .031 mmol $\times$ $L^{-1} \times mmHg^{-1}$. The modified Henderson-Hasselbalch equation describes the control of plasma pH by the bicarbonate buffering system.

Control of Blood pH

Blood pH is controlled by the ratio of $[HCO_3^-]$ to pCO_2, not the level of the individual components. Only when the ratio of $[HCO_3^-]$ to $[H_2CO_3]$ deviates from the usual value of about 20:1 is the pH abnormal. The bicarbonate concentration, controlled by the kidneys, is the metabolic component and pCO_2, controlled by the lungs, is the respiratory component of acid-base balance.

Buffering in RBCs depends on both the Hgb and bicarbonate buffer systems. The equilibrium reactions describing the Hgb buffering system and the coupling of the Hgb to the bicarbonate buffering system are

$$CO_2 + H_2O \longleftrightarrow H_2CO_3 \longleftrightarrow H^+ + HCO_3^-$$
$$H^+ + KHgb \longleftrightarrow HHgb + K^+$$

These reactions are driven by the CO_2 concentration, proceeding to the right in the tissues where CO_2 is produced and to the left in the lungs where CO_2 is excreted.

Hemoglobin buffering inside the RBC also is driven by pO_2 because oxyhemoglobin is a stronger acid than deoxyhemoglobin, that is, H^+ binds more tightly to deoxyhemoglobin than to oxyhemoglobin. Hence, as the release of O_2 in the tissues converts oxyhemoglobin to deoxyhemoglobin, there is an increased uptake (buffering) of H^+ by Hgb. This also drives the bicarbonate buffer equation to the right, consuming RBC CO_2 and promoting the diffusion of plasma CO_2 into the RBC. As O_2 binds with deoxyhemoglobin in the lungs, H^+ is released from the oxyhemoglobin formed, combines with HCO_3^- to produce CO_2, and CO_2 is then excreted. Some CO_2 is also reversibly bound directly to the Hgb molecule but this is a relatively small percentage. Figure 2-1 summarizes the buffering and CO_2 transport reactions that occur in the RBC and plasma.

Two interesting aspects of RBC buffering are the isohydric and chloride shift. The isohydric shift is the release or uptake of CO_2 by RBCs without a change in pH. An isohydric shift occurs because all of the H^+ ions produced in the RBCs after uptake of CO_2 are buffered by Hgb. At the same time, the bicarbonate ions produced by this process diffuse out of the RBCs with a compensatory influx of chloride ions, the chloride shift. These reactions are reversed in the lungs. The chloride shift, exchanging HCO_3^- for Cl^-, is responsible for the finding that the chloride level is lower in venous blood than in arterial blood.[9]

The primary renal mechanisms of acid-base control are the interrelated excretion of H^+ and resorption of HCO_3^-. Bicarbonate is filtered by the glomerulus and is reabsorbed mainly in the proximal but also in the distal renal tubule. For serum bicarbonate concentrations of up to about 24 mEq/L, nearly all the filtered bicarbonate is recovered. However, recovery of the filtered bicarbonate is not achieved by direct transport from the lumen into the tubular cells and from there to the plasma. Instead, carbonic anhydrase (CA) catalyzes the formation of H_2CO_3, which dissociates into H^+ and HCO_3^- in renal tubular cells (see Fig. 2-2, p. 23). The HCO_3^- produced is returned to the plasma, whereas the H^+ produced goes into the lumen, neutralizing the previously filtered bicarbonate in the tubular fluid.

Pulmonary and Cardiac Function • 15

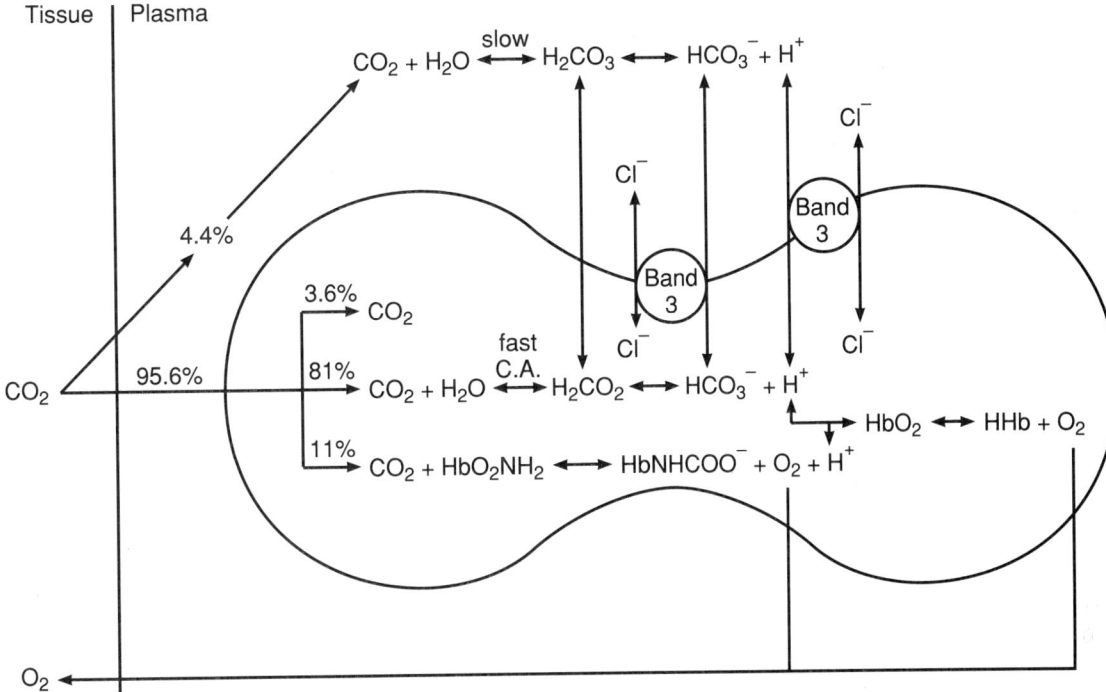

Fig. 2-1. Carbon dioxide (CO_2) transport and acidification of red blood cell (RBC) cytoplasm and plasma in tissue capillaries. Carbon dioxide produced in the tissues is transported in venous blood to the lungs as dissolved CO_2, bicarbonate, and carbamino groups of hemoglobin ($HgbNHCOO^-$). The more rapid hydration of CO_2 within the erythrocyte cytoplasm by carbonic anhydrases (CA) assures that the cytoplasm becomes more acid than capillary plasma. This gradient is dissipated by hydrogen ion (H^+) transport and by diffusion of H_2CO_3. The percentages shown are for the distribution of CO_2 transport in its several forms. (From Seldin and Gerhard,[8] with permission.)

Thus, there is a net movement of one HCO_3^- ion into the plasma.

The excretion of acid also utilizes the carbonic anhydrase mechanism. Acid is excreted as H^+ when intracellular H_2CO_3 dissociates and the resulting H^+ is either excreted directly or as NH_4^+ after combining with NH_3. For each H^+ excreted, one HCO_3^- ion is returned to the plasma, neutralizing one plasma H^+.

BLOOD GASES AND RELATED TESTS

Test: Arterial Blood Gases (ABG, Blood Gases)

Background

Clinical laboratory blood gas analyzers measure pO_2, pH, and pCO_2. The analysis is performed at atmospheric pressure and 37°C in a closed system. Additional acid-base parameters of interest are calculated from the measured values of pO_2, pH, and pCO_2. These include bicarbonate concentration ($[HCO_3^-]$), base excess (BE), and oxygen saturation (O_2 Sat).

Temperature and hematocrit correction for pH, pO_2, pCO_2, and O_2 Sat are available on modern blood gas instruments. The need to make these corrections for pH and pCO_2 is not essential for clinical purposes because even extreme variations in temperature result in relatively small changes for pH and pCO_2. Furthermore, recent experiments suggest that pH and pCO_2 measurements at 37°C accurately reflect the patient's acid-base status, even when extrapolated to other temperatures. Temperature correction is considered necessary for the interpretation of pO_2,[10,11] although the impact of temperature on O_2 transport and release is unclear because of multiple effects on O_2 transport and release mechanisms.

Selection

The measurement of ABG is indicated in the evaluation of any patient who is suspected of having a pulmonary and/or acid-base disturbance. This includes all patients with a change in consciousness, a change in respiratory status, or acute intoxication. Blood gases also are measured to determine baseline pulmonary function prior to thoracic or general surgery. Arterial blood gases are used to follow and manage patients on mechanical ventilation. Measurement of ABG is an essential part of in-hospital cardiopulmonary resuscitation to determine the adequacy of ventilation, perfusion, and the degree of metabolic acidosis. Serial blood gases also are measured to monitor the effects of therapy on an acid-base disturbance. Direct measurement of O_2 Sat is indicated when carbon monoxide poisoning, methemoglobinemia, or a Hgb variant is being considered as a cause of tissue hypoxia.

Logistics[12,13]

Blood gas analyzers require unclotted, whole blood that has not been in contact with room air and has not had time for metabolic activity to significantly alter the results. For collection of arterial blood, the artery chosen must have a collateral blood supply, as thrombosis occasionally occurs. In the upper extremities, the radial, ulnar, or brachial artery are each a good choice. The femoral artery is an acceptable alternative when necessary. Collateral circulation should be demonstrated using the Allen test.[14,15]

The preferred method of collection is from an arterial puncture into a heparinized glass syringe.[16] The amount of heparin in the syringe should be only enough to coat the inside of the syringe and fill the dead space. Plastic syringes are acceptable but are more permeable to O_2 at high concentrations and have a tendency to form more bubbles than glass syringes. After collection, the needle should be removed and discarded properly. Bubbles and dead space air should be forced out and the syringe capped immediately. The specimen should be placed on ice slush and delivered promptly to the laboratory for immediate analysis. The time needed to complete the collection, transport, and analysis should not exceed 20 minutes.[17]

If an arterial sample cannot be obtained, measurements can be made on "arterialized" capillary blood. Arterialized capillary blood is obtained by warming the skin at the sampling site for up to 40 minutes, thus increasing the flow into the area and the oxygenation of the capillary blood. A specimen can then be obtained by skin puncture.

Failure to use the proper procedure can lead to inaccurate results. Excess heparin can lead to decreased pCO_2.[18,19] If the blood is not chilled, the pH will decrease because of the glucose metabolized into lactate by RBCs and white blood cells (WBCs). Because room air has a pO_2 of approximately 160 mmHg (21.3 kPa) and a pCO_2 of approximately 0.25 mmHg (0.03 kPa), exposure of the specimen to room air or to bubbles left in the syringe can lead to an increase in the measured pO_2 and a decrease in the pCO_2.[20] If the patient is on O_2 therapy such that the pO_2 of the patient is greater than 160 mmHg (21.3 kPa), a decrease in the measured pO_2 will occur. In plastic syringes, changes may occur caused by diffusion of gases through the syringe wall but these are not considered to be clinically significant if the sample is processed correctly and rapidly.

Interpretation

Table 2-2 lists the reference ranges for blood gas tests.

Monitoring Respiratory Function

Partial Pressure of Oxygen. Abnormalities in pulmonary function can lead to decreased blood pO_2 (hypoxemia). Hypoxemia must be distinguished from hypoxia. Hypoxemia describes a low blood pO_2, whereas hypoxia describes inadequate delivery of O_2 to the tissues such that anaerobic pathways are activated. Although usually found together, it is possible to have one without the other. Hypoxemia can be measured directly using measurements of partial pressure of arterial O_2 (paO_2), whereas hypoxia is more a clinical than a laboratory finding.

Hypoxemia can be caused by decreased respiration, shunting, or increased O_2 consumption. Decreased respiration can occur because of a wide variety of condi-

Table 2-2. Reference Ranges for Arterial Blood Gas Parameters in Conventional and Système International (SI) Units

Test Name	Conventional Units	SI Units
pH	7.35–7.45	7.35–7.45
pO_2	75–105 mmHg	10.0–14.0 kPa
pCO_2	33–44 mmHg	4.4–5.9 kPa
HCO_3^-	22–26 mEq/L	22–26 mmol/L
BE	−2–+2 mEq/L	−2–+2 mmol/L
O_2 Sat	96–97%	96–97%

Abbreviations: pO_2, partial pressure of oxygen; pCO_2, partial pressure of carbon dioxide; BE, base excess; O_2 Sat, oxygen saturation.

tions that diminish alveolar ventilation or alveolar gas exchange (e.g., emphysema, pneumonia). This results in decreased oxygenation of the blood as it passes through the lungs because poor diffusion leads to a failure to reach equilibrium. Intra- and extrapulmonary shunting also can lead to hypoxemia. Intrapulmonary shunting occurs in alveoli that are not perfused or are underperfused relative to ventilation. This results in partially oxygenated blood mixing with fully oxygenated blood with the mixture having a low pO_2. Finally, low venous pO_2 caused by increased consumption can lead to a low paO_2.

Although hypoxemia is usually the cause of hypoxia, it is not the only etiology. Decreased cardiac output or severe anemia can lead to decreased O_2 transport to the tissues despite a normal pO_2. The shape and position of the Hgb dissociation curve affects O_2 transport and release. Abnormal Hgb with increased affinity to O_2 (P_{50}) such as Yakima, Rainier, and Olympia release less O_2 in the tissues, whereas Hgb with decreased affinities such as Hgb Seattle and Hgb Kansas release increased amounts of O_2.[21,22]

Partial Pressure of Carbon Dioxide. Abnormalities in pulmonary function can also lead to increased or decreased blood pCO_2 (hyper- and hypocapnia). As a measure of respiratory function, pCO_2 is considered to be directly related to ventilation. High rates of ventilation lead to low pCO_2 values and low rates of ventilation lead to high pCO_2 values. A low pCO_2 is commonly seen in anxious patients who are hyperventilating. Low pCO_2 also is seen frequently in patients who are being overventilated on a mechanical ventilator. Only in severe disturbances of respiration does pCO_2 start to become elevated owing to poor gas exchange.

Monitoring of pCO_2 in patients with acute or chronic pulmonary disorders may be needed to define the adequacy of ventilation, ventilatory reserves, and the disease trend. When an acute or chronic pulmonary disorder reaches the point at which ventilation can no longer be increased, the pCO_2 will begin to increase. This can be caused by fatigue, inadequate mechanical reserve, or inefficiency of increased respiratory effort. An increase in pCO_2 is a bad sign, indicating inadequate capacity of the pulmonary system to compensate further.

Bicarbonate Concentration. The bicarbonate concentration is readily calculated from the measured values of pH and pCO_2 using the modified Henderson-Hasselbalch equation. The calculated bicarbonate concentration is used in evaluating the metabolic component of a patient's acid-base status. Bicarbonate levels are controlled by renal reabsorption and production of bicarbonate. Increased levels are produced by the kidneys in response to acidotic states. Decreased levels usually represent the consumption of bicarbonate in the buffering of acids in an acidotic state. A decreased bicarbonate level also can be caused by the inappropriate loss of bicarbonate by the kidneys.

Base Excess. Base excess also gives an indication of the metabolic component of the acid-base status.[23] It represents the increase or decrease in the buffer base needed to achieve the measured acid-base status. A negative value for BE implies a decrease in available buffer base caused by increased acid production or increased alkali loss. Positive values for BE imply an excess of base for the measured acid-base status.

Oxygen Saturation (Calculated). Significant parameters for the evaluation of O_2 transport are the O_2 Sat and the O_2 dissociation curve of Hgb. Oxygen saturation is defined as

$$O_2 \text{ Sat} = \frac{\text{Oxyhemoglobin}}{\text{Total Hgb}} \times 100$$

and represents the percentage of Hgb carrying O_2. The higher the O_2 Sat, the larger the amount of O_2 being transported by Hgb. In healthy patients with a normal Hgb the O_2 Sat is greater than 95%.[3] Oxygen saturation is frequently reported as part of an ABG. However, the reported O_2 Sat result from a blood gas instrument is usually a derived value calculated assuming a normal O_2 dissociation curve.

Monitoring of Patients on Mechanical Ventilation. Blood gases are used extensively in the management of patients on mechanical ventilators. The level of pCO_2 is generally used to assess the adequacy of ventilation. The level of pO_2 measures respiration and is used to select the appropriate percentage of O_2 in the inspired gas. Increases in the percentage of inspired O_2 and the pressure of delivery of O_2 can be used to create a gradient across damaged alveolar membranes and an adequate blood pO_2. Generally, the percentage of inspired O_2 is kept as low as possible while maintaining a pO_2 of 100–150 mmHg (13.3–20.0 kPa). It is important to keep the pO_2 as low as possible so as to avoid O_2 toxicity in the lungs.[24,25] In premature infants, high pO_2 levels lead to retrolental fibroplasia.[26]

Acid-Base Balance

There are two etiologic categories of acid-base disturbances: respiratory and metabolic. Within each of these categories there can be an abnormal decrease (acidosis) or an abnormal increase (alkalosis) in pH. Thus, there are four primary types of acid-base disturbances: metabolic acidosis, respiratory acidosis, metabolic alkalosis, and respiratory alkalosis. Besides the four primary disorders, there are mixed disturbances in which a combination of more than one primary disorder occurs, that is, a patient can present with a respiratory acidosis and a superimposed metabolic acidosis.

Interpretation of blood gas data requires consideration of the sequence of events that take place to reach a particular state (Table 2-3). The sequence begins with an initiating pathologic event disturbing the normal acid-base equilibrium. This disturbance generates two responses, one immediate and one long-term. The immediate response is made by the respiratory system. Through the control of pCO_2 by increasing or decreasing the ventilation rate, alterations in the acid-base status can be rapidly compensated (Fig. 2-1). The long-term response is mediated by the kidneys. The ability of the kidneys to selectively increase or decrease acid and alkali excretion allow them to respond to the acid-base disturbances (Fig. 2-2). However, this response is slow, requiring hours to days to reach equilibrium.

The overall response may or may not be sufficient to correct the pH. If the response is adequate to correct the pH to within the reference range, the acid-base status is described as compensated. If the response does not bring the pH into the reference range, the acid-base status is described as uncompensated.

Metabolic Acidosis. Metabolic acidosis occurs when there is increased acid production or increased bicarbonate loss such that the blood pH decreases below the reference range. The initiating event is metabolic, causing a reduction in $[HCO_3^-]$ and thus in the $[HCO_3^-]:pCO_2$ ratio. Hence, as described by the Henderson-Hasselbalch equation, the decrease in the $[HCO_3^-]:pCO_2$ ratio leads to a decrease in the pH. The immediate response of the acid-base system is the increased excretion of acid by the lungs via increased excretion of CO_2. This is accomplished by increasing ventilation. The increased excretion of CO_2 causes a reduction of pCO_2 and an increase in the $[HCO_3^-]:pCO_2$ ratio, increasing the pH. The long-term response to metabolic acidosis is the increased excretion of H^+ by the kidneys accompanied by an increase in the production and retention of HCO_3^-. If these responses lead to a normal pH, the disorder is called a compensated metabolic acidosis. As the magnitude of the long-term response increases (over hours to days), the immediate response decreases, that is, the respiratory rate moves towards normal.

Table 2-4 lists the common causes of metabolic acidosis. There are three general pathogenic mechanisms. First, there are the conditions that lead to an increased acid load. This can occur either from endogenous or exogenous sources as in diabetic ketoacidosis or salicylate poisoning, respectively. This form of metabolic acidosis also is called increased anion gap acidosis because the added acid load leads to an increased anion gap caused by unmeasured anions. The second pathogenic mechanism is the decreased excretion of acid, as occurs in acute and chronic renal failure. Finally, there are the metabolic acidoses caused by bicarbonate loss in conditions such as renal tubular acidosis or chronic diarrhea (see Ch. 15, under Lactate).

Respiratory Acidosis. Respiratory acidosis is initiated by an increase in pCO_2 caused by either a lowering of the rate and depth of ventilation or by impairment of the CO_2 exchange. The increase in blood pCO_2 lowers the blood pH. The immediate physiologic response is increased ventilation. The long-term response is for

Table 2-3. Overview of Acid-Base Disturbances, the Abnormalities Induced, and the Immediate and Delayed Responses

Acid Base Abnormality	Initiating Event	Alteration in Acid-Base Balance	Immediate Response (Lungs)	Delayed Response (Kidneys)
Metabolic acidosis	↑ Acid production ↑ Alkali loss	↓ pH secondary to ↓ $[HCO_3^-]$	↓ pCO_2 by increasing ventilation	↑ Acid excretion ↑ $[HCO_3^-]$ retention
Respiratory acidosis	↓ Gas exchange in lungs	↓ pH secondary to ↑ pCO_2	↓ pCO_2 by increasing ventilation	↑ $[HCO_3^-]$ retention ↑ Acid excretion
Metabolic alkalosis	↑ Alkali gain ↑ Acid loss	↑ pH secondary to ↑ $[HCO_3^-]$	↑ pCO_2 by decreasing ventilation	↑ $[HCO_3^-]$ excretion ↓ Acid excretion
Respiratory alkalosis	↑ Gas exchange in lungs due to hyperventilation	↑ pH secondary to ↓ pCO_2	↑ pCO_2 by decreasing ventilation	↑ $[HCO_3^-]$ excretion ↓ Acid excretion

Table 2-4. The Common Causes of Metabolic Acidosis Listed by Type of Acid-Base Abnormality

Cause	Acid Produced
Increased acid production (increased anion gap)	
Diabetes mellitus	Acetoacetic, β-hydroxybutyric
Fasting	Acetoacetic, β-hydroxybutyric, lactic acid
Tissue hypoxia	Lactic acid
Alcohol	Lactic acid or ketoacids
Phenformin-induced	Lactic acid
Exercise-induced	Lactic acid
Salicylate overdose	Salicylic acid
Paraldehyde	Acetic acid
Methyl alcohol	Formic acid
Ethylene glycol	Oxalic acid, glycolic acid
Formaldehyde	
Hereditary organic acidoses	
Rhabdomyolysis	
Decreased excretion of acid (increased anion gap)	
Renal failure	
Loss of bicarbonate	
Carbonic anhydrase inhibitors	
Severe diarrhea	
Renal tubular acidoses	
Mineralocorticoid deficiency	
Hypoaldosteronism	
Small bowel or pancreatic drainage	

Table 2-5. The Common Causes of Respiratory Acidosis

Decreased excretion of CO_2 due to ventilatory effects
  Moderate to severe asthma with airway obstruction
  Drug-induced suppression (narcotics, sedatives, etc.)
  Emphysema with exacerbation of airway obstruction
  Flail chest
  Kyphoscoliosis
  Neurologic impairment
    Central nervous system—stroke, brain tumor, etc.
    Peripheral nervous system—myasthenia gravis, multiple sclerosis, etc.
Decreased excretion of CO_2 due to respiratory effects
  Severe congestive heart failure
  Pneumonia
  Respiratory distress syndrome
  Adult respiratory distress syndrome
  Interstitial diseases
  Emphysema with clogging or damage of alveoli
Increased CO_2 production
  Seizures
  Severe asthma with increased work of breathing
  Fever

---

the kidneys to increase the reabsorption of bicarbonate and the excretion of acid. This leads to an increase in $[HCO_3^-]$ that compensates for the increased pCO_2, thus increasing the pH towards or into the reference range. Table 2-5 lists the common causes of respiratory acidosis.

The three major mechanisms of respiratory acidosis are decreased ventilation, decreased respiration, and increased production of CO_2. Decreased ventilation or respiration leads to decreased CO_2 excretion and thus to increased pCO_2 in the blood. With decreased ventilation, the alveoli are not being cleared of CO_2 and there is an increase in the alveolar partial pressure of CO_2, ($pACO_2$). With decreased respiration, the $pACO_2$ can be normal but gas exchange is decreased and the blood pCO_2 is elevated. The high permeability of the alveolar membrane to CO_2 means that pCO_2 is often normal in congestive heart failure and pneumonia when there are only minor membrane damages. Only in severe cases with disruption or damage to the alveoli and/or alveolar membranes will a high pCO_2 be seen.

In the presence of a high blood pCO_2, the respiratory system attempts to increase ventilation. The increase in ventilation is achieved at the expense of increased work of breathing, generating increased CO_2. As the work of breathing increases, a point is reached where the increase in CO_2 caused by the increased work of breathing is greater than the decrease caused by increased ventilation.[23] At this point, increasing ventilation is ineffective and the pCO_2 cannot be decreased and may even be increased by the work of breathing.

Metabolic Alkalosis. Metabolic alkalosis occurs when increased intake or production of alkali or an increased rate of acid loss leads to a net increase in blood $[HCO_3^-]$ concentration. The immediate response is to slow the rate and depth of respiration such that the patient's pCO_2 increases.[27] This compensates for the increased $[HCO_3^-]$ and lowers pH. The long-term response is increased excretion of alkali by the kidneys leading to a decrease in $[HCO_3^-]$ and a decrease in pH towards normal.

Table 2-6 lists the common causes of metabolic alkalosis. As with metabolic acidosis, there are three major etiologic categories. An exogenous increase in blood alkali concentration can occur in the patient who overindulges in antacid or sodium bicarbonate consumption. Endogenous increases in alkali can occur from bicarbonate retention by the kidneys in patients on diuretic therapy or who are hypochloremic. Finally, increased rates of acid loss can be seen in patients who are vomiting and patients who are retaining sodium at the expense of K^+ and H^+.

Respiratory Alkalosis. Respiratory alkalosis is initiated by an increase in the rate or depth of ventilation, leading to a lower pCO_2 and an increase in the $pCO_2:[HCO_3^-]$ ratio. The immediate physiologic response should be to reduce ventilation but this does not occur because the etiology is an abnormality of ventilation. Thus, the primary corrective response is a decrease in the excretion of acid by the kidneys. The decrease in blood $[HCO_3^-]$ compensates for the decrease in pCO_2, moving the $[HCO_3^-]:pCO_2$ ratio towards normal, and lowering the pH towards or into the reference range.[28,29]

A wide variety of conditions can cause respiratory alkalosis (Table 2-7). Respiratory alkalosis is caused by a decrease in pCO_2 by increased ventilation. Increased

---

Table 2-6. The Common Causes of Metabolic Alkalosis

Exogenous increase in alkali
    Ingestion of sodium bicarbonate
    Milk-alkali syndrome
    Multiple blood transfusions
    Penicillin therapy
    Infusion of salts of organic acids (lactate, citrate, acetate)
Endogenous increase in alkali
    Recovery from respiratory acidosis[a]
    Potassium depletion[a]
    Increased levels of mineralocorticosteroids (e.g., Cushing syndrome, hyperaldosteronism)
    Diuretic therapy[a]
    Severe potassium depletion
Increased acid loss
    Vomiting[a]
    Diuretics[a]
    Contraction alkalosis[a]
Other
    Hypoproteinemia

[a] Chloride responsive metabolic alkalosis.

Table 2-7. The Common Causes of Respiratory Alkalosis

Increased excretion of CO_2 by the lungs
    Anxiety-induced hyperventilation
    Hypoxia
    Mechanical ventilation
    Interstitial lung disease
    Asthma, mild to moderate
    Pulmonary edema
    Pulmonary embolism
    Salicylate intoxication, early
    Fever
    Aminophylline
    Neurologic abnormalities
    Liver disease
    Delirium tremens
    Pregnancy
    Severe anemia

---

ventilation is driven by hypoxia, overstimulation of the respiratory control centers, or abnormal responses of the respiratory control centers to stimulation.

Mixed Acid-Base Disorders. In the discussion above, acid-base abnormalities were discussed as distinct entities with no overlap. However, mixed disorders occur with some frequency and must be recognized as such. The variations from normal are confined to distinct bands of values for pCO_2 and $[HCO_3^-]$. These bands are the result of the constraints that the Henderson-Hasselbalch equation places on these parameters at any given pH. Note that these regions represent the values after an equilibrium has been reached.

If a patient presents with an acid-base disorder outside the ranges established for the simple disorders, the patient most likely has a mixed acid-base disorder. However, mild mixed disorders or the counteracting effects of the simple disorders comprising a mixed disorder may give results within the ranges established for simple disorders or even those for healthy individuals. Careful evaluation of acid-base status with consideration of the expected findings of the simple disorders will usually reveal the presence and nature of a mixed disorder.

Summary of Acid-Base Evaluation. There are many approaches to evaluating ABG data to arrive at the patient's appropriate acid-base status. One of the easiest is to first look at the pCO_2, a measure of respiratory function (ventilation).

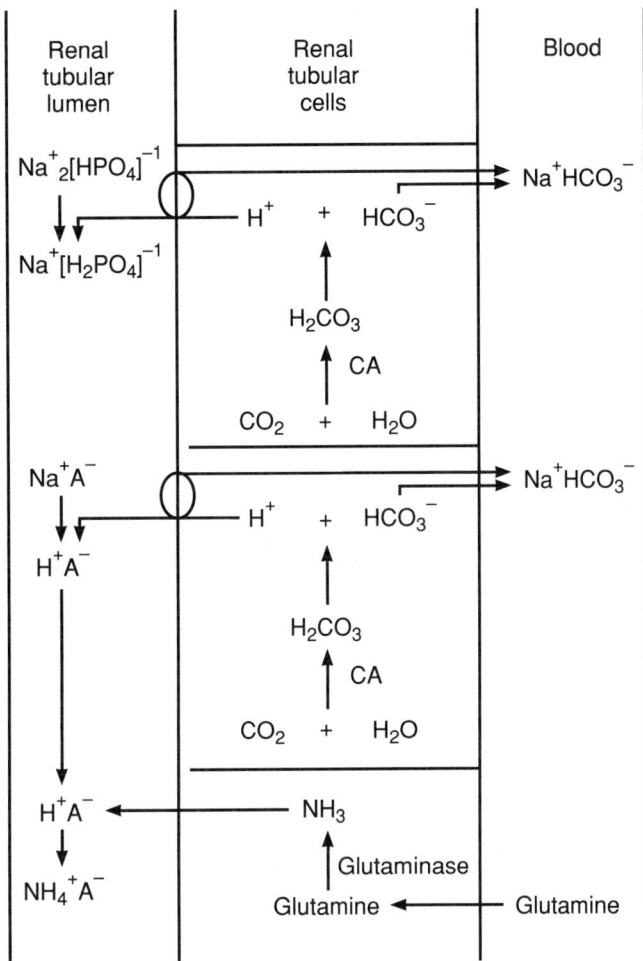

Fig. 2-2. Mechanisms of acid-base control by the renal tubular cells. Carbonic anhydrase catalyzes the formation of H_2CO_3 inside the cells, which then dissociates into the hydrogen ion (H^+) and HCO_3^-. The hydrogen ion is actively exchanged with sodium (Na^+) in the renal tubular lumen and HCO_3^- diffuses passively into the blood. The net effect of this process is the excretion of acid (H^+) and the reabsorption of HCO_3^- and Na^+. Likewise, NH_3 is formed in the renal tubular cells and enters the renal tubular lumen where it combines with H^+ to be excreted as NH_4^+.

A normal pCO_2 with an abnormal pH suggests an uncompensated metabolic disorder. If the pH is elevated, this would be a metabolic alkalosis, and if the pH is below normal, a metabolic acidosis.

If the pCO_2 is decreased, this suggests that hyperventilation is occurring either as a primary disorder or in response to a decrease in $[HCO_3^-]$. If the pH is elevated or greater than 7.40, this suggests respiratory alkalosis. When the pH is within the reference range but greater than 7.40, the status is likely to be a compensated respiratory alkalosis. If, however, the patient's pH is decreased or less than 7.40, this implies metabolic acidosis. If the pH is less than 7.40 but within the reference range, the status is a compensated metabolic acidosis.

Likewise, if the pCO_2 is increased and ventilation is decreased, the status is most likely to be either a primary respiratory acidosis or a response to a primary metabolic alkalosis. If the pH is decreased or less than 7.40, this would imply a primary respiratory acidosis. However, if the pH is increased or greater than 7.40, this would point to a primary metabolic alkalosis. Again, if the pH is within the reference range despite the abnormal pCO_2, the acid-base status is considered compensated.

Test: Transcutaneous and Continuous Arterial Blood Gas Monitoring

Background and Selection

Several methods have been developed for the direct and continuous measurement of pH, pCO_2, pO_2, and O_2 Sat. These methods include: pulse oximetry, transcutaneous O_2 monitoring, and intra-arterial optodes. All three techniques have the obvious advantage of not requiring an arterial puncture for each measurement although the third requires the placement of an intra-arterial line.

This test is indicated in most situations requiring ABG, but especially when continuous monitoring of blood gases is required.

Interpretation

Pulse Oximetry

The continuous measurement of O_2 Sat by pulse oximetry was one of the first transcutaneous methods for blood gas monitoring. A pulse oximeter consists of a small light source and spectrophotometer placed on the surface of the skin. Absorption of light passing through the skin is measured at two wavelengths (940 nm and 660 nm). These measurements are used to calculate the amount of reduced and oxygenated Hgb and thus the O_2 Sat of the blood below the skin surface.[30] The strength of the signal is enhanced by timing the measurements to occur during systole when arterial and capillary blood flow are at their maximums.

Pulse oximetry has been found to be accurate and reliable in a wide range of clinical applications[31-34] for O_2 Sat between 80 and 100%. For O_2 Sat below 80%, the accuracy diminishes but the measurements accurately reflect the trend of O_2 Sat.[9] Over the last several years, the pulse oximeter has gained acceptance as standard operating room equipment. It is also helpful in managing patients on O_2 therapy or mechanical ventilators. Due to its small size, about that of a clothespin, it has found acceptance in outpatient settings, including the transport of critically ill patients to the hospital.

The primary limitation of the pulse oximeter is the need for adequate perfusion at the measurement site. Hypovolemia, hypotension, hypothermia, and arrhythmias will prevent the pulse oximeter from functioning properly. The presence of carboxyhemoglobin (Hgb-CO), methemoglobin, or fetal hemoglobin (HgbF) can lead to inaccurate measurements because of alterations in absorbance or the shape of the O_2 Sat curve.[35] Severe anemia and certain arterial angiographic dyes can also alter results.[36] Measurements can also be distorted by electrical signals, excessive light, and motion.

The primary disadvantage of pulse oximetry is that it only measures O_2 Sat. The instrument cannot distinguish between pO_2 levels above 100 mmHg (13.3 kPa) because Hgb reaches 100% saturation at a pO_2 of about 100 mmHg (13.3 kPa).[37] This is of particular concern in the neonatal intensive care unit where hyperoxemia must be avoided to prevent retrolental fibroplasia. In this and other situations where elevated pO_2 levels must be avoided, pulse oximetry cannot totally replace ABG studies.

Direct Transcutaneous O_2 Measurement

It has been known for the last 100 years that there is gas exchange between the skin and the atmosphere. The transcutaneous O_2 monitor uses this principle to measure pO_2.[38,39] The transcutaneous monitor consists of a chemical membranous pO_2 sensor and heating element placed on the skin. The skin is warmed to 41°C by the heating element, increasing blood flow and the rate of diffusion of O_2 from the blood through the skin. The O_2 tension measured at the skin surface is proportional to that in arterial blood.[40] The transcutaneous O_2 monitor is noninvasive, can be calibrated on room air, and provides continuous, realtime information.[41]

The main disadvantage of this technique is that the sensor must be moved every 4 hours with a 30-minute equilibration period after each move. Burns can occasionally occur as the result of excess heating of the skin. Like the pulse oximeter, the transcutaneous O_2 monitor measures only one ABG parameter.

Intra-Arterial Optode

The instruments that hold the most promise for the future are the fluorescence based blood gas systems that directly measure pH, pCO_2, and pO_2 and that can be packaged small enough to pass through an arterial catheter.

Some fluorescent substances exhibit the property that stimulated fluorescent emission changes at a rate proportional to the presence of a substrate. In particular, certain fluorescent dyes exhibit a decrease in stimulated fluorescence directly proportional to the reversible binding of O_2 to the dye. The variation in stimulated emission over time can be used to measure changes in pO_2. Fluorescent dye binding systems are also available to measure pH and pCO_2. These systems are based on reversible equilibriums rather than on substrate consuming chemical reactions.[42]

The intra-arterial optode is a bundle of three optical fibers with a fluorescent dye contained in a semipermeable membrane at the end of each fiber.[43,44] The bundle is passed through a 20-gauge catheter that has been inserted into an artery. The dyes reversibly react with H^+, CO_2, and O_2 molecules that diffuse across the membrane until equilibrium is reached. The pH, pCO_2, and pO_2 are measured by stimulating the dyes with light transmitted to the tip of the optode via the optical fibers. The resulting fluorescent emission is transmitted back up the fibers and measured on an external device. The optode gives continuous data on all of the ABG parameters, pH, pO_2, and pCO_2.[45] The major disadvantage of the optode is that it is an invasive device.

Test: Oxygen Saturation (Measured)

Background and Selection

A co-oximeter is used to measure O_2 Sat directly.[46] The direct measurement of O_2 Sat is based on the principle that deoxyhemoglobin, oxyhemoglobin, Hgb-CO, and methemoglobin (oxidized Hgb where $HgbFe^{+2} \rightarrow HgbFe^{+3}$) each have a unique peak light absorption wavelength. A co-oximeter measures the absorption at each of these wavelengths simultaneously and calculates the concentration of each of the forms of Hgb. Oxygen saturation is calculated by taking the ratio of the concentration of oxyhemoglobin to total Hgb.

Oxygen saturation measures the oxygenation of Hgb and is thus a measure of the amount of O_2 being transported to the tissues. However, O_2 Sat does not measure O_2 release in the tissues. Oxygen release to the tissues is a function of the capillary-tissue O_2 gradient and the affinity of Hgb for O_2.

The O_2 dissociation curve is a plot of the percentage of O_2 Sat versus pO_2. The shape and location of the O_2 dissociation curve describe the affinity of O_2 to Hgb (Fig. 2-3), which determines the binding and release of O_2. A parameter used to describe the position of the O_2 dissociation curve is P_{50}, the pO_2 at which 50% saturation of Hgb is achieved. The higher the P_{50}, the higher the pO_2 required to achieve 50% saturation. This corre-

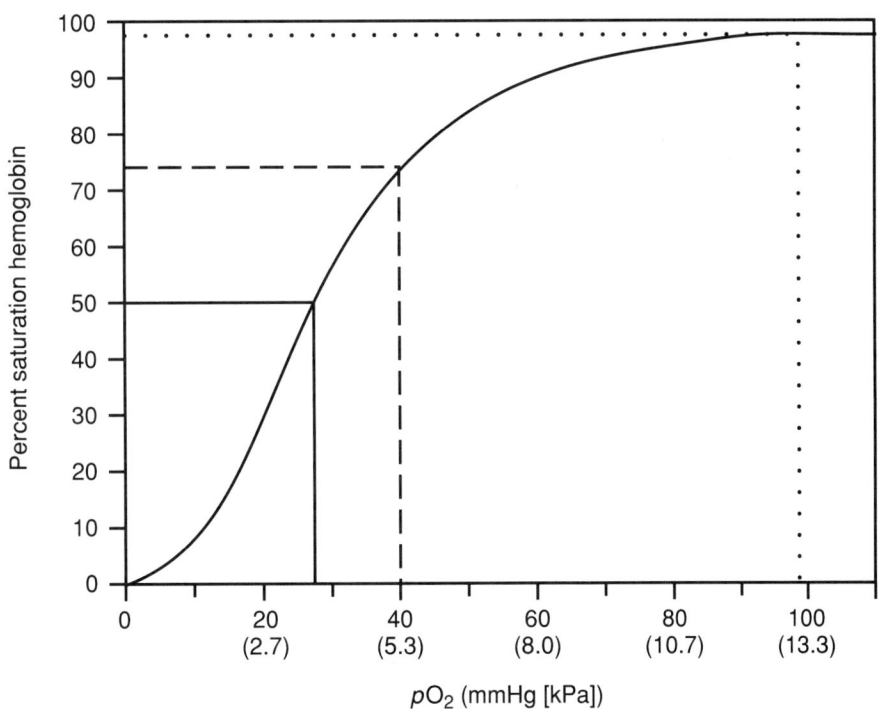

Fig. 2-3. The oxygen (O_2) dissociation curve of normal hemoglobin (Hgb). Marked on the curve are the partial pressures of O_2 (pO_2s) of P_{50} (27 mmHg [3.6 kPa]), venous blood (40 mmHg [5.3 kPa]), and arterial blood (97 mmHg [12.9 kPa]). Note the sigmoidal shape with arterial blood lying on a flat part of the curve and venous blood on the steep part of the curve. Dotted line, pO_2 of arterial blood; dashed line, pO_2 of venous blood; solid line, pO_2 at P_{50}.

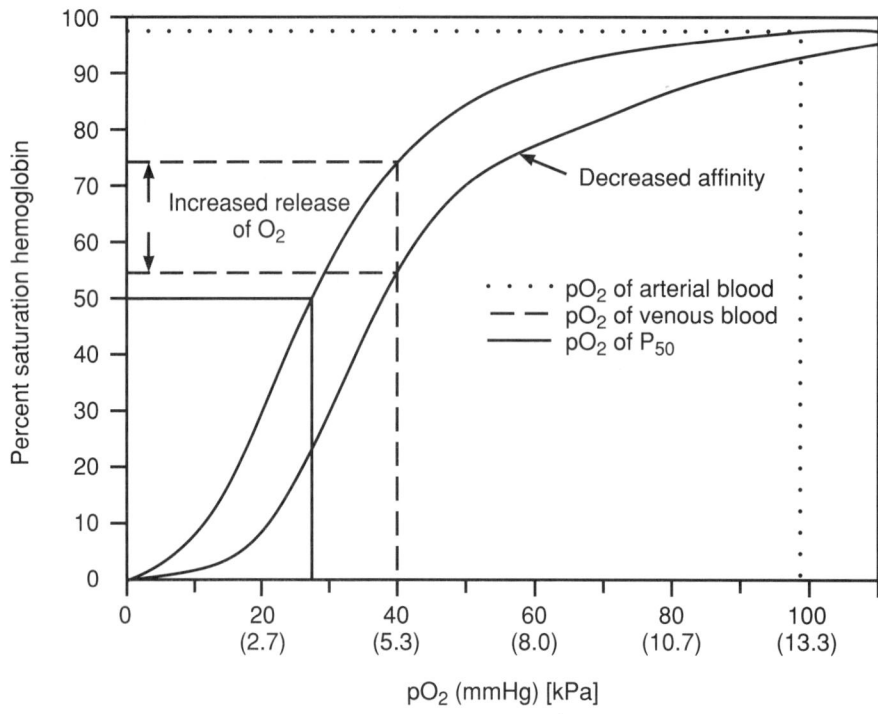

Fig. 2-4. (A) The oxygen (O_2) dissociation curve of hemoglobin (Hgb), where the curve is shifted relative to its usual position. The saturation difference between arterial and venous blood is increased such that more O_2 is released in the tissues at the venous partial pressure of O_2 (pO_2) despite a small decrease in arterial pO_2. *(Figure continues.)*

sponds to increased O_2 release in capillaries because of decreased saturation (increased desaturation).

Oxygen saturation is measured in patients when there is reason to suspect changes in the O_2 dissociation curve. This includes patients suspected of having Hgb-CO (from carbon monoxide poisoning) or other acquired or hereditary Hgb abnormalities.

Interpretation

Normal Hgb has a P_{50} of about 27 mmHg (3.6 kPa), is about 97% saturated in arterial blood, and is about 75% saturated in venous blood (pO_2 of 40 mmHg [5.3 kPa]).[47] This means that 22% of the O_2 carried by Hgb is released in the tissues.

The pO_2 of arterial blood lies on the flat part of the O_2 dissociation curve such that a decrease in pAO_2, and hence paO_2, initially has a small effect on O_2 Sat. The effect of decreased pO_2 on O_2 Sat does not become significant until the pO_2 decreases to as low as 60 mmHg (8.0 kPa). In contrast, the pO_2 of venous blood lies on the steep portion of the O_2 dissociation curve. A small decrease in pO_2 leads to a large decrease in Hgb saturation, which results in a large increase in O_2 release at the tissues.

Hemoglobin transport and release mechanisms respond to changing requirements by shifting the O_2 dissociation curve, thus increasing or decreasing P_{50}. Figure 2-4 illustrates the effect of increased or decreased affinity on the location of the O_2 dissociation curve, the P_{50}, and the delivery of O_2 to the tissues.

Decreased affinity results in an increased release of O_2 in the tissues because the O_2 Sat at any pO_2 is decreased (Fig. 2-4A). However, the decreased affinity is also present in the lungs, where a higher pAO_2 is required to achieve the same degree of saturation. As long as the increased release of O_2 in the tissues outweighs the decreased O_2 Sat seen in arterial blood, a decrease in affinity is the appropriate response to increased tissue O_2 requirements. This will occur as long as paO_2 is on the flat part of the curve and the venous pO_2 is on the steep part of the curve. Decreased affinity is seen with decreased pH, increased pCO_2, increased temperature, increased levels of RBC 2,3-DPG (2,3 diphosphoglyc-

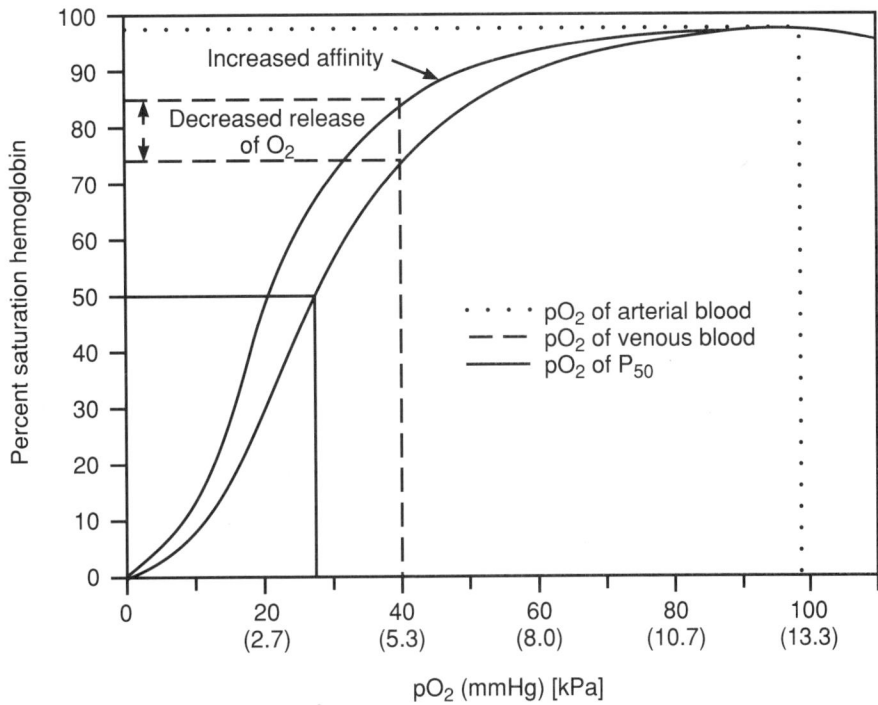

Fig. 2-4 *(Continued).* **(B)** The O_2 dissociation curve of Hgb where the curve is shifted to the left due to increased affinity of Hgb for O_2. The saturation difference between arterial and venous blood is decreased such that less O_2 is released in the tissues at the pO_2 of venous blood despite a slightly increased arterial saturation. Dotted line, pO_2 of arterial blood; dashed line, pO_2 of venous blood; solid line, pO_2 at P_{50}.

erate), and with some abnormal Hgb (such as Hgb Seattle, Kansas). The shift in P_{50} induced by these factors can cause the release of sufficient O_2 to prevent tissue hypoxia.

Conversely, increased affinity results in a decreased release of O_2 in the tissues because the O_2 Sat at any pO_2 is increased (Fig. 2-4B). This results in higher uptake and saturation in the lungs but a lower O_2 release in the tissues. Aside from abnormal Hgb (such as Hgb Yakima, Rainier, Olympia), increased pH, decreased pCO_2, decreased body temperature, decreased RBC 2,3-DPG, and the presence of methemoglobin or Hgb-CO cause increases in affinity.

TESTS FOR SERUM ENZYME AND CARDIAC DISEASE

Measurement of serum enzyme activity is important in the diagnosis of myocardial infarction. Although other enzymes have been used, the most important enzymes are creatine kinase (CK) and lactate dehydrogenase (LD).

Test: Creatine Kinase (CK, Creatine Phosphokinase, CPK)

Background and Selection

Creatine kinase is an enzyme found in high concentrations in skeletal muscle (2500 U/g), cardiac muscle (500 U/g), brain tissue (200 U/g), and in the smooth muscle of the colon, small intestine, uterus, prostate, lungs, and kidneys (less than 100 U/g).[48] In muscle, energy is stored as creatine phosphate. Creatine kinase is the enzyme that catalyzes the transfer of the phosphate group from creatine phosphate to adenosine diphosphate (ADP), forming adenosine triphosphate (ATP), the main source of usable energy.[49]

The test is used to diagnose myocardial infarction, infarct extension and size, and muscle disease such as myositis.

Logistics

Creatine kinase activity is normally measured in serum, although plasma from heparinized blood is acceptable. However, fluoride or citrate anticoagulants should not be used as they interfere with the enzymatic activity of CK. Severe hemolysis also can interfere with the measurement of CK activity because the lysis of RBCs releases adenylate kinase giving falsely elevated CK results.[50,51] Magnesium (Mg) can also interfere with both very low (needed as an enzyme cofactor) and very high Mg levels (interferes with enzyme activity) leading to a decrease in CK activity.

Creatine kinase activity decreases in specimens stored at room temperature for long periods because of both reversible oxidation of sulfhydryl groups and irreversible temperature degradation. Creatine kinase reagents contain a thiol reducing agent to reverse oxidative changes of CK that occur before analysis.[52] Specimens can be kept at room temperature for about 4 hours before CK values become unreliable. If chilled to 4°C samples can be kept for 10–12 hours, and if frozen to −20°C, they can be kept for 1–2 months. The CK-MM isoenzyme (see next section) is the most heat stable with CK-BB being the least heat stable; the stability of CK-MB is between that of CK-MM and CK-BB.[53]

Interpretation

The reference range for total CK activity is about 1–100 U/mL. Sex and racial differences are seen in the reference values for CK. Average CK levels are higher in men than in women.[54] The reference values for black men are up to twice those of white men. Athletic or muscular individuals may also have higher values, particularly after exercise.

The most important use of CK measurements is in the diagnosis and monitoring of patients with acute myocardial infarction. Creatine kinase is a sensitive indicator of cardiac muscle damage. It is the first of the cardiac muscle enzymes to be elevated and the first to peak after a myocardial infarction. Increased levels of CK are first noted from 0–12 hours after an acute myocardial infarction with peak levels occurring 12–24 hours after infarction (Fig. 2-5).[55]

Elevated CK levels are almost always seen in patients if measured within the first 24 hours after infarction. However, a patient who presents after a few days of chest pain may have a demonstrated infarction with a normal CK level. This occurs because the CK level has risen, peaked, and returned to normal before the first CK measurement.

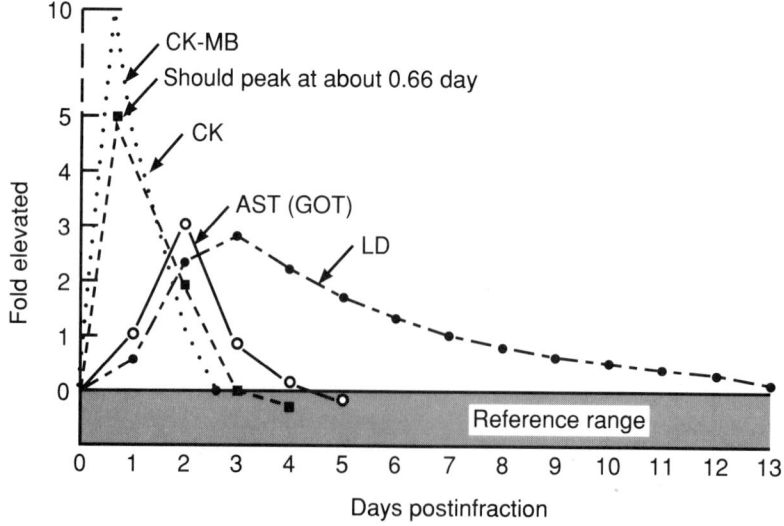

Fig. 2-5. Creatine kinase (CK), aspartate aminotransaminase (AST) (GOT), and lactate dehydrogenase (LD) levels after myocardial infarction. Note that the CK-MB rise is earliest, the LD rise is latest, and the LD elevations are present longer than those of CK-MB and AST.

Although CK is a sensitive indicator of myocardial damage, it is not very specific, with a false positive rate of up to 15%.[56] One study of hospitalized male patients found CK elevations in 52 of 100 patients, with twice normal levels occurring in about 25%.[57] Conditions that can cause elevated CK values include exercise, intramuscular injections, pregnancy, surgery, hypoxic shock, and trauma. High values of CK are seen in patients with myositis and some myopathies. Elevated CK levels also have been found in hypothyroidism, prostate, gastrointestinal, and bladder neoplasms, and after heavy alcohol consumption.[58]

Elevations of serum CK are not usually seen in patients with neurologic diseases such as strokes, tumor, or central nervous system infection. Increased levels of CK seen in these patients are generally derived from skeletal muscle.

The numerous causes of elevated CK levels make it difficult to rely on CK measurements alone for the diagnosis of myocardial infarction. However, in documented cases of myocardial infarction, CK can be used to diagnose extension of the infarct or reinfarction. A patient whose CK suddenly increases after having peaked or returned to normal is likely to be undergoing additional myocardial damage.

Many researchers have tried to use CK levels to determine the size of infarctions and predict outcome. There is a rough linear correlation between infarct size and CK levels.[59,60] However, it is difficult to apply these findings to specific patients to estimate infarct size or prognosis.

Test: Creatine Kinase Isoenzymes (CK Isoenzymes, Creatine Phosphokinase Isoenzymes, CPK Isoenzymes)

Background and Selection

Creatine kinase is a two chain molecule with three isoenzymes, CK-MM, CK-MB, and CK-BB, arising from the combination of two chain types, M and B (Table 2-8). The M chain derives its name from skeletal muscle and the B chain from brain tissue. Skeletal muscle contains almost exclusively the CK-MM isoenzyme (98–99%).[48,61] The only isoenzyme found in brain tissue is CK-BB (Table 2-9). Besides the brain, CK-BB is also found in the smooth muscle of the stomach, gastrointestinal tract, prostate, and bladder. The third isoenzyme, CK-MB, is a molecule combining one M

Table 2-8. The Isoenzymes of Creatine Kinase (CK), Their Structure, and Relative Distribution in Serum

Isoenzyme	Structure	% of Total Serum CK Activity
CK_1	B B	0
CK_2	M B	<5
CK_3	M M	>95

and one B chain. It is predominantly found in cardiac muscle, which is composed of 20–40% CK-MB; the rest is composed of CK-MM.[48,61] In contrast, skeletal muscle has only trace amounts of CK-MB. However, the mass of skeletal muscle is so much greater than that of cardiac muscle that most of the small amount of CK-MB measured in the blood of healthy patients is derived from skeletal muscle.

Two other forms of CK have been described, macro CK_1 and macro CK_2. Macro CK_1 is a CK-BB-IgG or CK-BB-IgA complex that electrophoretically migrates between the CK-MB and the CK-BB bands.[62] Macro CK_2 is a mitochondrial CK that migrates near the CK-MM band.[63] The clinical significance of the macro CKs is still being studied (see Ch. 12).

Three techniques can be used to measure CK isoenzymes: agarose gel or cellulose acetate electrophoresis, column chromatography, and immunochemical identification.[64–69] The method used can influence the interpretation of results. Electrophoretic methods separate and measure each of the three isoenzymes, whereas chromatographic and immunochemical methods separate CK-MM from CK-MB and CK-BB but usually do not separate CK-MB and CK-BB from each other. In the infrequent cases where CK-BB is present, most chromatographic and immunochemical methods will include CK-BB in the CK-MB fraction leading to falsely elevated values of CK-MB.

Test indications are the same as those for total CK.

Interpretation

Many conditions can present with elevated CK levels in the absence of myocardial infarction. In contrast to total CK, CK isoenzyme measurement is both sensitive and specific for the diagnosis of myocardial infarction.

Table 2-9. Creatine Kinase Concentration and Isoenzyme Patterns (Percent of Total Creatine Kinase Activity) in Human Tissues

Tissue	CK Activity (U/g wet tissue)	MM (%)	MB (%)	BB (%)
Skeletal muscle	2590	99	<1	<1
Heart muscle	380	77	22	1
Brain	157	0	0	100
Bladder	162	2	6	92
Ileum	161	3	1	96
Colon	137	4	1	95
Stomach	122	3	2	95
Uterus	39	2	2	96
Thyroid	32	15	1	85
Kidneys	18	8	0	92
Lungs	11	26	1	73
Prostate	9	4	3	93
Spleen	7	74	0	26
Salivary gland	6	44	0	56
Liver	4	90	6	4
Pancreas	3	14	1	85

(Modified from Tsung,[48] with permission.)

The isoenzyme CK-MM is found in the serum of healthy individuals with little (less than 2% of total CK activity) or no circulating CK-MB. In a patient who is having a myocardial infarction, measurement of serum CK isoenzymes will yield a pattern showing the presence of CK-MB (more than 5% of total CK activity) in addition to CK-MM. In contrast, most conditions leading to increased total CK activity represent abnormalities of skeletal muscle. Measurement of CK isoenzymes in these cases yields a pattern showing the presence of increased amounts of CK-MM with little or no CK-MB.

The CK-MB test approaches 100% sensitivity and specificity for the diagnosis of myocardial infarction in patients whose CK-MB levels are measured in the first 24 hours after infarction (Fig. 2-5).[70] The time course of elevation of CK-MB after myocardial infarction closely parallels that of total CK with an onset of elevation in the first 0–8 hours and peaking at 12–24 hours. Increased levels of CK-MB can be seen in patients whose total CK does not rise out of the reference range.[71] As with total CK measurements, CK-MB elevation may be absent if the patient presents after some delay rather than at the onset of chest pain.

Massive skeletal muscle damage may result in the presence of CK-MB in the serum in the absence of infarction, presumably caused by the small amount of CK-MB found in skeletal muscle. However, patients without infarction who undergo surgery show an increase in total CK and CK-MM, but do not show an increase in CK-MB. Patients undergoing open heart surgery frequently show elevated CK-MB levels such that this test is not diagnostically useful after cardiac surgery.

There are some cardiac conditions that occasionally produce elevations in CK-MB, even chronically, in the

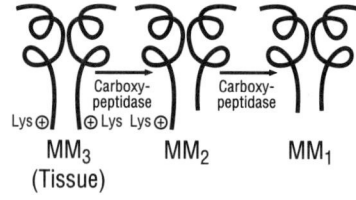

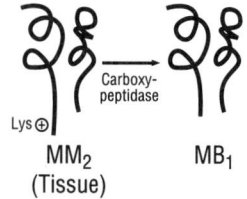

Fig. 2-6. CK-MM and CK-MB isoforms. Illustrated are the structure of the three CK-MM isoforms and the two CK-MB isoforms and the mechanism of their formation. N-Carboxypeptidase irreversibly cleaves a lysine from the M chain(s) of CK-MM and CK-MB. (Modified from Puleo,[93] with permission.)

absence of an acute myocardial infarction. These include: atrial fibrillation, cardioversion, angina, congestive heart failure, myocarditis, coronary angiography, and coronary angioplasty.[62] Additionally, noncardiac conditions such as idiopathic myoglobinemia, Reye syndrome, and Rocky Mountain Spotted fever can also occasionally cause an increase in CK-MB.[56,62]

CK-BB is the isoenzyme found in the brain and smooth muscle. Neurologic disease usually does not lead to the appearance of CK-BB in the blood although this can occur in cases of massive brain damage or breakdown of the blood-brain barrier.[61] Stroke patients may have elevated total CK, which is found to be CK-MM on electrophoresis. This is caused by the release of CK-MM from skeletal muscle that is denervated or traumatized, perhaps secondary to prolonged bed rest. Thus, elevated total CK seen in patients with stroke and other neurologic conditions is usually because of increased levels of CK-MM from skeletal muscle rather than from the release of CK-BB from brain tissue.

The unexpected presence of CK-BB in the blood suggests malignancy, most commonly prostatic, gastrointestinal, or breast (see Ch. 12, under Test: CK Isoenzymes).[61,63,72,73] Anoxia, labor and delivery, hypothermia, acute pancreatitis, prostatic or gastrointestinal surgery, malignant hyperthermia, and Reye syndrome can also account for the presence of CK-BB in the blood.

Test: Creatine Kinase Isoforms

Background and Selection

Creatine kinase isoforms are subforms of the CK-MM and CK-MB isoenzymes that can be distinguished on the basis of different isoelectric points. The isoforms are produced in the blood during the normal metabolism of CK isoenzymes released from muscle and are present in all human sera.

The CK-MM isoenzyme has three isoforms in blood, $CK-MM_3$, $CK-MM_2$, and $CK-MM_1$; the CK-MB isoenzyme has two, $CK-MB_2$, and $CK-MB_1$ (Fig. 2-6). Skeletal and cardiac muscles contain only the $CK-MM_3$ and $CK-MB_2$ isoforms.[74] After release into the blood, carboxypeptidase N acts to cleave a C-terminal lysine from the M chain.[75] This occurs at a fixed rate in a stepwise fashion converting $CK-MM_3$ to $CK-MM_2$ by the removal of one C-terminal lysine and then converting $CK-MM_2$ to $CK-MM_1$ by the removal of another.

$CK-MB_2$ is converted to $CK-MB_1$ in the same manner. $CK-MM_1$ is the dominant form in the blood implying that the rate of metabolism of $CK-MM_3$ to $CK-MM_1$ is greater than the rate of release of $CK-MM_3$ from muscle. When muscle damage occurs, $CK-MM_3$ is released into the blood ($CK-MB_2$ from cardiac muscle), resulting in an increase in the level of $CK-MM_3$ (or $CK-MB_2$) in the blood.

The indications for this test include the diagnosis of myocardial infarction, estimation of time of onset of myocardial infarction, and assessment of coronary artery reperfusion after thrombolytic therapy.

Logistics

Conversion of $CK-MM_3$ to $CK-MM_2$ and $CK-MM_2$ to $CK-MM_1$ proceeds at a relatively rapid rate in patient specimens. Storage at 4°C inhibits the rate of metabolism of the isoforms.[76] Collection of the specimen in a tube containing EDTA will inhibit carboxypeptidase N activity and block the conversion between isoforms.[76] This is desirable in order to prevent conversion between the time the specimen is collected and is processed or stored at 4°C in the laboratory.

There are three major methods of determining CK isoforms: electrophoresis, isoelectric focusing, and high performance liquid chromatography (HPLC).[77-81] Electrophoresis is the cheapest and uses electrophoresis equipment found in most hospital laboratories. However, it takes 30–90 minutes to do the assay. A high voltage electrophoresis system that gives rapid, sensitive isoform separation in less than 25 minutes has been developed.[82]

High performance liquid chromatography techniques can produce results in 30 minutes. However, the equipment is expensive and requires skilled personnel to operate it. It can only be used to measure the CK-MM isoforms because with current techniques the CK-MB fraction remains bound in the column.

Isoelectric focusing is the third method in common use. This method is expensive and difficult to perform and is used mostly as a research tool. Up to 21 bands can be separated with isoelectric focusing. The clinical significance of the additional bands is not yet known.

Chromatofocusing chromatography can also be used but it does not give the resolution of electrophoresis.[83,84] Monoclonal antibodies are also being studied.[85]

Interpretation

See Table 2-10 for reference values for CK-MM isoforms. Reference values for CK-MB isoforms are as follows: CK-MB$_2$, less than 1.2 U/L; CK-MB$_1$, less than 1.2 U/L; and CK-MB$_2$/CK-MB$_1$, less than 1.5.[91]

During the acute phase of a myocardial infarction the CK-MM and CK-MB isoenzymes are released from ischemic cardiac muscle as the tissue isoforms CK-MM$_3$ and CK-MB$_2$, respectively. This leads to a rise in serum CK-MM$_3$ and CK-MB$_2$ and an increase in the CK-MM$_3$/CK-MM$_1$ and CK-MB$_2$/CK-MB$_1$ ratios. The ratios decrease as normal metabolism converts CK-MM$_3$ to CK-MM$_1$ and CK-MB$_2$ to CK-MB$_1$.

The CK-MM$_3$/CK-MM$_1$ ratio is an early indicator of myocardial infarction and peaks before total CK-MB. The CK-MM$_3$/CK-MM$_1$ ratio can be used to reliably diagnose myocardial infarction by 6 hours after onset.[92,93] Moreover, since the rate of CK-MM$_3$ conversion is constant, the time since the onset of the infarction can also be estimated. This can all be done with a single blood sample.[87] In general, one finds that CK-MM$_3$ is the predominant form seen in plasma up to 10 hours after infarction. From 10–24 hours, one finds CK-MM$_2$ as the predominant form. After 24 hours, CK-MM$_1$ predominates. Thus, one can estimate the time since onset with CK-MM$_3$ indicating less than 10 hours, CK-MM$_2$ 10–24 hours, and CK-MM$_3$ greater than 24 hours since onset.

However, the CK-MB$_2$/CK-MB$_1$ ratio is the earliest indicator of myocardial infarction, peaking before total CK-MB and the CK-MM$_3$/CK-MM$_1$ ratio. A recent study showed that the CK-MB$_2$/CK-MB$_1$ ratio peaks at about 3.0 by 4–6 hours after infarction.[91] Furthermore, 100% of patients had an elevated ratio by 8 hours after infarction, with 92% positive by 6 hours. The specificity of the ratio was 95% at 8 hours. Despite the early peaking and high specificity, the CK-MB isoforms are not as widely used or studied as the CK-MM isoforms.

Although measurement of CK-MM isoforms is more sensitive than the measurement of the CK-MB isoenzyme and nearly as sensitive as measurement of the CK-MB isoforms in early detection of an acute myocardial infarction, it is not as specific as either of these tests. As with total CK, a false positive result can occur in any case of skeletal muscle injury or disease. Elevated levels of the CK-MM isoforms and the CK-MM$_3$/CK-MM$_1$ ratio are seen in chronic muscle diseases (e.g., Duchenne type muscular dystrophy), acute muscle trauma, and even exercise.[88,94,95]

Another major use of CK isoforms is in the evaluation and management of patients undergoing thrombolytic therapy for acute myocardial infarction. Current theory says that acute myocardial infarctions are caused by a fibrin clot that forms in a coronary artery already narrowed by atherosclerosis. If detected early enough, these clots can be eliminated by thrombolytic agents, angioplasty, or coronary artery bypass surgery.

However, both angioplasty and bypass surgery are invasive and expensive; thrombolytic therapy is both noninvasive and less costly. Thrombolytic therapy clears the coronary vessels by the intravenous administration of a thrombolytic agent that supplements the body's fibrinolytic system for breaking down clots. However, in order to be effective, these agents must be given within a few hours after the onset of the myocardial infarction.

Table 2-10. CK-MM Isoforms Measured in Serum of Healthy Subjects by Different Methods

Method	N	CK-MM$_1$	CK-MM$_2$	CK-MM$_3$	CK-MM$_3$/CK-MM$_1$
		Percent ± SD			Mean
Agarose electrophoresis[86]	20	56 ± 11	32 ± 5	12 ± 8	—
Isoelectric focusing[87]	8	47 ± 8	30 ± 4	18 ± 4	0.38
High performance liquid chromatography[80]	27	48 ± 12	35 ± 9	16 ± 5	0.30
Agarose electrophoresis[88]	15	54 ± 11	31 ± 8	15 ± 6	0.22
Cellulose acetate electrophoresis[89,90]	34	60 ± 8	24 ± 5	15 ± 6	0.27

(Modified from Panteghini and Colarco,[90] with permission.)

A means of diagnosing acute infarction, estimating the time of onset, and assessing the effectiveness of therapy are prerequisites for adequate treatment. Measurement of CK isoforms has the potential to provide information for all of these areas.

Once a myocardial infarction has been diagnosed, thrombolytic treatment can be given if the infarction is of recent enough onset. The Thrombolysis in Myocardial Infarction Study has shown that no matter which agent is used, the success of reperfusion decreases as the time from infarction increases.[96] Other studies have shown that if reperfusion is started within 3 hours of onset of an acute myocardial infarction, mortality is reduced by 20% at 21 days after infarction.[97] Another study has demonstrated that by 6 hours after an acute myocardial infarction, irreversible myocardial damage has occurred. This has led to a consensus that thrombolytic treatment must be started within 4 hours of onset of a myocardial infarction. Using CK isoforms for rapid 1 hour initial diagnosis of myocardial infarction, this time frame can be achieved.

The results of thrombolytic therapy need to be monitored. Cardiac catheterization and angiography can be used to assess reperfusion. However, by measuring the change in serum $CK-MM_3$ and the $CK-MM_3/CK-MM_1$ ratio over the 30–60 minutes after initiating thrombolytic therapy, the results of reperfusion can be accurately assessed noninvasively.[98] Patients undergoing successful reperfusion show an earlier increase and peak than those in whom reperfusion is unsuccessful. Therefore, CK isoforms allow for not only rapid detection of acute myocardial infarction but also for a noninvasive means of assessing coronary artery reperfusion after thrombolytic therapy.

Most studies have focused on the CK-MM isoforms. However, as mentioned before, measurement of the CK-MB isoforms might prove to provide more accurate information because of the specificity for cardiac muscle of CK-MB. So far, however, the CK-MB isoforms have been only partially studied.[99] It has been found that the $CK-MB_2/CK-MB_1$ ratio can detect reperfusion within 50 minutes, similar to the results seen from studying the CK-MM isoforms.[100]

Test: Lactate Dehydrogenase (LD, LDH)

Background and Selection

Lactate dehydrogenase is the catalytic enzyme for converting pyruvate to lactate under anaerobic conditions, a reversible reaction that goes in the opposite direction under aerobic conditions. The enzyme is found in high concentrations in several tissues including skeletal and heart muscle, the liver, RBCs, kidneys, and lungs. It can also be found in high concentrations in neoplastic tissues.

Logistics

Serum is the usual specimen for LD measurements. Oxalate, citrate, and fluoride preservatives interfere with LD activity and should not be used.[101,102] Heparin is acceptable if the platelets have been centrifuged off as they can cause optical interference.[103] It is also important that the plasma be removed from the RBCs within 2 hours of collection as the RBCs, having 100 times the LD concentration of serum,[104] can hemolyze and alter serum results.

Once separated from RBCs, samples for LD measurement are stable for 2–3 days at room temperature.[104] Samples for LD should not be frozen because the M subunit (see under Test: LD Isoenzymes, below) binds NAD^+ less than the H subunit after freezing. Therefore, freezing leads to a reduction of LD_4 and LD_5 relative to LD_1 and LD_2.

Interpretation

The reference range for serum LD activity is 90–200 U/L. The presence of LD in high concentrations in both cardiac and skeletal muscle leads to frequently elevated levels of LD in many pathologic conditions affecting muscle, the most important of which is myocardial infarction. Elevations of LD are seen in myositis and other forms of skeletal muscle damage.[105] Indeed, exercise and strenuous physical activity are the leading causes of unexpected LD elevations.[106] Elevated levels of the enzyme also can be seen after meals[107] and during pregnancy.[108]

Seasonal variations of reference values are seen, with average values higher in the summer and lower in the winter.[109] There is one other variant of LD, LD-X, that is found exclusively in sperm and has been used for forensic purposes.[110]

After myocardial infarction, LD peaks later and remains elevated longer than CK and aspartate aminotransferase (AST) (Fig. 2-5). Lactate dehydrogenase peaks about 48–72 hours after myocardial infarction and remains elevated for up to 14 days after the infarction. Although CK and CK-MB are more sensitive and specific markers for myocardial infarction than LD, LD values are more useful in some cases. In particular, LD is more useful than CK (or CK isoenzymes) in the patient who is first seen 2 days or later after myocardial

Table 2-11. The Five Isoenzymes of Lactate Dehydrogenase (LD), Their Structure, and Relative Distribution in Serum

Isoenzyme	Structure	% of Total Serum LD Activity
LD_1	H H H H	30
LD_2	H H H M	40
LD_3	H H M M	20
LD_4	H M M M	3
LD_5	M M M M	7

infarction. In this case, CK may have peaked and returned to normal whereas the LD would still be elevated.

However, total LD is not a specific indicator of myocardial disease because several related or frequently concurrent conditions can lead to elevated levels of LD. In particular, congestive heart failure without infarction can lead to elevations in total LD secondary to damage to liver tissue from passive congestion or to muscle damage secondary to hypoxia. Pulmonary embolism is another condition producing acute onset of chest pain that must be distinguished from myocardial infarction. Lung tissue contains relatively high concentrations of LD. Thus, a pulmonary embolism can lead to an elevated total LD. Likewise, a patient with an artificial heart valve can have an elevated total LD caused by valve-induced hemolysis. Finally, the presence of active liver disease, hemolysis from other causes, or neoplasm can negate the usefulness of total LD measurements in the diagnosis of myocardial infarction.

Test: Lactate Dehydrogenase Isoenzymes (LD Isoenzymes, LDH Isoenzymes)

Background and Selection

There are five isoenzymes of LD, each composed of four chains. The five isoenzymes of LD result from the combination of two chain types, H and M. The H and M subunits are coded by the LDHA and LDHB genes located on chromosomes 11 and 12, respectively. The H chain predominates in cardiac muscle and the M chain in skeletal muscle. The varying chain composition of the five isoenzymes is shown in Table 2-11.

All five isoenzymes are normally present in serum with LD_2 present in the highest concentration. The distribution of the isoenzymes in serum represents the relative leakage of the isoenzymes from the tissues in which they are present (Table 2-12).[111-114]

Most laboratories measure LD isoenzymes using agarose gel or cellulose acetate electrophoresis in a procedure similar to that used for CK isoenzymes. The patterns of isoenzyme activity rather than the amounts are used for diagnostic purposes. In particular, the presence of a relative increase in LD_1 suggests the presence of heart disease and/or the presence of hemolysis of RBCs. Determination of LD isoenzymes may be helpful in the diagnosis of myocardial infarction, particularly late in its course. The presence of a relative increase in LD_5 suggests hepatic or muscle damage.

The test is indicated for the diagnosis of myocardial infarction, particularly cases that present late, and for the evaluation of an elevated total LD.

Table 2-12. Lactate Dehydrogenase (LD) Activities and Isoenzymes Distributions (Percentage of Total Activity) in Human Tissues

Tissue	Total Activity (IU/g)	LD_1 (%)	LD_2 (%)	LD_3 (%)	LD_4 (%)	LD_5 (%)
Liver	156	<1	<1	1	4	94
Skeletal muscle	148	3	4	8	9	76
Kidneys	114	60	30	5	3	2
Spleen/lymph nodes	84	5	15	31	31	18
Brain	65	28	32	19	16	5
Erythrocytes	34	33	46	13	4	2
Lungs	27	10	18	28	23	21
Uterus	26	5	20	50	20	6
Serum	0.3	25	35	20	10	10

(Modified from Bissell,[104] with permission.)

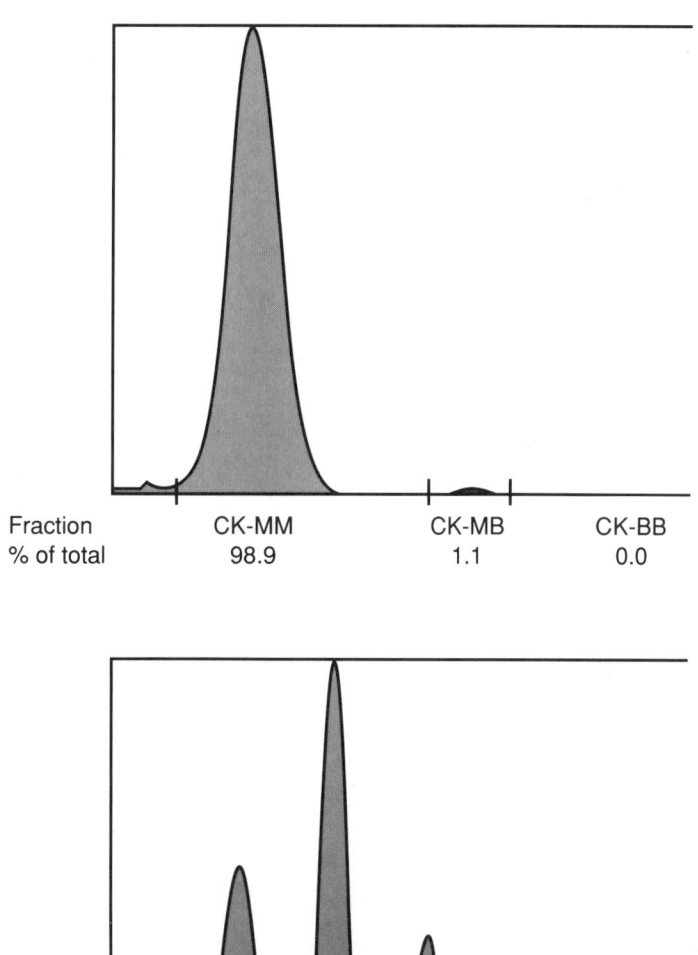

Fig. 2-7. Illustrated are the time course of creatine kinase (CK) and lactate dehydrogenase (LD) isoenzymes during an acute myocardial infarction. **(A)** Time of admission: the isoenzyme patterns are unremarkable with CK-MB less than 5% and LD_1 less than LD_2. This represents the early period before the CK and LD isoenzyme markers increase to abnormal levels. *(Figure continues.)*

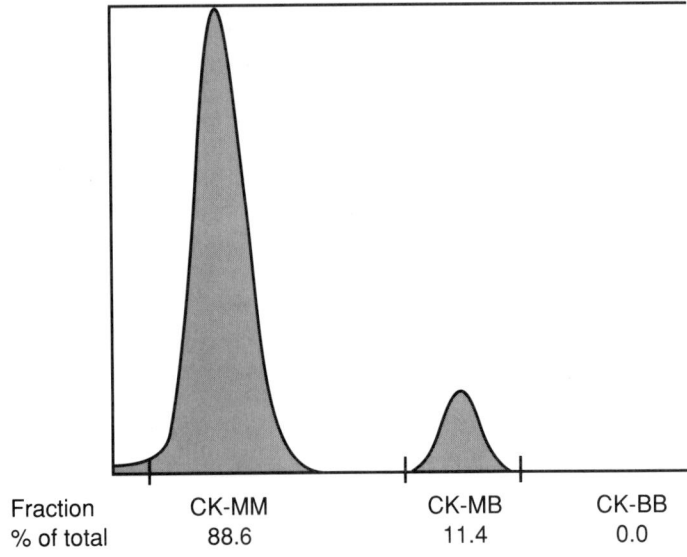

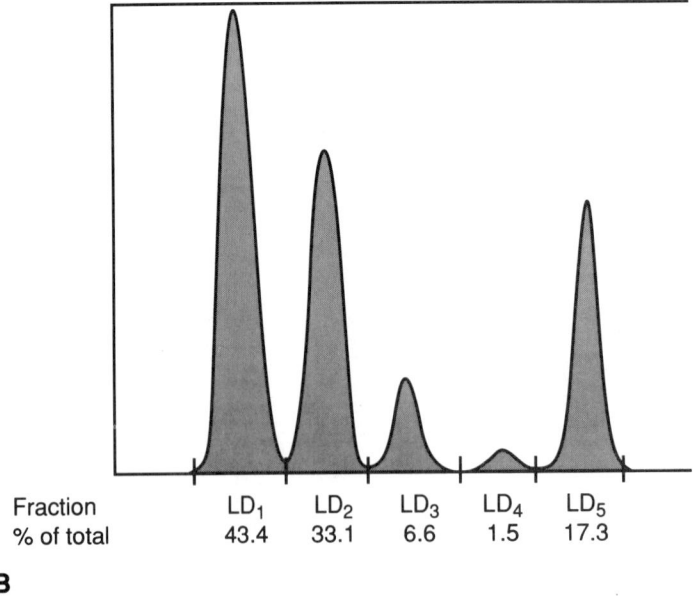

Fig. 2-7 *(Continued).* **(B)** Twenty-four hours after admission: the isoenzyme patterns show the typical changes seen during an acute myocardial infarction with CK-MB greater than 5% and LD$_1$ greater than LD$_2$. In addition, LD$_5$ is noted to be elevated as well, because of ischemic damage to liver and/or muscle. *(Figure continues.)*

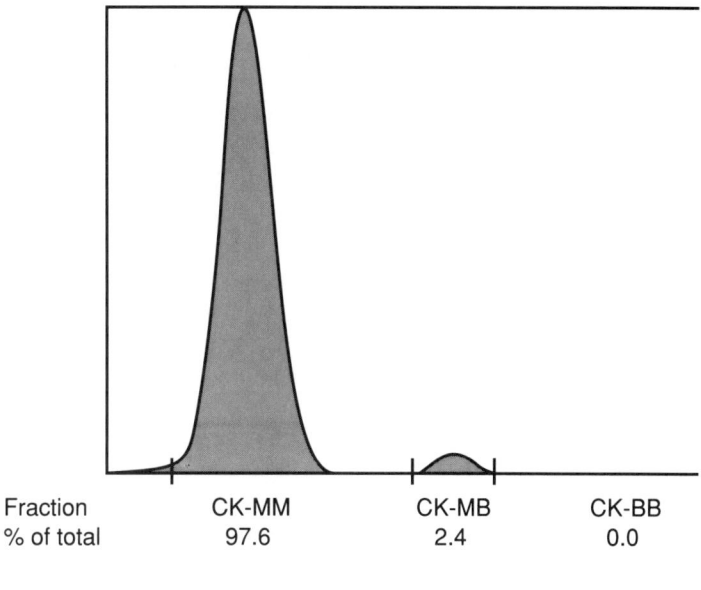

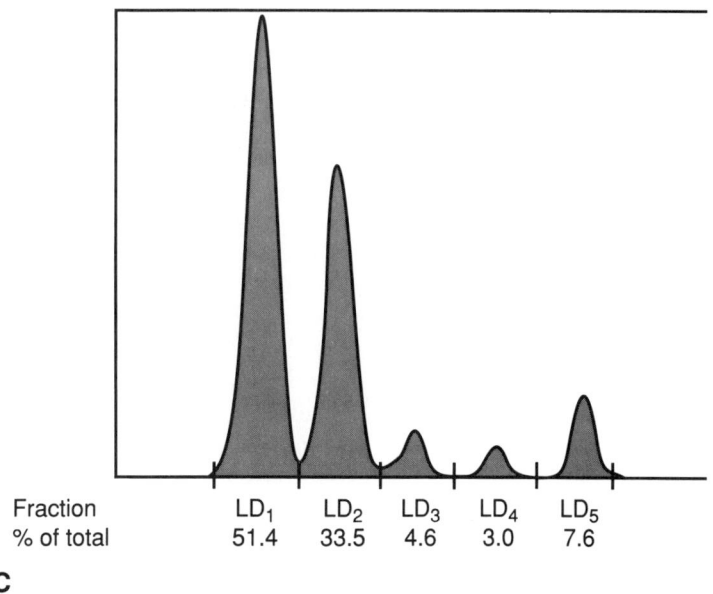

Fig. 2-7 *(Continued).* **(C)** Forty-eight hours after admission: the late isoenzyme pattern is seen where CK-MB is back to normal but the LD_1 greater than LD_2 "flip" remains. This will revert to the usual pattern seen in Figure A over the next 24–48 hours.

Logistics

Before the availability of electrophoretic techniques, two methods had been used in the clinical laboratory to obtain an estimate of LD_1, the predominant isoenzyme in cardiac muscle. In the first, it was noted that LD_1 was heat stable whereas the other isoenzymes were not. Thus the relative concentration of LD_1 could be determined by measuring the LD activity before and after heat denaturation. In the second method, an enzyme called HBD (α-hydroxybutyrate) was shown to be a marker for cardiac damage. α-Hydroxybutyrate activity is determined by measuring the conversion of α-ketobutyrate to α-hydroxyketobutyrate. However, further study showed that HBD is not a distinct enzyme but instead corresponds to the measurement of the activity of the H chain of LD across all the isoenzymes. These methods are not commonly used in clinical laboratories today.

Most laboratories measure LD isoenzymes using agarose gel or cellulose acetate electrophoresis in a procedure similar to that used for CK isoenzymes. The patterns of isoenzyme activity rather than the amounts are used for diagnostic purposes.

Interpretation

Reference ranges for the LD isoenzymes of a percentage of total LD are as follows: LD_1, 24-34%; LD_2, 35-45%; LD_3, 15-25%; LD_4, 4-10%; and LD_5, 1-12%.

As with total LD, there are many sources of LD isoenzymes. Evaluation of the isoenzyme pattern can help identify the tissue of origin and point towards a diagnosis.

Myocardial tissue has high concentrations of LD_1 and LD_2. Thus, in myocardial infarction, elevations of LD_1 and LD_2 occur. The isoenzyme elevations follow those for total LD, that is, they peak at 48-72 hours and can remain elevated as long as 14 days, although LD_1 usually returns to normal before total LD. Of more importance is the pattern of elevation. Although serum LD_1 and LD_2 are both elevated after myocardial infarction, the usual serum pattern of LD_2 being greater than LD_1 is reversed such that following an acute infarction, electrophoresis shows that LD_1 is greater than LD_2 (LD_1/LD_2 is greater than 1.0) (Fig. 2-7). This reversal in pattern has been labeled a "flipped LD"[115] and is considered diagnostic for myocardial infarction if other causes of LD_1 elevation have been ruled out. A flipped LD pattern within 48 hours of chest pain occurs in over 80% of patients with myocardial infarction.[116] Recent studies have concluded that an LD_1/LD_2 greater than 0.76 can be considered positive for myocardial infarction.[117]

The most important use of LD isoenzyme measurement is in the patient who presents with a normal CK and CK-MB after an event of indeterminate age. In these cases, the CK can return to normal before the patient is seen by a physician. The presence of a "flipped" LD would help make the diagnosis of myocardial infarction. In most cases where CK-MB is elevated, an elevated LD_1/LD_2 ratio is a confirmatory but unnecessary finding.

Red blood cells and renal tissue contain high concentrations of LD_1. Thus, renal infarction or hemolysis (in vivo or in vitro) can cause an elevated LD_1 and a noncardiac "flip." Indeed, some of the highest LD elevations with LD_1 predominating are caused by intramedullary hemolysis of RBCs in patients with megaloblastic anemia. High values of serum LD_1 are seen in patients with hemolysis secondary to a prosthetic cardiac valve. However, in the context of a patient with acute chest pain and no evidence of hemolysis, an abnormal LD_1/LD_2 ratio is diagnostic of myocardial infarction.

Elevated LD_3 is seen with lung damage. Pulmonary embolism, which might present with the acute clinical symptoms of a myocardial infarction, usually causes an elevation of the LD_3 fraction. The absence of an increase in the LD_1/LD_2 ratio would differentiate this condition from a myocardial infarction.

Cardiac failure or shock without acute infarction can lead to liver and/or hypoxic skeletal muscle damage. Liver and skeletal muscle contain high concentrations of LD_4 and LD_5. Thus, the LD isoenzyme pattern would distinguish cardiac failure from acute myocardial infarction by presenting with a pattern where LD_4 and LD_5 are elevated but the LD_1/LD_2 ratio is not elevated.[118] If the damage to liver and skeletal muscle is secondary to an acute infarction, one can see a mixed pattern where there is a "flip," (LD_1 is greater than LD_2) and also significant elevations of LD_4 and LD_5.

Malignancy can present with a variety of abnormal LD isoenzyme patterns but not usually with an increased LD_1/LD_2 ratio[119] (see Ch. 12, under Test: LD).

REFERENCES

1. Jones N, McHardy J, Naimark A et al: Physiological deadspace and alveolar-arterial gas pressure differences during exercise. Clin Sci 1966;31:19.

2. Christiansen D: Haldane. J Physiol 1914;48:244.
3. Koch G: Alveolar ventilation, diffusing capacity and the A-a PO$_2$ difference in the newborn infant. Respir Physiol 1968;4:168.
4. Davies C: The oxygen-transporting system in relation to age. Clin Sci 1972;42:1.
5. Mohler J, Collier C, Brandt W et al: Blood gases. p. 223. In Clausen JL (ed): Pulmonary Function Testing Guidelines and Controversies. Orlando, FL, Grune & Stratton, 1984.
6. Elkinton J: Acid-base disorders and the clinician. Ann Intern Med 1965;65:893.
7. Giebisch G, Berger L, Pitts R: The extrarenal response to acute acid-base disturbances of respiratory origin. J Clin Invest 1955;34:231.
8. Gunn R: Buffer equilibria in red blood cells. p. 63. In Seldin D, Gerhard G (eds): The Regulation of Acid-Base Balance. New York, Raven Press, 1989.
9. Shapiro B, Harrison R, Cane R et al: Clinical Application of Blood Gases. Chicago, Year Book Medical Publishers, 1989.
10. Ashwood E, Kost G, Kenny M: Temperature correction of blood gas and pH measurement. Clin Chem 1983;29:1977.
11. Andritsch R, Muravchick S, Gold M: Temperature correction of arterial blood-gas parameters: a comparative review of methodology. Anesthesiology 1985; 55:311.
12. Bruck E, Eichhorn J, Ray-Meredith et al: Approved Standard. Percutaneous Collection of Arterial Blood for Laboratory Analysis. Vol. 5:3. NCCLS, Villanova, PA, 1985.
13. Eichhorn J, Moran R, Cormier A: Proposed Guideline. Blood Gas Pre-Analytical Considerations: Specimen Collection, Calibration, and Controls. Vol. 5:11. NCCLS, Villanova, PA, 1985.
14. Peters K, Chapin J: Allen's test—positive or negative? Anesthesiology 1980;53:85.
15. Messick J: Allen's test—neither positive nor negative. Anesthesiology 1981;54:523.
16. Evers W, Racz G, Levy A: A comparative study of plastic (polypropylene) and glass syringes in blood gas analysis. Anesth Analg 1972;50:92.
17. Kelman G, Nunn J: Nomograms for correction of blood PO$_2$, PCO$_2$, pH and base excess for time and temperature. J Appl Physiol 1966;21:1484.
18. Bradley J: Errors in measurement of blood PCO$_2$ due to dilution of the sample with heparin solution. Br J Anaesth 1972;44:231.
19. Hamilton R, Corcket A, Alpers J: Arterial blood gas analysis: potential errors due to the addition of heparin. Anaesth Intensive Care 1978;6:251.
20. Scott P, Horton J, Mapleson W: Leakage of oxygen from blood and water samples stored in plastic and glass syringes. Br Med J 1971;3:512.
21. Miller D, Lichtman M: Clinical implication of altered affinity of hemoglobin for oxygen. In Weed RI (ed): Hematology for Internists. Boston, Little Brown, 1971.
22. Bellingham A et al: Regulatory mechanism of haemoglobin oxygen affinity in acidosis and alkalosis. J Clin Invest 1971;50:700.
23. Stern L, Simmons D: Estimation of non-respiratory acid-base abnormalities. J Appl Physiol 1969;27:21.
24. Steinberg H, Greenwald R, Moak S et al: The effect of oxygen adaptation on oxyradical injury to pulmonary epithelium. Am Rev Respir Dis 1983;128:94.
25. Kistler G, Caldwell P, Weibel E: Development of fine structural damage to alveolar and capillary lining cells in oxygen poisoned rat lungs. J Cell Biol 1967;32:605.
26. Biglan A, Brown D, Reynolds J et al: Risk factors associated with retrolental fibroplasia. Ophthalmology 1984;91:1504.
27. West J: Causes of carbon dioxide retention in lung disease. N Engl J Med 1971;284:1232.
28. Shapiro B, Cane R: Metabolic malfunction of the lung in noncardiogenic edema and adult respiratory distress syndrome. Surg Annu 1981;13:271.
29. Lucius H, Gahlenbeck H, Klein H: Respiratory functions, buffer system and electrolyte concentrations of blood during human pregnancy. Respir Physiol 1970;9:311.
30. Rasanen J, Downs J, Seidman P et al: Estimation of oxygen utilization by dual oximetry. Crit Care Med 1987;15:404.
31. Hess D, Kochansky M, Hassett L et al: An evaluation of the Nellcor N-10 portable pulse oximeter. Respir Care 1986;31:796.
32. Mihm F, Halperin K: Non-invasive detection of profound arterial desaturation using a pulse oximetry device. Anesthesiology 1985;62:85–87.
33. Fait C, Wetzel R, Dean J et al: Pulse oximetry in critically ill children. J Clin Monit 1985;1:232.
34. Ramanathan R, Durand M, Larrazabal C: Pulse oximetry in very low birth weight infants with acute and chronic lung disease. Pediatrics 1987;79:612.
35. Barker S, Tremper K: The effect of carbon monoxide inhalation on pulse oximetry and transcutaneous pO$_2$. Anesthesiology 1987;66:667.
36. Yelderman M, New W Jr: Evaluation of pulse oximetry. Anesthesiology 1983;59:349.
37. Sarnquist F: CE update—clinical chemistry I: clinical pulse oximetry. Lab Med 1988;19:417.
38. Lubbers D: Theoretical basis of transcutaneous blood gas measurements. Crit Care Med 1981;9:721.
39. Beran A, Tolle C, Huxtable R: Cutaneous blood flow and its relationship to transcutaneous pO$_2$/pCO$_2$ measurements. Crit Care Med 1981;9:736.
40. Van Duzee B: Thermal analysis of human stratum corneum. J Invest Dermatol 1975;65:404.
41. Halden L: Monitoring of optimal oxygen transport by the transcutaneous oxygen tension method. Acta Anaesthesiol Scand 1982;26:209.
42. Miller W, Gehrich J, Hansmann R et al: CE update—clinical chemistry: continuous in vivo monitoring of blood gases. Lab Med 1988;19:629.
43. Gehrich J, Lubbers D, Opitz N et al: Optical fluorescence and its application to an intravascular blood gas monitoring system. IEEE Trans Biomed Eng 1986;117.
44. Shapiro B, Cane R, Chemka C et al: Evaluation of a new intra-arterial blood gas system in dogs. Crit Care Med 1987;15:361.
45. Shapiro B, Cane R, Chemka C et al: Preliminary evaluation of a new intra-arterial blood gas system. Crit Care Med 1989;17:455.
46. Operator's Manual 482 Co-Oximeter. Boston, Instrumentation Laboratory Inc., 1987.
47. Brewer G, Eaton J: Erythrocyte metabolism: Interaction with oxygen transport. Science 1971;171:1205.
48. Tsung S: Creatine kinase isoenzyme pattern in human tissue obtained at surgery. Clin Chem 1976;22:173.
49. Lehninger A: The biochemistry of muscle and motile

systems. p. 767. In Lehninger A (ed): Biochemistry. 2nd Ed. New York, Worth Publishing, 1979.
50. Frank J, Bernes E, Bickel M et al: Effect of in vitro hemolysis on chemistry values for serum. Clin Chem 1978;24:1966.
51. Szasz G, Gerhardt W, Gruber W et al: Creatine kinase in serum. II. Interference of adenylate kinase with the assay. Clin Chem 1976;22:1806.
52. Post G: CK and CK isoenzymes: a review of methods. Am Soc Clin Pathol Check Sample 8, Chicago, 1987.
53. Bowie L, Griffiths J, Gochman N: The preferred method for creatine kinase. p. 121. In Griffiths J (ed): Clinical Enzymology. New York, Masson Publishing, 1979.
54. McNeely M, Berris B, Papsin F et al: Creatine kinase and its isoenzymes in the serum of women during pregnancy and peripartum period. Clin Chem 1977;23:1878.
55. Herlitz J: Time lapse from estimated onset of acute myocardial infarction to peak serum enzyme activity. Clin Cardiol 1984;7:433.
56. Lott J: Serum enzyme determinations in the diagnosis of acute myocardial infarction: an update. Hum Pathol 1984;15:706.
57. Nevins N, Saran N, Bright M et al: Pitfalls in interpreting serum creatine phosphokinase activity. JAMA 1973;224:1382.
58. Lee T, Coldman L: Serum enzymes in the diagnosis of acute myocardial infarction: recommendations based on quantitative analysis. Ann Intern Med 1986;105:221.
59. Horie M, Yasue H, Omote S et al: A new approach for the enzymatic estimation of infarct size: Serum peak creatine kinase and time to peak creatine kinase activity. Am J Cardiol 1986;57:76.
60. Grande P, Hansen B, Christiansen C et al: Estimation of acute myocardial infarct size in man by serum measurements. Am J Cardiol 1987;59:245.
61. Lang H (ed): Creatine Kinase Isoenzymes: Pathophysiology and Clinical Applications. Berlin, Springer-Verlag, 1981.
62. Pesce M: Diagnostic significance: Creatine kinase isoenzymes. Ill Med J 1985;167:370.
63. Lang H, Wurzburg U: Creatine kinase, an enzyme of many forms. Clin Chem 1982;28:1439.
64. Wolf P, Griffiths J, Koett J (eds): Interpretation of Electrophoretic Patterns of Proteins and Isoenzymes. New York, Masson Publishing, 1981.
65. Mercer D: Separation of tissue and serum creatine kinase by ion-exchange chromatography. Clin Chem 1974;20:36.
66. Wicks R, Usategui-Gomez M, Miller M et al: Immunochemical determinations of CK-MB isoenzyme in human serum: II. An enzymatic approach. Clin Chem 1972;28:54.
67. Kock T, Mehta W, Nipper H: Clinical and analytical evaluation of kits for measurement of creatine kinase isoenzyme MB. Clin Chem 1986;32:186.
68. Landt U, Vaidya H, Parter D et al: Semiautomated direct colorimetric measurement of creatine kinase isoenzyme MB activity after extraction from serum by use of a CK-MB specific monoclonal antibody. Clin Chem 1988;34:575.
69. Murthy V, Karmen A: Activity concentration and mass concentration (monoclonal antibody immunoenzymometric method) compared for creatine kinase MB isoenzyme in serum. Clin Chem 1986;32:1956.
70. Roberts R, Gmowda K, Ludbrook P et al: Specificity of elevated serum MB creatine phosphokinase activity in the diagnosis of acute myocardial infarction. Am J Cardiol 1975;36:433.
71. Hong T, Licht J, Wei J et al: Elevated CK-MB with normal total creatine kinase in suspected myocardial infarction: associated clinical findings and early prognosis. Am Heart J 1986;111:1041.
72. Wold L, Li D, Homburger H: Localization of the B and M polypeptide subunits of creatine kinase in normal and neoplastic human tissues by an immunoperoxidase technic. Am J Clin Pathol 1981;75:327.
73. Painter P, Dyer M, Hill D et al: Puzzling CK elevation. Lab Management 1988;11:48.
74. Wu A: Creatine kinase isoforms in ischemic heart disease. Clin Chem 1989;35:7.
75. Michelutti L, Falter H, Certossi S et al: Isolation and purification of creatine kinase conversion factor from human serum and its identification as carboxy peptidase N. Clin Biochem 1987;20:21.
76. Abendschein D, Fontanet H, Nohara R: Optimized preservation of isoforms of creatine kinase MM isoenzyme in plasma specimens and their rapid quantification by semi-automated chromatofocussing. Clin Chem 1990;36:723.
77. Chapelle J: Serum creatine kinase MM sub-band determination by electric focusing: a potential method for the monitoring of myocardial infarction. Clin Chim Acta 1984;137:273.
78. Schlabach T, Alpert A, Regnier F: Rapid assessment of isoenzymes by high performance liquid chromatography. Clin Chem 1978;24:1351.
79. Bostick W, Denton M, Dinsmore S: Liquid chromatographic separation and online bioluminescence detection of creatine kinase isoenzymes. Clin Chem 1980;26:712.
80. Wu A, Gornet T: Measurement of creatine kinase MM sub-types by anion exchange liquid chromatography. Clin Chem 1985;31:1841.
81. Escobar R, Gornet T, Wu A: Evaluation of an automated electrophoresis analyzer for cardiac isoenzymes. Clin Chem 1988;34:1284.
82. Puleo P, Guadagno P, Roberts R et al: Sensitive rapid assay of subforms of creatine kinase MB in plasma. Clin Chem 1989;35:1452.
83. Nohara R, Sobel L, Abendschein D: Quantitative analysis of isoforms of MM creatine kinase in plasma by chromatofocusing with online monitoring of enzyme activity. Clin Chem 1988;34:235.
84. Wagner G, Regnier F: Rapid chromatofocusing of proteins. Anal Biochem 1982;126:37.
85. Suzuki T, Tomita K: A monoclonal antibody inhibiting creatine kinase-MM_3, but not MM_1 sub-type. Clin Chem 1988;34:1279.
86. Falter H, Michelutti L, Mazzuchin A et al: Studies on the sub-banding of creatine kinase MM and the CK "conversion factor." Clin Biochem 1981;14:3.
87. Morelli R, Carlson C, Emilson B et al: Serum creatine kinase MM isoenzyme sub bands after acute myocardial infarction in man. Circulation 1983;67:1283.
88. Annesley T, Strongwater S, Schnitzer T: MM subisoenzymes of creatine kinase as an index of disease activity in polymyositis. Clin Chem 1985;31:402.
89. Panteghini M, Cuccia C, Malchiodi A et al: Isoforms of creatine kinase MM and MB in acute myocardial in-

farction: a clinical evaluation. Clin Chim Acta 1986;155:1.
90. Panteghini M, Calarco M: Serum isoforms of creatine kinase MM and MB in myocardial infarction. An appraisal of quantitative, clinical, and pathophysiological information. Scand J Clin Lab Invest 1987;47:235.
91. Puleo P, Guadagno P, Roberts R et al: Early diagnosis of acute myocardial infarction based on assay for subforms of creatine kinase MB. Circulation 1990;82:759.
92. Hashimoto H, Abendschein D, Strauss A et al: Early detection of myocardial infarction in conscious dogs by analysis of plasma MM creatine kinase isoforms. Circulation 1985;71:363.
93. Puleo P: Enzymatic methods for diagnosis of myocardial infarction and detection of reperfusion after thrombolysis. Practical Card 1989;15:50.
94. Apple F, Rogers M, Ivy J: Creatine kinase isoenzyme MM variants in skeletal muscle and plasma from marathon runners. Clin Chem 1986;32:41.
95. Clarkson P, Apple F, Byrnes W et al: Creatine kinase isoforms following isometric exercise. Muscle Nerve 1987;110:41.
96. Thrombolysis in Myocardial Infarction Study Group: Comparison of invasive and conservative strategies after treatment with intravenous tissue plasminogen activator in acute myocardial infarction: results of the thrombolysis in myocardial infarction (TIMI) phase II trial. N Engl J Med 1989;320:618.
97. Gruppo Italiano per lo Studio della Strepochinasi nell'Infarction Miocardico (GISSI): Effectiveness of intravenous thrombolytic treatment in acute myocardial infarction. Lancet 1986;1:397.
98. Devries S, Sobel B, Abendschein D: Early detection of myocardial reperfusion by assay of plasma MM creatine kinase isoforms in dogs. Circulation 1986;74:567.
99. Puleo P, Guadagno P, Roberts R et al: Sensitive, rapid assay of subforms of creatine kinase MB in Plasma. Clin Chem 1989;35:1452.
100. Christenson R, Ohman E, Clemmensen P: Characteristics of creatine kinase — MB and MB isoforms in serum after reperfusion in acute myocardial infarction. Clin Chem 1989;35:2179.
101. McComb R: The measurement of lactate dehydrogenase. p. 157. In Homberger H (ed): Clinical and Analytical Concepts in Enzymology. Skokie, IL, College of American Pathologists, 1983.
102. Lactate Dehydrogenase analysis. Kodak Ektachem Test Methodology. Rochester, NY, Eastman Kodak Co, 1984.
103. Peak M, Pejakovic M, Alderman M et al: Mechanism of platelet interference with measurement of lactate dehydrogenase activity in plasma. Clin Chem 1984;30:518.
104. Bissel M: Lactic dehydrogenase: review of methods. Am Soc Clin Pathol Check Sample 6, Chicago, 1987.
105. D'Angelo W: Diagnostic procedures and tests. p. 533. In Halsted J (ed): The Laboratory in Clinical Medicine. Philadelphia, WB Saunders, 1976.
106. Statland B, Winkel P: Sources of variation in laboratory measurements. p. 3. In Henry J (ed): Clinical Diagnosis and Management by Laboratory Methods. 16th Ed. Vol. 1. Philadelphia, WB Saunders, 1979.
107. Steinmets J, Panek E, Sourieau F et al: Influence of food intake on biological parameters. p. 193. In Siest G (ed): Reference Values in Human Chemistry. New York, S Karger AG, 1973.
108. Dambrosio F: Enzymes in pregnancy. Ann Obstet Gynecol Med Perinat 1965;87:163.
109. Winkelman J, Cannon D, Pileggi C et al: Estimation of norms from controlled sample survey. Clin Chem 1973;19:488.
110. Brewer M, Scott T: Concise Encyclopedia of Biochemistry. Berlin, Wlater deGruyter, 1983.
111. Diederichs F, Muhlhous K, Trautschold I et al: On the mechanism of lactate dehydrogenase release from skeletal muscle in relation to the control of cell volume. Enzyme 1979;24:404.
112. Cohen L, Morgan H, Morgan S et al: The effect of pH on enzyme leakage from isolated mouse heart. Res Comm Chem Pathol Pharmacol 1982;37:463.
113. Piper H, Hutter J, Spieckermann P: Relation between enzyme release and metabolic changes in reversible anoxic injury of myocardial cells. Life Sci 1984;35:127.
114. Piper H, Phahr R, Hutter J et al: Enzyme release and glycolytic energy production. Basic Res Cardiol 1985;1:143.
115. Galen R: The enzyme diagnosis of myocardial infarction. Hum Pathol 1975;6:141.
116. Ustegui-Gomez M, Wicks R, Warshaw M: Immunochemical determination of the heart isoenzyme of lactate dehydrogenase (LDH 1) in human serum. Clin Chem 1979;25:729.
117. Lee T, Goldman L: Serum enzyme assays in the diagnosis of acute myocardial infarction. Ann Intern Med 1986;26:148D.
118. Simmerman H, Henry J: Clinical enzymology. p. 266. In Henry J (ed): Clinical Diagnosis and Management by Laboratory Methods. 16th Ed. Vol. 1. Philadelphia, WB Saunders, 1979.
119. Friedman R, Anerson R, Entine S et al: Effects of diseases on clinical laboratory tests. Clin Chem 1980;26:148.

3 Renal Function

Denis O. Rodgerson

INTRODUCTION

Renal function, that is, the excretory role of the kidney as distinct from the endocrine role, is normal when both the glomerular filtration rate (GFR) and tubular function are normal. In the majority of cases of renal disease, both the glomeruli and the tubules are dysfunctional. A decrease in GRF causes the retention of nitrogenous end products (uremia), acidosis, hyperkalemia, and oliguria. Tubular damage results in acidosis, hypokalemia, hypophosphatemia, hypouricemia, and polyuria.

Tests to evaluate renal function can be divided into two broad categories. The first category relates to the assessment of a specific genetic disorder, which frequently causes a defect in the transport of one or more small molecules such as glucose, phosphate, water, amino acids, or hydrogen ions. The effects of heavy metals on renal transport, which can cause symptoms that mimic the transport defects seen in genetic disorders, are also evaluated by this group of tests. The second category relates to the assessment of the more common renal disorders caused by infection, immunoreactions, ischemia, and toxic agents. Although much variability is possible in the focus (glomerular or tubular) of the disease process and its speed of progression, the fundamental task is the assessment of the number of functioning nephrons. Testing may address the specific local functions of the nephron; but measurements of serum and urine levels of compounds cleared by the kidney are usually used to acquire an estimate of GFR, together with an assessment of glomerular permeability, as indicated by the quantity and type of protein appearing in the urine.

BASIC TESTS

Test: Urea Nitrogen (Blood Urea Nitrogen [BUN])

Background and Selection

Urea, the major product of protein catabolism, is synthesized in the liver, excreted by the glomeruli, and reabsorbed to a degree by the tubules. Measuring urea is probably the most popular laboratory procedure for assessing renal function. However, this test is limited by the fact that considerable glomerular destruction, perhaps as much as 70–80%, must occur before increases in the concentration of urea are seen in the serum. Furthermore, the concentration of urea in serum is a function of protein intake, endogenous protein catabolism from starvation, infection, fever or medication, and rate of urine formation. Low tubular flow rates may cause increased reabsorption of urea and hence a misleading elevation of serum values. As a result of these factors, the clearance of urea does not provide a valid measure of GFR, but rather a significant underestimation. It has been recommended that the utility of serum urea measurements is greatly enhanced when the results are considered together with the levels of serum creatinine. To this end, the ratio of urea nitrogen and creatinine in serum has been advocated. However, this indicator has also been criticized as being unreliable. As mentioned previously, these measurements do not have a high diagnostic specificity or sensitivity. Plasma urea nitrogen has a specificity of 91% and a sensitivity of 67% when the GFR is less than 75% of normal; comparable figures for plasma creatinine are 96% and 69%, respectively.[1]

Terminology

Current usage in the United States perpetuates the use of the descriptor BUN even though measuring urea in blood is seldom, if ever, performed. Furthermore, the Système Internationale d'Unités (SI system) recommends the use of urea, as opposed to urea nitrogen, expressed as mmol/L. The factor for converting mass units of urea nitrogen to mass units of urea is 2.14, whereas the factor for converting mg of urea nitrogen/dL to mmol urea/L is 0.166.

Logistics

The methods used for measuring urea nitrogen in physiologic fluids can, in general, be divided into direct and indirect procedures. In the latter, urea is hydrolyzed by urease into ammonium ion and carbon dioxide with subsequent quantitation of the ammonium by chemical, enzymatic, or electrochemical processes.[2,3] It should be noted that blood collected into fluoride must not be used in urease dependent methods. The direct methods are all variations on the Fearon reaction, in which urea reacts with a diacetyl to form a colored compound.[4]

Interpretation

The usually accepted adult reference range for serum or plasma urea nitrogen is 8–20 mg/dL (2.8–7.1 mmol/L), with serum urea nitrogen levels reported as being slightly higher in men than in women. Levels in children are significantly lower than adult values, with newborns having values approximately one-half the adult range. As children grow older, there is a progressive increase in plasma urea results until adult levels are reached at about age 2. The normal urinary excretion of urea nitrogen for adults ingesting an average protein diet is in the range of 17–20 g/24 h (610–710 mmol/d). Conditions that are known to increase or decrease the serum and urine levels of urea nitrogen are shown in Table 3-1.

Urea Clearance

As indicated above, serum urea concentration is a better indicator of nitrogen intake and the state of hydration than it is of renal function. However, the clearance of urea has, in the past, enjoyed some popularity as a measure of GFR.[5] Unlike creatinine, urea, after filtration at the glomeruli, is 40–50% reabsorbed in the tubules and the calculation of its clearance usually approximates 50–60% of the true GFR. However, considerable variability may be found. This is caused by the variability in serum urea nitrogen concentration and, more importantly, by the dependence of urinary urea nitrogen concentrations on the rate of urine flow. Nevertheless, the information obtained from the calculation of urea clearance may provide useful information (Table 3-2), especially when compared with data from the creatinine clearance.[6]

Test: Creatinine

Background and Selection

Creatinine is derived from the catabolism of creatine in skeletal muscle. Concentrations of creatinine in the serum and urine are governed predominantly by the lean body mass and are little affected by changes in diet or other factors. Thus, serum creatinine levels are remarkably stable, elevated by little other than renal disease and dehydration. Creatinine is removed from the blood by first-pass filtration in the glomeruli and is not reabsorbed in the tubules. These properties have made creatinine the most popular analyte for the determination of GFR (see Creatinine Clearance). There is, how-

Table 3-1. Conditions in Which Serum and Urine Urea Nitrogen Levels Are Outside the Reference Ranges

Serum increased	Chronic glomerular nephritis, pyelonephritis, other chronic renal diseases, acute or chronic renal failure; postrenal obstruction of urine flow, diarrhea, diuresis, excessive sweating; increased protein catabolism due to gastrointestinal hemorrhage, acute myocardial infarction, burns, sepsis, fever; high protein diet; congestive heart failure; tetracyclines; ketosis and dehydration of diabetes; corticosteroids; nephrotoxic drugs
Serum decreased	Pregnancy, low protein diet, intravenous feeding, acromegaly, severe liver disease, inappropriate secretion of antidiuretic hormone (SIADH), drug poisoning
Urine increased	Increased protein intake, postoperatively, hyperthyroidism
Urine decreased	Low protein diets, pregnancy, liver disease, toxemia, renal insufficiency

Table 3-2.	Reference Ranges for Urea Clearance[7]
Premature infants	3.5–17.3 mL/min/1.73 m² (0.06–0.30 mL/s/1.73 m²)
Newborn	8.7–33 mL/min/1.73 m² (0.15–0.55 mL/s/1.73 m²)
2–12 Months	40–95 mL/min/1.73 m² (0.67–1.59 mL/s/1.73 m²)
2 Years and over	52 mL/min/1.73 m² (0.88 mL/s/1.73 m²)

Table 3-3. Range of 24-Hour Urinary Excretion of Creatinine Expressed as Function of Body Weight

Age	Creatinine Coefficient mg/kg/24 h (mmol/kg/d)
6–66 Days (premature)	8.1–15.0 (7.2–13.3)
89–100 Days (full term)	10.4–19.7 (9.2–17.4)
1.5–7 Months	10.0–15.0 (8.8–13.2)
7–15 Years (males)	5.2–15.0 (4.6–13.2)
7–15 Years (female)	11.5–29.1 (10.2–25.7)

ever, some excretion of creatinine by tubular secretion, which is small at normal serum concentrations but significant at abnormally elevated serum creatinine levels. The concept of relating the urinary excretion of many solutes to the excretion of creatinine is common, although its validity has been challenged on numerous occasions, especially in relation to its use in children.[8]

Logistics

The Jaffé reaction (which depends on the formation of a red color), with an absorbance maximum at 485 nm by the reaction of creatinine with picrate in alkaline solution, remains the most widely used method for the quantitation of creatinine in serum or urine.[9] Unfortunately, this procedure is fraught with analytic difficulties. Of particular concern is the nonspecificity caused by the presence of chromogens in serum (but not in urine) that react to give identical color, thus causing an artifactual increase in the measured concentration. Although it is possible to remove or minimize these interferences by absorbing the noncreatinine compounds on to materials such as Fuller's earth (Lloyd's reagent),[10] this process is not compatible with modern clinical laboratories and has, in addition, been shown to be of variable efficaciousness. The validity of the picrate procedure for creatinine determinations has been significantly improved by the introduction of rate measurements as opposed to end point methods, although here the interference from bilirubin constitutes a major problem.[11,12] Other methods, including those based on the use of two creatinine cleaving enzymes, creatinine amidohydrolase and creatinine deaminase, and high performance liquid chromatography (HPLC), have found only limited acceptance.

Interpretation[9,13–15]

The range of serum creatinine concentration in children younger than 12 years old has been shown to be 0.3–1.0 mg/dL (26.5–88.4 μmol/L) with no significant difference between the sexes. For adults, because of the differences in lean body mass, reference ranges are segregated into male and female. For men, the range is 0.64–1.04 mg/dL (57–92 μmol/L); for women, the range is 0.57–0.92 mg/dL (50–61 μmol/L). It should be noted that these reference ranges were established using Jaffé procedures with Fuller's earth. Other methods would be expected to give higher values. The range of urinary excretion of creatinine for men is 1.0–2.0 g/24 h (8.8–17.7 mmol/d) and for women is 0.8–1.8 g/24 h (7.1–15.9 mmol/d). Because of the difficulty in obtaining valid urine measurements in small children, the reference ranges in Table 3-3 must be interpreted with caution.

Creatinine Clearance

The GFR is the most important clinical measurement of renal function. Simultaneous measurement in the serum and urine of the concentration of a substance that is removed from the serum by filtration at the glomerulus is required for this assessment. A further requirement is that the substance must neither be reabsorbed nor secreted by the tubules. These serum and urine concentrations are then used to calculate a number that is representative of the clearance of that compound from the blood and hence equal to the GFR. The equation for the calculation is, $C = UV/P$ (where C is the clearance expressed in milliliters of blood cleared per minute; U is the concentration of the substance in the urine; V is the volume of urine excreted per minute; and P is the concentration of the substance in plasma [serum]).

The calculated clearance can be corrected by an additional factor that is derived from a combination of the patient's height and weight to approximate the surface area of the patient relative to the standard surface area of an adult, taken as 1.73 m².

The GFR may be derived from the quantitation of any compound that meets the above criteria. However, creatinine is the only endogenous substance that comes close to satisfying these requirements, although it falls somewhat short. Foreign substances (such as inulin, see page 59), which must be infused to maintain a steady state plasma concentration, more nearly approach the ideal. Thus the GFR of healthy individuals assessed by creatinine clearance may exceed that measured by inulin clearance by as much as 30%.[16] Nevertheless, the ease with which a clinician can obtain a creatinine clearance has made this determination by far the most frequently requested procedure for evaluating renal function. The disadvantages of this test, as compared with those using agents that must be administered by injection, are that the accurate measurement of creatinine is difficult especially in serum, creatinine is secreted by the renal tubule especially at elevated serum levels, and that the urine specimen is frequently not collected with the degree of completeness necessary to avoid additional compromise of the final result.

It must be emphasized again that reference ranges[17-19] for creatinine clearance are influenced greatly by the type of methodology used for the estimation of urine and particularly serum creatinine concentrations. Table 3-4 indicates values obtained for individuals who were free from renal disease. The time for urine collection was 24 hours and all values were measured using a method in which dialyzable Jaffé reactive noncreatinine chromogens were also included in the quantitation.

The difficulty in collecting complete timed samples from children and infants render creatinine clearance determination in patients of these age groups of dubious value. In order to circumvent these difficulties, an estimate of the creatinine clearance may be obtained by the use of the following equation[20]:

$0.43 \times$ (height in centimeters/serum creatinine mg/dL)
= creatinine clearance mL/min

The use of the creatinine clearance or urinary creatinine as a reference for comparing the excretion of other substances is a common practice though it has been shown to have little justification.[15]

Test: Uric Acid (2,6,8-Trioxypurine, Lithic Acid) (See Ch. 6)

Background and Selection

In primates, uric acid is the end product of the metabolism of purines. Renal clearance of uric acid is approxi-

Table 3-4. Creatinine Clearance Measured at Various Ages in Normal Individuals

Age (years)	Results (mean ± 2 SD) in mL/min/1.73 m² Surface Area (mL/s/1.73 m²) Female	Male
17–36	74–154 (1.2–2.6)	49–185 (0.8–3.1)
20–29	57–133 (1.0–2.2)	64–156 (1.1–2.6)
30–39	53–153 (0.9–2.6)	19–175 (0.3–2.9)
37–56	74–134 (1.2–2.2)	56–163 (0.9–2.7)
40–49	29–133 (0.4–2.2)	44–132 (0.7–2.1)
50–59	26–122 (0.4–2.0)	39–123 (0.7–2.2)
57–76	38–150 (0.6–2.5)	58–130 (1.0–2.2)
60–69	33–93 (0.6–1.6)	28–116 (0.5–1.9)
70–79	30–78 (0.5–1.3)	34–94 (0.6–1.6)
80–89	18–74 (0.3–1.2)	17–77 (0.3–1.3)
90–99	23–55 (0.4–0.9)	16–52 (0.3–0.9)

Table 3-5. Conditions in Which Serum and Urine Uric Acid Levels Are Outside the Reference Ranges

Serum increased	Dehydration; acidosis; fasting or starvation; gout; renal failure; polycystic kidney disease; lead nephropathy; leukemia; polycythemia; multiple myeloma, lymphoma, and other disseminated neoplasias, especially following chemotherapy; toxemia of pregnancy; glycogen storage disease, type I; Lesch-Nyhan syndrome; Down syndrome; hypothyroidism; hypoparathyroidism; drugs including pyrazinamide, ethabutol, nicotinic acid, salicylates in low doses
Serum decreased	Fanconi syndrome; Wilson's disease, xanthinuria; acute intermittent porphyria; cystinosis; galactosemia; severe liver disease; drugs including corticosteroids, salicylates in high doses, allopurinol, probenicid, ticrynafen, and large amounts of ascorbic acid
Urine increased	Leukemia, gout, Lesch-Nyhan syndrome, Wilson's disease, polycythemia, sickle cell anemia
Urine decreased	Xanthinuria, folic acid deficiency, lead nephrotoxicity

mately 10% of the clearance of creatinine. The exact manner in which uric acid is handled in the kidney is still controversial. The current thinking leans toward a mechanism in which uric acid is filtered at the glomeruli, reabsorbed in the proximal convoluted tubule, followed by secretion in the lower portion of the proximal tubule, and further reabsorption in the distal tubule. Of the uric acid that appears in the urine of an individual on a typical diet, about 60% is derived from the catabolism of purine, whereas the remainder is from dietary sources.[21] Uric acid measurements are useful in patients suspected of having gout, but hyperuricemia may have other causes (Table 3-5). The renal picture in gout derives from the deposition of microcrystals of sodium urate in the renal medulla. These deposits evolve to frank tophi with giant cell association and fibrosis. Following these changes there is progression to pyelonephritis-type changes in the parenchyma without any indication of infection.[22,23]

Logistics

The preferred methods for the quantitation of uric acid are based on the reaction of the enzyme uricase with urates to form allantoin. The decrease in absorbance as urate is converted can be monitored spectrophotometrically or this reaction may be coupled to secondary indicator reactions to generate a chromophore with absorbance in the visible range. The other type of method commonly used relies on the reduction of phosphotungstic acid by urate in an alkaline buffer to produce a blue compound called *tungsten blue*. The phosphotungstic acid procedures are subject to many interferences including glucose, ascorbic acid, acetaminophen, salicylates, caffeine, and theophylline.[24]

Interpretation

Table 3-6 shows the reference ranges for uric acid. Asymptomatic individuals with serum uric acid levels (measured by the uricase method, Table 3-6) above 7.0 mg/dL (416 µmol/L) in males and 6.0 mg/dL (357 µmol/L) in females are viewed by most experts as candidates for long-term follow-up because many of these individuals are at risk for renal disease caused by hyperuricemia and hyperuricuria. In addition, many diseases, including renal disease and myeloproliferative disorders, can cause secondary hyperuricemia. Thus, all patients with gout have hyperuricemia with the associated manifestations of acute arthritis, tophaceous lesions, nephrolithiasis, and frequently, nephropathy; however, not all patients with hyperuricemia have gout. Hyperuricemia also can occur in Lesch-Nyhan syndrome, in which the enzyme hypoxanthine-guanine phosphoribosyltransferase is virtually deficient. This X-linked disorder is characterized by mental and physical retardation, self-mutilation, and choreoathetosis. There does not appear to be any renal complications with this disease.[26] In addition, several drugs including salicylates in doses below 2 g/d, diuretics, alcohol, and cytotoxic agents can lead to hyperuricemia with an associated increase in uric acid excretion.

Table 3-6. Reference Ranges for Uric Acid[26]

	Sex/Age	Reference Range
Serum		
Phosphotungstic acid method	Male (<60 y)	4.5–8.5 mg/dL (268–506 µmol/L)
	Female (<60 y)	3.0–6.5 mg/dL (178–387 µmol/L)
	Male (>60 y)	4.2–8.0 mg/dL (250–476 µmol/L)
	Female (>60 y)	3.2–7.3 mg/dL (190–434 µmol/L)
Uricase method	Child	2.0–5.5 mg/dL (119–327 µmol/L)
	Male (adult)	3.5–7.2 mg/dL (208–428 µmol/L)
	Female (adult)	2.6–6.0 mg/dL (155–357 µmol/L)
	Diet	**Reference Range**
Urine	Usual diet	250–750 mg/24 h (1.48–4.44 mmol/d)
	Purine free diet	
	Males	<420 mg/24 h (<2.50 mmol/d)
	Females	Slightly lower
	Low purine diet	
	Males	<480 mg/24 h (<2.86 mmol/d)
	Females	<400 mg/24 h (<2.38 mmol/d)
	High purine diet	<1000 mg/24 h (<5.95 mmol/d)

Test: Sodium

Background and Selection

The average diet provides between 8 and 15 g of sodium chloride per day. The body requires between 1 and 2% of the intake. Essentially all the excess is excreted in the urine. Between 60 and 70% of the filtered load is reabsorbed in the proximal tubules together with bicarbonate and water. A further 25–30% is reabsorbed in the ascending loop of Henle, thus only a small fraction of the original filter load is presented to the distal tubule. However, it is in the distal tubule that the most important aspect of sodium regulation occurs under the influence of the adrenocortical hormone, aldosterone (see Ch. 11). It is here that sodium is coupled to the exchange of potassium and/or hydrogen ions that ultimately determines the amount of sodium excreted in the urine.

Logistics

Ion-specific electrodes have now almost completely replaced flame photometry as the means to quantitate sodium in biologic fluids. It should be noted that in any situation where a dilution is required before measurement, an artifactual error can occur in hyperlipemic or, less commonly, in hyperproteinemic states. In these situations, the concentration of sodium or other analytes is underestimated because of the volume of serum water displaced by the lipid or protein. This has been referred to as the *electrolyte exclusion effect* or the *exclusion error*.

Interpretation

The primary reason for measuring sodium in patients with renal disease relates to its role as the most important cation in fluid and electrolyte balance, and because the kidney is the ultimate regulator of sodium homeostasis. Renal hyponatremia may be caused by decreased tubular reabsorption as a result of inappropriate diuretic therapy, primary or secondary hypoaldosteronism, or extreme polyuria. Hyponatremia is also common in tubular acidosis in which the exchange of sodium and hydrogen ions is impaired, in the so-called syndrome of inappropriate antidiuretic hormone secretion (SIADH) (see Ch. 11), and in any situation that results in alkaline urine. As might be expected, hypernaturia is frequently a concomitant feature of hyponatremia. Hypernatremia may be caused by hyperaldosteronism, Cushing syndrome, or nephrogenic diabetes insipidis. Table 3-7 shows the reference ranges for sodium.

Table 3-7. Reference Ranges for Sodium

Urine[a,b]	40–220 mEq/24 h
Serum[c]	mEq/L
Premature, cord	116–140
48 hours	128–148
Newborn, cord	126–166
Newborn	134–144
Infant	139–146
Child	138–145
Adult	136–146

[a] The excretion of sodium in the urine is markedly diet dependent.
[b] Conventional units are mEq/24 h; SI units are mmol/d. The numbers remain the same because the conversion factor is 1.
[c] Conventional units, mEq/L; SI units, mmol/L (the conversion factor is 1).
(Data from Tietz.[27])

Test: Potassium

Background and Selection

As with sodium, renal function constitutes the major mechanism for potassium homeostasis. Potassium is filtered at the glomerulus; however, approximately 90% is reasorbed in the proximal tubule and the ascending loop of Henle and about 10% of the filtered load reaches the distal tubule where the regulation of body potassium occurs through secretion in exchange for sodium under the influence of aldosterone. Owing to the establishment of a gradient from the renal cells to the filtrate in the distal tubules and collecting ducts, potassium is excreted. The secretion of potassium in exchange for sodium is a competitive process with hydrogen ions, thus a reciprocal relationship frequently exists between the excretion of potassium and that of hydrogen ions.

Logistics

Ion-specific electrodes have now almost completely replaced flame photometry as the means to quantitate potassium in biologic fluids. It should be noted that potassium may be raised artifactually by a number of causes. The most common cause is the disruption of the erythrocyte membrane due to mechanical forces (hemolysis) between the time of sampling and the time of centrifugation. Therefore, blood for potassium measurement must be handled as gently as possible. Even with such handling, serum potassium levels increase if the blood is not separated by centrifugation in a timely fashion. Serum potassium levels also may increase

Table 3-8. Reference Ranges for Potassium

Urine[a,b]	25–125 mEq/24 h
Serum[c]	mEq/L
Premature, cord	5.0–10.2
48 hours	3.0–6.0
Newborn, cord	5.6–12.0
Newborn	3.7–5.9
Infant	4.1–5.3
Child	3.4–4.7
Adult	3.5–5.1

[a] The excretion of potassium in the urine is markedly diet dependent.
[b] Conventional units are mEq/24 h; SI units are mmol/d (the conversion factor is 1).
[c] Conventional units, mEq/L; SI units, mmol/L (the conversion factor is 1).
(Data from Tietz.[28])

after blood drawing in specimens with grossly elevated leukocyte counts or with thrombocythemia.

Interpretation

Potassium depletion with hyperkaluria can occur in states of hypoalbuminemia, hyponatremia, hypochloremia caused by vomiting or nasogastric suctioning, and following the use of diuretic therapy, particularly with thiazides, mercurials, or acetazolamide. The question as to whether potassium depletion is caused by a renal or other condition may be answered by the result of a urinary potassium level. If the concentration of potassium in the urine is low (below 10 mEq/L [<10 mmol/L]) a renal cause can be virtually excluded, whereas a concentration of greater than 10 mEq/L (>10 mmol/L) is highly suggestive of renal wastage. Potassium loss caused by renal disorders occurs in the renal tubular dystrophies, occasionally in chronic renal failure, and in remission stages of acute tubular necrosis. Potassium depletion can itself cause vacuolar nephropathy.[19] Table 3-8 shows reference ranges for potassium.

Test: Chloride

Background and Selection

Chloride is the major anion involved in extracellular fluid balance and makes up about two-thirds of the inorganic anion in plasma. Excess chloride is excreted in the urine, and increased losses, such as from the gastrointestinal tract or through sweat, can lower urinary chloride. Chloride is measured routinely along with the other electrolytes, sodium, potassium, and carbon dioxide and results are used to calculate the anion gap. Urine chloride concentration is used to evaluate patients with metabolic alkalosis. Sweat chloride measurements are used to screen patients for cystic fibrosis.

Logistics

Methods are described for the measurement of chloride in serum or urine by titrimetric and colorimetric procedures that depend on the reaction of the ion with mercuric salts. However, these methods have been largely replaced in most laboratories by coulometric-amperometric or ion-selective electrode procedures.

Interpretation

The contribution of chloride measurement in renal disorders is limited to a few conditions. When chloride is selectively depleted, the patient develops a metabolic alkalosis characterized by hypochloremia, hypokalemia, hypokaluria, and paradoxical aciduria. The most common causes of this acidosis are vomiting, nasogastric suction, the use of silver nitrate for burns, and the diarrheas referred to as *chloridorrheas*. The laboratory findings are distinctive; in addition to an elevated pH, the anion gap is much increased, caused by a decrease in serum chloride concentration as compared with the serum sodium concentration. In hyperparathyroidism serum chloride is increased. Table 3-9 shows the reference ranges for chloride.

Test: Bicarbonate

The bicarbonate ion, HCO_3^-, is the chemical species that comprises almost all the CO_2 produced by the body. The total CO_2 of the plasma is made up of approximately 95% bicarbonate ions with the remainder

Table 3-9. Reference Ranges for Chloride

	Reference Range mEq/24 h (mmol/d)
Urine	
Infant	2–10 (2–10)
Child	15–40 (15–40)
Adult	110–250 (110–250)
Serum	
Infant	111–130 (111–130)
Adult	98–106 (98–106)

[a] The excretion of chloride in the urine is markedly diet dependent and has little, if any, clinical utility.
(Data from Tietz.[29])

Table 3-10. Reference Ranges for Bicarbonate[a]

Whole blood, arterial	19–24 mEq/L
Whole blood, venous	22–26 mEq/L
Plasma, venous	23–29 mEq/L
Plasma, capillary	
Premature, 1 week	14–27 mEq/L
Newborn	13–22 mEq/L
Infant	20–28 mEq/L
Child	20–28 mEq/L
Adult	22–28 mEq/L

[a] Conventional units are mEq/L; SI units are mmol/L. The numbers remain the same as the conversion factor is 1.
(Data for Tietz.[30])

present as carbonic acid (dissolved CO_2) or combined with amino acids (carbamino compounds). Bicarbonate ions are completely filtered by the glomeruli with approximately 90% reabsorption in the proximal tubule and a further 10% in the distal tubule. The threshold for this system is approximately 26 mEq/L (26 mmol/L); at concentrations above this level bicarbonate is excreted in the urine. The bicarbonate concentration of the blood may be obtained indirectly from measurment of blood pH and pCO_2 (blood gas parameters) by use of the Henderson-Hasselbach equation. Alternatively, bicarbonate may be measured (as total CO_2) in serum or heparinized plasma by ion-specific electrodes, enzymatically using phosphoenolpyruvate carboxylase, by the change in color of a pH indicator such as cresol red, or by a microgasometer. Specimens should be, but seldom are, handled anaerobically and separated by centrifugation at 37°C to prevent significant loss of CO_2 to the air. Bicarbonate concentration of the serum increases in metabolic alkalosis and in compensated respiratory acidosis.

Serum bicarbonate decreases in metabolic acidosis, compensated respiratory alkalosis, and situations where there is poor tissue perfusion as in dehydration or hypotension (see Ch. 2). Table 3-10 shows reference ranges for bicarbonate.

Test: Urinalysis

This somewhat unfortunate term has, by convention, come to mean the macroscopic and microscopic morphologic examination of urine for formed elements such as cells and casts and for crystals and amorphous material. This visual process is integrated with a chemical assessment of the urine that is now always achieved by the use of strips that carry dried reagents for multiple chemical tests (dipsticks). Both of these analytic processes have now been automated, although the majority of laboratories retain the conventional visual microscopic examination with manual or semiautomated chemical testing. In addition, it is common to measure and report the specific gravity of the urine sample. The procedure as a whole is fraught with problems of performance, precision, and interpretation. It should be viewed as a screening test useful in some situations, but of limited predictive value. The first morning specimen is the most concentrated and is therefore the specimen of choice for urinalysis.

Macroscopic Appearance of Urine

The tradition of reporting the color, appearance, and odor of urine is disappearing. However, Table 3-11 lists urine color and possible causes for those who may wish to continue this practice.

Microscopic Examination (See Appendix)

The urine specimen must be examined less than 6 hours after voiding and preferably within 2 hours, otherwise significant loss of formed elements may occur. The urine should be thoroughly mixed before centrifugation. The sediment may be stained with one of a number of supravital stains, although opinion is divided on the benefits of staining. It is probable that an experienced microscopist finds little benefit from staining. The inclusion of a microscopic examination as a component of all routine urinalyses has been challenged as being wasteful in the light of available test strip screening (e.g., leukocyte esterase) for pyuria. However, it appears that the preponderance of opinion believes this is not good practice, because of the errors of both specificity and sensitivity.

Cells

Erythrocytes

Usually erythrocytes are round biconcave discs about 7 μ in diameter that appear pale under the microscope. However, their characteristics may be greatly altered by the osmolarity of the urine and they may shrink, swell, become crenated, or even lyse. Thus, they may be easily missed in abnormal urine. The presence of a positive test for hemoglobin has been advocated as a more sensitive test for hematuria than microscopic evaluation.

Increased erythrocytes in the urine may derive from renal disease, diseases of the lower urinary tract, and

Table 3-11. Urine Color and Possible Causes

Urine Color	Possible Cause(s)
Yellow	The normal yellow color of urine is due to urochrome and other natural pigments
Yellow-to-Orange	Bilirubin, urobilin: an orange color may be imparted to urine by a number of nonpathologic substances such as carrots, food coloring dyes, rhubarb, senna, and a number of drugs including acriflavine, azo-gantrisin, pyridium, quinacrine, riboflavin, and sulfasalazine
White (Turbidity)	Chyle, leukocytes in large number, phosphates, and urates (note: urates usually have a pinkish color as compared with the white of phosphates)
Pink to red	Hemoglobin, myoglobin, porphobilin, porphyrins, erythrocytes in large numbers: these gradations of color may also be caused by a number of nonpathologic substances such as anthocyanins (derived from fruits and vegetables), food coloring dyes, senna, and by a number of drugs including amipyrine, antipyrine, sulfobromophthalein, diphenylhydantoin, methyldopa, phenacetin, phenolphthalein, phenothiazine, and pyridium
Red through brown to purple	Porphobilinogen, porphobilin, uroporphyrin
Brown through black	Bilirubin, homogentistic acid, indican, melanin, methemoglobin, myoglobin, phenol, p-hydroxyphenyl-pyruvic acid, porphyrins: these gradations of color may also be caused by a number of nonpathologic substances and drugs such as chloroquine, hydroquinone, iron compounds, levodopa, methyldopa, metronidazole, nitrofurantoin, quinine, and resorcinol
Blue through green	Biliverdin, *Pseudomonas* infections: these gradations of color may also be caused by a number of nonpathologic substances and drugs such as acriflavine, amitriptyline, azure A, creosote, Evan's blue, methylene blue, phenyl salicylate, thymol, tolonium, triamterene, and vitamin B complex

(Adapted from Graff,[65] with permission.)

from diseases unrelated to the kidneys or urinary tract such as acute appendicitis, salpingitis, diverticulitis, and tumors of the colon, rectum, and pelvis.[31] The reference range for erythrocytes in the urine is less than 3/high power field (hpf).

Leukocytes

In fresh urine, most leukocytes (principally neutrophils) appear as distinct granular spheres of about 12 μ diameter with well defined nuclear detail and frequently have a light greenish yellow coloration. Again, the osmolarity of the urine can have a profound effect on the appearance, which can lead to a loss of nuclear detail and even the disruption of the cells in a relatively short time. It can also lead to the development of so-called glitter cells which are characteristic products of hypotonic urine and are caused by Brownian movement within the leukocytes.

An increase in leukocytes in the urine (pyuria) is a much more reliable indicator of inflammation in the urinary tract than is the visual detection of bacteria in the urine (see below). Leukocytes, when seen in conjunction with leukocyte or leukocyte-epithelial casts, are most likely to be of renal origin. Large numbers of leukocytes (greater than 50/hpf) are suggestive of acute infection. The presence of leukocytes in more moderate numbers (5–50/hpf) is indicative of one or more localized inflammations that may be either bacterial or nonbacterial, acute or chronic. There have been suggestions that the differentiation of leukocytes in the urine, although rarely performed, has diagnostic benefits. The reference range for leukocytes in the urine is less than 5/hpf.

Reporting the Presence of Bacteria in Urine. It is generally agreed that the presence of bacteria in the urine is not a good indicator of urinary tract infection. Valenstein and Koepke[32] in a study of 1000 patients state that "the presence of bacteria or yeast in the urine sediment had little predictive value for urinary tract infection. The great majority of patients with bacteria in their urine sediment did not have significant bacteriuria (as judged by urine culture), were asymptomatic, and did not develop urinary tract disease during follow-up."

Wenk[33] showed that the specificity of a negative finding for bacteria in the urine sediment was only 53%, whereas that for leukocytes counted microscopically (normal, less than 10/hpf) was 90%. Musher[34] showed that the presence of less than 10 leukocytes/μL (<1 leukocyte/hpf) provides good evidence against urinary tract infection. In contrast, the finding of greater than 10 leukocytes/μL (<1 leukocyte/hpf) is consistent with, but not diagnostic of, urinary tract infections because other conditions such as inflammatory disease of adjacent genital organs, interstitial nephritis, or mycobacterial infections may be responsible.

In light of the great difficulty in obtaining uncontaminated specimens and because of bacterial multiplication after specimen collection, it is proposed that the presence of bacteria detected on the microscopic portion of routine urinalysis no longer be reported.

Renal Tubular Epithelial Cells

Renal tubular epithelial cells have a diameter of approximately 15 μ and contain a single large round nucleus. Papanicolaou's stain has been advocated as a useful aid in the sometimes difficult task of differentiating between renal tubular epithelial cells and other cells, especially certain lymphocytes. Renal tubular epithelial cells are found in increased numbers in situations where tubular damage has occurred, such as pyelonephritis, acute tubular necrosis, and following the ingestion of many drugs including salicylates. In addition, the number of renal tubular epithelial cells in the urine has been proposed as a useful indicator of the onset of rejection in renal transplants. However, because of the difficulty of absolute identification, these cells are considered by many to be of limited prognostic or diagnostic value.

Transitional Epithelial Cells

Transitional epithelial cells are cells that line much of the urinary tract and may derive from the ureter, bladder, upper urethra, or prostate. The cells are much larger than renal tubular epithelial cells having a diameter from 30 to 60 μ and may, on occasion, be binucleate. A few transitional epithelial cells are present in the urine of healthy individuals; when large numbers or sheets of cells are present, a full cytologic evaluation using the appropriate stains should be considered. Caudate cells are variants of transitional epithelial cells that show a typical tailed structure and are of no additional diagnostic value.

Squamous Epithelial Cells

Squamous epithelial cells are derived from the distal portions of the urethra, but in the urine of a female may be derived from the vulva or vagina. These are large cells with a small nucleus and large cytoplasmic area. Squamous epithelial cells have little diagnostic value, especially in the female.

Casts

Protein precipitation in the renal tubule, particularly in the distal convoluted tubule and collecting duct, forms a cast of the lumen and is then extruded, occasionally with damaged cells entrained, in the urine. The matrix of all casts is believed to be Tamm-Horsfall mucoprotein, but some serum may be included. Factors that contribute to cast formation include decreased urinary flow, lowered pH, the formation of concentrated urine, and the presence of proteinuria. Morphologically, casts reflect their origin with a cylindrical cross-section (approximately 25 μ), but considerable variation in length occurs. An increase in the number of casts in the urine has been called cylindruria.

Hyaline Casts

Composed only of protein, hyaline casts are the most frequently seen and the most simple. For this reason, they have a very low refractive index and are seen best with low levels of light. Hyaline casts are found in all forms of renal disease and have no value in differential diagnosis. Normal urine, with no detectable protein as assayed by conventional methods, may contain a few hyaline casts and this small number may increase significantly following exercise.

Red Blood Cell Casts

Red blood cell (RBC) casts are composed of erythrocytes in varying proportions to the protein matrix and range in color from brown to almost colorless. Their presence in the urine, detected under microscopic examination is one of the more important findings and is always considered pathologic. Red blood cell casts are usually diagnostic of glomerular disease, including acute pyelonephritis, lupus nephritis, subacute bacterial endocarditis, and renal infarction. When stasis has occurred in the nephron, the fine detail of the red cast may be lost and may take on a granular appearance; it is then called a hemoglobin or blood cast.

White Blood Cell Casts

White blood cell (WBC) casts are easy to recognize in their classical form because the leukocytes (usually polymorphonuclear neutrophils) and their nuclei are clearly defined. However, all too frequently, detail is lost and many WBC casts may be reported as granular casts. White blood cell casts usually indicate tubulo-interstitial disease, most commonly pyelonephritis; they also may be seen in lupus nephritis.

Tubular Epithelial Cell Casts

Tubular epithelial cell casts are rare casts that develop following tubular necrosis, which may be caused by a virus (e.g. hepatitis or cytomegalovirus) or by the nephrotoxic actions of heavy metals or drugs. The presence of this cast in the urine has been advocated as an indicator of renal allograft rejection. The epithelial cells within the cast may show a distinct parallel arrangement or may have a more random arrangement.

Granular Casts

Granular casts may be described as hyaline casts modified by the inclusion of plasma proteins or aggregated to form granules, or cellular casts in which the cellular architecture has been lost. Granular casts are described as fine or coarse depending on both the granule size and color, which ranges from gray or yellow to almost black as the granule size increases. The difference between fine granular casts and coarse granular casts is not diagnostically significant. The presence of either or both in the urine is highly suggestive of renal disease. For unknown reasons, there may be transient appearance of granular casts in the urine of healthy individuals who exercise vigorously or who partake of pure carbohydrate diets.

Waxy Casts

Waxy casts are highly visible casts believed to form when the granules of granular casts breakdown within the lumen of the tubule. They reflect a considerable increase in the time during which the cast remains in the tubule; therefore, the presence of these casts is suggestive of localized obstruction to urine flow or severe oliguria as seen in chronic renal failure or in allograft rejection. When waxy casts show a broadening of cross-section as compared with a hyaline cast, for example, this is presumed to indicate advanced tubular atrophy with dilatation and is a grave prognostic sign.

Fatty Casts

Fatty casts are casts that have incorporated variable amounts of fatty material. They may be seen in association with oval fat bodies (see below) and are indicative of a degenerative process in the tubular epithelial cells. The lipid that forms the inclusions is usually either cholesterol or triglyceride. Although differentiating between the two is not clinically important, it is easily achieved by viewing the cast under polarized light. Cholesterol is anisotropic showing a characteristic Maltese cross formation, whereas casts containing triglyceride stain with lipophilic stains such oil red O. Fatty casts are seen in the nephrotic syndrome, lipid nephrosis, chronic glomerulonephritis, diabetic glomerulosclerosis, and Kimmelstiel-Wilson syndrome. They also are seen in association with injuries that cause extensive damage to subcutaneous fat or that cause bone marrow to be released into the circulation.

Crystals

The presence of specific crystals in the urine, such as cysteine crystals, may have important diagnostic significance. However, crystals rarely provide substantial clinical information. It is important in the consideration of crystaluria to be aware of the effect of urine pH on the crystals. Urine temperature is also important; most crystals appear only after the urine has stood for a period of time and reached room temperature. Some crystals are present in the urine of individuals without disease and are reported only by convention. These crystals are calcium oxalate, uric acid, sodium urate, amorphous urate, calcium phosphate, triple phosphates, calcium carbonate, ammonium biurate, and amorphous phosphates.

Acid Urine

Calcium Oxalate. Calcium oxalate crystals also may be seen in neutral or even occasionally in alkaline urines. The almost colorless crystals are usually octahedral in shape with their two dimensional shape under the microscope appearing like that of an envelope. Rarely do they have an ellipsoidal or dumb-bell shape. These crystals appear in the urine in a variety of clinical situations, including idiopathic hypercalciuria, primary hyperparathyroidism and, in massive quantities, in primary hyperoxaluria.[35] However, the presence of calcium oxalate is not diagnostic of these conditions. More commonly the crystals arise from normal constituents of the diet, including spinach, tomatoes, rhubarb, garlic, oranges, asparagus, and tea; this excretion is greatly exacerbated following small bowel resection. In addition, because much of the usual amount of oxalate present in the urine is derived from the metabolism of ascorbate, increased ingestion of vitamin C may produce this crystaluria.

Uric Acid. Crystals of uric acid are deposited only from acid urine. As they crystallize, urinary pigments are incorporated causing the characteristic yellow to reddish color that varies in intensity with the thickness of the crystal. The crystals are most commonly diamond-shaped with rosettes occurring when several crystals aggregate. Occasionally barrel-shaped and hexagonal crystals occur. The crystals dissolve readily when the urine is alkalinized or heated to 60°C. Uric acid crystals, although normal constituents of urine, may increase in situations in which there is increased purine metabolism, such as gout or Lesch-Nyhan syndrome.

Sodium Urates. Sodium urates are colorless or pale yellow needle-like crystals without pointed ends that are frequently clustered in sheaves. They dissolve easily when the urine is heated to 60°C.

Amorphous Urates. Amorphous urates are mixed salts of sodium, potassium, magnesium, calcium, and uric acid present in the urine in a noncrystalline form. They usually have a yellow-red granular appearance and dissolve readily when alkali is added to the urine or when urine temperature is increased to 60°C.

Alkaline Urine

Calcium Phosphates. Calcium phosphate crystals are needle-shaped with a pointed end and are usually found in aggregates resulting in a rosette or star cluster, so-called stellar phosphates. Calcium phosphates dissolve readily when acetic acid is added to the urine.

Triple Phosphates. Triple phosphates are crystals of ammonium magnesium phosphate and may appear in the urine in two forms. The most common, the so-called coffin lid type, are prisms with oblique surfaces at each end, but a feathery fern-like variety also may be seen. It is believed that the most frequent reason for the formation of these crystals is the production of ammonium carbonate from urea by the action of bacterial urease either before or after urine has been voided.

Calcium Carbonate. Calcium carbonate crystals occur in dumb-bell or spherical forms. The crystals are small and may be difficult to distinguish from amorphous deposits. However, the edges of clumps of calcium carbonate crystal show better definition than do amorphous phosphates or urates. When acetic acid is added to the urine, the crystals dissolve with the evolution of bubbles of carbon dioxide.

Ammonium Biurate. Urine that contains bacteria may exhibit the thorn apple crystals of ammonium biurate. These are spherical crystals with long irregular spikes, usually yellow-brown in color. The crystals dissolve in acetic acid and on warming the urine. The addition of sodium hydroxide liberates ammonium.

Amorphous Phosphates. These phosphate salts are indistinguishable from amorphous urates described above; only the pH of the urine and their solubility in acid serve to differentiate them from the urates.

Crystals Associated with Abnormalities

Cystine. Cystine crystals are colorless hexagonal plates that appear singly or in clusters. They are soluble in alkali and mineral acids, but not in acetic acid or with heat. Cystine crystals may well be the most important products detected in urine. They are present in patients with all forms of the metabolic disorders, cystinosis and cystinuria. The presence of cystine in the urine should be confirmed by the cyanide-nitroprusside screening test. Patients with confirmed cystine crystals in the urine and a positive cyanide-nitroprusside test should be further evaluated to determine the pattern of amino acid excretion.

Leucine. Leucine crystals are yellow-brown spheres with concentric or radial striations and a high refractive index, so that the center of the crystal appears black. Leucine crystals redissolve in mineral acids, alkalies, and acetic acid. The presence of leucine crystals in the urine is of great significance because they are found in severe liver disease such as acute yellow atrophy and terminal cirrhosis. They also are found in two genetic diseases, oasthouse syndrome and maple syrup urine disease. Again, the presence of these crystals should be followed with an evaluation of the excretion of amino acids in affected patients.

Tyrosine. Tyrosine crystals appear as highly refractive tufts or sheaves of fine needles. They are soluble in mineral acids and alkalies but not in acetic acid. Tyrosine is frequently found in conjunction with leucine.

Sulfonamides. Years ago, it was quite common to observe clear to brown sheaves of needles in the urine of patients being treated with sulfa drugs. Now, however, this is a rare occurrence because of the advent of sulfonamides of much higher solubility.

Other Elements

Oval Fat Bodies

The term *oval fat bodies* is used to describe renal tubular cells that have become engorged with lipid and are becoming necrotic. Oval fat bodies may, on occasion, derive from cells of other types such as macrophages. The significance of these bodies is similar to that of finding fatty casts or free lipid droplets in the urine (see above).

Tumor Cells

Although routine urinalysis is not the appropriate test for the detection of renal and urinary tract tumor cells in the urine, such cells are seen on occasion. Such a finding, if unexpected, should initiate a full cytologic evaluation of the urine.

Mucus Threads

The occurrence of small amounts of mucus in the urine is a normal finding. However, there is a considerable increase following inflammation or local irritation of the urinary tract. Mucus appears as long threads of low refractive index, with occasional cells entrained in a mesh. Wider strands do occur and have been confused with hyaline casts.

Yeasts

Yeasts may appear in the urine as a result of infection of the urinary tract or as contaminants from the skin or from the air. Yeasts are similar in size and appearance to erythrocytes, with which they are frequently confused. The presence of budding forms of yeast is frequently the only way to distinguish between the two cells, although other discriminating tests are available.

Parasites

Parasites in the urine are frequently caused by contamination from the vagina or from fecal material. When this is suspected a fresh specimen should be requested. However, the finding of certain organisms may have important clinical significance.

Trichomonas vaginalis is probably the most commonly seen parasite. This protozoan may be mistaken for a leukocyte in some preparations, but in fresh preparations the flagella and the motility will allow positive identification.

Schistosoma haematobium is a trematode or blood fluke that inhabits the venous circulation of the bladder. The eggs of the female are discharged into the venules, which may rupture allowing the ova to pass into the urine together with red and white blood cells. This form of schistosomiasis is endemic to the Nile Valley, other parts of Africa, and the Middle East.

Enterobius vermicularis (pin worm) ova, which derive from the colon, may be found in the urine, especially in children, by transmission from the anus.

Contaminants

It is not unusual to find a variety of contaminants or artifacts in specimens submitted for urinalysis. These may include spermatozoa, starch granules, talc, and fibers from clothing, diapers, and toilet paper. The only significance of these entities is that they not be mistaken for elements of clinical importance.

Chemical Analysis as a Component of Urinalysis

It is now standard procedure to include in routine urinalysis a semiquantitative assessment of as many as nine analytes by the use of a reagent strip (dipsticks) or reagent tablets. The compounds measured have evolved less through clinical need than from the ability of manufacturers to formulate the necessary reagents in dipstick form. The usual tests performed are pH, protein, glucose, ketones, hemoglobin, bilirubin, urobilinogen, nitrite, leukocyte esterase and, occasionally, specific gravity by dipstick.

pH

The pH of a urine specimen can be determined with an accuracy of approximately one-half a unit by means of a dipstick with a reagent pad containing an acid-base indicator dye. Urinary pH is not only of importance as a measure of the acid-base status of the patient; it also signals urinary tract infection with urea-splitting bacteria. The pH of urine, taken in conjunction with blood pH, is an essential measurement in the recognition of hypokalemic, hypochloremic acidosis, in which the urine is paradoxically alkaline. As indicated previously a knowledge of the pH of a urine specimen is frequently a necessity in the identification of crystals.

Protein

Protein measurement is certainly the most important chemical evaluation performed during routine urinalysis. Indeed, some would argue that this test is the only one warranting inclusion in routine urinalysis. The test pad on the dipstick contains a buffered pH indicator that is sensitive to the protein concentration of the urine on the basis of the protein error of such indicators, whereby proteins can change the color of the indicator without a change in pH. The strip shows trace positivity at protein levels of approximately 100–200 mg/L, which is below the usually accepted upper limit of the reference range. The strip also has variable sensitivity to different proteins, for example, albumin shows better reactivity than the immunoglobulins and light chains (Bence Jones protein) may not react at all. Aside from the small amounts of protein arising from the urinary tract, such as the Tamm-Horsfall glycoprotein and some enzyme and cellular protein, the protein that appears in the urine is derived from the plasma by passage through the glomerulus. When the glomeruli are functionally intact, only about 0.1% of plasma albumin escapes from the plasma, most is reabsorbed in the proximal tubule. Proteins with a molecular mass larger than that of albumin are essentially excluded from the filtrate. Hence, the importance of the detection of abnormal quantities of protein in the urine. This can occur when the permeability of the glomerular filter is compromised as in the nephrotic syndrome, when there is decreased tubular reabsorption as in the Fanconi syndrome, in renal allograft rejection, or when the protein load presented to the glomeruli is excessive as in inflammatory or myeloproliferative diseases; proteinuria also can occur. The presence of significant amounts of protein in the urine may be missed because of dilution.

Glucose

The test pad for glucose on most dipsticks uses the glucose-oxidase-peroxidase system and shows positiveness at the trace levels of 750–3000 mg/L (4.16–16.65 mmol/L), depending on the physical properties (specific gravity, temperature, etc.) of the urine. Because the usual quantity of glucose in a person without disease is less than 100 mg/L (0.55 mmol/L), this represents a reasonable screening level. Increased glucose concentration in the urine occurs under two broad situations: hyperglycemia that exceeds the renal threshold for plasma glucose (about 180 mg/dL [10 mmol/L] in most individuals) or defective renal tubular reabsorption. Obviously, the former cause occurs most frequently in uncontrolled diabetes mellitus, whereas the latter may be caused by one of several congenital defects, or exogenous or endogenous toxins. It is important to note that the glucose oxidase method used on most dipsticks has a high specificity for glucose, and other sugars such as galactose, fructose, lactose, or the pentoses do not react. Because detection of the excretion of sugars other than glucose, especially galactose, is of importance especially in pediatric patients, other tests should be considered. Of particular utility in this respect are those tests (available in tablet form) that are based on the ability of many sugars to reduce cupric ions to cuprous ions with a change in color from blue to orange.

Ketones

This test is based on the reaction of sodium nitroprusside with acetoacetic acid. The test has a sensitivity of approximately 50 mg/L (490 μmol/L) (trace). Ketonuria occurs following starvation and in diabetes mellitus. The inclusion of this test in routine urinalysis has little clinical justification.

Blood

The presence of erythrocytes in the urine is an important finding as discussed above. The dipstick utilizes an o-tolidine test that actually detects hemoglobin or myoglobin with the assumption that positivity to hemoglobin is caused by the lysis of RBCs. This may not be the case because hemoglobin in the urine can reflect intravascular hemolysis and myoglobinuria occurs following skeletal or cardiac muscle injury. Both hemoglobinuria and myoglobinuria may occasionally be found following vigorous exercise. The usual dipstick test shows trace positivity at a hemoglobin concentration of approximately 0.2 mg/L (3.1 μmol/L). This level of hemoglobin is considerably below that produced by the 3 RBCs/hpf considered normal for the microscopic examination. On occasion, RBCs may be detected in conjunction with a negative dipstick result for hemoglobin. This can occur in a freshly voided specimen before lysis has occurred or due to the inhibition of o-tolidine reaction by the presence of ascorbic acid in the urine.

Bilirubin

Only the conjugated form of bilirubin is found in the urine because unconjugated bilirubin is insoluble. The test pad of the dipstick is impregnated with a stabilized diazotized 2,4-dichloroaniline that reacts with bilirubin to form a brown to purple chromogen. The test has a sensitivity of 0.5 mg/L (2.57 μmol/L), which is approximately twice the usual concentration of conjugated bilirubin in individuals without disease. Proposed as an indicator of occult liver disease the test is of little clinical value.

Urobilinogen

The urobilinogens are derived from conjugated bilirubin by bacterial action in the gut. As much as 50% of the urobilinogen is reabsorbed to be excreted in the urine. The dipstick contains a modified Ehrlich's reagent (p-dimethylamino-benzaldehyde). Urobilinogen is increased in the urine in any condition that causes an increased production of bilirubin. The test is sensitive to approximately 2 mg/L (3.4 μmol/L) of urobilin, which is about *one-half* the usual urinary concentration. The test is of little clinical value.

Nitrite

This test is based on the premise that if bacteria are present in the urine there will be reduction of the normally occurring nitrates to nitrites. Nearly all of the commonly occurring organisms that appear in the urine contain nitrate reductase enzymes; others such as *Streptococcus faecalis* do not. The basis of the test is the reaction of nitrite *p*-arsanilic acid to form a diazonium compound, which in turn complexes with 1,2,3,4-tetrahydrobenzoquinolinol to a pink compound. As indicated above, the examination of a urine specimen for bacteria, either directly or indirectly, is now believed to be a less satisfactory indicator of pyuria than is the finding of a significant number of leukocytes.

Leukocyte Esterase

This test is the most recent addition to the dipstick armamentarium. It is used to detect esterase released from many, but not all, white blood cells, and thus to indirectly establish pyuria. The dipstick is impregnated with a substrate for the esterase, 3-hydroxy-5-phenylpyrrole-N-tosyl-L-alanine ester, which is split to form a pyrrole alcohol that in turn reacts with a diazonium salt to give a purple color.

This test has been advocated as a prescreen test that, if negative, should negate the need for microscopy in routine urinalysis.[32] Although this proposal has found some support, most experts in the field are of the opinion that the high rate of error in both sensitivity and specificity (approximately 8%) make this approach clinically unacceptable.

Specific Gravity

The usual range of specific gravity in healthy individuals is 1.002–1.030. As a rough correlate with osmolality, determination of the specific gravity of urine is useful as an indicator of the concentrating ability of the kidneys and the hydration state of the patient. Most laboratories still measure or derive this entity by conventional methods such as the urinometer or total solids meter (refractometry). However, some newer test strips include a pad for the assessment of specific gravity. This is an indirect method that is based on the change in the pKa of a mixture of polymethylvinyl ether and maleic acid as a function of the number of ions in solution. This change may be visualized by the incorporation of an indicator, bromothymol blue, which changes color with the concomitant change in pH.

Summary

Positive results in some of the tests indicated above as having clinical importance should be confirmed by more rigorous analytic procedures.

The use of a 10% solution of ferric chloride added dropwise to a random urine specimen is a useful screening test for a variety of compounds as listed below[36]:

Ketonuria, salicylates, phenothiazines: red-purple
Phenylketonuria: green
Tyrosinemia: green
Homogentisuria: blue-green
Maple syrup urine: gray-green
Melanogens: brown to black

THE PORPHYRIAS

The porphyrins are formed by the linkage of four pyrrole rings to form the characteristic tetrapyrrole. This structure is the framework for the metalloporphyrins, which conjugated to specific proteins form many compounds of biologic importance, including the hemoglobins, cytochromes, myoglobin, and several enzymes. The prophyrin ring is synthesized from succinyl CoA (coenzyme A) and glycine by way of δ-aminolevulinic acid (ALA) and porphobilinogen (PBG). The porphyrias are a heterogenous group of genetic and acquired diseases. All the porphyrias are associated with overproduction or abnormal patterns of porphyrin or porphyrin precursor excretion caused by deficiency in, or inhibition of, an enzyme in the biosynthetic pathway. The porphyrias are subdivided into hepatic and erythropoetic porphyrias depending on the site of the metabolic defect (Table 3-12). The most widely used method for the fractionation of the porphyrins extracted from urine is high pressure liquid chromatography (HPLC) with fluorometric detection.[37,38] This procedure permits the quantitation of octacarboxyporphyrin (uroporphyrin), heptacarboxyporphyrin, hexacarboxyporphyrin, pentacarboxyporphyrin, tetracarboxyporphyrin (coproporphyrin), and dicarboxyporphyrin (protoporphyrin). The precursors of the porphyrins, ALA and PBG, are quantitated separately by column chromatography followed by reaction of the specific eluates with Erhlich's reagent.[39] Some aspects of this group of diseases are summarized below.

Hepatic Porphyrias

Acute Intermittent Porphyria (Pyrroloporphyria, Swedish Porphyria)

This is a genetic disease, inherited as an autosomal dominant, and characterized by neurologic and psychi-

Table 3-12. Classification of the Major Human Porphyrias

Classification	Deficient Enzyme	Inheritance	Photo-sensitivity	Neuro-visceral	Increased RBC Porphyrins	Increased Urine Porphyrins	Increased Stool Porphyrins
Congenital erythropoietic porphyria	Uroporphyrinogen III cosynthase	Autosomal recessive	Present (severe)	Absent	Uroporphyrin I (octacarboxyporphyrin) Coproporphyrin I (tetracarboxyporphyrin)	Uroporphyrin I (octacarboxyporphyrin) Coproporphyrin I (tetracarboxyporphyrin)	Coproporphyrin I (tetracarboxyporphyrin)
Erythropoietic protoporphyria	Ferrochelatase	Autosomal dominant	Present	Absent	Protoporphyrin III (dicarboxyporphyrin)	Usually absent Occasional excretion of hepta- and pentacarboxylporphyrins	Protoporphyrin III (dicarboxyporphyrin)
Acute intermittent porphyria	Porphobilinogen deaminase	Autosomal dominant	Absent	Present	Absent	Aminolevulinic acid Porphobilinogen	Absent
Hereditary coproporphyria	Coproporphyrinogen oxidase	Autosomal dominant	Present	Present	Absent	Aminolevulinic acid Porphobilinogen Coproporphyrin III (tetracarboxyporphyrin)	Coproporphyrin III (tetracarboxyporphyrin)
Porphyria variegata	Protoporphyrinogen oxidase or ferrochelatase	Autosomal dominant	Present	Present	Absent	Aminolevulinic acid Porphobilinogen Coproporphyrin III (tetracarboxyporphyrin)	Coproporphyrin III (tetracarboxyporphyrin) Protoporphyrin III (dicarboxyporphyrin)
Porphyria cutanea tardia	Uroporphyrinogen decarboxylase	?	Present	Absent	Absent	Coproporphyrin III (tetracarboxyporphyrin) Uroporphyrin III (octacarboxyporphyrin) Heptacarboxyporphyrin	Heptacarboxyporphyrin
Lead poisoning	Not applicable	Not applicable	Absent	Present	Protoporphyrin III (dicarboxyporphyrin)	Coproporphyrin III (tetracarboxyporphyrin) Aminolevulinic acid	Heptacarboxyporphyrin Coproporphyrin III (tetracarboxyporphyrin) Uroporphyrin III (octacarboxyporphyrin)

(Adapted from Kappas et al.,[66] with permission.)

atric dysfunction. As the name implies, there are periods of latency followed by the acute onset of abdominal pain, nausea, and neurologic impairment. There appears to be three precipitating factors for the attacks:

1. Drugs including barbiturates, sulfonamides, phenytoin
2. Steroids including estrogens and oral contraceptives
3. Stress including starvation and infection

Diagnosis is confirmed by increased levels of PBG and ALA in the urine, which often turns wine red on standing. The lack of other porphyrins in the urine is explained by the enzymatic defect that occurs at the step immediately following PBG (uroporphyrinogen-1-synthetase). There are no skin lesions associated with this porphyria.

Hereditary Coproporphyria

Hereditary coproporphyria is a genetic disease with autosomal dominant inheritance with many clinical similarities to acute intermittent porphyria. The defect is located in the liver at the enzyme coproporphyrinogen oxidase that causes the excretion of large quantities of tetra- and octacarboxyporphyrin in the urine and feces. Acute attacks may be precipitated by drugs as in acute intermittent porphyria. During acute attacks PBG may be increased in the urine and again the urine may turn red on standing. There are no skin lesions in this porphyria.

Porphyria Variegata (Protocoproporphyria hereditaria, South African Genetic Porphyria)

Porphyria variegata is a genetic disease with autosomal dominant inheritance, characterized by acute neurologic and psychotic attacks. The skin is sensitive to sunlight, the most apparent manifestation, and to mechanical trauma. The enzymatic lesion in this hepatic porphyria is thought to be in protoporphyrinogen oxidase or in ferrochelatase. The disease has high variability of expression with frequently a prolonged latent period with no symptoms appearing until the second or third decade of life. The excretion of abnormal amounts of the precursor(s) to the enzymatic block, namely tetracarboxyporphyrin and octa- and dicarboxyporphyrins, occurs mainly in the feces. It is only during the acute phase that octa-, hepta-, and pentacarboxyporphyrins appear in the urine together with porphobilinogen and aminolevulinic acid.

Porphyria Cutanea Tarda (Symptomatic Cutaneous Porphyria, Symptomatic Porphyria, Acquired Hepatic Porphyria, Constitutional Porphyria, Idiosyncratic Porphyria)

Porphyria cutanea tarda is the most common of the porphyrias. Although it is now established that it is a genetically inherited disease, it almost certainly requires the additional precipitating factor of concomitant liver disease. Otherwise, the condition exists in a subclinical or latent form. The clinical manifestations relate solely to chronic skin lesion with photosensitivity, hyperpigmentation, erythema, and ulcerative vesicles. The metabolic defect appears to be a partial block of the enzyme uroporphyrinogen decarboxylase. Increased amounts of all the porphyrins, especially octa-, hepta-, and tetracarboxyporphyrins, are excreted in the urine. There is usually no increase in PBG excretion: the urine may be pink or red due to the high concentration of porphyrins.

Erythropoietic Porphyrias

Congenital Erythropoietic Porphyria (Congenital Photosensitive Porphyria, Erythropoietic Uroporphyria, Gunther's Disease, Pink-Tooth Disease)

Erythropoietic porphyria is a rare genetic disease inherited as an autosomal recessive trait that presents in infancy. It is characterized by chronic sensitivity to sunlight with scarring and ulceration and by hemolytic anemia. Red urine is a typical finding, and red coloration of the skin and teeth may be observed. The defect occurs at the level of uroporphyrinogen III cosynthetase. The formation of uroporphyrinogen III is decreased, thus causing increased activity in ALA synthetase and a shunting of substrate into uroporphyrinogen I and coproporphyrinogen I. Coproporphyrinogen I cannot be metabolized further and hence accumulates in the tissues and is excreted in the urine and feces.

Erythropoietic Protoporphyria (Protoporphyria, Congenital Erythropoietic Protoporphyria)

A milder disease than congenital erythropoietic porphyria, erythropoietic protoporphyria is more common and is inherited as an autosomal dominant trait. The defect is located at the enzyme ferrochelatase, which is predominantly an erythrocyte enzyme responsible for the incorporation of iron into protoporphyrin IX to form heme. Although the symptoms of this porphyria are usually mild, photosensitivity with itching, eczema, and edema does occur with occasional moderate to severe liver disease. Diagnosis is confirmed by the presence of protoporphyrin in the erythrocyte. In general, urine findings in this disease are unremarkable with occasional increases in the excretion of hepta- and pentacarboxyporphyrins.

Related Disorders

A number of clinical entities can produce biochemical aberrations that may be indistinguishable from the porphyrias, that is, similar accumulation or excretion of porphyrins or porphyrin precursors occurs. The most common of these is lead poisoning, in which exposure to the metal inhibits a number of enzymes in the heme biosynthetic pathway leading to the excretion of excessive amounts of ALA and coproporphyrin (tetracarboxyporphyrin). Screening for the latter compound is a useful procedure for the detection of *chronic* lead poisoning. Coproporphyrinuria also may be seen in some rare diseases such as Dubin-Johnson syndrome and hereditary tyrosinemia; and in toxicities caused by a number of agents and drugs, including hexachlorobenzene, nitrous oxide, ethyl ether, barbiturates, choral hydrate, morphine, and some antibiotics.

Test: Porphyrins (See Ch. 15)

Depending on the disorder suspected, the specific porphyrin measurement(s) is ordered (see above and Table 13-12). Urine specimens are collected over 24 hours, refrigerated, and protected from light. The reference ranges for the porphyrins are found in Table 3-13.

Table 3-13. Reference Ranges for Porphyrins

Compound	Range
δ-Aminolevulinic acid	1.5–7.5 mg/24 h (11.4–57.2 µmol/d)
Porphobilinogen	<2 mg/24 h (<8.8 µmol/d)
Octacarboxyporphyrin (uroporphyrin)	<27 µg/24 h (<41.3 nmol/d)
Tetracarboxyporphyrin (coproporphyrin)	<72 µg/24 h (<110 nmol/d)
Heptacarboxyporphyrin	<6 µg/24 h (<9.2 nmol/d)
Hexacarboxyporphyrin	<3 µg/24 h (<4.6 nmol/d)
Pentacarboxyporphyrin	<5 µg/24 h (<7.6 nmol/d)

(Data from references 40 through 42.)

ENDOCRINE TESTS

Test: Cyclic AMP (Cyclic Adenosine Monophosphate, cAMP, 3^1,5^1-AMP)

Background and Selection

Cyclic AMP is a cyclic nucleotide that mediates the action of many hormones. Simply, it carries the hormonal message from the cell membrane to the nucleus and has thus been called the "second messenger." The measurement of urinary cAMP has been found to be useful in differentiating hypoparathyroidism from pseudohypoparathyroidism as causes of hypercalcemia since approximately 60% of the cAMP in the urine is derived from its excretion by the proximal tubule. This component is under the control of the parathyroid hormone. It has also been used in the differential diagnosis of primary versus nephrogenic diabetes insipidus. The assay of cAMP can be achieved by a radioimmunoassay using a phosphodiesterase inhibitor to prevent its breakdown during analysis.[43] It has been suggested that the simultaneous measurement of serum and urine cAMP permits the quantitation of the renal derived, as opposed to the serum derived and glomerular filtered, cAMP. This has been called the nephrogeneous cAMP; however, this determination has not found favor because of its complexity and large potential for error. Indeed, the usefulness of the more straightforward quantitation of urinary cAMP as compared with the assay of parathyroid hormone, remains to a large degree, unproven. This is especially true in patients who have any impairment of renal function, although the finding of elevated urinary cAMP with low serum parathyroid hormone levels has been thought to be indicative of malignancy.[44,45] The specimen required is a 24-hour or fasting morning urine that should be frozen if stored.

Interpretation

The reference range for cAMP is less than 3.3 mg/24 h or less than 1.64 mg/g creatinine (SI units are µmol/d or µmol/mol of creatinine with conversion factors of 3.04 and 344 respectively). (See Ch. 12.)

Test: Renin (See Ch. 11)

Background and Selection

Renin is a hydrolytic enzyme that is synthesized and stored in the cells of the juxtaglomerular apparatus.

The enzyme is a component of the renin-angiotensin-aldosterone system that regulates blood pressure, plasma volume, and electrolyte balance. The initiation of the regulator process occurs when receptors in the juxtaglomerular apparatus respond to decreased plasma volume, blood pressure, neural stimulation, or hyponatremia by releasing stored renin into the circulation. Renin converts plasma angiotensinogen into a 10 amino acid peptide, angiotensin I, which is cleaved to an octapeptide by a converting enzyme present in the endothelial cells of the vessels of the lung. Angiotensin II is the most powerful vasoconstrictor known, acting on the peripheral adrenergic neurons. It also has actions on the adrenal cortex stimulating the production of aldosterone, which results in the retention of sodium and water, the excretion of potassium in the distal convoluted tubule, and in the stimulation of the thirst centers of the brain. Angiotensin II regulates its own production by negative feedback on the production of renin.

Logistics

Blood for renin activity should be collected into an ethylenediaminetetraacetic acid (EDTA) container, centrifuged as soon as possible and the plasma frozen at −20°C or below. Because renin is an enzyme, two approaches have been taken to measure it in serum: by concentration and by activity. In general, the measurement of plasma renin activity (PRA) is now accepted as the test of choice. The procedure is a radioimmunoassay in which the production of angiotensin I from its endogenous substrate is measured. Commercially prepared kits are available; however, the assay is extremely difficult to standardize and control, making interlaboratory comparisons and the establishment of reference ranges very problematic.

Interpretation

Plasma renin activity is increased in some 15% of patients with essential hypertension and it is claimed that this group has a higher number of complications than the group with no elevation of renin and that they are more responsive to β-blockers.[46] Because PRA varies with the sodium load presented to the kidney, it has been shown to be helpful if measured renin is compared with the patient's sodium excretion.[47] Renin activity measurements have value in the assessment of hypertension due to renal ischemia or in the rare cases of a renin secreting tumor. Here the test can have excellent discriminatory power, particularly when the renin activity in the blood from the renal vein of the affected kidney is compared with the presumed normal contralateral kidney.[48-50]

Interpretation[51,52]

Quoting a reference range for PRA is fraught with dangers of misinterpretation caused by methodologic and interlaboratory variations. For patients whose sodium intake is less than 10 mmol/24 h a range of renin activity of 5-24 ng angiotensin I/mL/h (SI units are $\mu g \times h^{-1} \times L^{-1}$, with a conversion factor of 1) is frequently used. It should be noted that in addition to sodium intake, renin activity values may be affected by posture, hydration state, diuretics, antihypertensive drugs, and estrogen containing medications.

CLEARANCE TESTS

Test: Inulin Clearance

Background and Selection

Inulin is a polysaccharide with a molecular mass of approximately 5000 da. It is filtered completely at the glomeruli and is neither secreted nor reabsorbed by the tubules. There is good evidence, as described previously, that although creatinine clearance can provide valuable information in many patients, those with low GFR and/or grossly elevated blood creatinine causing tubular secretion of creatinine require a more dependable measurement of GFR. Inulin clearance provides a means of achieving this end without the use of radioactive compounds.

Logistics

The test is performed on a fasting patient who is encouraged to drink water to insure an adequate urinary flow. The patient is given a priming dose of inulin followed by a sustaining solution in order to maintain a constant plasma inulin level. Urine is collected over a timed period during which a blood sample is drawn. The quantitation of inulin in serum or urine is relatively straightforward, being based on the determination of fructose after the hydrolysis of the polysaccharide. The fructose is reacted with β-indolylacetic acid in acidic solution to form a purple-blue color. The GFR is then calculated by the same formula as given previously for creatinine clearance with appropriate correction for surface area. (SI units for this test are mL/s/m², the conversion factor is 0.00963.)

Table 3-14. Inulin Clearance Measured at Various Ages in Normal Individuals

Age (Months)	Range mL/min/1.73 m² Surface Area	
<1	29–88	
1–6	40–112	
6–12	62–121	

Age (Yrs)	Male	Female
1–20		
20–29	90–174	84–156
30–39	88–168	82–159
40–49	78–162	82–146
50–59	68–152	66–142
60–69	57–137	58–130
70–79	42–122	45–121
80–89	39–105	39–105

Interpretation[53-55]

The reference ranges for inulin are found in Table 3-14.

Test: Phenosulfonphthalein (PSP)

Various tests have been devised to quantitate the secretory function of tubules. Among these is the clearance of PSP, which is 95% cleared from the plasma by tubular secretion. The test is performed by giving an intravenous bolus of 1 mL of a 600 mg/dL sterile PSP solution. Urine samples are collected at timed intervals, usually 15, 30, 60, and 120 minutes after the dosing. The urine is then alkalinized and the PSP concentration determined spectrophotometrically. This test has now largely fallen into disuse. About 25–30% of the total excretion should be within the first 15 minutes after the injection of the dye (SI units are decimal fractions of the total excretion, conversion factor 0.01).[56]

MISCELLANEOUS TESTS

Test: Aluminum

Background and Selection

The widespread use of hemodialysis as therapy for uremia was followed by the recognition, in 1972, that patients on certain hemodialysis units were experiencing an epidemic of a usually fatal syndrome characterized by slurring and hesitancy of speech, followed by dysarthia, dyspraxia, and dysphasia.[57,58] Patients progressed to seizures, global dementia, microcytic anemia, and osteomalacia. The syndrome was named dialysis encephalopathy or dialysis dementia. Concentrations of aluminum found in the gray matter of the brains of patients dying of this disease led to the suggestion that the syndrome resulted from aluminum intoxication.[59] This hypothesis was confirmed when it was shown that the disease could be significantly reduced by removing aluminum from the water used to prepare the dialysate.[60] However, this did not eliminate the disease, as had been hoped, because a second source of aluminum was discovered, that of the aluminum containing phosphate-binding gels administered to many uremic patients to control their serum phosphate levels.[61] Aluminum absorption, and the factors that affect and regulate it, are poorly understood. However, it is known that little of the normal dietary intake of 3–5 mg/d is absorbed, perhaps only 15 μg. That which is absorbed is eliminated by renal mechanisms with the maintenance of a total body aluminum load of 30–40 mg. The regulator mechanisms appear to be altered in the presence of the antacid gels and that, together with compromised renal function can lead to elevation of aluminum concentrations.[62] The iron chelator, deferrioximine, has been used with some success to lower the body burden of aluminum in intoxicated patients.

Logistics

The measurement of aluminum in biologic material poses a considerable challenge to the analyst because of the low levels present, the ubiquitous distribution of the element, and the lack of reference materials. A variety of analytic techniques have been used but only two have found acceptance. The most commonly used technique is electrothermal atomic absorption spectrophotometry, although a more promising approach appears to be the use of inductively coupled plasma emission spectrometry.[58]

Interpretation

There are as yet no established reference ranges for aluminum in biologic material. There appears to be a consensus among workers in the field that the usual plasma aluminum concentration in nonuremic individuals is less than 10 μg/L (<0.37 μmol/L). Hemodialysis patients usually have plasma concentrations greater than 50 μg/L (>1.86 μmol/L), whereas those patients with concentrations greater than 100–150 μg/L (3.71–5.57 μmol/L) are at risk for aluminum toxicity.[58,59,61]

Test: Creatine (N-Methylguanidinoacetic Acid)

Background and Selection

Creatine is the substrate from which the high energy phosphate compound creatine phosphate is synthesized by the action of the enzyme creatine kinase (ATP, adenosine triphosphate; ADP, adenosine diphosphate):

$$\text{creatine} + \text{ATP} \xleftrightarrow{\text{creatine kinase}} \text{creatine phosphate} + \text{ADP}$$

This reaction occurs primarily in vertebrate muscle and nerve tissue. Creatine is synthesized in the kidney, liver, and pancreas and then transported in the blood to muscles and nervous tissue.

Logistics

Serum must be free from hemolysis because there is a high concentration of creatine in erythrocytes. Creatine is very unstable in urine. Timed specimens should be kept at 4°C until complete and then brought to neutral pH and stored frozen.

Interpretation[63,64]

The reference ranges for creatine in serum are as follows: males, 0.17–0.70 mg/dL and females, 0.35–0.93 mg/dL; and in urine: males, 0–40 mg/24 h and females, 0–80 mg/24 h. (The SI units for serum and urine are μmol/L and μmol/d, with conversion factors of 76.3 and 7.63, respectively.) The measurement of creatine in urine, useful for the diagnosis of muscular dystrophies and atrophic diseases, has been largely superseded by other assays that are more specific, such as the measurement of creatine kinase activity. Serum or urine creatine may be quantitated by conversion to creatinine by applying heat in acid conditions, with creatinine in the specimen measured before and after the conversion. The methods are fraught with difficulties and interferences, but because of the lack of clinical utility outlined above little effort has been expended to improve the methodology.

APPENDIX

SCHEMATIC DRAWINGS OF CELLS, CASTS, AND CRYSTALS AS THEY APPEAR IN URINE.

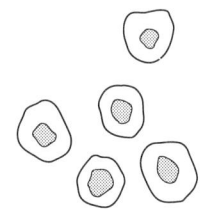

Fig. 3-1. White blood cells.

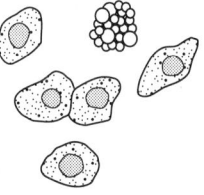

Fig. 3-2. Renal tubular epithelial cells.

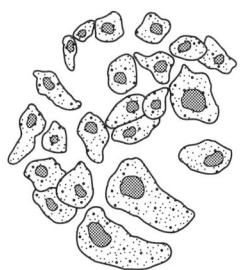

Fig. 3-3. Transitional epithelial cells.

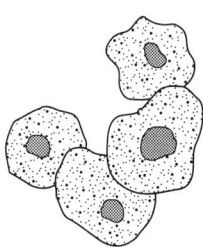

Fig. 3-4. Squamous epithelial cells.

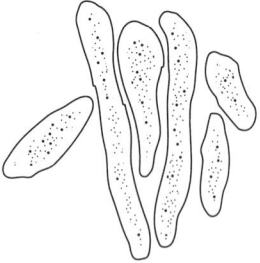

Fig. 3-5. Hyaline casts.

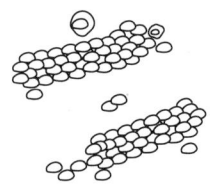

Fig. 3-6. Red blood cell casts.

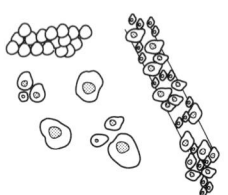

Fig. 3-7. White blood cell casts.

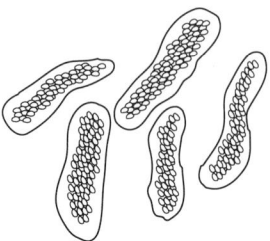

Fig. 3-8. Granular casts.

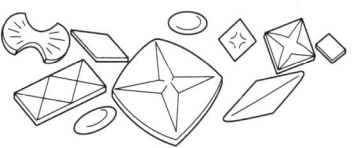

Fig. 3-9. Calcium oxalate crystals.

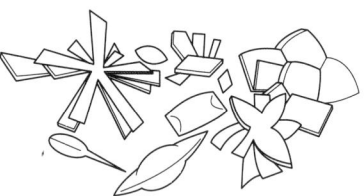

Fig. 3-10. Uric acid crystals.

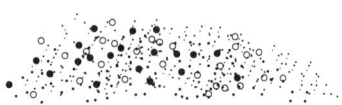

Fig. 3-11. Amorphous urates.

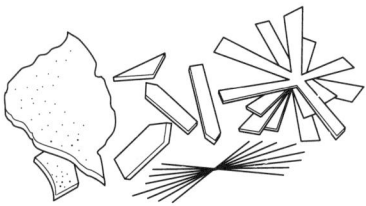

Fig. 3-12. Calcium phosphate crystals.

Renal Function • 63

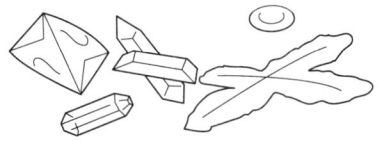

Fig. 3-13. Triple phosphate crystals.

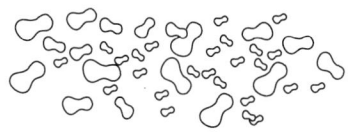

Fig. 3-14. Calcium carbonate crystals.

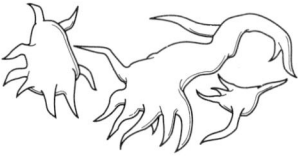

Fig. 3-15. Ammonium biurate crystals.

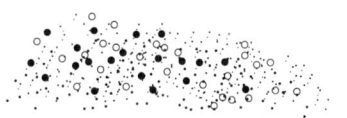

Fig. 3-16. Amorphous phosphates.

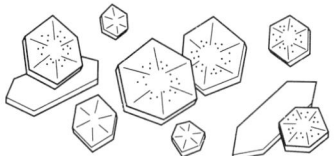

Fig. 3-17. Cystine crystals.

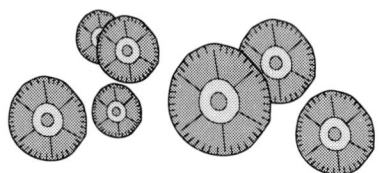

Fig. 3-18. Leucine crystals.

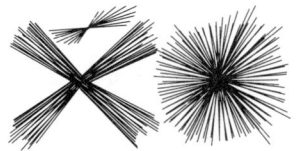

Fig. 3-19. Tyrosine crystals.

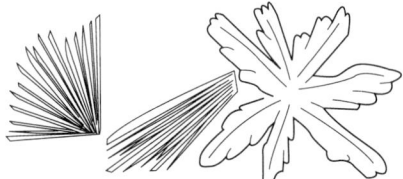

Fig. 3-20. Sulfonamide crystals.

REFERENCES

1. Baines AW: Disorders of the kidney and urinary tract. pp. 128–130. In Gornall AG (ed): Applied Biochemistry of Clinical Disorders. Hagerstown, Harper & Row, 1980.
2. Talke H, Schubert GE: Enzymatische Harnstoffbestimmung in Blut und Serum im optischen Test nach Warburg. Klin Wochenschr 1965;43:174–178.
3. Tiffany TO, Jansen JM, Burtis CA et al: Enzymatic kinetic rate and end-point analysis of substrate. Clin Chem 1972;18:829–840.
4. Di Giorgio J: Nonprotein nitrogenous constituents. pp. 511–522. In Henry RJ, Cannon DC, Winkelman JW (eds): Clinical Chemistry Principles and Technics. 2nd Ed. Hagerstown, Harper & Row, 1974.
5. Black DAK, Cameron JS: Renal function. pp. 483–514. In Brown SS, Mitchell FL, Young DS (eds): Chemical Diagnosis of Disease. New York, Elsevier Science Publishing, 1979.
6. Davies DP, Saunders R: Blood urea: normal values in early infancy related to feeding practices. Arch Dis Child 1973;48:563–565.
7. O'Brien D, Ibbott FA, Rodgerson DO (eds): Pediatric Microbiochemical Techniques. 3rd Ed. New York, Hoeber Medical Division, Harper & Row, 1968, p. 350.
8. Applegart DA, Ross PM: The unsuitability of creatinine excretion as a basis for assessing the excretion of other metabolites by infants and children. Clin Chim Acta 1975;64:83–85.
9. Narayanan S, Appleton HD: Creatinine: a review. Clin Chem 1980;26:1119–1126.
10. Haeckel R, Gadsden RH, Sherwin JE et al: Assay of creatinine in serum with use of fuller's earth to remove interferents. In Cooper GR (ed): Selected Methods of Clinical Chemistry. American Association for Clinical Chemistry, Washington, D.C. 1983;10:225–229.
11. Bowers LD: Kinetic serum creatinine assays. I. The role of various factors in determining specificity. Clin Chem 1980;26:551–554.
12. Bowers LD, Wong ET: Kinetic serum creatinine assays. II. A critical evaluation and review. Clin Chem 1980;26:555–561.
13. Meites S (ed): Pediatric Clinical Chemistry. 2nd Ed. Washington, D.C., American Association for Clinical Chemistry, 1981, pp. 171–173.
14. Murray RL: Creatinine. Nonprotein nitrogenous compounds. pp. 1247–1252. In Kaplan LA, Pesce AJ (eds): Clinical Chemistry: Theory, Analysis, and Correlation. St. Louis, CV Mosby, 1984.
15. O'Brien D, Ibbott FA, Rodgerson DO (eds): Pediatric Microbiochemical Techniques. 3rd Ed. New York, Hoeber Medical Division, Harper & Row, 1968, pp. 114–116.
16. Carrie BJ, Golbetz HV, Michaels AS et al: Creatinine: an inadequate filtration marker in glomerular diseases. Am J Med 1980;69:177–182.
17. Wibell L, Bjørsell-Ostling E: Endogenous creatinine clearance in apparently healthy individuals as determined by 24 hour ambulatory urine collection. Uppsala J Med Sci 1973;78:43–47.
18. Kampmann J, Siersbaek-Nielsen K, Kristensen M et al: Rapid evaluation of creatinine clearance. Acta Med Scand 1974;196:517–520.
19. Black DAK, Cameron JS. Renal function. pp. 453–524. In Brown SS, Mitchell FL, Young DS (eds): Chemical Diagnosis of Disease. New York, Elsevier/Science Publishing, 1980.
20. Szelid Z, Méhes K: Estimation of glomerular filtration rate from plasma creatinine concentration in children of various ages. Arch Dis Child 1977;52:669–670.
21. Boss GR, Seegmiller JE: Hyperuricemia and gout. Classification, complications and management. N Engl J Med 1969;300:1459–1468.
22. Pollard A: Disorders of purine and pyrimidine metabolism. pp. 335–344. In Gornall AG (ed): Applied Biochemistry of Clinical Disorders. Hagerstown, Harper & Row, 1980; pp. 335–344.
23. Wyngaarden JB, Kelley WN: Gout. pp. 1043–1114. In Stanbury JB, Wyngaarden JB, Fredricksson DS et al (eds): The Metabolic Basis of Inherited Disease. 5th Ed. New York, McGraw-Hill, 1983.
24. Rock RC, Walker WG, Jennings CD: Nitrogen metabolites and renal function. pp. 1284–1288. In Tietz NW (ed): Textbook of Clinical Chemistry. Philadelphia, WB Saunders, 1986.
25. Tietz NW (ed): Clinical Guide to Laboratory Tests. Philadelphia, WB Saunders, 1983, pp. 494–495.*
26. Kelley WN, Weingaarden JB: Clinical syndromes associated with hypozanthine-guanine phosphoribosyltransferase deficiency. pp. 1115–1143. In Stanbury JB, Wyngaarden JB, Fredricksson DS et al (eds): The Metabolic Basis of Inherited Disease. 5th Ed. New York, McGraw-Hill, 1983.
27. Tietz NW (ed): Clinical Guide, 1983, pp. 446–448.
28. Tietz NW (ed): Clinical Guide, 1983, pp. 398–400.
29. Tietz NW (ed): Clinical Guide, 1983, pp. 110–112.
30. Tietz NW (ed): Clinical Guide, 1983, pp. 96–98.
31. Bradley M, Schumann G, Ward PCJ: Examination of urine. pp. 559–634. In Henry JB (ed): Clinical diagnosis and Management by Laboratory Method. 16th Ed. Philadelphia, WB Saunders, 1979.
32. Valenstein PN, Koepke JA. Unnecessary microscopy in routine urinalysis. Am J Clin Pathol 1984;82:444–448.
33. Senk RE: Sediment microscopy, nitrituria and leucocyte esteraseuria as predictors of significant bacteria. Clin Lab Automat 1982;2:117–121.
34. Musher DM, Thorsteinsson SB, Airola VM: Quantitative urinalysis diagnosing urinary track infection in men. JAMA 1976;236:2069–2072.
35. Williams HE, Smith LH: Primary hyperoxaluria. pp. 204–228. In Stanbury JB, Wyngaarden JB, Fredricksson DS et al (eds): The Metabolic Basis of Inherited Disease. 5th Ed. New York, McGraw-Hill, 1983.
36. Hicks JM, Boeckx RL (eds): Pediatric Clinical Chemistry. Philadelphia, WB Saunders, 1984, pp. 665.
37. Ford RE, Ou C-N, Ellefson RD: Liquid-chromatographic analysis for urinary porphyrins. Clin Chem 1981;27:397–404.
38. Carlson RE, Sirasothy R, Dolphin D: An internal standard for porphyrin analysis. Anal Biochem 1984;140:360–365.
39. Fernandez AA, Jacobs SL: In MacDonald RP (ed): Standard Methods of Clinical Chemistry. Vol. 6. San Diego, Academic Press, 1970.

---

* References 27–30 refer to same text as reference 25; tabular data taken from pages cited.

40. Labbe RF, Lamon JM: Porphyrins and disorders of porphyrin metabolism. pp. 1589–1614. In Tietz NW (ed): Textbook of Clinical Chemistry. Philadelphia, WB Saunders, 1986.
41. Gornall AG: Porphyrins, the heme proteins, bile pigments, and jaundice. pp. 142–163. In Gornall AG (ed): Applied Biochemistry of Clinical Disorders. Hagerstown, Harper & Row, 1980.
42. Weinkove C, McDowell DR: Porphyrins, hemoglobin and related compounds. pp. 642–669. In Gowenlock AH (ed): Practical Clinical Biochemistry. Boca Raton, CRC Press, 1988.
43. Chiang CS, Kowalski AJ: cAMP radioimmunoassay without interference from calcium or EDTA. Clin Chem 1982;28:150–152.
44. Peck WA, Klahr S: Cyclic nucleotides in bone and mineral metabolism. pp. 90–130. In Greengard P, Robinson G (eds): Advances in Cyclic Nucleotide Research. Vol. 2. New York, Raven Press, 1980.
45. Orwoll ES, Belsey RE: The laboratory evaluation of osteopenia. Clin Lab Med 4984;4:763–774.
46. Watts NB, Keffer JH: Practical Endocrine Diagnosis. 3rd Ed. Philadelphia, Lea & Febiger, 1982.
47. Laragh JH, Sealey J, Brunner HR: The control of aldosterone secretion in normal and hypertensive man: abnormal renin-aldosterone patterns in low renin hypertension. Am J Med 1972;53:649–663.
48. Arakawa K, Masaki Z, Oside Y et al: Divided renal and peripheral venous renin as a means of predicting operative curability of renal hypertension. Clin Sci Mol Med 1973;45:311s–314s.
49. Wenting GJ, Tan-Tjiong HL, Derkx FHM et al: Split renal function after captopril in unilateral renal artery stenosis. Br Med J 1984;288:886–890.
50. Case DB, Laragh JH: Reactive hyperreninemia in renovascular hypertension after angiotensin blockade with saralasin or converting enzyme inhibitor. Ann Intern Med 1979;91:153–160.
51. Chattoraj SC, Watts NB: Endocrinology. pp. 1068, 1083–1084. In Tietz NW (ed): Textbook of Clinical Chemistry. Philadelphia, WB Saunders, 1986.
52. Freelender AE, Goodfriend TL: Renin and the angiotensins. pp. 889–907. In Jaffe BM, Behrman HR (eds): Methods of Hormone Radioimmunoassay. San Diego, Academic Press, 1979;889–907.
53. O'Brien D, Ibbott FA, Rodgerson DO (eds): Pediatric Microbiochemical Techniques. 3rd Ed. New York, Hoeber Medical Division, Harper & Row, 1968, pp. 191–193.
54. Meites S (ed): Pediatric Clinical Chemistry. 2nd Ed. Washington, D.C., American Association for Clinical Chemistry, 1981, pp. 291–292.
55. Tietz NW (ed): Textbook of Clinical Chemistry. Philadelphia, WB Saunders, 1986, p. 1833.
56. Cannon DC: Kidney function tests. pp. 1548–1551. In Henry RJ, Cannon DC, Winkelman JW (eds): Clinical Chemistry, Principles and Technics. 2nd Ed. Hagerstown, Harper & Row, 1974.
57. Alfrey AC, Mishell JM, Burks J et al: Syndrome of dyspraxia and multifocal seizures associated with chronic hemodialysis. Trans Am Soc Artif Intern Organs 1972;18:257–261.
58. Savory J, Berlin A, Courtoux C et al: The role of biological monitoring in the prevention of aluminum toxicity in man: aluminum analysis in biological fluids. Ann Clin Lab Sci 1983;13:444–451.
59. Alfrey AC, LeGendre GR, Kaehny WD: The dialysis encephalopathy syndrome: possible aluminum intoxication. N Engl J Med 1976;294:184–188.
60. Alfrey AC: Aluminum intoxication. N Engl J Med 1984;310:1113–1114.
61. Andreoli SP, Bergstein JM, Sherrard DJ: Aluminum intoxication from aluminum-containing phosphate binders in children with azotemia not undergoing hemodialysis. N Engl J Med 1984;310:1079–1084.
62. Alfrey AC: Aluminum. Adv Clin Chem 1983;23:69–91.
63. Rock RC, Walker WG, Jennings CD: Nitrogen metabolites and renal function. pp. 1271–1281. In Tietz NW (ed): Textbook of Clinical Chemistry. Philadelphia, WB Saunders, 1986.
64. Murray RL: Creatine. pp. 876–881. In Pesce AJ, Kaplan LA (eds): Methods in Clinical Chemistry. St. Louis, CV Mosby, 1987.
65. Graff L: A Handbook of Routine Urinalysis. Philadelphia, JB Lippincott, 1983.
66. Kappas A, Sassa S, Anderson E: The Porphyrias. pp. 1301–1384. In Stanbury JB, Wyngaarden JB, Frederickson DS et al (eds): The Metabolic Basis of Inherited Disease. 5th Ed. New York, McGraw-Hill, 1983.

4 Liver Function

Paul L. Wolf

INTRODUCTION

The liver regulates many important metabolic functions (Table 4-1). Diffuse, severe hepatic injury is associated with marked distortion of these metabolic functions and can be evaluated by determining serum concentrations of a relatively small number of analytes (Table 4-2). In general, only four groups of serum biochemical tests are necessary to assess hepatic abnormalities. These analytes are (1) alanine aminotransferase (ALT) and aspartate aminotransferase (AST), (2) alkaline phosphatase (AP), (3) bilirubin and its fractions, and (4) pseudocholinesterase or another analyte such as albumin or transferrin to measure hepatic synthetic function (Table 4-3). The aminotransferases are elevated with acute hepatic cell injury, in contrast to AP, which is elevated with cholestasis. Serum bilirubin is important in assessing the ability of the hepatic cell to conjugate and excrete an organic anion. Decreased serum pseudocholinesterase or albumin signifies decreased hepatic synthetic ability. The pattern of results from the above four test groups allows classification of liver disease into the broad categories of (1) acute hepatitis, (2) chronic hepatitis, (3) cirrhosis, (4) cholestasis, and (5) neoplasms (Table 4-4). In conjunction with other clinical parameters, the pattern of liver

Table 4-1. Metabolic Functions of the Liver

Metabolism and regulation
    Carbohydrates
    Amino acids and ammonia
    Proteins
    Cholesterol and other lipids
Synthesis
    Urea
    Serum proteins (e.g., albumin, coagulation proteins, carrier proteins, and acute phase proteins)
    Bile acids
Metabolism and degradation
    Proteins
    Drugs
    Hormones
    Endogenous substances (e.g., bilirubin)

Table 4-2. Important Analytes to Evaluate Liver Function

Alanine aminotransferase (ALT) (serum glutamate pyruvate transaminase [SGPT])
Alkaline phosphatase (AP)
Ammonia
Aspartate aminotransferase (AST) (serum glutamate oxaloacetate transaminase [SGOT])
Total bilirubin
    Unconjugated (indirect)
    Conjugated (direct)
    δ (delta)
γ-Glutamyl transferase (GGT)
Cerebrospinal fluid (CSF) glutamine
Lactate dehydrogenase (LD)
5′ Nucleotidase (5′ NT)
Pseudocholinesterase

Table 4-3. Information Obtained From Liver Function Analytes

Analyte	Indicator
Aspartate aminotransferase, alanine aminotransferase	Necrosis of liver
Alkaline phosphatase	Cholestasis
Bilirubin	Excretion defects
Pseudocholinesterase or albumin	Synthesis defects

Table 4-4. Classification of Liver Diseases

Hepatitis
  Acute
    Acute viral hepatitis, type A
    Acute viral hepatitis, type B
    Non-A, non-B
    Hepatitis associated with systemic viral infection
      Infectious mononucleosis hepatitis
      Cytomegalic virus hepatitis
    Alcoholic hepatitis
    Drug-induced hepatitis
      Toxic
      Idiosyncratic
    Chemical hepatitis
  Chronic
    Chronic active hepatitis
    Chronic persistent hepatitis
Cirrhosis
  Alcoholic
  Following viral hepatitis
  Following biliary obstruction: secondary biliary cirrhosis
  Secondary to passive congestion: congestive cirrhosis
  Unknown etiology
    Cryptogenic cirrhosis
Cholestasis
  Intrahepatic (no mechanical obstruction to bile flow)
    Acute
      Drug-induced
      Virus-induced
      Alcohol-induced
      Associated with neoplastic and other infiltration
    Recurrent cholestasis of pregnancy
  Intrahepatic (Mechanical obstruction to bile flow)
    Biliary atresia
    Infiltration of malignancy
    Primary biliary cirrhosis
  Extrahepatic
    Biliary atresia
    Choledocholithiasis
    Stricture
    Neoplasm
    Suppurative cholangitis
Neoplasms
  Primary
    Adenoma
    Hepatoma
  Secondary metastases

function test results is useful in classifying the type of liver disease present, following the course of hepatic disease, and predicting prognosis.

BASIC TESTS OF LIVER FUNCTION

Test: Alanine Aminotransferase (Serum Glutamate Pyruvate Transaminase [SGPT])

Background and Selection

Serum ALT results, which are useful for identifying inflammation and necrosis of the liver, are used to screen for blood donors for hepatic disease including possible viral hepatitis. An increase in ALT is found in acute hepatitis, especially acute viral hepatitis, and in cholestatic conditions. Serum ALT is useful for following the progression or regression of liver disease, especially viral hepatitis. The enzyme, which plays a role in nitrogen metabolism, has its highest concentration in the liver with lesser amounts in the kidney and skeletal muscle (Table 4-5). Alanine aminotransferase is located in the microsomal portion of the hepatic cell, in contrast to AST, which is found in hepatic cell mitochondria as well. Measurement of ALT often is used in conjunction with other enzymes to classify liver disease (see p. 69).

Terminology

In place of the term glutamate pyruvate transaminase, the preferred term is either alanine aminotransferase or alanine transaminase.

Interpretation

The usual reference range for serum ALT activity is markedly dependent on the method used for ALT analysis. Typical results are 25–65 IU/L for newborns and 10–40 IU/L for adults; the high values in newborns may reflect greater hepatocyte permeability. The reference range is skewed toward high values in healthy adults. In addition, a large number of conditions affect ALT; for example, men have higher results than women and obese individuals tend to have increased values. Additionally, strenuous exercise and moderate alcohol consumption increase results. These factors all

Table 4-5. Tissue Activities of Alanine Aminotransferase (ALT) and Aspartate Aminotransferase (AST) Relative to Serum

Tissue	ALT	AST
Liver	2750	7100
Kidney	1188	4550
Heart	444	7800
Skeletal muscle	300	4950
Pancreas	125	1400
Spleen	75	700
Lung	44	500
Erythrocytes	4	8
Normal serum	1	1

(From Lott and Wolf,[51] with permission.)

effect the ALT cutoff value that is used for exclusion of blood donor units.[1]

Decreases

Decreased ALT occurs in patients who are nutritionally deficient in pyridoxine (vitamin B_6). Decreased pyridoxine and low serum ALT activity also may be present in women taking oral contraceptives and in patients with renal failure who are undergoing hemodialysis.

Increases

Serum ALT is more useful in acute and cholestatic diseases, compared with AST, which is more helpful in chronic and infiltrative lesions. Because an increase in ALT is rarely seen in clinical conditions other than hepatic disease, ALT is more specific for liver disease than AST. Additionally, ALT remains elevated longer than AST, but in extensive necrotic injury of the liver AST exceeds ALT activity. Alanine aminotransferase results greater than 20 times the upper limit of the reference range usually indicate hepatic injury. In acute viral hepatitis without extensive necrosis, ALT exceeds AST, whereas AST exceeds ALT in alcoholic hepatitis owing to release of mitochondrial AST (m-AST).[2-4] Because it is elevated in hepatitis, serum ALT has been used as indicator for non-A, non-B hepatitis (hepatitis C) in donated blood. In hepatitis, ALT increases early and typically returns to the reference range in a few weeks, but the magnitude of the increase is not a reliable indicator of severity. Elevations lasting 6 months or more indicate chronic active or persistent hepatitis. In chronic active or chronic persistent hepatitis, ALT is minimally increased.

Serum ALT also is increased in intrahepatic and extrahepatic cholestasis. ALT activities in the heart and skeletal muscle are less than 10% of AST in these respective tissues, so ALT activities in disorders of the heart and skeletal muscle are within the reference range. Serum ALT is increased in about 30% of patients with acute myocardial infarction. Usually this increase is caused by hepatic congestion, but large infarcts can release measurable amounts of enzyme. Many drugs cause ALT elevations and ALT activity has been used to monitor drug toxicity.[1]

Test: Asparate Aminotransferase (Serum Glutamate Oxaloacetate Transaminase [SGOT])

Background and Selection

Measuring AST activity is useful for identifying inflammation and necrosis of the liver. Aspartate aminotransferase is located in the microsomal and mitochondrial portions of the hepatic cell and also is present in the epidermis of the skin, heart, skeletal muscle, pancreas, and kidneys. Red blood cells normally contain approximately 10 times more AST than serum. Agents such as ethanol, which induce liver cell mitochondrial necrosis, result in the release of m-AST. Viral hepatitis usually causes release of only microsomal AST, but fulminant viral hepatitis also may cause hepatic cell mitochondrial necrosis similar to alcoholic hepatitis. Measurement of AST activity is therefore used to screen for hepatic disease and is useful for determining the presence of chronic active or chronic persistent hepatitis. Serum AST measurements are often used in conjunction with other tests.

Interpretation

The reference range for serum AST activity is 25–65 IU/L for newborns and 10–40 IU/L for adults. Most often an abnormal serum AST result is associated with an acute abnormality of the heart, liver, or skeletal muscle.[5-6] The microsomal isoenzyme is the usual form of AST present in the blood. Mitochondrial AST, normally not detectable in blood, appears in some cases of extensive tissue destruction, such as with alcoholic hepatitis (Table 4-6). The cytoplasmic and mitochondrial forms can be separated electrophoretically.[7]

Decreases

Decreased AST is found in patients with poor nutrition accompanied by pyridoxine deficiency. Decreased plasma pyridoxine and low AST also occur in patients with chronic renal failure who are undergoing dialysis and in women taking oral contraceptives.

Table 4-6. Biochemistry of Cytoplasmic and Mitochondrial Aspartate Aminotransferase

	Cytoplasmic	Mitochondrial
Heat stability	Poor	Good
Inhibition by phosphate	No	Yes
Serum half-life of enzyme	Long	Short
DEAE chromatography with 8 mmol/L phosphate buffer, pH 7	Retained	Eluted
Present in normal serum	Yes	<12% of total
Electrophoretic mobility	Anodal	Cathodal

(From Lott and Wolf,[51] with permission.)

Increases

Serum AST is more sensitive in chronic and infiltrative lesions of the liver, whereas elevated ALT is associated with acute liver and cholestatic disease. In viral hepatitis, serum AST activity is typically 10–20 times the upper limit of the reference range, with AST usually above 1000 IU/L and ALT greater than AST. In patients with fulminant acute viral hepatitis, AST may decline rapidly to within or below the reference range because of marked hepatic necrosis and cellular exhaustion of the enzyme. In contrast to viral hepatitis without extensive necrosis in which ALT exceeds AST, serum AST exceeds ALT in extensive necrotic injury such as occurs in alcoholic hepatitis.[8,9] In patients with alcoholic hepatitis, serum AST is generally increased to the range of 300 IU/L with serum AST greater than ALT.

In alcoholic patients with or without liver disease, m-AST tends to be much higher than in healthy individuals. The m-AST/AST ratio may be superior to the AST/ALT ratio for identifying patients with alcoholism, because it is consistently abnormal in chronic drinkers. The increased m-AST suggests mitochondrial damage in alcoholic hepatitis and may distinguish alcoholic hepatitis from other types of liver disease. In contrast, in healthy individuals and patients with viral hepatitis, the m-AST/AST ratio is significantly lower than in alcoholics. Serum AST increases also can be seen in infectious mononucleosis, hepatobiliary obstruction, cirrhosis, primary and metastatic carcinoma of the liver, and in association with hepatic granulomas.

Although serum AST is increased in most patients with acute myocardial infarction, it is generally not used in the diagnosis of the disorder. In acute myocardial infarction, AST levels typically peak after creatine kinase (CK) but before lactate dehydrogenase (LD). Serum AST activity increases within 6–12 hours of infarction, peaks at 20–40 hours, and returns to normal within 4 to 5 days. Destruction of skeletal muscle is also accompanied by increases in AST, CK, and myoglobin.[10,11] Increased AST activity also has been reported in acute pancreatitis, hemolytic anemia, and kidney infection. Additionally, persistently elevated AST may occur when a macroenzymatic complex exists between AST and immunoglobulin.

Test: Alkaline Phosphatase (Orthophosphoric Monoester Phosphohydrolase) (Alkaline Optimum) (See Ch. 12)

Background and Selection

Alkaline phosphatase is useful for diagnosing hepatobiliary and bone disease. Liver AP localizes in the hepatic cell sinusoidal membrane, microvillus of the bile canaliculus, and portal and central vein endothelial cells. Bilirubin and liver AP have separate routes of exit from the hepatic cell; bilirubin must traverse the liver cell, whereas AP exists directly to the lumen of the biliary tree. Serum AP is especially useful for diagnosis, screening, and follow-up of cholestatic hepatobiliary lesions and osteoblastic bone diseases. In cholestatic hepatobiliary diseases, the highest elevations of serum AP occur in extrahepatic biliary tract obstruction.

Terminology

Although the various forms of AP usually are called isoenzymes, the term is not technically correct for some forms (see p. 73).

Logistics

False decrease in AP activity can occur if anticoagulants such as EDTA, oxalate, or citrate are used in blood collection, since various cations complexed by

Liver Function • 71

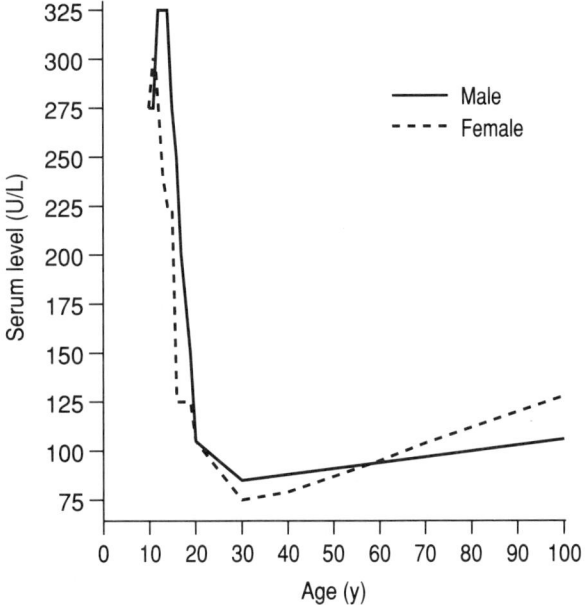

Fig. 4-1. Age- and sex-related upper limits for serum alkaline phosphatase.

these anticoagulants are important for the function of AP. Alkaline phosphatase specimens should be analyzed within 4 hours, as storage causes loss of CO_2 with an increase in pH and AP activity. Freezing causes a loss of AP activity, consequently serum should not be frozen. Blood specimens should be obtained during fasting because patients with blood type O or B who are secretors have elevations of serum AP after a meal owing to stimulation of intestinal AP release. Some pharmaceutical companies produce albumin for parenteral usage from blood that is extricated from human placentas. Because this product contains a large amount of AP, a prominent elevation in the level of serum AP develops in patients who receive intravenous albumin from this placental source.

Interpretation

For infants and children from 1–12 years old the reference range is 25–350 IU/L. For adults, the reference range is about 25–100 IU/L in men and 25–90 IU/L in women, but the reference range for women over 70 years of age is 29–120 IU/L (Fig. 4-1). Physiologic elevations of AP occur with bone growth and during pregnancy owing to AP that is derived from the placenta.[12] Placental AP is heat stable (90%) and inhibited by phenylalanine. Serum AP increases during pregnancy, late in the first trimester and is approximately twice the healthy adult level by the end of the third trimester, correlating with maturity of microvilli cyto-

trophoblast. Serum AP is lower in pregnant diabetic women when villous growth ceases. The level of AP may remain elevated in the serum for 1 month after termination of the pregnancy. Infarction of the placenta increases serum placental isoenzyme activity.

Decreases

Decreases in serum AP levels are seen in hypophosphatasia, hypothyroidism, pernicious anemia, and in anticoagulated oxalated specimens.[13,14] Hypophosphatasia is an inborn error of metabolism associated with defective mineralization of bone. In these patients, the AP level is reduced in tissues and serum and phosphoethanolamine is excreted in urine. Intestinal AP may not be affected by hypophosphatasia, thus variable amounts of intestinal AP appear in serum. Hypothyroid patients and patients who suffer from pernicious anemia have decreases in serum AP because thyroid hormone and vitamin B_{12} are required for osteoblastic function. Zinc and magnesium deficiency also causes a decrease in AP.

Increases

When serum AP is elevated in absence of physiologic causes, a pathologic lesion must be considered (Table 4-7). An elevated AP level may consist of a combination of various AP isoenzymes. For example, carcinomas

---

Table 4-7. Pathologic Lesions of Various Organs Associated With Elevated Serum Alkaline Phosphatase Level

Liver
    Cholestatic lesions
Bone
    Osteoblastic lesions
Heart
    Organization of infarct
    Cardiac failure
Lung
    Organization of infarct
Pancreas
    Acute pancreatitis
Gastrointestinal
    Giant peptic ulcer
    Erosive or ulcerative lesion of small intestine in malabsorption
    Acute infarction of small intestine
    Erosive ulcerative lesions of colon
Kidney
    Organization of acute infarction
Spleen
    Organization of acute infarction
Neoplastic ectopic production
    Regan isoenzyme
    Nagao isoenzyme

(From Nemesanszky,[53] with permission.)

may be metastatic to multiple organs including the liver and bone, thus resulting in elevation of AP isoenzymes in the liver and bone as well as ectopic production of AP by the carcinoma.[15]

Hepatic Disease. A variety of conditions leads to an elevation of the AP liver isoenzyme. These include acute hepatitis, cirrhosis, fatty liver, drug-induced liver disease, obstruction of biliary flow by carcinoma of the head of the pancreas, choledocholithiasis or bile duct structure, primary biliary cirrhosis, and metastatic carcinoma of the liver.[16] In acute hepatic necrosis, serum bilirubin increases with only minimal elevation of AP.

The increased serum AP level associated with liver disease results from decreased secretion of liver AP into the bile and regurgitation of AP into the circulation through the sinusoids. In addition, with cholestasis, biliary ductule cells increase synthesis of AP. Thus, an elevation of the liver AP level is a sensitive indicator of cholestasis. An increase in the liver AP level also is a sensitive indicator of hepatic infiltrate. The most common infiltrate is a primary or metastatic malignancy; however, AP elevations also are associated with other infiltrates, such as those caused by sarcoidosis, amyloidosis, tuberculosis, and bacterial abscesses.

With infiltrative disease of the liver, there is dissociation in elevation of serum bilirubin and AP. With localized obstruction, bilirubin, but not AP, can be excreted by nonobstructed areas in the liver. In partial obstruction, the level of AP increases more than bilirubin, whereas in complete obstruction, both bilirubin and AP levels increase together. Extrahepatic obstruction of the biliary tree, as is found with carcinoma of the head of the pancreas, causes an early and sharp elevation of the AP. Incomplete extrahepatic obstruction, as is found in bile duct stricture, causes an increase in the level of AP but not to the same degree as occurs in complete obstruction. Increased AP activity also occurs because of increased synthesis of the enzyme. The pattern of elevated AP and LD without an increase in bilirubin is indicative of a hepatic infiltrate but also may be seen in congestive heart failure with hepatic passive congestion.[17]

Typical elevation of AP levels associated with various types of hepatic diseases are listed in Table 4-8. Other conditions associated with extrahepatic biliary tract disease give variable enzyme patterns. For example, cholelithiasis is not associated with enzyme elevation, but acute cholecystitis may cause minimal AP, AST, and ALT elevations, especially if there is an associated cholangitis. Cholestatic liver disease is therefore associated with three types of AP isoenzymes: (1) liver, (2) bone, (3) intestinal. In the absence of physiologic and spurious causes, increased AP activity is most likely caused by a cholestatic liver lesion or an osteoblastic bone abnormality or both. Because liver disease frequently is associated with abnormal vitamin D absorption or metabolism, osteomalacia results. The presence of the intestinal isoenzyme is caused by increased production and absorption of intestinal AP or because the abnormal liver cannot convert intestinal AP to liver AP.[18]

Table 4-8. Types of Hepatic Disease Associated with Elevated Serum Alkaline Phosphatase Level

Twofold increase
    Acute viral hepatitis
    Acute toxic hepatitis
    Acute alcoholic hepatitis
    Cirrhosis
    Acute fatty liver
Fivefold increase
    Infectious mononucleosis
    Postnecrotic cirrhosis
Tenfold increase
    Drug cholestatic hepatitis
    Carcinoma of head of pancreas
    Choledocholithiasis
Fifteen- to twentyfold increase
    Primary biliary cirrhosis
    Metastatic or primary carcinoma

(From Nemesanszky,[53] with permission.)

Bone Disease. Various types of bone disease are associated with elevated AP including hyperparathyroidism (primary and secondary), osteomalacia secondary to decreased calcium absorption and increased calcium excretion, rickets, Paget's disease, primary or metastatic neoplasms of bone, acromegaly, and fractures. Alkaline phosphatase is usually within the reference range in osteoporosis.

Cardiac Disease. In acute myocardial infarction, serum AP is elevated during the reparative phase, which occurs 4–10 days after onset of the infarct. Serum γ-glutamyl transferase results also may increase concurrently. Presumably, both enzymes originate from vascular endothelium and are associated with the angioblastic proliferation, which is in turn associated with repair and organization of the necrotic myocardium. If the patient progresses to congestive heart failure, the level of serum AP may be increased on the basis of hepatic passive congestion.[19]

Pulmonary Disease. The reparative phase of an acute pulmonary infarct is similarly characterized by an elevation of the serum AP level.[20,21] Elevated AP occurs 1–2 weeks after onset of the infarct, because of the reparative phase of vascular endothelium. It has been established that AP is found in the capillaries of the lung, the adventitia of the pulmonary arteries, and the connective tissue of the bronchi. The AP derived from the lung is extremely heat labile, similar to the bone AP isoenzyme.[22]

Gastrointestinal, Renal, and Splenic Diseases. A number of gastrointestinal diseases are associated with an increase in the level of intestinal serum AP.[23] Acute infarction of the intestine causes release of intestinal AP from the mucosa. Large erosive or ulcerative lesions of the stomach, duodenum, other regions of the small intestinal tract, and colon may result in an elevation of the serum AP level. Small intestinal lesions are associated with an elevation of the serum intestinal AP only if there is an erosive or ulcerative mucosal lesion. An increase in the bone isoenzyme of AP occurs in patients with malabsorption because of osteomalacia that is induced by associated vitamin D deficiency. Acute infarction of the kidney or spleen causes an elevated serum AP because both of these organs are rich in AP; the increases occur approximately 7 days after the onset of the infarct.[24]

Neoplastic Disease (see Ch. 12). Ectopic production of AP is associated with a variety of neoplasms. The so-called Regan isoenzyme is heat stable and is inhibited by phenylalanine, characteristics similar to those exhibited by the placental isoenzyme. Because the Regan isoenzyme resembles the placental isoenzyme on electrophoresis, it also is known as carcinoplacental isoenzyme. In addition to lung cancer, other malignant neoplasms, such as breast cancer and carcinoma of the colon, can produce the Regan isoenzyme.[25] The highest incidence of Regan isoenzyme occurs with ovarian cancer or other gynecologic neoplasms such as carcinomas of the cervix. The Regan isoenzyme also may be present in conditions that predispose to neoplasia, that is, familial polyposis or ulcerative colitis. The Nagao isoenzyme is a variant of the Regan isoenzyme. This isoenzyme is associated with adenocarcinoma of the pancreas or bile duct. The Nagao isoenzyme is extremely heat stable and inhibited by phenylalanine, but differs from the Regan isoenzyme in that it is inhibited by L-leucine.

Miscellaneous. Increased synthesis of liver AP is associated with parenteral hyperalimentation, with glucose and with uncontrolled diabetes mellitus. Patients with uncontrolled diabetes mellitus can have a 40% elevation of AP.[26] In addition, drugs may cause intrahepatic cholestasis resulting in an elevation of AP of 2–20 times normal. Certain drugs produce a hepatitis-like picture, others a cholestatic one, and some a mixed pattern. In drug-induced hepatitis, the AP level is only slightly elevated in contrast to the marked elevation of AP in a cholestatic or a mixed cholestatic hepatitis-like condition.

Diagnostic Approach to Evaluating Elevated Serum AP Results. Two general approaches have been used to identify causes of AP elevations: (1) AP isoenzymes (see p. 71) and (2) analysis of other enzymes such as 5'-nucleotidase (5' NT), leucine aminopeptidase, and γ-glutamyl transferase (GGT) that increase with hepatobiliary disease, but do not increase with bone disease.

Isoenzymes. Various methods are available to identify the isoenzymes of AP including heating the serum at 56°C for exactly 10 minutes. The extremely heat-labile isoenzymes (90% labile) are derived from bone, the reticuloendothelial system, and vascular endothelium. The extremely heat-stable (90% stable) isoenzymes are produced by the placenta and malignant cells (Regan and Nagao isoenzymes).[27] The intermediate group of isoenzymes (60–80% stable) are derived from the liver and intestine. The intestinal, placental, and Regan isoenzymes are inhibited by phenylalanine, whereas the biliary, bone, and vascular isoenzymes are not (Tables 4-9 and 4-10). Amino acid inhibitors of AP prevent dephosphorylation of the enzyme substrates in which the amino acids form enzyme inhibitor substrate complexes and thus inhibit enzyme action.[28] Urea inactivation shows characteristics similar to the heat test

Table 4-9. Chemical Properties of Normal Alkaline Phosphatase Isoenzymes

Property	Biliary	Hepatic	Bone	Placenta	Intestine
Heat stability	Unstable	Unstable	Very unstable	Stable	Unstable
L-Phenylalanine inhibition	Weak	Weak	Weak	Strong	Strong
L-Homoarginine inhibition	Moderate	Strong	Strong	Weak	Weak
L-Leucine inhibition	Weak	Moderate	Moderate	Weak	Weak
Urea inactivation	Strong	Strong	Very strong	Moderate	Moderate
Electrophoretic mobility	α-1	α-2	α-2	α-2/β	β

(From Nemesanszky,[53] with permission.)

Table 4-10. Chemical Properties of Tumor-Associated Alkaline Phosphatase Isoenzymes

Property	Hepatoma	Kasahara	Nagao	Regan
Heat stability	Unstable	Stable	Very stable	Very stable
L-Phenylalanine inhibition	Moderate	Moderate	Strong	Strong
L-Homoarginine inhibition	Weak	Weak	Weak	Weak
L-Leucine inhibition	Weak	Moderate	Moderate	Weak
Urea inhibition	Moderate	—	—	Strong
Electrophoretic mobility	α-1	α-1	α-2/β	α-2/β
EDTA inhibition	Strong	—	Strong	Weak

(From Nemesanszky,[53] with permission.)

with the bone isoenzyme inactivated by urea.[29] In addition to phenylalanine, other amino acids such as L-leucine and homoarginine are used in inhibition studies. Furthermore, electrophoresis of the isoenzymes yields important information. The useful support media are acrylamide and cellulose acetate with Triton X-100 enhancing separation.[30] The liver phosphatase moves more rapidly toward the anode in contrast to the bone isoenzyme, which has a slower anodal mobility and may overlap the liver band. The intestinal isoenzyme moves more slowly than the bone isoenzyme.[31]

Test: Bilirubin

Background and Selection

Bilirubin is useful for diagnosis, screening, and follow-up of liver diseases and diseases such as hemolytic anemia. Bilirubin is useful as an indicator of liver excretory function. Unconjugated bilirubin is derived from heme, which in turn arises form the hemoglobin of senescent red blood cells, from bone marrow normoblasts, and from myoglobin and cytochrome. Albumin transports bilirubin to the liver where the hepatocyte conjugates bilirubin with glucuronic acid to form bilirubin monoglucuronides and diglucuronides that are excreted into the bile.[32] Decreased excretion of serum conjugated bilirubin into the biliary tract occurs with cholestasis or biliary obstruction owing to intrahepatic or extrahepatic lesions. (Table 4-11).

Interpretation

The reference ranges for total bilirubin is less than about 1.2 mg/dL (20.5 μmol/L). In healthy individuals, almost all bilirubin is unconjugated: conjugated bilirubin ranges up to about 0.2 mg/dL (3.4 μmol/L).

Hepatic Disorders

Patients with hepatic injury, as found in alcoholic, viral, or toxic hepatitis, have increased unconjugated bilirubin owing to their decreased ability to conjugate bilirubin to glucuronide. In addition, conjugated bilirubin is elevated in these conditions because of hepatic cell swelling that causes cholestasis. An elevated conjugated bilirubin also occurs in intrahepatic cholestasis (including that found in pregnancy), in postoperative patients, in viral and alcoholic hepatitis, and in extrahepatic cholestasis caused by extrahepatic bile duct lesions such as biliary calculi or malignancy. Dubin-Johnson syndrome, a genetic disorder of bilirubin or excretion, results in increased conjugated bilirubin as well. Table 4-12 lists the differential diagnosis for elevated levels of conjugated bilirubin.

Table 4-11. Differential Diagnosis of Jaundice

Elevated unconjugated bilirubin
    Hemolytic anemia
    Transfusions (especially of stored blood)
    Resorption of hematomas, blood in extravascular spaces
Hepatic dysfunction of elevated unconjugated and conjugated bilirubin
    Hepatitis-like picture
        Halothane anesthesia
        Drugs
        Shock
        Infection with hepatitis viruses
    Cholestatic picture
        Hypotension, hypoxemia
        Drugs
        Sepsis
Extrahepatic obstruction of elevated conjugated bilirubin
    Bile duct injury
    Choledocholithiasis
    Acute pancreatitis

Table 4-12.	Differential Diagnosis of Elevated Conjugated Bilirubin

Cholestasis, intrahepatic and extrahepatic
Postoperative intrahepatic and extrahepatic cholestasis
Recurrent intrahepatic cholestasis during pregnancy
Dubin-Johnson syndrome

Table 4-14.	Differential Diagnosis of Elevated Delta Bilirubin

Cholestasis, intrahepatic and extrahepatic
Neonates with physiologic jaundice
Gilbert syndrome
Crigler-Najjar syndrome
Hemolytic anemia

An elevated unconjugated bilirubin is associated with physiologic jaundice in the newborn as well as a number of other disorders (Table 4-13). Physiologic jaundice is associated with hemolysis and immaturity of hepatic conjugation of bilirubin by the newborn liver. In addition, deconjugation of conjugated bilirubin occurs in the newborn intestine because of the presence of β-glucuronidase in the absence of intestinal bacteria. Gilbert syndrome is a genetic condition associated with increased serum unconjugated bilirubin, which increases with fasting. During fasting in these patients, competition occurs between fatty acids and bilirubin for conjugation. Type I Crigler-Najjar syndrome is a fatal condition associated with absence of glucuronyl transferase whereas type II, which has a benign prognosis, is associated with the presence of hepatic glucuronyl transferase in reduced quantity.

Hemolytic Disease

Hemolysis and ineffective erythropoiesis cause hyperbilirubinemia with the unconjugated form of bilirubin predominating.

δ-Bilirubin

δ-Bilirubin is bilirubin covalently bound to albumin. High performance liquid chromatography (HPLC) can be used to resolve and quantitate the δ-bilirubin fraction. δ-Bilirubin is absent or found in only small amounts in healthy individuals, in neonates with physiologic jaundice, and in patients with Gilbert syndrome and hemolysis (Table 4-14).[33,34] In patients with a variety of hepatobiliary diseases, δ-bilirubin can account for more than 50% of total bilirubin. The formation of δ-bilirubin appears to require an active bilirubin conjugating process, but the exact mechanisms are unknown. δ-Bilirubin occurs in patients with intrahepatic or extrahepatic cholestasis who have elevated conjugated bilirubin. As cholestasis improves, δ-bilirubin increases in proportion to total bilirubin because it has a longer half-life and slower clearance than bilirubin.

Test: Pseudocholinesterase

Background and Selection

The role of pseudocholinesterase in evaluating liver function is primarily to assess hepatic synthetic function. Pseudocholinesterase activity in serum is decreased in patients with liver disease. Marked decreases of pseudocholinesterase are found in far advanced cirrhosis and fulminant acute viral hepatitis with marked hepatic necrosis.

Logistics

Hemolysis interferes with pseudocholinesterase measurements because of false increases owing to red blood cell (RBC) acetylcholinesterase (true cholinesterase). Dibucaine or fluoride inhibition is determined by performing concurrent assays in which dibucaine or fluoride is added to the substrate mixture. Percent inhibition is obtained by comparing results from the inhibited reaction with the noninhibited reaction.

Interpretation

The reference range for pseudocholinesterase activity is 8–18 IU/L. Serum pseudocholinesterase is useful for assessing the presence of end-stage cirrhosis in patients with hepatic disease. In fulminant acute viral hepatitis, decreases in serum pseudocholinesterase are caused by decreased synthesis. Genetic deficiency of the enzyme occurs, and insecticides such as parathion inhibit pseudocholinesterase, resulting in decreased levels.[35,36] Pseudocholinesterase deficiency also occurs as

Table 4-13.	Differential Diagnosis of Elevated Unconjugated Bilirubin

Gilbert syndrome
Crigler-Najjar syndrome
Hemolytic anemia
Resolving hematomas
Transfusion of blood that is old and has a short survival
Hemorrhagic pulmonary infarcts
Postoperative elevations

Table 4-15. Phenotype Differentiation by Pseudocholinesterase Measurements

Phenotype[a]	Dibucaine Number[b]	Fluoride Number[b]	Pseudocholinesterase Activity (IU/L)[b]
UU	84	49	13
UA	73	48	7.5
AA or AS	32	45	3.7
UF	81	34	6.8
AF	62	32	6.2
SS	—	—	0.02

[a] U, usual; A, abnormal; S, silent; F, fluoride deficiency.
[b] Approximate number or activity.
(From Sawhney and Lott,[54] with permission.)

the result of a suxamethonium overdose.[37,38] Dibucaine and fluoride inhibition studies are used to distinguish the presence and type of pseudocholinesterase enzyme defect. Results from a number of patients who are genetic variants are summarized in Table 4-15.

Test: Albumin (See Ch. 8)

Albumin, the most abundant protein in blood, is synthesized almost entirely by the liver. Its physiologic functions are to maintain osmotic pressure, transport endogenous and exogenous compounds, and to act as a protein reserve. Albumin is a source of amino acids for various tissues. If the functional synthetic tissue of the liver is decreased, the liver's ability to produce albumin and other proteins is diminished. The normal serum half-life of albumin is 17–26 days. Decreased serum albumin and prolonged prothrombin time are indicators of impaired synthetic function of the liver. Rapid decreases in serum albumin can be seen in hepatitis owing to decreased synthesis, and decreased serum albumin may indicate cryptogenic cirrhosis. Measuring serum albumin can be useful for assessing Wilson's disease and all types of liver necrosis including viral or alcoholic hepatitis. Low serum albumin in the absence of liver disease is seen in malnutrition, renal or intestinal albumin loss, severe infections, severe burns, pancreatitis, and exfoliative dermatitis. Serum albumin thus is a sensitive but nonspecific test for liver disease. It is rare to have a high concentration of albumin except in cases of dehydration and excessive intravenous administration of albumin.

Interpretation of Test Patterns

When liver function is evaluated, the four most important test groups are (1) the transaminase enzymes, AST and ALT, which are increased in patients with hepatic cell necrosis, (2) AP, increases of which indicate cholestasis, (3) total, conjugated (direct), and unconjugated (indirect) bilirubin, and (4) hepatic synthesis. Increased levels of unconjugated (indirect) bilirubin indicate hemolytic anemia or decreased conjugating ability of hepatic cells caused by hepatic injury or inherited defects, such as Gilbert syndrome. Increased levels of conjugated (direct) bilirubin (bilirubin glucuronide) indicate cholestasis. Decreased pseudocholinesterase activity, decreased levels of albumin or transferrin, and prolonged prothrombin time indicate decreased hepatic synthetic capacity.

Viral Hepatitis

In acute viral hepatitis, serum ALT is greater than AST with both frequently exceeding 100 IU/L. The AP activity is minimally increased, usually up to 200 IU/L. Unconjugated bilirubin is increased owing to hepatocellular damage and conjugated bilirubin is increased owing to intrahepatic cholestasis caused by hepatic cell swelling. Serum albumin is within the usual reference range. In a patient with fatal acute viral hepatitis that is fulminant, the AST may decline rapidly to normal or below normal because of marked hepatic necrosis and cellular exhaustion of enzyme. This type of patient had persistent or increasing jaundice. In acute hepatitis that is improving, AST and bilirubin decline concomitantly.

In chronic persistent hepatitis, AST and ALT activity vary between 40–200 IU/L with AP activity increasing minimally. Serum bilirubin is usually below 3 mg/dL (51.3 μmol/L). Both conjugated and unconjugated bilirubin are increased but total albumin is within the reference range. In chronic active hepatitis, the levels of AST and ALT are frequently above 400 IU/L with minimal increases in AP activity. In contrast to chronic persistent hepatitis, total bilirubin is above 3 mg/dL

(51.3 µmol/L) in chronic active hepatitis with increases in both conjugated and unconjugated bilirubin. Serum albumin is often decreased but the immunoglobulins are increased.

Alcoholic Hepatitis

Ethanol causes release of m-AST from injured hepatic cell mitochondria resulting in AST activity greater than ALT. The total level of AST usually does not exceed 300 IU/L but if it does, concomitant alcoholic rhabdomyolysis or alcoholic cardiomyopathy and congestive heart failure with ischemic damage of liver should be considered. Serum AP is minimally increased, usually up to 200 IU/L. Unconjugated bilirubin is increased owing to hepatocellular damage and conjugated bilirubin is increased owing to intrahepatic cholestasis caused by hepatic cell swelling. Serum albumin is within the usual reference range.

Drug-Induced Hepatitis

Some drugs cause hepatic cell necrosis, whereas others primarily cause cholestasis. For example, acetaminophen and isoniazid (INH) cause hepatic necrosis; in contrast, phenothiazines and oral contraceptives cause cholestasis. Drugs causing hepatic cell necrosis give rise to abnormalities in AST and ALT that resemble those found in alcoholic hepatitis with AST exceeding ALT results. Similarly, AP is minimally increased, and unconjugated and conjugated bilirubin elevations occur. Drugs that are associated with cholestasis cause a greater elevation of AP and conjugated bilirubin and a lesser elevation of AST than drugs that cause hepatitis.

Cirrhosis

Cirrhosis can be caused by alcohol, viral agents, biliary obstruction, or ischemia, or by a combination of these causative factors. The major laboratory abnormality in cirrhosis is a decrease in analytes related to hepatic cell synthesis. If the etiologic factor is persistent, other results, such as those for AST, ALT, AP, unconjugated, and conjugated bilirubin, remain elevated.

Cholestasis

The two major types of cholestasis are intrahepatic and extrahepatic. Intrahepatic cholestasis can occur with or without mechanical obstruction to bile flow. Drugs such as the phenothiazines; viruses such as hepatitis A, B, or non-A, non-B; alcohol; and hepatic malignant infiltrates may cause hepatic cell swelling or may directly affect the biliary canaliculi resulting in intrahepatic cholestasis. Obstructive causes of intrahepatic cholestasis within the portal triads include congenital biliary atresia of the intrahepatic bile ductules, infiltration by malignant cells such as leukemia or lymphoma, and autoimmune destruction of the bile ductules in primary biliary cirrhosis. Pregnancy also may induce recurrent intrahepatic cholestasis. Extrahepatic cholestasis may be caused by congenital atresia of the extrahepatic bile ducts, gall stones obstructing the common bile duct (choledocholithiasis), carcinoma of the common bile duct or ampulla of Vater, and suppurative cholangitis.

With cholestasis, the main abnormalities in liver function tests are an increase in serum conjugated bilirubin and AP. The conjugated bilirubin level is dependent on the degree of completeness of biliary obstruction. Extrahepatic biliary obstruction, if complete, may result in levels of conjugated bilirubin above 20 mg/dL (342 µmol/L). Intrahepatic cholestasis may result in an increased conjugated bilirubin between 1 mg/dL to 10 mg/dL (17.1 to 171 µmol/L). Alkaline phosphatase is about two to three times the reference range in intrahepatic cholestasis, in marked contrast to extrahepatic obstruction where AP activity is about 10 times the reference range. Cholestasis causes a mild elevation of AST and ALT because of regurgitation of AST and ALT into the systemic circulation. In addition, biliary obstruction results in increased synthesis of AST and ALT by the hepatic cell. Unconjugated bilirubin and albumin are within the reference range but may become abnormal if biliary cirrhosis occurs.

Neoplasms

Malignant lesions may be focal or they may diffusely infiltrate the liver. Frequently, hepatomegaly is present without the presence of clinical or biochemical jaundice. Conjugated bilirubin may increase minimally; however, AP, GGT, and 5′ NT are markedly elevated. Elevation of these enzymes may reach 10–20 times the reference range. The pattern of bilirubin within the reference range and a moderate to markedly elevated AP indicate neoplastic involvement of the liver. With slow infiltration of the liver by malignant cells, a small amount of normal and uninvolved liver tissue excretes the bilirubin into the bile. Enzymes such as AP and GGT, however, are regurgitated into the systematic circulation. If the neoplasm obstructs a major hepatic or bile duct, the patient becomes jaundiced with an elevation of conjugated bilirubin, a pattern consistent with a advanced malignancy. Elevation of AP suggests liver metastases; however, the pattern of dissociation of abnormalities in bilirubin and AP also is found in the hepatic disorder caused by congestive heart failure. In this condition, AST and ALT are minimally elevated and the albumin is decreased. Lactate dehydrogenase is moderately to markedly elevated with an AST and bilirubin within the reference range.

Ischemic Disease

With congestive heart failure, hepatocellular injury occurs especially in the central lobular zone of the liver. All other laboratory test abnormalities as described under Alcoholic Hepatitis (see p. 77) are present in ischemic hepatitis, but the total level of AST may exceed 1000 IU/L. The biochemical pattern of ischemic liver disease is somewhat similar to that of malignant liver disease. The pattern includes elevation of AST and ALT, which may be marked, elevation of AP, normal to minimal increase in bilirubin, and albumin within the reference interval. Elevation of LD activity occurs with the appearance of the LD-6 isoenzyme in seriously ill patients. In patients with arteriosclerotic cardiovascular disease and associated congestive heart failure, LD-6 is a sign of a serious hepatic circulatory disturbance (Fig. 4-2). Some investigators believe that LD-6 is not a true LD isoenzyme. They contend that anoxia of the hepatic lobule results in release of hepatic cell alcohol dehydrogenase into the circulation.

OTHER COMMONLY USED TESTS

Test: Ammonia

Background and Selection

Plasma ammonia is useful for diagnosis, screening, and follow-up of patients with hepatic encephalopathy. The most common cause for an increase in plasma ammonia is end-stage liver disease, causing a defective hepatic urea cycle and inability of the liver to metabolize ammonia to urea. Plasma ammonia is derived from several sources. Although some ammonia is derived from skeletal muscle metabolism, most of the ammonia is produced from bacterial production in the intestine and is transported to the liver where it is converted to urea. Some ammonia is derived from skeletal muscle metabolism.

Logistics

Specimens for ammonia should be drawn into EDTA or heparinized ammonia-free tubes. Following specimen collection, plasma should be separated and analyzed within a few minutes in order to avoid spurious increases in results.

Table 4-16. Etiology of Elevated Plasma Ammonia

Cirrhosis
Reye syndrome
Genetic urea cycle diseases
    Ornithine transcarbamylase deficiency
    Carbamyl phosphate synthetase deficiency
    Arginosuccinate synthetase deficiency
Organic acidemias
    Methylmalonic acidemia
    Propionic acidemia

Interpretation

Reye syndrome, characterized by hepatic injury with marked elevation of plasma ammonia, is associated with the use of aspirin during viral disease in children. Elevated plasma ammonia levels in neonates and children can be caused by a number of genetic disorders including urea cycle enzyme deficiencies such as carbamoyl-phosphate synthase or ornithine transcarbamoylase deficiency. Plasma ammonia also may become elevated in patients with certain congenital organic acidemias, notably methylmalonic and propionic acidemia (Table 4-16). The major cause for elevated plasma ammonia is end-stage cirrhosis leading to a defective hepatic urea cycle. Increased plasma ammonia is the associated development of hepatic encephalopathy in which there is decreased mental capacity and eventually stupor, coma, and death. Patients with hepatic disease have a higher risk for developing hepatic coma when various complications occur, such as gastrointestinal hemorrhage, metabolic alkalosis, and hepatorenal syndrome. Plasma ammonia increases in patients with gastrointestinal hemorrhage because of the production of ammonia by bacterial action on the blood protein and absorption of the ammonia from the gastrointestinal tract.[39] Hypokalemia, which leads to metabolic alkalosis, causes increases in production and absorption of ammonia. Renal failure caused by acute tubular necrosis or hepatorenal syndrome leads to excessive urea in the gastrointestinal tract. Bacterial action converts the urea to ammonia which then is absorbed, leading to elevated plasma ammonia.

Test: Lactate Dehydrogenase (see Chs. 2 and 12)

Although LD is not considered to be a liver function test, elevation of serum LD occurs in various types of liver disease, especially primary or secondary malignancies. Elevation of LD may occur in alcoholic, viral, or toxic hepatitis, whereas LD in cirrhosis and choles-

Table 4-17. Causes of Increased Serum Alkaline Phosphatase and Lactate Dehydrogenase Activities With Normal Serum Bilirubin

Congestive heart failure
Myocardial infarction without congestive heart failure
Liver infiltration (from carcinoma, and myeloproliferative and lymphoproliferative conditions)
Fracture plus hematoma
Pulmonary embolism and pulmonary infarction
Chronic renal failure
Malabsorption syndrome

tasis is usually within the reference range (Table 4-17).[40] Serum LD should not be considered a test of liver function because damage to other organs, such as heart, lung, spleen, pancreas, kidney, prostate, skeletal muscle, and hematopoietic and lymphoreticular system, is associated with serum LD elevations (Fig. 4-2).[41,42] The pattern of elevated LD, increased unconjugated bilirubin, and AP within the reference range is consistent with hemolytic disease. When serum LD is elevated as a result of hepatic disease, the most likely diagnosis is hepatic malignancy, which may occur in a variety of patterns (see Ch. 12). Hepatocellular injury caused by the infiltrating malignant cells leads to an increase in the LD-5 isoenzyme. In hepatic disease associated with malignancy, another cause for an elevated LD, particularly the LD-2 or LD-3 isoenzymes, is the release of LD from the malignant cells. Recently, isoenzyme LD-6 has been identified in association with hepatic disease caused by severe ischemic disease.[43]

Test: γ-Glutamyl Transferase (Gamma-Glutamyl Transpeptidase)

Background and Selection

γ-Glutamyl transferase is elevated in liver disease from a variety of causes. In identifying the presence of primary or metastatic malignancy involving the liver, GGT has the highest sensitivity of all of the hepatic enzymes. Another important use of GGT is in alcohol treatment programs because GGT elevation occurs rapidly in response to alcohol ingestion.

Interpretation

The reference range for GGT is up to 40 IU/L in males and up to 25 IU/L in females. γ-Glutamyl transferase is elevated in patients with hepatitis, liver neoplasms, and intrahepatic and extrahepatic cholestasis.[44] Of all the hepatic enzymes, GGT has the highest sensitivity for identifying liver disease, especially primary or metastatic malignancy. γ-Glutamyl transferase increases, especially in cholestasis, with the highest levels present with extrahepatic cholestasis. γ-Glutamyl transferase is elevated in alcoholics and is a sensitive indicator of both acute and chronic alcoholism. Because GGT elevation occurs early when an alcoholic begins drinking, the enzyme is a useful measure in alcohol treatment programs.

In spite of its extreme usefulness for detecting hepatobiliary disease, GGT elevations also may occur in other conditions namely pancreatitis, renal disease, diabetes mellitus, and carcinoma of the prostate (Table 4-18).

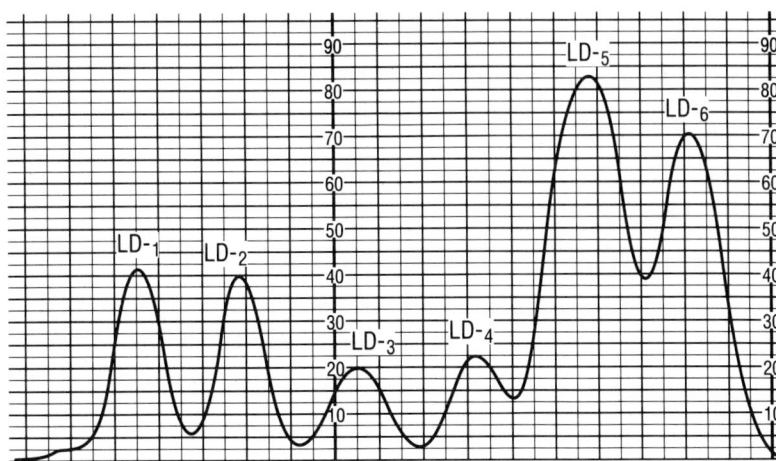

Fig. 4-2. Lactate dehydrogenase electrophoresis; flipped LD-1 to LD-2, increased LD-5, and presence of LD-6. Acute myocardial infarction with congestive heart failure with liver congestion with fatal outcome. Presence of LD-6 indicated a poor prognosis.

Table 4-18. Nonhepatobiliary Causes of Increased Serum γ-Glutamyl Transferase

	Magnitude of Increase[a]
Drugs	
Anticoagulants (e.g, coumarin)	Slight
Antihyperlipidemics (clofibrate)	Slight
Oral contraceptives (estrogens)	Slight
Analgesics (e.g., acetaminophen)	Moderate
Anticonvulsants (e.g., phenytoin)	Moderate
Antidepressants (tricyclics)	Moderate
Barbiturates	Moderate
Alcohol	Moderate to marked
Disorders	
Diabetes mellitus	Slight
Hyperthyroidism	Slight
Kidney diseases	Slight
Neurologic disorders	Slight
Obesity	Slight
Pulmonary diseases	Slight
Rheumatoid arthritis	Slight
Hyperlipidemia	Slight to moderate
Myocardial injury	Slight to moderate
Exocrine pancreatic diseases	Moderate to marked
Malignancy	Slight to marked

[a] Slight increase, serum GGT < 2 × upper reference limit (URL); moderate, > 2 and > 5 × URL; marked, > 5 × URL.
(From Lott et al.,[52] with permission.)

Thus, GGT is not entirely specific for hepatobiliary disease.[45] Additionally, certain drugs including phenobarbital and phenytoin cause GGT increases owing to enzyme induction.[46-49]

Test: Glutamine

Background and Selection

Plasma glutamine, which is the most abundant free amino acid in plasma, functions in the storage and transport of ammonia. Most ammonia is produced by bacteria in the intestine and is transported through the liver where it is converted to urea. The ammonia secreted by the kidney is derived from plasma glutamine. Elevated cerebrospinal fluid (CSF) glutamine occurs in neonates, in children with Reye syndrome, or is caused by genetic urea cycle enzyme deficiencies. Although CSF glutamine is thought to be more sensitive than plasma ammonia in assessing hepatic encephalopathy, it has the disadvantage of requiring a CSF specimen.

Interpretation

The reference range for CSF glutamine is less than 20 mg/dL (less than 1.4 mmol/L). Elevations of CSF glutamine have the same implications as elevated plasma ammonia, but CSF glutamine may be more sensitive for identifying patients with hepatic encephalopathy. The disadvantage of CSF glutamine is the specimen requirement; lumbar puncture represents a particular problem in liver disease patients with coagulation defects. In certain congenital organic acidemias (e.g., methylmalonic and propionic acidemia), CSF glutamine is increased. Additionally, CSF glutamine is increased in urea cycle enzyme deficiencies such as cambamoyl-phosphate synthase and ornithine transcarbamoylase deficiency.

Test: 5'-Nucleotidase

The phosphatase 5' NT is widely distributed in tissue. Enzyme activity is markedly increased in hepatobiliary disease whereas an increase in bone disease occurs only rarely. Measurement of 5' NT activity is therefore useful for identifying the presence of hepatobiliary disease. The reference range for 5' NT is up to 12 IU/L. The two main causes for increases in serum AP activity are hepatobiliary disease and osteoblastic lesions of bone. Because 5' NT is specific for hepatobiliary disease,[50] measuring its activity is useful for differentiating the cause of increases in serum AP.

MISCELLANEOUS TESTS OF LIVER FUNCTION

Test: α-Fetoprotein (AFP) (See Chs. 12 and 15)

α-Fetoprotein is a fetal globulin that appears between albumin and $α_1$-antitrypsin (AAT) on cellulose acetate electrophoresis. Normally AFP is produced by the fetal liver, gastrointestinal tract, and yolk sac. It reaches a maximum concentration in serum at approximately 12 to 15 weeks' gestation, then decreases to an undetectable concentration at about 5 weeks after birth.

In most patients with primary carcinoma of the liver (hepatoma), the tumor cells revert to the fetal function of synthesizing and excreting AFP. Therefore, AFP is useful as a marker for hepatoma and for following the course of the disease. Markedly increased adult serum concentrations occur in hepatocellular carcinoma, choriocarcinoma, embryonal carcinoma of the testis or ovary, and in some cases of carcinoma of the pancreas, stomach, colon, and lung. Moderate to slight or transient increases in AFP may be detected in other liver diseases such as alcoholic liver disease, cirrhosis, hepatitis, and tyrosinemia. Increased concentrations of AFP have been associated with inflammatory bowel disease and ataxia-telangiectasia.

Test: Anti-Smooth Muscle Antibodies (See Ch. 30)

Patients with chronic active hepatitis may develop autoimmune antibodies that are directed against smooth muscle. These antibodies are usually of the IgG type and less frequently of the IgM type. Measuring anti-smooth muscle antibodies has become an important serologic test for the detection of chronic active hepatitis: 40–70% of the patients have a positive test with the indirect immunofluorescent procedure. About 50% of patients with primary biliary cirrhosis test positive by the same method, whereas only 28% of those with cryptogenic cirrhosis test positive. An antibody titer of 1:320 or greater indicates the patient may have chronic active hepatitis. Other conditions in which antismooth muscle antibodies are found include viral hepatitis, infectious mononucleosis, asthma, yellow fever, and malignancy.

Test: Antimitochondrial Antibodies (See Ch. 30)

Antimitochondrial antibodies are present in plasma of patients with primary biliary cirrhosis as well as in those with chronic active hepatitis.

Test: Bile Acids

Background and Selection

The primary bile acids, cholic, (a trihydroxy acid) chenodeoxycholic (a dihydroxy acid), are synthesized in the liver by the catabolism of cholesterol. They are conjugated with glycine and taurine forming glycocholates and taurocholates before entering the gallbladder for storage. After a meal, the primary bile acids enter the intestinal lumen where they emulsify fats yielding a greater surface area for pancreatic lipase action. They also promote the aggregation of free fatty acids released by fat breakdown. The micelles thus formed maintain a concentration gradient of free fatty acids allowing rapid absorption. Secondary bile acids are formed by bacterial deconjugation and chemical alteration of the conjugated bile salts; deoxycholic and lithocholic acids are two prominent forms. Both the primary and secondary bile acids are reabsorbed almost completely from the bowel by passive and active reabsorption into the enterohepatic pathway where they are re-extracted from the blood by the hepatocytes and re-excreted into the bile. Bile salt metabolism is so well controlled that the total body content of 4 g may be cycled twice during a meal. Hepatic bile salt uptake and serum bile salt concentrations are sensitive indicators of hepatocellular dysfunction and decreased or altered blood flow in the enterohepatic pathway.

Logistics

Postprandial specimens for measuring bile acids are superior to specimens drawn during fasting because of the endogenous loading of the system after eating. Exogenous loading, that is, infusing bile acids extravenously and then determining hepatic removal capability, also is used as a liver function test. Bile acid tests are not used extensively because of technical difficulties with the measurement.

Interpretation

The reference interval for total bile acids in serum is 3–30 mg/L (0.8–8.0 μmol/L) (about 0.8 g/d is excreted in the feces. Total bile acids are increased in acute, chronic, and alcoholic hepatitis, cirrhosis, and cholestasis. One method used to differentiate excretory blockage from hepatocellular jaundice is to determine the trihydroxy/dihydroxy bile acid ratio. In excretory blockage, the conjugation to the trihydroxy form continues to occur, thus a greater amount of the trihydroxy form is found than in hepatocellular jaundice.

Test: Ceruloplasmin (See. Chs. 8 and 10)

Ceruloplasmin is a metalloprotein synthesized in the liver and released into the blood stream after the incorporation of copper. Only trace amounts of ceruloplasmin normally can be found in the liver. In Wilson's disease, an inherited metabolic disorder, tissue copper concentrations in the liver are usually markedly increased, but serum levels of ceruloplasmin and copper are decreased. Even when other liver function tests are within the reference interval, the most constant biochemical findings in Wilson's disease are decreases in serum ceruloplasmin and copper. Although hypoceruloplasminemia can be seen in patients with nephrotic syndrome, kwashiorkor, tropical sprue, and in infants with Menkes syndrome, these four conditions should be differentiated from Wilson's disease.

As an "acute phase reaction" protein, serum concentrations of ceruloplasmin are affected by a number of conditions. Elevated serum concentrations have been reported in hepatitis, biliary cirrhosis, and liver diseases characterized by intrahepatic or extrahepatic biliary tract obstruction. Although the majority of patients with liver disease have elevated levels, very low serum concentrations of ceruloplasmin have been found in a few patients with fatal hepatitis. Patients with active Hodgkin's disease often have very high serum ceruloplasmin results.

Test: Indocyanine-Green Excretion (ICG)

Indocyanine-green (cardiogreen) is a water soluble tricarbocyanine dye that is metabolized by liver cells in a manner similar to Bromsulphalein (BSP). The dye, which is virtually completely protein-bound, mainly to albumin, is rapidly excreted by the liver without significant extrahepatic removal. The dye is excreted into the bile without conjugation. Currently, the major medical use for ICG as an indicator is for dilution studies during cardiac catheterization. Following rapid intravenous injection of the dye, the plasma fractional disappearance rate, or half-life, of plasma retention at 20 minutes is used to estimate ICG clearance. The plasma concentration of ICG is determined spectrophotometrically. Although no serious allergic reactions to the dye itself have been reported, the usual preparation contains small amounts of sodium iodide; therefore its use in patients with an iodide sensitivity requires caution. Because ICG is free of the complications of tissue necrosis and anaphylaxis, which may occur occasionally with BSP, the use of plasma ICG disappearance curves has advantages over BSP as a test of liver function. In healthy individuals, the plasma ICG disappearance rate is appreciably faster than BSP.

Test: Ornithine Carbamoyltransferase (OCT)

Background and Selection

Ornithine carbamoyltransferase, also known as ornithine carbamoyl transferase and ornithine transcarbamoylase, catalyzes the second enzymatic reaction in the urea cycle. The enzyme is located almost exclusively in the liver mitochrondia. In addition to its presence in liver, OCT is found in the intestinal mucosa and leukocytes at 1% of the activity of liver OCT. Perhaps because of initial difficulties in assaying the enzyme, OCT measurements are usually not included in the standard battery of liver function tests. Serum OCT activity, however, is both specific and sensitive for hepatocellular injury.

Interpretation

The upper reference value in serum is about 20 μ/L. Elevated serum OCT may be found in acute viral hepatitis, liver necrosis, obstructive jaundice, cirrhosis, metastatic liver carcinoma, and congestive heart failure with ischemic liver disease. Transient elevations have been reported in women taking oral contraceptives during the sixth and ninth months after initiation of contraceptive use.

Deficiency of OCT has been reported as a primary inborn metabolic defect transmitted as a sex-linked dominant trait. The presentations of males and females with OCT deficiency differ. Typically, homozygous males have little or no hepatic OCT activity (0–2% of normal), and hyperammonemia develops within hours to days after birth, with death occurring within several weeks. A few rare cases of late onset manifestations (up to 8 years of age) of OCT deficiency have been reported in males, suggesting a pathologic mechanism secondary to a hepatocellular lesion. In heterozygous females and in those rarely reported cases of late-onset males, the severity of the symptoms of OCT deficiency depends on the number of functional hepatocytes. The signs and symptoms are secondary to hyperammonemia and include vomiting, drowsiness, acute encephalopathy, failure to thrive, developmental retardation, convulsions, headaches, irritability, ataxia, slurring of speech, and altered consciousness. Orotic aciduria occurs secondary to the defect in the urea cycle.

Test: Retinol-Binding Protein (RBP) (See Ch. 10)

Retinol-binding protein is one of two proteins responsible for transporting vitamin A in human blood. It is synthesized and secreted by the parenchymal cells of the liver and circulates in serum as a protein-protein complex with prealbumin. The kidneys play a major role in the catabolism of RBP. Although plasma proteins other than enzymes have been considered too insensitive, nonspecific, or cumbersome to be useful in monitoring the degree of hepatic injury, RBP is probably one of the most sensitive indicators of hepatocyte function found to date. In most patients with liver diseases, concentrations of serum RBP are markedly decreased, which is believed to represent a reduction in synthesis. Low concentrations occur in acute viral hepatitis, chronic active hepatitis, and cirrhosis (alcoholic, primary biliary, and cryptogenic). Other causes of decreased synthesis include hyperthyroidism, cystic fibrosis, infection, and kwashiorkor. In alcoholic fatty liver and hepatitis, RBP concentrations are increased. Besides alcoholic liver disease, the only other disorder known to cause elevated RBP levels is chronic renal disease.

REFERENCES

1. Steele BW, Wimsch CD: Alanine aminotransferase (ALT), review of methods. ASCP Check Sample (Care Chemistry) 1989;5:1–6.
2. Gitnick G, Weiss S, Overby LR et al: Non-A, non-B hepatitis: a prospective study of a hemodialysis outbreak with evaluation of a serologic marker in patients and staff. Hepatology 1983;3:625–630.
3. Eriksen J, Olsen PS, Thomsen AC: Gamma-glutamyltranspeptidase, aspartate aminotransferase, and erythrocyte mean corpuscular volume as indicators of alcohol consumption in liver disease. Scand J Gastroenterol 1984;19:813–819.
4. Cushman P, Jacobson G, Barboriak JJ et al: Biochemical markers for alcoholism: sensitivity problems. Alcoholism (NY) 1984;8:253–257.
5. Panteghini M, Falsetti F, Chiari E et al: Determination of aspartate aminotransferase isoenzymes in hepatic diseases-preliminary findings. Clin Chim Acta 1983;128:133–140.
6. Panteghini M, Malchiodi A, Calarco M et al: Clinical and diagnostic significance of aspartate aminotransferase isoenzymes in sera of patients with liver diseases. J Clin Chem Clin Biochem 1984;22:153–158.
7. Lum G: Aspartate aminotransferase (AST), review of methods. ASCP Check Sample Core Chemistry 1978;3:1–7.
8. Spech HJ, Liehr H: Of what value are SGOT/SGPT, GGT/AP and IgG/IgA ratios in the differential diagnosis of advanced liver diseases? Z Gastroenterol 1983;21:89–96.
9. Silverstein MD, Mulley AG, Dienstag JL: Should donor blood be screened for elevated alanine aminotransferase levels? JAMA 1984;252:2839–2845.
10. Lott JA, Speicher CE, Ayers LW: Typhoid fever toxemia with associated destruction of skeletal muscle. Clin Chem 1980a;26:1361–1362.
11. Lott JA, Landesman PW: The enzymology of skeletal muscle disorders. CRC Crit Rev Clin Lab Sci 1984;20:153–190.
12. Birkett DJ, Done J, Neale FC et al: Serum alkaline phosphatase in pregnancy: an immunological study. Br Med J 1986;1:1210–1212.
13. Warshaw JB, Littlefield HW, Fishman WH et al: Serum alkaline phosphatase in hypophosphatasia. J Clin Invest 1971;50:2137–2142.
14. Van Dommelen CKV, Klaassen CHL: Cyanocobalamin-dependent depression of the serum alkaline phosphatase level in patients with pernicious anemia. N Engl J Med 1964;271:541–544.
15. Stolbach L, Krant M, Fishman W: Ectopic production of alkaline phosphatase isoenzyme in patients with cancer. N Engl J Med 1969;281:757–762.
16. Zimmerman HJ: Serum enzymes in the diagnosis of hepatic disease. Gastroenterology 1964;46:613–618.
17. Ewen LM, Griffiths J: Patterns of enzyme activity following myocardial infarction and ischemia. Am J Clin Pathol 1971;56:614–622.
18. Barakat M, Grubb MN, Goyal RK et al: Intestinal alkaline phosphatase in patients with liver disease. Am J Dig Dis 1972;16:1102–1106.
19. Betro MG: Significance of increased alkaline phosphatase and lactate dehydrogenase activities coincident with normal serum bilirubin. Clin Chem 1972;18:1427–1429.
20. Nikkila EA: Serum alkaline phosphatase activity in pulmonary infarction. Scand J Clin Lab Invest 1959;11:405–406.
21. Dijkman JH, Kloppenborg PWC: Increased serum alkaline phosphatase activity in pulmonary infarction. Acta Med Scand 1966;180:273–281.
22. PetitClerc C: Quantitative fractionation of alkaline phosphatase isoenzymes according to their thermostability. Clin Chem 1976;22:42–48.
23. Yong JM: Cause of raised serum alkaline phosphatase after partial gastrectomy and in other malabsorption states. Lancet 1966;1:1132–1134.
24. Gault MH, Steiner G: Serum and urinary enzyme activity after renal infarction. Can Med Assoc J 1965;93:1101–1105.
25. Nathanson L. Fishman W: New observations on the Regan isoenzyme of alkaline phosphatase in cancer patients. Cancer 1971;27:1388–1397.
16. Belfiore F, Vecchio L, Napoli E: Serum enzymes in diabetes mellitus. Clin Chem 1973;19:447–452.
27. Fishman WH, Inglis NR, Stolbach LL et al: A serum alkaline phosphatase isoenzymes of human neoplastic cell origin. Cancer Res 1968;28:150–154.
28. Byers DA, Fernley HN, Walker PG: Studies on alkaline phosphatase: inhibition of human placental phosphoryl phosphatase by L-phenylalanine. Eur J Biochem 1972;29:197–204.
29. Birkett DJ, Conyers RAJ, Neale FC et al: Action of urea on human alkaline phosphatases, with a description of some automated techniques for the study of enzyme kinetics. Arch Biochem Biophys 1967;121:470–479.
30. Fishman L: Acrylamide disc gel electrophoresis of alka-

line phosphatase of human tissues, serum, and ascites fluid using Triton X-100 in the sample and the gel matrix. Biochem Med 1974;9:309–315.
31. Smith I, Perry JD, Lightstone PJ: Disc electrophoresis of alkaline phosphatase: mobility changes caused by neuraminidase. Clin Chem Acta 1969;25:17–19.
32. Schmid R: Bilirubin metabolism, state of the art. Gastroenterology 1978;74:1307–1312.
33. Sundberg M, Auff J, Weiss J et al: Estimation of unconjugated, conjugated, and delta bilirubin fractions in serum by use of two coated thin films. Clin Chem 1984;30:1314–1315.
34. Weiss J, Gautam A, Lauff J et al: The clinical importance of a protein-bound fraction of serum bilirubin in patients with hyperbilirubinemia. N Engl J Med 1983;309:147–150.
35. Hodgkin WE, Giblett ER, Levine H et al: Complete pseudocholinesterase deficiency: genetic and immunologic characterization. J Clin Invest 1965;44:486–493.
36. Belin JS, Chow I: Biochemical effects of chronic low-level exposure to pesticides. Res Commun Chem Pathol Pharmacol 1974;9:325–336.
37. Liddell J: Cholinesterase and anesthesia. Clin Biochem 1979;12:221–222.
38. Schuh FT: Serum cholinesterase: Effect on the action of suxamethonium following administration to a patient with cholinesterase deficiency. Br J Anaesth 1977;49:269–272.
39. Corless J, Middleton H: Normal liver function, a basis for understanding hepatic disease. Arch Intern Med 1983;143:2291–2294.
40. Prabhakaran V, Henderson AR: Unusual increases in serum lactate dehydrogenase isoenzyme-5 activity caused by severe congestive cardiac failure: two case reports. J Clin Pathol 1979;32:86–89.
41. Bruns DE, Savory J, Wills MR: More on "flipped" lactate dehydrogenase patterns in myocardial infarction. Clin Chem 1984;30:1881–1882.
42. von Eyben FE, Skude G: Lactate dehydrogenase and its isoenzyme, LDH-1, in serum are markers of testicular germ cell tumors. Clin Chem 1984;30:340–341.
43. Wolf PL: Lactate dehydrogenase-6: a biochemical sign of serious hepatic circulatory disturbance. Arch Intern Med 1985;145:1396–1397.
44. Goldberg DM: The diagnoses of hepatobiliary disease. Structural, functional and clinical aspects of gamma-glutamyltransferase. CRC Crit Rev Clin Lab Sci 1980;12:1–58.
45. Burlina A: Improved method for fractionating gamma-glutamyl transferase by electrophoresis on cellulose acetate. Clin Chem 1978;24:502–504.
46. Rosalki SB, Rau D: Serum gamma-glutamyl transpeptidase activity in alcoholism. Clin Chim Acta 1972;39:41–47.
47. Moussavian SN, Becker RC, Piepmeyer JL et al: Serum gamma-glutamyl transpeptidase and chronic alcoholism. Influences of alcohol ingestion and liver disease. Dig Dis Sci 1985;30:211–214.
48. Rosalki SB, Tarlow D, Rau D: Plasma gamma-glutamyl transpeptidase elevation in patients receiving enzyme-inducing drugs. Lancet 1971;2:376–377.
49. Acheampong-Mensah D: Activity of gamma-glutamyl-transpeptidase in serum of patients receiving anticonvulsant or anticoagulant therapy. Clin Biochem 1976;9:67–70.
50. Bodansky O, Schwartz M: 5′-Nucleotidase. Adv Clin Chem 1968;11:277–328.
51. Lott JA, Wolf PL: Alanine and aspartate aminotransferase (ALT and AST). pp. 111–138. In Lott JA, Wolf PL (eds): Clinical Enzymology. New York, Field Rich and Associates, 1986.
52. Lott JA, Wolf PL, Nemesanszky E: Gamma glutamyltransferase (GGT). pp. 199–211. In Wolf PL, Lott JA: Clinical Enzymology. New York, Field Rich and Associates, 1986.
53. Nemesanszky E: Alkaline phosphatase (AP). pp. 47–73. In Lott JA, Wolf PL (eds): Clinical Enzymology. New York, Field Rich and Associates, 1986.
54. Sawhney AK, Lott JA: Acetylcholinesterase and cholinesterase. pp. 1–26. In Lott JA, Wolf PL (eds): Clinical Enzymology. New York, Field Rich and Associates, 1986.

Pancreatic and Gastrointestinal Function

5

Lee H. Hilborne
John H. Eckfeldt

PANCREATIC FUNCTION

INTRODUCTION

The literature on acute pancreatitis is confusing and often contradictory. Except for surgical and autopsy specimens from patients with very severe pancreatitis, there is little histopathologic material available for examination. Furthermore, rarely is the pancreas examined by laparotomy when acutely inflamed. At present, much of the information on the anatomy of the pancreas during acute pancreatitis is limited to indirect observation of the gland with abdominal x-rays, ultrasound, endoscopic retrograde cholangiopancreatography (ERCP), and computed tomography (CT) scans. A 100% reliable, independent assessment of the presence or absence of pancreatitis (a "gold standard") is simply not available. In spite of the fact that much has been written on the subject,[1-5] the actual clinical sensitivity and specificity of all biochemical tests for pancreatitis are really not known.

Pancreatitis was originally classified as acute, relapsing acute, chronic relapsing (chronic pancreatitis with acute exacerbations), or chronic.[6] With acute pancreatitis and with the acute exacerbations of relapsing and chronic pancreatitis, the most consistent symptom is abdominal pain. Other clinical signs and symptoms are shown in Table 5-1. Histopathologically, acute pancreatitis has been further subclassified into edematous pancreatitis (mild edema with signs of cellular inflammation) and hemorrhagic pancreatitis (microscopic and gross pancreatic necrosis). Hypotension, Grey-Turner's and Cullen's signs (respectively, flank and periumbilical bluish discoloration from retroperitoneal hemorrhage), and subcutaneous fat necrosis are found almost exclusively with hemorrhagic pancreatitis, where the mortality exceeds 80%. Edematous pancreatitis is only rarely fatal.

Two recent symposia, the first in Cambridge[7] and the second in Marseille,[8] reviewed progress on pancreatitis over the previous 20 years. These two conferences reduced the number of pancreatitis classifications from four to two: acute and chronic. The following is a working definition of acute pancreatitis.[9]

> An acute condition typically presenting with abdominal pain usually associated with raised pancreatic enzymes in blood or urine, due to inflammatory disease of the pancreas.

As can be deduced from the above definition, biochemical analysis of serum or urine for pancreatic enzymes is a mainstay for the diagnosis of the disease.

Chronic pancreatitis is a more indolent disease as defined below.[9]

> A continuing inflammatory disease of the pancreas characterized by irreversible,

Table 5-1. Frequencies of Symptoms and Signs in Acute Pancreatitis

Symptom or Sign	Percent
Abdominal pain	95–100
Epigastric tenderness	95–100
Nausea and vomiting	70–90
Low-grade fever	70–85
Hypotension	20–40
Grey-Turner's or Cullen's sign	<5
Subcutaneous fat necrosis	<1

morphologic change typically causing pain and/or permanent functional impairment.

Patients with chronic pancreatitis may have recurrent acute attacks of pain, or the condition may be entirely painless, leading only to fibrosis, with the first evidence of disease being pancreatic insufficiency demonstrated as maldigestion or diabetes mellitus.[9] The primary pathophysiologic process in chronic pancreatitis is destruction of endocrine and exocrine parenchymal cells. In general, patients with chronic pancreatitis do not have serum pancreatic enzyme elevations, and in fact may have subnormal values. Varying degrees of pancreatic duct dilation may develop, leading to pseudocysts. Patients with pancreatic pseudocysts usually have chronic serum pancreatic enzyme elevations.

Introduced in 1929, measuring serum amylase was the first biochemical test for diagnosing pancreatitis. Since then, several additional tests including lipase and trypsin have been proposed, but none of these newer tests has totally replaced serum amylase. This is due largely to uncertainty in the actual diagnostic sensitivity and specificity of amylase and other biochemical tests for pancreatitis. With these limitations, diagnostic tests for acute pancreatitis are discussed. Chronic pancreatitis is discussed later in this chapter in the context of maldigestion, one of the causes of malabsorption.

TESTS OF PANCREATIC FUNCTION

Test: Amylase

Background and Selection

The term *amylase activity* refers to an enzyme's ability to hydrolyze internal α-1,4 starch linkages. The pancreas has the highest amylase concentration and largest total amount of amylase of any organ in the body. Unfortunately, other tissues, particularly the parotid salivary glands, also contain large quantities. Pancreatic or salivary amylase is not absorbed by intact gut mucosa, and normal serum amylase activity levels are relatively low. Any amylase that is present presumably comes from enzyme leakage directly into the blood from the ascinar cells or via lymphatics draining the glands. With ductular obstruction and/or inflammation of either the pancreas or parotid glands, enzyme leakage directly into the blood or via the lymphatics increases. In rare situations gut permeability changes, as in ischemic bowel disease or frank perforation, whereby a large quantity of amylase leaks into the peritoneal fluid and is eventually delivered via the thoracic duct into the circulation causing hyperamylasemia.

As mentioned above, amylase was the first biochemical test for the diagnosis of pancreatitis. For many clinicians, it is still the principle or only test used: a patient with abdominal pain and elevated serum or urine amylase has pancreatitis, one with clinically identical pain and a normal amylase does not, although this is clearly not always the case. False positive and false negative results occur. The false negative rate for serum amylase for diagnosis of pancreatitis may be as high as 32%.[10] This figure appears extraordinarily high and may reflect a large percentage of patients in that particular study who had acute exacerbations of chronic pancreatitis, where serum pancreatic enzyme elevations are less consistently observed and less dramatic. Another consideration is when the blood was collected relative to the onset of pain (see below).

Logistics

With resolving pancreatitis, serum amylase returns to within the reference range more rapidly than other serum biochemical tests (Fig. 5-1). In patients with acute pancreatitis, lactescent serum from hypertriglyceridemia may cause spuriously low amylase results. The exact prevalence of, or analytic reason for, triglyceride inhibition of serum amylase activity is unclear.

Interpretation

The serum amylase reference range varies widely depending on the substrate being used. The diagnostic specificity of amylase for pancreatitis has been extensively investigated. Spechler et al.[10] found that 32% of patients diagnosed with pancreatitis by pancreatic ultrasound or CT scan on "clinical grounds" had amylase within the reference range. However, many of these patients may not really have had acute pancreatitis.

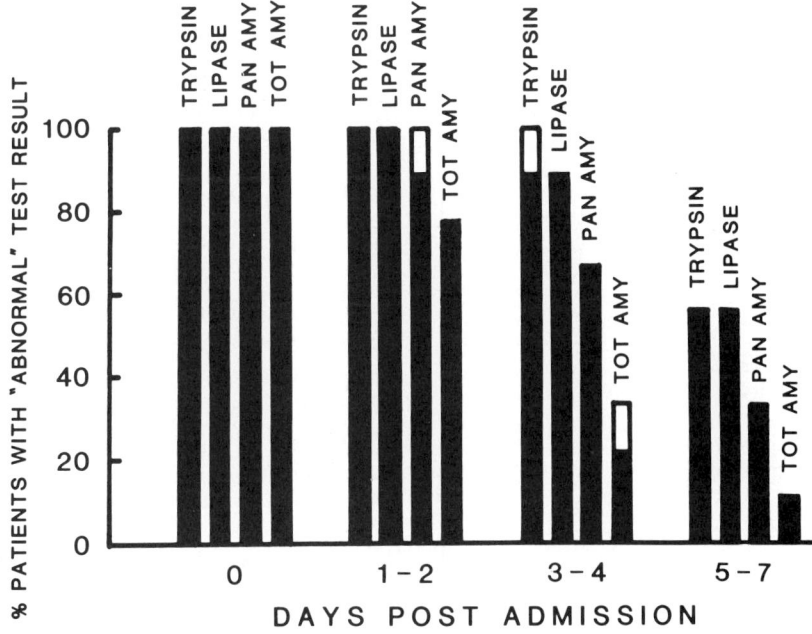

Fig. 5-1. Clinical sensitivity of serum immunoreactive trypsin, lipase, pancreatic isoamylase, and total amylase versus time after hospital admission for nine patients with well documented acute pancreatitis. Total bar represents sensitivity using blood donor mean + 2 SD and solid portion of bar sensitivity using blood donor mean + 3 SD for "cutoff" between "normal" and "abnormal." (From Eckfeldt et al.,[21] with permission.)

This raises the gold standard question alluded to previously. More typical figures for serum amylase diagnostic sensitivity for acute pancreatitis are 95–98%, at least during the first 12–24 hours of pain.[2–5,11] Salt and Schenker[12] compiled an extensive list of conditions associated with hyperamylasemia (Table 5-2). For many of these conditions, the amylase does not originate from the pancreas. Serum amylase elevations in excess of 20-fold the upper reference limit strongly suggest metastatic tumors that produce ectopic amylase, rather than pancreatitis.

Test: Amylase Isoenzymes

Pancreatic and salivary amylase are both glycoproteins (GP) with similar molecular weights (i.e., 55,000) and similar antigenicities of the protein portion. However, their carbohydrate content differs significantly.[1] Various physicochemical techniques have been used to distinguish pancreatic from salivary isoamylase. Specific plant isoamylase inhibitors and monoclonal antibody techniques employing antibodies specific to salivary isoamylase have been described.[1–3,16] All isoamylase methods seem to give reasonably consistent answers and differentiate pancreatic from salivary-type amylase activity. The amylase activity in the fallopian tube, normal lung, and liver appears to be very low. Amylase from these organs and elsewhere has the physicochemical characteristics of salivary amylase, and the term *salivary-type* amylase is used to include all nonpancreatic sources of amylase. Rarely malignant tumors, especially from the lung, ovary, and pancreas, produce and release large quantities of amylase into the circulation. Tumor-produced amylase has the physicochemical properties of salivary isoamylase in nearly all cases.

Test: Amylase/Creatinine Ratio

Background and Selection

Urinary amylase is derived from plasma amylase. Low molecular weight proteins (less than 35,000) are freely filtered by the glomeruli, nearly as rapidly as creatinine, whereas large proteins such as albumin (68,000) are only minimally filtered. Amylase (55,000) lies between these extremes. In the normal kidney, amylase is cleared only approximately 3% as rapidly as creatinine: the normal creatinine clearance is about 100 mL/min, and the amylase clearance is approximately 3 mL/min.[17] Based on its nonspecificity (see below), most

Table 5-2. Conditions Associated With Hyperamylasemia	
Condition	Type of isoamylase
Pancreas	
Pancreatitis of any etiology	P
Carcinoma of pancreas	P
Obstruction of pancreatic drainage	P
Trauma	P
Blunt or penetrating abdominal injury	
ERCP	
Complications of pancreatitis	
Pseudocyst, ascites, or abscess	P
Excessive secretin and/or CCK stimulation	P
Salivary gland	
Trauma	S
Infection (mumps, etc.)	S
Radiation	S
Salivary-type hyperamylasemia of unknown origin	S
Renal insufficiency	P & S
Nonpancreatic intra-abdominal conditions	
Perforated peptic ulcer	P
Mesenteric infarction	P
Bowel obstruction	?
Acute appendicitis	?
Lung disease	
Pneumonia?	S
Tuberculosis?	S
Carcinoma	S
Malignant tumors	
Ovary	S
Prostate	S
Lung	S
Pancreas	S
Colon	S & P[a]
Breast	P[b]
Miscellaneous	
Diabetic acidosis	Usually S
Other acidosis	Usually S[c]
Cerebral trauma	?
Thermal burns	P & S
Postoperative state	P or S
Prostate disease?	?
Pregnancy	?
Ruptured ectopic pregnancy	S
Ovarian cyst	S

Abbreviations: CCK, cholecystokinin; ERCP, endoscopic retrograde cholangiopancreatography.
[a] See Berk et al.[13]
[b] See Weitzel et al.[14]
[c] See Eckfeldt et al.[15]
(Adapted from Salt and Schenker,[12] with permission.)

authorities now believe that the amylase/creatinine clearance ratio has relatively little diagnostic advantage over other pancreatitis tests.[18] However, a low clearance ratio is useful for diagnosing macroamylasemia.

Interpretation

In healthy individuals, the amylase-creatinine clearance ratio is approximately 2–4%. In patients with pancreatitis, this clearance ratio may exceed 10%. Urinary amylase, in terms of amylase units per hour, increases with pancreatitis for two reasons. First, pancreatitis causes increased plasma amylase, which increases the amylase filtered by the glomeruli. Second, some of the amylase that is filtered by the glomeruli is reabsorbed by the renal tubules. In pancreatitis, however, the tubules fail to reabsorb as much amylase, resulting in even more amylase reaching the urine. This increased clearance is consistent with the clinical observation that urinary amylase stays elevated a few days longer than serum amylase as an attack of acute pancreatitis subsides. Elevated amylase/creatinine clearance ratios also occur in other conditions including diabetic ketoacidosis, multiple myeloma, thermal burns, and renal failure.

In macroamylasemia, normal serum amylase is bound to an abnormal serum protein, either an immunoglobulin or nonimmunoglobulin glycoprotein, preventing normal renal amylase clearance. Patients with this condition have persistent hyperamylasemia. If they have an episode of abdominal pain, in all likelihood unrelated to the pancreas, they are suddenly labeled as having pancreatitis when the elevated amylase is discovered. Because the large macromolecular complex is very poorly filtered by the glomeruli, in macroamylasemia the amylase/creatinine clearance ratio is less than 1%. Another rapid method has recently been described[19] for detecting the large macroamylase complex using polyethyleneglycol precipitation of serum amylase activity. Unequivocal identification of macroamylase requires molecular sizing by gel filtration or ultracentrifugation, procedures not routinely available in most clinical laboratories.[2]

Test: Lipase

Background and Selection

The only organ containing significant lipase activity is the pancreas. Thus, elevated serum lipase should be more specific for pancreatitis than elevation of total amylase activity.

Logistics

Until recently, serum lipase assays have never gained widespread clinical use because of analytic problems. Many of the early assays were technically very demanding, requiring several hours, and many had very poor reproducibility within and between laboratories. Attempts to simplify the assay using synthetic substrates that produce spectrophotometrically detectable products led to better analytic precision, but often to poorer clinical utility because serum esterases of nonpancreatic origin could hydrolyze such substrates. Recently, the role of colipase, a small pancreatic protein that is required at the oil/water interface for pancreatic lipase activity, has been elucidated. Colipase appears to be important in ameliorating the inhibitory effects of bile salts on pancreatic lipase activity.

Interpretation

The reference range for serum lipase varies with the substrate and assay used. Several commercial lipase kits have incorporated porcine colipase (see above) into their reagents. These technical advancements may improve the lipase assay's clinical performance enough that it becomes the test of choice for routine diagnosis of pancreatitis in the near future.[20]

Test: Trypsin (Immunoreactive)

Background and Selection

Trypsin originates only from the pancreas. Thus, its use is theoretically attractive for diagnosing acute pancreatitis. Enzymatically inactive precursors of trypsin are found in the pancreatic gland in two isoforms, cationic and anionic. When exposed to proteolytic enzymes in the intestine, cationic and anionic trypsinogens are cleaved to form cationic and anionic trypsins, which play major roles in digestion of dietary protein. Assays for tryptic activity in duodenal contents and in stool have been used for a long time for diagnosing maldigestion, but assays for trypsin in the serum have only recently been developed.

Terminology

Enzymatically active trypsin can activate several factors of the coagulation cascade leading to an intravascular clotting. To prevent this occurrence in vivo, active trypsin released into the blood is rapidly inactivated by α_1-antitrypsin (AAT) and α_2-macroglobulin. Consequently, serum trypsin assays have used immunologic detection methods, specifically radioimmunoassay, to diagnose pancreatitis; hence, the term *immunoreactive trypsin*.

Logistics

As tracer and standard, most commercially available immunoreactive trypsin assays use human cationic trypsin that has been covalently inactivated with one of several serine protease inhibitors. These assays cross-react approximately 100% with cationic trypsinogen, which is the primary form of immunoreactive trypsin in normal human serum. They also cross-react 20–40% with the cationic trypsin/AAT complex, but only slightly or not at all with the cationic trypsin/α_2-macroglobulin complex.

Interpretation

The reference range for immunoreactive trypsin is about 17–65 ng/mL (17–65 µg/L). Immunoreactive trypsin is a very sensitive and fairly specific indicator for pancreatitis.[1,5,21] However, whether it is really superior to other tests for pancreatitis, such as lipase or pancreatic isoamylase, is questionable. Furthermore, at present, immunoreactive trypsin requires radioimmunoassay technology, preventing its availability on a 24 h/d basis.

Test: Other Pancreatic Enzymes and Proteins

Assays for other pancreatic enzymes and proteins including chymotrypsin, elastase, ribonuclease, phospholipase, and pancreatic secretory trypsin inhibitor have been developed and proposed for diagnosis of pancreatitis.[1,2] In general, clinical experience with these tests by investigators other than those who developed them has been very limited. No doubt the concentrations of many of these proteins are elevated in the presence of acute pancreatitis when compared with healthy control subjects. However, whether or not they are elevated in sick patients with nonpancreatic disease, thereby decreasing their specificity and severely limiting clinical utility, has not been carefully addressed.

INTERPRETATION OF PANCREATIC TEST RESULT PATTERNS

Diagnosing pancreatitis remains one of the many medical areas that relies more heavily on clinical judgment and the art of medicine, than on objective science. A physician's confidence in the diagnosis of acute pancreatitis varies from very likely, through possible, to unlikely. The quality of clinical signs and symptoms shown in Table 5-1 help differentiate pancreatitis from other abdominal conditions. Classic severe, acute pancreatitis usually presents as follows: acute abdominal pain that is severe and constant, not intermittent; pain that radiates to the left upper quadrant or back; pain that reaches maximum intensity in 0.5–6 hours; vomiting that does not alleviate the pain; abdominal rigidity or guarding that is less than one might expect considering the severity of the pain; and diminished, but not absent, bowel sounds. Despite the presence of most or all of the above features, the clinical diagnosis of pancreatitis usually depends on finding an elevated serum amylase or lipase. The higher the pancreatic enzyme elevation, the more likely that the diagnosis will be pancreatitis. Pancreatitis secondary to temporary pancreatic duct obstruction by gallstones may have relatively severe symptoms, but only minor pancreatic edema and inflammation. In such patients, the serum amylase and lipase usually return to normal within 24–48 hours, concordant with rapid resolution of symptoms. In patients with alcoholic pancreatitis, the serum amylase and lipase resolve more slowly, but usually within 7–10 days. Failure to normalize within this period suggests pancreatic pseudocyst development, pancreatic ascites, or a nonpancreatic etiology.

Physicians must always keep in mind several conditions that mimic pancreatitis but require immediate surgical intervention, namely, gut perforation and infarction. With these conditions, the patient has abdominal pain and hyperamylasemia; without prompt surgical intervention, the clinical outcome is often death. Radiographic signs, such as free air under the diaphragm, can be used to diagnose perforation. Diagnosis of bowel infarction is far more difficult, directly relating to its mortality of more than 80% in most medical centers. Clinicians should consider the possibility of loss of gut integrity as the cause of the hyperamylasemia, rather than pancreatitis, with abdominal signs or symptoms that continue for more than 48 hours; bacteremia; only moderate (less than threefold the upper reference limit) amylase or lipase elevation; continued deterioration despite standard medical therapy; or a normal pancreas CT scan in a patient who appears clinically to have reasonably severe pancreatitis.[2] Sorting out the etiology of clinically less severe abdominal pain in patients with only modest elevations (less than threefold) of serum amylase is difficult. A large percentage of such patients are alcoholics who are at significantly increased pancreatitis risk. However, between 10–40% of acutely intoxicated alcoholics have amylase elevations, which in nearly half is due solely to salivary isoamylase elevations,[22,23] rendering the total serum amylase relatively unreliable for diagnosis of pancreatitis in such patients. Pancreatic isoamylase, lipase, or immunoreactive trypsin will confirm the pancreas as the source of the amylase elevation. An abdominal CT scan may also be helpful. Return of the serum pancreatic enzymes to the reference range with resolution of the pain is reasonably good evidence for acute pancreatic inflammation.

Patients with abdominal pain and renal failure pose a particular problem. Renal failure causes decreased clearance of all small proteins including amylase, lipase, and immunoreactive trypsin. Thus, modest elevations (less than threefold) of all these serum pancreatic enzymes can be found in patients with renal failure in the absence of pancreatic disease. However, serum amylase, lipase, or immunoreactive trypsin greater than threefold the upper reference limit is reasonably good evidence for pancreatitis, even in patients with renal failure.

Asymptomatic patients with chronic serum amylase elevation tend not to have pancreatic disease.[24] Macroamylasemia and salivary hyperamylasemia are far more likely. In such patients, serum pancreatic isoamylase or lipase should be measured to document pancreatic involvement before embarking on extensive and expensive radiologic investigations of the abdomen and pancreas.

MALABSORPTION

INTRODUCTION

Disorders of digested nutrient assimilation may be caused by an inability to break down complex macromolecules (maldigestion) or to absorb those nutrients across the intestine once digested (malabsorption). Since either situation results in an inability to properly absorb nutrients, they are grouped under a general category, malabsorption.

Malabsorption is a complex and, at times, clinically difficult process to diagnose. Malabsorption refers to a large number of biochemically and physiologically unrelated processes, each manifested by the inability to

Table 5-3. Signs and Symptoms of Malabsorption
Diarrhea
Protein-calorie malnutrition
Anemia
Amenorrhea
Glossitis
Tetany, paraesthesias, and weakness
Edema

Table 5-4. Classification of Malabsorption

I. Inadequate digestion
   A. Deficiency or inactivation of pancreatic lipase
      1. Exocrine pancreatic insufficiency
         a. Chronic pancreatitis
         b. Pancreatic carcinoma
         c. Cystic fibrosis
         d. Pancreatic resection
      2. Ulcerogenic tumor of the pancreas (Zollinger-Ellison syndrome, gastrinoma)[a]

II. Reduced intestinal bile salt concentration (with impaired micelle formation)
   A. Liver disease
   B. Abnormal bacterial proliferation in the small bowel
      1. Fistulas
      2. Blind loops
      3. Multiple diverticula of the small bowel
      4. Hypomotility states (diabetes, scleroderma, intestinal pseudo-obstruction)
   C. Interrupted enterohepatic circulation of bile salts
      1. Ileal resection
      2. Ileal inflammatory disease (reginal ileitis)
   D. Drugs (by sequestration or precipitation of bile salts)
      1. Neomycin
      2. Calcium carbonate
      3. Cholestyramine

III. Inadequate absorptive surface
   A. Intestinal resection or bypass

IV. Lymphatic obstruction
   A. Intestinal lymphangiectasia
   B. Lymphoma

V. Cardiovascular disorders
   A. Constrictive pericarditis
   B. Congestive heart failure
   C. Mesenteric vascular insufficiency
   D. Vasculitis

VI. Primary mucosal absorptive defects
   A. Inflammatory or infiltrative disorders
   B. Biochemical or genetic abnormalities
      1. Nontropical sprue (gluten-induced enteropathy): celiac sprue
      2. Disaccharidase deficiency
      3. Hypogammaglobulinemia
      4. Abetalipoproteinemia
      5. Hartnup disease
      6. Cystinuria
      7. Monosaccharide malabsorption

VII. Endocrine and metabolic disorders
   A. Diabetes mellitus
   B. Hypoparathyroidism
   C. Adrenal insufficiency
   D. Hyperthyroidism
   E. Zollinger-Ellison syndrome, gastrinoma
   F. Carcinoid syndrome

[a] Malabsorption caused by multiple defects.

absorb essential food elements. The pathologic process may be confined to one specific nutrient class (e.g., protein, carbohydrate, fat, vitamins, minerals), a particular nutrient within a class, or a process resulting in the inability to absorb a broad range of nutrients in several or all classes. Malabsorptive diseases also may be subclassified by whether they are inherited (e.g., cystic fibrosis, celiac disease) or acquired (e.g., surgical bowel resection, chronic relapsing pancreatitis).[25-27]

The clinical presentation of malabsorption may be obvious (e.g., fat malabsorption with malodorous stools) or subtle (e.g., vitamin B_{12} malabsorption with megaloblastic anemia) (Table 5-3). Generally the differential diagnosis is limited by the presenting signs and symptoms, the patient's age, and any pertinent history (e.g., recent travel, family history of similar disorders). The most frequent causes of malabsorption are listed in Table 5-4. Once the differential diagnosis is narrowed by the history and physical examination, laboratory testing may be used to help distinguish among the remaining diagnoses.

PANCREATIC EXOCRINE FUNCTION TESTS

Test: Secretin

Background and Selection

Secretin is a duodenal mucosa hormone that is released in response to gastric acid entering the duodenum. Secretin promotes pancreatic water and electrolyte secretion. Pancreatic electrolyte and fluid output following secretin stimulation is believed to be directly related to the functional mass of exocrine pancreatic tissue present. Although increased enzymes are found in the duodenal lumen initially following stimulation, this appears to be a "wash-out" phenomenon because enzyme concentrations return to near reference levels with continued stimulation.

The secretin test is used in the evaluation of patients with abdominal pain, weight loss, and steatorrhea when the clinical presentation suggests the possibility of chronic pancreatitis or a pancreatic neoplasm. The test is contraindicated when the patient has clinical or laboratory evidence of acute pancreatitis.

Logistics

Patient preparation for the test requires an overnight fast; consequently, the test is best performed in the morning. It is essential to ascertain the patient's past medical history since prior vagotomy, Crohn's disease, and anticholinergic therapy may produce low bicarbonate levels without concurrent pancreatic disease.

Multiple lumen tubes are used to separately collect gastric and duodenal contents with additional lumina communicating with balloons to occlude the pylorus and distal duodenum. To overcome the problems with duodenal content recovery, nonabsorbable marker compounds are introduced into the lumen but they often do not mix well with its contents. Because recovery is variable, technique comparison is difficult; 85% recovery of the marker substance is considered adequate for assessment of pancreatic secretions corecovered.[28]

After positioning the multiple lumen tube under fluoroscopic guidance, gastric secretions are aspirated with a 25–40 mmHg suction for 10–20 minutes. This duodenal fluid represents the basal secretion. Following intravenous administration of secretin (1 clinical unit [CU]/kg), four consecutive 20-minute specimens are collected by continuous suction. Each collection volume should be recorded and the specimens kept on ice before processing.

It is difficult to compare secretin test studies because the hormone product varies, as does the method (i.e., rapid intravenous, continuous intravenous, and subcutaneous injection) and amount of administration.[28] Plastic syringes and infusion sets bind secretin, reducing the effective hormone dose. Dissolving secretin in albumin abolishes this phenomenon.

Interpretation

Bicarbonate secretion into the duodenal lumen is conventionally used as the analyte to measure secretin response. The test is poorly standardized and is technically difficult to perform uniformly. A major problem is duodenal contents contamination by gastric juice and loss of secretions into the jejunum or reflexively into the stomach. Expected findings include a volume greater than or equal to 2 mL/kg in 80 minutes; a bicarbonate concentration of 80 mEq/L (80 mmol/L) or more; and a bicarbonate output of 10 mEq (10 mmol) or more in 30 minutes. Results outside these reference intervals are considered abnormal and suggest pancreatic dysfunction. Inadequate separation or aspiration of gastric contents may acidify the duodenal contents, decreasing the bicarbonate level. Failure to collect the entire duodenal sample leads to a falsely low estimation of pancreatic volume secretion.

Test: Secretin-Cholecystokinin

Background and Selection

Secretin's main biologic function is the stimulation of water and electrolyte secretion from the pancreas. To better study pancreatic enzyme output, cholecystokinin (CCK) may be added to the infusion because CCK is identical to the enzyme pancreozymin (PZ) and has the main function of stimulating pancreatic enzyme secretion. Using the combined secretin-CCK test, pancreatic enzyme production including amylase, lipase, trypsin, and chymotrypsin can be assessed in addition to pancreatic water and electrolyte output.[26,28,29]

Logistics

See Test: Secretin.

Interpretation

The duodenal levels of amylase, lipase, trypsin, and chymotrypsin vary widely following stimulation; considerable overlap exists between the reference population and patients with exocrine pancreatic insufficiency. Markedly decreased enzyme output, however, is highly suggestive of severe pancreatic disease. Because intubation is uncomfortable and in some patients impossible, the study of fecal enzymes as an alternative to duodenal enzyme analysis has been suggested. Generally the technique is less sensitive than the duodenal aspirate. Chymotrypsin fecal output correlates better than trypsin with duodenal aspirate enzyme levels.[30]

Test: Bentiromide (Tripeptide Hydrolysis Test)

Background and Selection

The secretin and secretin-CCK tests are difficult to standardize and require luminal intubation for specimen collection. A simpler, indirect pancreatic function test is the bentiromide test, also known as the tripeptide hydrolysis test, which measures the ability of intraluminal chymotrypsin to hydrolyze the orally administered synthetic peptide bentiromide (N-benzoyl-L-tyrosyl para-amino benzoic acid [Bz,Ty-PABA]).[29,31,32] Chymotrypsin, when present, hydrolyzes Bz,Ty-PABA to Bz, Ty and PABA. The amount of PABA appearing in the serum or urine is therefore directly related to the amount of chymotrypsin present in the small bowel and indirectly related to pancreatic enzyme production. This test appears to be safe and reliable for studying patients with suspected pancreatic insufficiency. The test is easier to perform and standardize compared with the intubation tests previously described.

Logistics

The patient is tested following an overnight fast. Nonessential medications should be withdrawn for 24 hours to avoid possible interference with pancreatic function. Sulfonamides, thiazides, furosemide, acetaminophen, and chloramphenicol may interfere with the spectrophotometric determination of PABA. Foods containing hippurate precursors (e.g., prunes, cranberries) should be discontinued before commencing this test. A 1-hour urine control sample is collected before oral administration of bentiromide. The patient is given the synthetic peptide orally followed by adequate fluids to ensure diuresis. Urine is collected for 6 hours in EDTA tubes, centrifuged, and frozen until analyzed. Conventionally, urinary PABA is assayed.

Interpretation

The expected amount of PABA excreted is roughly 60% (range 48–72%) of the orally administered dose. In patients with pancreatic insufficiency, PABA excretion is significantly less. The patient must have adequate gastrointestinal absorptive ability and renal function because the inability to absorb PABA from the gut or excrete it into the urine will lead to a falsely low urinary value.

Test: Fecal Fat

Background and Selection

The fecal fat test for malassimilation was first described in 1949 by van de Kramer et al.[33] and it remains, with few modifications, the gold standard for the diagnosis of these diseases. As initially described, the test collection period ranged from one to several days and the dietary fat intake was constant. The test has become more standardized in the intervening years. Steatorrhea first appears when pancreatic lipase output falls below 10% of the reference value.[34]

Logistics

Patients are placed on a normal fat diet (50–150 g/d) several days before specimen collection.[35] Some investigators have recommended a fixed diet containing 100 g of fat but this regimen is unpleasant, poorly tolerated, has poor compliance, and appears to offer little over a routine diet with adequate fat (70–100 g/d).[36]

Stool is then collected over at least a 3-day period. Perhaps the most difficult problem with the fecal fat test, when performed by a reliable laboratory, is the esthetic problem of stool collection, leading to less than perfect patient compliance and an underestimation of fecal fat output. There is good (94%) agreement between results obtained from 1-day and 3-day fecal fat collections.[37,38] Some have recommended the 1-day collection as a screening test. The 3-day collection, however, remains the standard for analysis and should be used when steatorrhea is a serious consideration.

Interpretation

Generally the mean daily fat excretion (grams per day) and mean fat concentration in the stool (grams of fat per 100 g of wet stool) are determined from the collected stool. Fecal fat excretion of 7 g/d and a fecal fat concentration of 5 g/100 g wet stool (5 g%) discriminate well between patients with malassimilation and those individuals in the reference population. Test efficiency at this discrimination level is 90%. Fecal fat results may suggest further assessment because patients with maldigestion have higher fecal fat levels than those with malabsorption. Using mean fat concentration as an indicator, fecal fat values between 5 and 10 g% are often associated with malabsorption and values greater than 10 g% more likely suggest maldigestion.

Test: Lundh

Background and Selection

This test, an alternative to the secretin-CCK/PZ test, is considerably simpler and less costly than the secretin-CCK test. There are varying reports discussing the sensitivity of this test compared with the secretin-CCK test, some investigators showing correlation and others disagreement.[39–43] The test is adequately sensitive when pancreatic function is reduced to a level that produces steatorrhea (10%). One study found the Lundh test to have a high diagnostic rate for chronic pancreatitis (90%) and pancreatic carcinoma (79%).

Logistics

This test requires the ingestion, following small bowel intubation, of a 300 mL test meal containing 6% fat, 5% protein, and 15% carbohydrate.[44] Duodenal contents are collected either for 2 hours, total, or as four 30-minute collections.

Interpretation

Generally two enzymes, trypsin and lipase, are measured. Although the Lundh test may be preferred to the secretin-CCK test because it requires fewer resources and is more physiologic, there are certain limitations. Because the Lundh test requires endogenous secretin and CCK-PZ release from the duodenal mucosa, the mucosa must be intact for the test to be reliable. Similarly, secretin release requires that acid enter the small intestine; the test is therefore unreliable in patients with achlorhydria or previous gastric resection.

Test: ^{14}C-Triolein Breath

Background and Selection

Although fecal fat measurement continues to be the gold standard for steatorrhea diagnosis, the test is poorly tolerated for reasons discussed above. The ^{14}C-triolein breath test is a reliable method to initially evaluate patients for fat malabsorption. The reagent used is a ^{14}C labeled triglyceride that is hydrolyzed in the small bowel by pancreatic lipase to free fatty acids and monoglycerides. The free fatty acids are then absorbed and metabolized to $^{14}CO_2$ and H_2O. The generated $^{14}CO_2$ appears in expired air with respiration. Several triglycerides have been tried, but triolein appears to confer the best sensitivity and specificity when compared with fecal fat quantitative tests.[45-47]

Logistics

Patients are instructed to fast overnight before the ingestion of labeled triglyceride contained in a test meal with 20 g of fat. No further food is ingested during the test. Expired air is collected in a trapping solution, then the quantity of $^{14}CO_2$ is measured hourly for 6 hours.

Interpretation

The $^{14}CO_2$ is expressed as a percentage of the total dose expired per hour and peak values are used to establish the expiration amount for comparison with reference values. The reference cutoff has been reported as a peak of 3.4% of the dose per hour.[45] Most peak values occur 4 to 6 hours following ingestion. When compared with fecal fat quantitative tests, the triolein breath test has a sensitivity of 100% and a specificity of 96%. Several considerations are important when evaluating patients with the ^{14}C-triolein breath test. Other disease processes may influence the results. Obese patients have delayed excretion of $^{14}CO_2$. Delayed gastric emptying, metabolic imbalances (e.g., hyperlipidemia, diabetes mellitus, liver failure) and respiratory insufficiency may similarly influence the results. The test is, however, a reasonable, safe, and efficient alternative to fecal fat determination in the assessment of misassimilation patients.

Since malabsorption and maldigestion will both lead to a decrease in $^{14}CO_2$ expired, test refinements have been advocated to discriminate between steatorrhea of pancreatic origin and that from other causes. Patients with decreased $^{14}CO_2$ expiration may be rechallenged with the same dose of triolein accompanied by pancreatic enzymes. Those without adequate pancreatic function should respond with a $^{14}CO_2$ expiration within the reference interval, whereas patients with malabsorption from other causes should continue to have low $^{14}CO_2$ expiration.[48] An alternative uses simultaneous triglyceride and free fatty acid administration, each labeled with a different radioactive tracer, followed by quantitation of serum tracer.[38] Appearance of only the free fatty acid tracer (conventionally ^{3}H) suggests pancreatic enzyme insufficiency, whereas absence of both tracers suggests other causes of malabsorption.

Test: Fatty Meal

Background and Selection

The difficulties associated with fecal fat collection have prompted investigators to look for alternative screening methods. The fatty meal test challenges the patient with a high fat meal that is followed by assay of the patient's serum for triglycerides and chylomicrons.[49]

Logistics

The patient, following an overnight fast, is given a 50 g fat load (50% butter, 50% margarine) followed by assay of serum triglycerides and chylomicrons hourly for 5 hours.

Interpretation

The reference population shows an increase in triglycerides of at least 100 mg/dL (1.11 mmol/L) or 100% above fasting levels and chylomicrons exceed 7% of the lipoprotein content. Using these criteria, Goldstein et al.[49] observed a 96% sensitivity and a 95% specificity as compared with the fecal fat test. Although some have suggested a 2-hour test, peak absorption occurs at 3 hours in most healthy individuals. This test, like others requiring intestinal absorption, assumes normal intestinal absorptive capacity.

Test: D-Xylose Absorption

Background and Selection

This test, described in 1937 by Helmer and Fouts,[50] and by Fourman[51] in 1948 is used to study the absorptive capacity of the proximal small bowel mucosa. The test uses the pentose D-xylose, which is 60% absorbed by the proximal small bowel and excreted unchanged into the urine. Because the sugar is not metabolized, the amount appearing in the urine is a reflection of the intestinal absorptive capacity.

Logistics

The patient should fast overnight and begin the test with an empty bladder. The patient ingests a specific xylose quantity, usually 5 or 25 g, followed by blood sampling 2 hours later and collection of urine for 5 hours. The D-xylose absorption test may be used in children with the ingested dose based on the child's weight (0.5 g/lb [15 μmol/kg]).

Interpretation

The appearance of D-xylose in the blood suggests absorption has occurred, and some recommend a 1- or 2-hour serum assay be performed rather than an assay for urine xylose.[52,53] With the 5-g dose, one expects the 2-hour level to be greater than 20 mg/dL (>1.33 mmol/L) and the urine 5-hour quantity excreted to be greater than 1.2 g (>8 mmol). Similar values for the 25-g dose are greater than 25 mg/dL (>1.67 mmol/L) and greater than 4.0 g (>26.64 mmol) for the blood and urine excretions, respectively. Although some suggest the 25-g dose better separates patients with malabsorption from the reference population, Haeney et al.[52] find equal sensitivity between the two methods. The lower dose is associated with less gastrointestinal discomfort from the sugar load.

The reference interval for urinary xylose excretion in elderly individuals is less than that of a younger population, because of the usual decrease in renal clearance. Although the D-xylose absorption test is useful for diagnosing malabsorption, it has limitations. The test requires adequate renal function for the sugar to be cleared in 5 hours. Vomiting, gastric stasis, dehydration, myxedema, ascites, edema, and bacterial overgrowth may yield false positive results.[54] False positive results may be associated with medications including diuretics, anti-inflammatory drugs, and antibiotics.[55]

Test: Breath Hydrogen Test for Carbohydrate Intolerance

Background and Selection

Although intestinal mucosa can absorb monosaccharides directly into the blood, most carbohydrates consumed are polysaccharides and disaccharides. Pancreatic and salivary enzymes convert polysaccharides to disaccharides. Intestinal epithelium disaccharidases split disaccharides into monosaccharides. Specifically, lactase splits lactose into glucose and galactose, sucrase splits sucrose into glucose and fructose, and maltose is split by maltase into two glucose molecules. The relative deficiency or lack of one or more enzymes leads to retention of its sugar substrate within the intestinal lumen. Excess sugar produces an osmotic diarrhea and, when the sugar reaches the large intestine, it serves as a nutritional source for intestinal flora. Bacterial sugar metabolism produces hydrogen gas (H_2), which is absorbed systemically and subsequently appears in expired air.

Interpretation

Breath H_2 increases 30–90 minutes following ingestion of 50 g of a nonabsorbable sugar.[56] The H_2 breath test is the most reliable indicator of carbohydrate enzyme deficiency.[57] Because detection of H_2 gas in a patient's breath requires sugar fermentation by intestinal bacteria, gastrointestinal sterility may rarely produce false negative findings.[57] In addition to being useful in the diagnosis of carbohydrate intolerance, the test may also be used to study small bowel transit time when a nondigestable sugar is ingested, because fermenting bacteria are normally found only in the large intestine.[58] Small intestine bacterial overgrowth may be sus-

Table 5-5. Carbohydrate Malabsorption	
Malabsorption	Diseases
Lactose	Congenital lactase deficiency Transient lactase deficiency in premature infants Acquired lactase deficiency Lactase deficiency with diseases of the small bowel
Starch	Congenital α-amylase deficiency not known Secondary deficiency of α-amylase with pancreatic insufficiency Physiologic malabsorption of starch
Trehalose	Congenital trehalase deficiency Trehalase deficiency with diseases of the small bowel
Sucrose	Congenital sucrase-isomaltase deficiency Sucrase-isomaltase deficiency in diseases of the small bowel
Maltose, maltotriose, α-limit dextrins	Congenital maltase deficiency not known Deficiency of α-glucosidases in diseases of the small bowel
Glucose, galactose	Congenital glucose-galactose malabsorption Intestinal hurry or bacterial overgrowth with diseases of the small bowel
Fructose	Congenital transport defect not known

pected when the H_2 breath test is positive following ingestion of a normally absorbable sugar (e.g., glucose) that would not be expected to reach the colon.[58,59] Although lactase deficiency is the most common cause of carbohydrate malabsorption, many others occur (Table 5-5).

Test: For Disaccharidase Deficiency

Background and Selection

The digestion and absorption of disaccharides are normally reflected by a rise in serum glucose, thus glucose measurements following disaccharide ingestion are used to assess disaccharidase deficiency.

Logistics

Following an overnight fast, the patient is given 50 g of a suspect disaccharide followed by serum glucose assays every half hour for 2 hours.

Interpretation

Normally a rise in serum glucose exceeding 20–30 mg/dL (>1.1–1.7 mmol/L) over the fasting glucose level occurs. A rise of less than 20 mg/dL (<1.1 mmol/L) suggests disaccharidase deficiency.[60] A positive finding (failure of serum glucose to rise 20 mg/dL [1.1 mmol/L]) should be confirmed by a subsequent glucose tolerance test. A normal rise following glucose ingestion and an abnormal response to the ingested disaccharide confirms the disaccharidase deficiency.

Test: Vitamin B_{12} Malabsorption (Schilling Test) (See Ch. 10)

Background and Selection

Vitamin B_{12} (cobalamin) is an essential cofactor for DNA synthesis. Primary dietary B_{12} sources include meat and dairy products. Intestinal flora synthesize vitamin B_{12}, but the amount is inadequate to prevent deficiency that manifests itself by megaloblastic anemia and neurologic damage. The vitamin requires gastric parietal cell synthesis of intrinsic factor (IF) for absorption across the ilial mucosa. Causes of vitamin B_{12} deficiency include decreased IF, chronic pancreatitis, small bowel bacterial overgrowth causing competition for the vitamin, and ilial disease (e.g., Crohn's disease).[61] Inadequate IF is the most common cause of vitamin B_{12} malabsorption, but about 40% of chronic pancreatitis patients and almost all cystic fibrosis (CF) patients have the deficiency. The pathophysiology of the latter remains somewhat obscure.

Logistics

In 1953 Schilling[62] described a test to discriminate vitamin B_{12} deficiency from a lack of IF and other intestinal processes. After an overnight fast, ingested radiolabeled vitamin B_{12} (0.5 μg [0.4 μmol]) absorption is measured by quantitating its appearance in serum, feces, or urine, most often the latter. When the test begins, the patient is given 1000 μg (750 μmol) of unlabeled vitamin B_{12} intramuscularly to saturate all available binding sites and promote urinary vitamin excretion.

Interpretation

The reference population excretes more than 8% of the ingested dose in a 24-hour urine collection, whereas patients with pernicious anemia excrete less than 7%. Patients with IF deficiency correct their response when vitamin B_{12} is administered with IF, whereas no response is observed in patients with malabsorption of other etiologies. To obviate the need for a second test, a dual tracer method may be used, one labeling vitamin B_{12} bound to IF and the other free vitamin B_{12}.[63]

Test: β-Carotene and Carotenoids (See Ch. 10)

Background and Selection

Carotenoids are a family of approximately 600 pigments found in all photosynthesizing plants.[64] Of these pigments, approximately 50 serve as precursors for mammalian vitamin A (retinol).[65] Only β-carotene, representing approximately 25% of serum carotenoids, can form two vitamin A molecules from one precursor. The majority of β-carotene is converted to vitamin A in the small intestine, yet the process is incomplete and both vitamin A and β-carotene are found in serum. Determinants of serum β-carotene levels are many and include dietary uptake, gastrointestinal destruction, absorption efficiency, metabolism, and rate of tissue uptake.[66] Once in the circulation, β-carotene is transported by lipoproteins with 80% bound to low density lipoprotein (LDL), 8% bound to high density lipoprotein (HDL), and 12% bound to very low density lipoprotein (VLDL).

In addition to being a precursor for vitamin A, carotenoids (β-carotene in particular), are antioxidants that inactivate potentially dangerous reactive chemicals within tissues including toxic free radicals.[67] As such, β-carotene has been postulated to reduce the risk of neoplasia.[68,69] Intestinal absorption of carotenes, in contrast to vitamin A, appears to be relatively nonspecific. While the serum level of vitamin A is more a reflection of intestinal regulation, serum carotene more closely reflects nutritional availability and intestinal absorption. Total body carotenoid storage is not appreciable; consequently, serum levels reflect recent changes in dietary intake and intestinal function.[65]

Although vitamin A is toxic when taken in high doses, pure β-carotene does not result in hypervitaminosis A and has not been shown to be toxic in doses 60 times the recommended daily allowance.[65] Excessive ingestion of β-carotene will cause a yellow pigmentation of the skin that suggests hyperbilirubinemia. However, high doses of β-carotene do not produce scleral icterus, which is prominent in patients with jaundice.

Logistics

Specimens for β-carotene should be obtained following an overnight fast. Serum should be separated from clotted blood, protected from excessive exposure to light, and stored frozen before analysis.

A β-carotene absorption test is often utilized for evaluating malabsorption. Following collection of a fasting baseline sample the patient is given 15,000 U of β-carotene orally tid with meals for 3 days. A second fasting collection is obtained on the morning following the third day.

Interpretation

The reference interval for β-carotene, determined by high pressure liquid chromatography, is 20–40 μg/dL (0.37–0.74 μmol/L).[65] The reference interval for total serum carotenoids, determined by spectrophotometry following petroleum ether extraction, is approximately 60–200 μg/dL (1.12–3.72 μmol/L). Most assays that measure total serum carotenoids using spectrophotometric techniques report their result as β-carotene for convenience. Serum β-carotene levels tend to inversely correlate with the number of cigarettes smoked per day.[70] Although not statistically significant, males tend to have a lower serum β-carotene level than do females.[70]

β-carotene levels rise following meals, peaking after 4–5 hours in patients with normal digestion. Carotenoid levels are increased in hypothyroid patients secondary to decreased conversion to vitamin A and in patients with hyperlipidemia, diabetes mellitus, and in pregnant women. Increased levels may also be found in patients ingesting increased quantities of natural and synthetic carotenoids. Serum levels are decreased in patients with malabsorption and malnutrition. Severe fat malabsorption is associated with carotenoid levels below 30 μg/dL (<0.56 μmol/L).

When malabsorption is suspected, a β-carotene absorption test is more reliable than a single β-carotene level. The reference population will show an increase of at least 35 μg/dL (≥0.65 μmol/L) between the initial fasting and after loading determinations.

Test: Abnormal Iron Absorption

Hemochromatosis is a serious disorder of iron metabolism that includes the clinical spectrum of liver disease (greater than 80%), diabetes mellitus (30–80%), skin pigmentation (80–90%), and cardiac, neurologic, and arthritic manifestations. Untreated, hemochromatosis has nearly a 70% mortality. Diabetes mellitus results from pancreatic atrophy and fibrosis that accompanies the disease but no direct correlation between the amount of islet cell iron deposition and the severity of glucose intolerance exists. Iron absorption is regulated in part by intestinal absorption; one theory regarding hemochromatosis pathogenesis suggests the disease is due to a disorder of intestinal iron absorption. Regulation of iron metabolism, serum iron, iron binding capacity, transferrin, and ferritin are discussed in greater detail elsewhere (see Ch. 17).

TESTS FOR CYSTIC FIBROSIS

Test: Sweat Chloride (See Ch. 15)

Background and Selection

Cystic fibrosis (CF) is the most common autosomal recessive disease. Organ systems most often involved are the sweat glands, lungs, and pancreas. Although many CF patients previously died from pancreatic insufficiency, pancreatic enzyme replacement has significantly reduced the morbidity and mortality from this cause. Most patients now succumb to opportunistic pulmonary infections, particularly *Pseudomonas aeruginosa*.

The sweat glands in healthy individuals initially produce isotonic sweat that is subsequently rendered hypotonic by active electrolyte resorption in the sweat duct. Patients with CF produce increased sweat sodium apparently owing to a resorptive transport mechanism defect.[71] This transport defect serves as the basis for the sweat chloride test that is the gold standard for CF diagnosis.

Logistics

Patient sweat is collected on preweighed gauze or paper following stimulation with pilocarpine and a low electric current. Test reliability requires the collection of at least 100 mg of sweat. Care must be taken to avoid collection surface contamination before and after the test. The patient's skin should be clean and dry before the test begins. Sodium chloride depleted CF patients may have sweat electrolyte values within the reference interval.

Interpretation

Healthy individuals have sweat chloride levels between 5 and 35 mEq/L (5 and 35 mmol/L), whereas CF patients typically have sweat chloride levels between 60 and 160 mEq/L (60 and 160 mmol/L). Using 60 mEq/L (60 mmol/L) as the discrimination value, the sweat chloride test has a 98% sensitivity for CF diagnosis.[72] Sweat sodium may alternatively be measured. Sweat sodium ranges from 10–40 mEq/L (10–40 mmol/L) and 70–190 mEq/L (70–190 mmol/L) in the reference and CF populations, respectively. Sweat electrolyte elevations have been reported in adrenal insufficiency, hypothyroidism, ectodermal dysplasia, malnutrition, mucopolysaccharidosis, fucosidosis, nephrogenic diabetes insipidus, glucose 6-phosphatase deficiency, familial cholestasis, and several other uncommon diseases.[73] These diseases, however, are clinically distinct from CF and do not pose a serious diagnostic problem.

Test: Restriction Fragment Length Polymorphism (RFLP) (See Ch. 15)

The basic genetic defect of CF is now known. In about 70% of individuals with CF, the phenylalanine residue at position 508 is deleted in the protein called cystic fibrosis transmembrane conductance regulator (CFTR). Before the specific CF gene was known, genetic information in close proximity was identified using RFLP. A mutant gene is indirectly located through its genetic proximity (linkage) to another well characterized nucleotide marker. These markers constitute 0.1–1% of DNA, are naturally occurring variations in the nucleotide DNA sequences, and are not phenotypically expressed. Nucleic acid alteration in these pleomorphic sequences alters their susceptibility to a group of bacterial enzymes, known as restriction endonucleases, that split DNA molecules at unique nucleotide series.

The laboratory obtains peripheral or neonatal blood, extracts the DNA, and digests it with a specific endonuclease, yielding DNA restriction fragments. The fragments are separated based on size by electrophoresis, transferred to a nitrocellulose or other solid support, and hybridized with a probe detecting a pleomorphic site genetically linked to the CF locus. Generally, hybridization is detected by autoradiography although new sensitive nonisotopic detection systems are being advanced.[74]

Using RFLP analysis, the CF gene has been localized to chromosome 7.[75,76] The specificity and sensitivity of the technique increases with additional probes for different linked loci.[77] As the technique becomes more refined and more closely linked markers are identified, its value in the diagnosis of CF and many other genetic diseases will expand.

GASTRIC FUNCTION

INTRODUCTION

The stomach is divided into four regions, the cardia, fundus, body, and antrum, each with unique functions. Cardiac mucosa secretes only mucin, whereas fundic and body glands contain acid and IF-secreting parietal cells and pepsinogen-secreting chief cells. Antral pyloric glands produce the most gastrin. Endocrine cells throughout the stomach produce a variety of peptide and amine hormones including serotonin, somatostatin, gastrin, vasoactive inhibitory peptide, adrenocorticotrophic hormone (ACTH)-like peptide, and enkephalin.[78]

Gastric acid secretion is proportional to parietal cell mass and is stimulated by the presence, smell, or taste of food; the presence of food in the stomach promotes neural (vagus nerve) and hormonal (gastrin) mediated secretion and intraluminal digested proteins. Gastric acid secretion is not stimulated by fat or glucose. In the presence of stomach acid and already activated pepsin, pepsinogen is quickly converted to its active proteolytic form, pepsin. Pepsinogen secretion is promoted by neural (vagal) and hormonal (gastrin, secretin, and CCK-PZ) stimulation. Gastric inhibitory peptide, anticholinergics, histamine antagonists, and vagotomy oppose pepsinogen secretion.[54]

Gastrin is produced mainly by the antral G cells although production also occurs in the small intestine and pancreas. Gastrin is transported via the circulatory system to its target organs including the stomach, which promotes acid secretion, release of pepsinogen, and IF; the small intestine, which releases secretin; and the pancreas, which is stimulated to produce bicarbonate. Three active forms of gastrin commonly exist naturally, with 34 amino acids (G-34, big gastrin), 17 amino acids (G-17, little gastrin), and 14 amino acids (G-14, mini gastrin). Segments of the peptide as small as four amino acids retain some biologic activity.[54]

TESTS FOR GASTRIC FUNCTION

Test: Gastric Acid Secretion

Background and Selection

Gastric acid analysis is useful for assessing patients with Zollinger-Ellison syndrome (gastrin secreting neoplasm) and recurrent peptic ulcer disease; for evaluating hyperacidity and pre- and postoperative acid output; following surgery (i.e., vagotomy, partial gastrectomy) for confirming the diagnosis of achlorhydria (i.e., atrophic gastritis); and evaluating patients with recurrent postoperative ulcer symptoms.[79] Gastric acid stimulation is contraindicated in patients with gastrointestinal bleeding or severe peptic ulcer disease. The presence of delayed gastric emptying, infection, and bleeding may be detected by gastric analysis.

Logistics

Gastric acid stimulation is facilitated by pharmacologic agents such as Histalog (3-β- aminoethylpyrazol). The patient is generally premedicated with an antihistamine 30 minutes before Histalog administration. Acid output peaks 1.5–2 hours after injection. Rare cases of anaphylaxis have been reported; the patient should be carefully observed during and following injection. Gastrin and pentagastrin may be used to stimulate acid secretion. Gastrin is the most potent gastric acid stimulator; synthetic pentagastrin has a less intense but similar effect. Pentagastrin is administered subcutaneously, producing a reliable response; it is currently the standard gastric acid stimulation agent. Gastric acid production tests are conducted following an overnight fast. Medications that may alter gastric secretion (e.g., antihistamines, H_2 antagonists, cholinergics, anticholinergics, tranquilizers, antidepressants, and carbonic anhydrase inhibitors) should not be taken in the 24 hours before the test is scheduled.

Interpretation

After 12 hours, gastric residue in the reference population is less than 100 mL. Increased volume suggests pyloric obstruction, regurgitated duodenal contents, or increased secretion. The residue is usually clear but may be slightly discolored by bile. A brown-red color suggests blood; blood in the gastric fluid suggests ulceration, neoplastic disease, or severe gastritis. Reference population gastric residue free acid does not exceed 40 mEq/L (40 mmol/L). Roughly 5% of healthy, young individuals have no free acid in the gastric residue and this likelihood increases with age. Therefore, the diagnosis of hypochlorhydria or achlorhydria should only be made after the results of a gastric acid stimulation test have been obtained. The residue pH ranges from 1.5–3.5 in the reference population.

A complete gastric analysis includes determination of the basal, peak, and maximum acid outputs. The basal acid output (BAO) can either be calculated from an overnight 12-hour or a 30-minute collection. In either case, acid output is determined by titration and reported in mEq/h (mmol/h). The peak acid output (PAO) is determined following administration of a gastric acid stimulator, followed by gastric secretion collection in 15-minute intervals for 90 minutes. Maximum acid output is defined as the average per hour output obtained from the first hour's collections. Peak acid output is the average of the two fractions with the highest free acid. The BAO/PAO ratio is useful for test interpretation.

Basal acid outputs less than 5 mEq/h (<5 mmol/h) and PAO between 5 and 20 mEq/h (5 and 20 mmol/h) are within the reference interval, although they may also be associated with gastric ulcer disease. Duodenal ulcer is suggested by a BAO between 5 and 15 mEq/h (5 and 15 mmol/h). A PAO between 20 and 60 mEq/h (20 and 60 mmol/h) suggests gastrointestinal pathology (such as duodenal ulcer, Zollinger-Ellison syndrome) even though some healthy individuals may have outputs in this range. Basal acid outputs greater than 20 mEq/h (>20 mmol/h) and PAO greater than 60 mEq/h (>60 mmol/h) are highly suggestive of Zollinger-Ellison syndrome and should prompt further diagnostic evaluation. The reference population has a BAO/PAO ratio less than 0.20; ratios between 0.20 and 0.40 suggest duodenal or gastric ulcer disease, 0.40–0.60 suggest duodenal ulcer disease or Zollinger-Ellison syndrome, and ratios greater than 0.60 highly suggest Zollinger-Ellison syndrome (Table 5-6).

Test: Gastrin

Background and Selection

Serum gastrin may aid in the differential diagnosis of gastric diseases (Table 5-7). Gastrin levels may be appropriately increased in physiologic response to hypoacidity (e.g., following gastric resection). In gastrin-producing cells, hyperplasias and neoplasias, gastrin production is not responsive to usual feedback control mechanisms, thus hypergastrinemia is considered inappropriate.

Gastrinomas are found in 0.1% of duodenal ulcer patients and in 1–2% of those with recurrent ulcers following surgical treatment. Most gastrinomas are pancreatic (85%) with most remaining neoplasms arising in the duodenum. The malignancy risk is about 60–65%; pancreatic neoplasms have a higher malignancy risk, whereas intestinal lesions have a lower risk. Gastrinoma presents clinically as Zollinger-Ellison syndrome. The clinical laboratory confirms the diagnosis by measuring serum gastrin and gastric acid output.

Logistics

Serum gastrin should be collected following an overnight fast and the specimen stored frozen before it is assayed because gastrin immunoreactivity quickly de-

Table 5-6. Gastric Acid Analysis

	BAO	PAO	Ratio BAO/PAO
Reference population	<5 mEq/h[a]	5–20 mEq/h	0.20
Gastric ulcer	<5 mEq/h	5–20 mEq/h	0.20
Duodenal ulcer	5–15 mEq/h	20–60 mEq/h	0.40–0.60
Zollinger-Ellison syndrome	>20 mEq/h	>60 mEq/h	>0.60

Abbreviations: BAO, basal acid output; PAO, peak acid output.
[a] Conventional units are mEq/h; SI units are mmol/h; the conversion factor is one.

Table 5-7. Conditions Associated With Increased Gastrin Levels

Gastrinoma
Antral G-cell hyperplasia
Retained antrum following gastric resection
Postvagotomy
Atrophic gastritis
Pyloric obstruction
Chronic renal failure
Elderly individuals
Rheumatoid arthritis
Cirrhosis

---

clines with refrigerator storage. Care should be taken to avoid freezing and thawing, which may occur in conventional frost-free freezers. Plasma analysis is unacceptable.

Interpretation

The reference range for gastrin levels as measured by radioimmunoassay is up to 100 pg/mL, values up to eight times this concentration are observed in 15% of elderly individuals. Daily cyclic variation exists, with lowest levels early in the morning. Increased gastrin levels should prompt further investigation of the pathologic processes listed in Table 5-8.

Table 5-8. Serum Gastrin Concentrations

Healthy (30–100 pg/mL)

Low (<30 pg/mL)
　Hypothyroidism, administration of oral acid, streptozotocin, phenformin

Minimal elevations (100–500 pg/mL)
　Ingestion for food, insulin administration, malignant carcinoma of the stomach, pheochromocytoma, hyperthyroidism, hyperparathyroidism, peptic ulceration, gastritis, cirrhosis of the liver, renal failure, rheumatoid arthritis, Zollinger-Ellison syndrome (unusual), pernicious anemia (unusual)

Significant increase (500–1000 pg/mL)
　Food ingestion, insulin administration, pheochromocytoma, hyperparathyroidism, renal failure, pernicious anemia, Zollinger-Ellison syndrome

Dramatic increase (>1000 pg/mL)
　Zollinger-Ellison syndrome, pernicious anemia, parietal cell antibody-positive chronic atrophic gastritis

Test: Pepsinogen

Background and Selection

Most pepsinogen (99%) secreted by chief cells enters the stomach where it is activated to pepsin. A small fraction of the inactivated pepsinogen diffuses back into the circulation making it available for analysis. Some pepsinogen is excreted into the urine.

Logistics

Radioimmunoassay and biochemical methods exist to measure pepsinogen, with varying reference ranges depending on the test system used. The test should be performed on fasting subjects; pepsinogen levels exhibit a diurnal pattern.[54]

Interpretation

Elevated pepsinogen is found in patients with increased gastric output, gastrinoma, duodenal ulcers, and acute gastritis.[54] Patients with pepsinogen levels below the reference interval include those with gastritis, gastric neoplasia, gastric resection, Addison's disease, and myxedema.

TESTS FOR GASTROINTESTINAL NEUROENDOCRINE NEOPLASMS

It was recognized in the 1960s that many cells, including those in the digestive tract, share the ability to take in amine precursors and decarboxylate them to amines and peptides that are subsequently stored as cytoplasmic granules.[80,81] These cells belong to the amine precursor uptake and decarboxylation (APUD) group.

Neuroendocrine neoplasms may occur anywhere in the gastrointestinal tract, most frequently in the pancreas. These neoplasms may produce specific peptide products causing characteristic disease patterns. The histologic appearance of these tumors makes differentiating benign from malignant processes difficult; furthermore, long-term survival is observed with many malignant processes. These neoplasms often show familial clustering when associated with the multiple endocrine neoplasia (MEN) syndrome. Some "apudomas" produce multiple hormones that may be found by direct serum assay (e.g., gastrin in gastrinoma) or by indirect assay for hormonal function (e.g., glucose in insulinoma). Immunohistochemistry may identify specific hormones in biopsy and resection specimens.

Test: Insulin (See Ch. 7)

Patients with insulin-secreting neoplasms usually manifest hypoglycemic symptoms (i.e., fatigue, weakness, sweating, tachycardia, and tremor) and there also may be associated emotional and behavioral changes. Classic insulinoma findings described by Whipple[82] and Higgins[83] include fasting hypoglycemic attacks, a fasting glucose less than 50 mg/dL (<2.75 mmol/L), and symptomatic relief following carbohydrate ingestion.

Because fasting normally suppresses insulin secretion, immunoreactive insulin levels within or above the reference interval (6 μU/mL or more) during fasting suggest inappropriate secretion. An immunoreactive insulin (μU/mL) to glucose (mg/dL) ratio greater than 0.3 during prolonged fasting suggests neoplastic insulin production.[84]

Most insulinoma patients have elevated serum proinsulin, usually greater than 0.25 ng/mL. The percentage of circulating insulin that is proinsulin is generally over 20%.[85] Measurement of the C-peptide is useful for diagnosing insulinoma in patients receiving exogenous insulin and for excluding factitious hyperinsulinemia (see Ch. 7). Because C-peptide is not present in exogenously administered insulin preparations the C-peptide test is useful for diagnosing insulinoma. At glucose levels of 40 mg/dL (2.2 mmol/L), endogenous insulin production, measured by the C-peptide, is suppressed by 50–70%.

The C-peptide suppression test has a sensitivity of approximately 90% for the diagnosis of insulinoma. Calcium infusion is a safe test to evaluate patients for insulinoma. Following calcium gluconate infusion, the insulinoma patient's glucose to insulin ratio decreases to less than or equal to 1.5 within 1 hour. Most insulinomas are solitary and benign. Within 1 hour following surgical resection, at least a 30 mg/dL (1.65 mmol/L) rise in serum glucose is usually observed.[82]

Test: Vasoactive Intestinal Peptide (VIP)

Vasoactive intestinal peptide is distributed throughout the gut and nervous system with the greatest concentration in the distal small bowel and large bowel. The hormone mediates fluid and electrolyte secretion from the small bowel and pancreas. The volume of small bowel intestinal secretion overwhelms the colon's absorptive capacity in patients with VIP producing neoplasms, leading to fluid loss of 5–10 L/d. The clinical entity is known as Verner-Morrison syndrome or pancreatic cholera and is characterized by watery diarrhea, hypokalemia, and achlorhydria.[86] Clinical findings of hypokalemia include muscle fatigue and listlessness. Hypercalcemia, hyperglycemia, and vasodilation (flushing) commonly accompany this syndrome.[87,88] The neoplasm is most often pancreatic in adults and accompanies ganglioneuroma in children.[88] Adult pancreatic neoplasms are malignant in at least 50% of patients.[87,88]

The clinical laboratory diagnosis of VIPoma employs sensitive and specific radioimmunoassay techniques for VIP. The reference range for plasma VIP is 0–170 pg/mL. Plasma VIP levels in VIPoma patients are reported between 225 and 6000 pg/mL.[54,87] Because VIP may not always be increased in VIPoma patients, a single value within the reference interval does not exclude the presence of this disease. In addition, VIP may be used as a tumor marker to follow patients after surgical resection. Increased VIP is associated with hepatic dysfunction in cirrhosis because the hormone is cleared via the liver.

Test: Hormonal Assays for Other Endocrine Neoplasms

Other hormones secreted by endocrine neoplasms include glucagon,[89] somatostatin,[90] pancreatic polypeptide,[91] growth factor releasing factor,[92] and secretin.[82] The diagnosis is made by plasma assay for the specific hormone product. Hormonal assays may subsequently be used to evaluate patients for disease persistence or recurrence.

REFERENCES

1. Goldberg DM: Enzymes and isoenzymes in the evaluation of diseases of the pancreases. pp. 31–55. In Hamburger HA (ed): Clinical and Analytical Concepts in Enzymology. Skokie, IL, College of American Pathologists, 1983.
2. Levitt MD, Eckfeldt JH: Diagnosis of acute pancreatitis. pp. 481–502. In Go VLW, Gardner JD, Brooks FP et al. (eds): The Exocrine Pancreas: Biology, Pathobiology, and Diseases. New York, Raven Press, 1986.
3. Lott JA: Inflammatory disease of the pancreas. CRC Crit Rev Clin Lab Sci 1982;17:201–228.
4. Moossa AR: Diagnostic tests and procedures in acute pancreatitis. N Engl J Med 1984;311:639–643.
5. Steinberg WM, Goldstein SS, Davis ND et al: Diagnostic assays in acute pancreatitis: a study of sensitivity and specificity. Ann Intern Med 1985;102:576–580.

6. Sarles H: Pancreatitis: Symposium at Marseille, 1963. Basel, Karger, 1965.
7. Sarner M, Cotton PB: Classification of pancreatitis. Gut 1984;25:756–759.
8. Singer M, Gyr K, Sarles H: Revised classification of pancreatitis: report of the Second International Symposium on Classification of Pancreatitis in Marseille, France. Gastroenterology 1985;89:683–690.
9. Sarner M: Pancreatitis: definitions and classification. pp. 459–464. In Go VLW, Gardner JD, Brooks FP et al. (eds): The Exocrine Pancreas: Biology, Pathobiology, and Diseases. New York, Raven Press, 1986.
10. Spechler SJ, Dalton JW, Robbins AH et al: Prevalence of normal serum amylase levels in patients with acute alcoholic pancreatitis. Dig Dis Sci 1983;28:865–869.
11. Kressel HY: Pancreatitis: through the looking glass. Dig Dis Sci, editorial 1984;29:285–286.
12. Salt WB, Schenker S: Amylase—its clinical significance: a review of the literature. Medicine (Baltimore) 1976;55:269–289.
13. Berk JE, Shimamura J, Fridhandler L: Tumor-associated hyperamylasemia. Am J Gastroenterol 1977;68:572–577.
14. Weitzel JN, Pooler PA, Mohammed R et al: A unique case of breast carcinoma producing pancreatic-type amylase. Gasteroenterology 1986;94:519–520.
15. Eckfeldt JH, Leatherman JW, Levitt MD: High prevalence of hyperamylasemia in patients with acidemia. Ann Intern Med 1986;104:362–363.
16. Mifflin TE, Benjamin DC, Bruns DE: Rapid quantitative, specific measurement of pancreatic amylase in serum with use of a monoclonal antibody. Clin Chem 1985;31:1283–1288.
17. Johnson SG, Ellis CJ, Levitt MD: Mechanism of increased renal clearance of amylase/creatinine in acute pancreatitis. N Engl J Med 1976;295:1214–1217.
18. Levitt MD, Johnson SG: Is the C_{am}/C_{cr} ratio of value for the diagnosis of pancreatitis? Gastroenterology 1979;75:118–119.
19. Levitt MD, Ellis CJ: A rapid and simple assay to determine if macroamylasemia is the cause of hyperamylasemia. Gastroenterology 1982;83:378–382.
20. Lott JA, Patel ST, Sawhney AK et al: Assays of serum lipase: analytical and clinical considerations. Clin Chem 1986;32:1290–1302.
21. Eckfeldt JH, Kolars JC, Elson MK et al: Serum tests for pancreatitis in patients with abdominal pain. Arch Pathol Lab Med 1985;109:316–319.
22. Berk JE, Fridhandler L, Webb SF: Does hyperamylasemia in the drunken alcoholic signify pancreatitis? Am J Gastroenterol 1979;71:557–562.
23. Dutta SK, Douglass W, Smalls UA et al: Prevalence and nature of hyperamylasemia in acute alcoholism. Dig Dis Sci 1981;26:136–141.
24. Levitt MD, Ellis CJ, Meier PB: Extrapancreatic origin of chronic unexplained hyperamylasemia. N Engl J Med 1982;302:670–671.
25. Cotran RS, Kumar V, Robbins SL (eds): The pancreas. pp. 981–1010. In Pathologic Basis of Disease. 4th Ed. Philadelphia, WB Saunders, 1989.
26. Greenberger NJ, Isselbacher KJ: Disorders of absorption. pp. 1252–1268. In Wilson JD, Braunwald E, Isselbacher KJ et al. (eds): Principles of Internal Medicine. New York, McGraw-Hill, 1991.
27. Toskes PR: Malabsorption. pp. 732–745. In Wyngaarden JB, Smith LH (eds): Cecil Textbook of Medicine. Philadelphia, WB Saunders, 1988.
28. Landisch PG: Exocrine pancreatic function tests. Gut 1982;23:777–798.
29. Arvantitakis C, Cooke AR: Diagnostic tests of exocrine pancreatic function and disease. Gastroenterology 1978;74:932–948.
30. Sale JK, Goldberg DM, Thjodleifsson B, Wormsley KG: Trypsin and chymotrypsin in duodenal aspirate and faeces in response to secretin and cholecystokinin-pancreozymin. Gut 1974;15:132–138.
31. Gyr K, Stalder GA, Schiffmann I et al: Oral administration of a chymotrypsin-labile peptide—a new test of exocrine pancreatic function (PFT). Gut 1976;17:27–32.
32. Weizman Z, Forstner GG, Gaskin KJ et al: Bentiromide test for assessing pancreatic dysfunction using analysis of para-aminobenzoic acid in plasma and urine. Gastroenterology 1985;89:596–604.
33. van de Kamer JH, ten Bokkel Huinink H, Weyers HA: Rapid method for the determination of fat in feces. J Biol Chem 1949;77:347–355.
34. DiMango EP, Go VLW, Summerskill WHJ: Relations between pancreatic enzyme outputs and malabsorption in severe pancreatic insufficiency. N Engl J Med 1973;288:813–815.
35. Watson WC: The malabsorption syndrome. pp. 92–125. In Gillespie I, Thomson TJ (eds): Gastroenterology: An Integrated Course. New York, Churchill Livingstone, 1983.
36. Pedersen NT, Halgreen H: Faecal fat and faecal weight: reproducibility and diagnostic efficiency of various regimens. Scand J Gastroenterol 1984;19:350–354.
37. Pedersen NT, Halgreen H, Worning H: Estimation of the 3-day faecal fat excretion and fat concentration as a differential test for malabsorption and maldigestion. Scand J Gastroenterol 1987;22:91–96.
38. Pedersen NT: Fat digestion tests. Digestion 37 (suppl 1), 1987;25–34.
39. Lurie B, Brom B, Bank S et al: Comparative response of exocrine pancreatic secretion following a test meal and secretin-pancreozymin stimulation. Scand J Gastroenterol 1973;8:27–32.
40. Moeller DD, Dunn GD, Klotz AP: Comparison of the pancreozymin-secretin test and the Lundh test meal. Am J Dig Dis 1972;17:799–805.
41. Gyr K, Agrawal NM, Felsenfeld O, Font RG: Comparative study of secretin and Lundh tests. Am J Dig Dis 1975;20:506–512.
42. Rolny P, Jagenburg T: The secretin-CCK test and a modified Lundh test. A comparative study. Scand J Gastroenterol 1978;13:927–931.
43. Braganza JM, Rao JJ: Disproportionate reduction in tryptic response to endogenous compared with exogenous stimulation in chronic pancreatitis. Br J Med 1978;2:392–394.
44. Lundh G: Pancreatic exocrine function in neoplastic and inflammatory disease: a simple and reliable new test. Gastroenterology 1962;42:275.
45. Newcomer AD, Hofmann AF, DiMango EP et al: Triolein breath test—a sensitive and specific test for fat malabsorption. Gastroenterology 1979;76:6–13.
46. Watkins JB, Klein PD, Schoeller DA et al: Diagnosis and differentiation of fat malabsorption in children using

^{13}C-labeled lipids: trioctanoin, triolein, and palmitic acid breath tests. Gastroenterology 1982;82:911–917.
47. Einarsson K, Bjorkhem I, Eklof R, Blomstrand R: ^{14}C-triolein breath test as a rapid and convenient test for fat malabsorption. Scand J Gastroenterol 1983;18:9–12.
48. Goff JS: Two stage triolein breath test differentiates pancreatic insufficiency from other causes of malabsorption. Gastroenterology 1982;83:44–46.
49. Goldstein R, Blondheim O, Levy E et al: The fatty test meal: an alternative to stool fat analysis. Am J Clin Nutr 1983;38:763–767.
50. Helmer OM, Fouts PJ: Gastro-intestinal studies. VII. The excretion of xylose in pernicious anemia. J Clin Invest 1937;16:343–349.
51. Fourman LPR: The absorption of xylose in steatorrhea. Clin Sci 1948;6:289–294.
52. Haeney MR, Culnak LS, Montgomery RD, Sammons HG: Evaluation of xylose absorption as measured in blood and urine: a one hour blood xylose screening test in malabsorption. Gastroenterology 1978;75:393–400.
53. Worwag EM, Craig RM, Jansyn EM et al: D-xylose absorption and disposition with moderately impaired renal function. Clin Pharmacol Ther 1987;41:351–357.
54. Tietz NW, Rinker AD, Henderson AR: Gastric, pancreatic and intestinal function. pp. 1434–1493. In Tietz NW (ed): Textbook of Clinical Chemistry. Philadelphia, WB Saunders, 1986.
55. Young DS, Pestaner LC, Gibberman V: Effects of drugs on clinical laboratory tests. Clin Chem 1975;21:1D.
56. Bond JH, Levitt MD: Use of breath hydrogen (H_2) in the study of carbohydrate absorption. Dig Dis 1977;22:379–382.
57. Newcomer AD, McGill DB, Thomas PJ, Hoffman AF: Prospective comparison of indirect methods for detecting lactase deficiency. N Engl J Med 1975;293:1232–1235.
58. Caspary WF: Breath tests. Clin Gastroenterol 1978;7:351.
59. King CE, Toskes PP: Comparison of the 1 gram [^{14}C]xylose, 10-gram lactulose-H_2 and 80 gram glucose-H_2 breath tests in patients with small intestine bacterial overgrowth. Gastroenterology 1986;91:1447.
60. Russell RI, Lee FD: Tests of small intestinal function-digestion, absorption, secretion. Clin Gastroenterol 1978;7:277–315.
61. Cotran RS, Kumar V, Robbins SL (eds): Nutritional diseases. pp. 435–438. In Pathologic Basis of Disease. 4th Ed. Philadelphia, WB Saunders, 1989.
62. Schilling RF: Intrinsic factor defects. J Lab Clin Med 1953;42:860–866.
63. Zuckier LS, Chervu LR: Schilling evaluation of pernicious anemia: current status. J Nucl Med 1984;25:1032–1039.
64. Olson JA: Provitamin A function of carotenoids: the conversions of β-carotene into vitamin A. J Nutr 1989;119:105–108.
65. Bendich A: The safety of β-carotene. Nutr Cancer 1988;11:207–214.
66. Parker RS: Carotenoids in human blood and tissues. J Nutr 1989;119:101–104.
67. Burton GW: Antioxidant action of carotenoids. J Nutr 1989;119:109–111.
68. Ziegler RG: A review of epidemiologic evidence that carotenoids reduce the risk of cancer. J Nutr 1989;119:116–122.
69. Shekelle RB, Lepper M, Liu S et al: Dietary vitamin A and risk of cancer in the Western Electric Study. Lancet 1981;2:1185–1190.
70. Comstock GW, Menkes MS, Schober SE et al: Serum levels of retinol, beta-carotene, and alpha-tocopherol in older adults. Am J Epidemiol 1988;127:114–123.
71. Welsh MJ, Fick RB: Cystic fibrosis. J Clin Invest 1987;80:1523–1526.
72. Davis PB, Hubbard VS, DiSant'Agnese PA: Low sweat electrolytes in a patient with cystic fibrosis. Am J Med 1980;69:643–646.
73. Shwachman H, Mahmoodian A: The sweat test and cystic fibrosis. Diagn Med 1982;5:61–76.
74. Thibodeau SN: Use of restriction fragment length polymorphism analysis for detecting carriers of "fragile-X" syndrome. Clin Chem 1987;33:1726–1730.
75. Tsui LC, Zengerling S, Willard HF, Buchwald M: Mapping of the cystic fibrosis locus on chromosome 7. Cold Spring Harbor Symp Quant Biol 1986;51:325–335.
76. Klinger KW, Winqvist R, Riccio A et al: Plasminogen activator inhibitor type 1 gene is located at region q21.3-q22 of chromosome 7 and genetically linked with cystic fibrosis. Proc Natl Acad Sci USA 1987;84:8548–8552.
77. Donis-Keller H, Barker DF, Knowlton RG et al: Highly polymorphic RFLP probes as diagnostic tools. Cold Spring Harbor Symp Quant Biol 1986;51:317–324.
78. Lewin KJ: The endocrine cells of the gastrointestinal tract: the normal endocrine cells and their hyperplasias. Pathol Annu 1986;21:1–27.
79. Powell DW, Drossman DA: Gastric analysis. pp. 53–61. In Drossman DA (ed): Manual of Gastroenterologic Procedures. New York, Raven Press, 1982.
80. Pearse AGE: Common cytochemical and ultrastructural characteristics of cells producing polypeptide hormones (the APUD series) and their relevance to thyroid and multibranchial C-cells and calcitonin. Proc R Soc Lond 1968;170:71–78.
81. Pearse AGE: The cytochemistry and ultrastructure of polypeptide hormone producing cells of APUD series and the embryologic, physiologic and pathologic implications of the concept. J Histochem Cytochem 1969;17:303–311.
82. Whipple AO, Frantz VK: Adenoma of islet cells with hyperinsulinoma. Ann Surg 1935;101:1299–1335.
83. Higgins GA: Pancreatic islet cell tumors: insulinoma, gastrinoma, and glucagonoma. Surg Clin North Am 1979;59:131–141.
84. Friesen SR: Tumors of the endocrine pancreas. New Engl J Med 1982;306:580–590.
85. Kaplan EL, Lee CH: Recent advances in the diagnosis and treatment of insulinomas. Surg Clin North Am 1979;59:119–129.
86. Verner JV, Morrison AB: Islet cell tumor and a syndrome of refractory watery diarrhea and hypokalemia. Am J Med 1958;29:374–380.
87. Debas HT: Clinical significance of gastrointestinal hormones. Adv Surg 1987;21:157–188.
88. O'Dorisio TM, Makhjian HS. VIPoma syndrome. pp. 101–116. In Cohen S, Soloway RD (eds): Hormone Producing Tumors of the Gastrointestinal Tract. New York, Churchill Livingstone, 1985.
89. Holst JJ: Glucagon-producing tumors. pp. 57–84. In Cohen S, Soloway RD (eds): Hormone Producing Tumors of the Gastrointestinal Tract. New York, Churchill Livingstone, 1985.
90. Boden G, Simoyama R: Somatostatinoma. pp. 85–101.

In Cohen S, Soloway RD (eds): Hormone Producing Tumors of the Gastrointestinal Tract. New York, Churchill Livingstone, 1985.
91. O'Dorisio TM, Vinik AI: Pancreatic polypeptide- and mixed peptide-producing tumors of the gastrointestinal tract. pp. 117–128. In Cohen S, Soloway RD (eds): Hormone Producing Tumors of the Gastrointestinal Tract. New York, Churchill Livingstone, 1985.
92. Frohman LA, Zabo M, Berelowitz M, et al: Partial purification of a peptide with GH releasing activity from extrapituitary tumors in patients with acromegaly. J Clin Invest 1980;65:43–55.

6 Body Fluids

Amin Nanji

INTRODUCTION

Body fluid analysis includes examination of the physical, chemical, and cellular elements in fluids derived from a variety of anatomic cavities. These fluids include cerebrospinal, synovial, pleural, pericardial, and ascitic fluids. Examination of body fluids is an important diagnostic maneuver: the commonly used tests are reviewed in this chapter by fluid source. Amniotic fluid tests are found in Chapter 15. Chapter 23 reviews the microbiologic aspects of fluids, except cerebrospinal fluid, which is covered in Chapter 27.

CEREBROSPINAL FLUID

Cerebrospinal fluid (CSF) is formed by the ultrafiltration of plasma in the highly vascular choroid plexus of the ventricles. It fills the subarachnoid space within and around the central nervous system (CNS) and is absorbed by the arachnoid sinuses. The total volume of CSF is about 150 mL; 500–600 mL is formed daily with the total CSF volume renewed every 5–7 hours.[1] The main indication for a spinal tap is suspected bacterial meningitis; CSF analysis is also used in the diagnosis of demyelinating diseases. There are a number of clinical contraindications for performing a spinal tap including papilledema, focal neurologic findings, and the presence of hemostasis disorders. Characteristics of normal CSF are given in Table 6-1.[2]

Normal CSF is clear and colorless, whereas abnormal CSF may appear cloudy, purulent, bloody, or pigmented. Leukocytosis is the most common cause of cloudy or turbid fluid. Xanthochromia refers to a pale pink to yellow color of the supernatant of a CSF specimen. The color usually represents the breakdown of cells, with three pigments contributing to xanthochromia: oxyhemoglobin, methemoglobin, and bilirubin. Plasma contamination from traumatic taps also can cause xanthochromia, for example, if the patient has hypercarotenemia. Xanthochromia is normal in the CSF from premature infants, because of the immaturity of the blood-brain barrier.[1]

A traumatic tap refers to local bleeding that can occur in up to 20% of patients who undergo lumbar punctures. In traumatic taps, the supernatant is clear, in contrast to the xanthochromic fluid that typically is associated with subarachnoid hemorrhage. Xanthochromia indicates that blood has been in the CSF for at least 1–2 hours.[3] Because lysis of red blood cells (RBCs) occurs in vitro within a few hours, the CSF specimen should be examined promptly to make the distinction between a traumatic tap and a subarachnoid hemorrhage. Cell counts also may be helpful in identifying traumatic taps (see Test: CSF Cell Count).

Routine laboratory examination of CSF usually includes determination of cellularity, total protein, and microbiologic studies. For a discussion of the latter as well as details regarding specimen collection see Chapter 27, Central Nervous System under Test: Cerebrospinal Fluid. For patients suspected of having bacterial meningitis, CSF glucose and lactate measurements also are frequently ordered.

Table 6-1. Characteristics of Normal Cerebrospinal Fluid

Volume	90–160 mL (adult)
Color	Colorless
Transparency (appearance)	Clear
Specific gravity	1.006–1.008
Glucose	40–70 mg/dL (60–80% of the blood glucose)
Protein	15–45 mg/dL
Lactate dehydrogenase	8–50 IU/L
Cells	0–5 mononuclear cells/mm^3 (chamber count method) or 0–5000 mononuclear cells/mL (membrane filtration method)

BASIC CEREBROSPINAL FLUID TESTS

Text: Cerebrospinal Fluid Cell Count

The CSF cell count is probably the most important indicator of bacterial meningitis. It varies with patient age, with total white blood cell (WBC) count in the healthy adult CSF ranging from zero to five mononuclear cells (lymphocytes and monocytes), with greater than 10/mm^3 considered abnormal. Pleocytosis of the monocytes can be graded as well. In healthy newborns, both mononuclear and granulocytic cells can be present: a cell count of up to 30/mm^3 is considered normal in both preterm and full term infants.[1] When a cytocentrifuge preparation is examined, an occasional polymorphonuclear cell can be seen in the CSF of healthy individuals.

If the initial CSF is bloody, both the first and the third tubes can be sent for a cell count and the results compared, but the actual WBC count of the CSF can be approximated by using a correction factor for contamination of the CSF with peripheral blood. If the peripheral counts are normal, the ratio of 1 WBC/700 RBC (for the normal ratio of WBC/RBC) can be subtracted from the CSF WBC count. The validity of this calculation has been questioned. A recent study, however, showed that if the observed WBC count was more than 10 times the WBC number indicated by the adjustment calculation, this indicated meningitis with a specificity of 90%.[4] Table 6-2 shows the causes of increased leukocytes in CSF.[5] Most patients with meningitis associated with malignancy have malignant cells in their CSF; other typical findings include elevated leukocyte counts, increased protein, and normal to decreased levels of glucose.[3]

Table 6-2. Causes of Increased Leukocytes in Cerebrospinal Fluid

Cell Type	Disease Process

Neutrophils	Infectious
	  Bacterial meningitis
	  Early tuberculous meningitis
	  Early viral meningitis
	  Early mycotic meningitis
	Noninfectious
	  Posthemorrhagic infarct
	  Subarachnoid hemorrhage
	  Intrathecal administration of medications, contrast media
	  Intracerebral hematoma

Lymphocytes	Infectious
	  Tuberculous and fungal meningitis
	  Partially treated bacterial meningitis
	  Viral encephalitis and meningitis
	  Measles
	  Subacute sclerosing panencephalitis
	Noninfectious
	  Multiple sclerosis
	  Polyneuritis
	  Chronic alcoholism and drug abuse
	  Periarteritis

Eosinophils	Infectious
	  Bacterial, viral, and fungal meningitis
	Noninfectious
	  Allergy
	  Intrathecal drugs and dyes
	  Acute polyneuritis
	  Periarteritis nodosa

Macrophages	Infectious
	  Tuberculosis, mycotic meningitis
	Noninfectious
	  Acute intracranial bleeding
	  Contrast media

Test: Cerebrospinal Fluid Glucose

The relationship between CSF and serum glucose is complex. Sudden changes in the serum level of glucose cause similar changes in the CSF. These changes, however, are not seen immediately because equilibrium between CSF and serum does not occur for at least 1–2 hours. With each incremental change in the serum glucose concentration, CSF glucose increases to a lesser degree because of saturation kinetics. At high serum glucose levels, the ratio of CSF/serum glucose is in the range of 0.4 as compared with the normal ratio of about 0.6.

The lower limit of normal for CSF glucose is in the range of 40–50 mg/dL (2.22–2.78 mmol/L) with a CSF/serum glucose ratio of 0.40:0.50.[6] The most important reason for measuring CSF glucose is in the diagnosis of bacterial meningitis. A low CSF level glucose (less than 40 mg/dL [<2.22 mmol/L]) is found in about 50–60% of patients with bacterial meningitis. A study evaluating the use of the CSF/serum glucose ratio showed that a ratio of less than 0.31 was found in 45 of 64 patients with meningitis, including 10 in whom the absolute CSF glucose was less than 40 mg/dL (<2.22 mmol/L).[7] The ratio was greater than 0.31 in 35 of 36 uninfected diabetic patients.

Because glucose results tend to be lowest in patients with the highest elevations in CSF cell counts and/or CSF protein, glucose measurements may not necessarily provide additional useful information in patients with bacterial meningitis.[8] Glucose also is decreased in a considerable percentage of patients with chronic infectious meningitis, subarachnoid hemorrhage, or malignant meningitis. Moreover, normal CSF glucose does not exclude the diagnosis of bacterial meningitis; glucose is decreased in only 50–60% of patients. After treatment for bacterial meningitis, CSF glucose returns to normal in most patients by the third day.[1]

Test: Cerebrospinal Fluid Protein

Background and Selection

Production of the CSF protein takes place by ultrafiltration, by diffusion of small proteins, and by pinocytosis of large proteins. However, much less protein is present in the CSF than in the serum and its composition shows relative increases in some of the low molecular mass components. This occurs because the blood-brain barrier acts as the molecular sieve at least to some extent. Because CSF protein is elevated in a variety of disorders, it is a useful indicator of CNS disease and is routinely measured. In cases of meningitis, CSF protein is usually increased.

Logistics

Because of the low protein concentration and relatively small sample volume available, usually a turbidometric procedure is used. The trichloracetic acid technique has been recommended because it is less sensitive to turbidity differences between albumin and globulins than is the sulfosalicylic acid method.

Interpretation

The amount of protein in CSF varies with the person's age and the site of CSF removal. The usual reference interval for fluid removed from the lumbar region in healthy adults is about 25 mg/dL (250 mg/L). By contrast, children tend to have lower levels, whereas newborns have higher concentrations, presumably caused by a poorly developed blood-brain barrier. Elderly persons have higher concentrations of CSF protein than younger adults. Fluid from the ventricular and cisternal regions generally has a lower protein content than fluid from the lumbar region. A traumatic tap can lead to elevations in CSF proteins, but a correction factor 1 mg/dL (10 mg/L) protein can be subtracted for every 1000 RBC.[1]

An increase in the level of total protein indicates CNS disease; however, a number of CNS diseases can cause elevation. Increased total protein levels can occur as a result of CNS abscesses, tumors, and hematomas, as well as from chronic inflammation, cerebrovascular disease, and intracranial obstruction. Often the total protein is measured in the setting of the suspected acute inflammatory conditions, especially meningitis. With the increased capillary permeability occurring in meningitis, total protein levels are increased. In most patients with meningitis, total protein is elevated along with an increased opening pressure and abnormal cell count.[8] In pyogenic and tuberculous meningitis, total protein concentrations tend to be higher than those in viral disease. Results of CSF protein measurements also are useful for confirming suspected chronic infectious meningitis and for detecting meningitis caused by malignancy. Elevated CSF protein with a normal WBC count occurs in about 20% of patients having meningitis caused by malignancy and in 10% of those individuals with fungal meningitis.[8] Typically, Guillain-Barré syndrome is associated with high CSF protein with the remainder of the CSF analyses within normal limits.[3]

Test: Cerebrospinal Fluid Lactate

Background

Sixty years ago Levinson drew attention to changes in the pH in the CSF of patients with pyogenic meningitis.[9] These changes were caused by increased lactate, as

Table 6-3. Summary of Studies Using Lactate Acid Measurement in Cerebrospinal Fluid to Distinguish Bacterial From Nonbacterial Meningitis

Study No.	CSF Lactate in Bacterial Meningitis (mmol/L)	CSF Lactate in Nonbacterial Meningitis (mmol/L)	Method of Lactate Measurement	Comments
1	3.0–30.2 (n = 38)	1.2–5.1 (n = 17)	GLC	Major overlap seen in lactate levels between bacterial and nonbacterial meningitis
2	>3.3	<2.8	Enzymatic	
3	>2.8 (60/62)[a]	<2.8 (299/299)[a]	GLC and enzymatic	Lactate levels decline with treatment; decline seen before the decrease in WBCs
4	>4.5 (14/15)	<4.5 (24/24)	Enzymatic	Levels of lactate in patients with partially treated meningitis overlapped with levels in viral meningitis
5	>2.2 (16/16)	<2.2 (26/26)	GLC	Within 48 hours of treatment, 12 of 16 patients with bacterial meningitis had levels in the nonbacterial range
6	>3.0 (27/29)	<3.0 (135/156)	Enzymatic	Misleadingly high values seen in patients with CNS malformations who have nonbacterial meningitis
7	>2.2 (68/68)	<2.2 (16/20)	Enzymatic	
8	>4.0 (66/66)	<4.0 (31/31)	Enzymatic	Lactate levels remained at 74.0 mmol/L in patients with bacterial meningitis until 4 days after start of therapy
9	3.5 (23/28)	<3.5 (104/121)	Enzymatic	
10	4.0 (46/46)	<4.0 (20/20)	GLC	
11	4.3 (5/5)	<4.3 (26/26)	Enzymatic	

Abbreviations: CSF, cerebrospinal fluid; GLC, gas liquid chromatography; WBCs, white blood cells; CNS, central nervous system.
[a] Number of patients with levels above or below stated lactate acid levels.
(Adapted from Nanji and Whitlow,[11] with permission.)

later confirmed by others. The cause of increased CSF lactate in bacterial meningitis is unclear, but appears to be dependent on the number of organisms present. However, only a small amount of lactate is produced by endotoxin-stimulated leukocytes and furthermore, high levels of lactate are seen in tuberculous meningitis and acute encephalitis, disorders in which few organisms and cells are present.

Other possibilities include the reduction of local blood supply in the presence of inflammation with a subsequent shift of metabolism from aerobic to anaerobic glycolysis. Also, increased intracranial pressure decreases cerebral blood flow.

Selection

Despite some shortcomings, the overwhelming evidence suggests that CSF lactate measurement is useful in the early diagnosis of bacterial meningitis.

Logistics

A decline in CSF lactate concentrations is seen in CSF specimens left at room temperature before measurement, with the decline being greater in specimens taken from patients with bacterial meningitis. To prevent misleading results for specimens that cannot be measured immediately, CSF specimens should be stored frozen at −20°C, at which temperature concentrations remain unchanged for up to 72 hours.[10]

Interpretation

If CSF lactate levels are to be used in the clinical diagnosis of bacterial meningitis, it is essential to determine the upper limit of the reference range carefully. When one examines the cutoff ranges in Table 6-3, the upper limit below which bacterial meningitis can be excluded ranges from 2.2–4.3 mEq/L (2.2–4.3 mmol/L) (see Ch. 27 under Test: Cerebrospinal Fluid Lactate).

Another major problem is the overlap in results between patients with bacterial meningitis and febrile patients with another site of bacterial infection, for example, the lungs. In one study, over one third of patients with bacterial infections at sites other than the meninges had increased CSF lactate levels in the range found in patients with bacterial meningitis. Similarly, elevated CSF lactate levels also were seen in more than one third of patients with head trauma or subarachnoid hemorrhage.

Recently, because of the ready availability of lactate measurements, there have been a large number of studies comparing lactate measurements between bacterial and other types of meningitis. Table 6-3 summarizes the data obtained from the various major studies.[11] Despite some shortcomings, the overwhelming evidence suggests that lactate measurement is useful in the early diagnosis of bacterial meningitis.

OTHER CEREBROSPINAL FLUID TESTS

Test: Cerebrospinal Fluid Lactate Dehydrogenase (LD)[12]

The distribution of LD isoenzymes in normal CSF is similar to those in serum, except that LD-1 is greater than LD-2. Increased levels of LD in neoplastic brain tissue are reflected in increased CSF LD activity, but the usefulness of LD as a marker for CNS neoplasms is controversial. Isoenzyme studies have shown that neoplastic changes in brain tissue result in a shift in the LD isoenzyme pattern from a predominance of isoenzymes 1 and 2 to a predominance of fractions 4 and 5. An increase in CSF LD-5 has consistently been observed in patients with leptomeningeal metastases, but a similar pattern is seen in patients with meningeal infections. Nonmalignant causes of increased CSF LD activity include hemorrhage, brain abscess, and cerebrovascular accident.

Test: Cerebrospinal Fluid Glutamine

See Ch. 4, Liver Function, under Test: Cerebrospinal Fluid Glutamine.

Test: CSF Immunoglobulin G (Including Derived Ratios)

Background and Selection

Immunoglobulins usually are not synthesized in the CNS, but enter the CSF via diffusion from the blood.[13] The concentration of immunoglobulins in the spinal fluid is determined largely by their molecular size and the relative impermeability of the blood-CSF barrier to large molecules. In CSF, the predominant immunoglobulin is IgG with very little IgA and IgM.

It is widely accepted that selective elevation (i.e., an increased percentage) of γ-globulin in the CSF signifies local production of the protein within the CNS. The concentration of CSF immunoglobulins may be increased for any one of three reasons.[14] First, CSF immunoglobulin can be increased by infection or other inflammation, tumor, or hemorrhage. Here the permeability of the normal blood-brain and blood-CSF barriers is increased or the anatomic barriers are destroyed, such that more blood constituents enter the CSF in a nonselective manner. The concentration of immunoglobulin along with other serum proteins increases; thus the amount of immunoglobulin relative to total protein or albumin does not change. Second, increases can occur as a result of chronic infections (outside the CNS) or connective tissue disease, when serum immunoglobulins are often diffusely increased. This increase in serum immunoglobulins in turn can lead to elevated immunoglobulin in the CSF through diffusion, but the proportion of immunoglobulin in the CSF relative to the serum is normal. Similarly, a monoclonal protein in the serum can appear in the CSF; this is readily detected by CSF protein electrophoresis. Third, increases can occur if antibody-producing cells are located within the CNS, that is, if there is local, endogenous synthesis of immunoglobulins. In this situation, the relative concentration of immunoglobulin in the CSF is increased compared with both other CSF proteins and serum immunoglobulin. For example, γ-globulin is increased in multiple sclerosis (MS), correlating weakly with extent, but not with the duration, activity, or course of disease. An increase in CSF γ-globulin occurs with a number of other diseases (see below).

Logistics

Numerous techniques including immunoprecipitation, radial immunodiffusion, and electroimmunodiffusion can be used for quantitation of CSF immunoglobulin. Electroimmunodiffusion (rocket electrophoresis) is used to measure both IgG and albumin, simultaneously. To distinguish between increased blood-brain barrier permeability and increased immunoglobulin synthesis in the CNS, CSF IgG can be expressed in relation to CSF protein or CSF albumin values. Abnormalities in CSF IgG concentrations have been expressed in a variety of ways including the IgG/total protein ratio, the IgG/albumin ratio, the IgG index [(IgG/albumin in CSF) ÷ (IgG/albumin in serum)], and the IgG synthesis rate. The CSF IgG index is a measure of CNS IgG synthesis and corrects for the effect of variations of serum albumin and IgG levels as well as blood-brain barrier damage. The IgG index, calculated as [CSF IgG/serum IgG] divided by [CSF albumin/serum albumin], tends to remain stable when serum IgG and serum albumin vary.[14]

Interpretation

The reference range for CSF γ-globulin is less than 12% of CSF protein and the reference interval for the CSF IgG index is less than 0.58.[15] Of patients with MS, 60–70% have an increased percentage of CSF γ-globulin.

The source of the immunoglobulins is believed to be increased local synthesis of IgG by lymphocytes within the CNS. Increased values for the IgG index occur in 80–90% of patients with definite MS. An increased IgG index also is seen with CNS infections and immunologic disorders. An increase in γ-globulins occur in a variety of other diseases such as neurosyphilis, acute Guillain-Barré syndrome, a variety of other acute neurologic disorders, and in some healthy individuals.

Test: Cerebrospinal Fluid Electrophoresis (Oligoclonal Banding)

Background and Selection

The electrophoretic pattern of normal CSF differs in relative concentrations of various proteins; for example, CSF has a prominent prealbumin band that migrates slightly faster than serum prealbumin. Electrophoresis of CSF specimens, however, is performed mainly to determine the presence of oligoclonal bands.

Logistics

Agarose is the most frequent CSF electrophoresis system used for demonstration of oligoclonal bands and has been shown to be superior to cellulose acetate and polyacrylamide gel. Cerebrospinal fluid is concentrated 50–80 times and runs in parallel with simultaneously drawn serum. Repeated freezing of specimens abolishes the oligoclonal bands. Isoelectric focusing is another available technique in which specimens are applied to thin-layer polyacrylamide gels with pH gradients. Although isoelectric focusing demonstrates the capacity for higher resolution of oligoclonal bands (up to 30), its clinical usefulness is limited because of a higher rate of false positive patterns and difficulty in interpretation. The use of isoelectric focusing should therefore be limited to cases where results by more conventional techniques are equivocal.

Interpretation

Electrophoresis of CSF showing two or more distinct bands in the immunoglobulin region is known as oligoclonal banding if the bands are found exclusively in the CSF or are more intense in the CSF than in the serum. Although more than 90% of patients with MS are said to have oligoclonal bands in the CSF at some time in their clinical course, the test has a lower sensitivity when used for diagnostic purposes. The sensitivity in this setting is about 70–80%.[16,17]

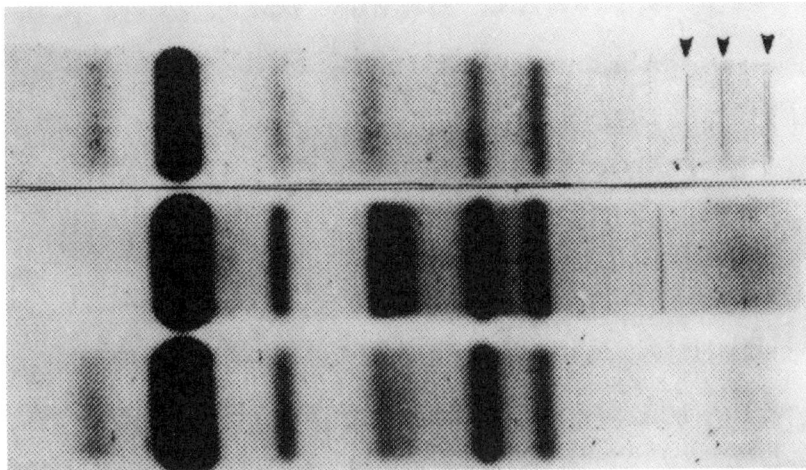

Fig. 6-1. Three channels of an agarose gel electrophoretogram are shown, with the anode on the left. The bottom channel is a sample of concentrated normal cerebrospinal fluid (CSF), with a heterogenous γ-globulin zone (no evidence of banding). The top channel is a sample of concentrated CSF from a patient with multiple sclerosis (MS); three homogenous bands (arrows) are present in the γ-globulin zone, representing an oligoclonal banding pattern. The middle channel is serum from the same patient, showing the absence of homogenous band in the gamma globulin region. (Courtesy of American Association for Clinical Chemistry.)

Figure 6-1 shows an electrophoretogram of CSF with oligoclonal banding compared with a control. Oligoclonal bands in the γ-region have been reported in a variety of diseases other than MS including myasthenia gravis, relapsing polyneuropathy, Alzheimer's disease, chronic encephalitis, meningitis, subacute sclerosing panencephalitis, herpes simplex encephalitis, CNS tumors, and acute cerebrovascular disease.[17]

It is thought that the oligoclonal reaction in some of these disorders reflects polyclonal B-cell activation within the CNS following brain tissue damage.

Test: Myelin Basic Protein (MBP)

Background and Selection

Central nervous system myelin contains approximately 70% lipid and 30% protein. Two proteins make up 80% of the total protein content of myelin. The larger protein (mass 24,000) is called proteolipid protein, and the smaller one (mass 18,500) is called myelin basic protein, because of its solubility in acid solution. The sensitivity and specificity of MBP in patients with MS is shown in Table 6-4.[18]

Table 6-4. Measurements of Myelin Basic Protein (MBP) in Patients with Multiple Sclerosis (MS) and in Control Subjects[a]

		No. of Patients With Detectable MBP[b]			
		Total Patients			Controls
Study No.	Molecular Species	Active (%)	Inactive (%)	Chronic (%)	(% Specificity)
1	MBP	21/22 (95)			
2	MBP	117/117 (100)	2/93 (2.2)	61/103 (60.1)	9/626 (98.6)
3	MBP (fragment 43–88)	23/33 (70)	1/71 (1.4)		29/425 (93.0)
4	Component III	23/23 (100)			
5	MBP (fragment 89–169)	27/28 (96)	16/25 (64)	9/19 (47)	3/23 (87)

[a] (1) Study showed the presence of a factor in the cerebrospinal fluid from patients with MS that inhibited the binding of human basic protein to α-macroglobulin or basic protein antibodies; (2) antibody specificity not defined with respect to MBP fragments; (3) measurements of MBP done within 15 days of disease exacerbation, in active group; and (4) measurements of MBP done within 15 days of disease exacerbation in active groups, after 15 days in inactive group.
[b] Shown in parentheses is the % sensitivity.
[c] Nondemyelinating neurologic diseases.
(Modified from Gupta,[18] with permission.)

Logistics

Sensitive radioimmunoassay methods can be used to quantitate nanogram amounts of CSF MBP. More recently, enzyme-linked immunosorbent assays that have better sensitivity than radioimmunoassays have been introduced. Different molecular species of MBP have been identified in CSF and can cross-react with most polyclonal antisera. Three components of MBP have been identified: component I is intact MBP, component II is proteolytic fragments of MBP, and component III is a larger protein.[19] It is thought that component III is specific for MS. The presence of these fragments complicates the measurement of MBP using polyclonal antisera; comparison of results from one assay to another also is made difficult.

Interpretation

Increases in MBP appear to be associated only with active phases of MS (Table 6-4). Release of MBP into CSF, however, is not specific for MS and is found in a variety of disorders in which myelin breakdown occurs. These include acute cerebrovascular injury, necrotizing leukoencephalopathy, postneurosurgery, encephalitis, Guillain-Barré syndrome, CNS lupus erythematosus, vasculitis, and peripheral neuropathy.[20,21] In patients with human immunodeficiency virus (HIV) infection, oligoclonal bands are found even when patients are asymptomatic.[22]

Cerebrospinal Fluid Markers of Malignancy[23]

A number of investigators have looked for biochemical markers for malignancies of the CNS. β_2-Microglobulin (B2M) as a tumor marker has been the subject of several investigations. β_2-Microglobulin, an 11,800 da protein subunit of the histocompatibility antigens found on the surface of nucleated cells, is normally present in the CSF. Cerebrospinal fluid B2M has been found to be increased when CSF contained malignant cells from solid tumors and hematologic malignancies. Minor elevations are also seen with epidermal and parenchymal metastases from solid tumors. Cerebrospinal fluid B2M also is elevated in some patients with solid tumors and hematologic malignancies without CNS involvement.

Other markers commonly measured in the CSF to detect meningeal metastases include β-glucuronidase, carcinoembryonic antigen, α-fetoprotein, and human chorionic gonadotropin (hCG). Large studies have shown that at least one of these markers is abnormal in 75–90% of patients with leptomeningeal metastases.

PLEURAL FLUID

Pleural effusions result from an imbalance or disruption in the hemostatic forces that control movement of fluid across cell membranes. Pleural effusions may have local or systemic causes and usually are categorized as transudates or exudates. Pleural fluid transudates are commonly associated with systemic edema, whereas exudates are caused by an inflammatory process. In addition, other types of fluid accumulation in the pleural space may occur. For example, localized disease, such as malignancy, may disrupt the blood vessels, resulting in hemorrhagic fluid. Some diseases may cause the accumulation of fluid by more than one mechanism; for example, malignant lymphatic obstruction may cause a transudate in addition to an exudate owing to malignant infiltration.

PLEURAL FLUID TESTS

Test: Pleural Fluid Protein

The first step in the evaluation of a pleural effusion is to determine if it is an exudate of a transudate. It is generally believed that a pleural fluid protein of 3.0 g/dL (30 g/L) or less indicates a transudate, a value greater than 3.0 g/dL (>30 g/L) indicates an exudate. However, approximately 15% of patients can be misclassified based on pleural fluid protein alone. A summary of the sensitivity, specificity, positive, and negative predictive values of pleural fluid protein in distinguishing exudates from transudates is shown in Table 6-5.

Test: Pleural Fluid Cell Count[24]

In determining the source of the effusion, the presence of RBC and WBC is useful in selected cases. Cellular characteristics of pleural fluid in different disorders are shown in Table 6-6. Blood tinged pleural effusion is of limited diagnostic value, because this can be caused by about 1 mL of blood in the pleural space. About 15% of transudates and 40% of exudates are blood tinged (equivalent to RBC count between 5000–100,000/mm^3). Whether blood was introduced via thoracentesis or was there previously can be resolved by use of the Wright stain. Previous presence of blood in the pleural space is indicated by the presence of macrophages con-

Table 6-5. Sensitivity, Specificity, and Predictive Value of Specific Gravity and Protein Determination in Differentiating Exudative and Transudative Pleural Effusions

Test	Sensitivity (%)	Specificity (%)	Predictive Value Positive	Predictive Value Negative
Specific gravity 1.1016	78	69	93	69
Protein 3 g/dL	93	85	95	78
Pleural fluid (protein ÷ serum protein = 0.05)	92	93	97	83
Protein ration combined with LD ratio	99	98	99	98

Abbreviation: LD, lactate dehydrogenase.

taining hemoglobin (Hgb) inclusion bodies. A grossly bloody effusion indicates trauma, malignancy, or pulmonary embolism.

Total pleural fluid WBC count is of limited value, but a differential count may be useful. Large numbers of polymorphonuclear leukocytes occur in white acute inflammatory processes. Small lymphocytes account for over 50% of the cells in the pleural fluid. An increase in the percentage of small lymphocytes is seen with tuberculosis and malignancy. Mesothelical cells, which line the pleural cavity, are 12–30 μm in diameter and may be confused with malignant cells. Their absence occurs with tuberculous effusions.

Table 6-6. Characteristics of Pathologic Pleural Fluid

Diagnostic	Gross Characteristics	RBC/μL	WBC/μL	Comments
Transudates				
Congestive heart failure	Clear, straw colored	<1000	<1000	Mononuclear cells predominate
Cirrhosis	Clear, straw colored	<1000	<500	Mononuclear cells predominate
Exudates				
Malignancy	Rubid, bloody	5000–100,000	1000–10,000	Mononuclear cells predominate; Cytologic examination is diagnostic in >60% of cases of malignancy
Parapneumonic	Rubid, bloody	5000–100,000	5000–100,000	Polymorphonuclear cells predominate
Pulmonary embolism	Straw colored	100–200,000	100–50,000	Both polymorphonuclear and monocytic cells are present
Pancreatic	Serosanguineous	1000–100,000	1000–50,000	Polymorphonuclear cells predominate
Collagen vascular disease	Turbid/yellow	<1000	1000–20,000	Mononuclear or polymorphonuclear cells may predominate
Tuberculosis	Straw colored	<10,000	<5000	Polymorphonuclear cells predominate early in disease; mononuclear cells predominate later on

Abbreviations: RBC, red blood cell; WBC, white blood cell.

Test: Pleural Fluid Glucose[25]

The pleural fluid glucose levels parallel those of serum. A pleural fluid glucose level of less than 60 mg/dL (<3.3 mmol/L) occurs in the following conditions: (1) parapneumonic effusions that are secondary to an infective process; (2) rheumatoid effusions that are secondary to rheumatoid disease and (3) in 15% of malignant pleural effusions. Very few patients with tuberculosis have a low pleural fluid glucose. Etiologic diagnosis of pleural effusions in the absence of other supporting evidence is unreliable.

Test: Pleural Fluid Amylase

Pleural fluid amylase is considered to be increased when results are greater than the upper limit of the serum reference interval or greater than results in a simultaneously obtained serum specimen. Pleural fluid amylase is increased in patients with acute pancreatitis, but increased activity also is seen with malignancy and esophageal rupture into the pleural cavity. Amylase isoenzymes may be of use in distinguishing the various conditions.

Test: Pleural Fluid pH and Lactate

The measurement of pleural fluid pH in patients with malignant pleural effusions provides important information.[26] A low pleural fluid pH (less than 7.2) indicates extensive involvement of the pleural space by tumor and fibrosis reflecting the terminal stage of the disease. The cause of the low pH is probably related to the accumulation of lactic acid.

Lactate measurements have been taken in patients with nonmalignant pleural effusions. A level of more than 5 mEq/L (>5 mmol/L) is found with bacterial and tuberculous effusions, while a level of less than 5 mEq/L (<5 mmol/L) is seen with other causes such as congestive heart failure, cirrhosis, trauma, and nephrosis.

Miscellaneous Tests

Pleural fluid cytology is positive in 90% of patients with pleural malignancy. A major problem is the difficulty in interpretation because mesothelial cells (which normally line the pleura) undergo marked variations in response to inflammation. Other tests that have been used include carcinoembryonic antigen (CEA), α-fetoprotein, rheumatoid factor, and lupus erythematosus (LE) cells, but most of these tests have little diagnostic value.

PERICARDIAL AND ASCITIC FLUIDS TESTS

Analysis of pericardial fluid obtained by needle pericardiocentesis and by surgical pericardiotomy is helpful in determining the cause of pericardial effusion and guiding the management of patients with this condition. One way of distinguishing a bloody pericardial effusion from an intracardial myocardial puncture is the immediate measurement of pericardial fluid pH.[27] A pH of less than 7.1 suggests that the fluid accumulation had an inflammatory cause such as bacterial pericarditis or systemic lupus erythematosus. Other measurements such as WBC count and glucose level also are useful.

Careful evaluation of ascitic fluid is also useful for distinguishing the cause of ascites formation. A recent study showed ascitic fluid cytology to be extremely sensitive for detection of peritoneal carcinomatosis.[28] However, not all patients with malignancy-related ascites have peritoneal carcinomatosis. Those patients with liver metastases and no other cause for ascites formation have low ascitic fluid protein and high alkaline phosphate.

SYNOVIAL FLUID

Laboratory studies of fluid obtained from joint effusions are used to differentiate noninflammatory disease from inflammatory and septic disorders. Examination of synovial fluid is particularly important in differentiating gout and pseudogout.

SYNOVIAL FLUID TESTS

Test: Synovial Fluid Examination

Background

Synovial fluid is a dialysate of plasma plus hyaluronic acid, a mucopolysaccharide produced by synovial cells. Normal synovial fluid (Table 6-7) is clear and pale yellow with a specific gravity of 1.010, similar to plasma. Synovial fluid normally is quite viscous and has a pH that approximates that of serum. The protein concentration is much less than that of serum. The large molecular weight proteins such as fibrinogen, α-2-macroglobulin, and IgM are present in small amounts, whereas albumin and glycoproteins are present in greater concentrations.

Table 6-7. Characteristics of Normal Synovial Fluid

Characteristics	Mean	Range
Volume (mL in knee)	1.2	0.13–4
Viscosity at 25°C	150	5.7–1160
pH	7.39	7.2–7.6
Total protein (g/dL)	1.9	1.3–3.0
Immunoglobulins		
IgG (mg/dL)	453	33–850
IgA (mg/dL)	74	27–177
IgM (mg/dL)	37	0–84
Fibrinogen	0	0
Erythrocytes (cells/μL)	160	0–2000
Leukocytes (cells/μL)	63	13–180
Polymorphonuclear cells (%)	6	0–25
Lymphocytes (%)	25	0–78
Monocytes (%)	48	0–71
Macrophages (%)	10	0–26
Synovial cells (%)	4	0–12

(Data from Cohen[34] and Glasser.[35])

Selection

Routine studies include mucin determination (mucin clot test), culture, WBC count and differential, and crystal examination. Although the cell count and WBC differential are not specific diagnostic parameters, they are important in classifying different types of synovial fluid. Special studies may include glucose and lactate estimation, antigen detection, complement, and CH_{50} determinations.

Logistics

Although normally synovial fluid does not clot, clots occur in association with inflammatory changes that cause fibrinogen exudation within the joint cavity. Synovial fluid is collected in a tube containing anticoagulant, preferably ethylenediamine tetraacetic acid (EDTA). Saline diluent is used; use of an acid diluent causes precipitation of hyaluronate that traps WBCs, resulting in a reduction of up to 50% in the WBC count. Fat globules (sometimes seen after trauma) may cause a "pseudoleukocytosis" when cells are counted on automated cell counters. Characteristics of synovial fluid including the color, turbidity, and viscosity of the fluid should be noted.

Interpretation

Cell Count

Presence of RBCs indicates either trauma of aspiration, traumatic bleeding, or hemorrhagic effusion into the joint. Causes of hemarthrosis include bleeding disorders, anticoagulant therapy, and benign and malignant tumors. Quantitative and qualitative changes in WBCs allow for a classification of fluid into the following categories: noninflammatory, noninfectious mild

Table 6-8. Pathologic Classification of Synovial Fluid

Classification	Leukocyte Count (cells/μL)	Neutrophil Percentage
Normal	180	25
Noninflammatory	200–2000 (almost never exceeds 5000)	30
Degenerative joint disease		
Neuroarthropathy		
Traumatic		
Osteochondromatosis		
Noninfectious, mild inflammatory	2000–5000	30
Systemic lupus erythematosus		
Scleroderma		
Hemorrhagic villonodular synovitis		
Hypertrophic pulmonary osteoarthropathy		
Noninfectious, severe inflammatory	5000–50,000	75
Gout		
Pseudogout		
Rheumatic fever		
Rheumatoid arthritis		
Reiter's disease		
Infectious	>50,000	75

inflammatory, noninfectious severe inflammatory, infectious, and hemorrhagic (Table 6-8).[29]

There are, however, several exceptions to the broad classifications shown in Table 6-8. One study showed that a synovial fluid leukocyte count of greater than 50,000 cells/μL (50 × 10^6 cells/L) was present in 70% of patients with bacterial arthritis, 13% of patients with gout, 10% of patients with calcium pyrophosphate dihydrate disease (pseudogout), and 4% of patients with rheumatoid arthritis.[30] Also of note is that 30% of patients with bacterial arthritis at initial presentation had a synovial fluid leukocyte count of 50,000 cells/μL (50 × 10^6 cells/L). Repeat analysis after 24 hours showed a much greater leukocytosis. Other cells in synovial fluid may offer additional diagnostic clues (Table 6-9).

Mucin Clot (Fig. 6-2)

Mucin is necessary for joint lubrication and changes in its character and concentration interfere with normal function. The formation of a mucin clot with the addition of 2% acetic acid to synovial fluid depends on the interaction of acid, hyaluronate, and protein. The quality of the clot is graded as good, fair, or poor and reflects the degree of polymerization of hyaluronic acid. In general, the poorer the mucin clot, the higher the leukocyte count, which suggests a lesser degree of hyaluronate polymerization in inflamed joints.

Crystals

The identification of crystals in synovial fluid often allows a definitive diagnosis. Although several methods are available for crystal identification, the most common method used in clinical practice is polarizing microscopy. A drop of synovial fluid (not collected in oxalate or lithium heparin because both will form birefringent crystals) is required. Crystals identified in synovial effusions together with their characteristic appearance are shown in Table 6-10 and Figures 6-3 to 6-7.[29,31]

Lactate[11]

Septic arthritis must be diagnosed early because untreated infection can rapidly destroy a joint. In patients with mild signs and symptoms, the diagnosis may be easily missed. Furthermore, it is difficult to distinguish septic arthritis from other inflammatory arthropathies. Gram stain of synovial fluid is often negative and awaiting culture results usually entails a delay in diagnosis of 24–48 hours. Thus, a method has been sought that would provide rapid diagnosis of septic arthritis. In the rapid differentiation between septic and nonsep-

Table 6-9. Presence of Other Cells in Synovial Fluid

Cell Type	Disease Process	Comments
LE Cells	Systemic lupus erythematosus	
Malignant Cells	Metastatic cancer	Reported in patients with gastrointestinal and lung cancer, leukemia
"Reiter's Cell"	Rheumatoid arthritis Septic arthritis Gout Calcium pyrophosphate dihydrate disease	"Reiter's cell" refers to a mononuclear cell phagocytizing a neutrophil
Eosinophils	Metastatic carcinoma to synovium Acute rheumatic fever Irradiation Infections Allergy Postarthrography	
Monocytes	Rubella Arbovirus Hepatitis Systemic lupus erythematosus Scleroderma Sickle cell disease	

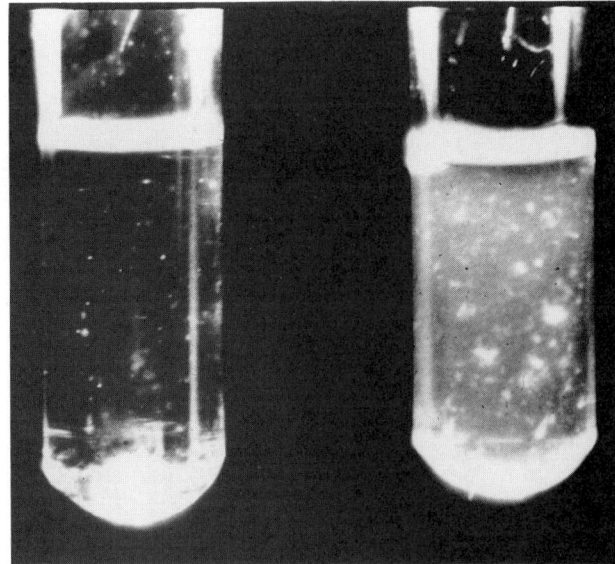

Fig. 6-2. Mucin clot test. The addition of acetic acid to normal joint fluid produces a firm white clot of mucin (left). In synovial fluid obtained from patients with septic arthritis and inflammatory joint disease, the mucin clot forms a flocculent precipitate and the surrounding solution becomes cloudy (right).

tic arthritis, synovial fluid lactate appears to be a useful adjunct to established methods such as Gram stain and WBC count (Table 6-11). In most studies, lactate measurement was more sensitive and specific than either Gram stain or WBC count and may be useful when antibiotics have already been given before testing the synovial fluid. Another potential use for synovial fluid lactate is in the follow-up treatment of septic arthritis. Lactate levels decline with treatment and correlate with clinical improvement.

The reason for the lactate increase in septic arthritis is uncertain. The presence of synovial inflammation leads to relative hypoxia resulting in a switch from

Table 6-10. Crystals Seen in Synovial Fluid

Crystal	Appearance/Comments
Monosodium urate (see Figs. 6-4 and 6-5)	Crystals are about 3–20 μm long. In acute gouty arthritis, they are most intraleukocytic and distend the cytoplasm of the neutrophil. Crystals are strongly negatively birefringent. With a first order red compensator, crystals will be blue and yellow in horizontal and vertical directions depending on the alignment of the first order red compensator. A yellow color is seen when the crystal axis is parallel to the slow ray of the compensator.
CPPD (see Fig. 6-6)	Plate-like, rhomboid, rod- or needle-shaped, and weakly positively birefringent. They exhibit colors opposite to those of monosodium urate using the first order red compensator (i.e., they are blue when parallel to the slow ray).
Hydroxyapatite	Small needle-shaped crystals less than 1-μm long and 75–250°A in diameter. They are too small to be seen with light microscopy and usually require electron microscopy for identification. Aggregated lumps may be birefringent.
Cholesterol (see Fig. 6-7)	Appear as large, extremely bright, square, or rectangular plate-like crystals often with a notch in the corner. Rarely they may be rod- or needle-shaped and negatively birefringent. Not usually phagocytized by neutrophils.
Corticosteroids	May be positively or negatively birefringent. Pleomorphic. Usually from intra-articular crystalline injections.
Lithium heparin	Pleomorphic positively birefringent crystals.

Abbreviation: CPPD, calcium pyrophosphate dehydrate crystal.

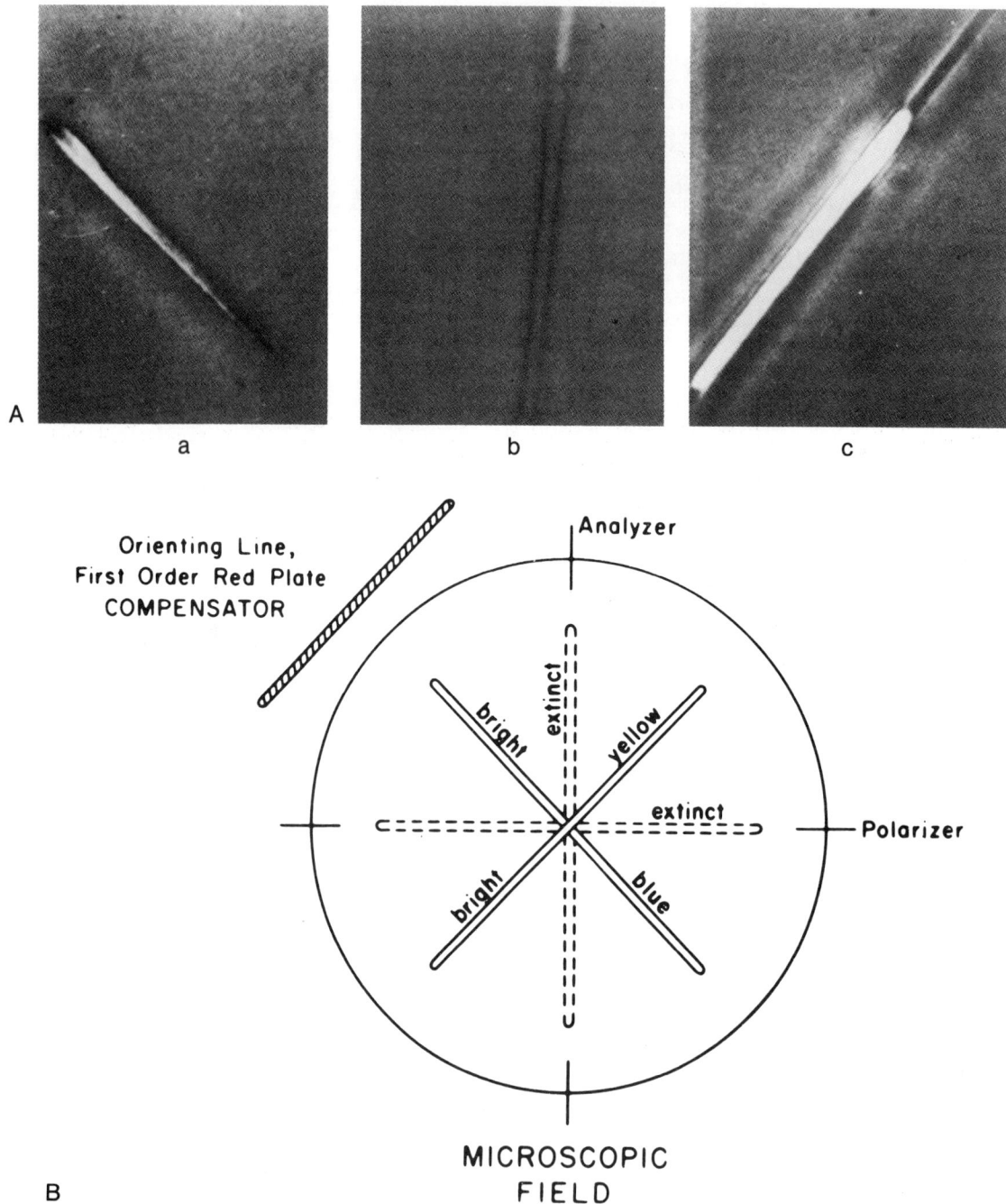

Fig. 6-3. (A) The same urate crystal is shown here under compensated polarized light in three different positions: *(a)* on the left, a strongly birefringent monosodium urate monohydrate crystal bright blue when perpendicular to the orienting line of the compensator; *(b)* the center frame shows the same crystal is extinct on axis of the polarizer; and *(c)* on the right, the urate crystal is now bright yellow when parallel to the slow vibration orientation of the compensator. (B) This is an illustrative representation of the urate crystal under compensated polarized light microscopy shown in Figure 6-3A.

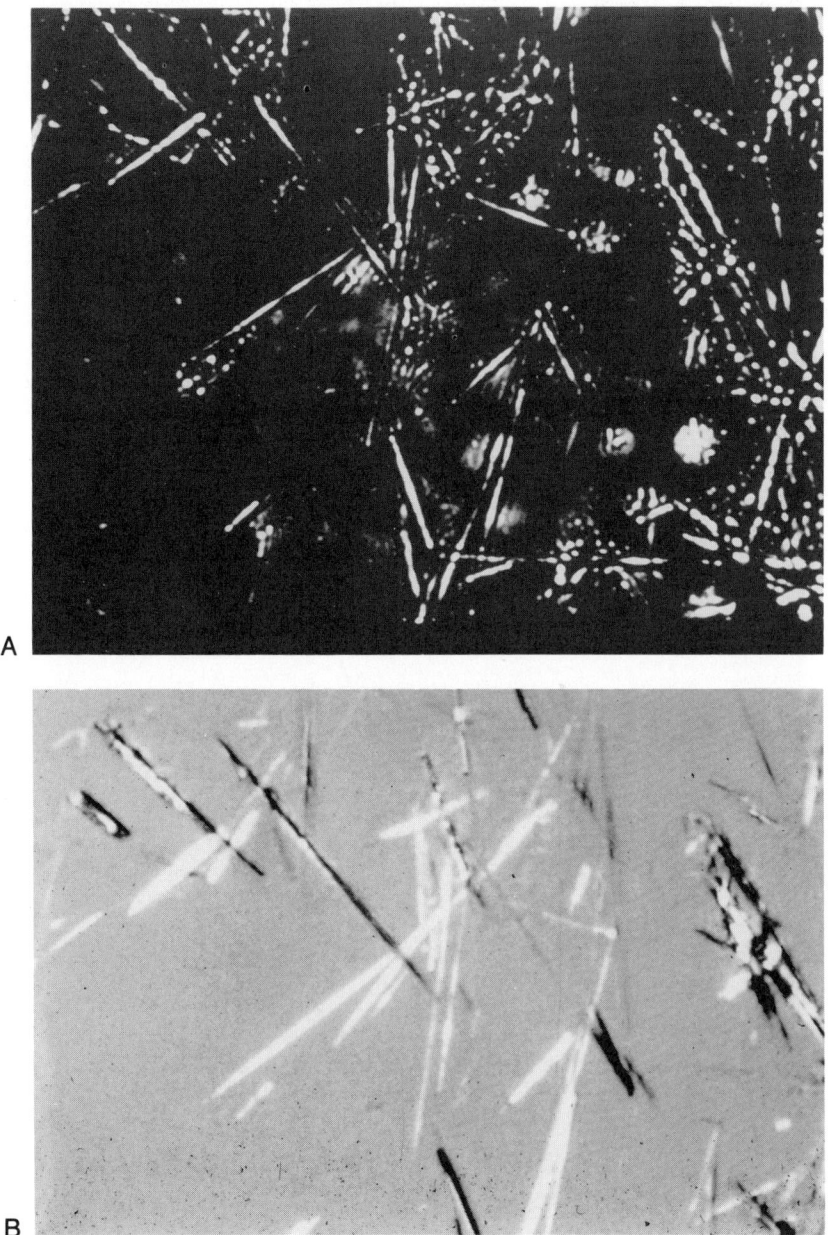

Fig. 6-4. (A) Urate crystals viewed under high power ordinary light microscopy. The crystals are very weakly refractile. (B) Urate crystals from the same field using high power compensated polarized light microscopy. The monosodium urate monohydrate crystals are strongly negatively birefringent. They are bright yellow when parallel to the orienting line and bright blue when perpendicular to this line.

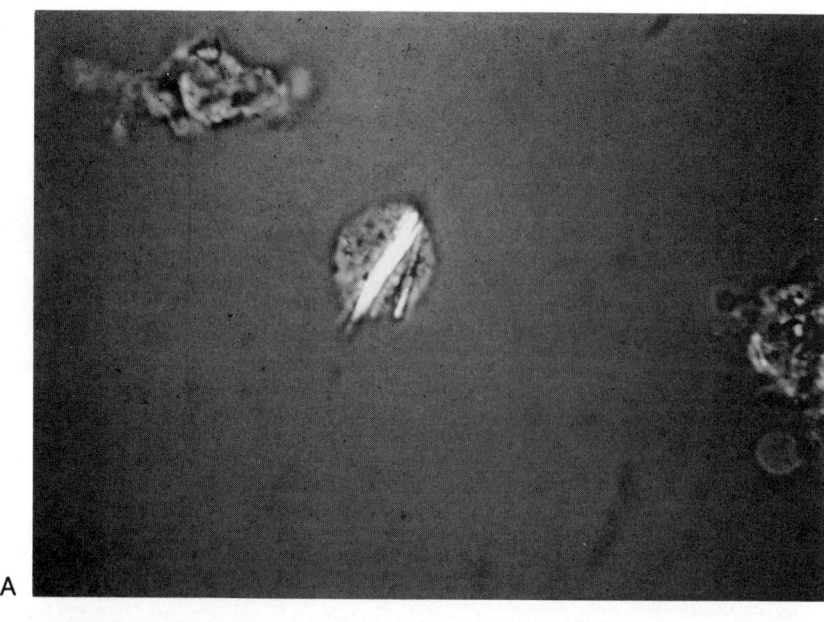
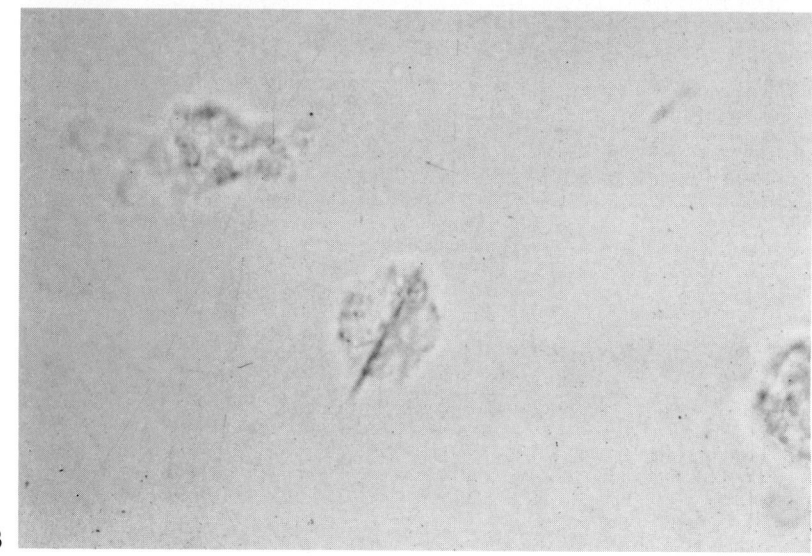

Fig. 6-5. Monosodium urate crystals phagocytosed by a polymorphonuclear leukocyte. **(A)** Two crystals with compensated polarized light. **(B)** The same field with ordinary light where only one of the crystals is identifiable.

mainly aerobic to anaerobic glycolysis. Furthermore, bacterial endotoxin stimulates glucose utilization and lactate production.

SEMINAL FLUID

Semen analysis is used in the study of the infertile couple where it is a predictor of male infertility. Semen analysis is important in determining the normalcy of spermatogenesis and the patency of the reproductive tract.

SEMEN TESTS

Test: Semen Analysis (Sperm Analysis)

Background

Spermatogenesis, the maturation of germ cells to mature spermatozoa, takes 72 days and requires an intact hypothalamic-pituitary-testicular access. Luteinizing hormone causes synthesis of testosterone from the Leydig cell, which diffuses to the tubular cells where it

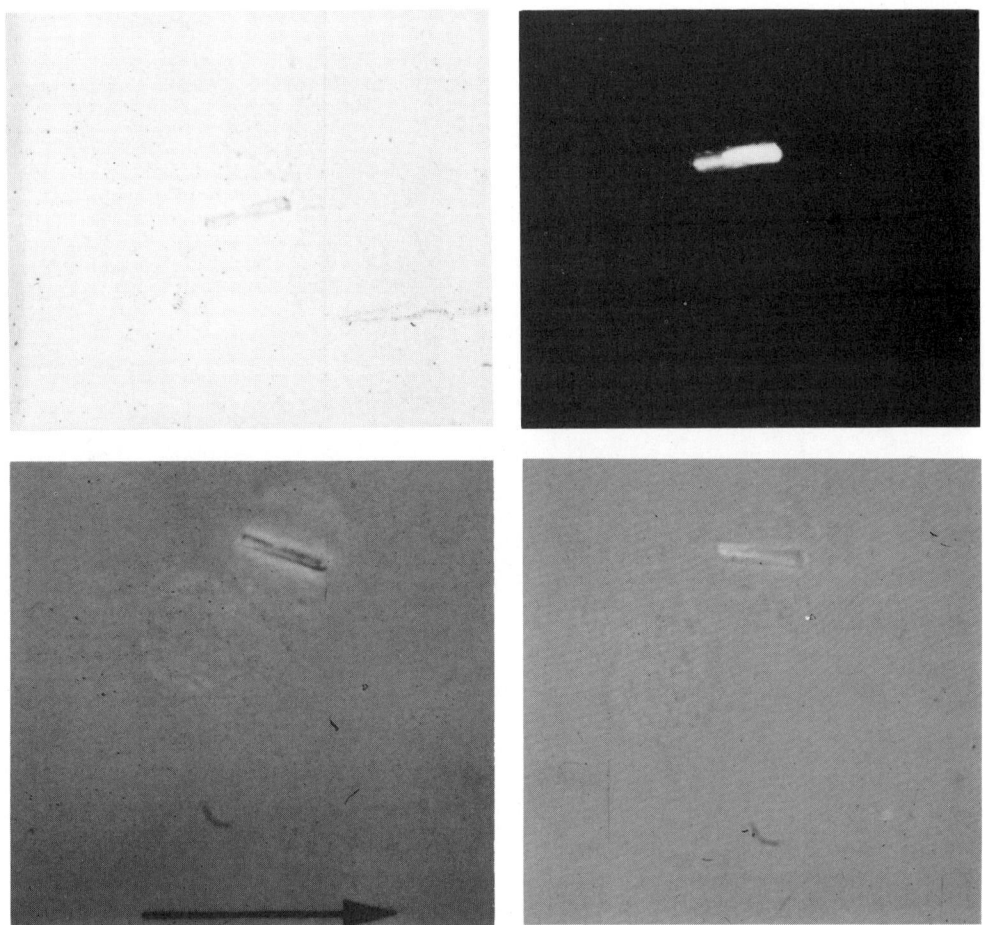

Fig. 6-6. Calcium pyrophosphate dehydrate crystal being engulfed by a leukocyte. The crystal is shown with regular light microscopy in the upper left view and with the addition of polarized lenses in the upper right panel. In the two lower panels, compensated polarized light microscopy is used with crystal parallel to the place of the compensator (arrow) and perpendicular on the right. The crystal has weak positive birefringence.

affects spermatogenesis either directly or indirectly through Sertoli cell function. The Sertoli cells function as a matrix for the germ cells. Follicle-stimulating hormone also is required to produce spermatozoa and acts directly on the Sertoli cells.

Complete semen analysis consists of at least five determinants: volume, density, motility, quantitative sperm movement (forward progression), and morphologic characteristics. Human semen contains many abnormal sperm cells with abnormalities involving many structural components of the sperm. These abnormal cells probably are not functional, and clinical assessment of semen has been aimed at quantifying normal spermatozoa. Whereas traditional morphologic characteristics incorporate subjective measurements, newer techniques are now being used to evaluate motility.

Selection

Semen analysis is useful in the evaluation of infertility and validating the effectiveness of vasectomy.

Logistics

Specimens are collected after 3–5 days of sexual abstinence and should be examined within 1 hour after ejaculation. If infection or severe stress occurred during the previous 90 days, the collection should be deferred. The specimen should be collected in glass containers because plastic containers can be spermaticidal. The spec-

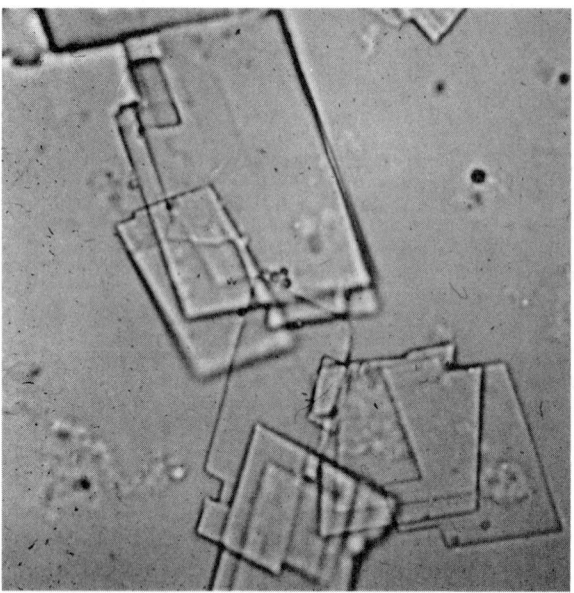 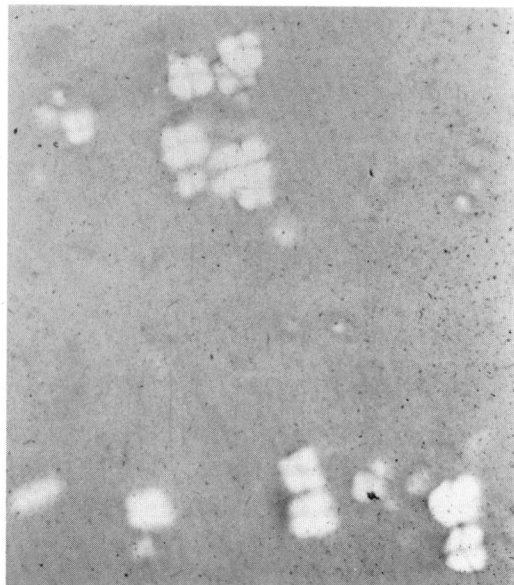

Fig. 6-7. On the right is synovial fluid viewed under polarized microscopy in which there is contamination with starch shed from a glove. Starch gives the appearance of Maltese crosses under polarized light. On the left are cholesterol crystals seen with regular light microscopy.

imen should not be subject to cold and if carried by a patient from a distant site to the laboratory the temperature should be maintained by storing the container in an inside pocket. Multiple specimens may be required if an abnormality is found on initial examination.

Interpretation

Semen analysis is only a gross estimate of testicular damage. Although the lower end of the reference range determined as 95th percentile of the population is considerably higher, most clinicians accept 20 million sperm/mL as the lower limit of the reference range. However, only when the sperm count decreases to 5 million/mL is fertility affected. The median sperm count in infertile men is 60 million/mL and over 80% of infertile men have counts greater than 20 million/mL. Alterations in serum volume also affect fertility; but only when the volume falls below 1 mL or exceeds 5 mL is fertility affected. In postvasectomy specimens, no sperm should be present if the vasectomy is complete.

Azoospermia, or the absence of sperm, occurs in primary testicular failure of the Leydig cells and germinal elements, although germinal tubular failure alone occasionally causes azoospermia. Other causes are retrograde ejaculation or obstruction of the ejaculatory system. Oligospermia (lower sperm count) occurs from damage to the germinal epithelium, although hypothalamic or pituitary disease is a frequent cause. During the summer, the concentration of sperm decreases by over 25% of values during the winter.[32]

Motility

The lower limit for the presence of motile sperm is 50%, whereas 40–50% is considered borderline. Sperm motility also is judged on a scale of 0–4+ in terms of how fast and how straight they swim. Severe motility defects, in which less than 10% of sperm are motile, occur with structural defects such as acrosome-less spermatozoa, macrocephalic sperm, and absence of the postacrosomal sheath. A number of newer methods such as time exposure photomicrography, videomicrography, and multiple exposure photomicrography are now used but these methods are poorly standardized.

Morphology

New techniques use sperm head morphometry to categorize sperm. With only a few exceptions, the classification of abnormal forms under the light microscope has not been useful.[33]

Based on the findings of the analysis, three categories of patients can be identified: (1) patients with normal semen quality and no evidence of infertility; (2) patients with marginal semen quality and possible infertility; and (3) patients with abnormal semen quality and likely infertility. Because of the variability of re-

Table 6-11. A Summary of Studies Using Synovial Fluid Lactate (SLac) to Distinguish Septic From Nonseptic Arthritis

Study No.	SLac in Septic Arthritis[a]	SLac in Nonseptic Arthritis	SLac in Gonococcal Arthritis	Method of SLac Measurement
1	15/15 patients had SLac >8 mmol/L	35/37 patients had SLac <8 mmol/L	—	GLC
2	6/6 patients had SLac >10 mmol/L	10/10 patients had SLac <10 mmol/L	—	Enzymatic
3	25/27 patients had SLac >5.5 mmol/L	37/45 patients had SLac <5.5 mmol/L	12/12 patients had SLac <5.5 mmol/L	GLC
4	5/5 patients had SLac >10 mmol/L	48/48 patients had SLac <10 mmol/L	7/7 patients had SLac <10 mmol/L	GLC
5	9/10 patients had SLac >8 mmol/L	33/33 patients had SLac <8 mmol/L	2 patients had SLac >8 mmol/L	Enzymatic
6	14/14 patients had SLac >10 mmol/L	19/19 patients had SLac <10 mmol/L	3 patients had SLac <6 mmol/L	—

Abbreviation: GLC, gas liquid chromatography.
[a] Excludes gonococcal arthritis patients.

sults, the patients in the latter two categories require additional semen analysis to substantiate the abnormalities.

REFERENCES

1. Conly JM, Ronald AR: Cerebrospinal fluid as a diagnostic body fluid. Am J Med 1983;75(1B):102–108.
2. Schumann GB, Crisman LG: Cerebrospinal fluid cytopathology. Clin Lab Med 1985;5:275–302.
3. Martin KI: The spinal tap: a new look at an old test. Ann Intern Med 1986;104:840–848.
4. Mayefsky JH, Roghmann KJ: Determination of leukocytosis in traumatic spinal tap specimens. Am J Med 1987;82:1175–1181.
5. Dougherty JM: Cerebrospinal fluid. Emerg Med Clin North Am 1986;4:281–298.
6. Donald PR, Malan C, van der Walt A: Simultaneous determination of cerebrospinal fluid glucose and blood glucose concentrations in the diagnosis of bacterial meningitis. J Pediatr 1983;103:413–414.
7. Powers WJ: Cerebrospinal fluid to serum glucose ratios in diabetes mellitus and bacterial meningitis. Am J Med 1981;71:217–220.
8. Hayward RA, Shapiro MF, Oye RK: Laboratory testing on cerebrospinal fluid. Lancet 1987;1:1–4.
9. Levinson A: The hydrogen-ion concentration of CSF. J Infect Dis 1917;21:556–570.
10. Brook I: Stability of lactic acid in cerebrospinal fluid specimens. Am J Clin Pathol 1982;77:213–216.
11. Nanji AA, Whitlow KJ: Clinical utility of lactic acid measurement in body fluids other than plasma. J Emerg Med 1984;1:521–526.
12. Wasserstrom WR, Schwartz MK, Fleisher M, Posner JB: Cerebrospinal biochemical measurements in central nervous system: a review. Ann Clin Lab Sci 1981;11:239–251.
13. Cutler RWP: Cerebrospinal fluid—a selective review. Ann Neurol 1982;11:1–10.
14. Hart RG, Sherman DG: The diagnosis of multiple sclerosis. JAMA 1982;247:498–503.
15. Epstein DJ: CSF protein analysis in multiple sclerosis. Check Sample Clin Chem 1982;22:1–5.
16. Ebers GC: Oligoclonal banding in multiple sclerosis. Ann NY Acad Sci 1983;436:206–212.
17. Che AB, Sever JL, Madden DL et al: Oligoclonal IgG bands in various neurological diseases. Ann Neurol 1983;13:434–439.
18. Gupta MK: Myelin basic protein and demyelinating disease. CRC Crit Rev Clin Lab Sci 1987;24:287–314.
19. Carson JH, Barbarese E, Braun PE, McPherson TA: Components in multiple sclerosis cerebrospinal fluid that are detected by radioimmunoassay for myelin basic protein. Proc Natl Acad Sci USA 1978;75:1976–1982.
20. Biber A, Englert D, Dommasch D, Hempel K: Myelin basic protein in cerebrospinal fluid of patients with multiple sclerosis and other neurologic diseases. J Neurol 1981;225:231–237.
21. Whitaker JN, Lisak RP, Bashir RM et al: Immunoreactive myelin basic protein in neurologic disorders. Ann Neurol 1980;7:58–64.
22. Grimaldi LME, Castagna A, Lazzarin A et al: Oligoclonal IgG bands in cerebrospinal fluid and serum during asymptomatic human immunodeficiency virus infection. Am Neurol Assoc 1988;24:277–279.
23. Malkin MG, Posner JB: Cerebrospinal fluid tumor markers for the diagnosis and management of leptomeningeal metastases. Eur J Cancer Clin Oncol 1987;23:1–4.
24. Light RW: Pleural effusions. Med Clin North Am 1977;61:1339–1352.
25. Light RW, Ball WC: Glucose and amylase in pleural effusions. JAMA 1973;225:257–260.
26. Sahn SA, Good JT: Pleural fluid pH in malignant effusions. Ann Intern Med 1988;108:345–349.
27. Kindig JR, Goodman MR: Clinical utility of pericardial fluid pH determination. Am J Med 1983;75:1077–1079.

28. Runyon BA, Hoefs JC, Morgan TR: Ascitic fluid analysis in malignancy related ascites. Hepatology 1988;8:1104–1109.
29. McCarty DJ: Arthritis associated with crystals containing calcium. Med Clin North Am 1986;70:437–454.
30. Krey P, Bailen DA: Synovial fluid leukocytosis. A study of extremes. Am J Med 1979;67:436–442.
31. Schumacher HR: Crystals, inflammation and osteoarthritis. Am J Med 1987;83,suppl 5A:11–16.
32. Overstreet JW, Katz DF: Semen analysis. Urol Clin North Am 1987;3:441–449.
33. Levine RJ, Mathew RM, Chenault CB et al: Differences in the quality of semen in outdoor workers during summer and winter. N Engl J Med 1990;323:12–16.
34. Cohen AS: Laboratory Diagnostic Procedures in the Rheumatic Diseases. Orlando, FL, Grune & Stratton, 1985, p. 6.
35. Glasser L: Body fluids. III. Reading the signs in synovia. Diagn Med 1980;Nov/Dec:39.

7 Carbohydrates

Peter J. Howanitz
Joan H. Howanitz

INTRODUCTION

Carbohydrates are compounds composed of carbon, hydrogen, and oxygen, usually with hydrogen and oxygen present in a proportion of 2 hydrogen atoms to 1 oxygen atom, as in water. These carbohydrates or "carbon hydrates" have the general formula $C_n(H_2O)_n$. The carbohydrates that are important medically include hexoses, glucose, fructose, and galactose and the disaccharides, lactose and sucrose. Lactose is hydrolyzed to glucose and galactose, whereas sucrose is hydrolyzed to glucose and fructose.

The average adult diet in the Western hemisphere is about 45% carbohydrate, 45% fat, and the remainder protein. Almost 60% of the carbohydrates are consumed as starch, originating from grains, vegetables, and legumes such as rice, wheat, corn, and potatoes. Fruits and cane sugar account for 30%, almost entirely as sucrose. The remainder of the dietary carbohydrates come from milk and milk products as lactose and from fruits, which contain glucose and some pentoses. Animal sources contain less than 1% glycogen, thus they account for a negligible portion of dietary carbohydrates. Salivary and gastrointestinal tract enzymes cleave starch, disaccharides, and other polysaccharides to monosaccharides, which are then absorbed in the small intestine by active transport and simple diffusion. Glucose accounts for almost all the saccharides in the blood with only a small portion made up of fructose, galactose, and other simple sugars. The hexoses are taken up by the hepatic cells through simple diffusion and are metabolized as shown in Figure 7-1. Glucose, the most important carbohydrate, enters the cells under the influence of insulin and is converted to glucose 6-phosphate by the enzyme hexokinase.

Glucose 6-phosphate is at a key location in the glycolytic scheme, because it can be converted along a number of metabolic paths back to (1) glucose, through the hexose monophosphate shunt to (2) triose phosphate and the production of CO_2, (3) to fructose 6-phosphate and then on through triose phosphate, and (4) to glycogen. Intermediary metabolism is portrayed as a simple scheme in Figure 7-1, but is exceedingly complex. In this figure, a number of enzymes and intermediates involved in many of the glycolytic reactions are depicted as a single step.

Glucose is stored as glycogen in animal tissue such as the liver and is highly branched with the glucose moieties connected by α1-4 and 1-6 linkages. With excessive feeding, glucose is converted to glycogen for storage. Under conditions of fasting, glycogen is converted through a series of complex enzymatic steps to glucose 6-phosphate and then metabolized through the glycolytic scheme.

During the fasting state, plasma concentrations of glucose are maintained by two compensatory mechanisms, glycogenolysis and gluconeogenesis. Glycogenolysis occurs in minutes and involves the conversion of existing glycogen ultimately to glucose. Gluconeogenesis takes hours to initiate and involves the transformation of nonsugars to carbohydrate, for example, the

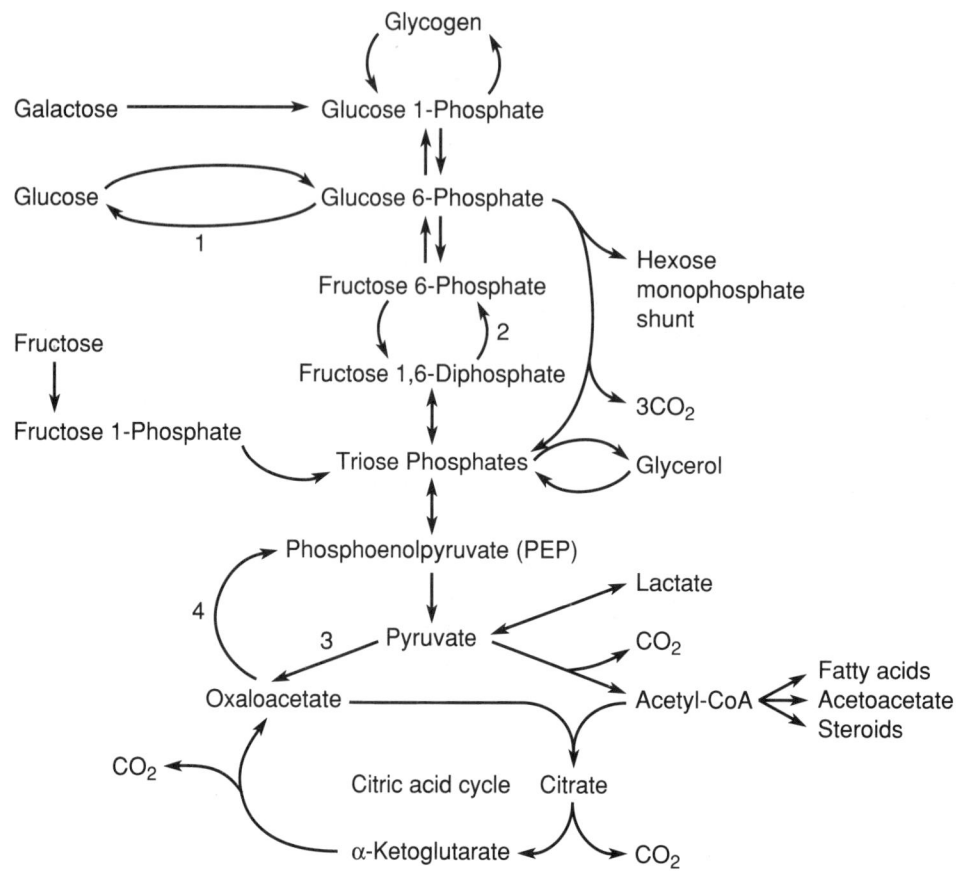

Fig. 7-1. Simplified scheme for metabolism of carbohydrates. Reversible enzymes are indicated by bidirectional arrows. Nonreversible enzymes are indicated by unidirectional arrows. Important irreversible gluconeogenic enzymes are (1) glucose 6-phosphatase, (2) fructose 1,6 diphosphatase, (3) pyruvate carboxylase, and (4) PEP carboxykinase.

conversion of fuels such as protein and amino acids to glucose.

A number of hormones also play important roles in the regulation of blood glucose concentration. Insulin and glucagon are ultimately involved in the minute to minute regulation of plasma glucose. Other hormones, such as growth hormone, have antagonistic actions on insulin and are responsible for raising plasma glucose concentrations. Glucocorticoids also stimulate gluconeogenesis, whereas epinephrine, secreted by the adrenal gland, stimulates glycogenolysis. Thyroid hormones stimulate glycogenolysis and also increase the rate of glucose absorption from the intestine. It is not surprising that conditions of growth hormone, thyroid hormone, glucocorticoid, or epinephrine excess occurring in acromegaly, hyperthyroidism, Cushing syndrome and pheochrocytoma, respectively, cause hyperglycemia (see Table 7-2).

Lactate, formed under anaerobic conditions from pyruvate by the enzyme lactate dehydrogenase, is another one of the key metabolic intermediates commonly measured in clinical situations. When anaerobic conditions predominate, pyruvate is formed from lactate (see Ch. 15).

ROUTINE TESTS

Test: Random Glucose

Background and Selection

Glucose values obtained without regard to patient preparation are used for screening individuals for hyperglycemia, hypoglycemia, diabetes mellitus, and to identify when patients should have a more sensitive diagnostic procedure such as measuring fasting glucose levels or administering a glucose tolerance test.

Logistics

Specimen

The usual specimen obtained for glucose analysis is venous blood, but occasionally capillary blood is used. In fasting individuals, capillary glucose results usually are less than 5 mg/dL (<0.3 mmol/L) higher than those obtained with venous samples. During carbohydrate ingestion such as glucose tolerance testing, however, capillary glucose values may be up to twofold higher than venous glucose results.[1]

After collection, the concentration of glucose in the specimen begins to decrease immediately, because of the glycolytic action of erythrocytes, leukocytes, platelets, and any bacterial contamination. Various methods have been used to delay glycolysis including the addition of preservatives such as sodium fluoride, sodium oxalate, or sodium iodoacetate. Usually the specimen is centrifuged and the glucose measurement performed using plasma or serum, allowing for measurement of glucose that is independent of hematocrit. If serum is used, the serum should be separated from the cells within 30 minutes. However, if erythrocytosis, leukocytosis, and bacterial contamination are absent, clinically acceptable results are found even if the serum and cells are not separated within 90 minutes. At temperatures of 4°C, glucose is stable as plasma or serum and can be stored for up to 48 hours. Even with storage at $-20°C$, glucose values gradually continue to decrease with time.

Methods

Although in the past, chemical methods were used for glucose measurements, the most widely used methods today are enzymatic. With the chemical methods, lack of analytic specificity produces results generally 5–20 mg/dL (0.3–1.2 mmol/L) higher than enzymatic methods. The common enzymatic methods are glucose oxidase, hexokinase, and glucose dehydrogenase. Glucose oxidase catalyzes the following reaction:

$$\text{D-Glucose} + O_2 \xrightarrow{\text{glucose oxidase}} \text{D-gluconic acid} + H_2O_2$$

This reaction is quantitated either manometrically or colorimetrically. In the manometric technique, glucose is determined by measuring the rate of oxygen consumption using an oxygen electrode. The H_2O_2 formed by the reaction is removed by catalase and iodide plus molybdate without yielding oxygen.

In one of the first modifications of this method, H_2O_2 reacts with an oxygen acceptor, such as ortho-dianisidine, phenylamine-phenazone (Trinder's reagent), or other chromogenic oxygen acceptors. The reaction is catalyzed by peroxidase to form a colored product that is quantitated.

$$H_2O_2 + \text{chromogenic } O_2 \text{ acceptor} \xrightarrow{\text{peroxidase}} \text{oxidized chromogenic} + H_2O$$
$$\text{(uncolored)} \qquad\qquad\qquad\qquad \text{(colored)}$$

Glucose oxidase is highly specific for β-D-glucose and any glucose present in the α form must be converted to the β form by addition of the enzyme mutarotase. Ascorbic acid causes spuriously decreased values. This technique commonly is used for urine "dip stick" testing (see Ch. 3, Renal Function; Urinalysis; Chemical Analysis).

The production of H_2O_2 by the glucose oxidase also can be measured amperometrically by oxidation of the H_2O_2 on a platinum electrode. Reports suggest acetaminophen interferes with this method by giving an electrochemical response. Glycolytic inhibitors such as sodium iodoacetate also interfere with this method.

Because of its specificity, the hexokinase glucose method has been proposed as the reference method for glucose estimation. The method couples the hexokinase reaction with glucose 6-phosphate dehydrogenase (G-6-PD) and the change in the concentration of nicotinamide-adenine dinucleotide phosphate (NADP) or reduced NADP (NADPH) is measured; ATP, adenosine triphosphate; ADP, adenosine diphosphate.

$$\text{Glucose} + \text{ATP} \xrightarrow[\text{Mg}^{2+}]{\text{hexokinase}} \text{glucose 6-phosphate} + \text{ADP}$$

$$\text{Glucose 6-phosphate} + \text{NADP} \xrightarrow{\text{G-6-PD}} \text{6-phosphogluconolactone} + \text{NADPH} + H^-$$

The main disadvantage of hexokinase is its cost. However, data from a large number of studies reveal that this method is essentially free of interferences.

The most recently developed enzymatic method uses glucose dehydrogenase. This enzyme has a high specificity for β-D-glucose, and nicotinamide-adenine dinucleotide (NAD) and mutarotase are auxiliary enzymes that are included to decrease the reaction time required. Only high concentrations of xylose and mannose have been reported to interfere.

Comparisons of glucose results made with various instruments in clinical laboratories are made routinely and over time differences between methods have been minimized. With widespread use of a variety of small instruments used in locations such as the physician's office laboratory and the lack of extensive comparison programs for these methods, surprisingly large differences in glucose results from these different locations occur.[2] In addition, large errors sometimes occur in results generated at these sites, because some of these instruments are prone to operator errors. For further information, see Burrin and Price,[3] who recently reviewed measurements of blood glucose.

Interpretation

The serum glucose concentration at birth is approximately 75% of the maternal serum glucose level: during the first few hours of life it ranges from 30–80 mg/dL (1.7–4.4 mmol/L), with a mean value of 50 mg/dL (2.8 mmol/L). After 72 hours the mean value is 65–80 mg/dL (3.8–4.4 mmol/L) and by 4–10 days, values comparable to adults are reached.

Up to the age of 2 months, low birth weight infants have lower serum glucose concentrations with a range of 20–100 mg/dL (1.1–5.5 mmol/L). In healthy adults, serum glucose concentrations vary only slightly throughout the day and generally range between 45 and 130 mg/dL (2.5 and 7.3 mmol/L). In persons older than 65 years, serum glucose may reach 180 mg/dL (10.0 mmol/L). Oscillations in glucose concentrations in the healthy occur only after meals and are rarely more than 10–15 mg/dL (>0.6–0.8 mmol/L). A seasonal difference in serum glucose has been shown, with highest values occurring during the winter. Results in the winter are approximately 10 mg/dL (0.6 mmol/L) higher than the lowest values, which occur in the spring. Obese people and those who are aged have increased glucose oscillations, and diabetics may have fluctuations in glucose as great as 150 mg/dL (8.3 mmol/L).

Values outside the reference range are unusual in adults under the age of 45 and warrant investigation. Glucose values below 45 mg/dL (<2.5 mmol/L) in adults may be indicative of an insulinoma, but commonly are seen in individuals who are fasting (see below). Glucose results above 200 mg/dL (>11.2 mmol/L) are diagnostic of diabetes mellitus, a common cause of hyperglycemia. However, for evaluation of gestational diabetes, random plasma glucose determinations have a low predictive value; therefore, 1 hour screening following a 5 g load is recommended.[4]

Test: Fasting Glucose (Fasting Blood Sugar, [FBS])

Background and Selection

The diagnosis of diabetes mellitus can be made by measuring plasma glucose when the patient has been fasting overnight for 12–14 hours. Measurement of fasting plasma glucose also is used in managing diabetes mellitus. Although other procedures are used for definitive diagnosis of hypoglycemia, occasionally fasting plasma glucose measurements are helpful.

Terminology

Fasting blood sugar is an archaic term that refers to the measurement of reducing sugars, among them glucose, galactose, mannose, lactose, maltose, sucrose, and fructose quantitated by chemical methods in whole blood specimens.

Logistics

Ideally plasma specimens collected after a 12–14 hour overnight fast should be used because they show less variation in glucose as compared with specimens collected at other times. Serum specimens also are acceptable with the appropriate precaution (see Test: Random Glucose).

Interpretation

An overnight fasting glucose level of 50–110 mg/dL (2.8–6.2 mmol/L) is accepted by most workers as being within the reference interval.

Decreases

Hypoglycemia is a syndrome characterized by low plasma glucose and an associated group of symptoms that are relieved by ingestion of food or carbohydrates. Overnight fasting plasma glucose levels below 45 mg/dL (<2.5 mmol/L) are clearly abnormal, whereas those above 55 mg/dL (>3.0 mmol/L) usually are accepted as within the reference interval.

Fasting values also should be interpreted in relationship to the patient. For instance, Felig et al. have shown that fasting healthy individuals when exercised to exhaustion commonly have plasma glucose values that

Table 7-1. Common Causes of Hypoglycemia
Reactive
Idiopathic
Large glucose load ingested on an empty stomach
Alcohol intake after prolonged fast
Alcohol and glucose on an empty stomach
Postgastrectomy hypoglycemia
Hereditary fructose intolerance
Galactosemia
Sudden cessation of tube feeding
Insulinoma/nesidioblastosis
Fasting
Hepatic disease
Adrenal, thyroid insufficiency
Extrapancreatic tumors
Autoimmune mechanism
Factitious hypoglycemia
Pharmacologic; excess insulin, etc.
Renal insufficiency
Burns

Table 7-2 Common Causes of Hyperglycemia
Primary
Insulin-dependent diabetes mellitus
Noninsulin-dependent diabetes mellitus
Impaired glucose tolerance
Secondary
Hyperglycemia resulting from disease of the pancreas
Inflammation
Acute pancreatitis (rare)
Chronic pancreatitis
Pancreatitis due to mumps
? Cell damage due to coxsackievirus B infection
? Autoimmune disease
Pancreatectomy
Pancreatic infiltration
Hemochromatosis
Tumors
Trauma to pancreas (rare)
Hyperglycemia related to other major endocrine diseases
Acromegaly
Cushing syndrome
Thyrotoxicosis
Pheochromocytoma
Hyperaldosteronism
Glucagonoma
Somatostatinoma
Hypoglycemia caused by drugs
Steroids
Thiazide diuretics, propranolol, phenytoin, and diazoxide
Oral contraceptives
Alloxan and streptoxotocin
Hyperglycemia related to other major disease states
Chronic renal failure
Chronic liver disease
Infection
Miscellaneous hyperglycemia
Pregnancy
Related to insulin receptor antibodies (acanthosis nigricans)
Abnormal insulin

are considered hypoglycemic; some of these results were lower than 35 mg/dL (<1.9 mmol/L). Others have attempted to define the criteria for the laboratory diagnosis of hypoglycemia during extended fasting. Merimee and Tyson,[6] in a group of healthy subjects who fasted for 24 hours, noted the lower reference limits of plasma glucose as 55 mg/dL (3.5 mmol/L) in men and 35 mg/dL (1.9 mmol/L) in young women. Men who could continue to fast for 72 hours had plasma glucose values as low as 50 mg/dL (2.8 mmol/L). In premenopausal women who have fasted more than 36 hours, they concluded it was virtually impossible to define a reference plasma glucose that was meaningful for discrimination of hypoglycemia. In the studies of plasma glucose levels in healthy women who fasted 72 hours, the levels were as low as 15 mg/dL (0.8 mmol/L). These and other studies have raised the question of the definition of hypoglycemia. Classification of the common causes of hypoglycemia are seen in Table 7-1.

Increases

A large number of syndromes and diseases are associated with inappropriately high fasting plasma glucose levels, some of which are listed in Table 7-2. For the diagnosis of diabetes mellitus, a plasma glucose level of 140 mg/dL (7.7 mmol/L) or greater is considered abnormal; if the concentration of plasma glucose is abnormal on two or more occasions, the diagnosis of diabetes mellitus can be made in accordance with the criteria of the National Diabetes Data Group (NDDG).[7] If results are less than 140 mg/dL (<7.7 mmol/L) and diabetes mellitus is still suspected, a glucose tolerance test is recommended (see Test: Glucose Tolerance). Measurement of fasting plasma glucose is a highly specific, but insensitive test for the diagnosis of diabetes mellitus. For the management of diabetes, the goal is a value at the upper end of the reference interval.

Test: 2-Hour Postprandial Glucose (2-Hour PP)

Background and Selection

Two-hour PP glucose levels have been used to screen patients for diabetes mellitus before the application of more specific tests and to monitor glucose control.

Logistics

The test usually is performed following a breakfast high in carbohydrate and requires the subsequent measurement of plasma glucose 2 hours later. After receiving a glucose load, plasma glucose levels peak between 60–90 minutes and by 2 hours approximate fasting values peak. For use in diagnosis of diabetes, 2-hour values are part of the criteria developed following a standardized procedure and described under glucose tolerance testing. In these circumstances, the conditions of test performance are rigidly controlled.

Interpretation

The routine use of the 2-hour PP value is limited by the lack of rigidly controlled conditions such as the amount of carbohydrate, preparation of the patient, and the size and content of the glucose challenge. When used as a screening test, a value greater than 140 mg/dL (>7.8 mmol/L) is used as the indication for performing more specific and standardized procedures. A 2-hour PP glucose value obtained during a glucose tolerance test cannot be used by itself for the diagnosis of diabetes mellitus; however, this value is the most specific and sensitive of those obtained during the test (see Test: Glucose Tolerance Test). The management goal for control of diabetes has been accepted as a 2-hour plasma glucose value of less than 140 mg/dL (<7.8 mmol/L), although a value of 175 mg/dL (10.8 mmol/L) occasionally is used.[8]

Test: Whole Blood Glucose (Blood Glucose, Whole Blood Sugar)

Background and Selection

Substantial improvements in diabetic control have been achieved with self monitoring of whole blood glucose and subsequent insulin dosing by patients at home. Specimens obtained by finger prick are placed directly on reagent strips and quantitation performed using small portable reflectance colorimeters. Because of erratic results, most whole blood glucose measurements have been abandoned in favor of serum or plasma glucose measurements. However, for pragmatic reasons including patient convenience, whole blood specimens are used for home monitoring. These measurements are too inaccurate for use in diagnosing diabetes mellitus.

Logistics

Specimens are usually obtained from finger sticks although venous whole blood or serum obtained from the arm can also be used for measurement. Fasting glucose values in specimens obtained from a finger stick are slightly higher than values in a simultaneously obtained specimen from a venous site. Following ingestion of food or glucose during a glucose tolerance test, values become widely discrepant with finger stick results up to twice that of venous specimens.

Glucose oxidase methodology (reagent strips) is used in home glucose monitors (see Test: Fasting Glucose). Major problems in instrument use can occur if individuals are improperly trained and do not understand instrument operation. Major operator errors include misuse of lot-specific instrument calibration strips, and use of inadequate or excess amount of specimen. Some instruments show extreme sensitivity to errors in timing blood reagent strip reactions and color development time prior to measurement.[9]

Because glucose is contained in the aqueous phase and red blood cells (RBC) and plasma are 73% and 93% water, respectively, whole blood glucose values vary with the hematocrit. At low hematocrits, whole blood glucose better approximates plasma values than at higher hematocrit values. With this method, ascorbic acid, acetaminophen, salicylic acid, and gentistic acid can cause increased results, whereas hyperuricemia can cause lower values.

Interpretation

Whole blood glucose values are approximately 15% lower than plasma glucose values, assuming the hematocrit is 45%, but this difference may range from 7–47%. In some systems, the plasma portion of the whole blood specimen may react with the reagent strip. Thus, in reality, results with a RBC free ultrafiltrate, are more analogous to plasma than whole blood. This may explain why results obtained using whole blood are higher than plasma in some circumstances.

Whole blood glucose values are usually compared with plasma (or serum) results obtained by clinical laboratories: those that differ by less than 20% are considered accurate for patient monitoring.

A situation has been described in which diabetics, using these instruments to monitor glucose control for presentation to physicians, fabricate their own results by consciously transcribing values much lower than those measured or log in values without actually making any measurements. This can be overcome by using instruments containing electronic memory chips so all glucose measurements made are stored and electronically retrieved at the time of the physician office visit.

GLUCOSE TOLERANCE TESTING

Test: Glucose Tolerance Test (GTT)

Background and Selection

During the past 30 years, much controversy has existed over performance and interpretation of glucose tolerance testing for the diagnosis of diabetes mellitus. Part of the confusion has occurred because a variety of protocols for test performance have been used, over 20 criteria for interpretation of results have been applied, and lack of adherence to established protocols was common place. Although there has been recent agreement on the size of the glucose load (75 g) for most patients, diagnosis of gestational diabetes still requires a 100 g load. Interpretation criteria have been promulgated by organizations or medical societies such that agreement of patient classification from test results no longer is a local issue. Despite these advances, test logistics still differ for diagnosis of diabetes in pregnant and nonpregnant individuals and international disagreement exists on evaluation criteria.

Glucose tolerance testing is widely accepted for the diagnosis of diabetes mellitus, but is not recommended for diagnosis of hypoglycemia.[10] Simultaneous sampling for glucose and growth hormone determinations are used in the diagnosis of acromegaly (see Ch. 11, Hormones; Test: Growth Hormone).

Logistics

For nonpregnant individuals, a 2-hour test using a 75 g load is used, whereas for gestational diabetes a 3-hour test with a 100 g load is recommended. Patient preparation was standardized in 1969,[11] but frequently these requirements are ignored, thereby jeopardizing proper interpretation of results.

The preparatory phase preceding the test requires a diet of at least 150 g of carbohydrate per day for 3 days, a testing delay of at least 2 weeks after an acute illness, discontinuance of all drugs proven or believed to influence the GTT for at least 3 days, fasting for 8–16 hours, and test postponement when unexpected illness or improper patient preparation occurs.

A list of over 125 drugs or medical conditions interfering with glucose tolerance testing has been developed.[7] The test is conducted between 0700 hours and noon. Between 0700 and 0900 hours and after 30 minutes of rest, blood for a baseline glucose determination is obtained. The patient then ingests the glucose load. Because pure glucose is extremely unpalatable, commercial products such as Glucola, consisting of hydrolyzable saccharide of corn syrup and carbonated water with cola, grape, or cherry flavoring, frequently are used. Seven ounces of commercial product is equivalent to 75 g of glucose. The glucose load is ingested over 5 minutes and the first blood specimen drawn at a specific time after the baseline depending on the criteria

Table 7-3. Diagnostic Criteria for Glucose Tolerance Testing

Classification	Glucose Load	Fasting		Other		2 Hour
		\multicolumn{5}{c}{Plasma Glucose mg/dL (mmol/L)}
NDDG	75 g					
Normal[a]		<115 (<7.8)	and	<200 (<11.1)[c]	and	<140 (<7.8)
IGT		<140 (<7.8)	and	≥200 (≥11.1)[c]	and	140–199 (7.8–11.1)
Diabetes		≥140 (≥7.8)	or	≥200 (≥11.1)[c]	and	≥200 (≥11.1)
Nondiagnostic		All other combinations of fasting, midtest, and 2-hour values				
WHO	75 g					
Normal[a]		<140 (<7.8)		—	and	<140 (<7.8)
IGT		<140 (<7.8)		—	and	140–199 (7.8–11.1)
Diabetes		≥140 (≥7.8)		—	or	≥200 (≥11.1)
O'Sullivan[b] (pregnancy)	100 g					
Normal		<105 (5.8)				
Gestational diabetes (2 Values abnormal)		≥105 (5.8)	or 1 hour or 3 hour	>190 (10.6) >145 (8.1)	or	165 (9.5)

Abbreviations: IGT, impaired glucose tolerance; NDDG, National Diabetes Data Group; OGTT, oral glucose tolerance test; WHO, World Health Organization.
  [a] Although WHO does not define a "normal" OGTT, the term is used here to include subjects who do not meet criteria for diabetes or IGT.
  [b] Two of four criteria exceeded for diagnosis of diabetes.
  [c] $\frac{1}{2}$, 1, and $1\frac{1}{2}$ hour midtest specimens obtained.

used for interpretation (Table 7-3). If nausea, fainting, sweating, or other autonomic nervous system activities occur, a specimen for glucose should be drawn immediately and the procedure discontinued. All specimens should be drawn as antecubital venous specimens.

Interpretation

Although a number of criteria have been used for the diagnosis of diabetes mellitus using a GTT, those developed in 1979 by the NDDG[7] are widely used in the United States. Still, differences occur because the World Health Organization (WHO) also has promulgated recommendations.[12] Both recommend a 2-hour, 75-g oral glucose tolerance test if the fasting plasma glucose concentration on a previous occasion was less than 140 mg/dL (<7.8 mmol/L). However, two main differences occur in the classification of patients depending on test results. These criteria are seen in Table 7-3. The NDDG defines a "normal" fasting glucose level as less than 115 mg/dL (<6.4 mmol/L), whereas WHO does not stipulate a cut-off value, but implies it must not exceed 140 mg/dL (7.8 mmol/L). For the test recommended by the NDDG, five plasma glucose values are required, whereas WHO requires only two.[7,12] Both require fasting and 2-hour postprandial values, but only NDDG recommends additional specimens at ½, 1, and 1½ hours after the challenge. To confirm the diagnosis of diabetes mellitus, both criteria require fasting glucose levels of 140 mg/dL (7.8 mmol/L) or more and 2-hour values between 140 and 199 mg/dL (7.8 and 11.1 mmol/L). If criteria for diabetes mellitus, impaired glucose tolerance, or "normal" are not fulfilled, the test results are placed in the category "nondiagnostic," a category not used in the WHO criteria. Almost 90% of patients are classified similarly by both criteria. However, the major difference is patients classified as nondiagnostic by the NDDG. Also, the impaired glucose tolerance group defined by WHO criteria is approximately twice the size of the NDDG group. A minor problem has been rounding errors introduced by the conversion of units of measure from mg/dL to mmol/L. The WHO system represents a simpler and more practical system for patient testing; however, uncertainty exists as to which criteria is more predictive of the development of diabetes or its complications.

Gestational diabetes has been identified by the presence of an abnormal 3-hour GTT after a 100-g glucose load. O'Sullivan and Mahaw[13] established reference values during pregnancy as a fasting plasma glucose value of up to 105 mg/dL (≤5.8 mmol/L), and a 1-, 2-, and 3-hour level up to 190, 165, 145 mg/dL (≤10.6, 9.2, and 8.1 mmol/L), respectively. If two of these values are exceeded, then the diagnosis is diabetes mellitus (Table 7-3).

Pregnant women needing the 3-hour GTT usually are identified by a screening test performed between the 24th and 28th week, consisting of 50 g of oral glucose given without regard to time of the last meal or time of day (see page 135).

Test: Glucose Tolerance Test, 5 Hour (5-Hour GTT)

Background and Selection

Occasionally the 5-hour glucose tolerance test is used for the diagnosis of postprandial hypoglycemia; however, it is far from satisfactory for this purpose. Neither the glucose nadir during the GTT nor the hypoglycemic index (the fall in glucose during the 90 minutes before reaching the nadir divided by the value of the glucose nadir) delineate hypoglycemia as the cause of the day-to-day symptoms of these patients.

Logistics

The test is performed using a 100-g glucose load and the usual standardized procedure, but sampling is extended to include specimens obtained at 4 and 5 hours.

Interpretation

Symptoms of reactive hypoglycemia appear within about 4 hours after eating or drinking or less commonly after cessation of intravenous infusions. Table 7-1 lists the usual causes of hypoglycemia. To ascribe a patient's complaints to hypoglycemia, the following criteria must be met:

1. Adrenergic or neuroglycopenic symptoms (Table 7-4).

Table 7-4. Symptoms and Signs of Hypoglycemia

Adrenergic	Neuroglycopenic
Irritability	Headache
Sweating	Mental dullness
Palpitations	Fatigue
Hunger	Confusion
Tremulousness	Amnesia
Anxiety	Seizures
	Loss of consciousness

2. Glucose levels that are abnormally low when the patient is experiencing these symptoms.
3. Relief of symptoms when glucose levels are no longer abnormal.

Although the upper reference interval for glucose tolerance testing is standardized internationally, there is no agreement concerning clinical significance of lower values during the test. In a large recent study of the 5-hour test using a 100-g load, 10% of patients had plasma glucose nadirs of 47 mg/dL (2.6 mmol/L) or below and 2.5% had values of 39 mg/dL (2.2 mmol/L) or less. However, the 5-hour GTT often evoked symptoms resembling hypoglycemia when plasma glucose was well above 60 mg/dL (3.3 mmol/L). In addition, in many individuals who were not suspected of having any disorders of glucose metabolism nor any spontaneous symptoms resembling hypoglycemia, the GTT caused brief reactive hypoglycemia.

An expression of glucose results from the GTT as the hypoglycemic index has been advocated. Values above 0.8 have been found in symptomatic patients; however, a recent study showed the hypoglycemic index valueless in diagnosis of functional hypoglycemia.[10] For these reasons, the 5-hour GTT is not recommended for the diagnosis of hypoglycemia.

Test: Intravenous Glucose Tolerance Tests

Background and Selection

A number of modifications of the intravenous glucose tolerance test have been used for the diagnosis of diabetes mellitus, but there is little scientific evidence to support routine use of these procedures.

Logistics

The advantage of intravenous glucose tolerance testing is the avoidance of the vagaries of gastrointestinal absorption that affect oral tests. The most commonly used test is one in which a 25-g bolus of glucose is given over 2 minutes as 50 mL of a 50% glucose solution. After equilibrium of approximately 15 minutes, specimens are obtained at intervals of approximately 5 minutes for 30–45 more minutes. Results are plotted on semilog paper and a line of best fit drawn through the series of values. The K value, or the percent rate of fall per minute, is calculated from this line.

It should be noted that infiltration of a high concentration glucose solution at the site of the injection is quite irritating.

Interpretation

Except in the elderly, K values below 1.0 are abnormal. When compared with the oral GTT, 40% of patients are classified differently with this test. Because of poor reproducibility, lack of standardization, technical problems of test performance, and difficulty of interpretation, this test has little clinical utility. For further information see West.[14]

Test: 1-Hour Postprandial Glucose (1-hour GTT)

The 1-hour PP glucose value has been used in screening for gestational diabetes mellitus. There is widespread agreement that all pregnant females between 24 and 28 weeks of pregnancy should undergo screening for gestational diabetes. For the screening test, a 50-g glucose load, irrespective of time since the last meal, is given. Patients with plasma glucose values greater than 140 mg/dL (>7.8 mmol/L) at 1 hour are referred for routine oral glucose tolerance testing for the diagnosis of gestational diabetes.[15] Those patients with glucose values above 182 mg/dL (>10.0 mmol/L) have more than a 95% probability of the diagnosis of diabetes by the GTT, whereas those with values below 135 mg/dL (<7.4 mmol/L) have been shown to have less than a 1% chance.[16]

MONITORING DIABETIC CONTROL

Test: Glycohemoglobin (Glycated Hemoglobin: Glycosylated Hemoglobin [GHb], Fast Hemoglobin, Hemoglobin A$_{1c}$)

Background and Selection

Classic methods of assessing diabetic control include frequent measurement of blood, plasma, and urine glucose. These measurements reflect acute changes and are not indicators of long-term aspects of diabetic control. To assess diabetic control for the previous 3 months, a single measurement of glycohemoglobin (GHb) is adequate. When control is poor and mean plasma glucose values are elevated, GHb values are elevated; with improving control, glucose and GHb values decrease. Use of GHb measurements have not proven useful for diagnosis of diabetes mellitus or hypoglycemia.

Terminology

When hemolysates of human red blood cells are separated by charge, at least three small, more negatively charged peaks called hemoglobin A_{1a}, A_{1b}, and A_{1c} are found before the main hemoglobin A peak. These three hemoglobins, sometimes called the "fast hemoglobins" because of the elution or electrophoretic migration in relation to hemoglobin A, are made by postsynthetic modification of hemoglobin A at a slow rate directly dependent on the glucose concentration within the RBC. Subsequently identified as glycoproteins, they were referred to as glycosylated hemoglobins, but when the glucose-hemoglobin linkage was identified as carbohydrate-protein, they were more correctly called glycohemoglobins. Studies have shown that formation of hemoglobin A_{1c} is a two-step process with initial formation of an aldimine (Schiff base), which then undergoes molecular rearrangement to form the ketoamine hemoglobin A_{1c} (Fig. 7-2). Glycohemoglobin is modified by glucose at the α- and β-chain amino terminal valine resulting in altered electrophoretic change. Although glucose is attached at the amino group of lysine of hemoglobin A_{1c} as well, no change in isoelectric point occurs. A major component of hemoglobin A is also glycated, hence called A_0, but because the charge properties are not altered, it continues to separate with hemoglobin A. The reactivity of various fractions in GHb assays is seen in Figure 7-3.

Logistics

Anticoagulated capillary and venous whole blood specimens give comparable results that are unaffected by recent food, exercise, or even previously administered antidiabetic drugs. The validity of hemoglobin A_{1c} measurements depends in part on the method used. Methods differ in the measurement of hemoglobin A_1 (A_{1a}, A_{1b}, A_{1c}) or A_{1c}, a pre-A_1, or pre-A_{1c} as well. Pre-A_{1c} is a labile form of GHb containing glucose attached by aldimine linkages at the β-chain terminal valine residue. If measurement of pre-A_{1c} is excluded from measurement, hemoglobin A_{1c} is stable at 4°C for many months. At temperatures above 4°C, hemoglobin A_{1a} and A_{1b} show steady increases with storage that are time and temperature dependent; hemoglobin A_{1c} is only minimally affected. Thus, methods that determine hemoglobin A_1 will show falsely increased values if specimens are not handled properly before assay.

The most common methods include electrophoresis, colorimetry, ion exchange chromatography, or affinity chromatography. Interferences include aldimine intermediates (pre-A_{1c}), hemoglobinopathies, and nonglucose adducts of hemoglobin with all of the above methods except affinity chromatography. Removal of the labile fraction of GHb is crucial in making the assay an accurate index of chronic metabolic control. A number of methods to exclude pre-A_{1c} are used including incubation of erythrocytes in a saline solution or lysis of blood specimens in a low-pH buffer. Some hemoglobins such as F, J, N, and Wayne separate with fast hemoglobin and increase apparent levels whereas others such as

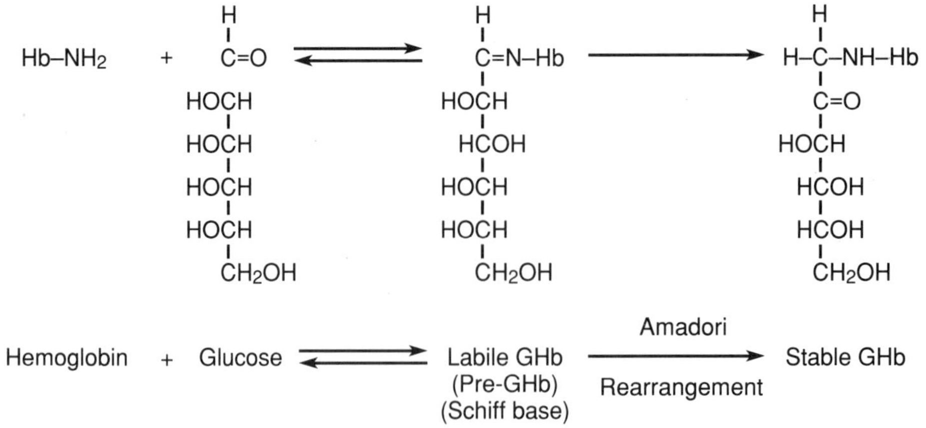

Fig. 7-2. Reaction of glucose with hemoglobin forming glycated hemoglobin. Hb, hemoglobin; Hb-NH_2, N terminal end of hemoglobin; GHb, glycated Hb.

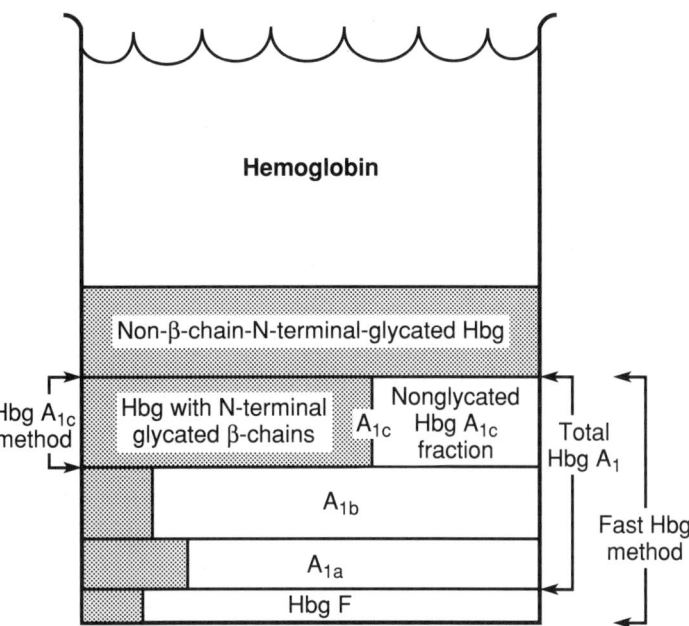

Fig. 7-3. Relationships and measurements of various glycohemoglobin fractions. Affinity chromatography measures fractions shaded.

S, C, D, E, G, or O falsely lower test results. A variety of other substances other than sugars form adducts with hemoglobin, thereby altering its charge characteristics and cochromatograph with the GHb. This occurs in opiate addiction, lead poisoning, uremia, alcoholism, and salicylate treatment. Lactescence increases GHb measurements by ion exchange chromatography by cochromatographing with the hemoglobin A_1 peak. Because affinity methods are based on chemical reactivity of hydroxyl glucose groups rather than charge, they are usually unaffected by these interferences. There is still no consensus on a GHb standard although some attempts to compare methods have occurred.

Interpretation

Reference intervals vary depending on the method employed with affinity chromatography values being the highest. For this method, nondiabetic children and adults have values of 5.5–8.5%, and uncontrolled diabetics in the range of 12–20%. Well controlled diabetics have values that are slightly higher than the upper end of the reference interval; a diabetic whose values are within the reference range usually has experienced frequent episodes of hypoglycemia. Studies have shown that a 1% increase in GHb represents a 35 mg/dL (1.9 mmol/L) increase in plasma glucose. With shortening RBC survival, as in hemolytic anemias, phlebotomy, and pregnancy, GHb values are decreased. In iron deficiency, results were reported as increased because of extended RBC survival but this is now disputed because of methodologic considerations. A few patients with essential fructosuria, galactosemia, and G-6-PD deficiency also have been reported to have elevated values.

Other procedures, which have been used to monitor diabetic control, include plasma or blood glucose measurements, urine glucose measurements, and glycosylated albumin and protein.

Test: Fructosamine (Serum Glycoproteins, Glycated Serum Proteins, Glycosylated Serum Proteins, Ketoamines)

Background and Selection

With increasing recognition of the importance of strict glycemic control for prevention or delay of diabetic complications, there is much interest in monitoring control of blood glucose concentration. Glycosylated or glycated hemoglobin has been used to monitor glucose control over the previous 120 days but because the half-life of serum proteins is much shorter then hemoglobin, measurement of serum glycoproteins reflects glucose control over the previous 1–3 weeks. Serum glycoprotein measurement also provides a means of assessing the effects of changes in diabetes management and indicates deterioration of control earlier than does GHb.

Serum glycoproteins are estimated by a number of methods, the most widely used of which quantitates fructosamines. Ketoamines, also known generally as fructosamines, are formed in an Amadori rearrangement of the condensation products between glucose and the amino groups of proteins. Fructosamine is a reductant under alkaline conditions, a property used in quantitation of serum glycoproteins in which such proteins reduce the dye nitroblue tetrazolium.

Logistics

The main practical advantages compared with GHb measurements are the use of unmodified stable serum specimens, ease of analysis, assay precision, and suitability of adequate standards and control. Expression of results in mmol/L precludes easy comparison with GHb results expressed as a percentage.

Interpretation

The reference range is approximately 37–58 mg/dL (1.5–2.3 mmol/L) and is lower in maternal serum during pregnancy. For children younger than 3 years, fructosamine concentration is 15% lower than in adults, but increases with age, reaching adult values by age 6. Albumin is the major component affecting the procedure, although IgM and IgG are the most highly glycated protein fractions. Therefore, interpretation of changes in fructosamine concentrations depend on the half-life of albumin being constant. However, all major serum proteins contribute to the overall result.[16] The test is sensitive to variations in specific proteins, and almost completed unaffected by labile fractions. For example, in patients receiving only parenteral nutrition, the test fluctuates widely despite stable plasma glucose results. Severe hypoproteinemic states when the serum albumin is less than 3.0 g/dL (<30 g/L) may falsely lower serum fructosamine concentrations.

There is a 1.3% increase in fructosamine for every 3 g/L increase in total protein concentration. Hemoglobin, ascorbic acid, and ceruloplasmin inhibit fructosamine generation.

INSULIN AND RELATED PEPTIDE TESTS

Test: Insulin (See Ch. 5)

Background and Selection

Insulin is a peptide with a mass of about 6000 da consisting of an α-chain of 20 amino acids connected by two disulfide bonds to a β-chain of 30 amino acids. A precursor of insulin, preproinsulin, is synthesized as a long single chain with a mass of about 9000 da. During storage within the pancreatic β-cell, two disulfide bonds are formed within the molecule forming proinsulin, which then is converted to a double chain molecule by a proteolytic process that removes the 31 amino acid C-peptide and other small peptides (Fig. 7-4). Equimolar concentrations of C-peptide and insulin are secreted into the portal blood, but because the liver extracts a large and variable amount of insulin, the ratio of both analytes in peripheral blood is unpredictable.

The major use of insulin measurements is to identify patients with insulin-producing tumors. Insulin levels are not recommended during glucose tolerance testing.

Logistics

Usually fasting plasma or serum insulin levels are obtained. Although in the past, specimens for insulin measurements were separated immediately and stored at $-20°C$, recent evidence indicates that whole blood specimens are stable for a few hours and plasma is stable for 3 days at $20°C$.

Interpretation

Insulin usually is measured by immunoassay with the usual reference concentration in fasting individuals of less than $25 \mu U/mL$. Insulin is released in seven to eight pulses per day including three postmeal pulses reaching almost $100 \mu U/mL$. With many immunoassays, insulin concentrations lower than $5 \mu U/mL$ cannot be detected even though quantitation in this range may be clinically relevant.

Fasting insulin levels are inappropriately high in patients with insulinoma or those who have chlorpropamide toxicity. In patients who have circulating insulin antibodies caused by use of nonhuman insulin, immunoassay values may be either factitiously high or low depending on the type of separation step used in the immunoassay procedure. Because accurate measure-

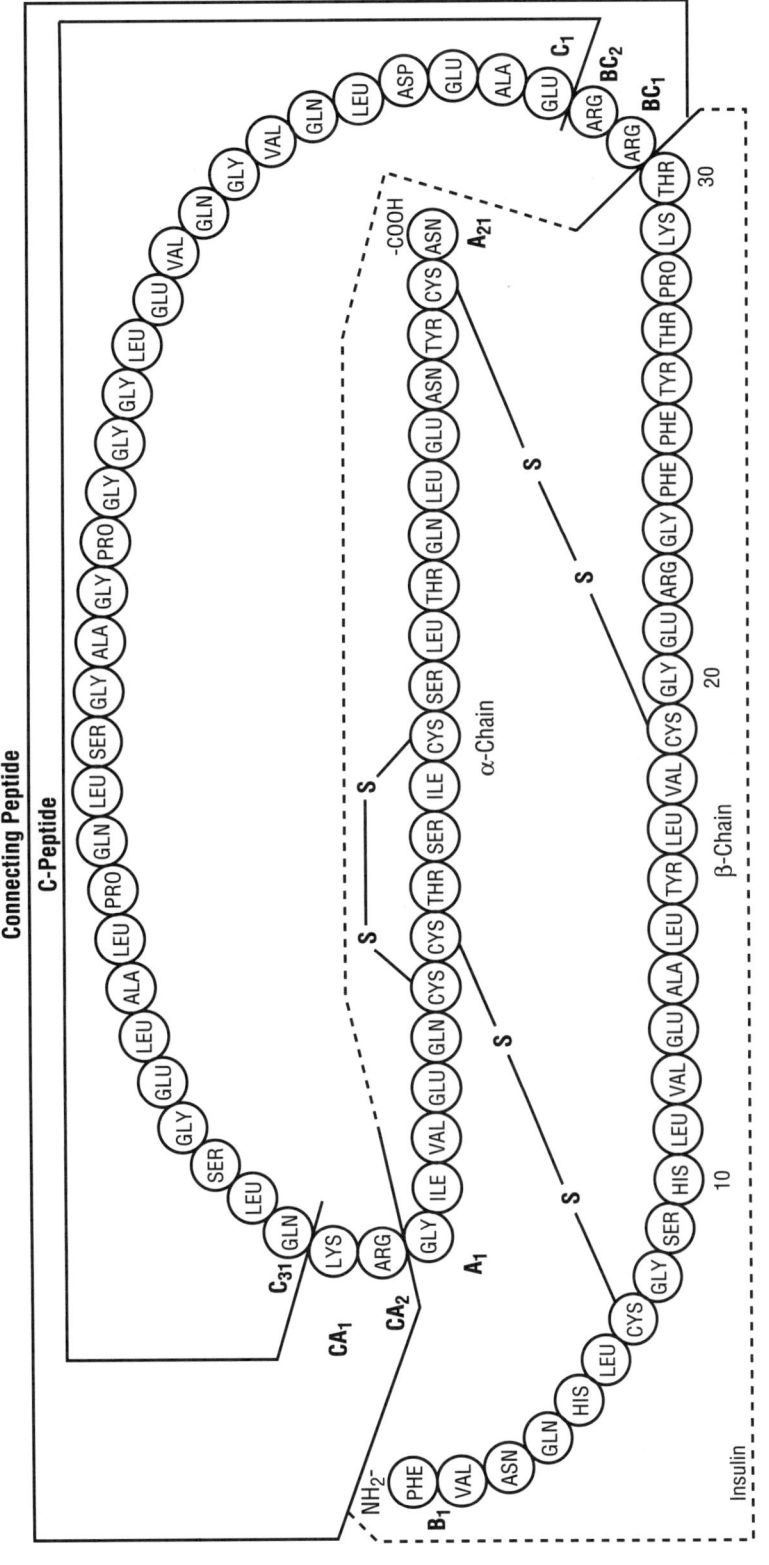

Fig. 7-4. Human proinsulin. The two amino acids at each end of the connecting peptide are ultimately cleaved to yield insulin (broken line) and C-peptide.

ment of insulin levels is hampered by insulin antibodies in insulin treated diabetics, free (unbound) insulin can be measured after separating the insulin antibodies and the antibody bound insulin from the unbound insulin. Proinsulin has a minor effect on insulin measurements. Proinsulin concentrations are approximately 15–35% of insulin levels and reactivity with reagent antibody is 40–60% that of insulin depending on the assay used. In a few patients, abnormal insulin has been identified as leading to elevated insulin immunoassay concentrations. These measurements have been validated using research techniques such as radioreceptor assays and high performance liquid chromatography.

Insulin values are frequently expressed in relationship to plasma glucose.[17] In healthy individuals, insulin (μU/mL) to glucose (mg/dL) ratios are usually less than 0.4, except in obesity and other states of insulin resistance. The numerical value for the immunoreactive insulin to glucose ratio depends on the techniques employed to measure plasma glucose and insulin. Because hypoglycemia suppresses insulin secretion and insulin levels are detectable when glucose is less than 30 mg/dL, an "amended" insulin to glucose ratio is used according to the following formula: insulin (μU/mL) $\times$ 100/glucose (mg/dL) $-$ 30 (mg/dL). This amended ratio provides better discrimination between those with insulinomas from those with other causes of hypoglycemia. A value of 50 discriminates those with elevated ratios (insulinoma or surreptitious sulfonylurea usage) from the reference population.

Test: C-Peptide

Background and Selection

Insulin and C-peptide are secreted simultaneously in equimolar quantities into the portal blood. During the first-pass circulation, a considerable and variable proportion of insulin is extracted by the liver, whereas almost all C-peptide secreted enters the systemic circulation intact. Most C-peptide is degradated in the kidney, but a small proportion of the intact peptide is excreted in the urine unchanged.

C-peptide is measured by radioimmunoassay, but differences exist in assay standards, the label of assay preparations, and antibody reactivity. Koskinen[18] concluded that variations between methods precluded transferability of results among methods and thus reference ranges are dependent on the specific method used. At least four different components have been identified in sera that react with reagent antibodies.

Table 7-5. Clinical Indications for C-Peptide Measurement

Hypoglycemic states
    Diagnosis of insulinoma
    Diagnosis of surreptitious injection of insulin
Euglycemic states
    Demonstration of remission phase or "recovery" from diabetes
Hyperglycemic state
    Follow-up evaluation after pancreatectomy
    Evaluation of the "brittle" diabetic patient

Reported molar crossreactivity of proinsulin with antisera used in C-peptide measurements varies between 3 and 80%.

The most important application of C-peptide measurement is for the diagnosis of surreptitious injection of insulin resulting in factitious hypoglycemia. C-peptide also is used to measure insulin secretion in individuals with diabetes mellitus and to aid in the diagnosis of insulinoma. Although urine C-peptide has been used as a measure of insulin secretion, it is only of limited value because considerable variability occurs in the percent excreted among subjects and in the same subject studied on different occasions.[19] Many other uses have been proposed (Table 7-5).

Test: Proinsulin

Proinsulin is formed within the β-cell with approximately 95% cleaved to insulin and C-peptide and 5% secreted directly into the circulation. Because proinsulin is cleared from plasma much more slowly than insulin, the concentration of proinsulin in human plasma is 15–35% that of insulin.

Because proinsulin contains the sequence of both insulin and C-peptide and is present in much lower concentrations than either of these, crossreactivity is a major problem in the immunoassay for proinsulin. Plasma proinsulin concentrations are often increased in patients with insulin-producing tumors.

Fasting proinsulin levels are frequently below 1 pmol/L, whereas limits of detection of proinsulin immunoassays are 1 pmol/L. Thus many healthy individuals have nondetectable fasting levels. Insufficient evidence exists as to whether proinsulin is elevated in patients with islet cell hyperplasia and nesidioblastosis; the preliminary evidence indicates it may not be.[17]

PROVOCATIVE TESTS OF INSULIN SECRETION

Test: Prolonged (72 Hour) Fast

Background and Selection

The prolonged (72 hour) fast has been reported as the best test for the diagnosis of an insulinoma.

Logistics

After the evening meal, the patient begins fasting, drinking only water or other caloric-free drinks. For the first 24 hours, plasma specimens are obtained every 6 hours for glucose, insulin, and C-peptide determinations. In some patients, profound symptoms of hypoglycemia occur and require termination of the test by administration of carbohydrate or food following sampling. If no symptoms occur during the first 24 hours, the frequency of plasma specimens should be increased to every 4 hours; if individuals are still asymptomatic, they should be exercised prior to specimen collection.

Interpretation

Most individuals with fasting hypoglycemia will not tolerate a 72-hour fast. Most patients with insulinomas develop symptomatic hypoglycemia and inappropriate hyperinsulinemia within the first 24 hours of the test and almost all of them develop both by 72 hours.

The appropriateness of the insulin concentration to the hypoglycemia during a prolonged fast has been evaluated in a number of ways. Most commonly, insulin and glucose determinations are expressed as a ratio (see Test: Insulin). For further information see Field.[20]

Test: Calcium Infusion

The infusion of calcium (4 mg/kg/h) over 2–4 hours has been reported to induce hyperinsulinism and hypoglycemia in some patients with islet cell tumors. Specimens are obtained for serum insulin and plasma glucose measurement while the patient is fasting and every 30 minutes thereafter during the infusion. In healthy individuals or individuals with reactive hypoglycemia, hypercalcemia has no significant effect on either plasma glucose or insulin levels. Although initially reported that this test could discriminate between benign and islet cell tumors, substantiation has not occurred. Others have not found changes in insulin and glucose in patients following calcium infusion.[20]

Test: Tolbutamide Tolerance

Background and Selection

The tolbutamide tolerance test has been used to separate individuals with an insulinoma from those with other conditions.

Logistics

Following the procurement of a specimen for baseline measurements in fasting adults, the rapid intravenous administration of 1 g of tolbutamide is given and plasma specimens for glucose and insulin are obtained at 1, 15, 30, 60, 90, and 120 minutes thereafter. Administration of tolbutamide may produce severe symptomatic hypoglycemia requiring termination of the test and administration of carbohydrate.

Interpretation

In healthy individuals, plasma glucose reaches a nadir at 30 minutes that may exceed 50% fasting, but then returns to reference range at the end of 2 hours. In contrast to changes in glucose, the insulin response is very rapid, attaining a maximum almost immediately. In healthy individuals, insulin levels peak at 2 minutes and rarely exceed 150 μU/mL. In patients with islet cell tumors, insulin response usually is greater. Insulin results in healthy individuals are within the reference interval at 60 minutes postinfusion, in contrast to patients with insulinomas who usually have elevated values. For further information on interpretation of results see Field[20] and Fajans and Vinik.[17]

Patients with hypopituitarism, adrenocortical insufficiency, liver disease, renal disease, or malnutrition may have plasma glucose responses to tolbutamide indistinguishable from those of individuals with islet cell tumors. However, only those with insulinomas have exaggerated plasma insulin levels.

Test: C-Peptide Suppression Test

Infusion of insulin causes suppression of C-peptide in healthy subjects, but not in the majority of patients with insulin-secreting pancreatic β-cell tumors. Simultaneous measurements of plasma levels of human C-peptide at frequent intervals during the infusion have been used as a diagnostic test. Because some healthy individuals may have abnormal test results, this test is not widely used.

Test: C-Peptide-Glucagon Test

Intravenous injection of 1 mg of glucagon and subsequent measurement of C-peptide 6 minutes later has been used as a measure of pancreatic β-cell function. If the patient has undetectable C-peptide concentrations in plasma after stimulation, this indicates that β-cell destruction is so extensive that exogenous insulin is required to maintain life. In those patients in which the C-peptide concentration exceeds a certain level, acceptable glycemic control can be obtained without exogenous insulin injections. The discrimination level is dependent on the immunoassay used. For further information, see Rönnemaa.[21]

REFERENCES

1. Larsson-Cohn U: Differences between capillary and venous blood glucose during oral glucose tolerance tests. Scand J Clin Lab Invest 1976;36:805–808.
2. Gerson B, Figoni MA: Clinical comparison of glucose quantitation methods. Arch Pathol Lab Med 1985;109:711–715.
3. Burrin JM, Price CP: Measurement of blood glucose. Ann Clin Biochem 1985;22:327–342.
4. Editorial: Glucose tolerance in pregnancy—the who and how of testing. Lancet 1988;2:1173–1174.
5. Felig P, Cherif A, Minagawa A, Wakren J: Hypoglycemia during prolonged exercise in normal men. N Engl J Med 1982;306:895–900.
6. Merimee TJ, Tyson JE: Stabilization of plasma glucose during fasting: normal variations in two separate studies. N Engl J Med 1974;291:1275–1278.
7. National Diabetes Data Group: Classification and diagnosis of diabetes mellitus and other categories of glucose intolerance. Diabetes 1979;28:1039–1057.
8. Kilo C: Value of glucose control in preventing complications of diabetes. Am J Med 1985;79(Suppl 2B):33–37.
9. Brooks KE, Rawal N, Henderson AR: Laboratory assessment of three new monitors of blood glucose: Accu-Chek II, Glucometer II, and Glucoscan 2000. Clin Chem 1986;32:2195–2200.
10. Lev-Ran A, Anderson RW: The diagnosis of postprandial hypoglycemia. Diabetes 1981;30:996–999.
11. Klimt CR, Prout TE, Bradley RF et al: Standardization of the oral glucose tolerance test: report of the committee on statistics of the American Diabetes Association. Diabetes 1969;18:299–307.
12. Harris MI, Hadden WC, Knowler WC, Bennett PH: International Criteria for the diagnosis of diabetes and impaired glucose tolerance. Diabetes Care 1985;8:562–567.
13. O'Sullivan JB, Mahaw CM: Criteria for the oval glucose tolerance test in pregnancy. Diabetes 1964;13:278–285.
14. West KM: Diagnosis of diabetes mellitus. pp. 103–108. In Rifkin H, Raskin P (eds): Diabetes Mellitus. Vol. 5. Bowie, MD, Robert J Brady, 1981.
15. Singer DE, Samet JH, Coley CM, Nathan DM: Screening for diabetes mellitus. Ann Intern Med 1988;109:639–649.
16. Zoppi F, Mosca A, Granata S, Montalbetti N: Glycated proteins in serum: effect of their relative proportions on their alkaline reducing activity in the fructosamine test. Clin Chem 1987;33:1895–1897.
17. Fajans SS, Vinik AI: Insulin-producing islet cell tumors. Endocrinol Metab Clin N Am 1989;18:45–71.
18. Koskinen P: Nontransferability of C-peptide measurements with various commercial radioimmunoassay reagents. Clin Chem 1988;34:1575–1578.
19. Tillil H, Shapiro ET, Given BD et al: Reevaluation of urine C-peptide as measure of insulin secretion. Diabetes 1988;37:1195–1201.
20. Field J: Hypoglycemia: definition, clinical presentations, classification, and laboratory tests. J Clin Endocrinol Metab 1989;18:27–43.
21. Rönnemaa T: Practical aspects in performing the glucagon test in the measurement of C-peptide secretion in diabetic patients. Scand J Clin Lab Invest 1986;46:345–349.

8 Amino Acids and Proteins

James H. McBride

AMINO ACIDS

INTRODUCTION

Amino acids are carboxylic acids that also contain an amino ($-NH_2$) group in the molecule and have the general formula RCH (NH_2) COOH. The majority have an amino group in the α-position with respect to the carboxyl group. With the exception of glycine, all α-amino acids are asymmetric, a property that gives rise to D and L optical isomers although the L-isomer predominates in proteins found in higher organisms.[1]

There are at least 21 amino acids commonly found in proteins of the body and these are listed in Tables 8-1 and 8-2. Most of these are essential in the sense that all must be present in order for protein synthesis to occur. Humans can biosynthesize only about one-half of those required, and the remainder, which must be supplied by the diet, are termed nutritionally essential amino acids. Proteins that contain all the essential amino acids (complete proteins) are usually of animal origin, whereas plant proteins often lack one or more of the essential amino acids. It is therefore not surprising that diet plays an important role in diseases caused by essential amino acid deficiencies.

Properties of Amino Acids

Amino acids are amphoteric in that they can serve as both acids and bases in aqueous solutions. The acid-base properties depend on the amino group, which can accept a proton to become $-NH_3^+$, and the carboxyl group, which can lose a proton to form $-COO^-$, and the basic or acidic functional groups present on the R group of the amino acid.

In the pH range of 7.35–7.45, amino acids become ionized with coexistent negative and positive charges and are said to be dipolar ions or ampholytes (formerly Zwitter ions). Also the pH at which all molecules of an amino acid exist in the ampholyte form (zero net charge) is called the isoelectric point (pI). If the pH is greater than the pI, excess OH^- groups in solution remove the proton from the $-NH_3^+$ group on the amino acid to give a net charge of -1 on the remaining ion. However, if the pH is less than the pI, excess protons (H^+) protonate the COO^- group to give a resultant charge of $+1$ on the ion.[2]

The R groups associated with amino acids may be aliphatic carbon chains, aromatic carbon rings, heterocyclic imino rings, or amides and give rise to hydrophobic amino acids with nonpolar R groups and hydrophilic amino acids with uncharged polar R groups. These groups account for the majority of amino acids; however, aspartic and glutamic acids belong to the dicarboxylic amino acids group with acidic R groups capable of losing two protons in solutions at high pH forming an amino acid anion with a charge of -2. The amino acids lysine, arginine, and histidine contain additional amino groups belonging to the basic amino acid group where at low pH, the amino acids can gain an additional proton to form a cation with a charge of $+2$.

Table 8-1. Nutritionally Essential Amino Acids

Name	Abbreviation	Biochemical Features	Reference Range mg/dL	Reference Range µmol/L
Arginine	Arg	174 da; necessary for urea synthesis	0.5–2.5	30–145
Histidine	His	155 da; imidazole group important physiologic buffer	0.5–1.7	30–110
Isoleucine	Ile	131 da; ketogenic	0.5–1.3	40–100
Leucine	Leu	131 da; ketogenic, deranged metabolism in maple syrup urine disease	1.0–2.3	75–175
Lysine	Lys	147 da	1.2–3.5	80–240
Methionine	Met	149; methyl group transfer mechanisms	0.1–0.6	5–40
Phenylalanine	Phe	165 da; found in excess in PKU	0.6–1.5	35–90
Threonine	Thr	119 da	0.9–2.5	75–210
Tryptophan	Trp	204 da; precursor of serotonin and melatonin	0.5–2.5	25–125
Valine	Val	117 da; ketogenic	1.7–3.7	145–315

Abbreviation: PKU, phenylketonuria.

The differing solubilities and acid-base properties of amino acids provide the basis for their separation by various methods in the clinical laboratory and differences in the chemical nature of the various R groups permit detection by color reactions.

Amino Acid Metabolism

Dietary protein is the primary source of amino acids for endogenous protein synthesis. Initially proteolytic enzymes in the gastrointestinal tract act on proteins to release amino acids, which are absorbed via the jejunum into the blood to become part of the body pool of amino acids. Plasma, intracellular, and structural proteins are then synthesized in the liver and other tissues. Amino acids may be interconverted in the liver and kidneys by the biochemical process of transamination, and degradation is usually carried out by deamination. Blood amino acids are filtered through the glomerular membrane but are readily reabsorbed in the renal tubules by an active transport system.

TESTS FOR AMINO ACIDS

Test: Amino Acids

Background and Selection

The term aminoaciduria as used clinically may denote either the appearance of an abnormal quantity of a normal constituent amino acid or the appearance of an abnormal amino acid in the urine. Aminoacidurias may be primary or secondary in nature. Primary aminoacidurias result from a mutation in the DNA sequence that codes for the amino acid sequence of a particular enzyme. Thus, a defective enzyme is produced that causes a block in the metabolic pathway of its substrate resulting in substrate accumulation or diversion into another metabolic pathway. The principal aminoacidurias inherited as autosomal recessive disorders are given in Table 8-3. As these diseases are uncommon and frequently present with nonspecific symptoms, it is desirable to detect and quantify individual amino acids as soon as possible after a problem is suspected. Certainly a baby who appears well initially but deteriorates after a few days of increased protein intake should be evaluated for a suspect inherited aminoaciduria.[3]

Logistics

Specimen Requirements

In the investigation of aminoacidurias, the patient should be on a normal diet and blood and urine specimens should be collected simultaneously. Because plasma amino acid concentrations vary during the day by about 30% (highest in midafternoon, lowest in early morning), specimen collection times must be kept in mind when investigating patients who are suspected of being heterozygotous for the inherited disorders of amino acid metabolism.[4] For infants, specimens are usually obtained 48 hours after birth because 2 days of protein intake are required to accumulate an abnormal concentration of an amino acid such as phenylalanine.

Table 8-2. Nutritionally Nonessential Amino Acids

Name	Abbreviation	Biochemical Features	Reference Range mg/dL	Reference Range µmol/L
Alanine	Ala	89 da; substrate for alanine aminotransferase (ALT)	2.2–4.5	245–500
γ-Aminobutyric acid	GABA	103 da; metabolite of Glu; a neurotransmitter	0.1–0.2	10–20
Asparagine	Asn	132 da; storage form of ammonia in tissues	0.5–0.6	35–45
Aspartic acid	Asp	133 da; used in pyrimidine biosynthesis cosubstrate for asparate aminotransferase (AST)	0.0–0.3	0–20
Citrulline	Citr	175 da; intermediate in urea synthesis	0.2–1.0	15–55
Cysteine	Cys	121 da; responsible for disulfide bridges in peptides and proteins	—	—
Cystine		Molecule is dicysteine	0.2–2.2	10–90
Glutamic	Glu	147 da; cosubstrate with Ala for ALT and with Asp for AST	6.0–10.0	420–700
Glutamine	Gln	146 da; supplies amido nitrogen in purine and pyrimidine biosynthesis	6.1–10.2	420–700
Glycine	Gly	75 da; optically inactive, required in biosynthesis of purines and porphyrins	0.9–4.2	120–560
Hydroxylysine	Hyl	164 da; found in collagen	0.5–1.0	38–76
Hydroxyproline	Hyp	131 da; appreciable amounts found in collagen; indicator of bone matrix metabolism	0–Trace	0–Trace
Ornithine	Orn	132 da; intermediate in urea synthesis	0.4–1.4	30–400
Proline	Pro	155 da; required for connective tissues e.g., collagen and elastin	1.2–3.9	105–340
Serine	Ser	105 da; active center of many enzymes	0.8–1.8	75–170
Taurine	Tau	125 da; inhibitor of nerve impulse transmission, conjugates with bile acids	0.3–2.1	25–170
Tyrosine	Tyr	181 da; intermediate in the synthesis of thyroxine, melanin, and catecholamines	0.4–1.6	20–90

For the quantitation of amino acids in urine, a 24-hour collection (acidified to pH 2–3 with 6.0 mol/L HCl) is preferred. The collection should be kept refrigerated, total volume recorded, and a 50-ml aliquot forwarded for analysis. Quantitation also may be performed on a random urine specimen. Serum or plasma may be used and the specimen should be sent to the laboratory as quickly as possible where the serum or plasma should be frozen immediately. Further, it is essential that nonhemolyzed plasma or serum specimens be used, because cells have amino acid concentrations about 10 times that of plasma.[4] Also the amount of amino acids visible in a chromatogram is influenced not only by the disease process, but also by the volume of fluid applied during chromatography. The sample volume is therefore standardized by reference to its total nitrogen content in serum (or plasma) or the amount of creatinine in a specified volume of the urine specimen.

Analysis

Initial Diagnostic Screening Tests. Screening tests include thin-layer or paper chromatography, urine color tests, or Guthrie microbiologic tests.

Chromatography. In chromatographic analysis of amino acids, most biologic fluids are first deproteinized with sulfosalicylic acid or some appropriate protein-precipitating agent. Following centrifugation to remove the proteins, the supernatant is desalted usually by electrodialysis. The sample is then applied to the chromatography stationary phase, which may be silica,

Table 8-3. Aminoacidurias Inherited as Autosomal Recessive Disorders

Condition	Defective Enzyme	Biochemical Features	Clinical Features	Treatment
Albinism Incidence 1:13,000	Deficiency of tyrosinase	Lack of melanin in skin, hair, and eyes	Photophobia, nystagmus, carcinomata of the skin	None known
Alkaptonuria Incidence 1:250,000	Absence of homogentisate oxygenase	Urinary excretion of homogentisic acid	Degenerative arthritis, cartilage pigmentation	None known
Argininosuccinic aciduria	Argininosuccinate lyase	Urinary excretion of argininosuccinc acid, high blood and CSF ammonia levels, normal urea excretion	Mental retardation, convulsions, hair abnormalities, ammonia intoxication	Diet low in protein
Branched chain ketoaciduria maple syrup urine disease Incidence 1:250,000	Deficiency of branched-chain keto acid decarboxylase	Leucine, isoleucine, and valine accumulate in blood, CSF; urinary excretion of the 3 keto acids and related compounds	Cerebral degeneration, usually early death, mental retardation	Diet low in leucine, isoleucine, and valine
Citrullinemia	Argininosuccinate synthetase	High blood and urinary levels of citrulline, blood ammonia increased	Mental retardation, epilepsy, vomiting, ammonia intoxication	Diet low in protein
Cystinosis	Cystine reductase	Cystine is deposited in reticuloendothelial system, aminoaciduria, proteinuria, phosphaturia	Dwarfism, photophobia, renal acidosis, hypokalemia, vitamin-resistant rickets	Palliative, potassium salts, vitamin D; diet low in cystine and methionine
Cystinuria Incidence 1:13,000	None. Primary renal aminoaciduria	Excess of lysine ornithine, arginine and cystine in urine	Defective transport mechanism in jejunal mucosa and proximal renal tubules	D-penicillamine, high fluid intake
Hartnup disease Incidence 1:18,000	None. Primary renal aminoaciduria	Excessive excretion of all neutral amino acids	Psychiatric symptoms and dermatitis	Nicotinamide with adequate protein diet
Histidinemia	Histidine ammonialyase	Urinary excretion of β-imidazolylpyruvic acid and related compounds	Speech defects, mental retardation in some cases	Diet low in histidine
Homocystinuria Incidence 1:200,000	Cystathionine β-synthetase	Urinary excretion of homocystine	Mental retardation, retinal defects, dislocated lenses, malar flush, thromboses	Diet low in methionine, high in cystine, pyridoxine
Hyperphenylalaninemia (phenylketonuria) type I Incidence 1:10,000	Absence of phenylalanine hydroxylase	Phenylalanine accumulates in blood, CSF etc; urinary excretion of phenylpyruvic acid and related compounds	Severe mental deficiency, epilepsy, abnormal EEG, eczema, behavioral disorders	Diet low in phenylalanine beginning early in life
Hyperphenylalanine (variant) type II Incidence 1:14,000	Deficiency of phenylalanine hydroxylase	Variable excretion of phenylalanine in urine	Mild retardation	Diet low in phenylalanine beginning early in life
Hyperprolinemia type I & type II	Pyrroline-5-carboxylate reductase	Hyperprolinemia, urinary excretion of proline, glycine and hydroxyproline	Mental retardation convulsions, renal disease, deafness	None known
Tyrosinemia Incidence 1:150,000	Absence of fumarylacetoacetate hydrolase	Accumulation of tyrosine and methionine in blood	Hepatic cirrhosis, retinal damage	Dietary restriction of phenylalanine, tyrosine, and methionine

paper, or cellulose, and developed using a solvent system. Usually two-dimensional thin-layer chromatography is employed, which requires rotating the chromatography media through 90 degrees to achieve more distinct separation of the amino acids. In the first dimension, a solvent mixture contains ammonia to increase the mobility of basic amino acids and the second dimension uses a second solvent mixture with formic acid to increase the mobility of dicarboxylic amino acids.[5]

Upon development, the chromatography plate is dried and stained usually with ninhydrin-collidine. The colors and R_f values (relative migration distance; see Ch. 14) of the relative spots are compared with those obtained by separating standard mixtures on the same type of chromatographic system. Each amino acid is then identified and the depth of staining assessed either visually or by direct comparison to the standards run in the system. Usually a normal urine chromatogram shows five prominent amino acids: alanine, glutamine, glycine, histidine, and serine; when pediatric urines are analyzed, moderate amounts of glutamic acid, lysine, taurine, threonine, and β-aminoisobutyric acid may be detected. Asparagine and cystine also may be detected.

Color Tests. It is not unusual for the laboratory to supplement amino acid chromatography with a number of qualitative screening tests for urine samples. In hyperphenylalaninemia (HPA), the ferric chloride test for phenylpyruvic acid in urine may be used although it is no substitute for measurement of blood phenylalanine as the test is both insensitive and nonspecific. Type I tyrosinemia may be detected by the Millon reaction or the nitrosonaphthol test, both of which detect a wide variety of substituted phenolic compounds in urine. These tests are not specific for p-hydroxyphenylpyruvic acid and also will detect tyrosine and its metabolites. In other disorders related to tyrosinemia, Thormählen's test may be used for detecting urinary melanin or melanogens and is considered to be specific and sensitive. Melanogens may be detected in urine with the ammonical silver nitrate test, which can also be used to demonstrate homogentisic acid (alkaptonuria) in urine. In homocystinuria, the cyanide-nitroprusside test for cystine and homocystine may be used, whereas the silver nitroprusside test can differentiate between cystine and homocystine. During the test, urinary cystine remains in the nonreactive form but homocystine reacts. Further, branched chain ketoaciduria (maple syrup urine disease) may be detected by testing urine with 2,4-dinitrophenylhydrazine for the presence of α-keto acids arising from the accumulation of the branched-chain amino acids and their corresponding α-keto acids in the body.

Guthrie Test. The Guthrie test, useful in neonatal screening, utilizes bacterial spores *(Bacillus subtilis)* that are added to an agar medium containing a competitive growth inhibitor specific for the amino acid in question. Urine or blood specimens are applied to the agar plate by filter paper and the plate is incubated and examined for bacterial growth. Growth is observed if the effect of the inhibitor is overcome by the presence of elevated concentrations of the amino acid under investigation.[6]

Amino Acid Quantitation. Amino acid quantitation includes the use of ion exchange chromatography, high performance liquid chromatography (HPLC), or gas liquid chromatography (GLC).

Urine or plasma may be applied to an ion exchange column and after separation of the amino acids by varying the column pH, detection is usually facilitated by a spectrophotometric or fluorometric technique. As compared with ion exchange chromatography, HPLC is somewhat more sensitive and analysis time is shorter. With HPLC, sample purification may be necessary in some cases as a number of interfering substances may be detected in the ultraviolet range. Although GLC has reasonable sensitivity and speed, it suffers from the low volatility of amino acids at temperatures required with this technique. Derivatization of samples is usually required before analysis.

Interpretation

The only amino acids that appear in the urine of normal individuals in significant quantities are alanine, glycine, serine, histidine, and taurine. Excretory rates for all of these exceed 60 mg/d in the average adult. Of the other amino acids, only a few milligrams are excreted in 24 hours, even though between 1 and 5 g/d of each are filtered. During pregnancy when the renal threshold for many substances is lowered, it also is not uncommon to detect phenylalanine and tyrosine. Further, premature babies present with a physiologic renal aminoaciduria and full term babies display an elevated aminoaciduria when compared with values for healthy adults.[3]

Aminoaciduria can be classified as:

1. *Overflow aminoaciduria without primary renal disease.* These conditions are either acquired secondary to other conditions or caused by an inborn error of metabolism.

Generalized aminoaciduria regularly occurs to a mild extent in cirrhosis and other chronic liver diseases and to a marked extent in acute hepatic necrosis. Slight aminoaciduria occurs in wasting diseases, eclampsia, tissue damage, and after infusion of protein hydrolysate. In contrast, a considerable number of congenital disorders are caused by enzyme defects in which one or more normal or incompletely degraded amino acids pass in abnormal amounts into the plasma and are excreted in excess in the urine. Among the best known are alkaptonuria, branched chain ketoaciduria (maple syrup urine disease), cystinuria, and phenylketonuria (PKU) (see below).

2. *Renal aminoaciduria due to diminished tubular reabsorption.* This disorder either can be acquired as secondary to some renal tubular damage or caused by inborn specific or nonspecific disorder of the renal tubular reabsorptive mechanisms. Acquired aminoaciduria can occasionally occur in the nephrotic syndrome, but is commonly due to exogenous toxins (e.g., heavy metal poisoning) or to abnormal metabolites (e.g., galactosylphosphate).

Aminoacidurias

Alkaptonuria. In patients with alkaptonuria, homogentisic acid accumulates owing to deficiency of homogentisic acid oxidase, the enzyme required in the major catabolic pathway that converts tyrosine to fumarate and acetoacetate. Homogentisic acid oxidizes readily to benzoquinone acetic acid, which polymerizes and has a special affinity for collagen-containing tissues. Eventually connective tissue breakdown occurs leading to the most serious clinical manifestation of the disorder, degenerative joint disease and pigmentation of cartilage. Alkaptonuria is usually not diagnosed until middle age when ochronosis and arthritis act as indicators of the disorder. Although there is no satisfactory treatment for alkaptonuria, a beneficial effect may be seen by dietary restriction of tyrosine or phenylalanine if the diagnosis is made early in life. The condition may be diagnosed by observing the slow darkening of urine on standing, exposure to air, or on adding alkali. The color formation, however, must be distinguished from darkening due to melanuria, phenols, gentisic acid, or indoxyl-sulfate (indican).

Branched Chain Ketoaciduria (Maple Syrup Urine Disease). An inherited defect of the oxidative decarboxylation of α-keto acids derived from leucine, isoleucine, and valine results in the accumulation of the branched-chain amino acids and their corresponding α-keto acids in blood, urine, and cerebrospinal fluid (CSF). In this disorder, which has an incidence of approximately 1 in 250,000, there is a deficiency of branched-chain keto acid decarboxylase. Classic manifestations of the condition are an infant appearing normal at birth but symptoms such as the infant failing to thrive, feeding poorly, and vomiting appear by the end of the first week. Neurologic signs such as convulsions and generalized rigidity appear with stupor, hypotonia, and irregular respirations soon following. An odor, described as that of maple syrup or curry, is often noted particularly in urine. The untreated patient becomes progressively more lethargic, becomes comatose, and dies. Plasma concentrations of branched-chain amino acids are persistently elevated more than 10-fold (isoleucine is greater than 40 mg/dL [>3.1 mmol/L], leucine is greater than 85 mg/dL [>6.5 mmol/L].[7] Also excessive urinary keto acids give a positive reaction in the dinitrophenylhydrazine test and a gray-blue color in the ferric chloride test. The Guthrie test, with 4-aza-leucine as inhibitor, may be used for neonatal screening and prenatal diagnosis may be made by assaying the decarboxylase in cultured amniotic cells.

Treatment of patients with this disease is difficult because of its neonatal clinical onset, acute course, and the involvement of three essential amino acids. However, treatment is by dietery restriction of leucine, isoleucine, and valine: follow-up should include frequent urine testing and monthly amino acid assays. A few cautions have been voiced concerning dietary restriction treatment. Attention has been called to the risk of folic acid deficiency if proprietary multivitamin preparations are substituted for the vitamins suggested in the Synderman diet.[8] Also hyperchloremic acidosis has recently been reported during the management of an affected newborn infant. The cause of the acidosis may have been the ingestion of a large amount of chloride-containing amino acid salts (lysine, arginine, and histidine) in an infant unable to excrete the acid load because of immature renal function.[9]

Cystinuria. This is the most common inborn error of amino acid transport and it is characterized by increased urinary excretion of cystine, lysine, arginine, and ornithine. The disorder, which is transmitted as an autosomal recessive trait, is caused by defective amino acid transport affecting the epithelial cells of the renal tubule and gastrointestinal tract. The heterozygous state may reflect true recessive or incompletely recessive inheritance. In the latter state, the affected amino acids are excreted in the urine in quantities greater than those excreted by healthy individuals but less than those with the homozygous state. Using a sensitive genetic marker, three types of cystinuric homozygotes can be defined and the evidence is that these types result from allelic mutations.[10]

Cystinuria is expressed clinically as urinary tract calculus disease. About 1–2% of all urinary tract stones are composed of cystine. Radiopaque cystine stones are formed and hexagonal cystine crystals appear in the urine. Stones generally form at cystine excretion rates of greater than 300 mg (1.26 mmol) cystine/1 g (8.8 mmol) of creatinine in acidic urine. Calculi can form in the renal pelvis, ureters, and bladder resulting in obstruction and infection. Renal insufficiency occasionally occurs. Treatment is directed at reducing the concentration of cystine in urine by increasing urine volume, increasing cystine solubility by alkalizing the urine, and reducing cystine excretion by use of D-penicillamine. D-Penicillamine, although very effective, is not without risk[11] and should be reserved for patients who fail to respond to conservative therapy.

Homocystinuria. Cystathionine β-synthetase deficiency is the most frequently encountered cause of homocystinuria. This deficiency is caused by a block in the conversion of homocysteine to cystathionine resulting in homocysteine and methionine accumulation in body fluids accompanied by a decrease in the usual metabolites, cysteine and cystine. In these patients, homocystine is detectable in plasma and methionine may increase up to 30 mg/dL (≤ 2.0 mmol/L) and their urine contains homocystine, methionine, and other sulfur-containing amino acids.[3]

More than 350 cases of proved or presumptive cystathionine β-synthetase deficiency have been described. Dislocation of the optic lens, osteoporosis, thinning and lengthening of the long bones, mental retardation, and thromboembolism affecting large and small arteries and veins are the most common features, although affected patients vary widely in the extent to which they manifest these abnormalities.

With routine screening programs, newborns with cystathionine β-synthetase deficiency are currently being detected with a worldwide frequency of approximately 1 in 200,000 live births in which hypermethioninemia is the initial diagnostic criterion. Treatment by dietary restriction of methionine, supplements of cystine, or large doses of the cofactor pyridoxine can be started early in life.

Phenylalaninemias. Hyperphenylalaninemia (HPA) is clinically and biochemically a heterogeneous condition. The most severe form is referred to as classic PKU and the most benign form, which does not require treatment, is referred to as benign HPA. The disorder involving the enzyme phenylalanine hydroxyase has been operationally defined as follows:

1. *Classic PKU.* Persons with classic PKU exhibit serum phenylalanine concentrations of greater than or equal to 20 mg/dL (≥ 1210 μmol/L), tyrosine results within the reference range, and excessive phenylalanine metabolites in the urine while on a normal diet. Little or no phenylalanine hydroxylase is present.
2. *Variant PKU.* Generally persons with variant PKU have serum phenylalanine concentrations between 10 and 20 mg/dL (605 and 1210 μmol/L), but may not have phenylalanine metabolites present in their urine unless ingesting excessive amounts of protein in their diet. Tyrosine levels are within the reference range and phenylalanine hydroxylase activity is definitely present.
3. *Benign HPA.* Benign HPA is applied to persons with serum phenylalanine concentrations between 4 and 10 mg/dL (242 and 605 μmol/L). The urine usually does not have metabolites of phenylalanine and serum tyrosine results are within the reference range. Patients with benign HPA may be identified by newborn screening, but because they have normal intelligence and are clinically asymptomatic they often may escape detection. Phenylalanine hydroxylase activity is present in significant amounts.

The Collaborative Study for the Treatment of Children with PKU[12] accepted the following three biochemical parameters, each of which must be met in the diagnosis of PKU: (1) two measurements of serum phenylalanine levels greater than 20 mg/dL (>1210 μmol/L) made 24 hours apart while the patient is on a normal diet; (2) serum tyrosine levels of less than 5 mg/dL (<303 μmol/L); and (3) the presence of metabolic excretion products of phenylalanine in urine. More recently molecular genetic methods are being applied in the detection of classical PKU, but these are not in general use.[13] Also an oral protein challenge may be used in the differential diagnosis of classic and variant PKU. The oral protein challenge is defined as feeding protein to equal 180 mg (1.1 mmol) phenylalanine per kilogram of body weight (mg phe/kg). Baseline studies of serum phenylalanine and tyrosine determinations, while the patient is on a restricted diet, as well as the usual urinary metabolites of phenylalanine are performed. Over a 72-hour period, 180 mg/kg/24 h (1.1 mmol/kg/d) of phenylalanine in natural protein is given and serum phenylalanine levels are obtained daily with repeat measurements of serum tyrosine and urinary metabolites on the third day. The classical PKU response is demonstrated by a sharp increase in serum phenylalanine (20–40 mg/dL) (1210–2420 µmol/L) and a concomitant rise in urinary metabolites of the amino acid (i.e., greater than 3000 mg [18.3 mmol] of phenylpyruvic acid/1 mg [88.4 mmol] of creatinine). The tyrosine level remains unchanged and may even decrease. The variant PKU patient demonstrates urinary metabolites of phenylalanine present in diminished amounts with increased serum tyrosine levels. These subjects have significant amounts of phenylalanine hydroxylase present in the liver (5–10%) and demonstrate levels of up to 20 mg/dl (≤1210 µmol/L) of phenylalanine during the test.[14]

Early detection is the best treatment for PKU and dietary restriction of the amino acid phenylalanine is necessary if mental retardation is to be avoided. Indeed, the most recent data indicate that intellectual ability and academic achievement are adversely affected when serum phenylalanine levels are persistently greater than 15 mg/dL (>908 µmol/L) before the age of 6 years.[15] Monitoring serum phenylalanine and dietary control should continue indefinitely although there has been much discussion concerning the length of dietary restriction. Dietary restriction is particularly important for women because a high level of serum phenylalanine in pregnancy has disastrous effects on the fetus (cardiac defects, anencephaly, retardation). To avoid maternal HPA, dietary phenylalanine and synthetic peptide sweetners must be restricted before conception and throughout pregnancy.[16]

To test for the heterozygote or carrier state for PKU, the suspected carrier is given an oral dose of 100 mg/phe/kg body weight after which blood specimens are obtained at hourly intervals for 4 hours and phenylalanine measured. The noncarrier is demonstrated by a fasting phenylalanine concentration of 1.5 mg/dL (91 µmol/L) to a value of 9–10 mg/dL (545–605 µmol/L) at approximately 90 minutes and a decrease to 5 mg/dL (303 µmol/L) by 4 hours. In heterozygotes, the phenylalanine concentration rises from within the reference interval to a value of approximately 18 mg/dL (1090 µmol/L) by the first hour and falls more slowly than in healthy individuals.

Tyrosinuria. There are several forms of tyrosinemia, each of which is accompanied by tyrosinuria and phenolic aciduria. There are two types of inherited tyrosinemia. Type I (tyrosinosis), which has principally been observed in isolated French-Canadian areas of Quebec, probably is caused by defective fumarylacetoacetate (FAA) hydrolase resulting in liver damage and renal tubular failure. Type II tyrosinemia arises owing to a deficiency of tyrosine aminotransferase, which is necessary to convert tyrosine to p-hydroxyphenylpyruvic acid (PHPPA).[17] Clinical symptoms include blindness and dermatologic involvement principally of the palms and soles. With both types of tyrosinemia, there are high levels of tyrosine in the blood and urine. Type I patients display high serum levels of methionine and a urinary excretion of PHPPA up to 1.5 g/24 h (≤8.2 mmol/d) (20 times normal).

Albinism is found when there is an absence or severe deficiency of tyrosinase, an enzyme that is necessary for the conversion of tyrosine to 3,4-dihydroxyphenylpyruvic acid and hence melanin. There is a lack of melanin in skin, hair, and eyes. Patients presenting with this disorder demonstrate a high incidence of carcinoma of the skin in later life.

PROTEINS

INTRODUCTION

All proteins have a basic structure that is constructed from amino acid residues linked by peptide bonds. Peptide bond formation is a condensation reaction between the nucleophilic lone pair of electrons on the amino group with the electrophilic carbonyl carbon on the other reacting amino acid. A water molecule is lost when the resulting peptide bond is formed. Polypeptides contain 6–30 peptide bonds, whereas polypeptides with 40 or more peptide bonds are often called proteins.

The primary structure of a protein molecule is based on the sequence, number, and type of amino acid residues making up the protein. Hence the primary structure is based on the peptide bonds linking 30,000–50,000 amino acid residues of the various proteins. The secondary structure of proteins is related to the helix formation that occurs due to hydrogen bonding between amino acid residues on a single peptide chain.

Weak intramolecular forces between amino acid residues on the peptide chain cause the molecule to fold, loop, and twist about itself. The tertiary structure is due to weak interaction between R side chain groups. Further, quaternary structure is seen when two or more peptide chains are linked together to form the protein.

Proteins may be classified as fibrous or globular. The basic structural organizations of fibrous proteins are the α-helix and the β-sheet. The molecules of fibrous proteins tend to be longer than they are wide and include collagen and elastin or proteins of connective tissue such as keratin, fibrin, and myosin. Globular proteins usually include mixtures of helical and sheet formation; they tend to be compact, spherical, and soluble in physiologic fluids. Examples of globular proteins include most enzymes, plasma proteins (excluding albumin), and hemoglobins.

In plasma, more than 300 proteins have been identified, but they differ greatly in concentration and only the clinically relevant ones are considered. Table 8-4 lists the principal plasma proteins according to their migration during electrophoresis.

The biologic functions of proteins are numerous, varied, and important. Enzymes catalyze biochemical transformations essential to metabolism: protein, polypeptide, and oligopeptide hormones regulate metabolism; antibodies and components of the complement system protect against infection. Further, plasma proteins maintain the oncotic pressure of plasma, and transport hormones, minerals, vitamins, and drugs, often serving as reservoirs for their release and utilization; apolipoproteins solubulize lipids; hemoglobin carries oxygen; and protein coagulation factors affect hemostasis. There are structural and contractile proteins and storage proteins such as ferritin. In addition, chromosomal histones are protein in nature.

Because any method of studying proteins first involves a separation step before quantitation, experimental techniques for classifying proteins differ mainly in the property difference used to separate various proteins in plasma. Techniques for separating proteins include the following:

1. *Solubility*. Variations in size and shape of protein molecules and the presence of ions or dehydrating solvents in the solution enable proteins to be separated.
2. *Electrophoresis*. Different ionic charges on proteins in alkaline buffers allow separation and, to a lesser extent, the size and shape of proteins influence electrophoretic separation (more acidic proteins tend to migrate faster owing to the increased negative charges on the protein in alkaline solution).
3. *Ultracentrifugation*. Protein separation is based on variation in molecular mass.
4. *Chromatography*. Protein separation is based on differences in size, shape, polarity, and differential affinity for fixed and mobile phases. Ion exchange chromatography may be used to separate proteins often on the basis of protein acidity in cation exchange chromatography and basicity in anion exchange chromatography. Gel filtration chromatography uses the principle that smaller proteins get trapped in a molecular polymer, whereas large proteins do not and hence can be easily separated.
5. *Immunoprecipitation (or fixation)*. Protein separation is based on unique antigenic determinants on specific proteins.
6. *Adsorption*. Proteins may be adsorbed onto finely divided inert materials that offer large surface areas for interaction with proteins. Adsorption on polar substances such as silica or hydroxyapatite depends on ionic interactions or hydrogen bonding; these substances can be used with buffer elution in chromatographic separation.

BASIC TESTS

Test: Albumin

Background and Selection

The main biologic functions of albumin include (1) transport of various ligands (bilirubin, long chain fatty acids, calcium, cortisol, sex steroids, thyroid hormones, and drugs); (2) maintenance of plasma oncotic pressure; and (3) serves as a source of endogenous amino acids.

Albumin, which is the most abundant protein in human plasma representing some 55–65% of the total protein,[18] is produced in the liver and has a half-life of approximately 4 weeks. Because of its relatively small size, albumin is a useful indicator of the integrity of glomerular and other membranes.

Albumin quantitation is useful in the management of dehydration and in other conditions such as (1) excessive protein loss due to renal damage (nephrotic syndrome, chronic glomerulonephritis, diabetes mellitus, severe hemorrhage, or burns); (2) impaired synthesis as seen in hepatic disease, toxemia of pregnancy, and genetic disorders; (3) increased catabolism as a result of tissue damage and inflammation; (4) reduced absorption of amino acids caused by malabsorption syndromes or malnutrition; and (5) altered distribution as in ascites where pressure in the portal circulation results in the movement of albumin into the peritoneal fluid.

Logistics

Specimen Requirements

For analysis, serum is the specimen of choice, but heparinized plasma also can be used if precautions are taken to prevent heparin interference. Specimens may be stored for up to 5 days at 4°C but if analysis is to be delayed, serum should be frozen at −20°C. Venostatis must be avoided during venipuncture as hemoconcentration increases the concentration of plasma proteins. Albumin concentration is approximately 0.3 g/dL (3 g/L) higher when the patient is ambulatory.

Analysis

Electrophoresis is considered by many to be the reference method for albumin determination although it is a labor intensive technique. In addition, no dye has been demonstrated to bind to all serum proteins equally or to have a binding strength that is linear with the concentration of all serum proteins.[18] Thus electrophoretic procedures tend to overestimate albumin, because albumin tends to bind the stains most avidly. Elution of the proteins from the membrane support make the procedure even more labor intensive.

Routinely, albumin estimation is based on its binding with the anionic dyes bromcresol green (BCG) or bromcresol purple (BCP). The BCG method is usually used because (1) the dye specifically binds albumin in the presence of other proteins; (2) there is high affinity binding between the dye and albumin, and small changes in ionic strength and pH will not disrupt the dye-protein complex; and (3) bilirubin and hemoglobin do not absorb at the absorption maximum of the dye-albumin species at 628 nm.[19]

Albumin also can be measured by reaction with antialbumin antibody and monitored by turbidimetric or nephelometric means. The antibody-albumin complexes that form increase the absorption (turbidometry) or the scattering (nephelometry) of incident light, which can be related to albumin concentration and measured using an automated instrument.[20]

Interpretation

The usual reference range for serum albumin is 3.5–5.0 g/dL (35–55 g/L). The most severe hypoalbuminemia is caused by protein loss by way of urine or feces. When plasma albumin levels are below 2.5 g/dL (25 g/L), edema results as the low plasma oncotic pressure allows water to move out of the blood capillaries and into the tissues. In situations of hemodilution, such as inappropriate secretion of antidiuretic hormone (ADH) due to carbamazepine therapy, levels of albumin may reach 2.0 g/dL (20 g/L). Albumin levels of less than 2.0 g/dL (<20 g/L) may also be seen in situations of deficient amino acid supply (e.g., malabsorption syndrome due to chronic pancreatitis), alcoholic liver disease, and protein-losing enteropathy (e.g., carcinoma of the stomach). Because of its relatively small size, albumin is a useful indicator of the integrity of glomerular and other membranes. Albumin that is filtered through the renal glomeruli is absorbed by the proximal tubules, degraded by lysosomal enzymes, and fragments are returned to the circulation. Changes in circulating albumin concentration affect the relative amounts of the bound and free ligands. Thus, the metabolism of analytes such as calcium is uniquely tied to circulating albumin concentrations. When interpreting serum protein electrophoresis (SPE) profiles, it should be kept in mind that there are 20–25 genetic variants of albumin that are not disease associated. These may present as a widening of the albumin band or two easily identifiable bands (bisalbuminemia). Analbuminemia (congenital absence of albumin) is asymptomatic except for causing occasional edema. The only known cause of hyperalbuminemia is that of hemoconcentration, which may arise through either improper collection (venous stasis) or any process that causes absolute or relative water loss from the vascular compartment. Certainly it is not unusual to see a patient with diabetic ketosis and dehydration having albumin levels up to 5.5 g/dL (55 g/L).

Test: Total Protein

Background and Selection

The total concentration of all proteins in plasma may vary because of changes in the volume of plasma water or in the amounts of individual proteins. Hyperproteinemia is seen in dehydration owing either to inadequate water intake or excessive loss of water, as in severe vomiting, Addison's disease, or diabetic ketosis. Hemodilution causes a decrease in the concentration of all proteins and occurs in water intoxication or salt retention syndromes, during massive intravenous infusions, and physiologically when a person is recumbent.

Logistics

Specimen Requirements

Serum, plasma, or other body fluids may be used for determining total protein concentration. Total protein is stable in serum and plasma for up to 48 hours at room temperature and for at least 1 month when refrigerated at 4°C.[21]

Analysis

The oldest approach to determining total protein in serum is to determine protein nitrogen using Kjeldahl's method. In this method, acid digestion converts nitrogen in the protein to the ammonium ion, and ammonia nitrogen is then evaluated by titration or nesslerization with correction of the final result for nitrogen contributed by nonprotein compounds. It should be stressed that this method provides a means of defining reference standards, but it is impractical for routine use especially for urinary protein measurements where urinary ammonia causes interference. The most frequently used method for determining total protein in serum is the biuret reaction. In this reaction, cupric ion reacts with the peptide linkages of protein in a basic solution to form a violet colored compound with an absorption maximum at 540 nm. The intensity of the color produced is proportional to the number of peptide bonds that are reacting and therefore to the number of protein molecules present in the reaction system. Thus the biuret reaction is suitable for the quantitative determination of total protein by spectrophotometry. Most biuret methods can detect between 1 and 15 mg of protein in the aliquot being measured, an amount present in 15–200 μL of a serum containing protein at 7 g/dL (70 g/L).

Another direct approach to the estimation of total protein relies on measuring the refractive index. Because the solutes present in greatest concentration in serum are proteins, the refractive index of serum provides a rapid, approximate measure of serum total protein concentration within the range 3.5–10.0 g/dL (35–100 g/L). Clinical refractometers are calibrated to read protein in g/dL and compensate for temperature changes in the range of 15–37°C, but significant errors may be caused by alterations in the albumin/globulin (A/G) ratio, azotemia, hyperglycemia, hyperbilirubinemia, and especially by lipemia.

Interpretation

The combined male (134 men) and female (97 women) reference interval established by the Doumas method (modified biuret) is 6.66–8.14 g/dL (66.6–81.4 g/L).[22] The subjects studied were healthy adults who had fasted for 10–12 hours and had been in the upright position for at least 2 hours before blood was collected without anticoagulant. This reference interval is similar to the one established by Reed et al.,[23] which was 6.6–8.3 g/dL (66.0–83.0 g/L) based on 1419 subjects. It is important to note that serum protein is lower when the patient is supine than when upright. A recumbent position decreases the total protein concentration by 0.3–0.5 g/dL (3.0–5.9 g/L), whereas ambulatory patients have slightly higher protein concentrations because of shifts of vascular water to the extravascular space. Increase in plasma water volume (hemodilution) causes a decrease in the concentrations of all proteins. Hypoproteinemia occurs in water intoxication, nephrotic syndrome, or salt retention syndromes; during massive intravenous infusions; and physiologically when a person is recumbent. In contrast, decrease in the volume of plasma water (hemoconcentration) causes increased concentration of all the proteins to the same degree. Hyperproteinemia thus is seen in dehydration because of either inadequate water intake or excessive loss of water as in severe vomiting, Addison's disease, or diabetic acidosis.

Test: Albumin-Globulin Ratio

By subtracting the albumin level obtained from the SPE profile from the total protein level, an indirect estimate of globulin can be obtained. Division of the albumin level by the globulin level gives a new parameter called the A/G ratio. Ratios are useful and usually present a more sensitive indicator for detection of disease than either measurement used independently when (1) increases in γ-globulin are directly proportional to the presence and severity of the disease and (2) levels of albumin are inversely proportional to the presence and severity of the disease.

Levels of the A/G ratio range from 1.5–2.5 in healthy individuals. The A/G ratio is a good indicator of liver disease, because liver disease causes a decreased albumin and an increased γ-globulin level. Low A/G ratios also are seen in burns, malnutrition, diarrhea, nephrosis, myelomas, lymphomas, and granulomatous disease. Figure 8-1 shows the A/G ratio calculated for a healthy patient and Figure 8-2 shows the A/G ratio for a patient with a monoclonal gammopathy in whom the A/G ratio is 1.19.

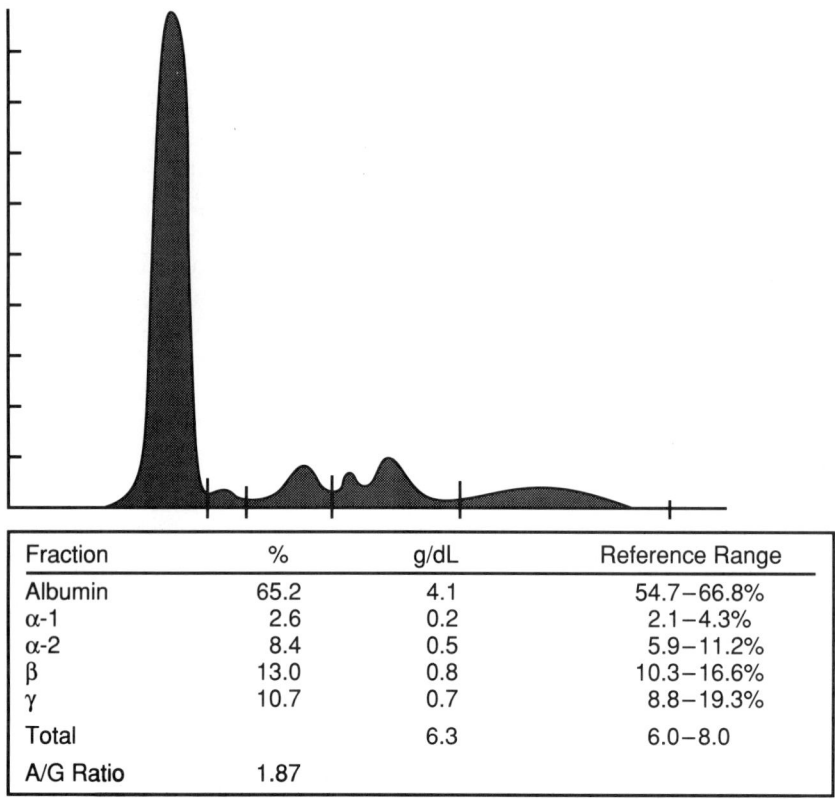

Fig. 8-1. Normal serum protein electrophoresis using agarose gel. Note the albumin-globulin (A/G) ratio is 1.87.

SPECIAL PROTEIN ANALYSIS

Test: Serum Protein Electrophoresis

Background and Selection

The physicochemical environment determines the number of positive and negative changes carried by a particular protein. At an alkaline pH, most proteins possess an overall negative charge, but the excess of negative over positive depends on the amino acid residue structure of each protein.

If a mixture of different proteins in a buffer solution of pH 8.6 is placed on an inert support such as cellulose acetate and a direct electric current is applied for a fixed time, most of the proteins migrate towards the positive electrode. The distance traveled by each protein species largely depends on the amount of negative charge carried. After such electrophoresis, the proteins can be fixed in position by precipitation, stained for visualization, and the relative amounts estimated by measuring the density of each stained area of protein.

Many disease processes cause distinctive electrophoretic patterns, and so requesting an SPE can aid in the diagnosis of various diseases, especially those listed in Table 8-4.

Logistics

Specimen Requirements

Serum is the specimen of choice, because of the fibrinogen band produced in the electrophoretic pattern by plasma. Urine and CSF also can be analyzed if their protein content is sufficient or increased by ultracentrifugation, dialysis, or other concentration techniques. As with total protein measurements, serum submitted for SPE is stable for at least 1 month when refrigerated at 4°C.

Analysis

Serum protein electrophoresis can be performed by use of a variety of supporting media that include polyacrylamide, starch, and agarose gels, paper, and cellulose acetate. Polyacrylamide support medium has served to establish the existence of over 100 serum proteins; how-

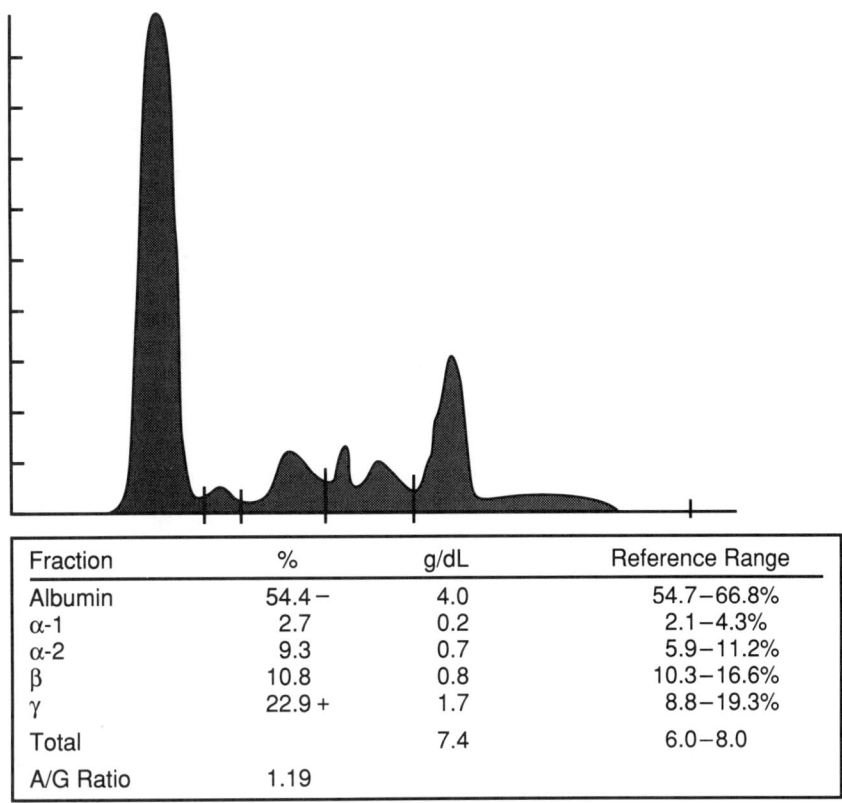

Fig. 8-2. Serum protein electrophoresis demonstrating a monoclonal gammopathy (band in the β to γ regions). Note the albumin-globulin (A/G) ratio is 1.19.

ever, the many bands seen with these techniques present a complex picture that is difficult to interpret.

With cellulose acetate, only five bands are evident (albumin, α_1, α_2, β, and γ); the abnormal electrophoretic patterns of these proteins as seen in various diseases are listed in Table 8-5. Serum protein electrophoresis with cellulose acetate or agarose yields five bands, as shown in Figure 8-1.

Agarose gel gives sharper resolution of the protein bands than does cellulose acetate, and adsorption is minimal. Because of its more consistent performance and ease of handling, agarose gel has become the preferred method.[24] Most commercially prepared agarose plates are 0.5-mm thick and contain 10 g/L agarose in barbital buffer, pH 8.6.

Interpretation

In general, reference values for the five well defined fractions are as follows: albumin, 3.2–5.0 g/dL (32–50 g/L); α_1, 0.1–0.4 g/dL (10–40 g/L); α_2, 0.6–1.0 g/dL (6–10 g/L), β, 0.6–1.3 g/dL (6–13 g/L); and γ, 0.7–1.5 g/dL (7–15 g/L). When one considers protein levels of a healthy population throughout life (8–95 years), no significant age-related variations are seen with prealbumin, ceruloplasmin, and IgM. Albumin concentrations remain constant until individuals reach 50 years of age, after which they tend to decrease. Levels of acid-1-glycoprotein increase until 30 years of age in the male and after 40 years of age in the female. Although haptoglobin levels increase with age, a pronounced decrease is seen in α_2-macroglobulin until 40 years of age after which levels increase. Young females exhibit an increase in transferrin followed by a decrease after age 30, in contrast to males, who show a decrease in transferrin values until 40 years of age.[25] Complement C3 levels in males increase with age while in females they decrease until about age 30 after which levels increase. Immunoglobulin (IgA) levels increase throughout life, but the increase tends to diminish at about 35 years of age. Until about 50 years of age, IgG values decrease, but then increase thereafter.

Serum protein electrophoresis with cellulose acetate or agarose is a technique that is helpful for establishing a diagnosis of monoclonal gammopathies, liver cirrhosis, renal failure, hypogammaglobulinemia, and multiple myeloma. Various and often distinct electrophoretic

Table 8-4. Major Serum Proteins (Electrophoretic Fractions)

Protein	Function	Increased	Decreased	Reference Range mg/dL (g/L)
Prealbumin (54,500 da)	Transport protein for T₃ & T₄; Useful in assessment of protein malnutrition	Hodgkin's disease	Inflammation, Malignancy, Cirrhosis	20–40 (0.20–0.40)
Albumin (66,000 da)	General transport protein; Controls fluid balance between intra- and extravascular compartments	Dehydration	Liver disease, Kidney disease, Neoplasms, Chronic infection, Hemorrhage, Starvation	3,500–5,000 (35–50)
α₁-Region α₁-Antitrypsin (45,000 da), APR	Neutralization of trypsin (derived from leukocytes) and plasmin	Inflammatory reactions	Lung disease, Deficiency leads to emphysema	80–200 (0.80–2.0)
α₁-Lipoprotein (200,000 da)	Transport of cholesterol and fat-soluble vitamins	Hyperlipidemia	Liver disease, particularly Tangier disease	170–320 (1.7–3.2)
α₁-Glycoprotein (44,100 da), APR	Protein-polysaccharide in tissues and mucus secretions	—	Decreased in certain inborn errors of metabolism	50–150 ng/dL (0.5–1.5 μg/L)
Thyroid-binding globulin (36,500 da)	Transport protein for thyroid hormones in blood	Pregnancy, use of contraceptive pills	Nephrosis, Methyltestosterone therapy	1.5–3.4 (0.015–0.034) Pregnancy, 3rd trimester, 5.0–10.5
Prothrombin (72,000 da)	Factor II, necessary for blood clotting, converted to thrombin by factor V	—	Liver disease	—
α₂-Region α₂-Macroglobulin (820,000 da)	Protease inhibitor; Neutralizes trypsin, plasmin, kallikrein	Nephrotic syndrome, Emphysema, Diabetes mellitus, Pregnancy, Down syndrome	Rheumatoid arthritis, Myeloma	120–400 (1.2–4.0)
Haptoglobin (85,000–1 million da) APR	Hemoglobin binding protein; Hgb-HAP complexes preserve iron stores	Acute and chronic inflammation, Neoplasms, Myocardial infarction, Hodgkin's disease	Liver disease, Hemolytic anemia, Megaloblastic anemia	30–220 (0.3–2.2)
Ceruloplasmin (13,200 da) APR	Copper-binding serum protein; bound copper is nontoxic	Pregnancy, oral contraceptives	Wilson's disease (CER not produced)	20–50 (0.2–0.5)
α₂-Lipoproteins	Transport of lipids	Hyperlipidemias	Severe liver disease	—
Erythropoietin (30,000 da)	Hormone essential for normal erythropoiesis	Certain anemias	Kidney disease, Certain autoimmune diseases	—
β-Region Transferrin (80,000 da), APR	Transport iron protein (e.g., shuttles iron from liver to bone marrow)	Iron-deficiency anemias	Liver diseases, Nephrosis, Malignant neoplasms	200–350 ng/dL (2.0–3.5 μg/L)
β-Lipoproteins (3 × 10⁶ da)	Transport of cholesterol, phospholipids, and hormones	Nephrosis, Hyperlipidemia	Starvation	—
C3 and C4 (185,000–417,000 da), APR	Two components of complement system	Acute phase	Immune disease (e.g., SLE and autoimmune hemolytic anemia)	C3: 90–200 (0.9–2.0) C4: 15–45 (0.15–0.45)

(Continued)

Table 8-4. Major Serum Proteins (Electrophoretic Fractions) (Continued)

Protein	Function	Increased	Decreased	Reference Range mg/dL (g/L)
Hemopexin (80,000 da)	Specific heme-carrying serum protein	Acute and chronic inflammation Neoplasms Myocardial infarction	Liver disease Hemolytic anemia Megaloblastic anemia	50–120 (0.5–1.2)
B$_2$-Microglobulin (11,800 da)	Found on surface of all nucleated cells associated with β-chain of HLA Indicator of renal tubular function	Renal failure Inflammation Neoplasms (B cells)	—	0.1–0.45 (1.0–4.5)
γ-Region IgG (150,000 da) IgA (180,000 da) IgM (900,000 da) IgD (170,000 da) IgE (190,000 da)	Immunoresponse	Hypergammaglobulinemia Liver disease Chronic infections SLE Multiple myeloma (mono- & polyclonal) Waldenström's disease Lymphoma	Age Induced by drugs Chronic lymphocytic leukemia Light chain disease Agammaglobulinemia Hypoimmune syndrome	IgG 525–1650 (5.25–16.5) IgA 40–390 (0.4–3.9) IgM 25–310 (0.25–3.1) IgD 0–8 (0–0.08) IgE 0–390 IU/mL

Abbreviations: APR, acute phase reactant (response to acute inflammation, e.g., postsurgery, myocardial infarction, infections, or tumors); CER, ceruloplasmin; Hgb-HAP, hemoglobin-haptoglobin; HLA, human leukocyte antigen; SLE, systemic lupus erythematosus.

patterns are seen in diseases affecting protein production, catabolism, or excretion. As changes in globulin fractions may be obscured by an increase or decrease in another protein migrating in the same fraction, great care and experience are required for proper interpretation of electrophoretic patterns.

When interpreting SPE, it should be remembered that many of the individual proteins are too low in concentration to manifest as distinctly stained bands. Furthermore, they may be overshadowed by proteins of higher concentrations that migrate near them as in the case with ceruloplasmin, which is masked by haptoglobin and α$_2$-macroglobulin. Also it should be stressed that some proteins, such as glycoproteins and lipoproteins, stain poorly with the commonly used stains. When comparing a patient's SPE pattern, it should be compared with that of a normal control serum analyzed at the same time. Any abnormalities of the SPE pattern can be investigated further by immunochemical determination of the specific protein under investigation. Direct visual interpretation of SPE membranes can prevent errors in interpretation owing to artifacts on membranes interpreted as monoclonal proteins.[26]

Serum Protein Electrophoresis

1. The SPE should be inspected for multiple bands, decreased or absent bands, and normal bands displaying different points of migration that can be caused by genetic variants, for example, transferrin in the β-region and haptoglobin in the α$_1$-region. Further the binding of increased amounts of fatty acids and bilirubin to albumin in-

Table 8-5. Abnormal Electrophoretic Patterns Seen in Various Disease States

	Albumin	α$_1$	α$_2$	β	γ	Comment
Acute phase reaction	↓	↑	↑			
Chronic infection	↓		↑		↑	
Cirrhosis	↓				↑	β-γ Bridging
Nephrosis	↓	↓	↑		↓	
α$_1$-antitrypsin deficiency		↓↓				
Myeloma	None or ↓				↓	M band present

creases the mobility. Drugs such as salicylates and penicillin also cause an alteration in the mobility of albumin. Figure 8-1 is an SPE performed on sera from a healthy individual.

2. The appearance of sharp narrow bands occurring in the β to γ-regions is suggestive of a monoclonal gammopathy (Fig. 8-2), where the exact position of the band depends on the type of immunoglobulin (or fragment thereof). Albumin and other immunoglobulins are decreased with this pattern.

3. A band not normally seen between albumin and α_1-region may become evident on SPE: this may be the result of increased α-fetoprotein associated with certain tumors. Also during the acute phase reaction, a large increase in C-reactive protein may result in a faint band in the γ-region.

4. Decreased albumin and α-bands along with an increased α_2-band suggest selective proteinuria such as that seen in nephrotic syndrome. An acute phase reaction is also suggested by an increase in the α_1- and α_2-bands that contain α_1-antitrypsin (AAT), α_1-acid glycoprotein, and haptoglobin, respectively.

5. Other features to be mindful of include an increase in α_1-components, which may be seen as acute phase reactions, chronic hepatitis, estrogen therapy, or pregnancy. Increases in the α_2-band can be observed in immunocomplex diseases and rheumatoid arthritis, whereas an increase in the α_1- band suggests iron deficiency anemia in which case transferrin is usually increased.

In conditions such as cirrhosis, respiratory infections, and rheumatoid arthritis, there is usually an increase in plasma IgA, which may be demonstrated on SPE by bridging of the β- and γ-bands. An overall increase in the γ-band suggests a polyclonal γ-globulin increase resulting from liver disease, chronic inflammatory disease, neoplasia, or an immunoreaction, whereas a decrease or absence of the γ-band suggests immunodeficiency.

The term *acute phase reaction proteins* describe a group of unrelated proteins whose concentrations alter in a characteristic way following trauma to the body. Some of the common disorders that lead to these changes are myocardial infarction, surgery, burns, major infection, and inflammation. The plasma levels of some of the acute phase proteins increase after injury probably caused by tissue damage releasing factors that stimulate synthesis by the liver. Most of the proteins show a rise of up to twice their usual plasma concentrations, except C-reactive protein, which may rise 20- to 30-fold from barely detectable levels, and albumin, which may fall as much as 20%. The overall effect of these changes probably reflect one part of the complex response to injury, that is (1) minimizing blood and fluid loss; (2) salvaging important components; (3) minimizing further damage by releasing lysosomal enzymes from damaged cells; (4) removing damaged cells; and (5) repairing the damage. Measuring acute phase reactants has no diagnostic value in the context of trauma, but care should be taken to determine if any of these are measured for other reasons 10–12 days following a traumatic event.

Test: High Resolution Serum Protein Electrophoresis

Background and Selection

High resolution electrophoresis (HRE) is a very sensitive electrophoretic method that resolves a protein pattern into multiple zones. As many as 15 proteins are readily identified by their location and appearance, but several others are recognized when found in abnormal concentration. To achieve high resolution, agarose gel is used as the electrophoretic medium and higher voltage is coupled with a cooling system in the apparatus and the system's buffer is modified.

Proteins seen in an HRE pattern can increase or decrease in concentration in disease states and thus will appear more or less dense than a reference pattern. Our clinical knowledge of protein metabolism is limited to about 25–30 relatively high concentration components of plasma, CSF, urine, and other body fluids. Of these, approximately 15 can be visualized by use of HRE and they have been studied in a variety of disease states. Thus HRE can be used as a screening technique and in particular it can be used to screen for abnormalities in the immunoglobulin fractions.

Logistics

Specimen Requirements

Serum is used because plasma contains fibrinogen which will be identified on the HRE pattern in the mid-γ_1-region as a small band of restricted mobility.

Hemolyzed specimens should be avoided, as the formation of haptoglobin-hemoglobin complexes results in a cathodal shift and an increase in the haptoglobin fraction of HRE. Serum for HRE can be stored up to 72 hours at 4°C, otherwise the C3 component of the complement system, usually detected in the β_2-region of the HRE pattern, will result in a decrease in this region appearing as a faint band in the γ_1-zone.

Analysis

To achieve high resolution of serum proteins, a 1% concentration of agarose is used in 75 mmol/L, pH 8.6 barbital buffer containing 2 mmol/L calcium lactate.[27] Commercially available agarose slides have a uniformly thin (1 mm) layer of agarose on an inert plastic support.

The application of the patient's sample to the gel is critical to achieving proper separation and reproducible results. It is essential that the specimen be applied to the gel surface in a very narrow band; usually this is done by using a plastic mask with uniform 1-mm × 14-mm slits. Most HRE systems in agarose run with an electrical field of about 20 V/cm (a setting of 200 V for each 10-cm length of agarose) and a current of 100–120 mA. Under these conditions, the typical run lasts 30–50 minutes.

On completion of electrophoresis, the agarose sheet is placed into an acetic acid-picric acid solution to fix the proteins. After washing in 5% acetic acid, the gel is dried and stained with Coomassie brilliant blue. An agarose gel HRE of normal human plasma is shown in Figure 8-3; note the presence of the fibrinogen band.

Recently, newer preparations of cellulose acetate membranes and staining techniques have allowed the clinical laboratory to perform HRE on cellulose acetate membranes. It is still a matter of controversy as to whether the resolution on this type of system is equal to that seen with agarose systems; however, the technique can separate serum proteins into 12 fractions that are useful for clinical diagnosis.[26]

Interpretation

Monoclonal Gammopathies

Monoclonal gammopathies are characterized by an uncontrolled proliferation of a single clone of plasma cells at the expense of other clones. This dysfunction often leads to the synthesis of large amounts of one homogeneous immunoglobulin or immunoglobulin subunit

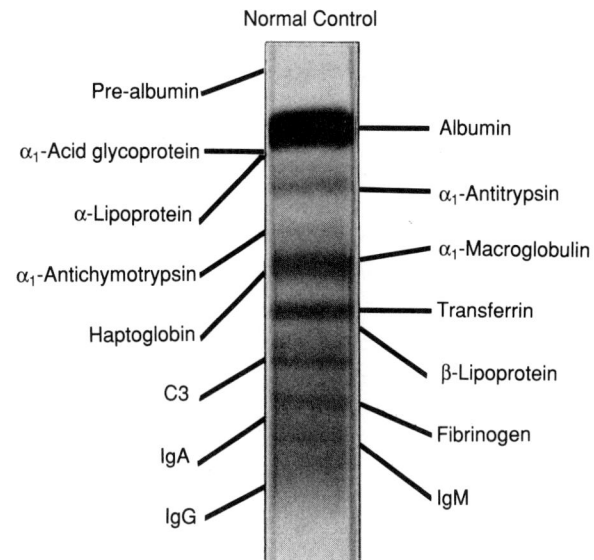

Fig. 8-3. High resolution electrophoresis of normal human plasma indicating 15 major proteins. (Courtesy of Helena Laboratories, Beaumont, Texas).

with decreased levels of normal immunoglobulins. Electrophoretic patterns and immunoglobulin test results can be abnormal in patients with multiple myeloma and other B-cell related neoplasms. Thus HRE has been a valuable tool for diagnosing and monitoring these lymphoproliferative diseases. However, it is important to remember that nearly 30% of patients with immunochemical evidence of monoclonal gammopathy are asymptomatic. Also some patients may show symptoms with no apparent abnormal protein pattern with HRE.

Other circumstances that can lead to problems in interpretation of HRE include production of more than one immunoglobulin subunit (complete molecules plus free or heavy chains), polymerization of the monoclonal protein as is seen sometimes with IgA, and depolymerization in the case of IgM. These situations can result in multiple bands on HRE and can present as diffuse increases.

HRE also can aid in the diagnosis of light chain disease, a monoclonal gammopathy in which only κ or λ monoclonal light chains or Bence Jones proteins are produced. Light chain disease comprises 10–15% of monoclonal gammopathies ranking behind IgG myeloma (about 60%) and IgA myeloma (about 15%) in incidence and occurring about as often as Waldenström's macroglobulinemia. As little as 50 mg/dL (0.5 g/L) of the monoclonal protein can be detected visually, and HRE allows the small light chains to be resolved from other proteins, especially when they migrate away from the γ-region on the agarose gel.

In suspected cases of light chain disease, HRE of serum and urine should be performed, as urine specimens with total protein results within the reference interval still may contain Bence Jones protein.

In general monoclonal gammopathy evaluation should include an initial workup as follows:

1. Serum and urine HRE
2. Quantitative serum immunoglobulins
3. Serum and urine immunoelectrophoresis (IEP)
4. Serum and urine immunofixation (IFE) if conventional IEP fails to identify anomalous band(s); also, immunofixation is useful in situations of low levels of monoclonal proteins as it is highly sensitive and interpretation does not depend on small deviations in the shape of precipitation arcs as in the case of IEP

Genetic Variations

When evaluating HRE patterns, each fraction should be closely compared with the reference serum for concentration, electrophoretic mobility, and heterogeneity. Heterogeneity indicates hereditary (genetic) alterations, which on HRE can be seen as double bands, deficiencies or changes in protein migration in albumin, AAT, haptoglobin, transferrin, and C3. Obviously whenever abnormal bands are present, IFE should be performed to rule out immunoglobulin involvement.

The most common genetically altered protein is haptoglobin, and its many different phenotypes often cause it to have an altered electrophoretic mobility compared with a reference HRE on normal serum. Bilirubin, drugs, and so forth can bind to various proteins, which also alter electrophoretic mobility. In general, most genetically altered proteins do not cause pathologic conditions unless the normally found protein is not produced at all.

Inflammatory Response

The inflammatory response pattern (acute phase changes) represents the most common abnormality seen on HRE, particularly in hospitalized patients. The intensity and duration of the protein changes vary with the stage of inflammation.

The pattern changes detected by HRE during an inflammatory response include increases in the intensity of the stained band for AAT, haptoglobin, and C-reactive protein. Decreases are observed in prealbumin, albumin, transferrin, and α-lipoprotein. Immunoglobulins may be increased in chronic inflammatory states, and C-reactive protein often will appear as a band at the cathodal end of the γ_2-region. As monoclonal bands of immunoglobulin origin also can appear in this region, an IFE should be performed to rule this out. Often the α_1-acid glycoprotein will appear diffuse giving a blurred edge to the α_1-band. A decreased transferrin fraction may be masked on HRE by a coexisting iron deficiency in the patient.

Hypogammaglobulinemia

Hypogammaglobulinemia is a very frequent finding in electrophoresis and may involve all or selective immunoglobulin classes. Deficiencies may be caused by (1) defective synthesis, (2) pathologic loss of immunoglobulins, or (3) increased catabolism. Immunodeficiency diseases include X-linked hypogammaglobulinemia, transient hypogammaglobulinemia of infancy, acquired hypogammaglobulinemia, immunodeficiency with hyper-IgM, selective class and subclass deficiencies, and deficiencies associated with drugs and protein-losing states.

The situation can be identified by a decrease in density of the generalized staining in the β-region and/or γ-region. Polyclonal IgA decreases appear as decreases in the β- and γ_1-areas. To verify the decreases seen on HRE, quantitative immunoglobulin measurements should be performed. When interpreting hypogammaglobulinemia of infancy, care should be taken to assess the patient's HRE pattern against a normal reference pattern from the same age group.

Hypergammaglobulinemia

Hypergammaglobulinemia or polyclonal gammopathy is a generalized diffuse elevation of immunoglobulins. Usually all classes of immunoglobulins are involved, but the elevation may be representative of a single class. Polyclonal gammopathy is seen in autoimmune or collagen disease such as lupus erythematosus, rheumatoid arthritis, in liver disease such as hepatitis, and in infections.

HRE may reveal one or more narrow bands in the γ-region. A single restricted band may represent an increase in a single subclass while multiple bands may indicate the early immunoresponse from several small clones of plasma cells. Also oligoclonal bands are seen sometimes in viral infections or in diseases with high concentrations of immunocomplexes. Since oligoclonal bands may be marked by high increases in polyclonal immunoglobulins, samples with protein concentrations greater than 8 g/dL (>80 g/L) should be diluted and repeated to further characterize the appearance of the γ-zone.

Liver Diseases

High resolution electrophoresis can be useful for diagnosing and treating chronic hepatocellular disease and cirrhosis. Advanced liver disease can lead to abnormalities in acute phase reactants, transport proteins, complement components, and immunoglobulins, all of which may be apparent when studying HRE serum patterns.

When liver damage is chronic and severe, both the ability of the liver to synthesize proteins and the effectiveness of Kuppfer cells to process antigens can be impaired. Commonly a pattern includes diffuse increases in IgG with greater increases in IgA and sometimes in IgM. Increased levels of acute phase reactant AAT is the most sensitive indicator for hepatocellular disease while C-reactive protein and fibrinogen are usually slightly increased. Haptoglobin may be decreased as a result of hemolysis, increased red blood cell (RBC) turnover, or reduced hepatic blood flow while α_1-acid glycoprotein may be normal or decreased. Prealbumin, albumin, α-lipoprotein, and transferrin show decreases, with prealbumin displaying as a very sensitive indicator of hepatic function in cirrhosis. Typically, α_2-microglobulin and ceruloplasmim are elevated in cirrhosis while C3 is decreased.

The various forms of hepatitis are associated with the acute phase inflammatory response in the early stages and diffuse elevations in one or more of the immunoglobulins with chronic disease. In general HRE is not a useful adjunct for diagnosing hepatitis.

Glomerular and Mixed Proteinuria

Glomerular proteinuria results from increased glomerular permeability of proteins such as albumin, transferrin, AAT, and α_1-acid glycoprotein. Typically, the corresponding serum pattern shows decreases in these proteins, and large molecular weight proteins, such as α_2-macroglobulin and β-lipoprotein, are selectively retained and may show increases in the corresponding serum pattern.

Where glomerular damage is suspected, both serum and urine HRE should be performed, with the urine sample requiring concentration to $\times 50$ before electrophoresis. If light chain disease is suspected, an IFE should be performed on a concentrated urine sample to rule out light chains in the β- or γ-regions.

Mixed proteinuria is described in situations where there is some glomerular and some tubular damage or glomerular damage plus overflow proteinuria. Significant amounts of albumin, α_1-proteins, and transferrin are indicative of glomerular proteinuria, whereas the presence of α_2-microglobulin (double band) and β_2-microglobulin indicate tubular damage. Thus HRE can aid in the differentiation of glomerular and mixed proteinuria. Also when α_1-proteins are present along with several bands in the α_2- region (antichymotrypsin and Zn-α_2-glycoprotein), inflammation is suggested.

Cerebrospinal Fluid Oligoclonal Banding

High resolution electrophoresis is useful for defining the presence of oligoclonal banding in CSF samples. The multiple, dense, highly restricted bands characteristic of this banding are found in the γ-region and represent immunoglobulins (usually IgG) produced locally within the central nervous system (CNS). In general they define multiple myeloma but can be found in viral and bacterial infections of the CNS and in some lymphoproliferative disorders.

When using HRE to examine CSF samples, the CSF should be concentrated approximately $\times 100$ and run in parallel with the patient's serum. If both the serum and CSF demonstrate monoclonal or oligoclonal bands, it can be deduced that they are of serum origin. When bands are present in the CSF but not in serum, this may be indicative of demyelinating disease (multiple sclerosis) or sometimes a CNS infection. Usually oligoclonal bands, as a result of an infection, will gradually disappear, but they are maintained in cases of demyelinating disease (see Ch. 6).

Test: Immunofixation Electrophoresis (IFE)

Background and Selection

Another technique becoming more prominent in the diagnosis of hyperimmunoglobulinemias is IFE,[28] a combination of zone electrophoresis and antibody-antigen interaction.

Immunofixation uses either cellulose acetate or agarose gel as a supporting medium. The proteins are first separated by zone electrophoresis, and strips of paper, each soaked in a monospecific antiserum (IgG, IgA, IgM, κ, and λ), are laid over the zone occupied by the protein to be identified. After approximately 1 hour at room temperature, the strips are removed. Excess protein is washed from the plate and the remaining precipitation band may be stained. In monoclonal gammopathies, the IFE pattern yields a distinct, sharply defined, precipitin band with one heavy chain and one light chain antiserum. These bands match the location of the paraprotein spike seen on SPE. In polyclonal gammopathies, there are diffuse precipitin bands with both light chain antisera and one or more heavy chain antisera. When compared with high resolution protein electrophoresis or quantitation of κ or λ light chains for identification of monoclonal serum proteins, IFE has a greater sensitivity.

Interpretation

A typical IFE pattern is shown in Figure 8-4 in which the patient is clearly demonstrated to have a monoclonal gammopathy of the IgG λ type. Thus IFE is a useful adjunct in the protocol for evaluating monoclonal gammopathy, particularly if Bence Jones proteins and free light chains may be present in serum, urine, or both. The technique also is useful for defining gammopathies in which more than one band may be present.

Advanced gammopathies are often associated with the asynchronous production of the components of the immunoglobulin molecule. This may result in synthesis of an intact monoclonal immunoglobulin plus excess monoclonal light chains. Monoclonal IgA molecules have a tendency to dimerize, and the resulting dimer often has a mobility different from the monomer parent molecule. The pentameric IgM molecule can break down to 7s subunits, which are defined on HRE as one or more monoclonal bands. Also the possibility may exist in which more than one clone could be producing monoclonal immunoglobulins, that is, a true biclonal gammopathy. IFE offers the opportunity to clearly define these situations.

Immunofixation also may be used for diagnosing heavy chain disease, which is characterized by the presence of monoclonal proteins composed of the heavy chain portion of the immunoglobulin molecule. Monoclonal proteins may be detected in urine, serum, or both. When heavy chain disease is suspected, nonspecific anti-Fab antisera should be used for definitive testing. Further, the sample should be tested against κ and λ light chain antisera to exclude prozoning as a result of antigen excess.

Immunofixation may be used to define monoclonal proteins in CSF, which result as a leakage of the protein from the plasma across the blood-brain barrier. In some research studies IFE has been used to demonstrate that oligoclonal bands seen in CSF protein patterns are composed primarily of IgG. The characterization of the

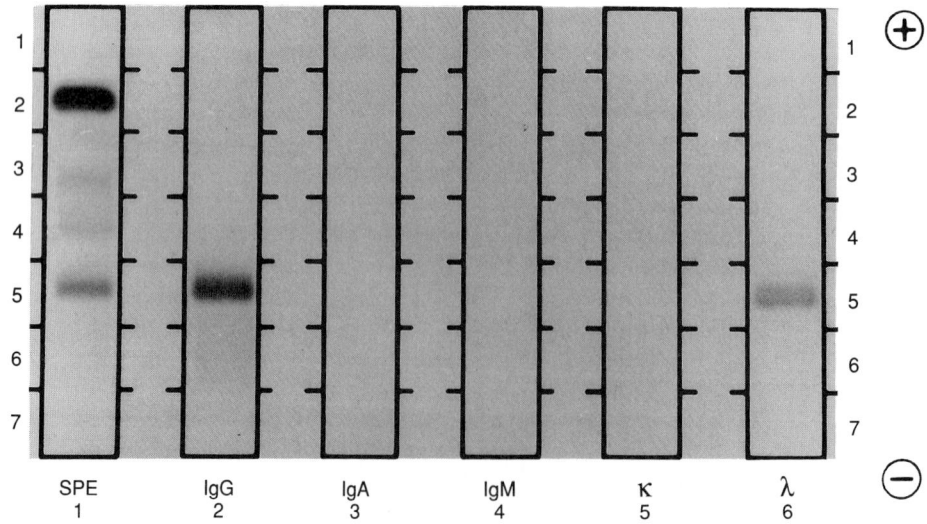

Fig. 8-4. Beckman Paragon immunofixation gel. Immunofixation (IFE) on serum from the patient whose immunoelectrophoresis is given in Figure 8-5. Note the presence of a monoclonal gammopathy (IgG λ type). Lane 1 shows serum protein electrophoresis, lanes 2–4 contain IgG, IgA and IgM heavy chain antisera applications and lanes 5 and 6 contain κ and λ light chain antisera applications.

immunoglobulin in the bands does not significantly improve the diagnostic usefulness of the test.

Test: Immunoelectrophoresis

Background and Selection

Immunoelectrophoresis is a sensitive semiquantitative procedure used to identify paraproteins. It is used in conjunction with serum or urine protein electrophoresis or quantitative immunoglobulin measurements with IFE. Following separation of various protein components by electrophoresis, antiserum to a protein of interest is placed in a trough parallel and adjacent to the electrophoresis specimen. Simultaneous diffusion of the protein from the specimen and the antibody from the trough results in the formation of the precipitin arc, the shape and position of which are characteristic of each protein. In addition, specimens are compared visually with those of healthy individuals and interpreted.

Interpretation

When interpreting IEP patterns, the presence of the monoclonal protein can be detected by one or more of the following: distortion of the curvature of the precipitin arc, difference in the arc electrophoretic mobility when compared with the control, and inhibition of arc formation (Figs. 8-5 and 8-6). A normal polyclonal arc is the combination of products from many different clones of plasma cells, and as such the arc represents chemically heterogenous groups of antibodies with no one clonal product predominating. Thus, the arc is an asymmetric, wide semicircle. As a monoclonal arc represents a large amount of chemically homogenous antibody from one clone, a monoclonal protein results in a precipitin arc with a bowing or humping effect and is asymmetric in appearance. Figures 8-5 and 8-6 show IEPs of serum and urine of an individual with a monoclonal protein.

Whereas monoclonal antibodies vary in size as compared with normal antibodies of the same immunoglobulin class, abnormal proteins compared with control antibodies may have different electrophoretic mobility. In particular Bence Jones proteins, because they are light chains, often produce an arc with greater mobility with λ or κ antiserum. Identification of a protein can be performed by use of monospecific antibody for that protein; the precipitin arc should have the same mobility as the arc for control material. Table 8-6 lists some conditions associated with monoclonal immunoglobulins.

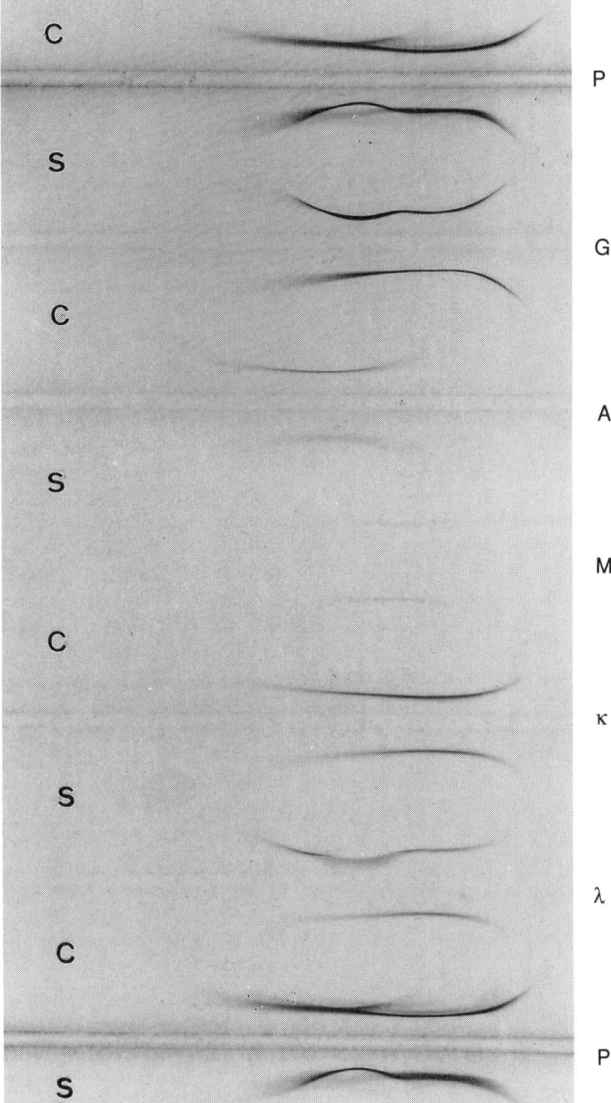

Fig. 8-5. Serum immunoelectrophoresis (IEP) on a patient with a monoclonal gammopathy IgG λ type, also IgA and IgM are decreased. P, G, A, M, κ, and λ denote antiserum against polyvalent serum, IgG, IgA, IgM, κ and λ light chains respectively. C and S represent the positions of normal control and patient serum.

Problems with IEPs include length of time required (3 days), lack of sensitivity or detection of smaller monoclonal gammopathies, frequent inability to detect biclonal gammopathies, and the occurrence of the *um-*

164 • Laboratory Medicine

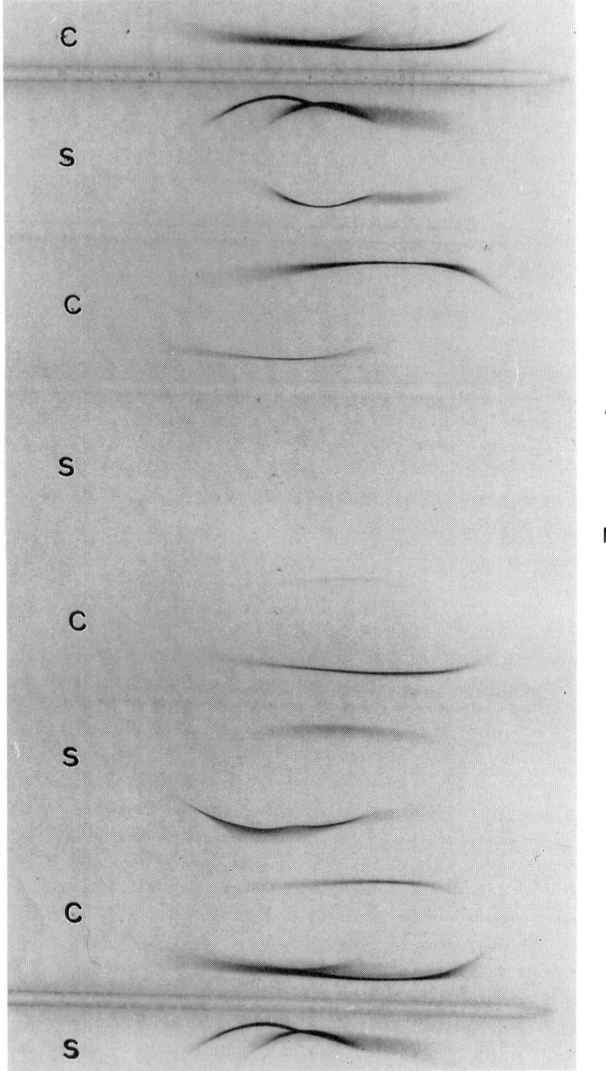

Fig. 8-6. Immunoelectrophoresis on concentrated (×15) urine from the patient whose immunofixation (IFE) and immunoelectrophoresis (IEP) are given in figures 8-4 and 8-5 respectively. Note the presence of IgG and abnormal λ light chain confirming the finding of a monoclonal gammopathy. Concentrated urine has been applied in those troughs usually reserved for serum (S) whereas normal control is denoted by C.

brella effect. The umbrella effect is the masking of IgM gammopathies by polyclonal IgG molecules. This occurs because IgGs comparatively smaller mass allows for more rapid diffusion through agarose, which in turn results in more IgG than IgM molecules reacting with antiserum.

In instances where an IEP presents difficulty in interpretation, an IFE can usually resolve problems in identification of a particular protein.

Table 8-6. Conditions Associated with Monoclonal Proteins

Multiple myeloma
Waldenström's macroglobulinemia
Chronic lymphocytic leukemia
Other leukemias
Lymphomas
"Benign" monoclonal gammopathy
Systemic capillary leak syndrome
Amyloidosis
Chronic liver disease
Autoimmune disorders, including rheumatoid arthritis, systemic lupus erythematosus, thyroiditis, pernicious anemia, polyarteritis nodosa, Sjögren syndrome
Various diseases
Malignancy types

Summary of Disorders

Multiple Myeloma

This is a malignant neoplasm of a single clone of plasma cells of the bone marrow. Although multiple myeloma usually is diffuse, it may present as a single tumor, called a plasmacytoma. Most myelomas involve excessive production of intact Ig molecules along with increased production of peptide fragments of Igs. In light chain disease, increased numbers of light chain fragments of Igs are produced and released and readily filtered in the urine. These chains are detected as Bence Jones protein. Franklin's disease is a myeloma involving the overproduction and release of heavy chain fragments.

About 50% of myelomas are of the IgG type (60% incidence of Bence Jones proteinuria), 25% of the IgA type (70% incidence of Bence Jones proteinuria), and IgD and IgM types account for 2% and 1%, respectively.[29] Only about 20% of patients have Bence Jones proteinuria. The incidence of this disease increases rapidly with age especially beyond the 60th year. The patient may present initially with nonspecific symptoms such as weight loss, anemia, hemorrhages, repeated infections, or renal failure. While these patients may have destructive bone lesions, serum alkaline phosphatase levels are within the reference range. Other aids in diagnosis include neoplastic cells in bone marrow, radiologic evidence of osteolytic lesions, and identification of the associated paraprotein in the serum or concentrated urine.

κ and λ Light Chains

Light chains may be bound to immunoglobulin or freely circulating (unbound). When light chains are free, they have been released from cells before they are able to bind to the heavy chains of the Ig. Usually an increase in free light chains is indicative of a more malignant tumor. The ratio of κ to λ light chains, which is usually between 2:1 and 3:2, also may be an index of the severity of the disease. In a polyclonal gammopathy, this ratio will be markedly elevated, whereas in a monoclonal gammopathy it will be decreased.

Waldenström's Macroglobulinemia

In this disorder, proliferating cells resembling B lymphocytes produce IgM, a high molecular weight protein that causes markedly increased viscosity. The increased viscosity reduces circulation encouraging thrombosis and cold intolerance. Although Bence Jones proteinuria may occur, the disease is less malignant than multiple myeloma and is usually treated by plasmapheresis.

SPECIFIC PROTEIN ANALYSIS

Test: Prealbumim

Background and Selection

Prealbumin, which migrates ahead of albumin on electrophoresis (hence its name), is synthesized by the liver. Prealbumin measurements are useful when assessing protein intake status and liver dysfunction, since its half-life makes it sensitive to changes. Because synthesis is decreased in a number of disorders, prealbumin measurements are helpful in patients with inflammation, malignancy, cirrhosis of the liver, and protein-wasting diseases of the gut or kidney.

Interpretation

The adult reference range for prealbumin as measured by nephelometry or radial immunodiffusion is 20–40 mg/dL (0.2–0.4 g/L), and healthy children usually present with levels of about one-half of those of adults. Serum prealbumin levels fall to 5–10 mg/dL (0.05–0.1 g/L) in malignancy and cirrhosis of the liver, whereas slight increases are observed in Hodgkin's disease. Prealbumin levels are useful for assessing the nutritional status of a patient, because the concentration of the protein decreases rapidly wherever there is a sudden decrease in protein synthesis. Decreases in prealbumin to less than 5 mg/dL (<0.05 g/L) preceeds the final, irreversible collapse of the malnourished patient. In patients presenting with zinc deficiency, measurement of prealbumin and transferrin are good indicators of the degree of deficiency. In situations of zinc deficiency, prealbumin concentrations return to the reference range after a short period, usually 2–4 days, of zinc supplementation.

Test: Albumin

See under "Basic Tests."

Test: α_1-Acid Glycoprotein (Orosomucoid)

Background and Selection

α_1-Acid glycoprotein is mainly used to monitor acute phase reactions and malignancy.

Interpretation

The reference range for α_1-acid glycoprotein, as measured by radial immunodiffusion or nephelometry with the antisera employed capable of detecting all of the polymorphic forms of α_1-acid glycoprotein, is 50–150 mg/dL (0.5–1.5 g/L). The concentration of the protein tends to increase until age 30 in males and after 40 in females. The most useful application of α_1-acid glycoprotein is in the acute phase reaction when there is a rapid increase, a maximum level at about 5 days, and a partial return to the reference range by 3 weeks.[28] After uncomplicated surgery, the protein begins to rise by 8–10 hours and reaches a maximum at levels of approximately 200–250 mg/dL (2–2.5 g/L) within 48–72 hours. Levels of up to 10-fold the reference range may occur in malignancy.

Test: α_1-Antitrypsin (See Ch. 15)

Background and Selection

α_1-Antitrypsin is an acute phase reactant protein that inhibits proteolytic enzymes including trypsin, leukocyte proteases, elastases, and collagenases. During the inflammatory process, AAT is especially important in inhibiting leukocyte proteases, whereby it protects the lung from proteolytic damage. Because AAT is a fairly small molecule, it can pass from capillaries into tissue fluid and subsequently into the intravascular fluid. α_1-Antitrypsin levels are decreased in patients with either the homozygous or heterozygous form of AAT deficiency. The usual AAT protein produced by the majority of the U.S. population is called M protein, with normal heterozygotes having the genotype MM. Although the ability to inhibit proteases is directly related to the concentration of M protein, two other proteins called Z and S occur. Considering relative activities, individuals with the genotypes ZZ, SS, MZ, and MS represent 15, 60, 56, and 80% respectively of MM activity.

Indications for measurement include monitoring patients with AAT deficiency as well as those with suggestive signs and symptoms, such as neonatal respiratory distress syndrome progressing to emphysema, neonatal hepatitis, and protein-losing conditions.

Logistics

Older methods of analysis of AAT include an assay called trypsin inhibitory capacity, which has been displaced by nephelometry as specific antisera against the M protein have become available.

Interpretation

The usual reference range for AAT is 80–200 mg/dL (0.8–2 g/L). Elevations of AAT greater than 200 mg/dL usually are seen in acute phase reactions and also in chronic infection, pregnancy, and estrogen administration. A level of AAT less than 60 mg/dL (<0.6 g/L) is usually associated with a phenotypic variant, and typing as to whether the variant is MZ, MS, and so forth can be performed easily by isoelectric focusing.[30] Levels as low as 20–30 mg/dL (0.2–0.3 g/L) are seen in neonatal cirrhosis, emphysema in young adults, and in patients with severe protein-losing conditions.

Test: α_2-Macroglobulin

The usual reference range for α_2-macroglobulin is 120–400 mg/dL (1.2–4.0 g/L) and females typically show higher values than males.[31] In nephrotic syndrome, increases up to 800 mg/dL (≤8.0 g/L) may be observed possibly because of increased synthesis caused by feedback stimulation by reduced levels of other proteins. In nephrosis α_2-macroglobulin, because of its large size, is not filtered by the kidney as rapidly as smaller proteins.

α_2-Macroglobulin is increased in patients with emphysema, diabetes mellitus, cirrhosis, pregnancy, rheumatoid arthritis, and multiple myeloma. It is significantly increased in cirrhosis, where values up to 600–700 mg/dL (≤6–7 g/L) may be seen.[32]

Test: Haptoglobin

Background and Selection

Haptoglobin is composed of two nonidentical chains linked by disulfide bonds. On electrophoresis normally three main phenotypes can be identified, but a small percentage of black and Asian adults have no detectable haptoglobin. The main function of haptoglobin is in the irreversible binding of free hemoglobulin mainly through the α-chain of the globin moieties of hemoglobins A, F, S, or C, and haptoglobin. After such binding, the haptoglobin-hemoglobin complex is taken up by reticuloendothelial tissue and catabolized, thus ensuring salvage of iron and amino acids. Haptoglobin also is an acute phase reactant; haptoglobin measurements, especially on serial samples, thus are useful for monitoring acute phase reactions and hemolytic states. The protein also may be useful as an index of liver function and neoplasms.

Interpretation

The usual reference range for haptoglobin is 30–220 mg/dL (0.3–2.2 g/L). Low levels are associated with intravascular hemolysis, hemolytic anemias, transfusion reactions, and malaria. After a severe episode of hemolysis that may deplete haptoglobin, plasma levels can be expected to return to the reference range within 7–10 days. Haptoglobin also is decreased in liver disease (less than 20 mg/dL or 0.2 g/L) because of reduced synthesis. Haptoglobin is increased in acute phase reactions; in conditions such as burns and nephrotic syndrome, results up to 400 mg/dL (≤4.0 g/L) occur.

Test: β_2-Microglobulin

Background and Selection

β_2-microglobulin, which is a subunit of the human leukocyte antigen (HLA),[33] is a protein of molecular mass 11,800 da found on the surface of all cells except erythrocytes and the trophoblastic layer of the placenta. As β_2-microglobulin has been demonstrated on the surface membranes of both T and B lymphocytes, it is also a subunit of the histocompatibility Y-chromosome antigen as well as tumor-associated transplantation antigens.[34] These tumor-associated antigens include antigens associated with melanoma, hepatoma, and adenocarcinomas of the colon, breasts, and ovaries. β_2-Microglobulin levels are useful for monitoring renal failure, inflammation, and neoplasms, especially those associated with B lymphocytes.

Logistics

Urine specimens should be collected at high diuresis and converted to alkaline pH (pH 7.4), after which they may be stored for 2 days at 2–8°C or for up to 2 months at −20°C. This treatment of urine samples is essential because β_2-microglobulin is extremely unstable in urine, even with a pH as high as 6.0. Where overnight urine collections are taken, specimens should be collected every 3 hours and alkalinized.

Interpretation

The serum reference range for β_2-microglobulin is 0.1–0.45 mg/dL (1.0–4.5 g/L), and the urine reference range is 10–30 µg/dL (100–300 µg/L). Levels are independent of body mass and sex, but may increase slightly in the elderly. β_2-Microglobulin is especially useful for assessing renal tubular function particularly in renal transplant patients because rejection of the transplanted kidney is manifested by reduced tubular reabsorption.

Test: Transferrin

Background and Selection

Transferrin measurements are useful in the differential diagnosis of anemia and for monitoring treatment. Assay of this protein also may be useful in inflammation and malignancy and may be of interest in chronic liver disease, nephrotic syndrome, and malnutrition.[35]

Interpretation

The reference range for transferrin is 200–350 mg/dL (2.0–3.5 g/L). Decreased levels of transferrin are usually seen in chronic infections, malignancy, iron poisoning, nephrosis, kwashiorkor, and thalassemia where levels down to 100 mg/dL (1.0 g/L) are not uncommon. In congenital atransferrinemia, levels less than 50 mg/dL (<0.5 g/L) may occur and are associated with iron overload and severe hypochromic anemia.

In anemias caused by a problem in the incorporation of iron into the erythrocytes, levels of transferrin are usually within the reference interval. In iron deficiency or hypochromic anemia, levels up to 800 mg/dL (≤0.8 g/L) may be seen. Transferrin also is elevated in late pregnancy, viral hepatitis, and estrogen administration. Because transferrin correlates with the serum total iron-binding capacity, a rough estimate of transferrin concentration may be made by multiplying the total iron-binding capacity value by 0.7. This calculation tends to overestimate transferrin because it assumes that all plasma iron is bound only to transferrin and neglects the influence of other binders such as albumin.

Test: Complement Proteins (See Ch. 30)

Background and Selection

Of all the 20 or more protein components of the complement system, only C1, C1 esterase inhibitor, C3, C4, and C3 proactivator will be considered. The proteins of this system are synthesized by the liver, are present as inactive molecules, and act through both *classic* and alternative pathways with antigen-antibody complexes to destroy viruses and bacteria. They also play a role in autoimmune disease. The classic pathway involves C1 to C5 proteins and is initiated by IgG or IgM bound to antigen or by complexed C-reactive protein. The alternative pathway is initiated by nonantibody factors and involves complement proteins C3 to C5. Both pathways lead to the action or conversion of C5 to C9 with final lysis of the virus or bacteria in question. Exquisite control is exerted on this whole system through the interaction of specific inhibitory proteins. Three distinct protein molecules, C1q, C1r, and C1s, present in the ratio 1:2:2 make up C1, which is responsible for the sequence of complement reactions when binding to an antigen-antibody complex occurs. Measurements of C3 and C4 are useful for assessing systemic diseases (systemic lupus erythematosus, subacute bacterial endocarditis, and cryoglobulinemia) and renal diseases (acute poststreptococcal glomerulonephritis and membranoproliferative glomerulonephritis types I and II). Lupus erythematosus involves both the classic and alternate pathways.

C4 and C1 esterase inhibitors also are useful for detecting inherited angioedema. Other inherited deficiencies of C1, C4, and C2 occur, and these specific proteins or total complement (referred to as CH50 or CH100 depending on the method) can be measured.

Logistics

Specimen Requirements

For measurement of C3, serum should be used and stored frozen as soon as possible after separation from the blood clot, because C3 will break down into split products at room temperature leading to spuriously elevated values. The same precautions should be observed with other complement proteins, and specimens other than blood, such as pleural and synovial fluids, should be treated in a similar manner.

Analysis

Nephelometry or radial immunodiffusion can be used for assays of C3, C4, and C3 proactivator, although radial immunodiffusion presents problems from breakdown products. Immunochemical methods also are available for C1q and C1 esterase inhibitors. The CH50 test for total complement involves addition of complement in the presence of Mg^{2+} and Ca^{2+} to cause lysis of sheep RBCs coated with antibody. The amount of hemolysis is evaluated quantitatively and compared with known controls. The CH100 test involves radial diffusion in agarose gel. The specimen is delivered to a well on the gel that has been impregnated with sheep RBCs sensitized with specific rabbit antibody. As complement diffuses radially through the gel from the well, cytolysis of the sensitized RBCs occurs leaving a clear zone of hemolysis. The zone diameter is proportional to the concentration of active complement.

Interpretation

The reference range for C3 is 90–200 mg/dL (0.9–2.0 g/L), C4 is 15–45 mg/dL (0.15–0.45 g/L), and C3 proactivator is 17–40 mg/dL (0.17–0.40 g/L). During acute phase reactions, any or all three of these proteins may be elevated.

In active lupus erythematosus and other immunocomplex diseases with reduced function of both the classic and alternative pathways, C3, C4, and C3 proactivator are greatly reduced. In diseases in which the alternative pathway is affected (diffuse intravascular coagulation, membranoproliferative glomerulonephritis, gram-negative bacteremia, and paroxysmal nocturnal hemoglobinemia), C4 levels are within the reference range. In contrast, C3 levels are usually less than 60 mg/dL (0.6 g/L), and C3 proactivator levels are less than 12–15 mg/dL (0.12–0.15 g/L).

Bacterial endocarditis associated with glomerulonephritis, acute glomerulonephritis, malaria, and severe chronic liver disease all have reduced classic pathway function, and, as such, C3 proactivator is within the reference range, although both C3 and C4 levels are lower than normal. When reduced serum complement is caused by proteolytic activation, both C3 and C4 proactive levels are within the reference range, but C3 is usually less than 60 mg/dL (0.6 g/L). This is seen in conditions such as gram-negative bacteremia with shock, rheumatoid vasculitis, acute glomerulonephritis, tissue damage, temporal arteritis, and hepatitis B.

In mixed cryoglobulinemia, vivax malaria, hereditary angioedema, and anaphylactoid purpura, C4 is usually less than 10 mg/dL (0.1 g/L), whereas both C3 and factor B are within their reference intervals.

Test: Immunoglobulin (Quantitative Immunoglobulin) (See Ch. 30)

Background and Selection

The assessment of immunoglobulin concentration in serum is usually required when immunoglobulin deficiency and polyclonal or monoclonal hyperimmunoglobulinemia is suspected. When a narrow, sharply discrete spike is seen in the β- or γ-region, on SPE, the investigation of a patient's immunoglobulin status is particularly useful. Of the various components of the immunodefense mechanism, both humoral antibodies of the B lymphocytes and the complement system are plasma proteins that may be readily measured.

Interpretation

The reference ranges for serum immunoglobulins are given in Table 8-4. It should be remembered, however, that reference ranges for IgG and IgM in various adult populations differ worldwide, due to the great differences encountered in antigenic stimulation. It appears that IgA levels are unaffected by environmental factors. In the neonate, circulating IgG represents IgG that has been transferred across the placenta. Adult levels of immunoglobulins are achieved at about 1 year of age for IgM, 3 years of age for IgG and IgA, and after about 12–14 years of age for IgE and IgD.

Decreases

In immunoglobulin deficiency, there is a marked reduction or absence of the γ-band on electrophoresis. Overall, the deficiency may be caused by the nephrotic syndrome, a primary inherited defect in immunoglobulin synthesis, or it may be secondary to lymphoid malignancy or multiple myeloma. Quantitative estimation of immunoglobulins is important in monitoring replacement therapy. This is particularly important in infants who are at risk for immunodeficiency as IgG levels can fall to very low concentrations. However IgA deficiency is the most common of all immunodeficiencies.

Increases

Spikes arise as the result of production of protein by a clone (monoclone) of plasma cells that is multiplying and producing immunoglobulin molecules with identical structures. A monoclonal gammopathy is a proliferative disease, often malignant, the cause of which should be followed closely by requesting quantitative immunoglobulin analysis as well as typing of the particular immunoglobulins involved. Monoclonal protein also is referred to as an "M" or as "paraprotein" electrophoretic band. Biclonal and triclonal gammopathies also may occur.

In hyperimmunoglobulinemia, a polyclonal increase in serum immunoglobulins is observed mainly as a normal response to infection. In autoimmune responses, IgG increases are mainly seen, whereas IgA predominates in skin, gut, respiratory, and renal infections. Increases in IgM are usually associated with viral infection. An overall increase in all serum Igs is usually seen in chronic bacterial infections with a broad diffuse band on SPE in the β-γ-region.

To evaluate the significance of the appearance of a monoclonal M band in an electrophoresis study, other laboratory tests should be requested. These may include (1) typing of the exact immunoglobulin or fragment and assessing the κ to λ light chains in serum and urine; (2) quantitation of IgG, IgA, and IgM to quantitate either increases or suppression in production; and (3) bone marrow examination.

A monoclonal spike (M band or paraprotein) observed on SPE usually is caused by multiple myeloma, macroglobulinemia (and other malignant lymphoproliferative diseases), Franklin's disease (heavy chain disease), and idiopathic or benign M spike. These monoclonal immunoglobulins may be polymers, monomers, or fragments of immunoglobulin molecules. The fragments that occur usually consist of light chains (Bence Jones proteins) but rarely may be composed of heavy chains or half immunoglobulin molecules. Polyclonal γ-globulin increases are an indication of many different clones of cells producing immunoglobulin in response to antigenic stimulation and, as a result, the immunoglobulins will vary in molecular structure. A polyclonal gammopathy caused by infection or liver disease leads to production of a broad, diffuse band on electrophoresis in the β-γ-region.

OTHER PROTEIN TESTS

Test: Ceruloplasmin (CER) (See Chs. 5 and 10)

Background and Selection

Interest in ceruloplasmin has centered mainly around its role in copper metabolism, in which copper absorbed from the intestine is incorporated into the CER apoprotein in the liver. In the circulation, copper is 95% bound to CER. As additional copper is absorbed, CER is synthesized thus avoiding potential copper toxicity.[36] The primary role of CER measurements is diagnosing and managing Wilson's disease, otherwise known as hepatolenticular degeneration because of the combination of liver and neuronal involvement that occurs. Wilson's disease is mainly a result of a decrease in the rate of incorporation of copper into the CER apoprotein and a reduction in the biliary excretion of copper. Additionally, CER measurements also are of interest in patients with biliary cirrhosis, malabsorption, and malnutrition.

Interpretation

The usual reference range for CER is 20–50 mg/dL (1.3–3.3 μmol/L). In Wilson's disease, CER usually is less than 10 mg/dL (0.7 μmol/L) with considerable increases in free copper. Wilson's disease is an autosomal recessive gene defect that occurs in 1:50,000 to 1:100,000. Unless treated, usually by administration of copper chelators, Wilson's disease is always fatal. Copper is deposited in the kidneys, liver, and brain resulting in tissue damage. Kayser-Fleischer rings also are evident on eye examination, owing to excessive deposits of copper in the cornea. Further, the disease may be confirmed by administration of radioactive copper followed by the measurement of plasma radioactivity at regular intervals. In healthy subjects, radioactivity increases, then falls, then rises again due to CER production. In Wilson's disease, the secondary rise in radioactivity is not observed because there is a defect in the incorporation of copper into the protein. In biliary cirrhosis, malabsorption, and malnutrition, CER levels are usually less than 10 mg/dL (1.3 μmol/L), whereas serum concentration of up to 70 mg/dL (4.7 µmol/L) may be observed in extreme exercise, pregnancy, and estrogen administration. (For further information see Ch. 10.)

Test: C-Reactive Protein (CRP)

Background and Selection

The first acute phase reactant to be discovered was C-reactive protein, which is synthesized in the liver. The "C" of C-reactive protein is derived from earlier studies that demonstrated that serum from acutely ill individuals contained a substance that precipitated with the C form (termed C-polysaccharide) of the cell wall of pneumococci. Structurally, CPR has five identical polypeptide subunits and can activate the classic complement pathway, initiate opsonization, phagocytose, lyse foreign cells, and act as a detoxification agent. Increased results occur in inflammatory diseases (e.g., rheumatoid arthritis, rheumatic fever, and vasculitic syndromes such as hypersensitivity vasculitis), infections (especially neonatal and postoperative, infections as well as intercurrent infections in leukemia and pyelonephritis), and neoplastic diseases. Additionally, C-reactive protein is increased in neoplasia including Burkitt's lymphoma and tissue injury such as myocardial infarction, embolism, and transplant rejection.

Interpretation

The reference range for CRP is less than 800 µg/dL (<8.0 mg/L). In the many clinical situations noted above, it is not unusual to find CRP concentrations of up to 2000 times the reference range with peak levels achieved at 24–48 hours. In the differential diagnosis of certain diseases, CRP measurements are especially useful. For example, systemic lupus erythematosus patients usually have less CRP in serum than rheumatoid arthritis patients. In Crohn's disease, CRP levels are much lower than in ulcerative colitis, and levels are usually up to 1000 times higher in pyelonephritis than in cystitis (less than 1000 µg/dL [less than 10 mg/L]). Patients with bacterial infections have higher levels than those with viral infections, and asthma patients have results one-half those seen with acute bronchitis. In monitoring the course of bacterial meningitis, CRP measurements can be used with results returning to the reference range within 7 days. In contrast, CRP does not rise at all in patients with viral meningitis or meningoencephalitis.[37,38] Also, CRP measurements can be applied to the prediction of chorioamnionitis in premature rupture of membranes, because it has been demonstrated that CRP has a sensitivity of 88% and a specificity of 96% for predicting chorioamnionitis.[39] Because of cathodal electrophoretic migration on high resolution serum protein electrophoresis, high concentration may cause the formation of a band confused with a monoclonal IgG.

Test: Cryoglobulins

Cryoglobulins, which tend to precipitate at temperatures lower than body temperature, are a result of polymerization of immunoglobulins. The condition is seen in people over 60 years of age and is caused by polymers of IgM (most common), IgG, or IgA and hence are frequently seen in myeloma and macroglobulinemia. Cryoglobulins also may be polyconal and are seen in rheumatoid arthritis, systemic lupus erythematosis, and other autoimmune diseases. Mixed cryoglobulin complexes deposit in vessel walls and fix complement causing inflammation. The resulting vasculitis can lead to renal damage and neurologic disease. Monoclonal cryoglobulin is more commonly associated with Raynaud's phenomenon or vascular purpura. In interpreting electrophoresis patterns in the diagnosis of cryoglobulinemia, it is essential to check that a temperature of 37°C was maintained, not only for blood collection but also for serum separation, to prevent the precipitation of cryoglobulins at lower temperatures.

Test: Viscosity (Blood and Serum)

Background and Selection

Hyperviscosity of blood may be due to elevated plasma or serum viscosity, to elevated numbers of cells (polycythemia or leukemia), or to increased resistance of cells to the deformation required to accommodate to the varying size and shape of the blood vessels (sicklemia or spherocytosis). Blood viscosity measurements are particularly useful during hyperviscosity in the neonatal period and after splenectomy in adults when blood viscosity is increased. Serum measurements are used to evaluate hyperviscosity syndromes associated with monoclonal gammopathy states.

Logistics

For blood viscosity measurements, heparinized whole blood is required, and clotted or hemolyzed specimens should be rejected. Serum or plasma may be used for other viscosity requests and specimens may be stored for up to 2 days at 4°C before analysis.

Blood and serum viscosities are usually measured at room temperature or 37°C using a viscometer (e.g., Coulter Harkness Viscometer). Water and plasma flow times are determined with the use of a viscometer RBC or white blood cell pipette and stopwatch. The relative viscosity is expressed as a ratio of plasma flow time to water flow time.

Interpretation

The usual reference range for neonatal viscosity is derived from a nomogram displaying viscosity (measured in centipoise) plotted against hematocrit for two shear rates, usually 106 and 11 seconds^{-1}. Viscosity normally rises with an increase in hematocrit and is lower with lower shear rates. Neonatal hyperviscosity may present with polycythemia plethora, hypoglycemia, lethargy, and seizures. Whole blood viscosity measurements can be used to follow exchange transfusion therapy in cases of neonatal hyperviscosity syndrome.

The normal reference range for serum viscosity is 1.4–1.8 relative to water, and the test is useful for evaluating hyperviscosity syndromes associated with monoclonal gammopathies, rheumatoid arthritis, systemic lupus erythematosus, and hyperfibrinogenemia. Hyperviscosity is most commonly associated with IgM monoclonal gammopathy (Waldenström's macroglobulinemia) where relative viscosity measurements of 6 to 7 are not uncommon. IgA and IgG myelomas also increase serum viscosity.

Wright and Jenkins[40] studied 20 myeloma-macroglobulinemia patients, 5 with hypogammaglobulinemia had serum viscosity values within the normal reference interval. The 16 IgG myeloma patients had values from 1.2–12.4, 5 IgA myeloma patients ranged from 1.9–13.0, and 3 IgM subjects ranged from 2.2–4.8.

REFERENCES

1. Harper HA, Rodwell A: Amino acids and proteins. pp. 24–48. In Harper HA (ed): Review of Physiological Chemistry. 15th Ed. Los Altos, CA, Lange Medical Publications, 1976.
2. Blick KE, Liles SM: Proteins. pp. 227–265. In Blick KE, Liles SM (eds): Principles of Clinical Chemistry. New York, John Wiley & Sons, 1985.
3. Grant GH, Silverman LM, Christenson RH: Amino acids and proteins. pp. 291–345. In Tietz NW (ed): Fundamentals of Clinical Chemistry. Philadelphia, WB Saunders, 1987.
4. Silverman LM, Christenson RH, Grant GH: Amino acids and proteins. pp. 519–618. In Tietz NW (ed): Textbook of Clinical Chemistry. Philadelphia, WB Saunders, 1986.
5. Smith I: Chromatographic and Electrophoretic Techniques. pp. 185–190. Vol. 1. 3rd Ed. London, Heinemann Medical Publishers, 1969.
6. Guthrie R, Susi A: A simple phenylalanine method for detecting phenylketonuria in large populations of newborn infants. Pediatrics 1963;32:338–343.
7. Langenbeck, U, Wendel U, Mensch-Hoinowski A et al: Correlations between branched-chain amino acids and branched chain α-keto acids in blood in maple syrup urine disease. Clin Chim Acta 1978;88:283–291.
8. Levy HL, Truman JT, Ganz RN, Littlefield JW: Folic acid deficiency secondary to a diet for maple syrup urine disease. J Pediatr 1970;77:294–296.
9. Foreman JW, Yudkoff M, Berry G, Segal S: Acidosis associated with dietotherapy of maple syrup urine disease. J Pediatr 1980;96:62–64.
10. Segal S, Thier SO: Cystinuria. pp. 1774–1791. In Stanbury JB, Wyngaarden JB, Fredrickson DS et al. (eds): The Metabolic Basic of Inherited Disease. 5th Ed. New York, McGraw-Hill, 1983.
11. Fawcett NP, Nyhan WL, Anderson WW: Thrombocytosis during treatment of cystinuria with penicillamine. J Pediatr 1966;69:976–977.
12. Williamson ML, Dobson JC, Koch R: Collaborative study of children treated for phenylketonuria: a study design. Pediatrics 1977;60:815–821.
13. Woo SLC: Prenatal diagnosis and carrier detection of classic phenylketonuria by gene analysis. Pediatrics 1984;74:412–423.
14. Koch R, Weng E: Phenylketonuria. pp. 117–135. In Olson RE, Beutler E, Broquist HP, (eds): Annual Review of Nutrition. Palo Alto, CA Annual Reviews, 1987.
15. Holtzman NA, Kronmal RA, Van-Doorninck W et al: Effects of age at loss of dietary control on intellectual performance and behavior of children with phenylketonuria. N Engl J Med 1986;314:593–598.
16. Lenke R, Levy HL: Maternal phenylketonuria and hyperphenylalaninemia. N Engl J Med 1980;303:1202–1208.
17. Goldsmith LA: Tyrosinemia and related disorders. pp. 287–293. In Stanbury JB, Wyngaarden JB, Fredrickson DS et al (eds): The Metabolic Basis of Inherited Disease. 5th Ed. New York, McGraw-Hill, 1983.
18. Peters T Jr: Serum albumin: recent progress in the understanding of its structure and biosynthesis. Clin Chem 1977;23:5–12.
19. Doumas BT, Biggs HG: Determination of serum albumin. Stand Methods. Clin Chem 1972;7:175–188.
20. Dito WR: Rapid immunonephelometric quantitation of eleven serum proteins by centrifugal fast analyzer. Am J Clin Pathol 1979;71:301–308.
21. Cannon DC, Olitzky I, Inkpen JA: Proteins. pp. 405–502. In Henry RJ, Cannon DC, Winkelman JW (eds): Clinical Chemistry: Principles and Technics. Hagerstown, MD, Harper & Row, 1974.
22. Doumas BT, Bayse DD, Carter RJ et al: A candidate reference method for determination of total protein in serum. I. Development and validation. Clin Chem 1981;27:1642–1650.
23. Reed AH, Cannon DC, Winkelman JW et al: Estimation of normal ranges from a controlled sample survey. I. Sex and age-related influence on the SMA 12/60 screening group of tests. Clin Chem 1972;18:57–66.
24. Patel S, Lott JA: Serum protein electrophoresis. pp. 1309–1315. In Kaplan LA, Pesce AJ (eds): Clinical

Chemistry: Theory, Analysis and Correlation. St. Louis, CV Mosby, 1984.
25. Lyngbye J, Kroll J: Quantitative immunoelectrophoresis of proteins in serum from a normal population: season-, age-, and sex-related variation. Clin Chem 1971;17:495–500.
26. Aguzzi F, Jayakar AD, Merlini G, Petrine C: Electrophoresis: cellulose acetate vs. agarose gel, visual inspection vs. densitometry. Clin Chem 1981;27:1944–1945.
27. Johansson BG: Agarose gel electrophoresis. Scand J Clin Lab Invest 1972;29(suppl)124:7–21.
28. Alper CA, Johnson AM: Immunofixation electrophoresis: a technique for the study of protein polymorphism. Vox Sang 1969;17:445–452.
29. Grant GH, Silverman LM, Christenson RH: Amino acids and proteins. pp. 291–345. In Tietz NW (ed): Fundamentals of Clinical Chemistry. Philadelphia, WB Saunders, 1987.
30. Jeppsson JO, Franzen B: Typing of genetic variants of α_1-antitrypsin by electrofocusing. Clin Chem 1982;28:219–225.
31. Weeke B, Krasilnikoff PA: The concentration of 21 serum proteins in normal children and adults. Acta Med Scan 1972;149:1972–1976.
32. LoGrippo GA, Anselm K, Hayashi H: Serum immunoglobulins and five serum proteins in extrahepatic obstructive jaundice and alcoholic cirrhosis. Am J Gastroenterol 1971;56:357–363.
33. Forman DT: Beta-2 microglobulin: an immunogenetic marker of inflammatory and malignant origin. Ann Clin Lab Sci 1982;12:477–452.
34. Peterson PA, Rask L: Highly purified papain-solubilized HLA antigens contain β_2M. Proc Natl Acad Sci USA 1974;71:35–39.
35. Rajamaki A, Irjala K, Aitio A: Immunochemical determination of serum transferrin. Scand J Haematol 1979;23:227–231.
36. Gutteridge JMC, Stocks J: Ceruloplasma: physiological and pathological perspectives. CRC Crit Rev Clin Lab Sci 1981;14:257–329.
37. Peltola HO: C-Reactive protein for rapid monitoring of infections of the central nervous system. Lancet 1982;1:980–982.
38. Morley JJ, Kushner I: Serum C-reactive protein levels in disease. Ann NY Acad Sci 1982;389:406–418.
39. Hawrylyshyn P, Bernstein P, Milligan JE et al: Premature rupture of membranes: the role of C-reactive protein in the prediction of chorioamnionitis. Am J Obstet Gynecol 1983;147:240–246.
40. Wright DJ, Jenkins DE Jr: Simplified method for estimation of serum and plasma viscosity in multiple myeloma and related disorders. Blood 1970;36:516–522.

9 Lipids, Lipoproteins, and Apolipoproteins

Paul C. Fu

LIPIDS

INTRODUCTION

Lipids, a term generally referring to a heterogeneous group of organic compounds, tend to be insoluble in polar environments, but are readily extractable by nonpolar, organic solvents. They are major precursors in energy metabolism and are important structural constituents of cellular membranes. The major lipids include fatty acids, triglycerides, cholesterol, phospholipids, and glycolipids. Because of their hydrophobic properties, they are transported by a group of specific proteins and albumin. The resulting complex of various lipids and protein macromolecules (apolipoproteins) are called lipoproteins. These include chylomicrons, very low density lipoproteins (VLDLs), low density lipoproteins (LDLs), intermediate density lipoproteins (IDLs), and high density lipoproteins (HDLs). The chemical and physical properties of the major lipids as well as various classes of lipoproteins are summarized in Table 9-1. In fact, one of the recent major advances in lipid biochemistry is a better understanding of the relationship among lipids, especially the roles of cholesterol and lipoproteins, in coronary heart disease (CHD).

ROUTINE TESTS

Test: Cholesterol

Background

Chemically, cholesterol is a steroid alcohol (sterol) containing a perhydrocyclopentanophenanthene skeleton with a hydroxyl group at carbon 3 of ring A and an aliphatic hydrocarbon chain at carbon 17 of ring D. The structure of cholesterol and its numbering system are illustrated in Figure 9-1. Cholesterol can be esterified with fatty acids through a hydroxyl group at carbon 3. About 70% of plasma cholesterol is esterfied with long chain fatty acids, especially linoleic acid as a predominant one, whereas the remainder exists in free form.

Cholesterol is an essential structural component of cell membranes, a precursor of bile acids and steroid hormones, and is synthesized in almost all animal tissues, except erythrocytes. The liver, intestine, adrenal glands, and gonads are the major sites of cholesterol biosynthesis. The conversion of acetoacetyl coenzyme

Table 9-1. Classification, Properties, and Composition of Human Serum Lipoproteins

Parameter	Chylomicron	VLDL	IDL	LDL	HDL
Hydrated density (g/mL)	0.93	0.97	1.003	1.034	1.121
Solvent density for isolation (g/mL)	<1.006	<1.006	1.006–1.019	1.019–1.063	1.063–1.21
Mass (da)	$(0.4–30) \times 10^9$	$(5–10) \times 10^6$	$(3.9–4.8) \times 10^6$	2.75×10^6	$(3.6–1.75) \times 10^5$
Diameter (nm)	>70.0	25.0–70.0	22.0–24.0	19.6–22.7	4–10
Electrophoretic mobility (paper, agarose)	Origin	Pre-β	Broad β (between β and pre-β)	β	α
Composition (% by weight)					
Cholesterol, unesterified	2	5–8	8	13	6
Cholesterol, esterified	5	11–14	22	49	13
Phospholipid	7	20–23	25	27	28
Triglyceride	84	44–60	30	11	3
Protein	2	4–11	15	23	50[a]
Apoproteins (% total apolipoprotein)					
A-I	7.4	Trace	—	—	67
A-II	4.2	Trace	—	—	22
B-100	Trace	36.9	50–70	98	Trace
B-48	22.5	Trace	Trace	—	—
C-I, C-II, C-III	66	49.9	5–10	Trace	5–11
E-II, E-III, E-IV	—	13.0	10–20	Trace	1–2
D	—	—	—	—	Trace
Synthesis	Intestine	Liver, intestine	Intravascular	Intravascular	Intestine, liver

Abbreviations: HDL, high density lipoprotein; IDL, intermediate density lipoprotein; LDL, low density lipoprotein; VLDL, very low density lipoprotein.
(From Stein,[1] with permission.)

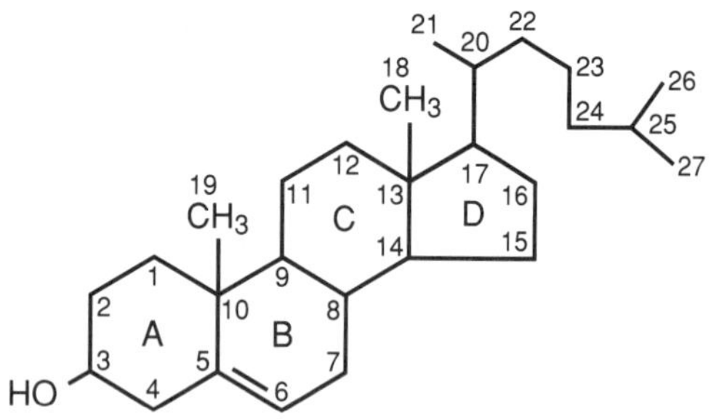

Fig. 9-1. Structure of cholesterol.

A (CoA) to 3 hydroxy-3-methylglutaryl-CoA (HMG-CoA) by HMG-CoA reductase is the major enzymatic rate limiting step in the endogeneous cholesterol synthesis. Feedback regulation exerted by cholesterol on this rate limiting step adjusts the rate of endogenous cholesterol synthesis to balance the dietary fat intake. Dietary cholesterol is first hydrolyzed by cholesterol esterase to free cholesterol before it is absorbed by intestinal mucosa. The absorption of free cholesterol requires the presence of bile salts and lecithin. Increased triglycerides in the diet tend to promote cholesterol absorption. Cholesterol in the intestinal mucosal cells is then incorporated into lipid protein macromolecular complexes known as chylomicrons, which are secreted into the circulation via the lymphatic system. After undergoing certain catabolic processes and exchange of lipid and apoprotein components, the resultant chylomicron remnants containing mostly the cholesterol ester, Apo B-48, and Apo E, are then taken up by the liver. When dietary cholesterol derived from the chylomicron remnants is insufficient, the liver synthesizes its own cholesterol by increasing the rate limiting enzymatic activities of HMG-CoA reductase. Intrahepatic cholesterol, triglycerides, and apoproteins are reassembled into lipoproteins called VLDL and released into circulation. In the circulation, VLDL undergoes several compositional changes by interacting with lecithin cholesterol acyltransferase (LCAT), HDL, and lipoprotein lipase (LPL). First, VLDL is transferred into IDL and then LDL after releasing or exchanging most of its triglycerides and apoproteins. The LDL contains almost all cholesterol ester in the core and Apo B-100 on the surface. Low density lipoprotein delivers cholesterol to all peripheral tissues and cells with LDL receptors. Once cholesterol enters the cells, the cholesterol esters are hydrolyzed to free cholesterol by cholesterol esterases. When the supply of free cholesterol exceeds cellular metabolic requirements, the enzyme acyl-cholesterol acyltransferase (ACAT) is activated to esterify free cholesterol to cholesterol ester for storage. In addition, the activity of the rate limiting enzyme for cholesterol synthesis of HMG-CoA reductase is inhibited.

Selection

The National Institutes of Health (NIH) Consensus Development Conference on lowering blood cholesterol held in 1984 concluded that the "elevation of blood cholesterol is a major cause of coronary artery

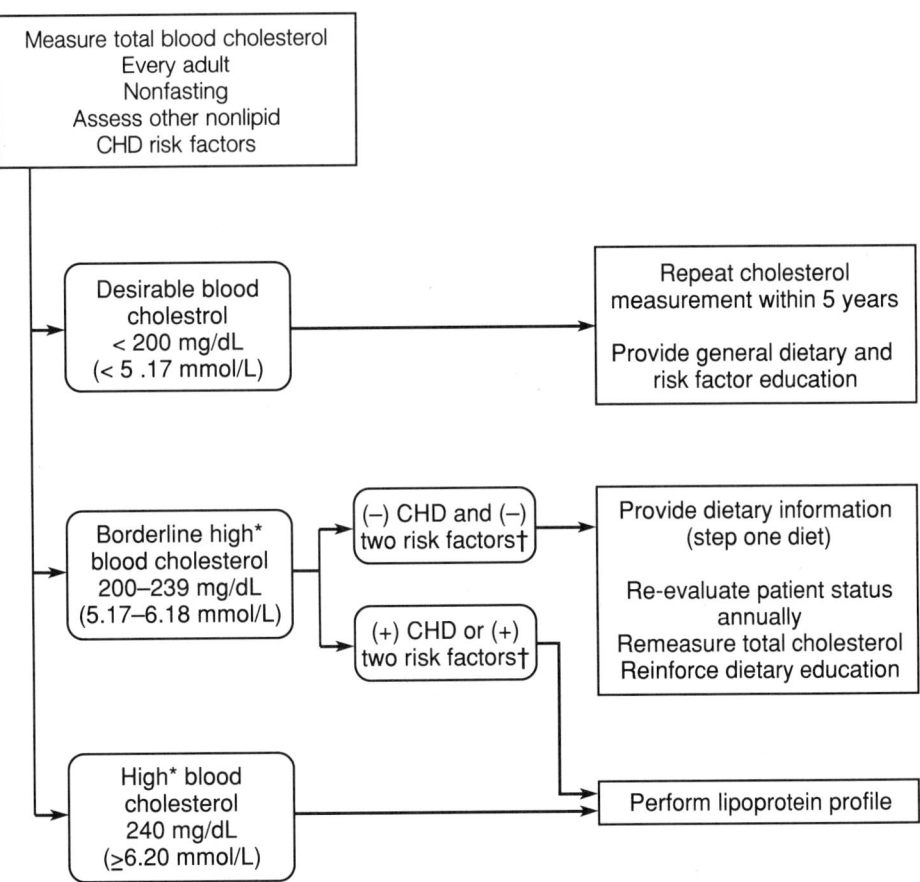

Fig. 9-2. Initial classification based on total cholesterol. *Must be confirmed by repeat measurement; use average value. † One of which can be male sex. CHD, coronary heart disease. (Adapted from The Expert Panel,[4] with permission.)

disease."[2] The Multiple Risk Factor Intervention Trial (MRFIT) provides further evidence connecting elevated cholesterol levels with increased incidence of coronary artery disease.[3] The expert panel on the detection, evaluation, and treatment of high blood cholesterol in adults (Adult Treatment Panel), convened by the National Cholesterol Education Program (NCEP) of the National Heart, Lung and Blood Institute, has recommended cholesterol testing for all American adults over the age of 20.[4] Others recommend screening all 5- to 8-year-old children as part of a school-based health program.[5] The panel further developed a detailed algorithm for initial classification of patients and follow-up treatment based on total cholesterol as shown in Figure 9-2.[4] Patients with cholesterol levels less than 200 mg/dL (5.17 mmol/L) should have the test repeated within 5 years. It is recommended that patients who have CHD or two other CHD risk factors, patients who have borderline high cholesterol levels between 200–239 mg/dL (5.17–6.18 mmol/L), and patients who have cholesterol levels greater than 240 mg/dL (6.20 mmol/L) should undergo further testing (see Figure 9-3). In contrast, the European Consensus Conference uses a serum cholesterol target of 200 mg/dL (5.17 mmol/L).[4,6]

Logistics

Specimen Requirements

Proper patient preparation and specimen collection are essential components of optimal lipid analysis. If only total cholesterol is measured, fasting or nonfasting specimens may be used. Although no significant increase of the cholesterol level was reported in the nonfasting specimen,[7] a fasting specimen is still strongly recommended. It is well known that increased triglyceride levels after meals tend to promote the cholesterol absorption in vivo. In addition, nonfasting specimens often exhibit turbidity caused by an increase of VLDL and chylomicrons, which in turn may cause in vitro interference with the measurement of cholesterol and in the examination of the specimen's physical appearance.

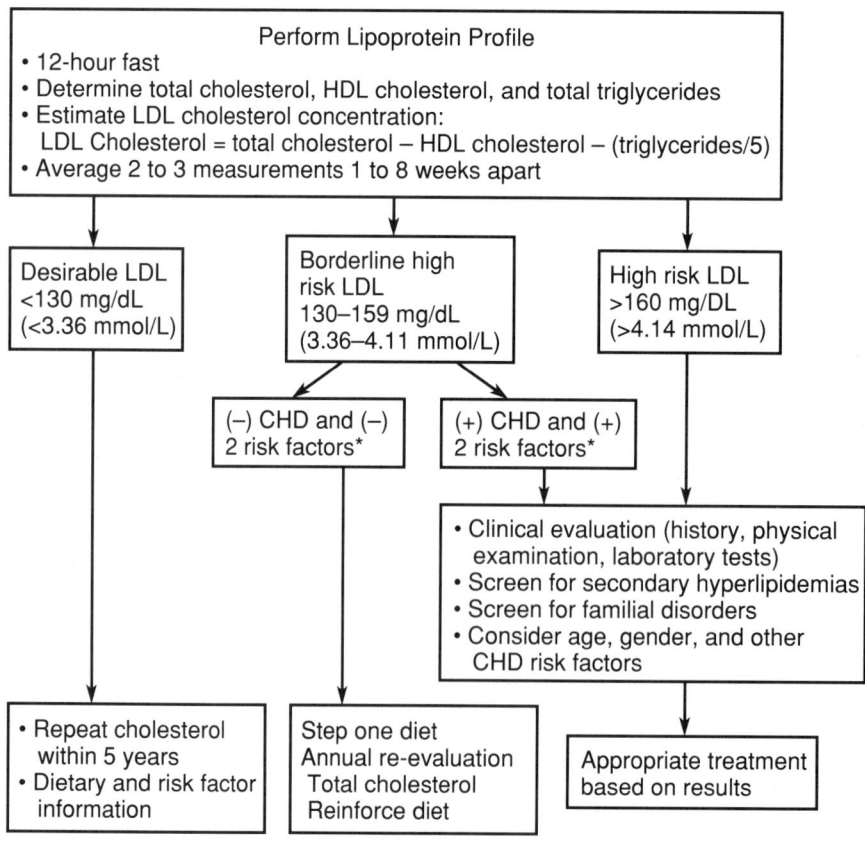

Fig. 9-3. Algorithm summarizing the approach to evaluating plasma lipoproteins in patients with high or borderline high serum cholesterol concentrations. *One of which can be male sex. CHD, coronary heart disease. (Modified from The Expert Panel,[4] with permission.)

Many factors effect cholesterol results, including blood collection techniques. If possible, the patient should be in the sitting position for about 5 minutes before venipuncture to avoid changes in cholesterol caused by redistribution of water between vascular and extravascular compartments. The apparent concentration of cholesterol varies whether the measurement is made using serum or plasma. Plasma derived from anticoagulant (such as citrate or oxalate)-treated specimens is not recommended, because of large losses of water from red blood cells (RBCS) to plasma that result in dilution of plasma components. Cholesterol results in EDTA plasma specimens are about 3% lower than those of comparable serum specimens. The Adult Treatment Panel recommendations for classification of patients reflect cholesterol results based on *serum* cholesterol. According to recent reports, on site screening measurements for cholesterol in venous samples were found to be more reliable than those in capillary blood samples.[8,9]

There is an average biologic variation in serum cholesterol of as much as 6–7%. Diurnal variation of up to 2–3% occurs, but larger variations can occur in those individuals who have high triglycerides. Seasonal variation accounts for changes in cholesterol of 3–5%, with values tending to be lower in the summer months and higher in the winter. Because of these factors, it is recommended that the average of the two results should be used in evaluating serum cholesterol elevation. The specimens should be obtained not less than 1 week or more than 2 months apart. If values differ by more than 30 mg/dL (0.78 mmol/L), a third analysis should be performed.

Serum cholesterol also varies with age, gender, diet, alcohol intake, and exercise. In addition to lipid-lowering drugs, various other drugs including antihypertensive medications and steroids can affect serum cholesterol concentrations. Cholesterol measurements should be deferred for at least 8 weeks after severe illness such as myocardial infarction or stroke.

Methods

Standardization of cholesterol assays to maintain accuracy is important, because physicians classify patients on the basis of the total cholesterol results using reference ranges as shown in Figure 9-2. Standardization is difficult, because some analytic systems are sensitive to the matrix of prepared materials including standards and quality control materials. The only universally reliable approach to demonstrating accuracy is to use fresh patient specimens. Results with these fresh specimens are compared directly with results using a standardized cholesterol method based on the National Reference Standard (NRS).

Many methods are used for measuring serum cholesterol. In laboratories of the Lipid Research Clinics (LRC) program, cholesterol is measured using automated continuous flow analyzers with the method based on isopropanol extract of total cholesterol and the Libermann-Burchard reaction. The Centers for Disease Control (CDC) reference method for cholesterol was based on the modified method of Abell et al.[10,11] Recently, the enzymatic method for cholesterol first described in Allain et al.[12] and Fu and Allain[13] has gradually replaced chemical methods as the routine procedure of choice for clinical laboratories. The recommended calibrator for the enzymatic procedure is the National Bureau of Standards (NBS) serum reference material (No. 909). With the appropriate cholesterol standard, the enzymatic method can be considered as a reference method for routine determination of total cholesterol. The isotope dilution–mass spectrometric method as established by the NBS is currently considered a definitive method for cholesterol measurement.[14]

Further information on standardization and preanalytical variation, as well as recommendations for precision goals can be found in "Recommendations for Improving Cholesterol Measurement": Special Cholesterol Education Program, U.S. Department of Health and Human Services, February 1990.[15]

Interpretation

Table 9-2 shows age- and sex-related reference ranges for plasma cholesterol.[16] The panel on detection, evaluation, and treatment of high blood cholesterol in adults (Adult Treatment Panel) recommends risks based on total cholesterol and LDL cholesterol as shown in Table 9-3.

The panel defines those individuals with cholesterol levels above the 75th percentile, but less than the 90th percentile, as having moderate risk. These individuals do not need further immediate evaluation or medical therapy in the absence of CHD or any two other CHD-related risk factors as shown in Table 9-4. However, these individuals should be given proper dietary information and be reevaluated annually.

High risk serum cholesterol levels are defined as results above the 90th percentile. The consensus panel further

178 • Laboratory Medicine

Table 9-2. The Age- and Sex-Related Reference Ranges for Total Cholesterol

Age (Yrs)	Total Cholesterol (mg/dL)[a] Percentiles				
	5	50	75	90	95
Male					
5–19	115	155	170	185	200
20–24	125	165	185	205	220
25–29	135	180	200	225	245
30–34	140	190	215	240	255
35–39	145	200	225	250	270
40–44	150	205	230	250	270
45–69	160	215	235	260	275
≥70	150	205	230	250	270
Female					
5–19	120	160	175	190	200
20–24	125	170	190	215	230
25–34	130	175	195	220	235
35–39	140	185	205	230	245
40–44	145	195	215	235	255
45–49	150	205	225	250	270
50–54	165	220	240	265	285
≥55	170	230	250	275	295

[a] For SI units (mmol/L) multiply mg/dL by 0.02586.
(From Levy,[16] with permission.)

Table 9-4. Risk Factors for Coronary Artery Disease

Male sex
Family history of premature CHD (definite myocardial infarction or sudden death before age 55 in a patient or sibling)
Cigarette smoking (>10 cigarettes/d)
Hypertension
Low HDL cholesterol concentration (<35 mg/dL confirmed by repeat measurement)
Diabetes mellitus
History of definite cerebrovascular or occlusive peripheral vascular disease
Vascular disease
Severe obesity (>30% overweight)

Abbreviations: CHD, coronary heart disease; HDL, high density lipoprotein.

classified hypercholesterolemia based on ages and cholesterol concentration with respect to the increased risk of CHD (Table 9-5).[17]

Hypercholesterolemia (type II$_a$ hyperlipoproteinemia [see below]) may be primary or secondary to other causes. The primary disorder appears to be inherited, and thus family screening is often useful. The classic inherited disorder is essential familial hypercholesterolemia, which occurs either in heterozygous or in homozygous forms. Secondary causes of hypercholesterolemia include diabetes mellitus, alcoholism, hypothyroidism, nephrotic syndrome, chronic renal failure, gout, liver disease, oral contraceptives, and steroid therapy. Lipid abnormalities often diminish when the underlying diseases or causes have been properly treated or corrected.

Test: Triglycerides

Background

Triglycerides are the major neutral fats found in mammalian tissues. Chemically, triglycerides are triesters of glycerol with fatty acids. Various fatty acids with differences in chain length and unsaturation are distributed among α, β, and α' positions: their typical structures are illustrated in Figure 9-4.

Triglycerides are mainly synthesized in the small intestine, liver, and adipose tissues, and are influenced by various metabolic and disease states. Transient hypertriglyceridemia occurs in healthy persons after meals rich in carbohydrate and fat content and in patients with uncontrolled diabetes mellitus. Triglycerides from

Table 9-3. Recommendations of the Adult Treatment Panel of the National Cholesterol Education Program for Classification of Patients

Risk Classification	Total Cholesterol (mg/dL) (mmol/L)	LDL Cholesterol mg/dL (mmol/L)
Desirable	<200 (<5.17)	<130 (<3.36)
Borderline high risk	200–239 (5.17–6.18)	130–159 (3.36–4.11)
High risk	>240 (>6.21)	>160 (>4.13)

Abbreviation: LDL, low density lipoprotein.
(Modified from The Expert Panel,[4] with permission.)

Table 9-5. Classifications of Hypercholesterolemia. NIH Consensus Conference on Cholesterol

Age (yr)	Moderate Risk (mg/dL) (mmol/L)	High Risk (mg/dL) (mmol/L)
2–19	>170 (4.40)	>185 (4.79)
20–29	>200 (5.17)	>220 (5.69)
30–39	>220 (5.69)	>240 (6.21)
>40	>240 (6.21)	>260 (6.72)

(Modified from the NIH Consensus Development Conference,[17] with permission.)

intestinal mucosal cells are transported via the thoracic lymph duct to systemic circulation mainly in the form of chylomicrons and to a small extent as VLDL. Chylomicrons contain about 84% triglycerides, 7% cholesterol, 7% phospholipids, and 2% proteins. The size of the chylomicrons or other lipoproteins often depends on the content of the triglycerides. Triglycerides synthesized in the liver are released to circulation as VLDL. Chylomicrons and VLDL are further catabolyzed by lipoprotein lipase to triglycerides, the chylomicron remnant, IDL and LDL. In addition, HDL found in the circulation also contains triglycerides. It has been shown that regulation of LPL activity by various hormonal factors plays an essential role in the turnover rate of triglycerides in the blood stream.

Selection

Clinical interest in the determination of triglycerides is based on its association with the differential diagnosis of primary or secondary hyperlipidemia and in the assessment of risk factors for acute pancreatitis. In hyperlipoproteinemia interpretation cannot rely on the triglyceride level alone; it is essential that other lipids and lipoproteins are taken into consideration. Recent studies have shown no substantial cause and effect relationship between the triglyceride level and CHD, and that triglyceride level is not an independent risk factor.[18] Commonly, triglyceride is ordered along with serum cholesterol. However, it has been suggested that triglyceride measurements may be useful only in patients with suspected primary metabolic lipid dysfunction. Routine screening for triglyceride level in asymptomatic patients is not recommended, but results are used to calculate LDL.

Logistics

Specimen Requirements

It is commonly recognized that proper patient preparation and specimen collection is critical in the laboratory evaluation of lipid disorders. In general, the patient should be on a stable diet for at least 3 weeks. Prior to specimen collection, the patient should fast for at least 12 hours and probably should not be taking any medications. An increase in circulating chylomicron triglyceride occurs after each meal and such an increase usually continues for several hours during intestinal absorption of fat. In addition, increased level of triglycerides in the diet may tend to promote cholesterol absorption. Because triglyceride concentrations are markedly elevated after meals, reaching a peak level at 4–6 hours, fasting specimens are particularly important for triglyceride determination. It is also recommended that the patient avoid alcohol ingestion for at least 72 hours before specimen collection. The patient's weight should be steady and specimen collection should be deferred for at least 2 weeks after a minor illness, and 2–3 months after an acute or major illness, trauma, or recent surgery.

Methods

Most of the methods for the determination of triglycerides are based on the amount of free glycerol occurring after chemical saponification or enzymatic hydrolysis of triglycerides. In the chemical procedure, glycerol is oxidized to formaldehyde in the presence of periodic acid. The formaldehyde can then be coupled to a number of reactants to form a distinctive chromophore. The Hantzsch condensation between formaldehyde, acetylacetone, and ammonium ion yields a yellow end product. The Hantzsch reaction and saponification step has been successfully automated, and this method is considered a candidate reference method.[19] In the enzymatic determination,[20] triglycerides are first enzymatically hydrolyzed by lipase in the presence of α-chymotrypsin to glycerol and fatty acids. Glycerol is then measured by coupled enzymatic reactions, including glycerol kinase and lactate dehydrogenase (LD).

$$H_2C\text{-}O\text{-}COR_1 \quad \alpha$$
$$HC\text{-}O\text{-}COR_2 \quad \beta$$
$$H_2C\text{-}O\text{-}COR_3 \quad \alpha'$$

R_1, R_2, R_3 Fatty Acids

Fig. 9-4. Common structure of triglycerides.

Table 9-6. Reference Ranges for Plasma Triglycerides (mg/dL)[a]

Age (yr)	Males Percentiles							Females Percentiles						
	5	10	25	50	75	90	95	5	10	25	50	75	90	95
5–9	28	34	39	48	58	70	85	32	37	45	57	74	103	126
10–14	33	37	46	58	74	94	111	39	44	53	58	85	104	120
15–19	38	43	53	68	88	125	143	36	40	52	64	85	112	126
20–24	44	50	61	78	107	146	165	37	42	60	80	104	135	168
25–29	45	51	67	88	120	141	204	42	45	57	76	104	137	159
30–34	46	57	76	102	142	214	253	40	45	55	73	104	140	163
35–39	52	58	80	109	167	250	316	40	47	61	83	115	170	205
40–44	56	69	59	123	174	252	218	45	51	66	88	116	161	191
45–49	56	65	88	119	165	218	279	44	55	71	94	139	180	223
50–54	63	75	94	128	178	244	313	53	58	75	103	144	190	223
55–59	60	70	85	117	167	210	261	59	65	80	111	163	229	279
60–64	56	65	84	111	150	193	240	57	66	78	105	143	210	256
65–69	54	61	78	108	164	227	256	56	64	86	118	158	221	260
70+	63	71	87	115	152	202	239	60	68	83	110	141	189	289

[a] For SI units (mmol/L) multiply mg/dL by 0.01129.
(From Stein,[1] with permission.)

Other enzymatic reactions involving diaphorase or the glycerol phosphate oxidase and peroxidase systems also have been used, but their indicator reactions are subjected to chemical interferences from other nonspecific reducing compounds. Because of its sensitivity and simplicity, the enzymatic method is considered the method of choice for the routine determination of triglycerides. Some of the major concerns regarding the enzymatic methods have been related to the uncertainty of complete enzymatic hydrolysis of triglycerides by lipase and the endogeneous level of glycerol in blood. Because the concentration of triglycerides is calculated against the glycerol standard and reported as a free triglyceride level, recovery studies should be done to check for completeness of hydrolysis. Enzymatic products can be extracted by organic solvents and examined by thin layer chromatography (TLC). In regard to the endogenous glycerol level, Whitlow and Gochman[21] reported that there were differences in the endogenous level of free glycerol from patients with a variety of clinical conditions, including diabetes mellitus, nephrotic syndrome, and obstructive liver disorders. It is recommended that glycerol blanking should be used to correct the total triglyceride level. Blanking based on a so-called correction factor is probably only appropriate for levels found in certain healthy individuals.[22] Standardization of the enzymatic triglyceride method is considered one of the major challenges in the optimization of these methods.

Interpretation

At all ages triglycerides are lower in females than in males. It is of interest that both cholesterol and triglyceride concentrations are higher in winter than in summer. The most extensive population studies on lipid reference ranges were conducted by the LRCs, involving 60,502 participants of 10 separate, well-defined North American populations. The triglyceride method used was the CDC's automated fluorometric procedure based on Hantzsch condensation reaction. Table 9-6 shows these reference ranges. To adopt such reference ranges, it is of the utmost importance to use standards that were calibrated by this reference CDC method. The fifth percentile is helpful to screen for individuals with lipoprotein deficiencies. Decrease of triglycerides are found in patients with a very rare clinical syndrome acanthocytosis (Bassen-Kanzwez syndrome), characterized by abetalipoproteinemia (deficiency of low density lipoprotein).

Table 9-7. Causes of Secondary Increases in Triglycerides

Alcoholism
Diabetes mellitus
Glycogen, storage diseases (types I, III, and IV)
Hypertension
Hyperuricemia
Hypothyroidism
Renal dysfunction (e.g., nephrotic syndrome)
Oral contraceptives
Other medications
    Cholestyramine
    Corticosteroids
    Estrogens
    β-blockers
Pancreatitis
Pregnancy

Table 9-8. Summary of Consensus Development Conference on Treatment of Hypertriglyceridemia

Definition	Triglyceride Level mg/dL (mmol/L)	Treatment
Definite	>500 (5.6)	Diet and drug
Borderline	250–500 (2.8–5.6)	Diet: drug if positive family history or other risk factors
Normal	<250 (2.8)	Diet and lifestyle change

(From Hunninghake,[23] with permission.)

The 90th percentile is often used to define hypertriglyceridemia. Primary hypertriglyceridemia is found in patients with hyperlipoproteinemias types I, IIb, III, IV, and V. Table 9-7 shows triglyceride increases that occur secondary to other diseases or medications. Summary of the Consensus Development Conference on Treatment of Hypertriglyceridemia is shown in Table 9-8.[23] The primary reason to treat patients with elevated triglycerides is to reduce the risk of pancreatitis.

TESTS FOR OTHER LIPIDS

Test: Fatty Acids

Background

Fatty acids are straight chain aliphatic carboxylic acids that can be either saturated or unsaturated with one or more double bonds. Their general structures are illustrated in Figure 9-5.

Fatty acids are classified according to the chain length, number of double bonds, and the position of double bonds. Several abbreviated designations have been devised to describe their unique compositions. Some of the most common fatty acids of metabolic or structural importance are listed in Table 9-9. In addition to the common and systematic (Geneva) names, the numbering system that labels the carbon atoms from the carboxyl terminal also is used commonly in the literature.

The amphipathic properties of fatty acids play a major biologic role in the structures of micelles formation,

$$CH_3(CH_2)_n COOH$$

$$CH_3(CH_2)_m-(CH_2CH=CH)_x-(CH_2)_n COOH$$

Saturated fatty acids

Cis unsaturated fatty acids

Fig. 9-5. General structures of fatty acids. m,n denotes the total number of —CH_2 units; x denotes the total number of —($CH_2CH=$)— units.

biomembranes, and lipid metabolism. Fatty acids are present as free fatty acids (FFA) or esterified form in triglycerides, phospholipids, and cholesterol esters. The properties of these lipids are influenced by the chain length and the number of double bonds in the fatty acid component. They vary among tissues and species. Most of the human fatty acids contain an even number of carbon atoms, the only uneven ones are those of the short chain metabolic intermediates. Free fatty acids (or nonesterified fatty acids) in plasma are mostly straight aliphatic chains. These include palmitic and steric acids, which are transported in the blood by albumin and prealbumin. It has been shown that albumin exhibits as many as seven binding sites for fatty acids and one molecule of albumin may carry 20 molecules of fatty acid. Mammalian systems generally do not synthesize unsaturated fatty acids, but derive them mainly from plant sources. These dietary fatty acids, including linoleic, linolenic, and arachidonic acids, are often called essential fatty acids. Of particular importance, arachidonic acid is the metabolic precursor of prostaglandin synthesis. Other common unsaturated fatty acids formed in both animal and vegetable tissues are palmitoleic and oleic acid. Metabolically, plasma FFA are the major sources of fuel. Any excess fatty acids are esterified into triglycerides by the liver and subsequently released into circulation as endogenous triglycerides.

Selection

Although fatty acids are vital in maintaining health, measurement of fatty acids is seldom requested or found to be useful for clinical purposes. Plasma concentration of FFA is affected directly by the blood glucose level; and in fasting, starvation, or in case of diabetes mellitus, plasma FFA are generally increased resulting from intracellular glucose deficiencies.

Logistics

The plasma FFA level can be determined by titrimetric and colorimetric procedures. The fatty acids profile is best analyzed by gas liquid chromatography (GLC).

Table 9-9. Some Common Fatty Acids

Common Name	Systemic Name	Numbering
Myristic	Tetradecanoic	14:0
Palmitic	Hexadecanoic	16:0
Palmitoleic	cis-9-Hexadecenoic	16:1(9)
Stearic	Octadecanoic	18:0
Oleic	cis-9-Octadecenoic	18:1(9)
Vaccenic	cis-11-Octadecenoic	18:1(11)
Linoleic	All cis-9, 12-octadecadienoic	18:2(9, 12)
Linolenic	All cis-9, 12, 15-octadecatrinenoic	18:3(9, 12, 15)
Arachidonic	All cis-5, 18, 11, 14-eicosatetraenoic	20:4(5, 8, 11, 14)

The patient should be fasting for at least 12 hours. Serum or plasma (heparin) is used for analysis. The specimen should be stored at −20°C if analysis is not done immediately.

Interpretation

The reference range for plasma FFA by the titrimetric method is 8–25 mg/dL (0.30–0.90 mmol/L). The reference ranges for fatty acid profile based on percentage (%) of total FFA are summarized in Table 9-10.[24]

The concentrations of plasma FFA are known to be influenced by dietary intake, medication, stress, glucose level, and various disease states. Elevated levels of fatty acids have been shown in fasting patients and those with diabetes mellitus, acute myocardial infarction, and other clinical conditions, but measurement is not considered a diagnostic test. In vitro interference has been shown by the presence of various organic acids (ketoacids), including acetic acid, acetoacetic acid, β-hydroxybutyric acid, lactic acid, and phospholipids.[24]

Table 9-10. Reference Ranges for Fatty Acid Profile

Profile	% Total FFA (by GLC)
Oleic acid	26–45
Palmitic acid	23–25
Stearic	10–14
Linoleic	8–16

Abbreviations: FFA, free fatty acid; GLC, gas liquid chromatography.
(From Tietz,[24] with permission.)

Test: Phospholipids

These complex conjugated lipids consist of two major classes, glycerophosphatides and sphingolipids. The major glycophosphatides are phosphatidyl choline (lecithin), phosphatidyl ethanolamine, phosphatidyl glycerol, and phosphatidyl inositol. Phosphatidyl choline represents 70% of the total phospholipids in sera. The major sphingolipid is sphingomyelin. Measurements of sphingomyelin in amniotic fluid have been used to assess fetal lung maturity (see Ch. 15 under Test: L/S Ratio). Plasma phospholipids are thought to play an active role in lipid transport. The plasma phospholipid level in healthy individuals is about the same as the plasma cholesterol concentration. Measurement of total plasma phospholipid has not yet been found clinically useful. Decreased levels are found in patients with Tangier's disease and abetalipoproteinemia. Increased levels are observed in patients with alcoholic and biliary cirrhosis, cholestasis, chronic pancreatitis, nephrotic syndrome, and deficiency of LCAT.

LIPOPROTEINS

INTRODUCTION

The plasma lipoproteins consist of five major classes: chylomicrons, VLDL, IDL, LDL, and HDL. Their physical and chemical properties are outlined in Table 9-1. A variety of methods can be used to separate lipoproteins into these classes including ultracentrifugation and precipitation with antibodies to their lipoproteins.

Classification of Lipoproteinemias

Lipid abnormalities have been classified using serum lipoprotein and lipid content as well as electrophoretic mobilities and physical appearance of the serum specimen. Lipoprotein electrophoresis is not suitable for quantitation, but can be used as a qualitative assessment of lipoproteins. Commonly, disorders of lipid transport have been classified using the Fredrickson

Table 9-11. Classification of Hyperlipoproteinemias

Lipoprotein Abnormality (Increase)	Plasma Appearance[a]	Total Cholesterol	Triglyceride	LDL Cholesterol	HDL Cholesterol	Apolipoprotein	Lipoprotein Electrophoresis	Lipoprotein Phenotype[b]	Clinical Association
Chylomicrons	Cream layer, infranate, clear or slightly turbid	Normal to moderately elevated	Markedly elevated	Normal	Normal to decreased	↑B-48 ↑A-IV ↓↑CH	Intense band at origin	Type I	Acute abdomen, pancreatitis
LDL	Clear, possible increase in yellow-orange tint	Usually elevated, occasionally within normal range	Normal	Elevated	Normal to decreased	↑B-100	Increased band in β-region	Type II-A	Markedly increased risk of CAD
LDL, VLDL	Clear to slightly turbid	Elevated, occasionally marginally so	Elevated	Elevated	Normal to decreased	↑B-100	Increased β- and pre-β-band	Type II-B	Increased risk of CAD
IDL	Turbid to opaque with thin creamy layer occasionally present	Elevated	Elevated	Normal to decreased	Normal to decreased	↑E-II ↓E-III ↓E-IV	Broad β-band	Type III	Increased risk of CAD
VLDL	Turbid to opaque	Normal to slightly elevated	Moderately to markedly elevated	Normal	Normal to decreased	↓↑C-II ↑B-100	Increased pre-β-band	Type IV	Increased risk of CAD
VLDL, chylomicrons	Creamy layer, infranate, turbid to opaque	Slightly to moderately elevated	Markedly elevated	Normal	Normal to decreased	↓↑C-II ↑B-48 ↑B-100	Intense band at origin plus increased pre-β-band	Type V	Pancreatitis, increased risk of CAD
HDL	Clear	Normal to moderately elevated	Normal	Normal	Elevated	↑A-I ↑A-II	Increased α-band	Hyper-α-lipoproteinemia	Decreased risk of CAD

[a] After 16 hours at 4°C.
[b] Fredrickson type.
Abbreviations: ↑, increase; ↓, decrease; HDL, high density lipoprotein; IDL, intermediate density lipoprotein; LDL, low density lipoprotein, VLDL, very low density lipoprotein; CAD, coronary artery disease. (From Stein,[1] with permission.)

Table 9-12. Classification of Hypolipoproteinemias

Lipoprotein Abnormality	Plasma Appearance[a]	Total Cholesterol	Triglyceride	LDL Cholesterol	HDL Cholesterol	Apolipoprotein	Electrophoresis	Lipoprotein Phenotype	Clinical Association
LDL	Clear	Markedly decreased	Decreased	Absent	Normal	↓↓B-100	Absent β-band and decreased pre-β-band	A-β-lipoproteinemia	Malabsorption; mental retardation; growth failure
LDL	Clear	Mildly to markedly decreased	Normal	Decreased	Normal	↓B-100	Decreased β-band	Hypo-β-lipoproteinemia	Decreased risk of CAD
HDL	Clear	Normal to decreased	Normal	Normal	Absent	↓↓↓A-I ↓↓A-II ?↓C-III	Absent α-band	A-α-lipoproteinemia	Increased risk of hypersplenism, CAD
HDL	Clear	Normal, decreased, or increased	Normal to increased	Normal to increased	Decreased	↓A-I ↓A-II	Decreased α-band	Hypo-α-lipoproteinemia	Increased risk of CAD

See Table 9-11 for explanation of abbreviations.
[a] After 16 hours at 4°C.
(From Stein EA and Glueck CJ: Lipids, lipoproteins, and apolipoproteins. p. 829. In Tietz NW (ed): Textbook of Clinical Chemistry. Philadelphia, WB Saunders, 1986, as adapted from Stein and Glueck,[58] with permission.)

classification as seen in Table 9-11 under the column labeled lipoprotein phenotype. However, many of the major syndromes now can be subclassified on the basis of inheritance patterns, abnormal proteins, or both.

Each of the lipoproteinemias can be either primary or secondary to another disorder and can be modified depending on the physical, nutritional, and clinical status of the patient. The diagnosis of primary (genotype) lipoproteinemia should not be made in the presence of acute illness or any known secondary causes. Screening of first degree relatives should be included in the routine investigation of lipoproteinemia testing, especially in the absence of secondary causes. The WHO classification of the hyperlipoproteinemias is listed in Table 9-11.

Hypolipoproteinemias as shown in Table 9-12 are generally uncommon and are related mainly to the deficiency or absence of LDL and HDL.[25] Again, these disorders may be inherited or may occur secondary to other diseases.

Laboratory Tests of Lipid Disorders

For practical purposes, measurement of total plasma cholesterol, triglycerides, HDL cholesterol, calculation of LDL cholesterol, and visual inspection of the physical appearance of the stored fasting plasma specimen after 12–16 hours at 4°C will provide useful diagnostic information to patients with suspected hyperlipoproteinemias. Lipoprotein electrophoresis is not recommended as an integral part of the routine lipid analysis because much of the information obtained is redundant.[26] In addition, phenotypes observed among hospitalized patients at acute care medical centers often result from secondary causes and medications. These lipoprotein patterns disappear as soon as the underlying diseases are corrected. However, lipoprotein electrophoresis is useful in the differential diagnosis of type III hyperlipoproteinemia, abetalipoproteinemia, and analphalipoproteinemia (Tangier disease). Although preparative ultracentrifugal analysis has been used extensively in the study of lipoprotein and hyperlipoproteinemia, its complexity, expense, and labor intensity have prevented it from becoming a routine procedure in the clinical laboratory. Preparative ultracentrifugation is useful for the diagnosis of certain dyslipoproteins, for example, type III hyperlipoproteinemia. A practical laboratory evaluation of lipid disorders is outlined in Figure 9-6.

TESTS FOR LIPOPROTEIN DISORDERS

Test: High Density Lipoproteins

Background

The physical and chemical properties of plasma HDL are shown in Table 9-1. The nascent HDL complexes synthesized by the liver and intestine contain 50% proteins and 50% lipids and can be isolated by preparative ultracentrifugation from plasma at densities between 1.063 and 1.21 g/mL or found in agarose electrophoresis with a mobility as α-globulin. The lipid is composed mainly of phospholipids (25–30%), cholesterol esters (15–20%), cholesterol (5%), and triglycerides (3%). The phosphatidyl choline (lecithin), which is the predominated phospholipid, serves as substrate for LCAT enzymatic reaction to form esterified cholesterol. The cholesterol ester then formed on HDL is transferred from HDL to VLDL and LDL, partly in exchange for the original triglyceride core of VLDL into cholesterol ester. HDL can be further subfractionated into HDL_2 and HDL_3 with densities ranging from 1.063–1.11 g/mL and 1.11–1.21 g/mL, respectively. Free cholesterol from peripheral tissues is transferred to HDL, then esterified by LCAT, enabling HDL to take up more free cholesterol. The proteins found in HDL composed of Apo A-I (70%), Apo A-II (20%), Apo C (5–11%), and Apo E (1–2%). Apoprotein in HDL is modulated as lipid content is changed. ApoE is the major apoprotein in nascent HDL, whereas Apo A becomes a predominant component in plasma HDL during circulation. These changes in composition may be associated with their specific metabolic functional role. Apo A-I is an activator for LCAT, whereas Apo C-II and Apo C-III act as activator and inhibitor for LPL, respectively. Uptake of Apo C-II from HDL by newly synthesized chylomicron and VLDL allows LPL to catalyze the hydrolysis of triglycerides resulting in triglyceride poor chylomicron remnant particles. The half-life of HDL apoproteins is 3–4 days.

Selection

Recent studies suggest that HDL plays a major role in transporting free cholesterol from peripheral tissues to the liver for removal through the bile, as well as a scavenger of lipids and apolipoproteins during catalytic degradation from chylomicrons and VLDL. Such reverse cholesterol transport diminishes the risk of lipid depositions on the arterial wall. Thus the HDL exhibits a reciprocal relationship with the prevalence of CHD: individuals with lower HDL level have a higher risk of

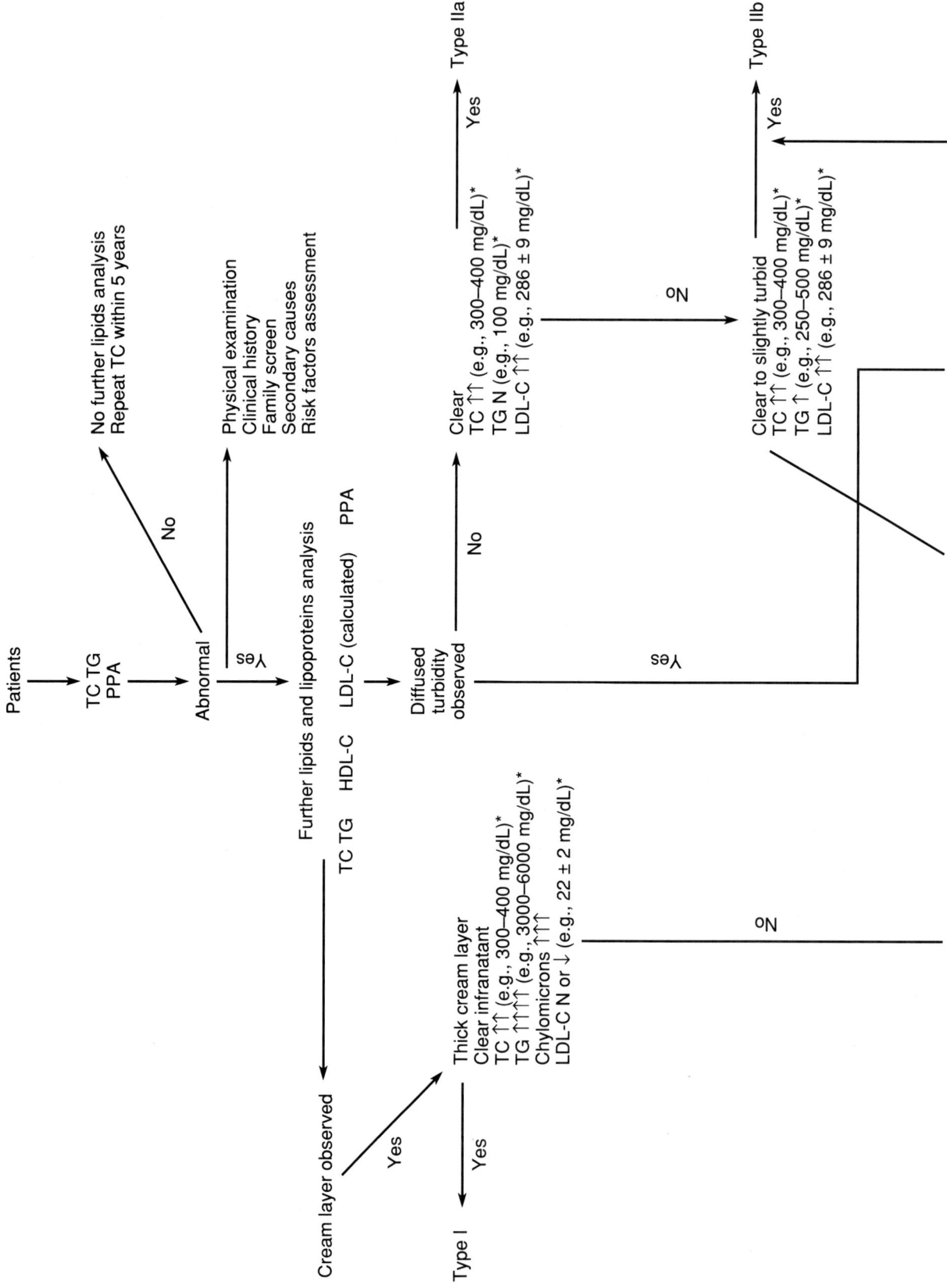

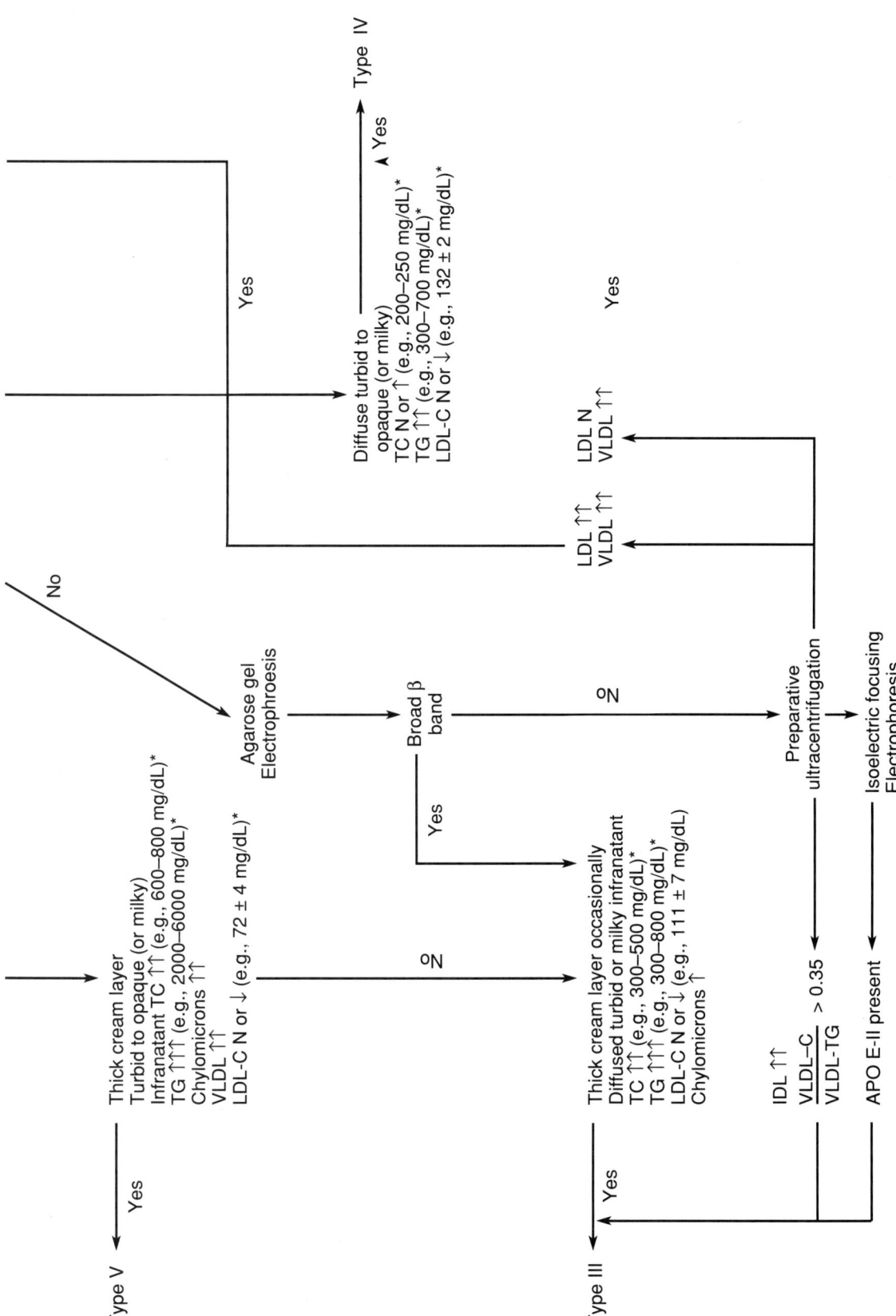

Fig. 9-6. Flow chart depicting the laboratory evaluation of hyperlipoproteinemias. ↑, increased; ↓, decreased; TC, total plasma cholesterol; TG, total plasma triglyceride; PPA, plasma physical appearance; HDL, high density lipoprotein; LDL, low density lipoprotein; C, cholesterol; N, normal; VLDL, very low density lipoprotein; IDL, intermediate density lipoprotein. * Typical ranges of results or examples to provide perspective, but other ranges are possible.

CHD. High HDL may exert a protective role in cardiovascular disease. Thus, HDL levels represent a risk factor for CHD (Table 9-4) and, additionally, HDL is used to calculate LDL results.

Logistics

HDL analysis should be performed as soon as possible, preferably the same day as collected, because prolonged storage (more than 7 days) at 2–8°C or frozen at −20°C causes significant changes in the lipid matrix of HDL. Long-term storage of specimens for measurement of HDL and its subfractions is preferable at −70°C.[27]

Methods

Direct measurement of HDL can be performed by ultracentrifugation or electrophoresis, but quantitation of HDL is routinely determined indirectly by its content of cholesterol. Most procedures require removal of VLDL, LDL, and other lipoproteins by differential precipitations with various polyanions followed by the determination of HDL cholesterol in the supernatant. Measurement of HDL cholesterol and total cholesterol should be done by the same procedure.

No recognized reference method exists for HDL. Any method adopted should provide an acceptable accuracy and precision within +3 mg/dL (0.08 mmol/L) or less than 8% for both interassay or intra-assay variance. Many methods of precipitation have been used including dextran sulfate, heparin-manganese chloride, and phosphotungstate magnesium chloride, with various advantages and disadvantages ascribed to each method.[28] Dextran sulfate/magnesium chloride as a precipitant has been recently shown to be compatible with the enzymatic determination of HDL cholesterol.[29] Dextran with a higher molecular weight (50,000) yields results closer to those obtained by heparin-manganese chloride. Subfractions of HDL_2 and HDL_3 can be separated by ultracentrifugation or polyanionic precipitations.[30] The HDL_3 cholesterol concentrations subtracted from total HDL cholesterol yield the HDL_2 cholesterol level. Methods for HDL_2 and HDL_3 need to be optimized and the clinical utility of results still require confirmation.

Interpretation

HDL cholesterol is an indirect measurement of HDL. There is an inverse relationship between low HDL cholesterol and the high prevalence of CHD in both men and women. This suggests that increased levels of HDL may retard the atherogenesis and measurement of HDL cholesterol may be a good predictor of risk for CHD. HDL cholesterol is higher in women than in men. Reference ranges for HDL cholesterol among men and women vary with age. The reference values derived from the LRC program have provided the most detailed information for the North American populations as shown in Table 9-13. Results less than 35 mg/dL (0.91 mmol/L) are considered to be associated with major risk of CHD. HDL_2 results are more closely correlated with CHD risk than either total HDL or HDL_3. For the assessment of CHD risk, studies by Naito[31] showed that ratios of HDL_2 cholesterol to HDL_3 cholesterol and HDL_2 cholesterol to HDL cho-

Table 9-13. Reference Values for HDL Cholesterol (mg/dL)[a]

	Males								Females						
Age (Yr)	Percentiles							Age (Yr)	Percentiles						
	5	10	25	50	75	90	95		5	10	25	50	75	90	95
5–9	38	43	49	55	64	70	75	5–9	36	38	48	52	60	67	73
10–14	37	40	46	55	61	71	74	10–14	37	40	45	52	58	64	70
15–19	30	34	39	46	52	59	63	15–19	35	38	43	51	61	68	74
20–24	30	32	38	45	51	57	63	20–24	33	37	44	51	62	72	79
25–29	31	32	37	44	50	58	63	25–29	37	39	47	55	63	74	83
30–34	28	32	38	45	52	59	63	30–34	36	40	46	55	64	73	77
35–39	29	31	36	43	49	58	62	35–39	34	38	44	53	64	75	82
40–44	27	31	36	43	51	60	67	40–44	34	39	48	56	65	79	88
45–49	30	33	38	45	52	60	64	45–49	34	41	47	58	68	82	87
50–54	28	31	36	44	51	58	63	50–54	37	41	50	62	71	84	92
55–59	28	31	38	46	55	64	71	55–59	37	41	50	60	73	85	91
60–64	30	34	41	49	61	69	74	60–64	38	44	51	61	75	87	92
65–69	30	33	39	49	52	74	75	65–69	35	38	49	62	73	85	96
70+	31	33	40	48	56	70	75	70+	33	38	45	60	71	82	92

[a] For SI units (mmol/L) multiply mg/dL by 0.02586.
(From Stein,[1] with permission.)

lesterol correlate far better than HDL cholesterol alone or the ratio of HDL cholesterol to total cholesterol. HDL cholesterol levels sometimes can distort total cholesterol concentration. A correction can be made by the formula:

Adjusted cholesterol concentration
= total cholesterol − (patient's HDL cholesterol − mean HDL cholesterol for men or women)

where the mean HDL cholesterol for men = 45 mg/dL (1.17 mmol/L); and the mean HDL cholesterol for women = 55 mg/dL (1.42 mmol/L).

The 5th and 10th percentiles are used to screen for individuals with HDL deficiency syndromes (e.g., hypoalphalipoproteinemia). This lipoprotein disorder may be primary or secondary to other underlying diseases and environmental agents. The complete absence of HDL in plasma has been shown in Tangier disease (analphalipoproteinemia), a rare autosomal recessive disorder characterized by the accumulation of cholesterol ester in the reticuloendothelial system and in other tissues. Other familial hypoalphalipoproteine-mias have been described in the literature, including Apo A-I (Milan),[32] fish-eye disease,[33] and others.[34] The 95th percentile is used to identify familial hyperalphalipoproteinemia. This disorder, which appears to be inherited as an autosomal dominant, is not associated with any distinctive clinical features and these individuals have a low incidence of CHD. Factors or diseases that are associated with abnormal levels of α-lipoproteins or HDL are summarized in Table 9-14.

Test: Low Density Lipoproteins (β-Lipoprotein)

Background

Low density lipoprotein particles have a fairly narrow density range (1.019–1.063 g/mL) and a diameter of 21–25 nm. Lipid moieties consist of about 50% cholesterol, 10% triglycerides, and the protein component is composed of Apo B (96%), with only trace amounts of Apo C and Apo A. The LDL Apo B is derived almost entirely from VLDL Apo B in plasma. Low density lipoproteins can be separated into two fractions, IDL and LDL_2, according to their densities. The characteristic β mobility of LDL on agarose electrophoresis is caused by the Apo B protein. Low density lipoproteins are catabolic remnants of intravascular VLDL and IDL. Usually more than 75% of plasma cholesterol is transported by LDL to the extrahepatic tissues. Catabolism of LDL occurs in both peripheral tissues and in the liver: LDL is taken up by highly specific receptors for Apo B on the target cell's surface. Bound LDL is then internalized by invagination into the cell liposomes, where Apo B is degraded and cholesterol esters are hydrolyzed to free cholesterol. Free cholesterol then exerts its negative feedback regulatory control on the rate limiting enzyme of HMG-CoA reductase, as well as on the modulations of the number of LDL receptors and on the activation of ACAT. Plasma LDL also can be categorized by nonreceptor scavenger cells such as macrophages. An excess accumulation of free cholesterol gives these cells the appearance of a "foam cell," a basic component of atherosclerotic plaques.

Selection

A deficiency of LDL receptors results in familial hypercholesterolemia. Evidence is convincing that LDL cholesterol is associated with increased risk for CHD. The ratio of LDL and HDL cholesterol also has been used to assess the relative risk factors as recommended by the Framingham study.[35] Recently, experts from the NCEP recommended that individuals with total

Table 9-14. Factors or Diseases Associated With the Abnormal Concentrations of HDL

Primary causes
   Increase
      Familial hyperalphalipoproteinemia
   Decrease
      Familial hypoalphalipoproteinemia
      A-1 Milano disease
      Apo A-1
      Fish-eye disease
      Lecithin cholesterol acyltransferase deficiency
      Tangier disease (absence)
Secondary causes
   Increase
      Exercise nutrition (polyunsaturated fatty acid)
      Alcohol intake
      Insulin-treated diabetes
      Estrogens
      Oral contraceptives
      Ascorbic acid
      Clofibrate
      Nicotinic acid
      Phenytoin
   Decrease
      Hypertriglyceridemia
      Coronary heart disease
      Uremia
      Diabetes (untreated)
      Malnutrition
      Acute or chronic liver disease
      Malabsorption
      Acquired immunodeficiency syndrome

plasma cholesterol above 200 mg/dL (5.17 mmol/L), or those patients with borderline high levels who also have definite CHD or at least two other risk factors for CHD require the determination of LDL cholesterol level. These guidelines are summarized in Figure 9-3. Laboratory assessment of LDL is based on the measurement of plasma total cholesterol, HDL cholesterol, triglycerides, and calculation of VLDL cholesterol.

Logistics

As previously described, patients should be on their usual diet without weight loss or medications for approximately 2–3 weeks before the test. Blood specimens should be collected after at least 12 hours of fasting. Direct measurement of LDL cholesterol is seldom performed in the routine clinical laboratory. Only when plasma triglycerides exceed 400 mg/dL (4.52 mmol/L) and an accurate LDL cholesterol level is required for the evaluation of hyperlipoproteinemia, then the method of preparative ultracentrifugal density of 1.006 g/mL is used to remove the VLDL and abnormal IDL fractions. The HDL cholesterol is determined in the supernatant after precipitation of the LDL fraction. The LDL cholesterol is obtained by subtracting the HDL cholesterol value from the total cholesterol of the bottom factions after ultracentrifugation. Excellent agreement of results for LDL cholesterol is obtained with the indirect calculated LDL cholesterol, based on the Friedwald formula. Calculated LDL is the method usually used in clinical laboratories. The formula is valid only if the concentration of triglycerides is less than 400 mg/dL (<4.52 mmol/L).[36] By measuring total cholesterol, triglycerides, and HDL cholesterol, LDL cholesterol can be calculated as follows:

$$\text{LDL cholesterol} = \text{total cholesterol} - (\text{HDL-C} + \text{triglyceride}/5)$$

Interpretation

The prevalence study of the LRC program has published detailed reference values of LDL cholesterol based on age and gender of a well-defined North American population (Table 9-15). It has been recommended by NIH guidelines to use the 75th percentile for LDL cholesterol as the upper limit to identify those individuals who are at high risk for CHDs. The 90th and 95th percentiles are often used to identify individuals with familial hypercholesterolemia type IIa and IIb. Desirable results for LDL are less than 130 mg/dL (<3.4 mmol/L), whereas high risk of CHD is associated with results greater than 160 mg/dL (4.1 mmol/L) (Fig. 9-4).

Familial hypercholesterolemia refers to a group of autosomal dominant disorders, most of which are caused by defects in the LDL receptor. There are at least 12 well characterized defects leading to variability in clinical presentation of the disorder. Patients with familial hypercholesterolemia usually present with elevated levels of total and LDL cholesterol with triglycerides within the reference range. In patients with homozygous familial hypercholesterolemia, LDL cholesterol usually exceeds 500 mg/dL (12.9 mmol/L) and can be in the range of 700–900 mg/dL (18.1–23.3 mmol/L). In patients with the heterozygous form, LDL cholesterol

Table 9-15. Reference Values for LDL Cholesterol (mg/dL)[a]

	Males								Females						
			Percentiles								Percentiles				
Age (Yr)	5	10	25	50	75	90	95	Age (Yr)	5	10	25	50	75	90	95
5–9	63	69	80	90	103	117	129	5–9	68	73	88	98	115	125	140
10–14	64	73	82	94	109	123	133	10–14	68	73	81	94	110	126	136
15–19	62	68	80	93	109	123	130	15–19	59	73	78	93	110	129	137
20–24	66	73	85	101	118	138	147	20–24	57	65	82	102	118	141	159
25–29	70	75	96	116	138	157	165	25–29	71	75	90	108	126	148	164
30–34	78	88	107	124	144	166	185	30–34	70	77	91	109	129	146	156
35–39	81	92	110	131	154	176	189	35–39	75	81	96	116	139	161	172
40–44	87	98	115	135	157	173	186	40–44	74	84	104	122	146	165	174
45–49	97	106	120	140	163	185	202	45–49	79	89	105	127	150	173	186
50–54	89	102	118	143	162	185	197	50–54	88	94	111	134	160	186	201
55–59	88	103	123	145	168	191	203	55–59	89	97	120	145	168	199	210
60–64	83	107	121	143	165	188	210	60–64	100	105	126	149	168	191	224
65–69	98	104	125	146	170	199	210	65–69	92	99	125	151	184	205	221
70+	88	100	119	142	164	182	186	70+	96	108	126	147	170	189	206

[a] For SI units (mmol/L) multiply mg/dL by 0.02586.
(From Stein,[1] with permission.)

Table 9-16. Secondary Causes of Increases and Decreases in LDL Cholesterol

Increases
    Hypothyroidism
    Nephrotic syndrome
    Gammopathies
    Hepatic disease; hepatic obstruction, viral hepatitis
    Porphyria
    Pregnancy
    Anorexia nervosa
    Diabetes mellitus
    Chronic renal failure
    Stress
    Drugs (e.g., estrogens, androgens, carbamazepine)
Decreases
    Malnutrition
    Intestinal malabsorption
    Chronic anemias
    Intravenous hyperalimentation
    Hyperthyroidism
    Severe hepatocellular dysfunction
    Acute severe stress (e.g., trauma, myocardial infarction)
    Myeloproliferative disorders
    Reye syndrome

(Modified from Stein,[1] with permission.)

is usually between 250 and 500 mg/dL (6.4 and 12.9 mmol/L). The diagnosis of familial hypercholesterolemia is based on xanthomas, premature coronary artery disease, and elevated LDL. Table 9-16 shows the secondary causes of increases and decreases of LDL cholesterol.

OTHER TESTS FOR LIPOPROTEIN DISORDERS

Test: Chylomicrons

Background

Chylomicrons are the largest and least dense of the lipoprotein particles with a density less than 0.95 g/mL. They float to the surface of stored plasma on standing or after preparative ultracentrifugation. Because of their rich content of uncharged lipid moieties, including 84% triglycerides, 7% phospholipids, 2% cholesterol and 5% cholesterol esters, and a very small amount of protein (2%), their mobilities on paper, agarose, and acrylamide gel electrophoresis are negligible. The major apoproteins contained in chylomicrons are A-I, A-II, B, C-I, C-II, C-III, and E. Chylomicrons are produced in the intestinal mucosa following the ingestion of fat-containing meals. The biosynthesis of chylomicrons requires the presence of Apo B protein. In abetalipoproteinemia, in which Apo B is lacking, the intestinal cells are filled with lipids because chylomicrons are not released into the blood stream via the thoracic duct. When traveling through the lymphatic system, chylomicrons acquire much of the cholesterol esters and Apo C-II from HDL in exchange for Apo A-I, Apo A-II, and small amounts of phospholipids as well as free cholesterol. Chylomicrons then are removed from the blood circulation by the adipose tissue and muscle capillary endothelial cells. Chylomicron triglyceride is rapidly changed to fatty acids and glycerol by extrahepatic LPL in the presence of activator Apo C-II. The fatty acids and glycerol can then be used for energy metabolism or the triglycerides can be resynthesized and stored. The resultant remnant particles containing mainly cholesterol esters, Apo B, and Apo E are rapidly cleared by the liver.

Selection

Laboratory assessment of hyperchylomicronemia is usually based on the physical appearance of stored serum and quantitation of triglycerides and cholesterol. Confirmation can be obtained using agarose gel electrophoresis or ultracentrifugation.

Logistics

The patient should fast for 12–16 hours prior to sampling. The presence of chylomicrons can readily be recognized as a thick homogeneous creamy layer floating on top of clear or slight turbid infratant after storage for 12–18 hours at 4°C. Because of the very low protein content, chylomicrons usually remain at the application point after electrophoresis either on agarose or polyacrylamide gel. Chylomicrons can be isolated by preparative ultracentrifugation at lower centrifugal forces ($30,000 \times g$ for 30 minutes).

Interpretation

In the fasting states, chylomicrons are usually absent, because in the healthy person, they are easily cleared from the circulation after an overnight fast of 12 hours. Marked increases of chylomicrons are found in primary or familial hyperchylomicronemia (Fredrickson type I hyperlipoproteinemia), which appears to be caused by a deficiency of LPL and mixed hyperlipoproteinemia (type V hyperlipoproteinemia). The plasma triglycerides in both these syndromes are greatly elevated with concentrations above 1000 mg/dL (11.29 mmol/L). Hyperchylomicronemia also occurs secondary to uncontrolled diabetes mellitus, acute pancreatitis, hypothyroidism, dysglobulinemia, systemic lupus erythematosus, and oral contraceptive medications. Increased chylomicrons are associated with the development of acute pancreatitis. Patients with hyperchylomicronemia do not have an increased risk of atherosclerosis and generally have a good long-term prognosis if their triglyceride levels are well controlled.

Test: Very Low Density Lipoprotein (Pre-β-Lipoprotein)

Background

Very low density lipoproteins are synthesized in the liver and intestine. These spherical particles have a density range of 0.95–1.006 g/mL, with diameters of 25–70 mm. Very low density lipoproteins contain about 44–60% triglycerides, 20–23% phospholipids, 11–14% cholesterol esters, 5–8% cholesterol, and 4–11% apoproteins. The apoproteins of VLDL are composed of at least five major distinct groups of polypeptides. They are Apo A with subfractions of A-I and A-II; Apo B with subfractions of B-100 and B-48; Apo C with subfractions of C-I, C-II, and C-III; Apo E with subfractions of E-II, E-III, and E-IV; and Apo D. C-I and C-II in VLDL serve as cofactors for LCAT and extrahepatic LPL, respectively. Very low density lipoproteins are catabolized rapidly to IDL and later to LDL and transport endogenously synthesized triglycerides from the liver and intestine to the peripheral tissues. In healthy individuals, VLDL represent about 22–33% of the total circulating lipoproteins. The half-life of VLDL is approximately 1–3 hours. Plasma specimens with high VLDL exhibit opalescence or turbidity, but no floating creamy layer on standing. Because of faster mobility than β-lipoproteins on agarose gel electrophoresis, they are called pre-β-lipoproteins.

Selection

Laboratory assessment of VLDL is generally based on measurement of serum cholesterol, triglycerides, and the physical appearance of the serum after standing for 12–16 hours at 4°C. Ultracentrifugation analysis is used only to differentiate among the suspected type II$_b$ and III hyperlipoproteinemias.

Logistics

The patient should fast at least 12–16 hours prior to specimen collection. Specimens with triglyceride-rich VLDL particles give a turbid appearance on standing in a refrigerator at 4°C for 12–18 hours. Very low density lipoproteins can be assessed directly by preparative ultracentrifugation and agarose electrophoresis. At a density less than 1.006 g/mL, VLDL will float to the top by ultracentrifugation at 100,000 $\times$ g for 16 hours. The amount of VLDL can be estimated indirectly by the measurement of cholesterol or triglyceride content. Very low density lipoprotein cholesterol also can be estimated as approximately ⅕ of the total triglycerides, provided that the total triglycerides level does not exceed 400 mg/dL (4.5 mmol/L). On agarose gel electrophoresis, the VLDL is resolved as pre-β-lipoproteins. Their quantity is estimated based on the staining intensities of the fat soluble dye.

Interpretation

Very low density lipoproteins increase in nonfasting specimens and increased VLDLs are found in types II$_b$, IV, and V hyperlipoproteinemia. Hyperprebetalipoproteinemia (familial hypertriglyceridemia or type IV hyperlipoproteinemia), characterized by an increase in VLDL without other lipoprotein abnormalities, is the most frequent type of hyperlipoproteinemia. Electrophoresis reveals a distinct pre-β-lipoprotein band with no other lipoprotein abnormalities and LDL cholesterol is within reference limits. The total cholesterol may be increased because of the VLDL level, and the triglyceride level is moderate to markedly elevated. On standing overnight at 4°C, the serum remains turbid and does not develop a creamy layer of chylomicrons. Increases of VLDL may occur secondary to a wide variety of diseases, drugs, and diets. Causes of a secondary increase in VLDL and chylomicrons are summarized in Table 9-17. If both VLDL and LDL cholesterol are increased, the disorder is type II$_b$ hyperlipoproteinemia. In type V hyperlipoproteinemia, both chylomicrons and VLDL are increased in the fasting state.

Table 9-17. Causes of Secondary Increases in VLDL and Chylomicrons

Alcoholism or excessive alcohol intake
Excessive food (especially simple carbohydrate) intake
Obesity
Juvenile diabetes mellitus
Hypothyroidism
Nephrotic syndrome
Uremia
Pregnancy (last trimester)
Pancreatitis (usually alcoholic)
Estrogen-progesteronal oral contraceptives
Steroid therapy (corticosteroids)
Glycogen storage diseases
Dysproteinemias (such as systemic lupus erythematosus)
Lipid storage diseases (Gaucher's, Niemann-Pick, lecithin cholesterol acyltransferase deficiency)

(From Stein,[1] with permission.)

Test: Intermediate Density Lipoprotein (Floating β-Lipoprotein)

Intermediate density lipoproteins are intermediate products of VLDL catabolism. Their particle size (22-24 nm) and relative mass are between VLDL and LDL, with densities ranging from slightly less than 1.006-1.019 g/dL. The IDL contain about equal amounts of cholesterol and triglycerides, Apo B (60%), Apo E (30%), and Apo C (10%). After taking up cholesterol ester from HDL, IDL undergo further catalytic conversions to LDL, which contain almost pure cholesterol esters in the core and Apo B on the surface. Deficiencies and variants of Apo E isoforms have been considered as the causes of IDL elevation in type III hyperlipoproteinemia. These IDL particles have a VLDL-like density, but β-lipoprotein mobility.

Laboratory assessments of IDL generally are based on the measurement of cholesterol, triglycerides, physical appearance of the serum specimen after standing for 12-16 hours at 4°C, lipoprotein electrophoresis, and ultracentrifugation. Both cholesterol and triglycerides are usually above 300-350 mg/dL (3.39-3.95 mmol/L), with a ratio of approximately 1. When chylomicrons are not present and a broad β-lipoprotein band occurs on electrophoresis, then the presence of IDL should be suspected. The presence of IDL should be confirmed by preparative ultracentrifugation at a density of 1.006 g/dL.

The marked accumulation of IDL is the dominant feature of Type III lipoproteinemia. In addition, type III hyperlipoproteinemia is suspected when the VLDL cholesterol/VLDL triglyceride ratio exceeds 0.35 or when the VLDL cholesterol/plasma triglyceride ratio exceeds 0.25. Type III hyperlipoproteinemia is a rare disorder and usually inherited. Secondary type III hyperlipoproteinemia is associated with hypothyroidism, gout, and diabetes mellitus, as well as with patients with acute renal failure on maintenance hemodialysis.

Tests: Lipoprotein (a) [Lp(a)] and Lipoprotein X (LpX)

Lipoprotein (a) is a variant of LDL and is found in the sera of 35% of the random population. Lipoprotein (a) has a density range of 1.050-1.090 g/mL with a lipid content identical to LDL and an electrophoretic mobility similar to pre-β-lipoproteins. The observed fast migration of Lp(a) is caused by the relatively large negative charge from its unique apoprotein, Apo Lp(a). Because of the close similarities between LDL and Lp(a), they can be differentiated only by immunologic methods.[38,39] Lipoprotein X has a density similar to LDL, but with a distinct protein and lipid composition. This very small protein moiety consist of albumin (40%), Apo C (50%), and small amounts of Apo E and Apo A-I (10%). The lipid components consist of unusually high concentrations of phospholipids (66%) and unesterified cholesterol (25%).

The functional role of Lp(a) is not clear, but it has been suggested to be very atherogenic. A recent study indicates that an increased concentration of Lp(a) is an independent risk factor for early myocardial infarction and the concentrations of Lp(a) and Apo B of LDL are under separate metabolic controls.[40,41] The concentrations of Lp(a) in serum are not affected by Apo E polymorphism. The presence of Lp(a) can introduce falsely elevated pre-β-lipoprotein levels in agarose electrophoretic patterns. LpX exhibits α/β mobility on most supporting electrophoretic media, except in agar gel electrophoresis where LpX moves toward the cathode at pH 8.6. This LpX is often found in patients with cholestasis and LCAT deficiency.

APOLIPOPROTEINS

TESTS FOR APOLIPOPROTEIN DISORDERS

Test: Apolipoproteins (Apoproteins)

There is strong evidence that variations in apolipoproteins are potential risk indicators of CHD. At least four major families of apolipoproteins have been identified and characterized from the human plasma lipoproteins. Each of the four major apolipoproteins A, B, C, and E consists of two or more immunologically distinct apoproteins. Their distribution among various lipoproteins fractions is listed in Table 9-1. Apolipoproteins have been shown to have significant roles in lipoproteins and lipid metabolism, as well as in the structural formations of lipoproteins. Most of the laboratory procedures were developed for Apo A-I and Apo B, because these two apolipoproteins have been shown to be more effective than lipid measurements as predictors of CHD.[42]

Logistics

There are no accepted reference methods or standards for standardization and validation of apolipoprotein assays.[43] Immunoassays are probably the most common quantitative methods for measuring apoproteins. Among these methods, radioimmunoassay (RIA) for both Apo A-I and Apo B could be considered as a candidate reference method, but nephelometric immunoassay (NIA) may be considered as the preferred routine method for clinical laboratory. With automation, NIA provides an acceptable precision. The intrinsic disadvantage as found in these procedures is the potential inferences from lipemic specimens. Lack of primary or secondary standards and homogeneous antisera are still the major challenges for the proper performance of apolipoprotein measurements.

Interpretation

Information regarding reference ranges for various apolipoproteins have been reported by using the many different procedures illustrated in Tables 9-18 through 9-20. However, an acceptable reference range has not yet been generally established and recognized. Examples of reference values for Apo A-1 and Apo B are tabulated in Table 9-19.[44,45] Increasing evidence in the literature has suggested that measurement of apoproteins may provide better assessment of risk for coronary artery disease, especially Apo A-I and Apo B, and their ratio.[31,46] Apo A-I is the major component of HDL and is associated with the decreased risk of CHD, whereas Apo B is generally characteristic of LDL and is associated with an increased risk of atherogenesis. The ratio reflects both a cholesterol lowering potential and an increased atherogenic risk. Apo A-I and Apo B distribution are different depending on age and gender. Higher Apo A-I levels are found in women. Studies show a good correlation between the ratio of Apo B/Apo A-1 and LDL/HDL cholesterol and suggest the following guidelines for interpretation of Apo A-I/Apo B based on rate immunonephelometic analysis as shown in Table 19-20.[47] Patients with coronary artery disease have lower Apo A-1, higher Apo B, and a ratio of Apo A-1/Apo B equal or less than 1. Several recent studies[48-50] have shown that measurements of Apo A-1 and Apo B are superior to the measurement of HDL cholesterol, LDL cholesterol, and total cholesterol. Many structural variants of apolipoprotein have been recently identified, but their roles in lipid metabolism and CHD are still far from clear. Some of the apolipoprotein profiles of patients with lipid disorders are summarized in Tables 9-11 and 9-12.

Apo A

Apo A-I and Apo A-II are the major apoproteins of HDL. Lecithin cholesterol acyltransferase is activated by Apo A-I. Recent studies show Apo A-1 is decreased in patients with CHD despite normal HDL cholesterol levels, thus Apo A-1 measurements are superior to the measurement of HDL cholesterol in assessing the risk of CHD.[48]

Apo B

Apo B is the major apoprotein of LDL and has been shown to be composed of two forms: Apo B-100 and Apo B-48. Apo B-100, which is synthesized in the liver, is the major Apo B protein in fasting plasma specimens and is found in both LDL and VLDL. Apo B-48 is not an integral part of Apo B-100. Apo B-48 is synthesized in the intestinal jejunum and is found in chylomicrons.

Table 9-18. Reference Ranges of Plasma Apolipoproteins in Adults (> 20 Years)[a]

Apolipoproteins	Males[b] mg/dL ± SD	Females[c] mg/dL ± SD
A-1	127 ± 23 (1270 ± 230)	147 ± 26 (1470 ± 260)
A-II	61 ± 11 (610 ± 110)	71 ± 16 (710 ± 160)
B	100 ± 27 (1000 ± 270)	92 ± 23 (920 ± 230)
C-1	7.4 ± 2.0 (74 ± 20)	10.4 ± 2.6 (104 ± 26)
C-II	3.3 ± 0.9 (33 ± 9.0)	3.6 ± 1.3 (36 ± 13)
C-III	8.1 ± 2.7 (81 ± 27)	8.8 ± 2.6 (88 ± 26)
D	9.4 ± 3.1 (94 ± 31)	8.1 ± 1.9 (81 ± 19)
E	10.9 ± 3.6 (109 ± 36)	11.7 ± 4.1 (117 ± 41)

[a] Method: Enzyme immunoassay.
[b] Males, N = 69.
[c] Females, N = 85.
(Modified from Alaupovic et al.,[44] with permission.)

Table 9-19. Reference Ranges for Apo A-1 and Apo B (mg/dL)

Method	Apo A-1 Male	Apo A-1 Female	Apo B Male	Apo B Female
NIA	127 ± 21	142 ± 25	82 ± 23	72 ± 21
EIA	132 ± 20	139 ± 17	83 ± 13	82 ± 12
EIA	127 ± 23	147 ± 26	100 ± 27	92 ± 23
RIA	130 ± 20	149 ± 30	81 ± 20	78 ± 19
RIA	119 ± 19	135 ± 26	83 ± 25	

Abbreviations: NIA, nephelometric immunoassay; EIA, enzyme immunoassay; RIA, radioimmunoassay.

Both Apo B-100 and Apo B-48 play an important functional role in the metabolism of LDL and chylomicron remnants. Sniderman et al.[49] reported Apo B was superior to total cholesterol and LDL cholesterol as a discriminator of angiographically documented coronary disease. Their study specifically showed that there are patients with CHD who have normal LDL cholesterol, but high concentrations of Apo B. This finding suggested that Apo B concentrations are a more effective predictor of LDL atherogenicity than the LDL cholesterol level. Naito[51] and Freedman et al.[52] further suggest the ratio of Apo A-I/Apo B provided a better indicator of assessing atherosclerotic risk than Apo A-I or Apo B alone.

Apo C

The "Apo C" family consists of three major apoproteins; Apo C-I, C-II, and C-III. These Apo C proteins have been found in all lipoproteins. Apo C-I and C-II are activators for LCAT and LPL. Patients with Apo C-II deficiency have severe hypertriglyceridemia and impaired plasma clearance of VLDL and chylomicrons (type I hyperlipoproteinemia). Apo C-III is the most abundant of the C apoproteins and exists in at least three polymorphic forms containing different amounts of sialic acid residues, including Apo C-III-O (no sialic acid), Apo C-III-1 (one sialic acid), and Apo C-III-2 (two sialic acids). The functional significance of Apo C-III and its polymorphic forms are not yet clear.

Apo E

Apolipoprotein E is found in all lipoprotein fractions and exists in three homozygous (E4/4, E3/3, E2/2) and three heterozygous (E4/3, E4/2, E3/2) phenotypes, of which E3/3 (E3) is the most common phenotype.[53] Patients with type III hyperlipoproteinemia have an increased frequency of the E2/2 phenotype.[54] Variants of Apo E as well as familial apolipoprotein E deficiency have also been associated with type III hyperlipoproteinemia.[55,56] Apo E has been shown to play a significant role in lipoprotein metabolism and in the uptake of chylomicron remnants as well as VLDL remnants by the specific receptors on hepatic or extrahepatic cellular membranes. Additionally, Apo E may exert a significant role in atherogenesis, because of the high affinity of Apo E for macrophages.[57]

Other

In addition to the above major apolipoproteins, several apoproteins such as Apo D, Apo E, Apo G, and Apo H are found in very small concentrations. Their physical, chemical as well as functional roles are not well defined or understood. The clinical significance of these minor apolipoproteins is still unknown.

REFERENCES

1. Stein EA: Lipids, lipoproteins and apolipoproteins. pp. 849, 857, 866, 881, 886, 890. In Tietz NW (ed): Text Book of Clinical Chemistry. Philadelphia, WB Saunders, 1986.
2. Consensus Conference: Statement on lowering blood cholesterol to reduce coronary heart disease. JAMA 1985;253:2080–2086.
3. Martin MJ, Hulley SB, Browner WS et al: Serum cholesterol, blood pressure, and mortality. Implications from a cohort of 361,662 men. Lancet 1986;2:933–936.

Table 9-20. Coronary Atherosclerotic Risk Based on the Apo A-1 and Apo B Ratio

Relative Risk	Apo A-1/Apo B Ratio Men	Apo A-1/Apo B Ratio Women
Average risk	1.4	1.6
Twice average risk	1.1	1.1
Thrice average risk	1.0	1.0

(From Maciejko et al.,[47] with permission.)

4. The Expert Panel: Report on the national cholesterol education program expert panel on detection, evaluation, and treatment of high blood cholesterol in adults. Arch Intern Med 1988;48:36–69.
5. Franklin FA, Brown RF, Franklin CC: Screening, diagnosis, and management of dyslipoproteinemia in children. J Clin Endocrinol Metab 1990;19:399–450.
6. Hoey JM: Detection and evaluation of dyslipoproteinemia. J Clin Endocrinal Metab 1990;19:311–320.
7. Cohn JS, McNamara JR, Schaefer EJ: Lipoproteins cholesterol concentrations in the plasma of human subjects as measured in the fed and fasted states. Clin Chem 1988;34:2456–2459.
8. Bachorik PS, Rock R, Cloey T et al: Cholesterol screening; comparative evaluation of on site and laboratory-based measurements. Clin Chem 1990;36:255–260.
9. Greenland P, Bowley NL, Meiklejohn B et al: Blood cholesterol concentration: fingerstick plasma versus venous serum sampling. Clin Chem 1990;36:628–630.
10. Abell LL, Levy BB, Brodie BB, Kendall FE: Simplified methods for the estimation of total cholesterol in serum and demonstration of its specificity. J Biol Chem 1952;195:357–366.
11. Cooper GR, Smith SJ, Duncan IW et al: Interlaboratory testing of the transferability of a candidate reference method for the total cholesterol in serum. Clin Chem 1986;32:921–929.
12. Allain CC, Poon LS, Chan CSG et al: The enzymatic determination of total serum cholesterol. Clin Chem 1974;20:470–475.
13. Fu P, Allain C: Automation and evaluation of a new enzymatic method for the determination of total serum cholesterol. Ann Clin Lab Sci 1974;4:201.
14. Ellerbe P, Meiselman S, Sniegoski LT et al: Determination of serum cholesterol by a modification of the isotope dilution mass spectrometric definitive method. Anal Chem 1989;61:1718–1723.
15. Recommendations for improving cholesterol measurement. NIH Publication No. 90-2964. Bethesda, MD, US Department of Health and Human Services, February, 1990.
16. Levy RI: Cholesterol and coronary artery disease. What do clinicians know? Am J Med 1986;80(2A):18–22.
17. The National Institutes of Health Consensus Development Conference: Lowering blood cholesterol to prevent heart disease. JAMA 1985;253:2080–2086.
18. Cambien F, Jacqueson A, Richard JL et al: Is the level of serum triglyceride a significant predictor of coronary death in "normocholesterolemic" subjects: The Paris prospective study. Am J Epidemiol 1986;124:624–632.
19. Kessler G, Lederer H: Fluorometric measurement of triglycerides. pp. 341–344. In Skeggs LT Jr et al (eds): Automation in Analytical Chemistry. Technicon Symposia 1965. New York, Mediad, 1966.
20. Bucolo G, David H: Quantitative determination of serum triglycerides by the use of enzymes. Clin Chem 1973;19:476–482.
21. Whitlow K, Gochman N: Continuous-flow enzymic method evaluated for measurement of serum triglycerides with use of an improved lipase reagent. Clin Chem 1978;24:2018–2019.
22. Stinshoff K, Weisshaar D, Staehler F et al: Relation between concentrations of free glycerol and triglycerides in human sera. Clin Chem 1977;23:1029–1032.
23. Hunninghake DB: Drug treatment of dyslipoproteinemia. J Clin Endocrinol Metab 1990;19:345–360.
24. Tietz NW: Clinical Guide to Laboratory Tests. WB Saunders, Philadelphia, 1983.
25. Steinmetz J, Dardaine T: HDL-cholesterol. pp. 196–208. In Siest G, Schiele F, Henry J et al (eds): Interpretation of Clinical Laboratory Tests. Reference Values and their Biological Variation. Foster City, CA, Biomedical, 1985.
26. Kuiterovich PO Jr, Sniderman AD: Atherosclerosis and apoproteins B and A-1. Prev Med 1983;12:815–834.
27. Nanjel MM, Miller NE: Evaluation of long term frozen storage of plasma for measurement of high density lipoproteins and its subfractions by precipitations. Clin Chem 1990;36:783–788.
28. Naito HK: Cholesterol: review of methods. ASCP Check Sample Core Chemistry 4:(5) Chicago, IL 1988.
29. Warnick GR, Benderson J, Albees JJ: Dextran sulfate-Mg^{++} precipitation procedure for quantitation of high density lipoprotein cholesterol. Clin Chem 1982;28:1379–1387.
30. Gidez LI, Miller GJ, Burstein M et al: Separation and quantitation of subclasses of human high density lipoprotein by a simple precipitation procedure. J Lipid Res, 1982;23:1206–1223.
31. Naito HK: The association of serum lipids, lipoproteins, and apolipoproteins with coronary artery disease assessed by coronary arteriography. Ann NY Acad Sci 1985;454:230–238.
32. Francheschini GR, Sirtori CR, Capurso A et al: A-1 milano apoprotein. Decreased high density lipoprotein cholesterol levels with significant lipoproteins modifications and without clinical atherosclerosis in an Italian family. J Clin Invest 1980;66:892–900.
33. Carlson LA, Phillpson B: Fish eye disease: a new familial condition with massive corneal opacities and dyslipoproteinemia. Lancet 1979;2:922–924.
34. Schaefer EJ, Heaton WH, Wetzel MG, Brewer HB Jr: Plasma apolipoproteins A-1 absence associated with a marked reduction of high density lipoproteins and premature coronary artery disease. Arteriosclerosis 1982;2:16–26.
35. Castelli WP, Anderson K: A population at risk, prevalence of high cholesterol levels in hypertensive patients in the Framingham study. Am J Med 1986;80(2A):23–32.
36. Friedwald WT, Levy RI, Fredrickson DS: Estimation of the concentration of low-density lipoprotein cholesterol without the use of the preparative ultracentrifuge. Clin Chem 1972;18:499–507.
37. Lipid Research Clinics program. The prevalence study. Vol. 1. In the Lipid Research Clinics. Population Studies Data Book. NIH Publication 80:1527. Bethesda, MD, US Department of Health and Human Services, 1980.
38. Gaubatz JW, Cushing GL, Morriset JD: Quantitation, isolation and characterization of human lipoprotein (a) [review]. Methods Enzymol 1986;129:167–186.
39. Labeur C, Michiels G, Bury J et al: Lipoprotein (a) quantified by an enzyme-linked immunosorbent assay with monoclonal antibodies. Clin Chem 1989;35:1380–1384.
40. Hoefler G, Harmoncourt F, Paschke E et al: Lipoprotein Lp(a), a risk factor for myocardial infarction. Arteriosclerosis 1988;8:398–401.
41. Sandkamp M, Funke H, Schulte H et al: Lipoprotein (a) is an independent risk factor for myocardial infarction at a young age. Clin Chem 1990;36:20–23.

42. Albers JJ, Brunzell JD, Knopp RH: Apoprotein measurements and their clinical application. Clin Lab Med 1989;9:137–152.
43. Albers JJ, Mascovina SM: Standardization of apolipoprotein B and A-1 measurements. Clin Chem 1989;35:1357–1361.
44. Alaupovic P, McConathy WJ, Fesmire J et al: Profiles of apolipoproteins and apolipoprotein B-containing lipoprotein particles in dyslipoproteinemias. Clin Chem 1988;34(B):13–27.
45. Kukita H, Hiwada K, Kokubu T: Serum apolipoprotein A-1, A-II and B levels and their discriminative values in relatives of patients with coronary artery disease. Atherosclerosis 1984;51:261–267.
46. Van Stiphant WAH, Hofman A, Kruijssen HACM et al: Is the ratio of ApoB/ApoA-1 an early predictor of coronary atherosclerosis? Atherosclerosis 1986;62:179–182.
47. Maciejko JJ, Levinson SS, Markyvech L et al: New assay of apolipoproteins A-1 and B by rate nephelometry elevated. Clin Chem 1987;33:2065–2069.
48. Maciejko JJ, Holmes DR, Kottke BA et al: Apolipoprotein A-1 as a marker of angiographically assessed coronary-artery disease. N Engl J Med 1983;309:385–389.
49. Sniderman A, Shapiro S, Marpole D et al: Association of coronary atherosclerosis with hyperabetalipoproteinemia (increased protein but normal cholesterol levels is human low density (B) lipoproteins). Proc Natl Acad Sci USA 1980;77:604–608.
50. Noma A, Yokosuka T, Kitamura K: Plasma lipids and apolipoproteins as discriminators for presence and severity of angiographically defined coronary artery disease. Atherosclerosis 1983;49:1–7.
51. Naito HK: The association of serum lipids, lipoproteins, and apolipoproteins with coronary artery disease assessed by coronary arteriography. Ann NY Acad Sci 1985;454:230–238.
52. Freedman DS, Srinivasan SR, Shear GL et al: The relation of apolipoproteins A-1 and B in children to parental myocardial infarction. N Engl J Med 1986;315:721–726.
53. Utermann G, Albrecht G, Steinmetz A: Polymorphism of apolipoprotein E.I. Methodological aspects and diagnosis of hyperlipoproteinemia type III without ultracentrifugation. Clin Genet 1978;14:351–358.
54. Ghiselli G, Schaffer EJ, Gascon F, Brema HB Jr: Type III hyperlipoproteinemia associated with apolipoprotein E deficiency. Science 1981;214:1239–1241.
55. Breslow JL, Zannis VI, SanGiacomo TR et al: Studies of familial type III hyperlipoproteinemia using as a genetic marker the ApoE phenotype E 2/2. J Lipid Res 1982;23:1224–1235.
56. Gregg RE, Ghiselli G, Brewer HB Jr: Apolipoprotein E Bethesda. A new variant of apolipoprotein E associated with type III hyperlipoproteinemia. J Clin Endocrinol Metab 1983;57:969–974.
57. Basu SK, Brown MS, Ho YK et al: Mouse macrophages synthesize and secrete a protein resembling apolipoprotein E. Proc Natl Acad Sci USA 1981;78:7845–7549.
58. Stein EA, Glueck CJ: Hyperlipoproteinemia: implications, diagnosis and therapy. pp. 677–695. In Fowler NO (ed): Cardiac Diagnosis and Treatment. 3rd Ed. New York, Harper & Row, 1980.

10 Metals, Vitamins, and Nutritional Factors

Robert De Cresce
Elizabeth Sengupta

TRACE ELEMENTS

INTRODUCTION

A trace element is one that has a concentration in the body of 1 µg/g of tissue or less (Tables 10-1 and 10-2). More recent sophisticated methods of analytic assay have permitted the study of elements present in even smaller quantities, that is, nomograms per gram or less. These elements have been dubbed ultratrace elements. An element is considered essential if a predictable deficiency state can be corrected only by the administration of that element. In addition, there must be a recognized biochemical basis for the element's essential function. The trace metals considered essential for proper health are zinc, copper, and iron. The ultratrace metals currently identified as essential are manganese, cobalt (only essential as a component of cobalamin), molybdenum, and chromium. Trace metals that have not yet been demonstrated to be essential are nickel, vanadium, arsenic, and silicon. Most of these elements act as cofactors in unique metalloenzymes. Well de-

Table 10-1. Body Content of Trace Metals

Metal	Safe and Adequate Daily Intake	Total Body Amount in the Adult
Chromium	50–200 µg[a] (960–3840 µmol)	4–6 mg (76.8–115 mmol)
Cobalt	Not recognized	1 mg (in cobalamin)
Copper	3.2–9.5 µg (5–15 µmol) intravenously 19.0–25.4 µg (30–40 µmol) orally (2–3 mg/24 h (31.5 µmol/d)	75 mg (1.18 mmol)
Manganese	2.5–5 mg/24 h (45.5–91.0 mmol/d)	12–20 mg (220–360 mmol)
Molybdenum	150–500 µg/24 h (1560–5200 µmol/d)	
Selenium	50–200 µg/24 h (630–2530 µmol/d)	
Zinc		
Adolescents and adults[b]	15 mg/24 h (230 µmol/d)	1.5–2.0 g (23.0–31 mmol)
Pregnant females	20 mg/24 h (310 µmol/d)	
Lactating females	25 mg/24 h (380 µmol/d)	
Infants 0–5 mo	3 mg/24 h (45.9 µmol/d)	
Infants 5–12 mo	5 mg/24 h (76.5 µmol/d)	
Children 1–10 yr	10 mg/24 h (150 µmol/d)	

[a] Data from clinical nutrition cases.[1]
[b] Data from Ronaghy.[23]

Table 10-2. Routes of Excretion for Trace Metals

	Bile	Urine	Feces	Sweat	Pancreatic Secretions
Chromium		++++			
Cobalt					
Copper	+	+	++	++	
Manganese	+++	+			
Molybdenum	+	+++			
Selenium		++++			
Zinc	+	+	+++	+	++

fined deficiency states are recognized for most of these metals, especially the trace metals. In addition, some of these elements are toxic when present in excess (Table 10-3). The essential trace and ultratrace metals, except for iron and magnesium, are discussed in this chapter.

Laboratory Analysis

No "gold" standards for clinical laboratory assessment of trace metal nutriture have been established. Many methods, often insensitive and nonspecific, have been used to measure concentrations of the metals in various body fluids and tissues. Because of the minute quantities of the metal present, contamination of the specimen with exogenous metal is a major problem encountered by laboratories. This contamination together with the variation of analytic methods largely account for the wide reference ranges for these metals.

Whole blood, serum or plasma, erythrocytes, urine, sweat, saliva, fingernails, and hair can be used as specimens, but blood is the most practical specimen in the

Table 10-3. Laboratory Determination of Trace Metal and Ultratrace Metal Status: Clinical Uses

	Deficiency	Toxicity	Specific Disease States	Comment
Chromium[a]	Documented in patients receiving hyperalimentation	Industrial exposure	None	? Role of chromium deficiency in diabetes
Cobalt[a]	Not of cobalt alone, but as part of cobalamin	Industrial exposure	None	? Cardiomyopathy in beer drinkers and people with renal disease
Copper[b]	Rare dietary deficiency in the general population	Yes	Menkes or kinky hair disease / Wilson's disease	
Ceruloplasmin[c]	Asymptomatic hyperuloplasminemia		Menkes or kinky hair disease / Wilson's disease	
Manganese[a]	Difficult to determine	Industrial exposure (manganism) and accidental ingestion		Other metals substitute for manganese
Molybdenum[a]	Not defined	Not defined	Inborn error of metabolism (see text)	
Selenium[a]	Not well defined but reported in China (see text)		? Keshan's cardiomyopathy	Deficiency syndromes are seen in animals
Zinc[b]	Yes (see text)	Industrial exposure and excess ingestion	Acrodermatitis enteropathica	Excess ingestion may be accidental or purposeful

[a] Ultratrace metals.
[b] Trace metals.
[c] Copper containing plasma protein.

clinical diagnostic setting. All specimens must be collected and processed with great care to avoid contamination with exogenous metal. Blood must be collected in evacuated tubes specified for trace metal analysis. These tubes must not have rubber stoppers since rubber is a common source of trace metal contamination. In lieu of specially designated tubes, plastic disposable syringes with stainless steel needles are adequate. For iron, zinc, and copper analysis hair should be cut with stainless steel scissors; the occipitonuchal region is the best sample site. The proximal 3–4 cm of a 0.3 g sample of hair is adequate for analysis.

Atomic absorption spectrophotometry (AAS), either flame or flameless, offers good sensitivity and specificity and is the method of choice for laboratories without more sophisticated instrumentation.

TESTS FOR TRACE METALS

Test: Chromium (Cr)

Background

Chromium, unlike other essential trace transition metals, is not present in the body as a metalloenzyme. As a potentiator of insulin action, chromium is purported to play a role in glucose tolerance as part of a trivalent chromium (CrIII) nicotinic acid complex called *glucose tolerance factor* (GTF). Because purification has not yet been accomplished, GTF, to this date, remains a somewhat nebulous entity with unknown structure.[1] Brewer's yeast is a good source of chromium, based on a high score when evaluated for biologic GTF activity. Deficiency, documented in patients receiving parenteral nutrition, results in weight loss, impaired glucose tolerance, encephalopathy, and peripheral neuropathy that improves only with chromium supplementation. Chromium deficiency appears to be a factor in the insulin resistance seen in noninsulin-dependent diabetes mellitus. Indeed, some evidence indicates that chromium supplementation improves insulin resistant glucose intolerance and decreases insulin requirement in patients receiving insulin. However, some investigators cite no benefit from supplementation. The positive chromium effect in such cases may require adequate levels of nicotinic acid.

Contact with chromates occurs in many industrial and occupational situations including electroplating, steelmaking, leather tanning, photography, dyeing, stainless steel welding, chrome ore processing, construction (cement handline), paint manufacturing, and chemical manufacturing. Exposure to chromium occurs in the form of fumes and dusts of chromates that irritate and enter the body through the skin, mucous membranes, gastrointestinal tract, and the bronchopulmonary system. This exposure may result in allergic reactions such as contact eczema or asthma; toxic eczema; conjunctivitis; nasal septal and skin ulceration; malignancy in the nose, paranasal sinuses, and lung; gastrointestinal irritation; and central nervous system abnormalities with convulsions.[2-4] Acute exposure, especially from dermal exposure to concentrated chromate solutions, can result in acute renal damage.[4] Hexavalent chromates (CrVI) are the most toxic. In contrast, CrIII has a low order of toxicity with an apparently wide margin of safety between supplementation to cure deficiency and toxicity.

Selection

Evaluation of chromium status is indicated only in rare situations, most often in industrial/environmental medicine. For biologic monitoring of chromate exposure, simultaneous measurements of plasma and erythrocyte levels are suitable. Plasma measurements best reflect environmental exposure, whereas erythrocyte chromium best reflects the carcinogenic risk.[3]

Logistics

Specimen Requirements

As with other trace metals, contamination control is critical in all phases of collection and analysis. Urine should be collected in plastic containers free of acid or preservative and checked for chromium contamination. Blood must be collected in all-plastic syringes free of measurable chromium. The siliconized "butterfly" type needles are acceptable for the venipuncture. Serum is the preferred specimen, prepared by direct centrifugation of the collection syringes. Plasma can also be analyzed if a sufficiently chromium-free anticoagulant is available. Erythrocyte levels of chromium also can be determined and, perhaps, most usefully reflect risk from the carcinogenic CrVI.[3]

Methods

Chromium levels are among the most difficult of the ultratrace metals to determine, simply because the concentration in body tissues and fluids is minute. Neutron activation analysis, mass spectrometry, and graphite furnace atomic absorption spectrometry (GFASS) are the methods presently available for chromium determination in biologic materials. Recent advances in GFASS technologicaly have made it possible to accurately measure concentrations in the biologic range, making it the method of choice.

Interpretation

Reference intervals for serum and urine have shown a downward trend as the methods for determination have gained sensitivity and specificity. Average plasma and urine levels in occupationally nonexposed persons are reported to be between 0.16–1.04 µg/L (3.07–20.0 nmol/L) and 0.18–1.60 µg/L (1.66–3.07 nmol/L), respectively.[3] According to a study from Germany,[3] urine and plasma levels of 40 and 10 µg/L (768 and 192 nmol/L), respectively, correspond to workplace exposure of 10 µg CrIII/m^3. In contrast, erythrocyte concentrations of greater than 0.60 µg/L (11.52 nmol/L) indicate chromate exposure greater than those recommended by the guidelines (e.g., the German technical guideline concentration or limit value for exposure).

Test: Cobalt (Co)

Background

Cobalt, an integral part of the essential vitamin cobalamin, is indirectly an essential metal. Free cobalt does not interact with the body pool of cobalamin nor is there any known function of cobalt in the body other than the role it plays in the cobalamin molecule. A cobalt deficiency per se, therefore, does not exist. It follows, however, that the total amount of cobalt in the body decreases when there is a deficiency of cobalamin.

Toxicity caused by excess cobalt ingestion has been reported in patients with chronic renal failure secondary to treatment with cobalt as an erythropoietic agent and in beer drinkers who consume large volumes of beer containing cobalt as a foam stabilizer. In both populations, fatal cardiomyopathies have been reported, but the underlying renal disease and alcohol toxicity possibly contribute substantially to the outcome. Hard-metal workers such as tungsten carbide workers and diamond polishers are exposed to aerosolized cobalt. This exposure has been linked to lung disease, such as diffuse interstitial fibrosis and bronchial asthma, cardiomyopathy, polycythemia, and allergic dermatitis.[5] A contact dermatitis in which one of the culprits is probably cobalt has also been reported in cement workers.

Selection

Assessing cobalt status is required only in the special setting of possible environmental exposure to the metal dust. Monitoring of persons in occupations who come in contact with cobalt dust can be accomplished by following urine and blood concentrations.

Logistics

As with analysis of other trace metals, care must be taken to avoid contamination. Analysis of cobalt in the urine or blood can be accomplished by numerous methods including flame or electrothermal AAS, atomic emission spectrometry, neutron activation analysis, chemiluminescence, and colorimetry. Although there is no standard technique for cobalt determination, AAS is the most rapid, versatile, and reliable method. Stainless steel needles and vacutainer tubes should be avoided. Siliconized stainless steel needles or Teflon-polyethylene intravenous cannulae and polypropylene syringes are recommended. The first several milliters of blood flowing through the infusion apparatus should be collected in a separate syringe and discarded.[6]

Interpretation

The reference ranges for serum and urine are 0.1–2 ng/mL (1.70–33.9 nmol/L) and 0.7–10 µg/24 h (11.9–169.7 µmol/d), respectively. There is a linear relationship between the concentrations of cobalt in blood and urine specimens and in the ambient air of the workplace. When exposure is curtailed, urine levels decrease rapidly, whereas blood levels fall slowly reflecting the body stores.[5] In one Japanese study,[5] the cobalt concentration with cobalt exposure of 100 µg/m (1.70 mmol/m) was found to be 5.7–7.9 ng/mL (96.8–134.1 nmol/L) in blood and 59–78 µg/L (1.0–1.3 nmol/L) in urine.

Test: Copper (Serum, Urine)

Background

Copper is a cofactor in many human enzymes including cytochrome oxidase, superoxide dismutase (also known as erythrocuprein), tyrosinase (monophenal monoxygenase), dopamine β-hydroxylase, lysyl oxidase, ceruloplasmin, and an unknown enzyme that cross-links keratin.[7] These enzymes have catalytic roles in the synthesis of melanin, cross-linking of collagen and elastin, iron metabolism, neuronal metabolism, and catecholamine conversions. From 40–60% of ingested copper is absorbed by the gut, transported to the liver, complexed to albumin and selected amino acids, and stored in hepatocytes primarily as a cuproprotein. Copper is released into the blood by the liver and incorporated mainly into the blue copper protein ceruloplasmin, the serum ferroxidase that oxidizes iron prior to its binding by plasma transferrin. Ceruloplasmin contains over 90–95% of the circulating copper, making it the major vehicle for copper transport. It is also an acute-phase reactant, perhaps consequent to its antioxidant function. The serum level of this protein correlates well with total plasma copper. Absorbed copper is primarily excreted through the biliary tract and gastrointestinal secretions. The renal tubules efficiently reabsorb most of the filtered copper making urinary excretion low. Abnormalities of copper metabolisms are summarized in Table 10-4.

Copper Deficiency

Nutritional copper deficiency has a low incidence in the general population, but it is occasionally seen in special situations. In infants and children, deficient copper nutriture is related to prematurity, low birth weight, malnutrition with chronic diarrhea, hyperalimentation, and prolonged feeding with copper-poor, total milk diets. Effects of the deficiency include the hematologic manifestations of neutropenia and hypochromic anemia responding to copper supplementation but not iron. Vacuolation of peripheral blood neutrophils and a maturation arrest of the bone marrow accompany the neutropenia. The anemia and neutropenia in premature and low birth weight babies is seen at about 3–4 months of age.[7] Osteoporosis and scurvy-like bone changes are also reported. Severe deficiency of the neonate may result in signs and symptoms similar to those seen in Menkes disease (see discussion below) such as hypopigmentation, apnea, hypotonia, and developmental retardation.[7] However, these findings are not the rule in nutritional deficiency. Because copper supplementation generally reverses these findings, monitoring of copper status with serum copper levels is warranted in the infant at risk.[8]

Hypocupremia due to dietary copper deficiency in older children and adults is associated with long-term parenteral nutrition with copper-poor hyperalimentation so-

Table 10-4. Abnormalities in Copper Metabolism

	Disease or Condition	Laboratory Values
Deficiency states	Premature infants Prolonged total milk diet in infants Long-term hyperalimentation in adults and infants Infants in association with malabsorption and chronic diarrhea Malabsorption syndromes Malnutrition Kwashiorkor and marasmus	Low serum copper, low serum iron
Hereditary hypocupremia	Menkes or kinky hair disease	Very low serum copper and ceruloplasmin; urinary copper may be normal
	Wilson's disease	Low ceruloplasmin; increased dialyzable (free) serum copper; increased urinary copper
Therapy related hypocupremia	Zinc therapy for sickle cell disease Penicillamine therapy	Low serum copper
Conditions associated with hypercupremia	Estrogenic oral contraceptives	Elevated serum copper and ceruloplasmin
	Pregnancy	Two- to threefold increase in serum copper
	Testosterone therapy	Increased serum copper
	Progesterone	Increased serum copper
	Addison's disease and hypopituitarism	Increased serum copper and decreased urinary copper
	Infection and inflammatory stress	Increase in ceruloplasmin
	Rheumatoid arthritis	May be increased in serum ceruloplasmin and joint fluid copper
	Liver disease: portal cirrhosis, biliary tract disease, hepatitis biliary cirrhosis; intrahepatic cholestasis	Increased serum copper
	Lymphomas, especially Hodgkin's disease	Elevated serum copper

lutions, chronic gastrointestinal disease, and protein-losing conditions. Because copper is removed during food processing, otherwise healthy persons whose diet consists primarily of processed rather than fresh foods may have suboptimal copper intake that may result in deficiency.[7] Iatrogenic conditions associated with copper deficiency are zinc therapy for sickle cell disease and treatment with chelating agents such as penicillamine for metal intoxication.[7] Excessive zinc ingestion interferes with absorption of copper and chelating agents bind most metals without preference for the one in excess.

A rare inherited defect in copper metabolism is the X-linked recessive disorder known as Menkes disease or kinky hair disease (trichopoliodystrophy). The disease has a calculated prevalence at birth of 1 in 35,000.[9] The defect, which has not yet been characterized, prevents incorporation of copper into the cuproapoenzymes producing an effective profound deficiency in copper although total body copper may be normal or increased. One of the biochemical features of the disease is the abnormal distribution of copper in the tissues. The symptoms that appear by 3 months of age include kinky or twisted hair (pili torti), depigmentation of skin and hair, growth retardation, hypotonia, hypothermia, seizures, and cerebral and cerebellar degeneration. The defect affects absorption of copper at the level of the gastrointestinal tract, and duodenal tissue will show accumulation of copper in the mucosa. In contrast to copper deficiency of other etiologies, neutropenia and anemia are not features of the disease. Intravenous administration of copper, but not oral therapy, returns the serum copper and ceruloplasmin to normal levels but does not alter the neurologic anomalies.[9] Life expectancy is about 3 years.

Copper Excess

Wilson's disease, or hepatolenticular degeneration, is an autosomal recessive disorder of copper overload with an undefined defect of copper metabolism. The incidence of this disease has been reported to range from 1:30,000–1:200,000. The hallmarks of the full-blown disease are liver cirrhosis, degenerative changes in the brain primarily in the lenticular nuclei (putamen and globus pallidus) with resultant movement disorders, and Kayser-Fleischer rings that encircle the periphery of the iris. These rings, resulting from deposition of copper in Descemet's membrane, are brown-green in color, may be unilateral, and may require slit-lamp microscopic examination for demonstration. Onset of the disease is variable ranging from 4–70 years. Clinical presentation is also variable,[9,10] requiring a high index of suspicion on the part of the physician. Rarely, persons with Wilson's disease have presented with anemia induced by release of stored copper into the bloodstream.[11] Recognition of this disease is important because it can be controlled with therapy.

The work-up for Wilson's disease and the carrier state includes eye examination for Kayser-Fleischer rings, determination of serum ceruloplasmin and urinary copper, liver biopsy to evaluate copper content and histopathology, and radioactive copper studies. Kayser-Fleischer rings, although showing a high specificity for Wilson's disease, are not present in all cases. Also, they are not pathognomonic for Wilson's disease as microscopic Kayser-Fleischer rings have been reported in cases of severe liver disease of other etiologies such as primary biliary cirrhosis, chronic active hepatitis, and cryptogenic cirrhosis.[9,10] Macroscopic Kayser-Fleischer rings have been seen in one case of monoclonal gammopathy.[9]

Copper toxicity can occur in various settings. Occupational exposure may occur in smelting or alloy production and from use of pesticides, fungicides, or algicides. Community exposure may be secondary to ingestion of acidic fluids prepared, stored, or fed through copper containers, tubes, or pipes. Copper coated intrauterine devices and copper in dialysis fluid are possible sources on an individual basis. Copper sulfate is also used as a poison for suicide or homicide in some countries. Hemolytic anemia with Heinz body formation accompanied by hemoglobinuria, hemoglobinemia, and reticulocytosis is the characteristic clinical presentation of occult copper poisoning. The onset of the anemia may take hours to days after acute exposure to copper sulfate or it may occur weeks to months after chronic exposure and copper storage in the tissues. Nonhematopoietic symptoms and signs of copper toxicity include abdominal pain, nausea, vomiting, diarrhea, oliguria, uremia, and contact and eczematous dermatitis.[11]

Selection

Copper studies must be undertaken in any patient with a clinical presentation suspicious for Menkes disease. Any patient between 5 and 50 years of age with unexplained liver disease (including fulminant hepatic necrosis), hepatosplenomegaly, a history of jaundice, signs of unexplained brain damage, or a psychiatric disorder in conjunction with hepatic or neurologic abnormality should be screened for Wilson's disease.

Copper studies also are warranted when dietary deficiency or excess is suspected (see above).

Routine clinical laboratory tests for copper status are total serum copper, serum ceruloplasmin, and urinary copper. Additional information is gained from hepatic biopsy for copper content and histology, radiocopper studies, and free (dialysable) copper. The usefulness of copper content in hair, claimed to be a good estimate of long-term copper intake, is hampered by the copper present in shampoos and hair sprays.[10]

Logistics

As with any metal, care must be taken to avoid contamination. Urine should be collected in an acid washed polypropylene container. Copper is one of the easiest elements to measure in biologic materials if AAS, either flame or electrothermal, is used.[12]

Interpretation

Decreases

In extreme deficiency, serum copper is less than 50 µg/L (8 µmol/L) making this one test sufficient for diagnosis.[7] However, demonstrating the existence of mild deficiency is difficult, partly because of the wide range of serum ceruloplasmin and hence serum copper in normocupric individuals. Also, urinary copper excretion is normally low and small changes in renal function can cause large changes in urinary copper excretion making this test a poor indicator of copper nutriture. Studies show that in patients receiving zinc therapy, monitoring using urine and plasma copper is very useful.[13]

Increases

In Wilson's disease, copper excretion in a 24-hour collection is nearly always significantly greater than the reference range, generally showing a greater than two- to threefold increase over the upper limit of normal of ~100 µg/24 h (16 µmol/d). However, an increase is also seen in severe proteinuria and cholestatic liver disease. After the diagnosis of Wilson's disease is made and treatment instituted, the efficacy of therapy must be monitored. The various methods presently utilized include copper balance, liver biopsy with determination of copper concentration, plasma copper levels, 24-hour urinary copper excretion, and eye examination. In the event that a patient with Wilson's disease is diagnosed, screening of close relatives for presymptomatic disease is mandatory.

Test: Ceruloplasmin (See Ch. 8)

Background and Selection

Indications are the same as for serum copper. It is suggested that measurement of ceruloplasmin levels before and after 3–4 days of a daily, physiologic dose of copper may provide the simplest method of determining copper status.[7]

Logistics

Ceruloplasmin levels can be determined photometrically by the oxidase reaction with dimethyl p-phenylenediamine (PPD oxidase activity) or by immunomethods such as immunonephelometry, radial immunodiffusion, or immunoelectrophoresis.

Interpretation

Diagnosis of Menkes disease is established by the laboratory findings of hypocupremia less than 63 µg/dL (<10 µmol/L) and hypoceruloplasminemia (less than 20 mg/dL [<200 mg/L]). If an immunoassay is used to determine ceruloplasmin levels, the concentrations may be within the reference interval because the antibody used in the assay may be raised against the apoceruloplasmin that may be present in usual concentrations. Low levels of ceruloplasmin also can be found in protein-losing conditions, malnutrition, malabsorption, severe liver failure of other etiologies, and in some carriers of Wilson's disease.[10]

Generally, ceruloplasmin levels in Wilson's disease are less than 20 mg/dL (<200 mg/L) (reference range 20–40 mg/dL [200–400 mg/L]), however, in 5% of patients the ceruloplasmin level is within the reference range falling in the lower end and almost never over 30 mg/dL (300 mg/L).[9,10] In others, the ceruloplasmin level may be raised to within the reference range because of synthesis of ceruloplasmin induced by various factors including hepatic disease caused by copper overload.[9,10] In addition, pregnancy and exogenous estrogen may increase ceruloplasmin levels in Wilson's disease.

In the copper deficient individual, the ceruloplasmin will rise significantly. In protein-losing conditions, however, the ceruloplasmin level may fail to rise even in the copper deficient state.

Test: Copper (Liver)

Confirmation tests for Menkes disease include determination of copper content in a needle biopsy of the liver and tissue culture of the patient's lymphocytes or fibroblasts. The copper content of the liver is lower than the usual range of 50–150 µg (0.8–2.4 µmol/g) dry weight found in early infancy. The cultured cells will demonstrate increased uptake and retention of copper. Antenatal diagnosis is accomplished by measuring the accumulation of copper in vitro by cultured amniotic or chorionic villus fibroblasts.[9]

Copper content in a liver biopsy sample will reveal concentrations significantly greater than the reference range (less than 50 µg/g [<0.8 µmol/g] dry weight) in Wilson's disease. Usually, untreated patients will have copper concentrations much greater than 250 µg/g (>3.9 µmol/g) dry weight, but an occasional patient with neurologic symptoms may have concentrations between 100 and 250 µg/g (1.6 and 3.9 µmol/g) dry weight.[10] Heterozygotes for the defective gene may have slight elevations of copper content, but not beyond 250 µg/g (3.9 µmol/g) dry weight. Slight elevations may also be present in patients with primary chronic liver disease with cholestasis. Children with Indian childhood cirrhosis may have hepatic copper content in the Wilson's disease range, but without hypoceruloplasminemia. Histologic examination of the liver is abnormal in the homozygote but normal in the heterozygote. However, the hepatic histopathology in Wilson's disease is nonspecific and, therefore, cannot unequivocally differentiate heptolenticular degeneration from other severe liver diseases such as Indian childhood cirrhosis. Hepatic copper levels are summarized in Table 10-5.

Test: Radiocopper Studies

The radiocopper studies, used when other parameters are equivocal or liver biopsy is contraindicated, involve intravenous or oral administration of radiocopper followed by timed measurements of plasma radioactivity. The intravenous route of radiocopper administration eliminates potential difficulties in interpreting the results of patients with poor intestinal absorption, such as those with severe malabsorption syndromes or Menkes disease. These studies evaluate the incorporation of radiocopper into ceruloplasmin, therefore they are of no value in the patient with low levels of this protein.[10] Normally, plasma shows a peak in radiocopper shortly after it is introduced. This peak is followed by a fall as the copper is taken up by the liver and then a second peak corresponding to the slow release of copper from the liver in newly synthesized ceruloplasmin. In Wilson's disease, there is impaired incorporation of copper into ceruloplasmin, thus there is an absence of the normal second peak resulting in a low 24:2 hour ratio of radiocopper activity (normal, greater than 0.8; heterozygote, greater than 0.5). This test reliably differentiates those patients with Wilson's disease showing ceruloplasmin levels within the reference interval from healthy persons and those with other liver diseases.[9,10] When oral zinc is used as maintenance therapy, oral radiocopper uptake also can be used because zinc impairs copper transfer into the bloodstream from the intestinal mucosal cells slowing the appearance of radioactive copper (^{64}Cu) into the blood.

Test: Free (Dialysable) Copper

See Diagnosis of Wilson's Disease below.

Diagnosis of Wilson's Disease

The differential diagnosis and steps in the diagnosis of Wilson's disease depend on the patient's signs and symptoms and are summarized in Figure 10-1 and Table 10-6. The initial step in patients presenting with neurologic or psychiatric dysfunction is the search for Kayser-Fleischer disease rings, which may be a feature in most or all cases of Wilson's disease with such a presentation. If rings are present, Wilson's disease is

Table 10-5. Hepatic Copper in Normal Individuals and Those With Various Disease States

Condition	Hepatic Copper µg/g [µmol/g] dry weight)
Normal adult	10–30 (0.16–50.0)
Normal infant	50–150 (0.79–2.36)
Wilson's disease	158–2950 (2.49–46.4)
Wilson's heterozygote	≤250 (≤3.94)
Primary biliary cirrhosis	
Assymptomatic	~100 (~1.57)
Active	~300 (~4.72)
Advanced	~1100 (~17.3)
Obstructive jaundice	
<6 months	<150 (<2.36)
>12 months	200–950 (3.15–15.0)
Indian childhood cirrhosis	53–5800 (0.83–91.3)
Menkes disease	<50 (<0.79)

(Adapted from Owen,[14] with permission.)

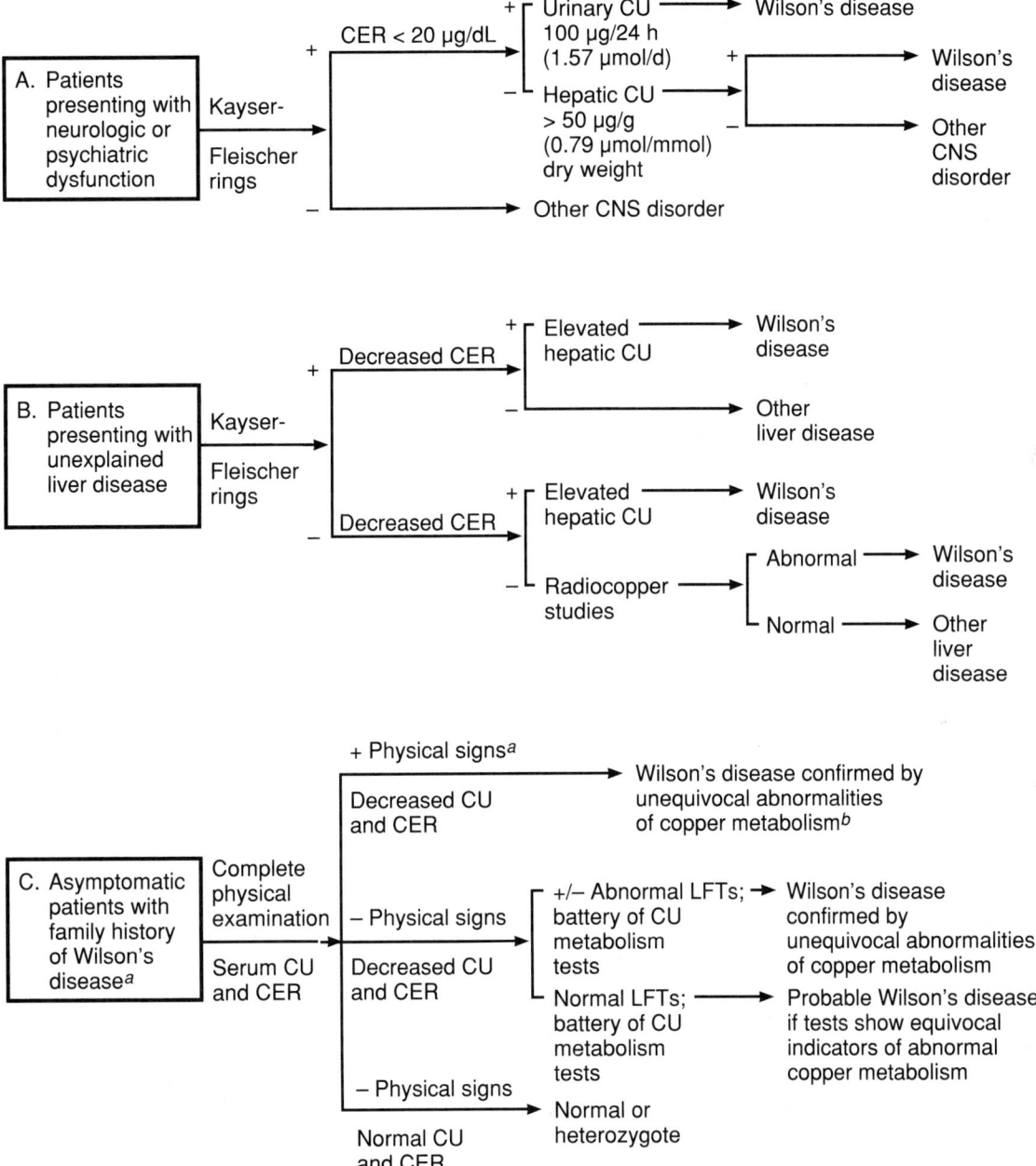

Fig. 10-1. Flow chart for diagnosis of Wilson's disease in different clinical settings. [a]Abnormal physical signs include the following: Kayser-Fleischer rings, CNS signs, hepatomegaly, splenomegaly; abnormal CT (cortical atrophy; abnormal basal ganglia). [b]Abnormal copper metabolism includes finding most or all of the following abnormal parameters: increased liver function tests (LFT); decreased CER; increased urinary copper; increased liver copper; abnormal liver histology; abnormal radiocopper test; decreased total and increased free serum copper. CU, copper; CER, ceruloplasmin; CNS, central nervous system; CT, computed tomography.

Table 10-6. Differential Diagnosis of Parameters Used in the Diagnosis of Wilson's Disease

	Ceruloplasmin	Urinary Copper	Kayser-Fleischer Rings	Hepatic Copper Content	Radiocopper Studies[a]
Wilson's disease	<20 mg/dL[b] (<200 µg/L)	>100 µg/24 h	Often present[c]	100->2000 µg/g (1.57–31.5 µmol/mmol) dry weight	Abnormal
Primary biliary cirrhosis	Normal to elevated	May be elevated	Seen rarely[d]	Elevated, variably	Normal
Cholestatic liver disease	Normal to elevated	May be elevated	Seen rarely[d]	Elevated, variably	Normal
Chronic active hepatitis	May be low	Elevated in proteinuria	Absent	Normal	Normal
Protein-losing diseases	May be low	Normal	Absent	Normal	Normal (intravenous route)
Indian childhood cirrhosis	Normal	Normal	Absent	May be in Wilson's disease range	Normal
Fulminant hepatitis	May be low	Normal	Absent	Normal	Normal
Menkes disease	<20 mg/dL (<200 µg/L)	Normal	Absent	<50 µg/g (0.79 µmol/mmol) dry weight[e]	Normal (intravenous route)

[a] Useful only in patients with normal ceruloplasmin.
[b] Five percent may have normal ceruloplasmin; others may have a low ceruloplasmin elevated to normal by a physiologic or exogenous factor.
[c] Seen in all Wilson's disease patients presenting with neurologic symptoms.
[d] Usually seen only by slit-lamp examination.
[e] This is lower than the normal range for age.

confirmed by abnormal levels of serum ceruloplasmin and urinary copper. If the rings are present but ceruloplasmin is within the reference range, a determination of the copper load in the liver is required to confirm the diagnosis. In a patient with low ceruloplasmin and in the absence of Kayser-Fleischer rings, a liver biopsy can provide laboratory evidence for heterozygosity. If doubt persists, a radioactive copper load test offers the final diagnostic choice.

The diagnosis of Wilson's disease in those presenting with liver abnormalities can be more difficult because the parameters used are not specific for Wilson's disease, that is, the parameters are often abnormal in severe liver disease of other etiologies. In patients with liver disease, low ceruloplasmin, Kayser-Fleischer rings, and increased urinary copper, the diagnosis of Wilson's disease is likely but must be confirmed by liver biopsy if biopsy is not contraindicated. In the absence of Kayser-Fleischer rings, a reduced ceruloplasmin value requires a liver biopsy to confirm diagnosis. Radioactive copper studies would not be helpful. If there are no Kayser-Fleischer rings and the ceruloplasmin level is within the reference range, a biopsy may not be diagnostic because liver copper content may be significantly raised because of severe cholestasis and not as a result of Wilson's disease. In this case radioactive copper studies should be diagnostic. Perhaps the most difficult diagnosis is when Wilson's disease presents as fulminant hepatic failure, because the serum copper level may be within the reference range and ceruloplasmin levels are uninterpretable. Clues to the diagnosis in such a situation are increased urinary copper levels, inappropriately small elevations in liver function tests, and hemolytic anemia.[9,10]

The diagnosis of Wilson's disease in presymptomatic patients with a positive family history requires a physical examination, liver function tests, and laboratory evaluation of copper metabolism. The initial investigation consists of the physical examination and measurement of serum copper and ceruloplasmin. On physical examination, careful search for Kayser-Fleischer rings, neurologic abnormality, and hepatosplenomegaly must be pursued. A computed tomographic examination looking for cortical atrophy and abnormal basal ganglia may also be useful. If any physical finding and/or the initial copper status determinations are suggestive of Wilson's disease, additional evaluations of copper metabolism must be performed. These tests include the remainder of the tests mentioned for the diagnosis of Wilson's disease in patients with liver or neurologic disease plus total and free serum copper and liver function tests. In Wilson's disease, total serum copper is decreased but free (dialysable) copper is increased. Most of the parameters of copper metabolism should be abnormal before the diagnosis can be confidently established. If copper metabolism is definitely within the range seen in Wilson's disease, with or without elevated liver function tests, Wilson's disease can be diagnosed with confidence. Difficulty arises when physical findings are absent and liver functions are within the reference range, serum copper and other parameters of copper metabolism are borderline, or ceruloplasmin is within the range seen in Wilson's disease. In these cases, Wilson's disease is probable but not firmly established.

Test: Manganese (Mn)

Background

Manganese is a cofactor for a number of enzymes including glycosyl transferases, arginase, and enzymes involved in cholesterol biosynthesis. The mineral is mainly excreted in the bile. Because other metals can substitute for manganese, a deficiency state is difficult to define and has been described in only one case. However, chronic manganese poisoning, manganism, has occurred in a number of industrial workers exposed to chronic inhalation of manganese dust including miners, smelters, foundry workers, welders, and workers manufacturing drugs, pottery, ceramics, glass, varnish, and food additives.[15] Manganism also has been reported after high oral intake of manganese from well water or from mineral supplements.

Schizophrenic-like behavior or psychosis similar to amphetamine-induced psychosis, termed manganese madness or *locura manganica* in Chilean manganese miners, occurs after acute manganese aerosol intoxication.[16] Neurologic abnormalities clinically similar to Parkinson's or Wilson's disease are seen in chronically exposed patients. Standard Parkinson's therapy is effective in some of those affected.[16] Acute pneumonia and pleurisy and chronic granulomatosis disease also have been associated with exposure.

Selection

Evaluation of manganese status is indicated in patients presenting with schizophrenic-like behavior or Parkinsonism with suspected toxic exposure to manganese.

Table 10-7. Reference Ranges for Manganese

Specimen	Upper Limit of Reference Range
Serum	1 μg/L or lower (18.2 mmol/L)
Whole blood	11.8 μg/L (214 mmol/L)
Plasma	1.7 μg/L (30.9 mmol/L)
Packed red blood cells	24.6 μg/L (448 mmol/L)

Values were determined prior to 1980 by furnace atomic absorption spectrophotometry and may contain contaminants.
(Data from Slavin.[18])

Logistics

Avoiding contamination is important in manganese determination, as it is with other trace metals. Levels can be determined in urine, serum, plasma, whole blood, packed red blood cells, and hair. Flame AAS has been widely used for manganese determination in the past. However, stabilized temperature platform furnace AAS (furnace AAS) is presently the method of choice for biologic materials.[17] An ultrasensitive colorimetric photo-oxidation assay recently has been described that may provide a convenient and inexpensive alternative to AAS.

Interpretation

Reference intervals determined using AAS are given in Table 10-7. Urine normally contains little manganese. Thus, the appearance of manganese in the urine may be diagnostically helpful. Levels are increased following industrial exposure, acute hepatitis or other hepatobiliary disease, and myocardial infarction. Increased levels have been found in patients with rheumatoid arthritis.

Test: Molybdenum

Molybdenum, occurring in trace amounts in nearly all biologic material, is an oxidation-reduction active metal present in three human metalloenzymes: xanthine oxidase, aldehyde oxidase, and sulfite oxidase. Neither molybdenum deficiency nor intoxication has been defined in humans, even though a probable autosomal recessive defect in the synthesis of molybdenum-pterin cofactor does occur. Neonates affected with this defect have dysmorphic features, feeding difficulties, bilateral dislocation of the lens, hypertonicity or hypotonicity, mental retardation, cerebral and cerebellar atrophy with encephalopathy, and generalized or partial epilepsy.

There is no need for a molybdenum assay in the clinical setting. The diagnosis of the inborn error of molybdenum metabolism is made by biochemical anomalies that include hypouricemia, xanthinuria, sulphituria, thiosulphituria, reduced urinary excretion of inorganic sulphate, and undetectable levels of hepatic sulphite oxidase and xanthine dehydrogenase.[19] Antenatal diagnosis can be made by finding the absence of sulphite oxidase activity in fibroblasts.

Test: Selenium (Se)

Background

Selenium is an essential trace metal acting as an integral component of the metalloenzyme, glutathione peroxidase (GSHPx), which acts as an antioxidant and detoxifies lipid hydroperoxide. This selenoenzyme works synergistically with vitamin E, another micronutrient with antioxidant activity. The protective properties of GSHPx help prevent Heinz body formation in erythrocytes, hemolytic anemia, hepatic damage by oxidative compounds, and may play a role in inhibiting cataract formation. Also, GSHPx in phagocytic cells protects the cell from auto-oxidation. The high concentration of the metal is found in platelets because the enzyme also plays a role in prostaglandin synthesis.

Human disease caused by selenium deficiency is not well defined but there are many deficiency syndromes in animals. In China, selenium deficiency has been associated with a specific endemic cardiomyopathy termed Keshan disease. However, the direct association between suboptimal intake of selenium and the disease has never been firmly established. There is an anecdotal relationship between the resolution of myalgia with selenium supplementation but no clear-cut relationship has been found experimentally except in one patient receiving total parenteral nutrition.[20] A possible link between low selenium levels and increased risk of myocardial infarction has been postulated but not proven.[21] Glutathione peroxidase deficiency is related to a number of clinical disorders including hemolytic anemia, Glanzmann's thrombasthenia, Hermansky-Pudlak syndrome, and carcinoma. However, neither GSHPx activity nor selenium levels play a role in the diagnosis of these disorders. A role for selenium in the pathogenesis of cancer has been suggested but not substantiated. An antithetical idea, also not documented, is the speculation that selenium derivatives of glutathione might play a role in cancer prevention by detoxifying carcinogenic substances.

Selection

Because no clear-cut relationship has been established between clinical symptoms and low selenium levels, selenium levels are rarely appropriate except for research and epidemiology purposes.

Logistics

Determination of selenium can be done on whole blood, erythrocytes, plasma, serum, platelets, urine, hair, and toenails. Hair has not been a useful specimen in most countries, because of the selenium content of some shampoos,[20] although hair was used in China to determine risk of deficiency. Glutathione peroxidase activity in whole blood and erythrocytes, reported as units per gram of hemoglobin, shows a direct relationship with selenium content of whole blood or erythrocytes up to a concentration of 1.3 and 1.8 μmol/L, respectively, providing a useful functional test of selenium status. Platelet GSHPx activity is also a valid indicator of selenium status.[20] However, a drawback in the use of GSHPx enzyme assays is the lack of a suitable enzyme standard, a necessity for interlaboratory comparisons. Other drawbacks to functional assays for estimating selenium are the many factors that interact with selenium including vitamins, trace and heavy metals, and dietary fat and fatty acids.[20]

The method of choice for determining static selenium in biologic matrices such as serum, urine, erythrocytes, serum or whole blood, feces, and hair is spectrofluorimetry. Flame AAS is useful for tissues with a high concentration of selenium. The definitive method, having both good detection limits and precision, is isotope dilution gas chromatography with mass spectrometry (GC/MS), but the required sample size is fairly large making it unsuitable for pediatric specimens. Other methods include GFAAS with the Zeeman correction and gas liquid chromatography with electron capture detectors. In the research laboratory neutron activation analysis has been used,[21] but this technology is not practical for clinical use.

Interpretation

Blood and tissue selenium levels vary by geographic area and reflect selenium content in the soil where food for that area originated. Certain areas in China, New Zealand, and Finland are especially low in this metal.[20,22] In the control group for a study in the Netherlands of the relationship between myocardial infarction and selenium status, the mean levels for plasma, erythrocyte, and toenail selenium measured by neutron

Table 10-8. Reference Ranges for Selenium

Parameter	Level
Plasma	104.2–109.4 ng/mol (156–1.64 μmol/L)
Erythrocytes	0.57–0.61 μg/g of hemoglobin (8.55–9.15 μmol/g)
Toenails	0.76–0.08 mg/kg (11.7–12 μmol/g)
Erythrocyte GSHPx activity	27.1–28.9 U/g

Abbreviation: GSHPx, glutathione peroxidase.
Controls were age and sex matched to patients (all under 75 years of age) who had suffered a first acute myocardial infarction. (Data from Kok et al.[21])

activation analysis and for erythrocyte GSHPx activity are given in Table 10-8.[21]

Abnormally low values have been reported in patients with gastrointestinal cancer and in protein-calorie malnutrition (PCM). The reported effect of pregnancy on selenium levels has been inconsistent.[22] Levels higher than reference levels have been observed in patients with reticuloendothelial neoplasms and young women taking oral contraceptives.[22]

Test: Zinc

Background

Zinc is quantitatively the second most important micronutrient, with a total body content about half that of iron. The metal is found in more than 20 human metalloenzymes as an integral, tightly bound cofactor, which often plays a direct role in the catalytic action of the enzyme. Among the more important of the zinc metalloenzymes are carbonic anhydrase, pancreatic carboxypeptidase A, thymidine kinase, RNA and DNA polymerases, thymidine kinase, alkaline phosphatase, and alcohol dehydrogenase. Zinc dependent enzymes are found in many tissues including the kidney, testes, bone, the choroid of the eye, and the esophagus. The enzymes play roles in numerous biochemical activities involving the cell membrane, immunosystem (lymphocyte maturation), collagen metabolism, and both RNA and DNA synthesis.

Zinc is absorbed in the distal small intestine, primarily carried by albumen, and excreted primarily into the gastrointestinal tract, urine, and sweat. A high concentration of zinc is found in breast milk.[23,24]

The ubiquitous nature of this metal in the body results in protean and nonspecific clinical features of deficiency. These include alteration in normal growth ranging from severe dwarfism to more mild growth retardation, alteration in sexual development ranging from hypogonadism to delayed sexual maturity, failure to thrive in infants, hepatosplenomegaly in patients with coexistent severe iron deficiency anemia, reduced taste and smell acuity, impairment of dark adaptation, poor wound healing, scaly dermatitis, diarrhea, and impairment of the immunoresponse. Zinc deficiency also is suggested as a possible cause of congenital malformation.[23,25,26] Many of these manifestations may reflect concomitant deficiencies of other essential metals or vitamins. Growth retardation and hypogonadism in zinc deficient patients definitely respond to zinc supplementation alone suggesting a direct relationship between deficiency and these disorders.

The most common cause of zinc deficiency is malnutrition, especially PCM, because the bioavailability of zinc is best in high protein foods. Population groups especially vulnerable to deficiency are infants, children during the rapid growth phases, and lactating or pregnant women. Pica can result in iron and zinc deficiencies, especially when the ingested material contains chelating agents. Other patients have a conditioned zinc deficiency as a result of a primary disease either leading to excessive excretion or decreased absorption. Included in this category are patients with chronic liver disease, chronic renal failure, diarrheal diseases (especially Crohn's disease and steatorrhea), and diabetes mellitus. The stress and tissue destruction of severe burns, surgery, and major fractures may also cause a zinc deficiency. Conditioned deficiency also can occur secondary to sickle cell anemia, neoplastic disease, parenteral nutrition, and various drugs including corticosteroids, metal chelating agents such as desferrioxamine and penicillamine, oral contraceptives, diuretics, and various chemotherapeutic drugs.[23]

Acrodermatitis enteropathica is a rare, autosomal recessive condition of zinc deficiency secondary to a defect in intestinal zinc absorption. The onset is generally in infancy, but rare cases present in adolescence or adulthood. The disorder is often clinically recognized in infants by a skin rash that shows a characteristic, symmetrical acral and circumorificial distribution. Other major presenting features are failure to thrive, anorexia, irritability, alopecia, and severe chronic watery diarrhea. The clinical course is often complicated by acquired immunodeficiencies. In patients with onset at a later age, chronic skin disorders, neuropsychiatric changes, or a history of abnormal pregnancies may be the presenting features.[25]

Acute toxicity from zinc salts secondary to accidental ingestion of excessive amounts manifests as gastrointestinal irritation with fever, nausea and vomiting, diarrhea, and abdominal pain. Onset is between 20 minutes to 10 hours postingestion. Accidental ingestion can occur with consumption of acidic foods or beverages prepared in galvanized iron containers. Purposeful ingestion of excess zinc by food faddists accounts for most of the reported cases of zinc intoxication. Bloody diarrhea, vomiting, loss of reflexes, tremors, paralysis, and ataxia are the signs and symptoms. Also a sideroblastic anemia and neutropenia may result indirectly from zinc-induced copper deficiency.[27] Swallowing of caustic zinc chloride solutions can result in erosive pharyngitis and esophagitis, whereas elemental zinc intake causes lethargy.[24]

Zinc is used in the manufacture of white paint, rubber, glazes, enamel, glass and paper, galvanized iron and brass, and it is used as a wood preservative. Acute poisoning from industrial exposure to zinc oxide fumes causes metal fume fever with chills, nausea and vomiting, and muscular aches and weakness usually resolving in 24–48 hours. Inhaled zinc oxide may also cause pulmonary edema with cyanosis and dyspnea, dermatosis, and ulceration of the nasal passages. Zinc oxide dust and zinc chloride may cause eczema and skin ulceration, respectively. There is no evidence that zinc oxide inhalation has chronic manifestations.[24] Therapeutic intravenous administration of pharmacologic doses of zinc has been reported to result in profuse sweating, blurred vision, and hypothermia.[23]

Selection

At present, plasma zinc levels, although not ideal, are the best single choice for determination of zinc status in suspected deficiency states. Urinary levels are perhaps adequate for detection of toxicity.

Determination of zinc nutriture can be used to diagnose acrodermatitis enteropathica, nutritional or constitutional zinc deficiency, or zinc toxicity. Evaluation of zinc also is useful in assessing necessity of zinc replacement in patients on hyperalimentation, corticosteroids, or chemotherapy, and those with burns, malabsorption, nutritional deficiency, renal failure (patients on dialysis), sickle cell anemia, impaired immunity, and poor wound healing or tissue repair. In patients at risk for zinc deficiency, evaluation of zinc status should be performed prior to surgery and, if deficiency is found, treated to maximize wound healing.[23]

Logistics

Specimen

Zinc status can be evaluated by direct determination of the zinc content of hair, urine, erythrocytes, saliva, plasma, and serum; by functional assays involving zinc dependent enzymatic reactions; and by assessment of taste acuity. Although zinc deficiency may be demonstrated using the tests mentioned, no one test has proved to be a definitive indicator of zinc status. Because zinc levels are influenced by factors other than the absolute content of body zinc, there is difficulty in establishing reference ranges. Plasma levels show both circadian and postprandial variation, with highest levels in the morning and before eating; therefore, blood collection timing should be standardized. Serum values are 15% higher than plasma from heparinized blood. Hair levels may represent long-term zinc intake; but, because trace element concentration in the hair is influenced by a number of largely uncontrollable variables, hair analysis has little place in the analysis of trace metals including zinc.[28]

Urinary excretion of zinc is decreased in zinc deficiency but some zinc deficiency states such as alcoholic cirrhosis, viral hepatitis, sickle cell anemia, postsurgical periods, and total parenteral nutrition often result in increased excretion. Urinary measurement also is hindered by exogenous zinc contamination in the 24-hour urine collection, difficulty with accurate sampling, and the lack of established standards. Erythrocyte zinc content is decreased in the deficient state and associated conditions, such as malnutrition and sickle cell disease, but may be within the reference range in others, such as hepatitis, postnecrotic cirrhosis, diabetes, and pulmonary tuberculosis. Therefore, erythrocyte zinc does not have an established role in zinc nutritional assessment. Assays of erythrocyte zinc are only useful in adults, because in childhood there is a progressive rise in erythrocyte levels.

Zinc, found in the taste mediating protein gustin, is important in taste. Zinc deficiency can lead to hypogeusia but not all patients with hypogeusia respond to zinc and patients with severe zinc deficiency do not invariably demonstrate taste impairment. Therefore, neither salivary zinc levels nor tests for taste acuity have proven useful for assessment of zinc nutriture.

A few zinc dependent enzymes are found in the circulation and activity assays of these enzymes, especially alkaline phosphatase, have been used as indices of zinc deficiency. Unfortunately, these assays are nonspecific and affected by a number of metabolic conditions unre-

Table 10-9. Zinc Status in Selected Diseases and Conditions

Disease or Condition	Serum	Urine	Erythrocyte
Nutritional deficiency	Decreased	Decreased	Decreased
Hepatic cirrhosis	Decreased	Increased	Normal
Pregnancy	Decreased		
Oral contraceptives	Decreased		Increased
Chronic infection or injury (loss of zinc from catabolized tissue)		Increased	
Nephrosis		Increased	
Hepatic porphyria		Increased	
Acrodermatitis enteropathica	Subnormal		

lated to zinc status. Serum alkaline phosphatase, however, may be useful in conjunction with plasma levels of zinc. The carrier protein, metallothionein, in serum, urine, or erythrocytes may prove useful as index of zinc status, but the protein is difficult to assay in body fluids although assays under development may prove useful.[28]

Analysis

Either flame or electrothermal AAS is the method of choice for routine zinc determination in biologic samples.[29] Specimen contamination, as expected, is a problem and care must be taken in collection. Metal-free acid washed polypropylene tubes and containers are used for blood and urine, respectively.

Interpretation

Reference ranges vary widely probably because of specimen contamination. The reference interval has been given as 0.50–1.50 µg/mL (7.7–23.0 µmol/L).[30] In one study, serum levels measured by neutron activation analysis ranged from 0.69–1.21 µg/mL (10.6–18.5 µmol/L).[31] The 24-hour urinary excretion rate ranges from 110–600 µg/L (1.7–9.2 µmol/L).[24]

A fasting, morning plasma level of less than 0.7 µg/mL (10.7 µmol/L) is considered evidence of deficiency.

Plasma and serum values, as with other parameters of zinc status, must be interpreted with caution.[25,28] The plasma or serum zinc level correlates with the major carrier protein albumin and thus both are low in conditions in which there is hypoalbuminemia: at present plasma or serum zinc values cannot be interpreted in the presence of decreased albumin.[28] Decreases in zinc also occur with stress, infection, pregnancy, and oral contraceptive use.

Plasma zinc concentration in acrodermatitis enteropathica is usually reduced, but subnormal levels of plasma zinc are not invariable in the condition. In addition, many pathophysiologic conditions, as reviewed above, result in lowered plasma zinc levels. Ultimate diagnosis, in the face of suggestive clinical findings, may require observing the resolution and then the reappearance of the clinical findings after administration and subsequent withdrawal of supplemental zinc. Monitoring of the plasma zinc concentration and alkaline phosphatase activity during this process can be of aid in the diagnosis.[25]

A 24-hour urinary excretion rate of greater than 800 µg/L (>12.2 µmol/L) indicated toxicity,[24] but conditions that cause increased zinc excretion via the kidneys must be kept in mind. Table 10-9 summarizes zinc concentrations in selected conditions.

VITAMINS

INTRODUCTION

Vitamins or vitamers, compounds that interconvert to a common functional form or that can substitute for one another, are organic compounds required in the daily diet in amounts ranging from micrograms to milligrams per day (Table 10-10). These compounds can be divided into two categories based on their solubility in water or fat. The fat-soluble vitamins essential to humans are vitamins A (A_1 and A_2), D (D_2 and D_3), E, and K (K_1 and K_2). The essential water soluble vitamins are thiamin (B_1), riboflavin (B_2), nicotinic acid (niacin), pantothenic acid, pyridoxine (B_6), biotin, folic acid, vitamin B_{12}, and ascorbic acid (C).

Table 10-10. Recommended Daily Intakes for Essential Vitamins

Essential Vitamins	Recommended Daily Intake	Essential Vitamins	Recommended Daily Intake
Biotin (adequate intakes)	30–60 μg/d	Riboflavin (3)[f]	
Infant	35 μg/d	Men	1.4–1.8 mg/d
Adult	200 μg/d		(0.8 mg/1000 kcal)
Vitamin A (1)		Women	1.2–1.3 mg/d
Adult male	700 RU[a]	Pregnant women	1.5–1.6 mg/d
Adult female	600 RU	Lactating women	1.7–1.8 mg/d
Pregnant female		Vitamin B_6	
First and second trimesters	600 RU	Men	2.2 mg/d[d]
Third trimester	800 RU	Women	2.0 mg/d
Lactating female		Pregnant and lactating women	2.5–2.6 mg/d
0–5.9 mo	1000 RU	Niacin	
6+ mo	920 RU	Men, women, and children	9–19 mg/d[e]
Infants		Pregnant women	+2 mg/d
0–1 yr	375 RU	Lactating women	+5 mg/d
Children		Infants	
1–1.9 yr	375 RU	0–1/2 yr	6 mg/d
2–5.9 yr	400 RU	1/2–1 yr	8 mg/d
6–9.9 yr	500 RU	Vitamin C (6)[f]	
Vitamin E		Male	
Adult male	10 mg[b]	10–11.9 yr	30 mg/d
Adult female	8 mg	12–70+ yr	40 mg/d
Males		Female	
11–14 yr	8 mg	10–70+ yr	30 mg/d
Pregnant female	10–11 mg	Pregnant female	
Lactating female	10–11 mg	0–2.9 mo	30 mg/d
Children	4–8 mg	3–5.9 mo	+5 mg/d
Vitamin K (2)[f]		6–9.0 mo	+10 mg/d
Infants		Lactating female	
0–1/2 yr	10 μg/d	0.5.9 mo	+25 mg/d
1/2–1 yr	10 μg/d	6+ mo	+20 mg/d
Children		Infants	
1–3 yr	15 μg/d	0–11.9 mo	25 mg/d
4–6 yr	20 μg/d	Children	
7–10 yr	25 μg/d	1–9.9 yr	25 mg/d
Adolescents		Vitamin D (7)[f]	
11–14 yr	30 μg/d	Children	
15–18 yr	35 μg/d	0–18 yr	10 μg/d
Men		Adult	
19–70+ yr	45 μg/d	19–22 yr	7.3 μg/d
Women		>22 yr	5 μg/d
19–70+ yr	35 μg/d	Pregnant and lactating female	+5 μg/d
Pregnant women	+10 μg/d[c]		
Lactating women	+20 μg/d		
Thiamin (B_1)			
Adults	0.5 mg/1000 kcal		
Pregnant women	0.9 mg/d		
Older women	1.0 mg/d		
Young men	1.5 mg/d		
Young infants	0.3 mg/d		

[a] RU: 1 retinol unit = 1 μg all-*trans*-retinol or 6 μg all-*trans* β-carotene or 12 μg of other provitamin A carotenoids or 3.33 IUa or 10 IUc.
[b] α-tocopherol equivalents are based on the abundance and activity of all the tocopherols and tocotrienols in a usual mixed diet relative to that of the most active d-α-tocopherol.
[c] Indicates additional requirement.
[d] These recommended daily intakes are based on a protein intake of 100 g/d; requirements increase with high protein intake.
[e] Niacin equivalents (in mg) take into account the dietary tryptophan as well as niacin.
[f] Requirement per 1000 kcal of metabolism.

Laboratory Analysis

Vitamin nutriture can be determined by various direct or indirect laboratory techniques. Direct assays measure the vitamer in the blood, urine, or tissue. Indirect assays include levels of urinary metabolites of the vitamer; blood or urine levels of abnormal metabolic products resulting from a deficiency; measurement of changes in blood components or enzyme activity related to the nutrient; and load, saturation, and isotopic tests.[32]

The specimens most often used for assay are blood or urine. Both have inherent disadvantages. The blood

Table 10-11. Reference Ranges for Vitamin Nutriture

Vitamin	Range
Vitamin A	
Newborns	35–75 µg/dL (1.22–2.62 µmol/L)
Children	30–80 µg/dL (1.05–2.79 µmol/L)
Adults	30–65 µg/dL (1.05–2.27 µmol/L)
Biotin (4)	
Blood	820–2700 ng/L (3.35–11.0 nmol/L)
Plasma	330–722 ng/L (1.35–2.95 nmol/L)
Urine	11–95 ng/mg (5.1–44.0 nmol/mmol) creatine
Vitamin E (total tocopherols)	0.5–1.2 mg/dL (11.6–27.9 µmol/L)
Thiamin (transketolase)	0.75–1.30 IU/g Hgb
Vitamin B_6	
Plasma PLP (by radioactive tyrosine and apodecarboxylase)	5–23 ng/mL (29.9–137.6 nmol/L)
Urinary 4-pyridoxic acid (by HPLC)	0.8 mg/24 h (4.8 nmol/d)
Urinary B_6 (by microbiologic assay)	>20 µg/g (>13.5 µmol/mmol) creatine
Tryptophan load test (oral dose of 2–5 g)	near 25 mg/24 h (121.8 mmol/d) of urinary xanthurenate
Niacin	
Urinary excretion ratio of metabolites pyridone to methylnicotinamide	1.3–4.0
Vitamin C	
Plasma	>0.30 mg/dL (>7.0 µmol/L)
Whole blood	>0.50 mg/dL (>28.4 µmol/L)
Leukocyte levels	>15 µg/dL (850 nmol/L)
Urine	
Adults	8–27 mg/24 h (45.4–153.3 µmol/d)
Children	35–54 mg/g (28.5–34.7 µmol/mmol) creatine
Vitamin D	
25-(OH)D	
Serum	
Children	2–8 ng/mL (5.2–20.8 nmol/L)
Adults	8–45 ng/mL (20.8–117 nmol/L)
1,25-$(OH)_2$D	
Serum	
Children	19–70 pg/mL (48.3–177.8 nmol/L)
Adults	15–40 pg/mL (38.1–101.6 nmol/L)
24,25-$(OH)_2D_3$	
Serum	1.9–10.3 ng/mL (4.74–26.2 nmol/L)

Abbreviation: PLP, pyridoxal-5′-phosphate.
[a] These values are not considered reliable.[37]

levels of a vitamer are generally a reflection of recent dietary intake rather than a true indication of total body stores. Although urine is an easily obtainable specimen, standardization is a substantial problem and the question of the type of sample—24-hour collection, random, first voided, timed collection—must be answered with compromise in some situations. In a clinical setting, the most useful information is generally obtained from a 24-hour collection. Widely quoted reference intervals are listed in Table 10-11.

Methods used for the various assays have changed over the years as technology has become more sophisticated. Some older indirect methods of vitamin assays, such as microbiologic assays and functional assays with or without in vitro addition of the vitamer being analyzed, are being replaced by direct measurements of vitamers after separation by high performance liquid chromatography (HPLC). The change is welcome because microbiologic assays are time consuming, hard to standardize, and badly reproducible; and functional assays have problems in reproducibility and standardization. Also, antibiotics may interfere with microbiologic assays and concurrent disease states may cause changes in enzyme activity independent of vitamin deficiency.

TESTS FOR FAT-SOLUBLE VITAMINS

Test: Vitamin A

Background

The fat-soluble vitamin A has two natural forms, retinol (A_1) and 3-dehydroretinol (A_2), which are absorbed in the small intestine. The provitamin A, β-carotene, can be cleaved in the intestinal mucosa to retinal, which is then largely reduced to retinol. Retinol is then esterified with long chain fatty acids in the mucosal cells and transported with chylomicrons to the liver, which is the major storage organ. The important role played by the vitamin A vitamers in the visual cycle has been well delineated. In addition, vitamin A is a key component in reproduction, normal epithelial differentiation and growth, prevention of xerophthalmia, and immunosystem integrity.

Deficiency of vitamin A is common in underdeveloped countries, especially in south and east Asia. In the United States, it is one of three essential vitamins most likely to be available in marginal amounts in the diet, especially among certain groups including Mexican-Americans and alcoholics. Certain patient groups are also prone to inadequate or deficient levels. These include patients with cirrhosis and malabsorption (celiac disease, sprue, cystic fibrosis, obstructive jaundice, gastrointestinal surgery), chronic users of mineral oil laxatives, and patients undergoing plasmapheresis. The elderly in poor health are especially predisposed to deficient intake, but children up to 5 years of age are the most often affected.

An early symptom of deficiency is night blindness (nyctalopia). Xerophthalmia and keratomalacia represent effects of severe deficiency and may result in blindness. Usually the eye changes are accompanied by skin changes characterized by dryness, roughness caused by atrophy of sebaceous and sweat glands with follicular hyperkeratosis, white papules, dull scalp (phrynoderma), and severe acne.

Hypervitaminosis A syndrome results from excess dietary ingestion (e.g., consumption of bear liver) or inappropriate therapy. Retinoids are now an accepted, highly effective treatment for severe acne and psoriasis; unfortunately they are not innocuous, the major side effect being vitamin A toxicity. Aqueous emulsions prompt more rapid symptoms than do oily preparations. Symptoms of acute toxicity as a result of a single massive dose begin within 4 hours and include abdominal pain, nausea and vomiting, anoxia, severe headaches, dizziness, sluggishness, and irritability, followed by desquamation of the skin. Recovery occurs within a few days. Chronic toxicity results in a wide range of symptoms and signs covering many organ systems: some of these are bone and joint pain, hair loss, and hepatomegaly. The reader is referred to Silverman et al.[33] for a thorough discussion of hypervitaminosis A. Therapeutic or large daily doses are teratogenic. High levels of carotenoids can cause discoloration of the skin, but are otherwise harmless.

Selection

Testing for serum vitamin A content is used in screening for malabsorption, evaluation of vitamin A nutriture, diagnosis of hypervitaminosis A, and determining response to oral supplementation in patients with malabsorption.

Logistics

Specimen Requirements

The proper specimen for determination of serum levels of vitamin A (retinol) and β-carotene is fasting blood free from hemolysis and protected from light with an aluminum foil wrapping. The blood should be centrifuged promptly and the serum separated as soon as possible. Vitamin A and β-carotene are stable for about 2 weeks if serum is frozen at 20°C and protected from light. Specimen determination of retinol in liver biopsies is the best estimate of body stores[34] but other, more easily obtainable specimens are more practical.

Analysis

One assay method for determining serum levels of vitamin A and β-carotene is the colorimetric Neeld-Pearson procedure using trifluoroacetic acid, but it is tedious, imprecise, and nonspecific. Newer methods include a direct spectrophotometric method, fluorimetry, gas chromatography, and HPLC by the procedure of Bieri et al.[35] The HPLC method has a number of advantages over the other techniques and allows the simultaneous measurement of vitamins A and E. A bidirectional gradient elution technique for separation of vitamin A and carotenoids from serum extracts of small samples has recently been described by Ohmacht et al.[36]

Interpretation

Reference ranges for serum levels of vitamin A are given in Table 10-11. Levels increase slightly with age and values for men are about 20% higher than those for women. Levels above 30 μg/dL (1.05 μmol/L) indicate adequate intake, whereas those below 10 μg/dL (0.35 μmol/L) signal probable depletion of liver stores and emergence of clinical signs of deficiency.[37] Depressed levels are seen with fever, chronic infection, liver disease, and sprue. Serum levels are elevated by hypothyroidism, nephrotic syndrome, oral contraceptives, and other disorders of lipid metabolism. Although the serum level of vitamin A reflects dietary intake, the relationship between intake and serum level is not linear. Nonlinearity occurs because the liver releases vitamin A, when needed, to maintain serum levels as long as stores are present. Thus β-carotene levels more directly relate to dietary intake and are less useful as a measure of total body stores.

The reference ranges for β-carotenoids assay by HPLC after extraction in petroleum ether and iso-octane are 60–200 and 50–300 μg/dL (1.12–3.72 and 0.93–5.58 μmol/L), respectively. Depletion is seen in dietary deficiency and many cases of steatorrhea making the tests a useful screen for malabsorption. Elevation is found in hypothyroidism, dietary excess, pregnancy, and in poorly controlled diabetes with hyperlipemia. Rarely is elevation secondary to the lack of the intestinal converting enzyme.

Because serum concentrations of vitamin A do not invariably reflect body stores, the relative dose response (RDR) test has been advocated as a more true indication of vitamin A nutriture.[34] Intravenous or oral (in the absence of malabsorption) retinol preparations are administered and the plasma retinol level after 5 hours is compared with the level prior to vitamin delivery. The RDR is the percentage increase (increase/5-h value × 100). An RDR greater than 20% indicates low body stores; an RDR less than 10% is normal; and a value between 10 and 20% indicates low body stores; an RDR less than 10% is normal; and a value between 10 and 20% is not diagnostic.

Absorption Test

To evaluate intestinal absorption, the vitamin A absorption test has been used. An oral dose of a large quantity of the vitamin in oil is given and blood levels of vitamin A are determined at timed intervals from time 0 (fasting) to 12 hours after the oral dose. The mean rise in mucoviscidosis, sprue, biliary obstruction or atresia, and pancreatic insufficiency is 20 μg (0.7 μmol) with an oral dose of 180,000 U in oil as compared with a mean rise of 120 μg/dL (4.2 μmol/L) in individuals with normal absorption. However, the test is tedious and gives no more information than other tests for malabsorption. Recommended diagnostic tests for malabsorption are the 72-hour quantitative fecal fat test and the d-xylose absorption test.

Screening Test

Impression cytology of the conjunctiva is a recently described procedure for indirectly assessing vitamin A status that may prove useful as a screening test in countries with a high incidence of blindness related to vitamin A deficiency. Vitamin status is estimated by staging the degree of squamous metaplasia in the specimen.[38]

Test: Vitamin D

Background

Vitamin D_2 (ergocalciferol) and vitamin D_3 (cholecalciferol), which differ only by one side chain, are the two forms of the steroid hormone vitamin D used by the human body. The two forms are of equal potency and have the same mechanism of action. In humans, cholecalciferol is produced by natural irradiation of the provitamin 7-dehydrocholesterol in the skin. The previtamin undergoes thermal isomerization to form the prohormone-like vitamin D. Ergocalciferol is manufactured commercially from the plant sterol ergosterol by similar reactions. Both vitamers are used as food supplements, but the pharmaceutical form is usually ergocalciferol. Vitamins D_2 and D_3 are fat-soluble vitamins readily absorbed in the normal jejunum and carried to the liver in the lymphatics bound directly to chylomicrons. In the liver, hydroxylation occurs producing 25-hydroxy-D, which circulates bound to an α-globulin, vitamin D-binding protein (DEP). A second hydroxylation by 25-hydroxy vitamin D-1-hydroxylase (1-OHase) occurs in the kidney to create the active form of the vitamin, 1 α-25-dihydroxy-D. The kidney also produces other metabolites of 25-hydroxy-D, the most important of which is 24,25-dihydroxy-D. The active vitamin is carried in the blood to the target organs by DEP.

The final step in the production of the active hormone is regulated closely by a number of factors, including parathyroid hormone, plasma calcium and phosphate, calcitonin, and metabolites of vitamin D. When conditions such as hypocalcemia, hyperparathyroidism, and hypophosphatemia call for calcium mobilization, or if vitamin D deficiency occurs, the enzyme 1-OHase is stimulated to catalyze the synthesis of 1,25-dihydroxy-D. Estrogens, progestins, testosterone, growth hormone, and prolactin can also stimulate the enzyme. When calcium levels are within physiologic range or elevated, the synthetic pathways are switched over to 24,25-dihydroxy-D, a compound that does not play a role in the functions of vitamin D_3.[39] In healthy individuals with normal calcium balance, the plasma ratio of 1,25-dihydroxy-D to 24,25-dihydroxy-D is low. When calcium intake is impaired, the ratio becomes higher due to the increase of 1,25-dihydroxy-D and the decrease of 24,25-dihydroxy-D.

The hormone, vitamin D, has several biologic functions involving calcium homeostasis. It stimulates active calcium absorption by the small intestine, calcium resorption from bone in concert with parathormone, calcium reabsorption from the distal renal tubules, and intestinal absorption of phosphate. In addition, it stimulates differentiation of a variety of cells perhaps including osteoclast precursors. The net effect of vitamin D is to increase total and ionized plasma calcium and inorganic phosphate concentrations and to increase urinary excretion of calcium (increase in the filtered load of calcium is greater than the enhancement of calcium resorption). Vitamin D, although apparently not having a direct effect on bone forming cells, aids in bone mineralization by maintaining plasma calcium and phosphorus at levels that are supersaturating. These calcium levels also prevent hypocalcemic tetany,[39] a life-threatening condition.

Selection

Vitamin D deficiency and vitamin D malabsorption in patients with chronic hepatobiliary or gastrointestinal disease cause defective mineralization expressed as rickets in children and osteomalacia in adults. Failure of the organic matrix to acquire the hydroxyapatite mineral results in soft, pliable bones.[39] Poor dietary intake, perhaps of calcium as well as of vitamin D, coupled with inadequate exposure to sunlight lead to deficiency. The deficiency disease is less common than formerly, especially in the Western world, but the poor are still at risk. Signs and symptoms in children include poor growth, lethargy, proximal muscle weakness, hypotonia, delayed tooth eruption, bowed limbs and swollen joints, and pathologic fractures. Adults may present with poorly localized, dull bone pain, muscle weakness generally in the proximal muscles, and pathologic fracture.

Logistics

Numerous methods for single as well as multiple metabolites of vitamin D have been developed. Most of these assays require three steps: (1) extraction, (2) separation by HPLC, and (3) radioligand (competitive binding assay), radioimmunoassay, or ultraviolet detection.[40] Methods to detect multimetabolites are not recommended because of complexity, technical difficulties, and problems with performing the assay on plasma containing D_2 metabolites. Some of the assays that measure metabolites directly have limitations. Determination of 24,25-$(OH)_2D_3$ in plasma by competitive protein-binding assay is not suitable if the patient is receiving large doses of vitamin D_2. The determination of vitamin D in plasma by ultraviolet detection is sensitive enough for patients receiving large doses of vitamin D but is not sensitive enough for patients who are not receiving therapeutic supplementation.[40]

Interpretation

Three stages of deficiency in children can be distinguished by laboratory parameters and bony changes on radiographs (Table 10-12).[41] The most practical parameter for confirmation of a clinical suspicion of deficiency is plasma 25-hydroxy-D, which is low or undetectable in all stages of vitamin D deficiency. Measurement of vitamin D metabolites is also useful to monitor compliance in patients being treated with vitamin D supplements and to determine vitamin D absorption and its half-life.

A number of inherited defects in vitamin D metabolism and function are known, most of which have abnormal

Table 10-12. Laboratory Evaluation of the Stage of Vitamin D Deficiency

Stage	TC	PTH	UP	PP	Amino-aciduria	1,25-(OH)$_2$D	25-(OH)D	Radiograph
I	D	N	N	N	—	N/I	LO	Minimal change
II	N	I	I	D	+	LO/—	LO/—	Classic lesions[a]
III	D	I	I	D	+	LO/—	LO/—	Widespread lesions

Abbreviations: TC, total calcium; PTH, parathyroid hormone; UP, urinary phosphate; PP, plasma phosphate; D, decreased; N, normal; I, increased; LO, low.

[a] Generalized rarefaction and increase in trabecular markings without involvement of the vetebral column; localized pseudofractures (Looser's zones).

levels of 1,25-dihydroxy-D. The diseases represent defects in conversion of the prohormone to the active hormone, end organ resistance to the hormone, overproduction of 1,25-dihydroxy-D, or end organ oversensitivity to 1,25-dihydroxy-D. These diseases include X-linked hypophosphatemic rickets in children or osteomalacia in adults, type I vitamin D dependent rickets, pseudohypoparathyroidism, type II vitamin D dependent rickets, osteopetrosis, tumoral calcinosis, hereditary hypophosphatemic rickets with absorptive hypercalciuria, and Williams syndrome. Comparison of the types of vitamin D dependent rickets is seen in Table 10-13.

Low levels of both major metabolites of vitamin D imply either dietary deficiency, lack of exposure to sunlight, or malabsorption. Vitamin D deficiency and osteomalacia also may occur in rheumatoid arthritis.[42] However, the diagnosis must be made by bone biopsy, because 25-hydroxy-D levels and other laboratory parameters of bone disease are not discriminatory. Low levels of 25-hydroxy-D and abnormal levels of calcium, phosphate, and alkaline phosphatase are common in nonosteomalacia rheumatoid patients.[42] Low levels of 25-hydroxy-D with 1,25-dihydroxy-D low or within the reference interval may be a feature of the nephrotic syndrome because of urinary loss of the DEP-vitamin D complex. Anticonvulsants, especially phenytoin, impair hepatic conversion to 25-hydroxy-D with or without bone disease. The 1,25-dihyroxy-D may be within the reference interval. Conditions that may cause a high 1,25-dihydroxy-D with 25-hydroxy-D within the reference interval are shown in Table 10-14.

Excessive exposure to sunlight or ultraviolet light and/or excessive intake of vitamin D may lead to toxicity from 25-hydroxy-D, which has hormonal action at high levels.[43] This occurs because the production of 25-hydroxy-D is unregulated, whereas regulatory mechanisms stabilize the levels of 1,25-dihydroxy-D. Also the monohydroxy vitamin has a much longer half-life than the dihydroxy form. Hypervitaminosis may result from unregulated conversion of vitamin D to its active metabolites as in lymphoma or sarcoidosis.[39,44] The result of hypervitaminosis D is hypercalcemia and abnormal bony mineralization (similar to osteomalacia).[45] Symptoms include skeletal pain, weakness, lethargy, headaches, nausea, and polyuria. Nephrocalcinosis and calcification in ligaments and tendons may occur.

Test: Vitamin E

Background

The most active form of vitamin E, d-α-tocopherol, is one of this vitamin's eight fat-soluble vitamers. The vitamin is absorbed from the small intestine with the aid of bile and transported from the intestine to the systemic circulation via the lymphatic system incorporated in chylomicrons and very low density lipoproteins. In the body, vitamin E is stored in diverse tissues, but especially adipose tissue, and acts as an antioxidant for polyunsaturated fatty acyl parts of membrane phospholipids, including red blood cell (RBC) membranes. The vitamin also plays an important role in the maintenance of normal neurologic structure and function.[46]

Table 10-13. Comparison of Vitamin D Dependent Rickets Types I and II

	Incidence	Genetics	25-(OH)D	1,25-(OH)$_2$D	Defect
Type I	Rare	Autosomal recessive	Normal	Decreased	1-OHase
Type II	Rare	Autosomal recessive	Normal	Raised	Cytosol receptor deficiency

Table 10-14. Vitamin D Metabolites in Disease

25-(OH)D	1,25-(OH)$_2$D	Diseases or Conditions
Low	Low	Deficient supply of vitamin D
		Malabsorptive intestinal disease
		Cholestatic liver disease
Low	Normal or low	Nephrotic syndrome
Low	Normal	Phenobarbital or phenytoin therapy
Normal	Low	1-Hydroxylase deficiency: (1) chronic kidney disease; (2) VDDR; (3) senile osteoporosis[39]
		Hypoparathyroidism
		Pseudohypoparathyroidism
		Tumor-induced hypophosphatemia
		Infantile hypercalcemia syndrome
		Osteomalacia associated with TPN
		Hypercalcemia of malignancy
Normal	Elevated	1,25-dihydroxy-D therapy
		Pregnancy[39]
		VDDR II
Normal	Elevated	Hyperparathyroidism
		Renal calculi
		Sarcoidosis[39]
		Lymphoma[39]

Abbreviation: VDDR, vitamin D dependent rickets; TPN, total parenteral nutrition.

Selection

Testing for vitamin E status is useful for identifying deficiency and monitoring therapy in chronic vitamin E deficient patients. In childhood and early adulthood, vitamin E status should be estimated in patients presenting with spinocerebellar syndromes to screen for selective vitamin E malabsorption.[46]

Logistics

Specimen Requirements

Serum collected for vitamin E determination must be protected from light with aluminum foil wrapping. Measuring RBC levels of α-tocopherol may be useful in the clinical setting for diagnosing a lipid abnormality, but are generally not more accurate than plasma levels. α-tocopherol levels in a needle biopsy of adipose tissue may also be measured in special settings.[47]

Analysis

Older methods for analyzing α-tocopherol include the Emmeric-Engel color reaction after thin-layer separation, fluorimetric analysis, and gas chromatography. Medications that fluoresce will interfere with fluorimetric assays. The recommended method for quantitation of α-tocopherol in serum or plasma is HPLC using a reverse-phase column for separation and an ultraviolet detector. A new, highly sensitive and rapid HPLC method that separates α-tocopherol and its five oxidation products has been described using a normal-phase column for the separation, and an ultraviolet detector.

Red Blood Cell Hemolysis. The RBC hemolysis test that measures the stability of the RBC membrane gives an excellent indication of vitamin E status. Hydrogen peroxide (H_2O_2) is most commonly used as the hemolytic agent. Another commonly used method of hemolysis is autohemolysis but it is less sensitive, slower, and uses more blood than hemolysis induced by H_2O_2.[48] In the H_2O_2 hemolysis procedure, RBCs are washed in a 2–2.4% H_2O_2 solution for 3 hours and the amount of hemolysis is compared with that produced in distilled water. The result is expressed as a percentage.[49] The H_2O_2 test must be done under carefully controlled conditions in regard to sample handling; time lag between collection and actual test performance; preparation of reagents; and incubation temperature.[49] Ideal evaluation would include assessment of the degree of erythrocyte hemolysis in addition to the measurement of plasma α-tocopherol.

Interpretation

Table 10-15 shows the reference ranges for serum α-tocopherol and red blood cell hemolysis. Vitamin E deficiency in premature infants with high polyunsaturated fatty acid intakes has been associated with hemolytic anemia occurring at 1–2 months of age. However,

Table 10-15. Vitamin E Data (Tentative Guidelines)

Vitamin E Status	Serum α-Tocopherol Level (mg/dL [mmol/L])	Red Blood Cell Hydrogen Peroxide Hemolysis (%)
Deficient	<0.50 (<0.12)	>20
Low	0.50–0.70 (0.12–0.17)	10–20
Reference	>0.70 (>0.17)	<10

(Adapted from Sauberlich et al.,[49] with permission.)

there is no clear evidence that vitamin E supplementation improves hemoglobin levels or lowers bilirubin in premature infants. With current feeding practices and formula formulations, vitamin E deficiency anemia is a rare problem and pharmacologic levels of vitamin E are not required for prevention of hemolytic anemia in the premature infant. Deficiency also can occur in children and adults with fat absorption disorders such as biliary atresia, cystic fibrosis, lymphangiectasis, and celiac disease. In abetalipoproteinemia, the vitamin is undetectable in plasma using routine methods of assay. The ataxia, absence of reflexes, posterior column dysfunction, and pigmentary retinopathy seen in conditions of malabsorption can be attributed to vitamin E deficiency.[46] A selective vitamin E deficiency state also occurs presenting with neurologic symptoms similar to those in abetalipoproteinemia.[46]

A variety of toxic effects associated with vitamin E administration have been noted in humans and other animals. These include irritation at injection sites, inhibition of platelet prostaglandin synthesis and decreased platelet aggregation, potentiation of coagulopathy due to vitamin K deficiency, inhibition of fibrinolysis, creatinuria, anti-inflammatory activity, and impaired wound healing. Toxicity, which develops from the intake of large quantities of vitamin E, has been seen in patients on anticoagulant therapy following myocardial infarction. The symptoms are malaise, intestinal distress, and ecchymoses. The pathophysiology of this effect of high vitamin E intake appears at least to be partly due to suppression of absorption of other fat-soluble vitamins, especially vitamins K and D.

Test: Vitamin K

Background

The fat-soluble, principal vitamers of vitamin K ("Koagulation" vitamin) are the phylloquinones (K_1 type) of plant origin and the menaquinones (K_2 type) of bacterial origin.[50] It is assumed that one-half of the body's supply of this vitamin originates from intestinal flora and the other half from the diet.[51,52] The recommended daily requirements take this assumption into account. The jejunum and ileum are the predominant sites of absorption. The presence of bile in the gut is required for absorption, as with other fat-soluble vitamins. The absorbed vitamin is transported primarily through the lymphatics bound to chylomicrons to the liver and then distributed systemically. Excretion is mainly in the bile as metabolites, but a small amount is eliminated through the urine.

Vitamin K is essential for the post-translational carboxylation of several γ-carboxyglutamic acid (Gla) containing proteins including the procoagulation factors prothrombin (II), proconvertin (VII), Christmas factor (IX), and Stuart-Prower factor (X); the thrombolytic factors, protein C and protein S[53]; and a bone protein, osteocalcin,[50,52] which may function in mineralization. The predominant sign of vitamin K deficiency, defective coagulation resulting in asymptomatic elevation of the prothrombin time or a hemorrhagic diathesis of varying degree, reflects its role in the synthesis of coagulation proteins.

Selection

In the face of a prolonged prothrombin time (see above), the differentiation of vitamin K deficiency from hypoprothrombinemia of liver disease is made on the basis of the prothrombin precursor which is elevated in vitamin K deficiency.[52]

Logistics

Vitamin K status is not conventionally assessed by direct measurement of the compound. Instead, an indirect measurement is done by assessing the activity of the vitamin K dependent coagulation factors VII, X, and II using the prothrombin time, a functional assay of the extrinsic coagulation pathway.

An alternative to measuring vitamin K is empirical treatment with vitamin K that will correct the prothrombin time if a deficiency rather than liver disease exists. Oral or intramuscular administration of 5–25 mg of K_1 should correct the prothrombin time within 8–24 hours, whereas slow intravenous infusion of 20–40 mg should correct it within 4–6 hours.[50]

Interpretation

Deficiency of vitamin K can arise in newborn infants resulting in hemorrhagic disease.[50–52] Newborns in the first few days of life are especially susceptible because the intestinal flora have not yet colonized the infant gut and early breast milk is low in vitamin K.[50,52] Also, newborns whose mothers are receiving hydantoin or other vitamin K agonists are especially at risk. Diarrhea and the antibiotics used to treat it exacerbate the deficiency. In adults, deficiency is uncommon in the general population requiring both dietary insufficiency and suppression of the intestinal flora or anticoagulation with a dicoumarol type anticoagulant. However, deficiency is common in the special settings of chronic fat malabsorption, obstructive jaundice, chronic diarrhea, long-term antibiotic or anticoagulant treatments, and cholestyramine therapy. Occasionally, depressed patients ingest vitamin K antagonists either surreptitiously to gain attention or in a suicide attempt.[50] As deficiency develops, factor VII and protein C activities decrease rapidly because of their short half-lives. The activities of IX, X, and II decrease more slowly.

Toxicity from the natural vitamin K vitamers apparently does not occur; however, the water soluble synthetic analog menadione (K_3) can lead to the formation of Heinz bodies in erythrocytes and hemolytic anemia. This can be a problem in newborns because of the potential for kernicterus.[50–52]

TESTS FOR WATER-SOLUBLE VITAMINS

Test: Biotin

Background

Biotin, also known as vitamin H, coenzyme R, protective factor X, bios II or IIB, and egg white injury preventative factor, is a slightly water-soluble vitamin that, in humans, is a prosthetic group of the following carboxylases: acetyl-coenzyme A (CoA), propionyl-CoA, 3-methylcrotonyl-CoA, and pyruvate. Therefore, biotin is important in fatty acid biosynthesis, propionic acid oxidation, leucine metabolism, and gluconeogenesis. Biotin forms a tight, stable, noncovalent bond with avidin, a protein found in egg whites. The avidin-biotin complex is presently used to advantage in numerous bioanalytic methods including immunoassay and gene probing, and the system is rapidly finding new usages in evolving technologies such as bioaffinity sensors, drug delivery, and nuclear imaging.

The symptoms of deficiency, whether dietary or enzymatic, are diverse but mainly involve central nervous system dysfunction and skin lesions. Symptoms include nausea and vomiting, anorexia, and pallor. Depression, hallucinations, somnolence, and a panic state may occur in adults. Infants may present with metabolic acidosis, organic aciduria, profound developmental delay, hypotonia, seizures, and ataxia. The skin manifestations in adults include dry scaly dermatitis around body orifices; dry, red oral mucosa; and glossitis. An unusual distribution of facial and subcutaneous fat (biotin deficiency facies)[54] may also occur. The skin in the early-onset inherited disorder presents as an ichthyosis or generalized seborrheic dermatitis. Diffuse skin lesions like arcrodermatitis enteropathica, scaly dermatitis, and alopecia, which may progress to alopecia totalis, characterize the skin findings in the late-onset type. The late-onset type of inherited disorder (see below) may also result in signs of an immunologic defect. The self-limiting seborrheic dermatitis in infants under 6 months of age that responds promptly to biotin therapy is due to a transient biotin deficiency.[55]

Selection

Measurement of biotin may be useful in patients on special diets (see below) or in those patients suspected of having an inherited defect. Biotin, widely present in nature, is found in many foods and is also available from the gut where it is synthesized by the intestinal flora. Therefore, dietary deficiency infrequently occurs, but may be seen in special situations including ingestion of large quantities of raw egg whites, chronic dialysis, and long-term administration of anticonvulsant medication.[56] Biotin deficiency is also the most common water-soluble vitamin deficiency associated with total parenteral nutrition. Inherited defects in the metabolism of biotin that are responsive to pharmacologic doses of biotin are of two types: neonatal or late-onset (onset around 3 months of age). Both are referred to as a biotin responsive multiple carboxylase deficiency.[56]

Logistics

Determination of biotin would rarely, if ever, be indicated, but there are several methods available. Quantitation using a tedious microbiologic assay involves addition of aliquots of hydrolyzed whole blood, serum, or plasma (to liberate the bound biotin) to a biotin deficient medium inoculated with a test organism. Growth is compared with standard curves developed from growth in controls containing known amounts of biotin. Standard values vary according to the method of hydrolysis and the organism used.[55] Other methods include isotopic dilution assays with avidin utilizing colorimetric determination[57] and the evolving technology of bioaffinity sensing.

Screening for biotinidase deficiency can be accomplished by a qualitative colorimetric functional assay of the enzyme in serum or on dried samples of whole blood spotted on filter papers. Further evaluation can be done by the quantitative determination of enzyme activity in peripheral blood leukocytes and fibroblasts by fluorescence detection, HPLC with fluorescent detection, or radioassay.[58]

Interpretation

The reference range for serum biotin is 200–500 pg/mL (819–2047 pmol/L). The neonatal disorder for biotin metabolism is caused by an abnormal holocarboxylase synthetase, whereas the late-onset type results from deficiency of the biotin recycling enzyme, biotinidase.[58] The two forms can be distinguished by clinical features, serum and urinary biotin levels, and by the fibroblast carboxylase activities[59] (Table 10-16). The late-onset type is inherited as an autosomal recessive trait with an incidence variably reported as 1:40,000–1:60,000.[58] Other inborn errors of metabolism that respond to biotin are β-methylcrotonylglycinuria and propionicacidemia.

Test: Niacin (Niacinamide)

Background and Selection

Niacin can be synthesized in humans using tryptophan as the precursor so daily requirement estimates take into account the dietary protein as well as the dietary niacin (Table 10-10). The bioavailability of niacin in foods such as cereals is questionable. The water-soluble vitamin is found in tissues as nicotinamide in nicotinamide adenine dinucleotide (NAD) and nicotinamide adenine dinucleotide phosphate (NADP). The excreted metabolites are N_1-methylnicotinamide (NMN or MNA) and N_1-methyl-2 pyridone-5 carboxamide (2-PYR). Numerous enzymes require either the coenzyme NAD or NADP. Most of these oxidoreductases are dehydrogenases. The glucose tolerance factor (GTF) also contains nicotinic acid (see discussion of GTF under cobalt). Niacin deficiency occurs in a variety of clinical situations including dietary deficiency or due to secondary causes such as Hartnup's disease (see below). Initial symptoms include the nonspecific complaints of anorexia, weight loss, abdominal discomfort, weakness, irritability, and inability to concentrate. As the deficiency continues the equally nonspecific manifestations of glossitis, stomatitis, soreness and pain in the mouth, and vaginitis appear. This is followed by a characteristic symmetrical, erythematous and scaling, chronic dermatitis occurring on sun exposed skin. Diarrhea and dementia, often with frank psychoses, also occur in those with advanced deficiency.[60]

Terminology

Niacin, nicotinic acid, and pellagra preventing factor all refer to the compound pyridine-3-carboxylic acid. Niacin also is used in a broader sense to mean nicotinic acid (NA) as well as nicotinamide and other active pyridine derivatives.

Table 10-16. Features Distinguishing Biotinidase Deficiency From Holocarboxylase Synthetase Deficiency

	Biotinidase	Holocarboxylase
Age on onset	3 Months	Newborn
Urine biotin	Normal	Low
Serum biotin	Normal	Low
Leukocyte carboxylase activities	Deficient	Deficient
Fibroblast carboxylase activities	Deficient	Normal

(Adapted from Wolf and Feldman,[59] with permission.)

Interpretation

The recommended test for niacin nutriture is a determination of the urinary excretion ratio of 2-PYR to NMN. This ratio is best determined by HLPC.[61] Normally, 20–30% of niacin in adults is excreted as NMN and 40–60% as 2-PYR; therefore, the normal ratio expected is 1.3:4.0. A value below 1.0 is considered an indication of deficiency. N_1-methylnicotinamide increases during pregnancy but is otherwise stable with age.[62]

Pellagra is the classic niacin deficiency disease traditionally associated with diets consisting primarily of corn, which is tryptophan poor and contains niacin in a bound state with poor bioavailability. The disease can be primary (caused by dietary insufficiency of niacin and tryptophan, usually in combination) or secondary (caused by the carcinoid syndrome or Hartnup's disease).[63] In the carcinoid syndrome, a large percentage of dietary tryptophan may be diverted for the synthesis of serotonin. Hartnup's disease is a genetic disorder with defective mucosal transport of several amino acids, including tryptophan. In addition, long-term alcohol abuse; treatment with isonicotinic acid hydrazide; some chemotherapeutic drugs, in particular 6-mercaptopurine; and excess dietary leucine or lysine can result in niacin deficiency, but is usually so mild as to be clinically inapparent.[60]

Pharmacologic levels of niacin are used to treat schizophrenia, other psychiatric disorders, and hyperlipidemia.[64] Intense flushing of the face and body and pruritus are reported in 90–100% of treated patients.[65] Also, hyperpigmentation and acanthosis nigricans may occur. Other effects include abnormal glucose tolerance, hyperuricemia, inflammatory bowel disease, and diarrhea. The drug is potentially hepatotoxic, generally causing mild increases in liver function tests, but fulminant hepatic failure has also been reported.[64] Acute toxicity to single large doses has also been reported to cause flushing and itching.[66]

Test: Riboflavin (Vitamin B_2)

Background

Riboflavin, also known as vitamin B_2, is a naturally fluorescent, heat-stable, light-labile compound that is an integral component of many flavoenzymes (i.e., coenzymes flavin mononucleotide [FMN] and flavin adenine dinucleotide [FAD]). Dietary flavins are converted to free riboflavin by intestinal enzymes before intestinal absorption, which occurs primarily in the proximal portion of the small bowel. The flavins are utilized in diverse oxidation-reduction reactions in metabolic pathways and in energy production via the respiratory chain.

Dietary deficiency of the vitamin is one of the most common vitamin deficiencies in the Third World especially where the staple is rice and the diet is poor in fresh vegetables, fruits, meat, and dairy products. The functional effects of this depletion are not known, but supplementation is recommended.[67] Negative nitrogen balance secondary to high carbohydrate, low protein diets can lead to increased urinary secretion and riboflavin deficiency. Riboflavin deficiency is often associated with deficiency of other water-soluble vitamins, thus symptoms of deficiency are not specific for this vitamin alone. An oculourogenital syndrome is described for the deficiency state, reflecting the location of the typical lesions. Angular cheilitis, atrophic glossitis (magenta tongue), conjunctivitis, and genital hyperpigmentation (resembling zinc deficiency) are typical lesions. Seborrheic dermatitis, although a less specific finding, can be seen around the nose, eyes, and ears. Anemia, usually microcytotic, is a late and somewhat variable finding. However, slow recovery of bone marrow following blood loss is seen in the early phase of deficiency. Anemia is probably not directly related to riboflavin deficiency, but rather to multiple interrelating deficiencies in which iron status and metabolism play a major role.[68] Personality deterioration and, with advanced deficiency, retarded intellectual development are also features of riboflavin deficiency. The flavins are generally free of toxic effects.

Selection

Riboflavin measurement, preferably the functional assay (see below), is indicated in patients suspected of having the vitamin deficiency.

Logistics

The vitamin is excreted in the urine primarily in the free form. Urinary excretion with either fasting, timed, or 24-hour collections can be determined either by direct fluorimetric measurement, HPLC-separation with fluorimetric detection, or by microbiologic assays. Erythrocyte riboflavin also can be determined by fluorimetry or microbiologic assay, although the sensitivity and interpretation of results is difficult because of the small difference between adequate and inadequate levels. Plasma levels using older techniques reflect recent intake and are too variable to be of much use, although a new method determining riboflavin as FAD and FMN by HPLC separation and ultraviolet quantitation has been described. This method measures riboflavin simultaneously with vitamins B_1 and B_6 in serum or whole blood.[69]

Interpretation

In adults with sufficient riboflavin intake, more than 120 μg/24 h (>320 μmol/d) or 80 μg/g (24.2 μmol/mmol) of creatinine is excreted. Results of urinary riboflavin measurement can be altered by physical activity, environmental stress, temperature, certain therapeutic drugs, and nitrogen balance making interpretation of the results difficult especially in the marginally deficient patient. Sensitivity can be somewhat improved by utilizing a load return test, if indicated. In adults given an oral 5 mg dose of riboflavin, less than 1000 μg/4 h (2660 μmol/4 h) and 1000–1399 μg/4 h (2660–3720 μmol/4 h) of urinary riboflavin indicates deficient and low body stores, respectively.[70] The load test should not be used without other parameters of riboflavin status. Erythrocyte riboflavin levels below 15 μg/dL (0.40 μmol/L) of cells certainly represent a low or deficient state.

Functional Assay

The most commonly used test, which is highly specific for variations in riboflavin status and requires only very small amounts of venous blood collected in heparin, is a functional assay. The assay is based on the determination of FAD dependent glutathione reductase activity in freshly lysed erythrocytes with and without addition of FAD. The results are reported in terms of erythrocyte glutathione reductase activity coefficients (EGRAC), which are calculated by dividing the activity with FAD by that without FAD (Table 10-17). An EGRAC of 1.0 means that addition of FAD failed to result in stimulation and, therefore, riboflavin is adequate. Although this measurement is the method of choice, it cannot be used in patients with glucose 6-phosphatase deficiency, because there is an increased affinity of the glutathione reductase for FAD in this disease. If indicated, a test evaluating another red blood cell flavin, pyridoxamine phosphate oxidase, can be used.[68] EGRAC values in adults, but not in newborns, with hypothyroidism are in the range associated with riboflavin deficiency.[71,72]

Test: Pyridoxamine (Vitamin B_6)

Background

Pyridoxine (pyridoxol), pyridoxamine, and pyridoxal are the three naturally occurring vitamers of the water-soluble vitamin B_6, each of which becomes phosphorylated in the tissues. Pyridoxal-5-phosphate is the most important compound, because it is the coenzyme form that participates in the numerous B_6 dependent reactions. The majority of the B_6 enzymatic reactions involve metabolism of amino acids (including tryptophan) and proteins, but some also participate in lipid and carbohydrate metabolism and in heme and sphingosine synthesis. All of the vitamers are excreted in the urine in small amounts, but the main catabolite, 4-pyridoxic acid, is found in high concentrations.

Possibly because of the diverse biologic activities of the coenzyme, there is not a well defined syndrome of B_6 deficiency. (Some of these are listed in Table 10-19.) Experimentally-induced deficiency results in a periorificial seborrheic dermatosis similar to that seen in zinc or vitamin B_2 deficiency.[71] Glossitis, cheilosis, dermatitis, and stomatitis may occur. In isoniazid associated deficiency, neuritis and diarrhea occur in adults, whereas anemia and seizures may develop in children. Markedly deficient patients may show irritability, weakness, depression, dizziness, peripheral neuropathy, and seizures. Infants and children typically present with diarrhea, anemia, and seizures. An increased risk of renal lithiasis occurs because of secondary hyperoxaluria produced by chronic vitamin B_6 deficiency. Pellagra-like manifestations may occur, because of a nicotinic acid deficiency induced by pyridoxine deficiency. Lack of response to nicotinic acid reveals the true diagnosis. Pyridoxine is not toxic at normally prescribed levels; however, a sensory neuropathy has been described in patients administered 2 g or more of the drug per day.

Logistics

Several methods for determining vitamin B_6 status are used (Table 10-18). The indirect measurement of the B_6 vitamers using a microbiologic assay reflects the

Table 10-17. Interpretation of Erythrocyte Glutathione Reductase Activity Coefficient

Reference range	<1.3%
Low	1.3–1.7
Deficient	>1.7

A value <1.4 has been used in evaluation of elderly patients.
(Adapted from Bates,[68] with permission.)

Table 10-18. Methods for Determination of Vitamin B_6 and B_6 Status

Method	Specimen	Compound Measured	Levels Indicating Deficiency	
Microbiologic assay: using *Saccaromyces uvarum*	24-h urine, un-hydrolyzed	Free B_6	Level µg/g Cr (µmol/mmol Cr)	Age (yr)
			<20 (<13.6)	Adult
			<30 (20.3)	13–15
			<40 (<27.1)	10–12
			<50 (<33.9)	7–9
			<75 (<50.8)	4–6
			<90 (<60.9)	1–3
Fluorimetric assay	24-h urine	4-Pyridoxic acid	<0.5 mg/24 h (<3.0 mmol/d)	
HPLC with fluorimetric assay	24-h urine		<0.5 mg/24 h (<3.0 mmol/d)	
L-Tyrosine apodecarboxylase assay (TDC assay)	Plasma	PLP	NL 5–23 ng/mL (20.3–93.2 nmol/L)	
Aminotransferase activity assay			Activity Coefficient[a]	
Aspartate (AST)	Blood		>1.5	
Alanine (ALT)	Blood		>1.25	
Tryptophan load test (net increase in excretion)		Xanthurenate	Load	Levels
	24-h urine		2 g L-tryptophan	>50 mg/24 h (245 mmol/d)
	6-h urine		5 g L-tryptophan	>25 mg/6 h (122.5 mmol/6 h)

Abbreviations: Cr, creatinine, HPLC, high performance liquid chromatography; PLP, pyridoxal-5'-phosphate; NL, normal.
[a] See text under riboflavin for explanation of activity coefficient.
(From Sauberlich et al.,[73] with permission.)

dietary intake but falls short of accurate estimation of vitamin B_6 nutriture and cannot be recommended for that purpose.[73] Fluorimetric assay or HPLC with fluorimetric detection of the major urinary metabolite, 4-pyridoxic acid can be performed. However, the excretion of the metabolite also varies considerably with age. This fact, plus analytic problems and inadequate investigation of the relationship between intake of vitamin B_6 and 4-pyridoxic acid make this test a poor choice as well. Pyridoxal-5'-phosphate concentration in plasma is usually determined by using the L-(1-14C) tyrosine apodecarboxylase enzymatic assay.

Interpretation

Table 10-18 shows the reference range for vitamin B_6 and related tests. Pure dietary deficiency is uncommon because vitamin B_6 is widely available in both plant and animal food sources, but food processing does cause vitamin loss. Hypovitaminosis B_6 does occur as a result of therapeutic use of certain drugs such as isoniazid (in genetically predisposed slow metabolizers of the drug), D-cycloserine, penicillamine, long-term L-dopa, and oral contraceptives. In addition, there are a number of vitamin B_6 dependency syndromes affecting specific vitamin B_6 dependent apoenzymes (Table 10-19). Patients affected by these syndromes do not manifest clinical or biochemical parameters of deficiency, but the conditions respond to administration of therapeutic doses of vitamin B_6. Measurement of erythrocyte alanine aminotransferase (ALT) or aspartate transferase (AST) activity provides a useful measure of B_6 nutriture, limited, however, by the wide variation in normal enzyme activity. In this indirect assay, an activity index or coefficient is calculated in order to minimize individual variation in transferase activity. This functional assay is similar to that used for riboflavin.

Tryptophan Load Test

The tryptophan load test involves oral loading of 2 or 5 g of L-tryptophan in adults (the larger dose increases the sensitivity) and 100 mg/kg body weight in infants and children. Metabolites of tryptophan excreted in the urine are then measured. Xanthurenic acid is the metabolite of choice because it is easy to measure. A 24-hour urine specimen is best but a timed 6-hour collection is adequate because most adults with an appre-

Table 10-19. Vitamin B₆ Dependent Syndromes

Condition	Defect
Pyridoxine dependent infantile convulsions	Poor affinity of apoenzyme glutamate decarboxylase for the coenzyme
Pyridoxine responsive hypochromic, microcytic anemia	Defect not well defined
Xanthurenic aciduria	Reduced affinity of mutant kynureninase for PLP
Primary cystathioninuria	Reduced affinity of mutant cystathionase for PLP
Homocystinuria	Decreased levels of cystathionine synthetase
Oxalosis[a]	Decreased carboligase (type I) or glyceric dehydrogenase (type II)

Abbreviation: PLP, pyridoxal-5′-phosphate.
[a] Pyridoxal decreases oxalic acid levels.

ciable deficiency excrete significantly high values in that time. Protein intake, exercise, lean body mass, individual variation, and circadian rhythm of tryptophan metabolism are all important variables that can affect the quantity of excreted metabolite in deficient subjects, but appear not to be factors in healthy individuals. Pregnant women and women on oral contraceptives may excrete abnormally high levels.[73]

Test: Vitamin B₁₂ (Cyanocobalamin)

Background

Cobalamin (Cbl), vitamin B₁₂, is carried in the blood bound to one of three proteins that migrate in the α-2 and α-2-β region on routine protein electrophoresis (see Ch. 17). These serum proteins are called transcobalamin I, II, and III. Transcobalamin II (TC II), which is derived from many sources probably including myeloblasts,[74,75] comes predominantly from the liver. It is probably an acute-phase reactant as well as the chief Cbl transport protein, binding 6–20% of the endogenous Cbl in a 1:1 ratio. This protein efficiently transports Cbl to the tissues from the gut or the liver. Transcobalamin I (TC I), primarily derived from granulocytes, appears to act as a passive reservoir. It carries 80–90% of the endogenous Cbl and slowly delivers Cbl from peripheral tissues to the liver. The function of the remaining carrier protein TC III, which is also derived from granulocytes, has not yet been well characterized but may also involve Cbl transport. The binders TC I, TC III, and Clb found in saliva, gastric juice, and amniotic fluid are collectively called cobalophilins (R-binders). They are immunologically identical but electrophoretically distinguishable.

Congenital deficiency of all the Cbl-binding proteins has been described but only TC II deficiency produces symptoms of clinical significance.[75] Congenital deficiency of TC II, transmitted as a recessive trait, has been proven in at least 27 cases.[76] Three different forms of the deficiency have been described by Frater-Schroder as listed by Rosenblatt et al.[77] These forms are (1) absence of endogenous B₁₂-binding capacity as well as low levels of immunoreactive TC II (the most common form); (2) lack of B₁₂-binding capacity associated with normal immunoreactivity; and (3) presence of TC II, which is capable of binding vitamin B₁₂ but which is nonfunctional. Initial symptoms, generally occurring within the first year of life, most often within the first month, include vomiting, pallor, and weakness. The patients generally have pancytopenia and megaloblastic anemia, but severe erythroid hypoplasia is present in a few patients. Neurologic disease including subacute combined degeneration of the spinal cord develops in some patients a few months after onset. In addition, some children have a severe immunologic deficiency[76] that responds to treatment with vitamin B₁₂ along with response of the hematologic and systemic symptoms.

Logistics

Levels of unsaturated vitamin B₁₂-binding capacity (UBBC), unsaturated TC I, II, and III, and total vitamin B₁₂-binding capacity (TBBC) are significantly lower in fluorinated plasma than in serum.[74] Also, heparin increases the apparent B₁₂-binding capacity of serum.[78] Parameters of serum Cbl binding proteins include TBBC, UBBC, and UBBC of the individual serum binders. Unsaturated vitamin B₁₂-binding capacity is a direct measure of the sites available for binding Cbl. Total vitamin B₁₂-binding capacity is generally a calculated number derived from the addition of serum vitamin B₁₂ to the UBBC.[74] Total UBBC levels can be determined by rapid charcoal assay as described by Gottlieb et al.[79] or by rapid, diethylaminoethyl (DEAE)-cellulose column chromatography as described by Retief et al.[80] The levels of the individual unsaturated binding proteins are assayed by a double batch separation technique described by Jacob et al.[74] Radioactive vitamin B₁₂ is used in these assays and measurements are done by γ scintillation. A radioimmunoassay kit for TC II is also available.[81] Cobalophilins from sources other than serum can be detected by gel filtration and DEAE-cellulose column chromatography.

Interpretation

Normally, the TBBC is approximately one-third saturated and the UBBC is 80% β-globulin (TC II) and the remainder, α-globulin (corresponding to the R-proteins).[78] Decreased levels of UBBC with normal or elevated serum Cbl are seen in chronic leukopenia, aplastic or hypoplastic anemia, and erythroid leukemia with leukopenia. In pernicious anemia, the percentage of unsaturated serum R-proteins is typically increased by about 15% to one-third of the total UBBC, but the TBBC is low and serum Cbl is markedly decreased. As seen in Table 10-20, elevated levels of UBBC and TBBC occur in late pregnancy, liver disease, uremia, leukocytosis, acute myelocytic leukemia (AML), and myeloproliferative disorders. In all these conditions, except for late pregnancy and leukocytosis, the serum Cbl levels are also generally increased.

In the myeloproliferative diseases (chronic myelocytic leukemia [CML], polycythemia vera [PV], myelofibrosis with myeloid metaplasia, erythroleukemia, AML, essential thrombocytosis), the increase in Cbl and the TBBC is roughly proportional to the degree of leukocytosis. The same relative elevations, but more pronounced, occur in the UBBC.[78] In CML, this correlation holds true during the chronic phase but not necessarily during the blast crisis.[75] In AML, there is wide variation in the Cbl binding parameters that seems to roughly correspond to the French-American-British classification, with the most consistent and highest levels being found in M3 (acute promyelocytic leukemia).[75] The elevation in UBBC in both CML and AML is generally due to elevated levels of either TC I or TC III[75] as would be expected, because these proteins are derived from granulocytes. In one study of patients with refractory anemia with hypercellular marrow,[75] UBBC and TC II levels were significantly increased, but the number of cases was small. The finding of elevated TC II in some of the cases studied by Ghosh et al.[75] gives validity to the belief that myeloblasts may be a source of this TC.

Elevation of UBBC can aid in the differential diagnosis of PV from relative polycythemia because it rises linearly with white blood cell count and/or with white blood cell turnover in the former condition. The UBBC will be elevated in the majority of PV patients because the disease causes proliferation of myeloid as well as erythroid elements. The degree of granulocyte proliferation in PV may also be estimated by the rise in UBBC and levels of UBBC may be used to evaluate effectiveness of therapy as the levels will fall with effective treatment.[78] Also, CML may be differentiated from myeloid metaplasia in the case of a true Philadelphia chromosome negative CML by being more markedly elevated in CML.[75]

A recent, as yet unconfirmed, study indicates that the finding of decreased holotranscobalamin II (TC II + Cbl) may prove useful as an early diagnostic sign of negative vitamin B_{12} balance as seen in very early pernicious anemia or advanced type A atrophic gastritis.[82]

Table 10-20. Vitamin B_{12}-Binding Proteins in Various Conditions

Condition	Serum B_{12}	UBBC	IBBC
Late pregnancy	D	I	I
Liver disease	I	I	I
Myeloproliferative disorders			
Polycythemia vera	I	I+	I
Myelofibrosis	I+	I++	I
CML	I++	I+++	I+++
Leukocytosis	D	I	I
Chronic leukopenia	NL or I	D	I
Aplastic anemia		D	
Erythroid leukemia (with leukopenia)	NL or I	D	D
AML	I	I+	I
Uremia	slightly I or NL	I	I
Pernicious anemia	D+	D	D

Abbreviations: UBBC, unsaturated vitamin B_{12}-binding capacity; TBBC, total vitamin B_{12}-binding capacity; CML, chronic myelocytic leukemia; AML, acute myelocytic leukemia; D, mildly decreased; D+, moderately decreased; I, mildly increased; I+, moderately increased; I++, greatly increased; I+++, markedly increased; NL, normal.

Use of R-binders plus or minus TC II as tumor markers in carcinoma of the gastrointestinal tract especially for gastric and primary hepatocellular carcinoma has been proposed but not yet of proven diagnostic validity. Also monoclonal antibodies raised against R-binders have been used to stain tissue sections of various carcinomas of the gastrointestinal tract. The results suggest that raised levels of serum TC I found in some carcinomas is secondary to synthesis of R-binders by the tumor cells. Also, because four of four cholangiocarcinomas and none of nine hepatocellular carcinomas stained positively, a role for the antibody as an aid in differentiating these two primary liver tumors on the tissue level is suggested. Increased levels of TC II have been found in sarcoidosis,[83] lymphoproliferative disorders,[83] malignant myeloma,[75,83] macroglobulinemia,[83] Gaucher's disease,[83] liver disease,[78,83] lupus erythematosus,[81] and essential mixed cryoglobulinemia with glomerulonephritis.[81] In most of these diseases there is no clinical usefulness in this fact either for diagnostic or monitoring purposes. However, it correlated with the activity of the renal involvement in essential mixed cryoglobulinemia in one small series and may prove helpful on further investigation.[81]

Test: Thiamin

Background and Selection

Thiamin, also called thiamine, vitamin B_1, aneurin, vitamin F, and antineuritic vitamin, is a water-soluble vitamin that is somewhat heat labile. The vitamin is absorbed by active and passive transport in the small intestine, and phosphorylated in the liver into the active coenzyme, thiamin pyrophosphate (TPP). This coenzyme is required for oxidative decarboxylation of α-ketoacids and formation of α-ketols as catalyzed by transketolase. As a coenzyme for transketolase, thiamin is a catalyst in the erythrocyte hexose monophosphate shunt. Thiamin and its derivatives are also found in skeletal muscle, heart, liver, kidneys, and nervous tissue. Deficiency causes a rapid loss of the vitamin from all the tissues except brain tissue. The loss of erythrocyte thiamin pyrophosphate is proportional to the decrease in other tissues making erythrocytes a reliable specimen for assessing thiamin nutriture. Thiamin and its numerous metabolites are excreted in the urine.

Chronic thiamin deficiency leads to the disease beriberi, which has signs and symptoms involving the cardiovascular and peripheral and central nervous systems (Table 10-21). Pure dietary deficiency results from thiamin-poor diets, such as diets with rice as the staple, and diets including raw fish with microbial thiaminases. The most common cause of thiamin deficiency in the United States is alcohol abuse, which combines low dietary intake of thiamin with the inhibition by alcohol, directly or indirectly, on absorption and storage of the vitamin.[84] Other patients susceptible to thiamin deficiency are those with diabetes, cancer and other chronic illnesses, patients enduring long-term hyperalimentation or dialysis, and elderly, demented patients. A recent study suggests that a higher than expected level of marginal deficiency may exist in the United States.[85] Several inborn errors of metabolism respond to thiamin administration (Table 10-22).[86-90]

Terminology

The current method of choice for evaluation of thiamin status is the measurement of whole blood or erythrocyte transketolase activity with or without the addition of thiamin pyrophosphate. Synonyms for the test are

Table 10-21. Body Content of Trace Metals

Nervous system (dry beriberi)
  Dementia
  Anorexia and weight loss
  Peripheral neuropathy
    Characteristic features
      Symmetrical foot drop
      Tenderness of muscles and mild sensory disturbance over the outer aspects of the legs, thighs, abdomen, chest, and forearms
    Features frequently present (especially in alcoholics) but are characteristic of chronic diabetic polyneuropathy, pellegra, etc.
      Ataxia with loss of position and vibratory sense
      Burning paresthesia in the feet
      Amblyopia
  Wernicke encephalopathy[a]
  Korsakoff psychosis[b]
Cardiovascular system (wet beriberi)
  Anasarca
  Tachycardia
  Cardiomegaly
  Cyanosis
  High output heart failure
Childhood beriberi
  Age: 2–4 months
  Aphonia or characteristic cry
  Cardiac failure
  Abnormal deep tendon reflexes

[a] Acute onset of vomiting, fever, ataxia, progressive mental confusion leading to coma, bilateral sixth nerve weakness—ophthalmoplegia, or gaze nystagmus.
[b] Korsakoff's psychosis is the sequel to Wernicke's encephalopathy characterized by impairment of short-term memory.

Table 10-22. Thiamin Responsive Inborn Errors of Metabolism

Thiamin responsive anemia syndrome
Lactic acidosis due to defect in pyruvate decarboxylase
Intermittent cerebellar ataxia associated with hyperpyruvic acidemia, hyperphenylalaninemia, and hyperalaninemia due to a defect in pyruvate dehydrogenase
Branched-chain ketoaciduria due to defect in branched-chain ketoacid dehydrogenase system[a]
Subacute necrotizing encephalomyelopathy with lack of thiamin triphosphate in neural tissue (Leigh syndrome)[b]

[a] One of the four currently distinguished phenotypes of maple-sugar-urine disease.[94,95]
[b] Leigh syndrome is a pathologic diagnosis syndrome associated with several defects of oxidative metabolism. Recently there has been controversy concerning its association with lack of thiamintriphosphate.

thiamin nutritional status, transketolase, red blood cell transketolase, and thiamin load test.

Logistics

In the past, 24-hour or random (fasting) urinary levels of thiamin, measured by the thiochrome method or by microbiologic assay with *Lactobacillus viridescens* were used as a measure of thiamin nutriture.[91] The thiochrome method entails oxidation of thiamin to thiochrome with quantification by direct fluorimetric measurement or by fluorescence detection following HPLC separation.[92] However, because thiamin is a water-soluble compound, many variables influence the amount secreted and the information gained is primarily an indication of thiamin intake levels. Better information about actual stores can be gained from the thiamin load test. But other more reliable methods to assess the state of deficiency or degree of depletion of body stores have been developed.[91,93] One new method to analyze blood or serum is separation of the B_1 vitamers by HPLC with detection by ultraviolet light.[92]

The test is indicated when there is a suspicion of deficiency especially in the alcoholic patient and among those patient populations at risk, including the elderly. The test, as modified by Jeyasingham[84] (see Interpretation), may have a role in determining prognosis in demented and alcoholic patients.

A tube of heparinized blood drawn prior to therapy and transported on ice is required for the transketolase test. The test, an assay of transketolase activity, entails hemolyzing a sample of blood, incubating the hemolysate with ribose-5-phosphate, and measuring the substrate remaining and the product formed at timed intervals. Transketolase activity can be determined in terms of rate of substrate conversion or rate of product (hexoses) appearance. The sensitivity can be improved by performing the assay before and after addition of thiamin pyrophosphate (TPP), which optimizes the enzyme activity. The increase in activity is the TPP effect (TPPE).

The thiamin load test involves determination of urinary excretion of thiamin in a 4-hour collection after an intravenous test load of 5 mg.

Interpretation

Normal transketolase activity is 850–1000 µg hexose/mL hemolyste per hour. Reference ranges for TPPE as given in Table 10-23 distinguish between normal, mar-

Table 10-23. Reference Ranges for Thiamin Nutriture

Test	Range
Transketolase test	
Red blood cell transketolase activity	850–1000 µg hexose/mL hemolysate/h
Thiamin pyrophosphate effect[a]	
Normal	0–14%
Marginally deficient	15–24%
Severely deficient (with clinical signs)	≥25%
Thiamin load test	
Acceptable	≥80 µg (≥0.24 µmol)
Low	20–79 µg (0.06–0.23 µmol)
Deficient	<20 µg (<0.06 µmol)

[a] Classification of Brun et al.[8]

ginally deficient, and severely deficient. No differences are found between male and female.

In a study of 50 demented patients, 36 acute alcoholics, and 7 brain damaged chronic alcoholics, Jeyasingham et al.[84] found some of the specimens showed an increase of transketolase activation when the TTP concentration was increased from the standard 0.3 mM to 3.0 mM suggesting the presence of a variant form of the apoenzyme. They used their data to define and calculate three parameters:

1. STZ: specific transketolase activity in units per gram of hemoglobin.
2. PAR: the ratio of activity in the presence of 0.3 nM of TPP to the activity without TPP added.
3. FAR: the ratio of activity with 3 mM TTP to that with 0.3 mM TTP.

They found that the two parameters, PAR and FAR, varied independently and speculated that patients with an abnormally high value of FAR might be at higher risk of brain damage. Deficient persons will secrete less than 20 μg of thiamin after a test load (Table 10-23).

Test: Vitamin C (Ascorbic Acid)

Background

Ascorbic acid or vitamin C (antiscorbutic vitamin) is a strong reductant that can be synthesized by plants and some animals, but not humans. This ketolactone, resembling sugar compounds in structure, is highly water soluble, heat labile, and susceptible to oxidation when in solution. It is destroyed by cooking and exposure to air. The first two thirds of the small intestine provide the predominant site of absorption. Some absorbed ascorbic acid is oxidized to another active vitamer, dehydroascorbic acid (DHAA), thus both vitamers are present in plasma. Ascorbic acid is found in most tissues and body fluids, but in widely varying concentrations. Very high concentrations are found in endocrine tissue, especially the adrenal and pituitary. Both ascorbate and dehydroascorbic acid are excreted into the urine along with other inactive catabolites such as 2,3-diketugluconic acid, ascorbate-2-sulfate, and oxalate, which are present in lesser amounts. The predominant, perhaps unique, function of ascorbic acid is as a cofactor for the oxygen requiring hydroxylations important in the synthesis of connective tissue matrix proteins. Other reactions in which ascorbic acid may play a role, but perhaps not a unique one, include the metabolism of tyrosine, folic acid, histamine, and some drugs; the synthesis of carnitine, norepinephrine, and 5-hydroxytryptophan; the release of corticosteroids; formation of bile acids; and transfer of iron to ferritin. Roles for ascorbate in the complex reactions involved in leukocyte function, immune response, wound healing, and allergic responses also have been proposed, perhaps only as an electron donating bystander rather than as an essential cofactor for the reactions.

The classic disease of vitamin C deficiency is scurvy. The disease is now rare, but it can still be seen in persons with diets completely lacking in vegetables and fruits. The populations most scurvy prone are elderly men living alone and the very young; other factors are also frequently associated (Table 10-24). The full-blown manifestations are primarily a reflection of the vitamin's function as a cofactor in matrix protein synthesis. Early on in experimental deficiency, only general malaise, lethargy, and weakness may be present. Later, dyspnea and nocturnal aching in bones, joints, and muscles occur. Increasingly numerous hyperkeratotic follicles enclosing fragmented, corkscrew-like hairs develop especially on the back, buttocks, upper arms, backs of thighs, calves, and shins. Perifollicular hemorrhages then develop around the hyperkeratotic follicles, especially on the legs. Petechiae and later purpura on all hair bearing parts follow and ecchymoses may develop at points of pressure or trauma. Gum changes develop after 6 months of deprivation. The changes begin as reddening, swelling, and tiny hemorrhages of interdental papillae and progress, in some, to a purplish, hyperplastic gingivitis with focal necrosis and bleeding. In later stages of experimental deficiency, wound healing is impaired. Other signs of scurvy in an experimental setting include the sicca syndrome, joint effusions, neuropathy, and marked edema.[94,95]

Infantile scurvy (Barlow's disease) generally presents in the second half of the first year of life when the gestational stores are depleted. The lack of vitamin C results in defective collagen, osteoid, and dentin lead-

Table 10-24. Factors Related to Low Vitamin C Levels

Smoking
Alcohol abuse
Obesity
Oral contraceptives
Male sex
Severe stress
Acute infection
Chronic inflammatory disease
Dietary iron overload

ing to abnormal growth of tissues rich in collagen, especially bone. Irritability, tenderness of the legs, and pseudoparalysis are the dominate presenting symptoms. Bleeding may occur from the gums but skin hemorrhages are not common. Costochondral beading and subperiosteal hemorrhages, especially at the distal end of the femur and proximal end of the tibia, may be palpated on physical examination. The radiographic changes seen at the sites of most active bone growth include cortical atrophy, a "ground glass" appearance and osteoporosis, widening of the zone of provisional calcification, and increased soft tissue shadows. Bleeding dyscrasias and rickets are in the differential diagnosis.[95]

Symptoms and signs in the deficient adult are similar to those seen in experimental deprivation. Additionally, hemorrhages deep in muscles and into joints, extensive splinter hemorrhages in the distal nail bed, and loss of teeth secondary to infection superimposed on the bleeding, friable gums can occur in the late stages. Also, osteoporosis may occur, which must be distinguished from other causes such as senile and endocrine osteoporosis, multiple myeloma, and metastatic malignancy.[96]

Selection

Certain groups are at risk for biochemical ascorbic acid deficiency, if not symptomatic deficiency. These include smokers, alcoholics, the obese, patients under stress, patients with acute inflammatory conditions such as tuberculosis and rheumatic fever, and those with many of the chronic inflammatory disorders.[94,97]

Logistics

Specimen Requirements

Ascorbic acid can be measured in serum, plasma, whole blood, leukocytes, or urine. Venous blood samples are not acceptable if hemolyzed. All specimens must be processed quickly by the laboratory to minimize oxidation. As a determinant of vitamin C status, serum levels are more sensitive than whole blood levels, because the leukocyte contribution to the total falls much more slowly in the deficient state than do the serum levels. The higher concentration of ascorbate present in leukocytes compared with that in plasma or serum reflects the closer relationship of leukocyte levels to the body stores, whereas the plasma level represents current intake. Leukocyte levels are more difficult to determine, however, and require larger specimens.

Analysis

Several methods are available for determining ascorbic acid levels. The most commonly used assays are based on the reductive properties of ascorbic acid or formation of colored or fluorescent complexes with DHAA, which can be measured spectrophotometrically or fluorimetrically. These methods are plagued by problems with the stability of the ascorbic acid and poor specificity caused by interfering reducing substances and metal cations. However, one fluorimetric method and a method using L-ascorbate oxidase to oxidize ascorbic acid to DHAA coupled to production of ferrous ions and subsequent formation of a chromogenic complex apparently show sufficient specificity and sensitivity to be acceptable.[98] High pressure liquid chromatography with ultraviolet, electrochemical, or fluorescent detection holds promise as a sensitive and specific method for determining ascorbic acid and its oxidation products, but the ideal procedure has not yet been developed.[98] The main advantage of the chromatographic methods is that ascorbic acid is measured directly, but its stability is still a problem. Ideally, chromatography should be the method of choice for separating and quantitating ascorbic acid and its oxidation products but the procedure is at present quite complicated.[98]

Interpretation

Both serum and leukocyte levels are more reliable than urinary levels for assessing ascorbic acid nurture in nutritional surveys, because the reference range for urine is wide and the levels represent immediate dietary intake (Table 10-25). However, in the scorbutic patient, the urinary excretion would be expected to be

Table 10-25. Interpretation of Serum, Blood, and Leukocyte Levels of Vitamin C

Fluid	Level mg/dL (μmol/L)
Plasma	
Acceptable (low risk)	≥0.30 (17.0)
Low (medium risk)	0.2–0.29 (11.4–16.5)
Deficient (high risk)	<0.2 (11.4)
Whole blood	
Acceptable (low risk)	≥0.50 (28.4)
Low (medium risk)	0.30–0.49 (17.0–27.8)
Deficient (high risk)	<0.30 (17.0)
Leukocyte	
Acceptable (low risk)	>15 (852)
Low (medium risk)	8–15 (454–852)
Deficient (high risk)	0–7 (0–398)

(Modified from Sauberlich et al.,[94] with permission.)

Table 10-26. Loading Tests to Establish Tissue Ascorbic Acid Deficit

Test Name	Oral Dosage	Specimen Required	Interpretation
Saturation test of Lowry[99]	0.5–2.0 g divided over 24 h × 4 d	24-h urine × 4 d	60–80% test dose recovered with normal ascorbic acid status
Tolerance test of Dutra de Olivei[94]	15 mg ascorbic acid/kg body weight	serum 3-h postdose	<0.25 mg/dL (<14.2 µmol/L)

below detectable levels.[94] Also, in a scorbutic patient, ascorbic acid loading tests can be helpful in establishing a diagnosis.[94,96] One of these procedures, that of Lowry,[99] involves administering 0.5–2.0 g of ascorbic acid daily in small divided doses over 4 consecutive days and measuring the ascorbic acid excreted in the urine each day. In those with normal tissue saturation, 60–80% of the test dose will be recovered. Another loading test developed by Dutra de Olivei[94] involves giving an oral dose of 15 mg ascorbic acid/kg body weight. Serum ascorbic acid is determined 3 hours later. In patients with scurvy, the ascorbic acid will not increase above 0.25 mg/dL (14.2 µmol/L). These loading tests are summarized in Table 10-26.

Leukocyte and plasma levels are reduced in women taking oral contraceptives and in men when compared with women, pointing to a possible role of sex hormones in vitamin C status.[94] Also, it must be kept in mind that, whereas all clinical cases of scurvy have low or undeterminable plasma ascorbic acid levels, low levels do not necessarily indicate scurvy, but probably do mean increased risk for clinical deficiency. Patients with glucose 6-phosphate dehydrogenase deficiency and premature infants may be at increased risk for Heinz body hemolytic episodes.[100] In addition, diabetics with hyperglycemia may have an intracellular deficiency due to the competition between sugars and ascorbate for the same transport mechanism.

Patients with iron overload secondary to ingestion of alcoholic beverages high in iron content are at increased risk for scurvy and osteoporosis probably because of dietary deficiency and functional deficiency owing to oxidation of the ascorbic acid by the iron.[95] Excessive ascorbic acid ingestion is generally nontoxic, as the low renal threshold for excretion assures elimination of excess vitamin and the establishment of an upper limit for body stores. Plasma (and serum) levels of ascorbic acid rise in a linear manner as dietary ascorbate increases to around 60 mg/24 h (3.4 µmol/d) and the renal threshold of 1.2–1.4 mg/dL (68–80 µmol/L) is reached.[94] As intakes increase over 60 mg/24 h (3.4 µmol/d), more and more of ingested unmetabolized ascorbic acid is lost in the urine. However, gastrointestinal symptoms may occur with excessive ascorbic acid ingestion, along with more serious consequences including enhancement of iron absorption and development of dependency. Also, increased production of oxalate compounds the risk of renal calculi in stone formers.[97] High intakes of ascorbic acid may interfere with copper availability leading indirectly to elevation of serum cholesterol[97] and increased risk for atherosclerosis. Absorption of nickle and manganese also is decreased with high ascorbic acid intake. Large doses of ascorbic acid may result in hyperglycemia and symptoms of diabetes due to inhibition of glucose uptake by the sugar-like ketolactone.

REFERENCES

1. Clinical nutrition cases: Is chromium essential for humans? Nutr Rev 1988;46:17–20.
2. Kanerva L, Estlander T, Jolanki R: Occupational skin disease in Finland. Int Arch Occup Environ Health 1988;60:89–94.
3. Angerer J, Amin W, Heinrich-Ramm R et al: Occupational chronic exposure to metals. I. Chromium exposure of stainless steel welders—biological monitoring. Int Arch Occup Environ Health 1987;59:503–512.
4. Rinehart WE, Gad SC: Current concepts in occupational health: Metals—chromium. Am Ind Hyg Assoc J 1986;47:696–699.
5. Ichikawa Y, Kusaka Y, Goto S: Biological monitoring of cobalt exposure, based on cobalt concentrations in blood and urine. Int Arch Occup Environ Health 1985;55:269–276.
6. Shapiro R, Martin MT: Determination of cobalt by atomic absorption spectrometry. Methods Enzymol 1988;158:344–351.
7. Danks DM: Copper deficiency in humans. Excerpta Medica 1980;79:209–225.
8. Soo TL, Simmer K, Carlson L, McDonald L: Copper and very low birthweight babies. Arch Dis Child 1988;63:79–81.
9. Aggett PG: Inborn errors of trace metal metabolism. Br J Hosp Med 1987;38:190–196, 200–201.
10. Marsden CD: Wilson's disease. Q J Med 1987;65:959–966.

11. Ringenberg QS, Doll DC, Patterson WP et al: Hematologic effects of heavy metal poisoning. S Med J 1988;81:1132–1139.
12. Evenson MA: Measurement of copper in biological samples by flame or electrothermal atomic absorption spectrometry. Methods Enzymol 1988;158:351–357.
13. Brewer GJ, Hill G, Prasad A, Dick R: The treatment of Wilson's disease with zinc. IV. Efficacy monitoring using urine and plasma copper (42499). Proc Soc Exp Biol Med 1987;184:446–455.
14. Owen CA, Jr: Copper and hepatic function. Excerpta Medica, 1980;79:267–282.
15. Scheinberg IH, Sternlich I: Metabolism of trace metals. pp. 1321–1334. In Bondy PK (ed): Duncan's Diseases of Metabolism: Endocrinology and Nutrition. 6th Ed. WB Saunders, Philadelphia, 1969.
16. Donaldson J: The physiopathologic significance of manganese in brain: Its relation to schizophrenia and neurodegenerative disorders. Neurotoxicology 1987;8:451–462.
17. Sandstrom B, Davidsson L, Cederblad A et al: Manganese absorption and metabolism in man. Acta Pharmacol Toxicol (Copenh) 1986;suppl. 7:60–62.
18. Slavin W: Atomic absorption spectrometry. Methods Enzymol 1988;158:138.
19. Johnson JL: Molybdenum. Methods Enzymol 1988;158:371–382.
20. Robinson MF: 1988 McCollum award lecture. The New Zealand selenium experience. Am J Clin Nutr 1988;48:521–534.
21. Kok FJ, Hofman A, Witteman JCM et al: Decreased selenium levels in acute myocardial infarction. JAMA 1989;261:1161–1164.
22. Heese H, Lawrence MA, Dempster WS et al: Reference concentrations of serum selenium and manganese in healthy nulliparas. S Afr Med J 1988;73:163–165.
23. Ronaghy HA: The role of zinc in human nutrition. World Rev Nutr Diet 1987;54:237–254.
24. Calesnick B, Dinan AM: Zinc deficiency and zinc toxicity. Am Fam Physician 1988;37:267–270.
25. Aggett PJ: Inborn errors of trace metal metabolism. Br J Hosp Med 1987;38:190–196, 200–201.
26. Clayton BE: Clinical chemistry of trace elements. Adv Clin Chem 1980;21:147–169.
27. Ringenberg QS, Doll DC, Patterson WP et al: Heavy metal poisoning. S Med J 1988;81:1132–1139.
28. Hambidge KM: Assessing the trace element status of man. Proc Nutr Soc 1988;47:37–44.
29. Falchuk KH, Hilt KL, Vallee BL: Determination of zinc in biological samples by atomic absorption spectrometry. Methods Enzymol 1988;158:422–434.
30. Henry JB: Clinical Diagnosis and Management. 17th Ed. WB Saunders, Philadelphia, 1984.
31. Versieck J: Neutron activation analysis. Methods Enzymol 1988;158:267–286.
32. Sauberlich HE, Dowdy RP, Skala JH: Laboratory tests for the assessment of nutritional status. Crit Rev Clin Lab Sci 1973;4:215–217.
33. Silverman AK, Ellis CN, Voorhees JJ: Hypervitaminosis A syndrome: A paradigm of retinoid side effects. J Am Acad Dermatol 1987;16:1027–1039.
34. Amedee-Manesme O, Mourey MS, Hanck A, Therasse J: Vitamin A relative dose response test: Validation by intravenous injection in children with liver disease. Am J Clin Nutr 1987;46:286–289.
35. Bieri JG, Tolliver TJ, Catignanci GL: Simultaneous determination of alpha-tocopherol and retinol in plasma or red cells by HPLC. Am J Clin Nutr 1979;32:2143–2149.
36. Ohmacht R, Toth G, Voigt G: Separation of serum carotenoids and vitamin A on chromsil-amino and -cyano phases by a bi-directional gradient elution technique. J Chromatogr 1987;395:609–612.
37. Sauberlich HE, Dowdy RP, Skala JH: Laboratory tests for the assessment of nutritional status. Crit Rev Clin Lab Sci 1973;4:215–217.
38. Natadisastra G, Wittpenn JR, West KP et al: Impression cytology for detection of vitamin A deficiency. Arch Ophthalmol 1987;105:1224–1228.
39. DeLuca HF: The vitamin D story: A collaborative effort of basic science and clinical medicine. FASEB J 1988;12:224–236.
40. Fraser D et al: Calcium and phosphate metabolism. pp. 1357–1368. In Tietz N (ed): Textbook of Clinical Chemistry. Philadelphia, WB Saunders, 1986.
41. Fraser D, Kooh SW, Scriver CR: Hyperparathyroidism as the cause of hyperaminoaciduria and phosphaturia in human vitamin D deficiency. Pediatr Res 1967;1:425–435.
42. Ralston SH, Willocks L, Pitkeathly DA et al: High prevalence of unrecognized osteomalacia in hospital patients with rheumatoid arthritis. Br J Rheumatol 1988;27:202–205.
43. Elsas LJ, McCormick DB: Genetic defects in vitamin utilization. Part I: General aspects and fat soluble vitamins. Vitam Horm 1986;43:103–144.
44. Papapoulos SE et al: 1,25-Dihydroxycholecalciferol in the pathogenesis of the hypercalcaemia of sarcoidosis. Lancet :628–629.
45. Davies M, Mawer EB, Freemont AJ: The osteodystrophy of hypervitaminosis D: A metabolic study. Q J Med 1986;61:911–919.
46. Muller DPR: Vitamin E—Its role in neurological function. Postgrad Med J 1986;62:107–112.
47. Traber MG, Kayden HJ: Tocopherol distribution and intracellular localization in human adipose tissue. Am J Clin Nutr 1987;46:488–495.
48. Muller DPR, Harries JT, Lloyd JK: The relative importance of the factors involved in the absorption of vitamin E in children. Gut 1974;15:966–971.
49. Sauberlich HE, Dowdy RP, Skala JH: Laboratory tests for the assessment of nutritional status. Crit Rev Clin Lab Sci 1973;4:288–294.
50. Cecil: Textbook of Medicine. Philadelphia, WB Saunders, 1988.
51. McLaren DS: The vitamins. pp. 1315–1317. In Bondy PK (ed): Duncan's Diseases of Metabolism: Endocrinology and Nutrition. 6th Ed. Philadelphia, WB Saunders, 1969.
52. Elsas LJ, McCormick DB: Genetic defects in vitamin utilization. Part I: General aspects and fat soluble vitamins. Vitam Horm 1986;43:103–144.
53. Litwiller RS, Jenny RJ, Mann KG: Identification and isolation of vitamin K-dependent proteins by HPLC. Anal Biochem 1986;158:355–360.
54. Mock DM, Johnson SB, Holman RT: Effects of biotin deficiency on serum fatty acid composition: Evidence for abnormalities in humans. J Nutr 1988;118:342–348.
55. Bonjour JP: Biotin in man's nutrition and therapy—A review. Int J Vitam Nutr Res 1977;47:107–118.

56. Sweetman L, Nyhan WL: Inheritable biotin-treatable disorders and associated phenomena. Ann Rev Nutr 1986;6:317–343.
57. McCormick DB, Roth JA: Specificity, stereochemistry, and mechanism of the color reaction between p-dimethylaminocinnamaldehyde and biotin analogs. Anal Biochem 1970;34:226–236.
58. Bankson DD, Martin RP, Forman DT: A qualitative assessment of biotinidase deficiency. Ann Clin Lab Sci 1987;17:424–428.
59. Wolf B, Feldman GL: The biotin-dependent carboxylase deficiencies. Am J Hum Genet 1982;34:699–716.
60. Barthelemy H, Chouvet B, Cambazard F: Skin and mucosal manifestations in vitamin deficiency. J Am Acad Dermatol 1986;15:1263–1274.
61. Shibata K: Microdetermination of N_1-methyl-2-pyridone-5-carboxamide, a major metabolite of nicotinic acid and nicotinamide, in urine by high performance liquid chromatography. J Chromatogr 1987;417:173–177.
62. Sauberlich HE, Dowdy RP, Skala JH: Laboratory tests for the assessment of nutritional status. Crit Rev Clin Lab Sci 1973;4:284–288.
63. Scriver CR, Mahon B, Levy HL et al: The Hartnup phenotype: Mendelian transport disorder, multifactorial disease. Am J Hum Genet 1987;40:401–412.
64. Naito HK: Reducing cardiac deaths with hypolipidemic drugs. Postgrad Med 1987;82:102–112.
65. Knodel LC, Talbert RL: Adverse effects of hypolipidaemic drugs. Med Toxicol 1987;2:10–32.
66. Bartlett PC, Glenn Morris UJ, Spengler J: Foodborne illness associated with niacin: Report of an outbreak linked to excessive niacin in enriched cornmeal. US Public Health Reports 1982;97:528–560.
67. Lucas A, Bates CJ: Occurrence and significance of riboflavin deficiency in preterm infants. Biol Neonate 1987;suppl. 1:113–118.
68. Bates CJ: Human riboflavin requirements, and metabolic consequences of deficiency in man and animals. World Rev Nutr Diet 1987;50:215–265.
69. Botticher B, Botticher D: A new HPLC-method for the simultaneous determination of B1-, B2-, and B6-vitamers in serum and whole blood. Int J Vitam Nutr Res 1987;57:273–278.
70. Sauberlich HE, Dowdy RP, Skala JH: Laboratory tests for the assessment of nutritional status. Crit Rev Clin Lab Sci 1973;4:244–249.
71. Cimino JA, Noto RA, Fusco CL, Cooperman JM: Riboflavin metabolism in the hypothyroid newborn. Am J Clin Nutr 1988;47:481–483.
72. Cimino JA, Jhangiani S, Schwartz E, Cooperman JM: Riboflavin metabolism in the hypothyroid human adult. Proc Soc Exp Biol Med 1987;184:151–153.
73. Sauberlich HE, Dowdy RP, Skala JH: Laboratory tests for the assessment of nutritional status. Crit Rev Clin Lab Sci 1973;4:251–263.
74. Jacob E, Wong K-TJ, Herbert V: A simple method for the separate measurement of transcobalamins I, II, and III: Normal ranges in serum and plasma in men and women. J Lab Clin Med 1977;89:1145–1151.
75. Ghosh K, Mohanty D, Tana KS et al: Plasma transcobalamins in haematological disorders. Folia Haematol (Leipz) 1986;suppl. 6:766–775.
76. Cooper BA, Rosenblatt DS: Inherited defects of vitamin B_{12} metabolism. Ann Rev Nutr 1987;7:291–320.
77. Rosenblatt DS, Hosack A, Matiaszuk N: Expression of transcobalamin II by aminocytes. Prenatal Diag 1987;7:35–39.
78. Herbert V: Diagnostic and prognostic values of measurement of serum vitamin B_{12}-binding proteins. Blood 1968;32:305–311.
79. Gottlieb C, Lau KS, Wasserman LR, Herbert V: Rapid charcoal assay for intrinsic factor (IF), gastric juice unsaturated B_{12}-binding capacity, antibody to IF, and serum unsaturated B_{12}-binding capacity. Blood 1965;25:875–884.
80. Retief FP, Gottlieb CW, Kochwa S et al: Separation of vitamin B_{12}-binding proteins of serum, gastric juice and saliva by rapid DEAE cellulose chromatography. Blood 1967;29:501–516.
81. Biosca M, Encabo G, Garcia-Bragado F, et al: Transcobalamin II. A specific marker of renal involvement in essential mixed cryoglobulinemia. Nephron 1987;45:255–256.
82. Herzlich B, Herbert V: Depletion of serum holotranscobalamin II: An early sign of negative vitamin B_{12} balance. Lab Invest 1988;58:332–337.
83. Selroos OBN: Biochemical markers in sarcoidosis. Crit Rev Clin Lab Sci 1986;24:185–218.
84. Jeyasingham MD, Pratt OE, Burns A et al: The activation of red blood cell transketolase in groups of patients especially at risk from thiamin deficiency. Psychol Med 1987;17:311–318.
85. Lonsdale D: Red cell transketolase studies in a private practice specializing in nutritional correction. J Am Coll Nutr 1988;7:61–67.
86. Rotoli B, Poggi V, De Renzo A, Robledo R: In vitro addition of thiamin does not restore BFU-E growth in thiamin-responsive anemia syndrome. Haematologica 1986;71:441–443.
87. Murphy JV, Craig LJ, Glew RH: Biochemical characteristics of the inhibitor. Arch Neurol 1974;31:220–227.
88. Rosenberg LE: Vitamin-responsive inherited diseases affecting the nervous system. Res Publ Assoc Nerv Ment Dis 1974;53:263.
89. Pincus JH, Solitare GB, Cooper JR: Thiamin triphosphate level and histopathology—Correlation in Leigh disease. Arch Neurol 1976;33:759–763.
90. van Erven PMM, Gabreels FJM, Ruitenbeek W et al: Familial Leigh's syndrome: Association with a defect in oxidative metabolism probably restricted to brain. J Neurol 1987;234:215–219.
91. Sauberlich HE, Dowdy RP, Skala JH: Laboratory tests for the assessment of nutritional status. Crit Rev Clin Lab Sci 1973;4:236–244.
92. Botticher B, Botticher D: A new HPLC-method for the simultaneous determination of B1-, B2-, and B6-vitamers in serum and whole blood. Int J Vitam Nutr Res 1987;57:273–278.
93. Barthelemy H, Chouvet B, Cambazard F: Skin and mucosal manifestations in vitamin deficiency. J Am Acad Dermatol 1986;15:1263–1274.
94. Sauberlich HE, Dowdy RP, Skala JH: Laboratory tests for the assessment of nutritional status. Crit Rev Clin Lab Sci 1973;4:227–236.
95. McLaren DS: The vitamins. pp. 1310–1314. In Bondy PK (ed): Duncan's Diseases of Metabolism: Endocrinology and Nutrition. 6th Ed. Philadelphia, WB Saunders, 1969.

96. Shamash R, Laufer D, Tulchinsky V: Scurvy—A disease not only of historical interest. Br J Oral Maxillofac Surg 1988;26:258–260.
97. Chalmers AH, Cowley DM, Brown JM: A possible etiological role for ascorbate in calculi formation. Clin Chem 1986;32:333–336.
98. Tangney CC: Analyses of vitamin C in biological samples with an emphasis on recent chromatographic techniques. Prog Clin Biol Res 1988;259:331–362.
99. Lowry OH: Biochemical evidence of nutritional status. Physiol Rev 1952;32:431–448.
100. Ballin A, Brown EJ, Koren G, Zipursky A: Vitamin C-induced erythrocyte damage in premature infants. J Pediatr 1988;113:114–120.

11 Hormones

Peter J. Howanitz
Joan H. Howanitz

THE ANTERIOR PITUITARY GLAND

INTRODUCTION

The anterior lobe of the pituitary gland secretes growth hormone (GH), adrenocorticotropic hormone (ACTH) (corticotropin), thyroid stimulating hormone (TSH) (thyrotropin), follicle stimulating hormone (FSH) (follitropin), luteinizing hormone (LH) (lutropin), and prolactin. Anterior pituitary hormone secretion is controlled by the hypothalamic region of the brain, which produces releasing and inhibiting hormones, and by feedback mechanisms operating at both the pituitary and hypothalamic levels. The posterior pituitary gland stores and releases antidiuretic hormone (ADH) (also called vasopressin) and oxytocin. β-Lipotropic hormone is secreted by the rudimentary intermediate lobe as well as the anterior lobe of the pituitary. Pituitary disorders may be manifested by hypo- or hypersecretion of one or more pituitary hormones. Although many disorders of the pituitary cause hyposecretion of pituitary hormones, pituitary hormones are commonly secreted by pituitary adenomas (Table 11-1) and are produced ectopically by various tumors.

Laboratory assessment of pituitary function most often involves measurement of serum pituitary hormones by immunoassay. Because of normally occurring fluctuations in pituitary hormone secretion, it is often impossible to use a single random determination to delineate whether a patient has abnormal pituitary function. Therefore, serum sampling following stimulation commonly is used to delineate hormone deficiency and following suppression to determine excess hormone secretion. In other cases, assays of multiple serum specimens obtained during specific time frames or secretory products stimulated by the hormone in question are measured. Growth hormone, prolactin, and the pituitary stimulatory tests are covered under Tests of Pituitary Function. The other pituitary hormones in this chapter are covered under the gland for which they act as tropic hormones. The hormones related to diabetes mellitus are addressed in Chapter 7 and the hormones of pregnancy are reviewed in Chapter 15. Because measurements of oxytocin and β-lipotropic hormone are not commonly performed, they are not reviewed.

TESTS OF PITUITARY FUNCTION

Test: Growth Hormone (Somatotrophin)

Background and Selection

Until recently, GH measurements have been the main laboratory parameter used for determining GH deficiency and excess. Classically, the diagnosis of GH de-

Table 11-1. Classification of Pituitary Adenomas by Endocrine Activity
Growth hormone-secreting adenomas[a]
Prolactin-secreting adenomas[a]
Adrenocorticotropic hormone-secreting adenomas
Thyroid stimulating hormone-secreting adenomas
Follicle stimulating hormone/luteinizing hormone-secreting adenomas
α-Subunit-secreting adenomas
Nonsecreting adenomas
Plurihormonal adenomas

[a] The most common pituitary adenomas are growth hormone-secreting and prolactin-secreting adenomas.

Table 11-2. Changes in Growth Hormone Secretion
Decreases
Hypercortisolism
Hyperglycemia
Hypothyroidism
Growth hormone deficiency
Pygmies
Increases
Acromegaly
Exercise
Fasting
Gigantism
Hypoglycemia
Laron dwarfs
Liver disease
Malnutrition
Newborns
Protein ingestion
Renal failure
Sleep
Stress
Uncontrolled diabetes mellitus

ficiency is made using GH measurements following pharmacologic stimulation and GH excess is confirmed by failure of serum GH suppression following an oral glucose load. Insulin-like growth factor I (IGF I) (formerly called somatomedin C), however, is finding increasing use in the diagnosis and follow-up of patients with GH excess and deficiency [see Test: Insulin-Like Growth Factor I (Somatomedin C)].

Logistics

Using routine immunoassays, serum GH is undetectable for most of the day in healthy, nonstressed individuals. Additionally, discrete GH spikes normally occur making a single GH result difficult to interpret. To distinguish GH abnormalities from secretory patterns occurring in healthy individuals, stimulation of GH secretion is performed for suspected GH deficiency and suppression for suspected GH excess. Multiple blood specimens taken over specific periods are important in the diagnosis of neurosecretory GH defects. Most GH assays are performed with serum specimens, but recently, highly sensitive assays that allow direct measurement of the low GH concentrations found in the urine have become available.[1]

Interpretation

For most of the day, serum GH levels in healthy, nonstressed individuals are in the range of 0.025–0.7 ng/mL (0.025–0.7 μg/L), levels that cannot be detected by most routinely used GH assays.[2] In healthy individuals, 70–80% of results are below 1 ng/mL (<1 μg/L), but secretory peaks reach 20–40 ng/mL (20–40 μg/L).[3] Thus, in a child with decreased growth velocity, a low or nondetectable GH result may indicate GH deficiency or it may be a normal finding. Before the diagnosis of GH deficiency is made, physiologic or pharmacologic agents are used to stimulate GH secretion. In addition, it is now recognized that patients with neurosecretory defects in GH secretion respond normally to pharmacologic stimuli, thus peak GH levels greater than 15 ng/mL (>15 μg/L) do not exclude GH deficiency. In addition to the usual discrete secretory episodes, a number of physiologic conditions cause changes in GH secretion (Table 11-2). Thus, suppression tests are necessary to determine GH excess, which is usually caused by a GH-secreting pituitary tumor. In most patients with active acromegaly, serum GH levels fail to suppress following an oral glucose load.

Decreases

There is no simple, reproducible test to delineate normal GH secretion. Growth hormone response following physiologic stimuli such as exercise or sleep is often used as an initial screening test. Although blood may be randomly sampled during sleep, specimens taken under electroencephalographic control improve results because GH secretion occurs during stage IV (slow wave) of sleep. If GH fails to increase to greater than 15–20 ng/mL (>15–20 μg/L) with physiologic stimuli, pharmacologic stimuli are indicated in children who are candidates for GH replacement therapy. If an inadequate response occurs with one pharmacologic test, a second, but different, pharmacologic test is performed. If the child fails to respond to the second test, the child is referred for GH therapy. Common pharmacologic stimuli used include insulin-induced hypoglycemia, arginine infusion, and clonidine administration. Many other stimuli of GH secretion have been advocated including propranolol, L-dopa (levodopa), glucagon, prostaglandin E_2, and bombesin. However, diagnostic accuracy of the various tests and combinations of tests have not been systematically evaluated.[4]

Classically, failure of serum GH to reach 7 ng/mL (7 µg/L) or greater in response to at least two pharmacologic stimuli is defined as total GH deficiency, whereas attaining peak serum GH levels of 7–15 ng/mL (7–15 µg/L) defines partial deficiency. Although treatment is based on well accepted values for peak GH levels, considerable variation in GH results exists depending on the immunoassay used for measurement and thus criteria for confirming the diagnosis must be established accordingly.[5] Most GH deficient children have only a partial deficiency and show a moderate response to physiologic and pharmacologic stimuli. Many short, slowly growing children have normal GH responses to pharmacologic stimuli. With the recent availability of synthetic GH and the realization that stimulatory tests do not reliably identify all the patients who respond to GH replacement, criteria used to determine treatment eligibility are changing.

The term *GH neurosecretory dysfunction* is used to describe children who show low growth velocity, normal response to GH stimulation tests, reduced endogenous GH output, and growth in response to GH administration. Additionally, in some of these children the GH secreted may be biologically inactive. Some investigators believe these groups have not been sufficiently characterized and consider these children under the broad group of non-GH deficient short stature.[6] Endogenous GH secretion is assessed by measurements of GH levels in serum specimens collected every 20 minutes for 24 hours with the mean calculated from the 72 GH results. Because of the expense and inconvenience of determining endogenous GH secretions by the 24 hour mean method, investigators have tried other methods to delineate these defects including a shortened sampling time, 24-hour integrated concentrations (continuously withdrawn, pooled specimens), urinary GH, and IGF I measurements. Plasma IGF I levels correlate well with mean 24-hour GH concentrations[7] and recently urinary GH measurements have been reported to reflect endogenous GH secretion.[1]

In patients with pituitary tumors, GH deficiency is the most common disorder that occurs and thus GH levels usually are measured during an insulin tolerance test (ITT) in individuals suspected of having pituitary lesions. Decreases in GH secretion also occur in hypothyroidism and in the presence of hypercortisolism.

Increases

Considerable overlap in GH results exists between healthy persons and patients with acromegaly, because of the GH secretory spikes that are part of the normal GH secretory pattern. In most patients with untreated acromegaly, however, GH levels remain above basal levels throughout the day ranging from 10–100 ng/mL (10–100 µg/L). Serum GH levels in excess of 50–100 ng/mL (>50–100 µg/L) are virtually never seen in nonacromegalic persons.[3] Occasionally, clinical acromegaly occurs in patients with GH levels in the 2–5 ng/mL (2–5 µg/L) range, whereas some acromegalic patients have results greater than 1000 ng/mL (>1000 µg/L).[2]

Most cases of acromegaly are caused by GH-secreting pituitary adenomas, but a few are caused by ectopic production of GH releasing hormone. Although generally larger adenomas are associated with higher GH levels, correlation between serum GH levels and acromegalic manifestations is poor in treated and untreated patients. Patients suspected of having GH excess are assessed by measuring serum GH levels during a glucose tolerance test (GTT). Most patients with active acromegaly do not show suppression of GH during the GTT (GH does not fall below 2 ng/mL [2 µg/L]). Other diagnostic maneuvers, including administration of thyrotropin releasing hormone (TRH), gonadotropin releasing hormone (GnRH), or L-dopa are sometimes used, but testing with these agents is usually reserved for equivocal cases.

The pituitary adenomas that cause acromegaly tend to be invasive and thus are difficult to treat. A true cure of acromegaly is not easily achieved and controversy surrounds the definition of a "true cure." In assessing cure, some investigators believe baseline GH levels are sufficient, whereas others regard determining reversal of paradoxic responses to provocative agents as essential. However, abnormal secretory responses to provocative testing do not occur in all acromegalics (e.g., only 60–70% show increased GH with TRH administration) and may occur with other conditions (suppression with L-dopa also occurs in hypothyroidism, renal failure, and a number of other disorders). Generally, little progression of acromegalic manifestations occurs when serum GH levels are less than 5 ng/mL (<5 µg/L), but most patients do not show normal GH regulation with basal GH levels above 2 ng/mL (>2 µg/L).[2] Measurement of plasma IGF I (somatomedin C), which reflects GH concentrations integrated over time, is finding increasing use in the diagnosis and assessment of treatment of acromegaly and correlates well with mean serum GH results in acromegalics.

Short stature can occur in the presence of elevated GH levels, for example, in Laron dwarfs who lack GH receptors, which in turn leads to IGF I deficiency and poor growth. Sustained elevations of GH without concomitant acromegalic manifestations occur as a response to starvation, in anorexia nervosa, and in malnutrition secondary to cancer or chronic disease. Serum GH also increases with emotional and physical stress as well as in cirrhosis, renal failure, and uncontrolled diabetes mellitus.[2] In contrast, acromegalic manifestations can occur in the absence of elevated GH or IGF I levels. The cause of this syndrome, called acromegaloidism, is unknown.[8]

Test: Insulin-Like Growth Factor I (Somatomedin C)

Background and Selection

Measurements of IGF I, also called somatomedin C, have found increasing importance in the diagnosis and monitoring of patients with GH deficiency and excess. Measurement of IGF I also has been used to predict response to long-term GH therapy, to ensure adequacy of GH therapy, and may prove useful in assessing patients with nutritional disorders.

Terminology

Insulin-like growth factor I is the recommended nomenclature for the GH dependent peptide that is structurally related to proinsulin. In the 1970s, the term *somatomedin* was proposed for serum GH dependent factors that were then known by the operational terms *sulfation factor* and *thymidine factor*. After it became apparent that these factors were similar or the same as nonsuppressible insulin-like activity in serum (NSILA-S), the term *IGF* was proposed to replace the term *NSILA-S*. Moreover, it was recognized that NSILA-S actually contains two peptides, IGF I and another less GH dependent factor, IGF II. In clinical literature, the term *somatomedin C* was used for the GH dependent peptide that in the research literature was known as IGF I. Eventually a dual system of nomenclature was used, namely, somatomedin C (SmC)/insulin-like growth factor (IGF) written as SmC/IGF I or IGF I/SmC. In 1987, the recommendation was made to use the term IGF I and to reserve somatomedin for use as a generic term for both IGF I and IGF II.[9]

Logistics

Serum (or plasma) IGF I is usually measured by immunoassay. In the circulation, IGF I is found as part of a GH dependent complex with binding proteins. The major problem with the immunoassays for IGF I is interference from these somatomedin-binding proteins, which may bind label or interfere with binding of unlabeled IGF I. To overcome these problems, IGF I is separated from its binding proteins, for example, by acid gel filtration chromatography. Others have used high affinity antibodies to measure IGF I in plasma directly: the fraction measured generally provides a reliable estimate of the total IGF I. Changes in the amount of IGF I binding occur in nonchelated plasma or serum specimen depending on the amount of time the specimen is exposed to temperatures greater than 4°C. For the direct assay method, therefore, it is crucial to use ethylenediaminetetraacetic acid (EDTA) plasma in order to inhibit the cation dependent protease that changes IGF I binding.[10]

Interpretation

The reference range for total serum IGF I by immunoassay is variable depending on age.[11] In healthy adults, the reference range for IGF I is about 10–180 ng/mL (10–180 μg/L). As compared with adults, IGF I levels are lower in children until the age of 5 or 6, and are higher during adolescence, when IGF I levels show a stronger correlation with pubertal development rather than with chronologic age. In the aging adult, IGF I levels decrease corresponding with the diminished GH secretion that occurs. There is little fluctuation in serum IGF I levels during the day, but an approximate 30% decrease occurs following the onset of sleep.

Generally, plasma IGF levels can be viewed as an index of plasma GH levels integrated over time. Circulating IGF I is bound to specific serum proteins that are under GH stimulatory control. Changes in these somatomedin transport proteins influence serum IGF I results, magnifying increases or decreases in GH secretion; however, the relationship of GH, active IGF I levels, and growth may be obscured, at least in some clinical situations. Total serum IGF I levels may fail to reflect the activity of the free IGF I or its local effects. In addition, GH nutritional status is a major factor controlling circulating IGF I levels. Moreover, it is likely that IGF I is not the sole and final pathway of GH action as indicated by a number of observations including pharmacologic doses of somatomedins that do not equal the growth response obtained with small doses of GH.[2]

Decreases

Low IGF I levels are compatible with but, not diagnostic of, GH deficiency. Recently, IGF I measurements have been used to screen for GH deficiency, because levels within the reference range in a short child are strong evidence against GH deficiency. Usually GH deficiency is delineated by measuring GH levels following provocative testing such as the ITT or arginine infusion, but it is now recognized that the usual tests for GH deficiency do not identify all individuals who respond to GH replacement therapy. In patients with GH deficiency, there is a spectrum in response to provocative GH stimuli that ranges from no response to results that are essentially normal. Patients with GH neurosecretory dysfunction have normal responses to GH provocative stimuli, but abnormal endogenous GH secretion as demonstrated by blood sampling for GH every 20 minutes for 24 hours. Because this multiple sampling procedure is costly and inconvenient, other means of identifying patients with neurosecretory defects have been sought. Although GH provocative testing frequently does not correlate with endogenous GH secretion, plasma IGF I results correlate well.[7] Serum IGF I measurements also have been used during short-term GH administration as a predictor of the response to long-term GH therapy. When children are grouped to eliminate the influences of age and puberty, there is good correlation between percentage of increase in IGF I levels within the first 10 days of GH therapy and the benefits of a course of GH treatment.[12] Decrease in IGF I occurs in a variety of other conditions (Table 11-3) and can coexist with high GH levels (e.g., in Laron dwarfs and patients with kwashiorkor).

Increases

Because IGF I results accurately indicate GH secretion, they are useful for diagnosing and monitoring the progress of patients with active acromegaly. Insulin-like growth factor I results are a sensitive indicator of even mild GH excess and are elevated early in the course of acromegaly. In patients with untreated acromegaly, mean levels of serum IGF I are from 5-10 times those of healthy individuals and correlate fairly well with clinical signs and symptoms. In patients with acromegaly, there is an excellent log dose-response correlation between mean 24 hour plasma GH and IGF I concentrations.[13] In patients treated for acromegaly, IGF I levels do not fall into the reference range until GH levels are below 2 ng/mL (<2 μg/L).[2] Using IGF I levels, it may be difficult to distinguish a child with gigantism from a normal adolescent because adolescents normally have elevated levels of IGF I as compared with adults.

Assessment of Nutritional Status

Insulin-like growth factor I values correlate well with intake of protein and calories. Thus, IGF I measurements may be a sensitive marker of malnutrition and may be useful in monitoring response to nutritional therapy.[14]

Test: Prolactin

Background and Selection

Serum prolactin is measured routinely in patients suspected of having pituitary tumors because of the frequency with which these tumors are associated with hyperprolactinemia. Usually the larger the prolactin-producing tumor, the higher the prolactin levels, but microadenomas may also give rise to hyperprolactinemia. Because gonadal dysfunction is associated with hyperprolactinemia in both men and women, serum prolactin also is measured as part of the work-up of infertility.

Logistics

Serum prolactin rises in response to many physiologic factors including sleep, ambulation, exercise, protein ingestion, stress, and pregnancy. During lactation,

---

Table 11-3. Changes in Serum Insulin-Like Growth Factor I

Decreases
    Advanced age
    Children to age 5 or 6 years
    Chronic renal failure (method dependent)
    Emotional deprivation syndrome
    Estrogens (pharmacologic doses)
    Growth hormone deficiency
    Hepatic failure
    Hypothyroidism
    Laron dwarfs
    Pygmies
    Starvation
Increases
    Adolescence
    Growth hormone excess (acromegaly, gigantism)
    Pregnancy (last 20 weeks)
    Prolactin-secreting tumors

prolactin results may be increased or within the reference range depending on the length of time after parturition, but values rapidly rise in response to suckling. Ambulation causes a particularly pronounced increase in serum prolactin in women and in men treated with estrogens.

Interpretation

The usual reference range for prolactin is approximately 15–20 ng/mL (~15–20 μg/L) in men and up to 20–25 ng/mL (≤20–25 μg/L) (1 ng/mL equals approximately 20 mU/L) in women, but the upper limit of the reference range varies considerably among laboratories. The variation appears to reflect differences in defining the reference range.[15] Because of the many physiologic causes of increased prolactin, two or three specimens obtained at different times are used to assess whether the patient has hyperprolactinemia. Serum prolactin is increased in patients with prolactin-producing pituitary tumors as well as in other pituitary tumor patients owing to compression of the pituitary stalk. In addition to pathologic causes, increased serum prolactin levels occur in response to physiologic stimuli and pharmacologic agents (Table 11-4).

Decreases

There is a lack of recognition of decreased serum prolactin levels, perhaps owing to lack of study. At least in the nonlactating woman, the role of prolactin is not fully known. In addition, there may be few cases of prolactin deficiency because in contrast to other pituitary hormones, compression or severing the pituitary stalk leads to increased levels of prolactin by decreasing prolactin-inhibiting factor (PIF).

Increases

Some of the causes of increased prolactin levels are shown in Table 11-4. At least 30% of all pituitary adenomas are prolactin-secreting.[16] The degree of prolactin elevation correlates with the likelihood of the presence and size of a prolactinoma. Some patients with prolactin-producing microadenomas (tumor less than 1 cm in diameter) have serum prolactin levels less than 100 ng/mL (<100 μg/L), whereas those persons with prolactin levels over 300 ng/mL (>300 μg/L) usually have a prolactinoma.[17] An exception to this is patients with macroprolactinemia in which the predominating prolactin form has a molecular weight greater than 100,000 ("big, big form" of prolactin), which has only about 15% of the receptor activity of monomeric prolactin.[18]

Stimulation of prolactin secretion with agents such as TRH and chlorpromazine as well as suppression with L-dopa and bromocriptine has been used to distinguish patients with prolactinomas from other causes of hyperprolactinemia. Considerable controversy exists regarding the diagnostic value of these dynamic tests and none of the provocative or suppression tests are sensitive or specific enough to warrant routine use in differentiating the cause of hyperprolactinemia.

Treatment with dopamine agonists such as bromocriptine has lessened the importance of distinguishing a microadenoma from a so-called functional hyperprolactinemia (high serum prolactin in the absence of physiologic or pharmacologic cause and without a demonstrable adenoma), because therapy restores fertility in both patient groups and causes shrinkage of prolactinomas.[19] However, great care must be used in assessing the etiology of hyperprolactinemia, because dopamine agonist therapy is likely to cause a reduction in size only in these patient groups. Elevated serum prolactin can be caused by interference with PIF levels

Table 11-4. Hyperprolactinemia

Causes	Example(s)
Physiologic	Pregnancy, nursing Stress, sleep, exercise, food ingestion
Drug-induced	Antiemetics and antihistamines (metoclopramide, cimetidine [intravenous], sulpiride) Antihypertensives (methyldopa and reserpine) Hormones (estrogens, thyrotropin releasing hormone) Other (verapamil) Psychotropic agents (phenothiazines, butyphenones, opiates)
Intracranial disorders	Acromegaly Compression of pituitary stalk Empty sella syndrome Hypothalamic disorders Prolactinomas
Other	Chronic renal failure Cirrhosis Functional Hypothyroidism Neurogenic Nipple stimulation

because of pituitary stalk compression and is sometimes also associated with the empty sella syndrome. It is important to rule out primary hypothyroidism, which is frequently associated with hyperprolactinemia and sometimes accompanied by pituitary hyperplasia. In addition, approximately 20–40% of patients with acromegaly have elevated serum prolactin; the tumor sometimes is capable of producing both GH and prolactin or the tumor may cause PIF inhibition by compressing the pituitary stalk. Prolactin-secreting adenomas are associated with multiple endocrine neoplasia type I.

PROVOCATIVE TESTS

Test: Insulin Tolerance Test

Background and Selection

The ITT is the standard provocative test used to assess GH and cortisol response. (See p. 261.)

Logistics

The test is performed by infusing insulin intravenously. Glucose, GH, and cortisol are determined on serum specimens obtained before insulin administration and at 15, 30, 45, 60, 90, and 120 minutes after intravenous insulin infusion. The amount of insulin administered varies depending on a number of clinical criteria, but an adequate degree of hypoglycemia must be obtained in order for the test to be valid. The usual definition of an adequate challenge is the reduction of serum glucose levels to less than 40 mg/dL (<2.2 mmol/L), but others report that a decrease to less than 50% of basal serum glucose levels also is acceptable.

Interpretation

For the interpretation of GH levels and cortisol in response to the ITT, see Test: Growth Hormone (Somatotrophin) and Test: Cortisol (Compound F), respectively. Serum prolactin levels also normally increase during an ITT.

Test: Arginine Infusion

Background and Selection

Arginine normally releases GH; the main use of the arginine infusion test is to assess GH function in children. The test is used alone or following an ITT (arginine-insulin test).

Logistics

Arginine is infused after obtaining a serum specimen for baseline GH measurement. After arginine infusion, serum specimens for GH are obtained at 15–30 minute intervals for 1–2 hours.

Interpretation

For the interpretation of the arginine infusion test, see Test: Growth Hormone (Somatotrophin). In addition to GH deficiency, abnormal GH response to arginine can occur in a variety of conditions including hypothyroidism, hyperthyroidism, obesity, diabetes mellitus, starvation, and cirrhosis.

THE THYROID GLAND

INTRODUCTION

In healthy individuals, thyroxine (T_4) is the main thyroid hormone released from the thyroid gland, although L-3,5,3′ triiodothyronine (T_3) is secreted as well (Fig. 11-1). Following release from the thyroid gland, the thyroid hormones circulate attached to plasma proteins. About 70% of T_4 is bound to thyroxine-binding globulin (TBG), 20% to thyroid-binding prealbumin (TBPA), and 10% to albumin. By contrast, most of the T_3 is bound to TBG. A small percentage of the thyroid hormones remains unbound to protein and presumably these unbound hormones, or so-called free fractions, are the major active hormonal forms. Thyroxine undergoes metabolism in the peripheral tissues giving rise to the majority of the serum T_3 by deiodination. A portion of the T_4 also undergoes deiodination to 3,3′,5′ triiodothyronine (reverse T_3 [rT_3]). Both T_3 and rT_3 are further metabolized by monodeiodination (Fig. 11-2). Thyroid stimulating hormone controls the synthesis and release of the thyroid hormones from the thyroglobulin contained within the colloid of the thyroid gland. Thyroid stimulating hormone, a glycoprotein hormone synthesized in the anterior pituitary gland, is in turn regulated by the hypothalamus via TRH and by negative feedback of the thyroid hormones.

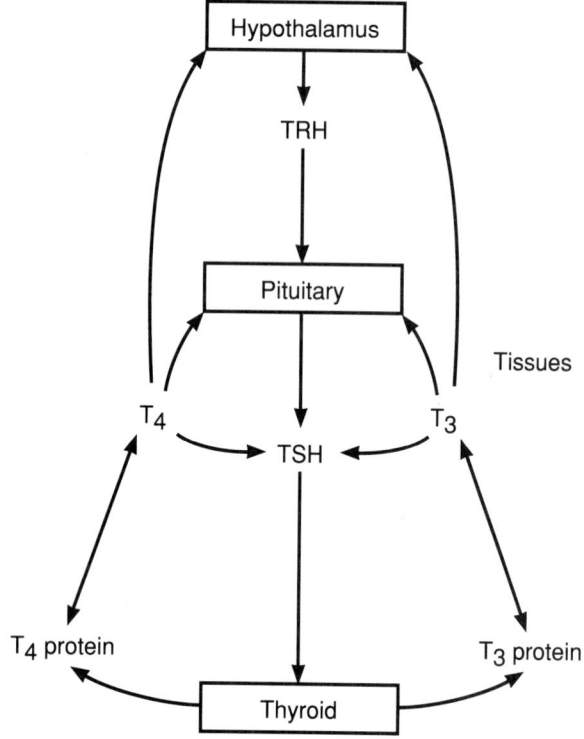

Fig. 11-1. Schematic diagram of the thyroid-pituitary axis. T_4, thyroxine; T_3, triiodothyronine.

Thyroid Disease

Depending on their metabolic status, patients with thyroid disorders can be classified into the functional categories of euthyroid, hyperthyroid, and hypothyroid. Patients with goiter as well as benign and malignant tumors of the thyroid gland often are euthyroid, that is, they have no metabolic abnormalities caused by an ex-

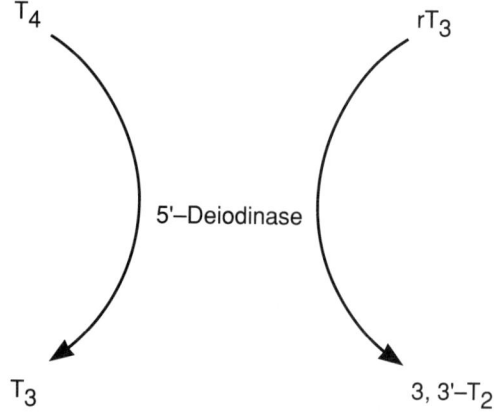

Fig. 11-2. Metabolism of thyroxine (T_4) and reverse triiodothyronine (rT_3) by 5'-deiodinase.

cess or deficiency of thyroid hormones. When tissues are exposed to excess thyroid hormone, hyperthyroidism results. Hyperthyroidism is most commonly associated with Graves disease, which is caused by circulating antibodies to TSH receptors. Hyperthyroidism also can occur in patients with multinodular goiter or adenomas and rarely is caused by TSH-secreting pituitary tumors. Hypothyroidism occurs when there is a lack of thyroid hormone action on tissue and most commonly results from a preceding, usually silent, thyroiditis. By destroying pituitary function, pituitary adenomas can cause inadequate secretion of thyroid hormones.

Screening Tests

Except in certain high risk populations, screening tests for thyroid disease are not recommended for persons who lack symptoms of thyroid dysfunction. When thyroid dysfunction is suspected, the clinician usually orders a thyroid screening test, which, until recently, has been the serum total T_4 test. Currently the most useful test to screen for thyroid dysfunction appears to be the so-called sensitive TSH assay, although patients with nonthyroidal illness (NTI) still present difficulties, and some clinicians suggest that this test is less cost-effective than other tests, such as total T_4. In certain clinical circumstances, serum T_4 levels are necessary for interpretation of TSH results. In most patients with hyperthyroidism, serum T_4, T_3, and free T_4 are increased, TSH levels as measured by sensitive immunoassays are suppressed, and the TRH test is blunted. In contrast, the opposite occurs in primary hypothyroidism, that is, serum T_4, T_3, and free T_4 are decreased, TSH is elevated, and there is hyperresponsiveness of TSH in response to TRH. A low TSH in an individual with clinical hypothyroidism strongly suggests a pituitary disorder (secondary hypothyroidism). A number of clinical situations can lead to difficulties in the interpretation of thyroid function tests. These include patients with abnormal protein binding of thyroid hormones and those taking drugs that can affect results of the thyroid function tests. However, the most important and common problem with thyroid function tests probably occurs in those individuals with various illnesses that do not directly involve the thyroid gland, so-called NTI.

Nonthyroidal Illness

A variety of illnesses not directly involving the thyroid or pituitary axis effect thyroid function tests. Although it is often particularly important to know the metabolic status of patients with NTI, thyroid function tests frequently fail to accurately reflect it. Serum T_3 levels are decreased in NTI (low T_3 syndrome), and in critically ill patients serum T_4 is decreased as well (low T_3, low T_4 syndrome). Free T_4 levels are variable depending on the severity of the illness and the method used for measurment. In patients with NTI, monodeiodination of rT_3 to T_2 is reduced leading to increased serum rT_3 results, but changes in rT_3 occur with thyroid disease as well. In individuals with NTI, TSH suppression occurs initially, then is followed by TSH rebound, with TSH levels finally returning to the reference range as the patient's clinical status improves. In some cases, the TSH rises above the reference range during the recovery phase. The situation is further complicated by a number of drugs that influence the various thyroid function tests (e.g., L-dopa suppresses TSH secretion).

Screening for Congenital Hypothyroidism

Screening programs have been developed for congenital hypothyroidism because of its relatively high incidence, lack of recognizible clinical features, and importance of early treatment. In developing screening tests, it must be recognized that thyroid function tests in the newborn yield results that differ from the adult reference ranges. Typically, TSH is elevated with the stress of birth and there are high circulating levels of T_4 and T_3 secondary to elevated TBG levels. In addition, results of thyroid function tests differ depending on the maturity of the infant; for example, premature infants tend to have lower serum T_4 results than full term infants (Fig. 11-3).[20]

The number of false positive results and the detection rate vary depending on the screening tests used and the timing of specimen collection. Because of the transient hypothyroxinemia of preterm infants, screening for congenital hypothyroidism with T_4 alone gives unacceptably high false positive rates of 2–3%. Because of the transient TSH elevation that peaks shortly following birth, early collection of blood specimens can cause false positive TSH screening test results.[21] Measurement of T_4 and TSH together have the advantage of detecting patients with pituitary and hypothalamic hypothyroidism, which represent about 3–5% of detected cases of congenital hypothyroidism.[22]

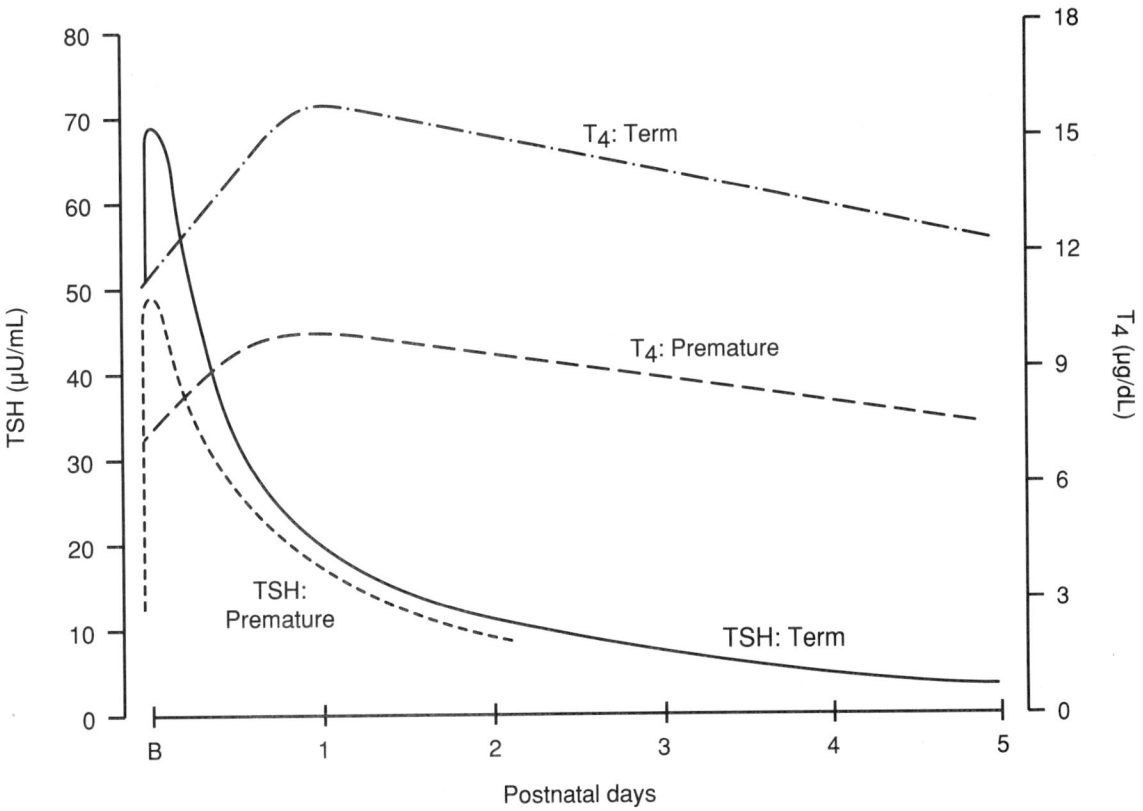

Fig. 11-3. Serum thyrotropin stimulating hormone (TSH) and thyroxine (T_4) concentrations in newborn infants during the first 4 days of life. (From Fisher and Klein,[20] with permission.)

Test: Thyroxine

Background and Selection

Serum T_4 commonly has been used to assess thyroid function and to follow patients treated for a variety of thyroid disorders. The popularity of serum T_4 in screening for thyroid dysfunction, however, has waned with the increasing recognition that abnormal test results occur in euthyroid individuals. Sensitive TSH assays are replacing T_4 as the screening test for evaluating thyroid function. In screening for neonatal hypothyroidism, serum T_4 is usually not used alone because of the unacceptable rate of false positive results (2–3%).[22]

Logistics

Because serum T_4 is usually measured by immunoassay, iodine does not directly interfere. It should be recognized, however, that iodine can cause changes in a patient's thyroid function. Depending on the immunoassay method used, autoantibodies to the thyroid hormones, which occur in patients with thyroid as well as nonthyroid diseases, cause falsely low or high results for T_4.[23] For detection of congenital hypothyroidism, thyroid hormones can be measured using dried blood spot specimens collected for phenylketonuria screening. Recently, T_4 in blood spots has been shown to decrease unless specimens are kept cold.[24]

Interpretation

The reference range for serum T_4 is about 5.5–12.5 μg/dL (71–161 nmol/L). In the absence of interfering physiologic and pharmacologic factors, serum T_4 results correlate well with degree of thyroid function.

Decreases

Thyroxine results are decreased in hypothyroidism with the decreases correlating well with the degree of hypofunction. Although serum T_4 measurements are helpful in confirming the presence of hypothyroidism, serum TSH measurements are necessary to distinguish primary hypothyroidism from secondary or tertiary forms. Serum T_4 levels are used to follow treatment in patients with hypothyroidism caused by TSH deficiency. In euthyroid individuals, low T_4 levels occur from a variety of causes, for example, TBG deficiency. An important cause of euthyroid hypothyroxinemia is NTI in which serum T_4 as well as serum T_3 levels are decreased in up to half of severely ill patients. The magnitude of serum T_4 decreases correlate with patient outcome; the mortality for patients with serum T_4 levels less than 3.0 μg/dL (<38.6 nmol/L) is 68% or greater.[25] Low or undetectable serum T_4 levels are found in patients treated for thyroid dysfunction with T_3 preparations.

Increases

Most patients with hyperthyroidism have elevated serum T_4 results that correlate well with the degree of thyroid dysfunction. A small percentage of thyrotoxic patients, however, have T_3 thyrotoxicosis in which T_4 levels are within the reference range, but serum T_3 is elevated. The findings of elevated serum T_3 levels, serum T_4 levels within the reference range, and clinical hyperthyroidism also can occur early in the course of hyperthyroidism and with relapse from treatment for hyperthyroidism. Hyperthyroidism with elevated serum T_4 and free T_4, but with serum T_3 levels within the reference range, is called T_4 thyrotoxicosis. So-called T_4 thyrotoxicosis is associated with iodine-induced thyrotoxicosis and thyrotoxicosis in patients with NTI.

Many individuals with elevated serum T_4 levels are not clinically hyperthyroid. There are many causes for this syndrome (Table 11-5), which is called euthyroid hyperthyroxinemia, and depending on the cause, the individual may have other thyroid test abnormalities in spite of their euthyroid metabolic status. For example, estrogen, which acts by raising TBG levels, causes increased binding of T_4 and T_3, resulting in increased serum levels of both these hormones. High serum T_4 levels occur in the newborn period because of the effects of estrogen on TBG as well as the TSH surge that occurs at birth. Other drugs such as narcotics, 5-fluorouracil, and clofibrate can cause less consistent increases in T_4 binding. Euthyroid hyperthyroxinemia also is caused by increased T_4 binding to TBPA or a high affinity binding site on albumin (dysalbuminemic hyperthyroxinemia). Because T_3 is not bound to TBPA or the high affinity albumin-binding site, patients with elevations in these binding proteins have elevated serum T_4, but their serum T_3 results remain within the reference range. In patients with familial dysalbuminemic hyperthyroxinemia, the T_3 uptake (T_3U) is within the reference range and the serum T_4 is high, thus these patients have an elevated free T_4 index (FT_4I). Generally, these patients have results for free T_4 by equilibrium dialysis within the reference range.[26] Individuals with peripheral resistance to thyroid hormones have elevated serum T_3 as well as elevated T_4 levels. Drugs such as iopanoic acid may cause euthyroid hyperthyroxinemia by reducing the peripheral conversion of T_4

Table 11-5. Causes of Euthyroid Hyperthyroxinemia and Hypothyroxinemia

Euthyroid hyperthyroxinemia (examples)
    Increased thyroxine-binding globulin
        Drug-induced (estrogens, heroin, methadone)
        Genetic
        Intercurrent illness (hepatitis)
        Physiologic (pregnancy, newborns)
    Increased thyroid-binding prealbumin (islet cell tumors)
    Increased albumin binding (familial dysalbuminemic hyperthyroxinemia)
    Peripheral resistance to thyroid hormones (Refetoff's)
    Nonthyroidal illness
    Drugs (amphetamines, iodine-containing contrast media, amiodarone)
    Autoantibodies to thyroxine (method dependent)
Euthyroid hypothyroxinemia (examples)
    Decreased thyroid-binding globulin
        Congenital
        Drug-induced (androgens)
        Intercurrent illness (hepatic failure)
    Decreased thyroid-binding globulin binding (renal failure)
    Decreased thyroid-binding prealbumin
    Nonthyroidal illness
    Drugs (phenytoin, carbamazepine)
    Autoantibodies to thyroxine (method dependent)

and T_3 and causing central stimulation of the thyroid axis. Amiodarone has multiple effects on thyroid function and there is a significant percentage of patients who develop hypothyroidism or hyperthyroidism.[27]

Test: Triiodothyronine

Background and Selection

Although high serum T_3 levels are a good index of hyperthyroidism, serum T_3 measurements usually are not needed to confirm the diagnosis. However, in patients who are clinically hyperthyroid and who have serum T_4 levels within the reference range, serum T_3 measurements are a helpful adjunct in diagnosis. Serum T_3 levels are not ordinarily indicated in patients with NTI or in patients suspected of having hypothyroidism.

Logistics

Usually no adjustments are made in specimen timing for the small diurnal variation in serum T_3 that occurs. Specimen timing for serum T_3 measurements is important, however, for patients treated with preparations containing T_3. Serum T_3 levels peak 2–4 hours after T_3 ingestion. Depending on the dose, peak serum T_3 reach levels approximately two to six times the reference range, returning to or near the reference range by 24 hours.[28]

Interpretation

The reference range for serum T_3 by immunoassay is about 60–160 ng/dL (~0.92–2.46 nmol/L). Because T_3 is bound to TBG, there are concomitant changes in T_3 levels with changes in TBG concentrations. Serum T_3 measurements are not a valuable indicator of hypothyroidism because levels within the reference range occur in a large percentage of patients. Moreover, low T_3 levels are found in many patients with clinical disorders unrelated to an underlying defect in the thyroid-pituitary axis, the so-called NTI.

Decreases

In about 15–30% of hypothyroid patients, serum T_3 is within the reference range in spite of low serum T_4 and elevated TSH. Low serum T_3 levels occur in severely hypothyroid patients, but are not uniformly decreased until patients have serum T_4 values less than approximately 2 µg/dL (<32 nmol/L).[29] Serum T_3 decreases rapidly with NTI; for example, serum T_3 levels drop to about 50% of initial values within several days following acute myocardial infarction.[30] Even if a patient is hyperthyroid, serum T_3 decreases with intercurrent illness. Most patients with NTI appear to be clinically euthyroid even though they have low serum T_3 levels as well as other thyroid function test abnormalities. In severely ill patients with various systemic illnesses, serum T_4 may be reduced as well (low T_3 and T_4 syndrome). Levels of T_3 also are low in cord blood of full term infants, but rapidly increase in the first few hours of life. In premature infants, serum T_3 levels also increase following birth, although not as dramatically as in the full term infant. In premature infants, T_3 decreases before a slow increase begins several days after birth. Serum T_3 levels also are decreased in states of calorie deprivation, after major surgery, and after administration of some drugs. In patients who have received propylthiouracil or oral cholecystographic agents, such as ipodate, decreased serum T_3 is caused by a block in the peripheral conversion of T_4 to T_3.

Increases

Most hyperthyroid patients have elevations in serum T_3 levels. In some patients, the increase occurs before, and to a greater extent than, the increase in serum T_4. In hyperthyroid patients, the mean serum T_3 is approximately four times the reference range, but wide variation in levels occurs. Elevated serum T_3 also is a reliable indicator of relapse in hyperthyroidism. Hyperthyroidism with elevated serum T_3, but without elevations of serum T_4, is called T_3 thyrotoxicosis. Only 1–4% of hyperthyroid patients have T_3 thyrotoxicosis, except in areas of iodine deficiency where T_3 thyrotoxicosis occurs in as many as 10–12% of hyperthyroid patients. Serum T_3 measurements are sometimes helpful in determining metabolic status in patients with types of euthyroid hyperthyroxinemia; for example, an elevated serum T_3 indicates hyperthyroidism in patients taking amiodarone. Serum T_3 levels are increased in patients with familial TBG excess and in those with familial thyroid hormone resistance (Refetoff's syndrome), but these patients do not have signs and symptoms of thyrotoxicosis. In patients treated with T_4 preparations, serum T_3 levels gradually increase after therapy is instituted, reaching stable levels several weeks after commencement of therapy. In patients treated with T_3 preparations, serum T_3 levels are above the reference range for most of the day, whereas serum T_4 concentrations are subnormal.

Test: Thyroid Stimulating Hormone (Thyrotropin)

Background and Selection

Serum TSH measurements are used to distinguish primary from secondary hypothyroidism as well as in following patients treated for primary hypothyroidism. Serum TSH alone or in combination with serum T_4 is used to screen newborns for thyroid dysfunction. So-called sensitive TSH assays have additional uses including diagnosis of hyperthyroidism and possibly in the assessment of patients treated with suppressive thyroid hormone therapy. Sensitive TSH assays also have been advocated as the single best test to screen for thyroid dysfunction, although this may not be true in all patient groups (see below). In addition to TSH, other thyroid hormone measurements are necessary to delineate conditions such as secondary hypothyroidism, thyroid hormone resistance, and TSH-producing tumors.

Logistics

The assay sensitivity is a critical factor in determining the uses of a TSH measurement. With most conventional TSH immunoassays, the lowest detectable concentration of TSH is about 1 μU/mL (~1 mU/L), a value close to the mean concentration in euthyroid individuals.[31] So-called sensitive TSH assays are 10 or more times more sensitive than conventional assays; the assays can detect TSH concentrations in the 0.1–0.2 μU/mL (0.1–0.2 mU/L) range, with some assays having minimal detectable doses as low as 0.02 μU/mL (0.02 mU/L). Using sensitive TSH assays, serum TSH levels show a circadian rhythm with a sleep-independent, nocturnal rise as well as bursts, although of relatively low magnitude, throughout the day.

Interpretation

Conventional TSH assays with a reference interval of less than about 5–7 μU/mL (<5–7 mU/L) yield undetectable results in 20% or more of euthyroid individuals. In contrast, sensitive TSH assays have a reference range of about 0.3–4.0 μU/mL (~0.3–4.0 mU/L),[32] but considerable variation has been reported depending on the assay used. Ideally, sensitive TSH assays can reliably discriminate between euthyroid and hyperthyroid individuals. High serum TSH results indicate primary hypothyroidism and suppressed values, as determined by sensitive TSH assays, indicate hyperthyroidism. Although serum TSH within the reference range generally excludes thyroid dysfunction, decreased or increased results do not always indicate a thyroid abnormality. For example, both decreased and increased TSH results have been reported in patients with NTI depending on the stage of illness (see below).

Decreases

Using appropriately sensitive TSH assays, hyperthyroid patients can be separated from eumetabolic persons. In hyperthyroid patients, low TSH is accompanied by increased T_4 and T_3 as well as clinical signs and symptoms of hyperthyroidism. In hyperthyroid patients, the mean TSH level is in the range of 0.05–0.11 μU/mL (0.05–0.11 mU/L) depending on the assay used.[33] In diagnosing hyperthyroidism, sensitive TSH assays appear to be superior to other tests such as free T_4 and the TRH test for a variety of reasons. In patients with overt hyperthyroidism, TSH results are usually below 0.005 μU/L (<0.005 mU/L).[34] A significant percentage of patients with suppressed TSH, however, do not have thyrotoxicosis.

Suppressed TSH is particularly prevalent in nonthyrotoxic patients with NTI or with drug therapy, especially glucocorticoids and dopamine. In patients with NTI, TSH appears to be low early in the course of the disorder, returning to the reference interval with resolution of the NTI (Fig. 11-4). In most patients with NTI, TSH is only marginally below 0.1 μU/L (<0.1 mU/L); there is considerable overlap in TSH results between mild hyperthyroidism and NTI.[34]

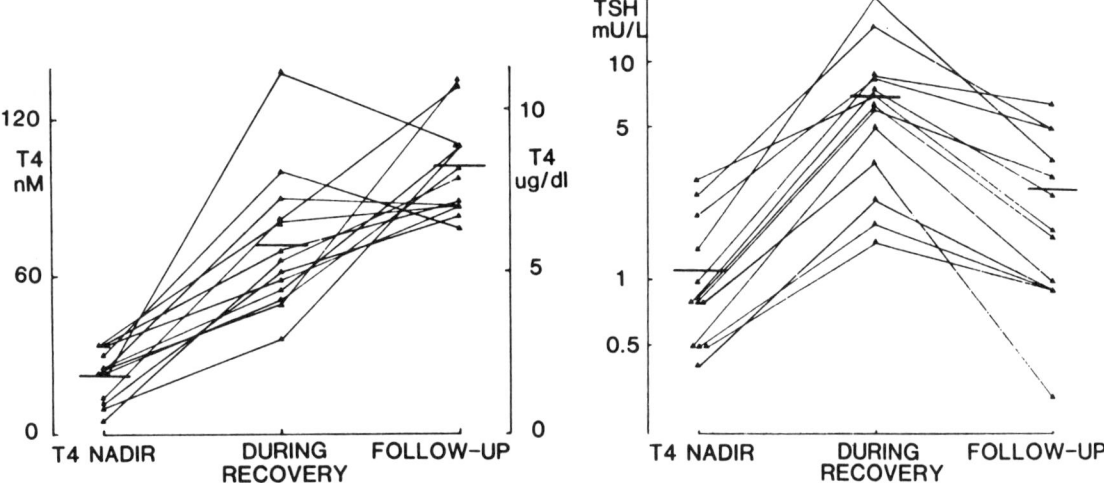

Fig. 11-4. Serum thyrotropin stimulating hormone (TSH) concentrations at the time of the thyroxine (T_4) nadir, during recovery (time of maximum TSH), and follow-up (after 4–20 weeks).

In patients treated with exogenous thyroid to suppress TSH secretion, TSH levels are in the range of those seen in hyperthyroid patients. In these patients, depressed basal serum TSH levels in the morning are associated with lack of a TSH surge at night and an absent TSH response to TRH.[35] Thus basal serum TSH, as measured by sensitive TSH assays, may be helpful for assessing adequacy of long-term, thyroid hormone suppressive therapy, although some investigators suggest adequate assessment of these patients await TSH assays with ever greater sensitivity. Patients on thyroid replacement therapy also can have suppressed TSH values. Although some of these cases may represent overreplacement, low TSH results may occur because of a postmedication surge in serum T_4.[36] Until thyroid hormone levels stabilize during the first few months of therapy, serum TSH measurements are of little value.

Increases

In a patient with signs and symptoms of hypothyroidism, TSH concentrations greater than 10.0 µU/mL (>10.0 mU/L) confirm the presence of primary hypothyroidism with few exceptions. Increases in serum TSH can occur in clinically euthyroid individuals with underlying thyroid disorders (compensated hypothyroidism) or in individuals living in areas of iodine deficiency. In these situations, the elevated TSH level maintains the patient's eumetabolic state. Elevated TSH results also occur in newborns during the first few days of life. In hypothalamic hypothyroidism, increased TSH results have been reported perhaps reflecting TSH that is immunoreactive, but not bioactive. In NTI, a decrease in TSH occurs early in the course of the disorder followed by a TSH increase in the recovery phase. In some patients recovering from NTI, TSH becomes elevated before returning to the reference interval.[25] Rarely, hyperthyroidism is produced by elevated serum TSH caused by a TSH-secreting pituitary tumor or hyperplasia, and adrenal insufficiency is associated with TSH elevation, which returns to within the reference range with corticosteroid therapy.

TESTS FOR FREE THYROID HORMONES

Free T_4 measurements have been used in the diagnosis of patients suspected of having either hypothyroidism or hyperthyroidism, especially where there are discrepancies between clinical findings and results of other thyroid function tests. Free T_4 measurements also have been used in screening for thyroid disease, but spurious results in patients with NTI have proved a problem. Free T_3 is not commonly measured, but may be useful in a few clinical circumstances (see below). The current trend is toward replacing free T_4 with sensitive TSH measurements in difficult diagnostic cases and for screening.

Test: Free Thyroxine

Background and Selection

Measurement of free T_4 is used for patients who are suspected of having binding protein abnormalities or it is used in clinical situations in which the patient's signs and symptoms of thyroid disease and thyroid function test results give an equivocal picture.

Logistics

Free T_4 may be quantitated using a variety of methods including equilibrium dialysis or several types of immunoassays based on different principles. A number of method dependent interferences occur, not only between measured and calculated free T_4, but also with various free T_4 methods. For example, hypoalbuminemia or high nonesterfied fatty acids can cause low free T_4 with certain methods.

Interpretation

The reference range for free T_4 is about 0.8–2.3 ng/dL (~10.1–29.6 pmol/L). Typically, hyperthyroid patients have elevated free T_4 levels, whereas free T_4 levels are decreased in hypothyroid patients. Increases or decreases in serum free T_4 without concomitant changes in metabolic state have been reported owing to a variety of causes; the most important, protein-binding changes and NTI, are discussed below.

Test: Free Thyroxine Index

Background and Selection

The FT_4I is indicated in patients with ambiguous signs and symptoms of thyroid dysfunction, especially in those patients in whom results of other thyroid function tests are equivocal.

Terminology

The results are calculated from total T_4 and T_3U and thus are sometimes called calculated free T_4 or T_7 or T_{12}.

Interpretation

The reference range for the FT_4I depends on the ranges of total T_4 and percent T_3U used in its calculation. In many clinical circumstances, the FT_4I appears to be an excellent approximation of the free T_4 concentration. Although the FT_4I is satisfactory in patients with small changes in TBG, it may not accurately reflect free T_4 concentrations in patients with marked abnormalities in binding proteins or with NTI.

Test: T_3 Uptake

Background and Selection

The T_3U is directly proportional to the degree of saturation of the patient's binding proteins by endogenous thyroid hormone. The T_3U is used in conjunction with total T_4 measurements to calculate the FT_4I.

Terminology

The T_3U is a measure of the unoccupied protein binding sites for the thyroid hormones. The term T_3 *uptake* is derived from the use of radioactive T_3 as the label. Although "T_3" in the uptake refers to the tracer used in the assay and not to the hormone T_3, the T_3U is sometimes confused with the measurement of total serum T_3. The confusion has led the Committee on Nomenclature of the American Thyroid Association to recommend changing the name of uptake tests to *thyroid hormone binding ratio* (THBR), but the term has not been widely adopted.

Logistics

A nonspecific binder such as charcoal or resin acts as a matrix, binding radioactive T_3 that does not attach to the patient's thyroid-binding proteins. Many methods have been used to calculate percent uptake but "normalized" values are preferred, that is, results are calculated by relating the count in the patient's serum to those of a euthyroid reference serum.

Interpretation

A typical reference range for the T_3U is 25–35% (0.25–0.35), but results vary significantly depending on the method used. The T_3U values normalized to that of a reference serum value yield the THBR, which has a normal variance of 1.00 ± 0.15%. The patient's total T_4 result is multiplied by the THBR to yield the FT_4I. See Test: Free Thyroxine Index for interpretation of the results.

Test: Free Triiodothyronine

Background and Selection

Free T_3 measurements are used in patients with elevated serum total T_3 who are suspected of having serum-binding protein abnormalities. Additionally, free T_3 has been advocated in monitoring thyroid hormone replacement therapy.

Logistics

Abnormal thyroid hormone binders can interfere with free T_3 assays in a manner analogous to free T_4.

Interpretation

The usual reference range for free T_3 is about 190–500 pg/dL (~2.9–7.7 pmol/L). Free T_3 normally appears to be increased in pregnancy and gestation, thus time-specific reference intervals are needed to appropriately interpret free T_3 results in pregnant patients. In euthyroid patients with TBG deficiency, free T_4 results are low and free T_3 results are high.[37] Because free T_3 levels tend to be markedly decreased in patients with NTI,[38] T_3 measurements have been advocated to delineate hyperthyroidism in patients with NTI. Free T_3 measurements also have been advocated in monitoring T_4 replacement therapy because T_3 is produced in patients taking T_4 by peripheral conversion and thus acts as a biologic indicator of this function.[39]

Summary of Important Method Dependent Problems

Results from direct measurement of free T_4 and calculated FT_4I (from total T_4 and a parameter of thyroid hormone binding) have the same theoretic interpretation, but considerable differences exist, especially in certain clinical circumstances such as changes in hormone binding and with NTI.

Changes in Hormone Binding

In situations in which there is a change in binding protein concentration or affinity, free T_4 results (measured or calculated) correlate, theoretically, more closely with the patient's clinical state. However, the relationship between TBG concentration and T_3U is nonlinear at very high or low concentrations of TBG; thus the FT_4I does not correct for extremes of TBG concentration.[40] In a recent study of patients with TBG excess and deficiency, neither the FT_4I nor T_4/TBG ratio reflected concentrations of serum free T_4.[41]

Discrepant results for free T_4 have been reported in persons with unusual T_4-binding proteins, most notably in patients with familial dysalbuminemic hyperthyroxinemia. In a patient with familial dysalbuminemic hyperthyroxinemia, the high affinity binding site on the patient's albumin leads to spurious assay results with some methods.

Serum albumin binds T_4 with abnormally high affinity, but the protein does not bind T_3, resulting in normal T_3U and an elevated FT_4I. Generally, these patients have free T_4 levels within the reference range as measured by equilibrium dialysis, but they have elevated levels when measured by many of the immunoassays.

Changes with Nonthyroidal Illness

Free T_4 methods also are variably affected by NTI. In patients with NTI, the free fatty acids released are suspected of competing with T_4-binding sites on serum proteins, but albumin concentration may be important in the expression of the effects of free fatty acids. Changes in prealbumin and TBG also have been implicated in the methodologic changes as well. In patients with NTI, free T_4 has been found to be increased, decreased, or within the reference range depending on the method used. The FT_4I is often decreased in patients with NTI who have low serum T_4. In NTI patients with the low T_3 syndrome only, free T_4 by immunoassay is within the reference interval or increased, but patients with the low T_3, low T_4 syndrome often show decreases in free T_4. In contrast, serum-binding inhibitors in critically ill patients can result in overestimates of serum free T_4 when measured by equilibrium dialysis.[38]

OTHER TESTS OF THYROID FUNCTION

Test: Protein Bound Iodine (PBI)

Background and Selection

Before the introduction of competitive protein binding and immunoassays for T_4, the PBI was used to estimate serum T_4, the major component of serum PBI. The PBI can be used to assess patients with iodine-induced thyroid disease or thyroid dyshormonogenesis, or it can be used as an indicator of thyroiditis.

Logistics

Interference with the PBI also occurs with large doses of organic iodine preparations or if at least 1 g of inorganic iodine per day has been administered.[42] Many iodinated compounds, especially radiographic contrast media, cause spurious elevation in the PBI.

Interpretation

The reference range for PBI is about the same as for total T_4. However, in addition to hormonal iodine, which comes mainly from T_4, the PBI measures iodoproteins, iodotyrosines, and inorganic iodine. Thyroglobulin and iodoalbumin also are estimated as PBI because they remain in the protein fraction. In patients exposed to large amounts of iodine, the PBI may be increased because of the iodine administered or because the iodine has led to formation of iodoproteins, including T_4. Iodotyrosines are the major source of the serum iodine in certain types of dyshormonogenesis, leading to elevated PBI in these cases. With thyroiditis, many iodinated proteins, which are measured by the PBI, are released; thus, a high ratio of PBI to T_4 is an indication of thyroiditis. However, abnormal amounts of iodinated protein have been found in association with simple goiter as well as with a number of other thyroid disorders.[42]

Test: Reverse Triiodothyronine

Background and Selection

Most rT_3 (3,3′,5′) is derived from extrathyroidal monodeiodination of T_4. Reverse T_3, which is calorigenically inactive, binds to the same serum thyroid hormone-binding proteins as T_4 and T_3, but with less avidity. Serum T_3 is rarely used clinically, but may be helpful in some patients with NTI.

Interpretation

The reference range for serum rT_3 is about 10–50 ng/dL (~0.15–0.77 nmol/L). Decreases in rT_3 occur in hypothyroidism, whereas increases occur in hyperthyroidism. Elevations of serum rT_3 also occur in newborns, with calorie deprivation, and in patients taking drugs resulting in low T_3 concentrations caused by impaired deiodination. Some patients with NTI have increased rT_3; those with the low T_4, low T_3 syndrome have higher values than those with the low T_3 syndrome. If the rT_3 level is high or within the reference interval in a patient with NTI, this weighs against the patient having hypothyroidism.[43]

Test: Thyroglobulin

Background and Selection

Thyroglobulin measurements are primarily used in the management of patients with differentiated thyroid carcinoma, but also are helpful in evaluating thyroid ablation and diagnosing thyrotoxicosis factitia.

Logistics

Because thyroglobulin is measured by immunoassay, the assays may yield spurious results in patients with circulating thyroglobulin antibodies, for example, in patients with Hashimoto's thyroiditis. The presence of thyroglobulin autoantibodies gives rise to falsely increased or decreased results depending on the properties of the endogenous antibody and the assay method used.[44] Generally, there has not been good correlation between antibody titer and thyroglobulin assay interference; thyroglobulin antibody levels, even below the detection limit of agglutination assays, can effect thyroglobulin assays.[39]

Interpretation

The reference range for serum thyroglobulin is about 1–30 ng/mL (~1.5–45 pmol/L). Values are slightly increased in the third trimester of pregnancy and are markedly increased in neonates, especially premature infants. Thyroglobulin levels rise in the first few hours of life remaining elevated for several days. Children have levels intermediate between neonatal and adults values.

Decreases

Thyroglobulin below the lower detectable limit of 1–2 ng/mL (1.5–3 pmol/L) occurs in about 15% or more of healthy subjects. Thyroglobulin is decreased in patients with thyroid agenesis, following ablative surgery of the thyroid, and in patients treated with thyroid hormone. In hyperthyroid patients, results that are low or within the reference range suggest thyrotoxicosis factitia.[45]

Increases

Thyroglobulin levels are a relatively sensitive index of thyroid gland activity and are increased in patients with hyperthyroidism. Patients with Hashimoto's thyroiditis or Graves disease sometimes also have circulating thyroglobin antibody and significant levels of thyroglobulin-antibody complex. In addition, serum thyroglobulin is increased in patients with thyroid adenomas and papillary thyroid carcinoma. Thyroglobulin levels also can be increased in patients with trophoblastic disease or renal failure.[44]

Because various thyroid diseases cause thyroglobulin elevation, measurements are not helpful preoperatively in patients suspected of having thyroid malignancy. After surgery, the combination of a serum thyroglobulin test and total body scan appears to be more sensitive than either test alone in separating out those patients who have residual metastatic disease. With successful treatment, thyroglobulin levels decrease in patients with papillary thyroid carcinoma, with thyroglobulin results greater than 10–15 ng/mL (>15.0–22.5 pmol/L) indicating metastases. Thyroglobulin measurements are more sensitive in detecting metastases when hormone therapy has been discontinued and TSH stimulation is used.[39,44]

Test: Thyronine

Background and Selection

Thyronine is a completely deiodinated derivative of T_4 produced by sequential monodeiodination. Measurement of urinary thyronine excretion may be helpful in differentiating patients with NTI from those with hypothyroidism.

Interpretation

Preliminary data indicate that the mean urinary thyronine excretion in healthy subjects has a range of 7–21 µg/g creatinine (2.9–8.9 nmol/mmol creatinine). When expressed in terms of creatinine excretion, urinary thyronine excretion is decreased in patients with hypothyroidism and increased in patients with hyperthyroidism or NTI.[46]

Test: Thyrotropin Releasing Hormone (TRH Test)

Background and Selection

The TRH test has been used for patients suspected of having thyroid dysfunction, but in whom other thyroid function tests yield equivocal results. For this use, the TRH test is being replaced by the so-called sensitive TSH assays. The TRH test also is used to assess TSH suppression especially in patients treated with thyroid hormone.

Logistics

The TRH test usually is performed by obtaining a specimen for baseline TSH measurements, administering TRH intravenously, and obtaining specimens at 20 or 30 minutes and 60 minutes for TSH administration. In addition to TSH, TRH releases prolactin and, in up to 60–70% of acromegalic patients, it also releases GH. Side effects of TRH administration include pressor effects, especially in hypertensive patients, and cardiac arrhythmias.[47]

Interpretation

The usual response to TRH is a rise in TSH to a maximum of 2–25 µU/mL (≤2–55 mU/L) above baseline.[48] The minimal response over baseline is considered to be 1–2 µU/mL (1–2 mU/L) with the exact result depending on the amount of TRH administered and the time of sampling. Because the TSH response to TRH correlates with the baseline TSH level (Fig. 11-5), the TRH test adds little information not yielded by sensitive TSH assays. The TRH test is useful in patients treated with suppressive doses of thyroid hormone. Both pituitary and hypothalamic disease can be associated with a delay in TSH peak of 45 minutes or more following TRH administration.[48] The TRH test thus cannot reliably separate the two groups of patients. The TRH test is blunted in individuals with hyperthyroidism, in patients treated with suppressive doses of thyroid hormone, and in those with functioning thyroid adenomas. In primary hypothyroidism, the TSH response to TRH is increased, but problems in defining hyperresponsiveness have made interpretation of results difficult.[49] There are a number of nonthyroidal cases of decreased or increased response of TSH to TRH (Table 11-6). Because blunted TSH response to TRH is found in a significant percentage of patients with depression, the TRH has been suggested as a diagnostic test for depression.

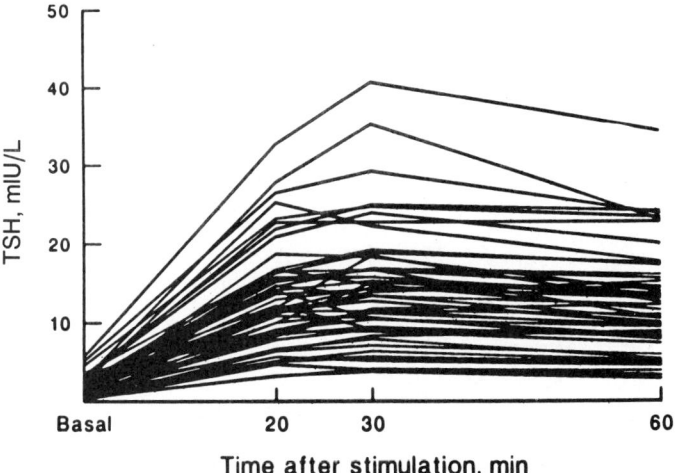

Fig. 11-5. Serum thyrotropin stimulating hormone (TSH) concentrations before and after stimulation with thyrotropin releasing hormone (TRH) in 50 healthy persons. (From Klee and Hay,[49] with permission.)

Table 11-6. Thyrotropin Releasing Hormone Test: Influence of Nonthyroidal Conditions
Decreased thyroid stimulating hormone
Anorexia nervosa
Depression
Drugs (dopamine antagonists, glucocorticoids, oral contraceptives)
Nonthyroidal illness
Increased thyroid stimulating hormone
Anorexia nervosa
Drugs (lithium, dopamine antagonists, iodine contrast materials)

(Modified from Kolesnick and Gershengorn,[48] with permission.)

Test: Thyroxine-Binding Globulin

Background and Selection

Thyroxine-binding globulin levels are useful in patients when there is a discrepancy between clinical findings and serum T_4 and/or serum T_3 results. Because TBG is the major thyroid hormone-binding protein, increases or decreases in serum TBG are reflected by concomitant changes in serum T_4 and serum T_3.

Logistics

Thyroxine-binding globulin generally is measured by electrophoresis in the presence of radioactive T_4 or by immunoassay. Depending on the specific method used, various drugs or abnormal binders may interfere. Polyacrylamide electrophoresis has been used to identify patients with familial dysalbuminenic hyperthyroxinemia (Fig. 11-6).[39]

Interpretation

The reference interval for TBG is about 12–28 µg/dL (~150–360 nmol/L). Measurement of serum TBG is helpful in patients suspected of having congenital TBG excess or deficiency. Inherited reduction or absence of TBG is more commonly reported than inherited increases. There are a number of varients of TBG that differ in their affinity and binding capacity for T_4. To date, all identified congenital TBG abnormalities, including TBG excess and deficiency, are inherited as X chromosome-linked traits.[50] Drugs such as estrogens and androgens cause consistent increase or decrease in TBG, respectively. In contrast, a number of drugs change binding of thyroid hormones; for example, high doses of glucocorticoid decrease T_4 binding to TBG, but increase its TBPA binding.

TESTS FOR AUTOANTIBODIES TO THYROID AND THYROID HORMONES

The thyroid contains three well characterized thyroid-specific autoantigens (Fig. 11-7): thyroglobulin, thyroidal microsomal antigen, and the TSH receptor. Autoantibodies to these thyroid antigens are used in the

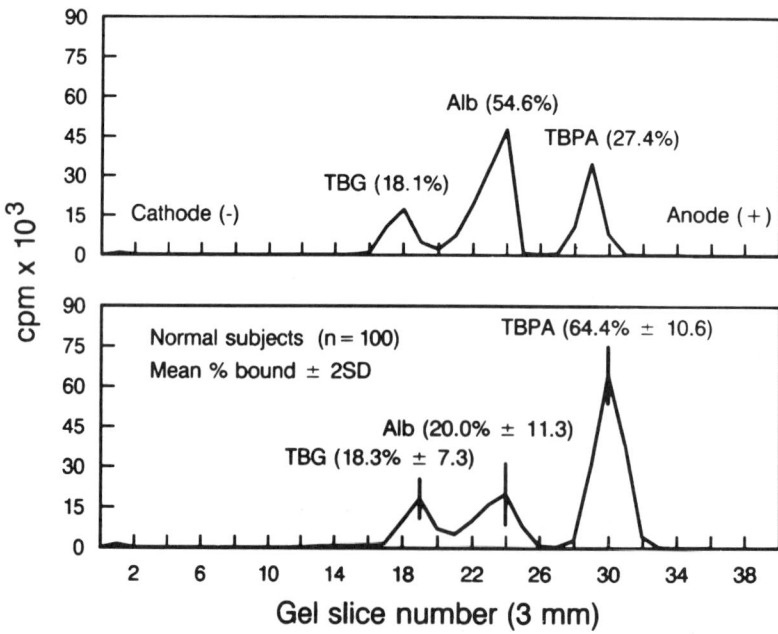

Fig. 11-6. Polyacrylamide gel electrophoresis of thyroxine-binding proteins. Upper panel shows a specimen from a patient with familial dysalbuminemic hyperthyroxinemia, and the lower panel shows normal adult values. TBG, thyroxine-binding globulin; Alb, albumin; TBPA, thyroid-binding prealbumin. (From Hay and Klee,[39] with permission.)

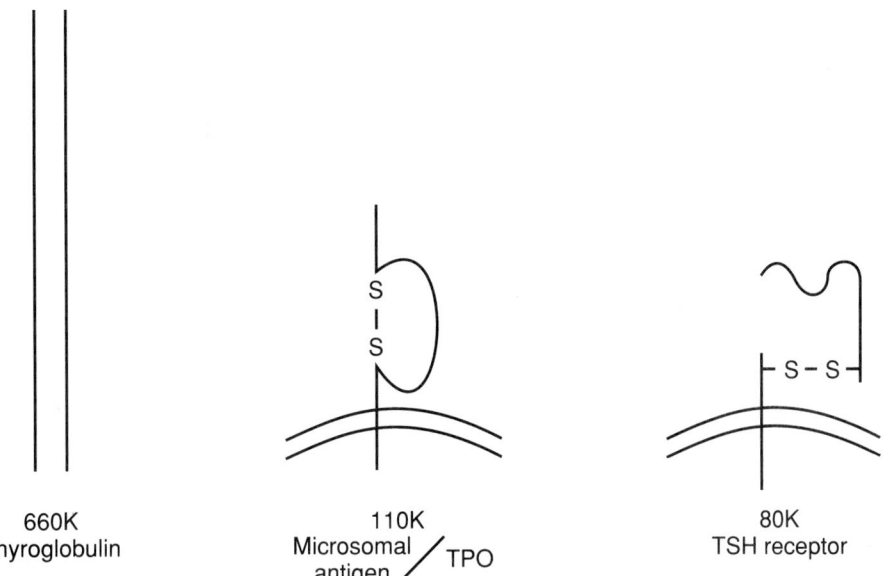

Fig. 11-7. Thyroid autoantigens. TPO, thyroid peroxidase; TSH, thyroid stimulating hormone. (From Smith et al,[51] with permission.)

diagnosis of a number of thyroid disorders. In addition, antibody to thyroid hormone or thyroid antigens can cause assay interference. Interference is manifested by results that fail to correlate with the patient's clinical picture. Autoantibodies against thyroid hormone have been reported in patients with a wide variety of thyroid disorders as well as in patients with autoimmune diseases and certain malignancies.[23] Depending on the specific assays in question, antibody to T_4 or T_3 can cause increases or decreases in T_4 (or T_3) results. Antibodies to thyroglobulin are important causes of interference with assays for thyroglobulin, and antibody to TSH interferes with assay for TSH-binding inhibitor immunoglobin.[52]

Test: Thyroglobulin Antibodies

Background and Selection

Measurement of thyroglobulin antibodies has been used in patients suspected of having Hashimoto's thyroiditis, but thyroid microsomal antibodies are more sensitive and specific for this disorder.

Interpretation

Although results are normally "negative," some apparently healthy individuals may have low titers of thyroglobulin antibodies. High titers of thyroglobulin antibodies are found in most patients with Hashimoto's thyroiditis. Most patients with thyroid microsomal antibodies have thyroglobulin antibodies, but thyroglobulin antibodies occur in a variety of conditions other than Hashimoto's thyroiditis. Thyroglobulin antibodies are frequently found in the serum of patients with antibody to thyroid hormones, with autoimmune disorders, or those taking amiodarone. Along with thyroid microsomal antibodies, thyroglobulin antibodies may predict prognosis in patients treated with drug therapy.[53] Additionally, thyroglobulin antibodies are often increased in drug treated Graves patients who develop hypothyroidism during remission from hyperthyroidism.[54]

Test: Thyroid Microsomal Antibodies

Background and Selection

Although they have a number of limitations, thyroid microsomal antibody assays are used in the laboratory to confirm the diagnosis of Hashimoto's thyroiditis and to predict its course. The thyroidal microsomal antigen is thyroid peroxidase, an integral membrane protein.[51]

Interpretation

Results of thyroidal microsomal antibody assays are usually "negative" in healthy individuals, although up to 20% of healthy middle-aged women have detectable microsomal antibody in their serum. Thyroid microsomal antibodies occur in almost all patients with Hashimoto's thyroiditis. However, it is now recognized that some patients with Hashimoto's thyroiditis may have thyroid microsomal antibody production in the thyroid, but have undetectable antibody in serum.[55] Although thyroid microsomal antibodies are fairly specific for Hashimoto's thyroiditis, they do occur in patients with Graves disease or with idiopathic myxedema.[55] Thyroid microsomal antibodies may predict prognosis in drug treated Graves disease patients.[55] Additionally, high titers of thyroid microsomal antibodies have been reported in drug treated patients who develop hypothyroidism during remission from the hyperthyroidism of Graves disease.[54] Patients with postpartum thyroid dysfunction and patients treated with amiodarone have been reported to have circulating thyroidal microsomal antibodies. A recent report indicates that there appears to be at least three kinds of thyroid microsomal antibodies; these are antibodies against (1) native, (2) denatured, or (3) denatured and reduced microsomal antigens. It appears that only antibodies to the latter two denatured forms lead to thyroid gland destruction.[56]

Test: Thyrotropin (Thyroid Stimulating Hormone) Receptor Antibodies (TRAb)

Background and Selection

Thyrotropin receptor antibody assays have been used to predict and assess neonatal thyroid dysfunction and to assess treatment strategies in patients with Graves disease. In patients with Graves disease, several types of antibodies to the TSH receptor exist including antibodies that activate cyclic adenosine monophosphate (cAMP) causing increased thyroid hormone production. The TSH receptor thus is stimulated leading to hyperthyroidism and Graves disease. A small percentage of patients with Graves disease have blocking antibodies that inhibit binding of TSH or thyroid stimulating immunoglobulins to the TSH receptors of the thyroid. These blocking antibodies may cause hypothyroidism, but in other cases lead to no clinical symptomatology. Antibodies to the TSH receptor cross the placenta and may cause neonatal thyrotoxicosis or in the case of blocking antibodies, neonatal hypothyroidism.[51]

Terminology

The term TSH receptor antibodies now is recommended for autoantibodies to the TSH receptor with the phrase "measured by assay __" to identify the type of assay performed. Previously, these antibodies were known by the generic terms, thyroid stimulating immunoglobulins (TSI) or human thyroid stimulator (HTS), or by assay-related terminology including long-acting thyroid stimulator (LATS) or human thyroid/adenylate cyclase stimulator (HTACS).[57] Antibodies that bind to the TSH receptor without causing stimulation were called "TSI-block" antibodies, TSH-binding inhibitor immunoglobulins (TBII), or LATS protector.

Logistics

There are two main categories of assays, those dependent on some index of thyroid stimulation and those that assess the ability of TRAb to inhibit binding of labeled TSH to its receptor. The ability of antibody to cause TSH-binding inhibition does not always reflect thyroid stimulating activity.[58]

Interpretation

With the newer assays, TRAbs of the agonist type are found only in serum of patients with Graves disease and in a small proportion of patients with autoimmune thyroiditis. In patients with Graves disease, assays for stimulatory antibodies have been used to assess drug treatment therapy. Detectable TRAb levels following a course of drug treatment predict relapse of thyrotoxicosis; however, negative receptor levels do not necessarily predict remission after antithyroid drug withdrawal.[51] Furthermore, TRAb assays may be helpful in assessing patients without clinically evident thyroid disease who are suspected of having Graves disease, for example, those who have eye signs or symptoms compatible with Graves ophthalmopathy. Although blocking antibodies are found mainly in patients with atrophic thyroiditis, they also occur in some patients with Hashimoto's thyroiditis and in some patients with hypothyroidism occurring after treatment for Graves disease. Measurement of TRAb of both the stimulatory and blocking types have been used to predict the risk of thyroid dysfunction in newborn infants. A highly positive result for TRAb in pregnant patients with Graves disease at about 28–30 weeks may lead to consideration of intrauterine hyperthyroidism and the possibility of therapeutic intervention.[58] Neonatal hypothyroidism caused by transplacental passage antibody with blocking activity may be transient; measurement of blocking antibody to confirm this situation may be warranted when the mother has a history of autoimmune thyroid disease.

THE HYPOTHALAMIC-PITUITARY-ADRENAL AXIS

INTRODUCTION: ADRENAL CORTEX

Three hormones play a major role in the function of the hypothalamic-pituitary-adrenal axis. The paraventricular nucleus of the hypothalamus secretes corticotropin releasing hormone (CRH), a 41 amino acid peptide. Secretion of CRH is increased in stressful conditions and in states of cortisol deficiency, whereas elevated concentrations of cortisol suppress its secretion. Corticotropin releasing hormone reaches the anterior pituitary by way of the hypophyseal portal system and acts on specific receptors coupled to adenylate cyclase causing corticotropin (ACTH) synthesis and release. Although the dominant role in regulating ACTH is CRH, other factors are important, among them arginine vasopressin (ADH), which has been considered an auxiliary ACTH secretagogue. Stress, interleukins, epidermal growth factor, lymphokines, and a number of other substances also have a stimulatory role at the pituitary, and some of these substances provoke a response at the hypothalamus as well.

Adrenocorticotropic hormone, a polypeptide with a mass of 4500 da, contains 39 amino acids and is secreted by the corticotrophs of the anterior pituitary. The main action of ACTH is the stimulation of adrenal growth and secretion of cortisol, but stimulation of aldosterone and androgen secretion and a number of other effects are also important. Adrenocorticotropic hormone secretion is regulated by three main factors: feedback mechanisms of cortisol, diurnal variation, and stress. Plasma cortisol, the most important hormone for controlling the secretion of ACTH, falls when ACTH secretion rises. The subsequently produced high circulating plasma cortisol levels ultimately suppress secretion of ACTH. Adrenocorticotropic hormone acts on the adrenal gland by binding to a specific receptor in the cell membrane resulting in stimulation of adenylate cyclase with a rapid production of cAMP. Other fragments of the ACTH precursor, such as pro-opiomelanocortin (POMC), also may have a tropic effect on the adrenals. Secretion of ACTH is episodic with 7–13 secretory spikes throughout 24 hours, most of which occur during sleep.

The adrenals are paired, highly vascular structures consisting of an outer cortex that comprises 90% of the gland surrounding the central medulla. The cortex is composed of three distinct areas, the outer zona glomerulosa, the zona fasiculata, and the zona reticularis, which adjoins the inner medulla. The venous circulation within the gland is complex and thought to play an important role in regulating steroid synthesis.

The adrenal cortex produces three major types of steroid hormones: mineralocorticoids, glucocorticoids, and androgens. The glomerulosa cells secrete the mineralocorticoids, aldosterone and desoxycorticosterone. The major factor controlling aldosterone secretion is angiotensin, but an increased plasma potassium concentration also is an efficient aldosterone-stimulating agent. The role of ACTH in stimulation of aldosterone is not as important in healthy individuals, except in those who are salt depleted.

Cortisol and androgens, synthesized by fasiculata and reticularis cells, respectively, arise mainly from hydrolysis of circulating cholesterol esters, but the novosynthesis of cholesterol is also an important source. These synthetic steps are controlled mainly by ACTH. The side chain of cholesterol is cleaved yielding pregnenolone, and increased concentrations of pregnenolone then lead to increased biosynthesis of cortisol, aldosterone, and androgens by the steps seen in Figure 11-8. Although the pathways are common to various steroids shown, specificity is achieved by location of specific enzyme systems. For instance, the glomerulosa cells lack 17-hydroxylase and do not participate in synthesis of cortisol or androgens for which this enzyme is essential. Conversely, the fasiculata and reticularis cells lack the enzyme 18-hydroxylase and thus cannot synthesize aldosterone.

Adrenal Hypofunction

Adrenal insufficiency includes all conditions in which the secretion of adrenocorticosteroids falls below body requirements. Adrenal insufficiency is characterized by the insidious onset of slowly progressive fatigability, weakness, nausea and vomiting, weight loss, cutaneous and mucosal pigmentation, and hypotension. Although the spectrum varies and the diagnosis is not difficult in patients presenting with fulminant glucocorticoid and mineralocorticoid deficiency, milder forms of the disorder often pose a diagnostic problem.

258 • Laboratory Medicine

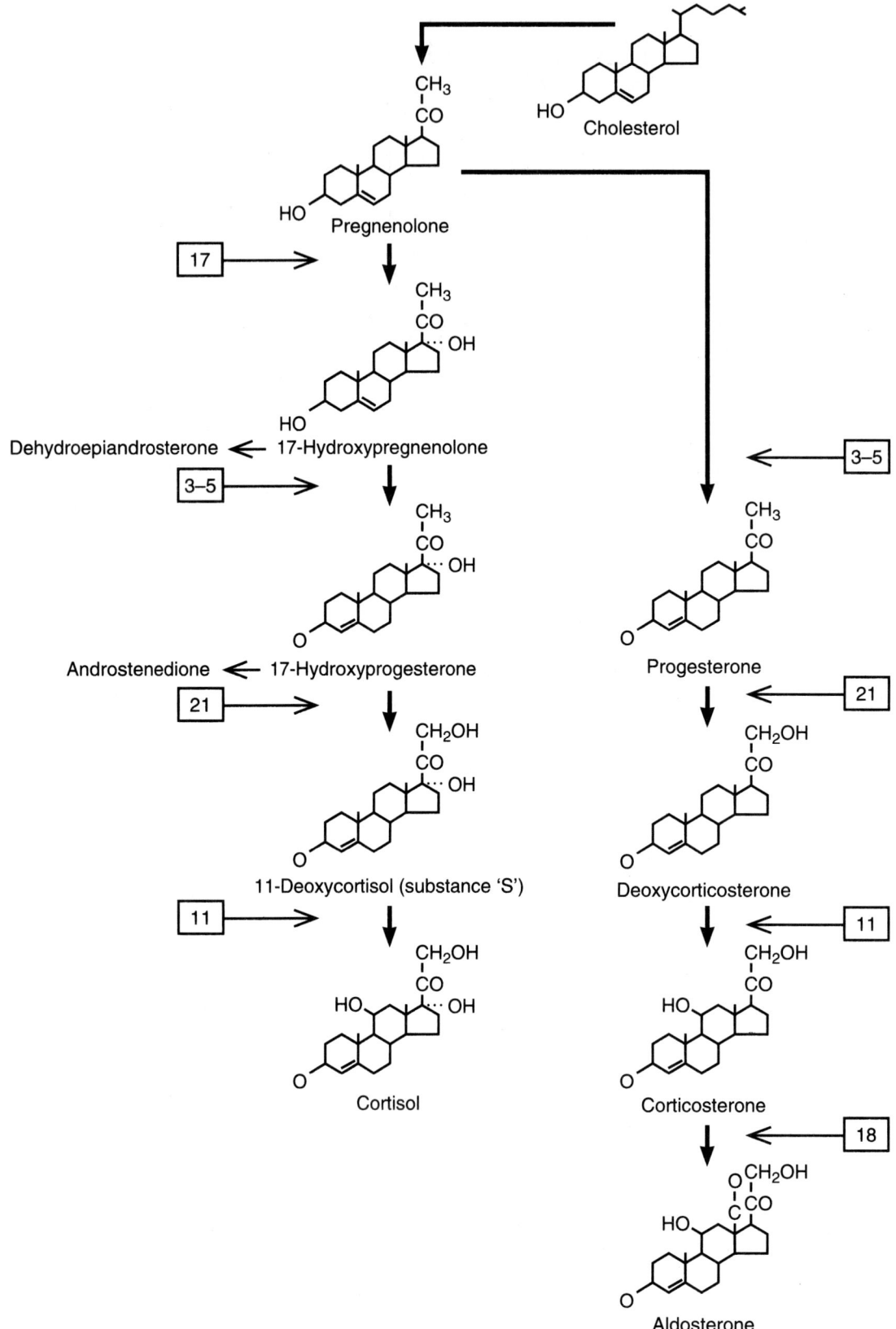

Fig. 11-8. Biosynthetic pathways and enzymes involved in the synthesis of glucocorticoids (cortisol) and mineralocorticoids from cholesterol precursor. The androgens, dehydroepiandrosterone and androstenedione, are precursors of the sex steroids, testosterone and estradiol. Enzymes are as follows: 3–5, 3-hydroxydehydrogenase and δ-5-isomerase; 11, 11-hydroxylase; 17, 17-hydroxylase; 18, 18-hydroxylase; 21, 21-hydroxylase.

Table 11-7. Frequent Causes of Primary Adrenal Insufficiency
Anatomic destruction of gland (chronic and acute)
"Idiopathic" atrophy (autoimmune)
Surgical removal (metastatic breast cancer)
Infection (tuberculous, fungous)
Hemorrhage
Replacement (metastatic disease)
Metabolic failure in adequate hormone production
Congenital adrenal hyperplasia
Enzyme inhibitors (metyrapone)
Cytotoxic agents (o,p -DDD)
Therapeutic agents (ketoconazole, etomidate)
Failure to increase replacement during illness

Adrenal insufficiency is divided into primary (or adrenal) and secondary (or pituitary) disorders. Secondary disorders are evaluated as part of the diagnostic procedures for pituitary function (see Test: Insulin Tolerance Test). The differential diagnosis of primary adrenal insufficiency or Addison's disease, is seen in Table 11-7. Tuberculosis (once the most common cause of adrenal insufficiency) and other infectious agents are becoming common causes of adrenal insufficiency in acquired immunodeficiency syndrome (AIDS) patients.

Although screening for adrenal insufficiency is usually accomplished by measuring baseline cortisol at 0800 hours, a more definitive procedure is the short ACTH (Cortrosyn) stimulation test.

Congenital Adrenal Hyperplasia

Congenital adrenal hyperplasia consists of a group of autosomal recessive enzymatic deficiencies affecting adrenal corticosteroid biosynthesis. For the most part, these deficiencies present at birth but a few instances of the so-called late-onset variety have been described as occurring later in life. Congenital adrenal hyperplasia is the most common cause of ambiguous genitalia, but adrenal insufficiency, virilization, and hypertension also occur frequently, depending on the enzymatic defect. Approximately 95% of the cases are attributed to 21-hydroxylase deficiencies, whereas at least five other forms account for the other 5% of cases (see Table 11-11). Because of the infrequency of these later forms, diagnostic tests have not been well described. In many circumstances, urine tests are still recommended because studies using serum steroid measurements have not yet been reported. For all causes of congenital adrenal hyperplasia, laboratory diagnosis is made by demonstrating decreased levels of hormones in the metabolic sequence beyond the defective enzyme and elevated levels proximal to the enzyme defect as seen in Figure 11-8. Recently, gene probes have been used for prenatal diagnosis, followed by treatment in the first trimester.[59]

TESTS FOR ADRENAL HYPOFUNCTION

Test: Adrenocorticotropic Hormone (Cortrosyn) Stimulation Test (Short ACTH Test, Rapid ACTH Test, Short Tetracosactrin Test)

Background and Selection

Several analogues of ACTH with steroidogenic action such as cosyntropin (Cortrosyn) have been synthesized and are readily available for diagnostic testing. They have actions very similar to native human ACTH. The short ACTH test is used to detect adrenal insufficiency and late-onset or nonclassical forms of congenital adrenal hyperplasia. One of these ACTH analogues is cosyntropin (Cortrosyn), a synthetic α-subunit of ACTH containing amino acids 1–24. For patients who are seriously ill, a 0800 hour cortisol value less than 12.7 µg/dL (<350 mmol/L) has been used to identify patients at risk for adrenal insufficiency and those who should have the ACTH stimulation test.

Logistics

For the diagnosis of adrenal insufficiency, usually the test consists of cortisol determinations with specimens obtained at baseline and at 30 and/or 60 minutes after the intravenous injection of 0.25 mg cosyntropin. Although there are no widely accepted recommendations for the time at which this test should be performed, some recommend 0900 hours if possible. At baseline, a specimen obtained for subsequent measurement of ACTH can help in distinguishing primary from secondary adrenal insufficiency. A variant of this procedure requires the intravenous administration of cosyntropin for 2 hours with subsequent cortisol measurements, but has no diagnostic advantage over the short test.

To test for 21-hydroxylase deficiency, specimens are collected for measurements of 17-hydroxyprogesterone (17-OHP) at basal state and 60 minutes after stimulation. Women should be tested in the follicular phase of the menstrual cycle.

Interpretation

Although some investigators have proposed criteria for adrenal insufficiency relying on the basal cortisol level, stimulated cortisol level, or their difference, the peak level after cosyntropin administration is the most valuable in judging test performance.[60] A peak cortisol level greater than or equal to 20 µg/dL (≥ 550 nmol/L) generally is accepted as the criterion for normal adrenal function. Unfortunately, a few patients who had an insufficient response on initial testing showed an adequate response on repeat testing. Patients with secondary adrenal insufficiency generally have inadequate responses, but occasionally they may have a normal response; therefore this test should not be relied on to exclude secondary adrenal insufficiency. Secondary adrenal insufficiency can be distinguished from primary adrenal insufficiency by measurement of ACTH in a specimen obtained in the basal state, although some favor use of the long ACTH test or the ITT for this purpose.[61]

This test appears less reliable than the ITT in assessing the hypothalamic-pituitary-adrenal axis in patients withdrawing from steroids and also in the first 14 days or so after pituitary surgery (the time taken for the responsiveness of the adrenal cortex to reset to a reduced ACTH concentration).[62] Treatment of patients with low doses of dexamethasone or other steroids for 24–36 hours before testing has been shown to result in inadequate responses. Patients with AIDS and pa-

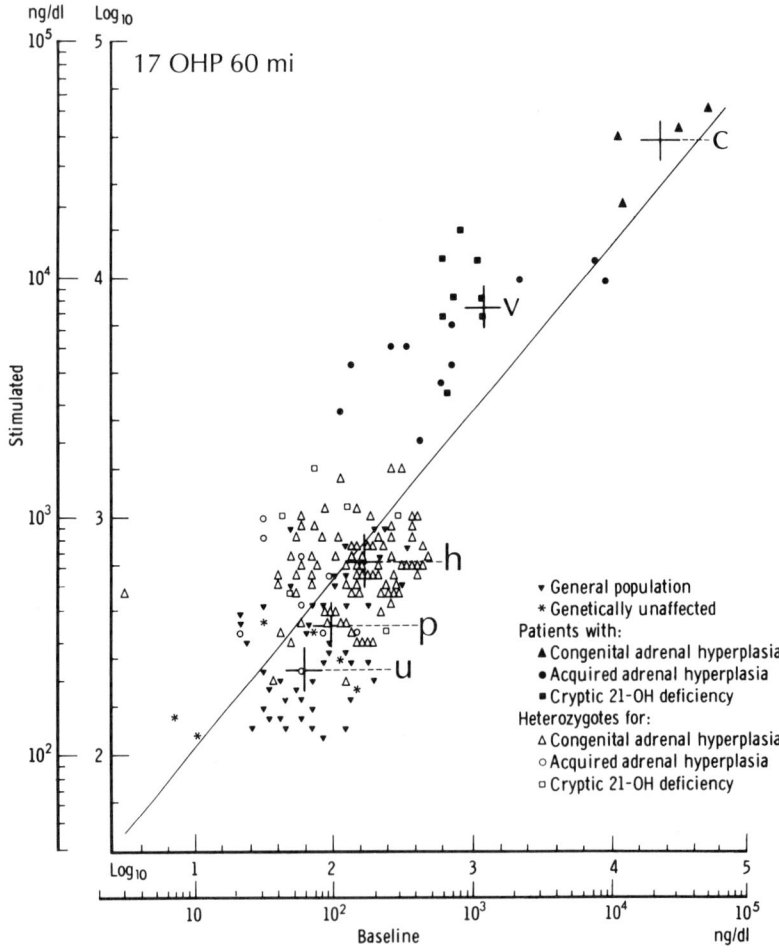

Fig. 11-9. Nomogram relating baseline to adrenocorticotropic hormone (ACTH) stimulated serum concentrations of 17-hydroxyprogesterone. A regression line for all data points is shown. The mean for each group is indicated by a large cross and adjacent letter: C, classical 21-hydroxylase deficiency; v, variant or nonclassical 21-hydroxylase deficiency; h, heterozygotes for all forms of 21-hydroxylase deficiency; p, general population; and u, known unaffected persons. OH, hydroxyl. To convert ng/dL to nmol/L, multiply ng/dL by 0.0303.

tients taking ketoconazole may also have inadequate responses.

For the identification of 21-hydroxylase deficiency, values are plotted on a nomogram that permits the assignment of individuals to classical, nonclassical, heterozygotes, or general population groups (Fig. 11-9). Basal 17-OHP levels greater than 200 ng/dL (>6.0 nmol/L) and above 1200 ng/dL (>36.3 nmol/L) following stimulation are consistent with 21-hydroxylase deficiency.[63]

Test: Long ACTH (Long Tetracosactrin Test)

This procedure has been used to distinguish primary adrenal insufficiency from secondary adrenal insufficiency. It is performed in a variety of ways ranging from the intravenous infusion of ACTH for a few days to the intramuscular injection of a depot ACTH analogue such as tetracosactrin. Serum cortisol or urine glucocorticoids are measured before and at the end of the procedure. Generally, patients with adrenal failure do not show a response or exhibit a minimal response, whereas patients with pituitary insufficiency show a brisk response. Adrenocorticotropic hormone immunoassays or the ITT are used much more frequently to aid in this differential diagnosis of primary versus secondary adrenal insufficiency.[60-62]

Test: Insulin Tolerance (ITT, Insulin Stress Test)

The ITT is used in the differential diagnosis of adrenal insufficiency or when pituitary insufficiency is suspected (see Test: Insulin Tolerance Test under The Anterior Pituitary Gland). Because patients with suspected adrenal insufficiency are not expected to respond to the hypoglycemic stress of the procedure, it is not recommended for diagnostic evaluation of primary adrenal insufficiency. During this procedure, specimens for cortisol determinations are obtained at baseline and at 60 minutes following an insulin bolus. Healthy individuals have an increment in serum cortisol greater than 7 µg/dL (>190 mmol/L) and a maximum level greater than 18 µg/dL (>500 mmol/L). If an adequate cortisol response occurs, the hypothalamic-pituitary-adrenal axis is assumed to be normal. A suboptimal response indicates secondary adrenal insufficiency if normal adrenal responsiveness to ACTH has been documented.[64] The ITT has been found to be superior to the short ACTH test in assessing the hypothalamic-pituitary-adrenal axis.[62]

Adrenal Hyperfunction (Cushing Syndrome)

Cushing syndrome is a clinical condition characterized by an inappropriate excess of glucocorticoids. Occasionally other endocrine manifestations may occur because of concomitant production of ACTH fragments or excess androgens. Because the first cases described by Cushing in 1932 were caused by pituitary adenomas, the disorder was named Cushing's disease. Subsequently, when a variety of other causes were identified, the clinical syndrome was called Cushing syndrome. The most frequent pathologic condition causing Cushing syndrome was thought, until recently, to reside within the adrenal; it is now believed that Cushing's disease (a pituitary tumor) is a much more frequent cause[65] (Table 11-8). Cushing syndrome also commonly results from therapeutic use of glucocorticoids or ACTH; however, iatrogenic Cushing syndrome usually is not a diagnostic problem. Alcohol-induced pseudo-Cushing syndrome is a rare disorder that is poorly understood and not predominantly ACTH dependent. Withdrawal of alcohol leads to remission of the biochemical abnormalities over a period of days, but the clinical signs take longer to abate.

A large number of laboratory procedures have been developed to evaluate patients for Cushing syndrome, and although many approaches have been suggested, the small numbers of patients in each series have not

Table 11-8. Differential Diagnosis of Cushing Syndrome

Cause	Approximate Incidence
Pituitary dependent (Cushing's disease)	60%
Ectopic Cushing syndrome	20%
ACTH and ACTH active peptides	Most cases
CRH-producing tumors	Few cases
Adrenal adenoma	10%
Adrenal carcinoma	5%
Alcohol-induced (Pseudo-Cushing)	1–3%
Iatrogenic	Rare[a]
Hypothalamic	Few cases

Abbreviations: ACTH, adrenocorticotropic hormone; CRH, corticotropin releasing hormone.

[a] Most common cause, but rarely a diagnostic problem.

made possible a consensus on an appropriate diagnostic work-up. When investigating patients with suspected Cushing syndrome, it is first necessary to confirm the presence of the syndrome, then identify its cause. The hallmark for diagnosis of Cushing syndrome is the loss of the diurnal pattern of cortisol, nonsuppressibility of the hypothalamic-pituitary-adrenal axis by dexamethasone, and elevated serum and urine cortisol concentrations.

BASIC TESTS FOR ADRENAL HYPERFUNCTION (CUSHING SYNDROME)

Test: Cortisol (Compound F)

Background

Cortisol is synthesized from cholesterol and secreted by the adrenal cortex in response to corticotropin (ACTH). At usual serum concentrations in healthy individuals, cortisol is 70–80% bound to corticosteroid-binding globulin (CBG or transcortin) and 10–20% bound to albumin, whereas only 5–10% remains nonprotein bound. Cortisol is metabolized rapidly in the liver with a half-life of approximately 2 hours. The double bonds and ketone groups are reduced, and about 60–70% is excreted in the urine conjugated with glucuronic acid. A small amount is excreted unchanged.

Selection

Isolated serum cortisol measurements provide little useful information about activities of the hypothalamic-pituitary-adrenal axis. Despite this precaution, low morning cortisol or inappropriately high evening cortisol (preferably midnight) are indicative of adrenal insufficiency or Cushing syndrome, respectively. Cortisol measurements also are useful in the diagnoses of depression.

Logistics

Immunoassay has replaced other methods such as competitive protein-binding or fluorimetry for routine measurement of serum cortisol. Few studies from research laboratories continue to use the older methods and generate values generally higher when compared with immunoassay results. Although many reports still describe measurements made on plasma, serum is the specimen of choice. Serum values are highest between 0600 and 0800 hours and lowest at midnight in persons with the usual sleep-wake patterns. Alterations in the sleep-wake pattern produce a change in the timing of this circadian rhythm. Superimposed on the circadian rhythm is an ultradian rhythm of 5–10 secretory bursts.

Interpretation

Early morning cortisol values range from 3–20 µg/dL (83–552 mmol/L) and by 2300 hours are less than 5 µg/dL (<138 mmol/L). Individuals who are under stress, as well as hospitalized patients, have elevated values, sometimes over 25 µg/dL (>700 mmol/L). A normal circadian rhythm has been defined as an evening value less than 75% of the 0800 hour value. The absence of a cortisol circadian rhythm may occur with stress, anorexia nervosa, obesity, emotional disturbances, and secondary to a variety of sedatives, stimulants, psychotropic, and antiepileptic drugs. Falling or persistently low cortisol values (less than 12.7 µg/dL [<350 mmol/L]) are indications of poor prognoses in patients in intensive care units.[66]

Isolated serum cortisol measurements mainly are used in screening for adrenal insufficiency or excess. However, the major use of serum cortisol measurements is in the diagnosis of adrenal disorders where serial determinations are made following stimulation or suppression testing (Table 11-9). Because increases in cortisol-binding globulin cause increases in serum cortisol, elevated values are seen following estrogen ingestion, in pregnancy, and in chronic active hepatitis.[67] In individuals with chronic renal failure, widely discrepant values are found by various immunoassays, because of variable assay reactivity with cross-reacting steroids, some of which may be glucuronides. Many immunoassay antibodies also react with steroids, which may be elevated in some relatively rare conditions, thereby producing spuriously elevated cortisol values. One of these steroids, 11-desoxycortisol, is elevated with the 11-hydroxylase enzyme deficiency in congenital adrenal hyperplasia and after metyrapone testing. Determination of serum cortisol is rarely indicated during acute corticoid therapy; when measured, intravenous, oral, and topical pharmaceutical steroid preparations, such as hydrocortisone hemisuccinate, hydrocortisol acetate, and fludrocortisone acetate (florinef), react in some cortisol immunoassays.

Test: Urinary-Free Cortisol (UFC, Urinary Free Corticoids)

Background

Free cortisol, which accounts for only 5–10% of the cortisol in serum of healthy individuals, is filtered through the glomerulus, but only partially reabsorbed by the renal tubules. The portion of cortisol that is filtered is relatively constant because only the nonpro-

Table 11-9. Serum Cortisol Measurements

Specimen Collection	Test Perturbation	Use
Baseline testing		
Morning value	None	Low result suggestive of adrenal insufficiency
Midnight value	None	High result suggestive of Cushing syndrome
0800 h and 2400 h	None	Midnight value <75% of morning value—loss of diurnal pattern
Stimulation tests		
Anytime	Following cosyntropin 30, 60 min	Diagnosis of adrenal insufficiency
0800 h	Following CRH	Testing for Cushing syndrome
Anytime	Following ITT	Diagnosis of pituitary insufficiency
Suppression tests		
0800 h	Following 1 mg dexamethasone, 2300 h	Screening for Cushing syndrome
0800 h	Following 8 mg dexamethasone, 2300 h	Diagnosis of Cushing syndrome
0800 h and 1600 h	Following 1 mg dexamethasone, 1300 h	Diagnosis of depression
1600 h on second day	0.5 mg Dexamethasone q6h, 2 days	Diagnosis of Cushing syndrome
1600 h on second day	2.0 mg Dexamethasone q6h, 2 days	Diagnosis of Cushing syndrome
Other		
Anytime		Prognosis in ICU patients

Abbreviations: CRH, corticotropin releasing hormone; ITT, insulin tolerance test; ICU, intensive care unit.

tein-bound serum fraction passes the kidney glomerulus and can be reabsorbed. Therefore, the UFC excretion rate reflects the prevailing serum concentration of free hormones. Fortunately, serum unbound cortisol rises disproportionately to total cortisol when transcortin (CBG) capacity is saturated, thereby magnifying UFC increases. Thus UFC measurements are particularly useful in conditions of cortisol excess such as in Cushing syndrome.

Selection

Urinary-free cortisol measurements are used for the diagnosis of Cushing syndrome, especially after dexamethasone suppression testing. They are of limited value in states of hypocortisolism such as Addison's disease.

Terminology

Depending on the antibody, cortisol and a variety of other corticoids may react in the assay causing some to call this measurement *urinary free corticoids* rather than UFC.

Logistics

Usually 24-hour urine collections are used for the procedure and immunoassay is carried out with an aliquot of the specimen. Urinary free cortisol measurements using random urine collections occasionally have been recommended, but other than in situations such as nocturnal hypoglycemia occurring in some patients with insulin treated diabetes random urine collections are of limited value.

Because UFC and creatinine clearance strongly correlate and are influenced minimally by body weight, UFC reference intervals are increased only trivially in the obese, the population most likely to be tested for Cushing syndrome. With renal failure sufficient to lower the glomerular filtration rate below 30 mL/min, UFC measurements are no longer valid.

Interpretation

In adrenal insufficiency, urinary corticoid values are low, but because of overlap, they fail to discriminate these patients from healthy persons. Urinary-free cortisol results of greater than approximately 100 μg/24 h (>278 mmol/d) are considered elevated. During a low dose (2 mg) dexamethasone suppression test, healthy persons have UFC measurements less than 20 μg/24 h (<52 mmol/d) on the second day of testing, whereas those with higher values are considered nonsuppressed. When the high dose (8 mg) dexamethasone suppression test is used, a 50% or more fall in UFC compared with the baseline is considered a positive response indicative of excess pituitary ACTH secretion as the origin of the patient's hypercortisolism. Although exceptions do occur, UFC results in patients with ectopic or adrenal tumors are rarely suppressed during the high dose dexamethasone test.

264 • Laboratory Medicine

Table 11-10. Urinary-Free Cortisol: Suppression With Dexamethasone

Condition	Basal	2 mg/d[a]	8 mg/d[b]
Normal	80–100 µg/24 h (222–278 mmol/d)	<20 µg/24 h (<52 mmol/d)	<50% initial value
Adrenal hyperplasia	Increased	Not suppressed	<50% initial value, occasional "paradoxical response"
Adrenal adenoma	Increased	Not suppressed	Not suppressed
Adrenal carcinoma	Markedly increased	Not suppressed	Not suppressed (rare exceptions)
Pituitary tumor	Markedly increased	Not suppressed	Not suppressed
Ectopic ACTH syndrome	Markedly increased	Not suppressed	Usually not suppressed

Abbreviation: ACTH, adrenocorticotropic hormone.
[a] Low dose.
[b] High dose.

Some investigators have expressed UFC concentrations in relation to urine creatinine, but others find the ratio valueless.[68] Urinary free cortisol is increased threefold in the second and third trimesters of pregnancy mainly because of a rise in serum of unbound cortisol and high concentrations of estrogens, which in turn increases transcortin. Urinary-free cortisol values also are increased in alcoholic pseudo-Cushing syndrome, depressive psychosis, starvation, and anorexia nervosa. Significant proteinuria also carries excess cortisol into the urine and may hinder reabsorption leading to spuriously increased results. When the affinity of CBG for cortisol is reduced, increased UFC values occur. Table 11-10 shows UFC results after dexamethasone suppression tests. With dexamethasone suppression testing, UFC has replaced 17-hydroxycorticosteroid and 17-ketogenic steroid measurements because it provides a more accurate estimate of overall cortisol secretion.

Test: Corticotropin (Adrenocorticotropic Hormone, Adrenocorticotropin)

Background

Corticotropin is a 39 amino acid single chain peptide that is synthesized as part of a precursor molecule of approximately 245 amino acids, POMC. The prohormone also is a precursor for endorphins, lipotropins, and melanotropins. A series of post-translational enzymatic modifications convert the intact prohormone into smaller active peptides (Fig. 11-10). Corticotropin releasing hormone causes the release of ACTH and β-endorphin in a coordinated, equal molar fashion.

Corticotropin is secreted episodically with a diurnal pattern. The lowest levels occur in evening with onset of sleep and peak values are found in the morning at time of awakening. Superimposed on the diurnal pattern are about 10 pulses per day of approximately 5 pg/mL (~1.1 pmol/L) in magnitude. These pulses are of increased amplitude in patients with Cushing syndrome, but are not always reflected with a concomitant pulse of cortisol secretion.

The primary function of corticotropin is its effect on the adrenal cortex, where it is the predominant regulator of adrenal glucocorticoid and androgen secretion and to a lesser extent mineralocorticoid secretion. Corticotropin binds to high affinity receptors in the adrenocortical membrane and stimulates steroidogenesis by activating the cell membrane adenylate cyclase system.

Selection

Corticotropin measurements are used in the differential diagnosis of Cushing syndrome, to substantiate the ectopic production of the ACTH, in the CRH stimulation test, and in monitoring compliance and treatment efficacy in patients with congenital adrenal hyperplasia.

Logistics

The corticotropin molecule is degraded easily by enzymes present in sera. Storage at room temperature for 24 hours results in a loss of 50–90% of activity. Specimens therefore should be collected as plasma in EDTA-containing tubes, immediately centrifuged at 4°C, and stored at −20°C until assay. Some corticotropin immunoassays show reactivity with 1–39 cortico-

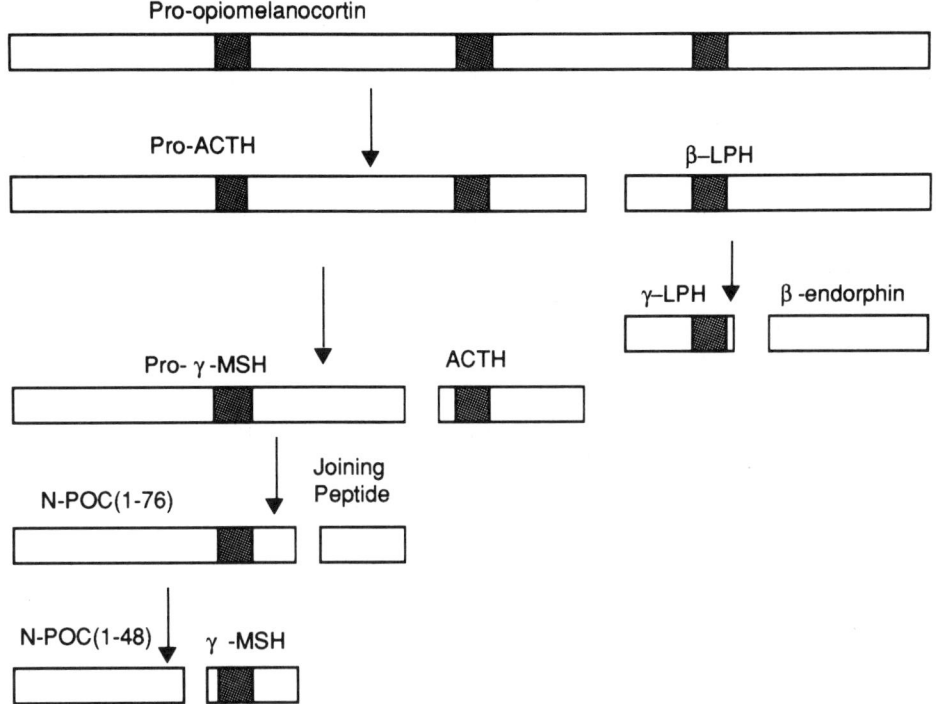

Fig. 11-10. Diagramatic representation of pro-opiomelanocortin (POMC) showing the major peptides released as a result of proteolytic cleavage. ACTH, adrenocorticotropic hormone; LPH, lipotropin; MSH, melanocyte stimulating hormone.

tropin, POMC, ACTH fragments, and pro-ACTH. Pro-ACTH, a 22,000 da molecule, is the major circulating component with corticotropin immunoreactivity in patients with ectopic ACTH syndrome, but is present in much lower amounts in healthy persons and patients with aggressive pituitary tumors (Fig. 11-10). Monoclonal immunometric assays show increased analytic specificity, but in some instances they may be too specific and not measure biologically active fragments of ACTH or "big" ACTH, which is detected by other less specific radioimmunoassays.[69] For this reason, monoclonal assays have slightly lower reference intervals than those using polyclonal antibodies. Because corticotropin is relatively a small molecule, it tends to stick to glass, but this can be minimized by using siliconized glass tubes or polystyrene tubes. Some recommend sampling for ACTH between 0800 and 0900 hours.

Interpretation

A typical reference interval for corticotropin is approximately 10–80 pg/mL (~2.2–17.8 pmol/L): results from early morning are usually 7–55 pg/mL (1.6–12.2 pmol/L). Plasma corticotropin levels greater than 250 pg/mL (>55.6 pmol/L) confirm the diagnosis of primary adrenal insufficiency, whereas values less than 50 pg/mL (<11.0 pmol/L) are consistent with pituitary corticotropin deficiency. In Cushing syndrome, suppressed levels of corticotropin, less than 20 pg/mL (<4.4 pmol/L), are diagnostic of primary glucocorticoid excess. Patients with pituitary Cushing syndrome have plasma ACTH levels within the reference interval to moderately elevated (40–200 pg/mL [8.8–44.4 pmol/L]). In contrast, patients with ectopic ACTH may have markedly elevated corticotropin levels in the range of 200–1000 pg/mL (44.4–222.2 pmol/L). Because of the overlap, corticotropin levels may not always distinguish patients with ectopic secretion of ACTH. Cosyntropin administration causes spuriously low ACTH values in some assays by binding to the reagent antibodies. Corticotropin is measured following infusion of CRH. For interpretation of results, see Test: Corticotropin Releasing Hormone (Corticotropin Releasing Factor [CRF]) Stimulation Test.

Correlating corticotropin results in specimens obtained under radiologic guidance from the petrosal sinus with results from peripheral specimens has been used to diagnose Cushing's disease. A central petrosal sinus to peripheral ratio greater than 2:1 is suggestive of Cushing's disease.[70] Corticotropin results have been used to monitor patients with treated adrenal hyperplasia caused by 21-hydroxylase deficiency; good control results are within the reference interval, whereas markedly elevated levels are associated with poor control.

STIMULATION AND SUPPRESSION TESTS FOR ADRENAL HYPERFUNCTION

Test: Corticotropin Releasing Hormone (Corticotropin Releasing Factor [CRF]) Stimulation Test

Background

Corticotropin releasing hormone, a 41 amino acid peptide produced by the hypothalamus, regulates the pituitary secretion of corticotropin (ACTH). The structure of human and ovine peptide differs by only seven amino acids, therefore both have been used in human testing. Corticotropin releasing hormone is found in the central nervous system, pancreas, stomach, duodenum, and placenta, as well as in a variety of tumors. After binding to receptors in the pituitary, CRH acts by activating the adenylate cyclase. Although concentrations are relatively low in body fluids, immunoassay techniques have made routine CRH measurement possible; however, the clinical significance of serum measurements has not yet been established.

Selection

The CRH stimulation test has been found to be useful in the differential diagnosis of Cushing syndrome. It is used also in preoperative localization of intrasellar ACTH-secreting tumors following placement of catheters under radiologic guidance for specimen collection.

Logistics

Intravenous administration of synthetic ovine CRH into healthy men and women results in a dose dependent increase in plasma corticotropin and serum cortisol unaffected by age and sex. The CRH test is performed by obtaining baseline corticotropin and cortisol, then administering an intravenous bolus of CRH. A dose of 1 µg/kg body weight or 100 µg of CRH is administered and specimens are obtained at 15, 30, 60, 90, and 120 minutes. Peak corticotropin levels are usually reached between 15 and 60 minutes.

For a given dose of CRH, the corticotropin response is inversely correlated with the initial cortisol level and dependent on the time of day when testing occurs. If CRH is administered in the evening, the incremental rise in corticotropin is greater than that in early morning. It is recommended that the test be performed at 0800 hours.

Venous sampling following administration of CRH has been used in localizing the cause of Cushing syndrome. Baseline specimens for plasma corticotropin are obtained simultaneously from each petrosal sinus and from peripheral veins 3, 5, and 10 minutes after the injection of ovine CRH.

Interpretation

Patients with Cushing's disease show normal to exaggerated response to CRH, whereas patients with ectopic ACTH secretion fail to respond.[71] Patients with the ectopic and adrenal Cushing syndromes have no increases in corticotropin and cortisol. The test appears to have similar sensitivity and specificity to the dexamethasone suppression test. False positive results have been seen in a few patients with adrenal hyperplasia and a single patient with carcinoid.[72]

When used for localizing the cause of Cushing syndrome, patients with intrasellar ACTH-secreting tumors have a ratio of at least 1:7 for petrosal corticotropin to that of peripheral corticotropin. This ratio rises to at least 3:1 or more following CRH administration. Patients with ectopic ACTH secretion do not show a central to peripheral step up or lateralization in the petrosal sinus specimens.

Although CRH has been used in the differential diagnosis of adrenal insufficiency, it remains a research tool at present. Patients with primary adrenal insufficiency have high ACTH levels and increased responses to ovine CRH, whereas patients with secondary adrenal insufficiency have normal to flat responses. However, a variety of corticotropin responses occur ranging from subnormal to levels approaching those seen in primary adrenal insufficiency. In response to CRH, patients with pituitary disease show little or no increase in corticotropin, whereas those with hypothalamic abnormalities have exaggerated and prolonged corticotropin responses.

Test: Dexamethasone Suppression Test (DST) (and Other Tests for Cushing Syndrome)

Background and Selection

Dexamethasone is a potent synthetic glucocorticoid that has been used to test the integrity of a hypothalamic-pituitary-adrenal axis. When given to healthy individuals, it decreases the production of cortisol and other adrenal steroids through the usual feedback mechanisms. In patients with Cushing syndrome, depression, and a variety of other conditions, suppression of the hypothalamic-pituitary-adrenal axis does not occur with the administration of dexamethasone. Dexamethasone is not measured in cortisol assays because of the low concentrations attained owing to dexamethasone's potency and because of the specificity of immunoassays. A variety of suppression tests have been used with differences in the quantity and duration of dexamethasone ingested and the timing and type of specimen collected.

When steroids are used therapeutically, such as beclomethasone for treating asthmatics, suppression of cortisol occurs. In contrast, many drugs that increase dexamethasone metabolism contribute to nonsuppression.

Logistics

A number of dexamethasone suppression tests are used. Some of the more frequent ones are listed below.

Overnight Screening Test for Cushing Syndrome

One milligram of dexamethasone is ingested at 2300 hours, and at 0800 hours cortisol values are obtained. Patients with values higher than 5 μg/dL (>38 mmol/L) are called nonsuppressors.

Persons who fail to suppress are candidates for further dexamethasone suppression testing. If cortisol is suppressed by dexamethasone, the person is considered healthy. Approximately 13% of obese and healthy individuals, however, fail to show suppression. Other conditions producing false positive tests include acute stress, high estrogen states, psychiatric disease, and drugs such as rifampin, phenytoin, and phenobarbital, which increase metabolism of dexamethasone. In hospitalized patients, the test does not distinguish among patient groups very well; 30% of patients without adrenal abnormalities fail to suppress normally. Nonsuppression also results from failure to ingest tablets supplied. False negative test results are exceedingly rare, but have been reported to occur in persons who metabolize dexamethasone at an abnormally slow rate. Because of few false negative results and ease of use for outpatients, the overnight dexamethasone suppression usually is the first test used for diagnosing Cushing syndrome (Table 11-9).

Low Dose (2 mg) Dexamethasone Suppression Test

This test is used to differentiate healthy individuals from those with Cushing syndrome. The patient ingests 0.5 mg of dexamethasone every 6 hours for 48 hours and on the second day, either urine is collected for UFC measurements or a 1600 hour plasma cortisol value is obtained. This dose of dexamethasone is equivalent to about four times the usual adrenal output of glucocorticoids. Healthy individuals show suppression of UFC results to less than 20 μg/24 h (<55.2 mmol/d) or serum cortisol to less than 5 μg/dL (<140 mmol/L) at 1600 hours on the second day.[73] Usually individuals who are obese show appropriate response to this suppression test. Patients who show nonsuppression of their results then undergo high dose (8 mg) dexamethasone testing.

High Dose (8 mg) Dexamethasone Suppression Test

This test is useful in delineating the cause of Cushing syndrome and usually is administered following the low dose test described above. The patients ingest 2 mg of dexamethasone every 6 hours for 48 hours and either UFC or serum cortisol is measured during the second day of testing. The usual response is a UFC level less than 50% of baseline, or a 1600-hour serum cortisol level of 10 μg/dL or less (≤280 mmol/L) on the second day of testing.[73]

A useful approach obviating the need to have patients hospitalized is, after a baseline 0800 hour cortisol measurement, the high (8 mg) dose of dexamethasone is administered at 2300 hours and cortisol remeasured at 0800 hours the next day.[74] A positive response (suppressibility) is a cortisol value of 50% or less of the baseline cortisol level. Suppression indicates pituitary origin of the cortisol excess, whereas lack of suppression occurs with adrenal or ectopic tumors.

Most patients with Cushing's disease show suppression, whereas most patients with ectopic production of ACTH or with adrenal tumors do not. Unfortunately, some patients with Cushing's disease do not show suppression and some patients with ectopic tumors or adrenal tumors show suppression, thereby complicating test interpretation. Occasionally, paradoxic increases occur in patients with Cushing's disease. This high dose overnight test compares favorably with the 2-day test.

Dexamethasone Suppression Test for Depression

One milligram of dexamethasone is given at 2300 hours and cortisol is measured at 0800 and 1600 hours the next day. Individuals who have a diagnosis of major depression have a value greater than 5 μg/dL (>140 mmol/L) in either specimen. Because compliance may be a problem in this procedure, some authors recommend that methylene blue be added to dexamethasone tablets and the urinary excretion of the dye monitored as an indicator of drug ingestion.

The specificity of the dexamethasone suppression test for depression is approximately 90%, whereas its sensitivity is about 45%. With this procedure, many patients with acute psychosis, mania, and dementia have nonsuppression of cortisol as well and are not differentiated from those with major depression.[75] If for practical reasons, sampling is limited only to the 1600-hour specimen, then there is about a 20% loss in procedure sensitivity.

Metyrapone Test

Metyrapone, a chemical inhibitor of the enzyme responsible for converting 11-desoxycortisol to cortisol, has been used for over 30 years in evaluation of Cushing syndrome. Originally in the standard test, patients received 3 g daily in divided doses for 2–3 days and on the last day of testing, urinary excretion of steroids was measured. Doubling the urinary steroids was defined as a normal response, indicating adequate pituitary reserve. Because this test results in the inhibition of residual cortisol production and thus is sometimes lethal in cortisol deficient patients, it has been recommended that this 2 or 3 day test be abandoned.

As currently used, 2–3 g of metyrapone is given between 2300 and 2400 hours and cortisol, 11-desoxycortisol, and ACTH are measured in the early morning. Baseline cortisol levels in the early morning specimen should decrease caused by inhibition of the enzyme required for cortisol formation. If in healthy persons cortisol does not decrease, an adequate enzymatic block has not been achieved, thereby invalidating the test. In healthy persons, 11-desoxycortisol increases after administration of metyrapone, because of an intact pituitary-adrenal axis. This response is usually preserved in persons with pituitary tumors. In patients with Cushing's disease, postmetyrapone 11-desoxycortisol values usually are greater than 10 µg/dL (>276 mmol/L), whereas patients with adrenal adenomas have 11-desoxycortisol results below 10 µg/dL (>276 mmol/L). When plasma corticotropin results after metyrapone administration are measured, healthy persons have a five- to ninefold increase in values, patients with pituitary disease have a smaller increase, and patients with adrenal adenomas show almost no increase.[70,76]

17-Hydroxycorticosteroids (17-OH Corticosteroids, 17-OH CS) Test

This procedure has been used to estimate glucocorticoids in a 24-hour urine collection. It lacks specificity because 11-desoxycortisol, cortisone (a metabolite of cortisol), and other metabolites are measured in addition to cortisol. The 17-hydroxycorticosteroid procedure has been abandoned in favor of the more specific UFC measurement or serum cortisol measurements.[77]

Interpretation

A myriad of tests are available for the diagnosis of Cushing syndrome; despite these tests, however, inaccurate diagnoses still occur. An approach to the diagnosis is seen in Figure 11-11. Perturbations of the dexamethasone suppression test include changing the dose size, timing of the dose, the specimen required for measurement, and the analyte measured. However, there is little evidence of diagnostic improvement with these measures.

TESTS FOR CONGENITAL ADRENAL HYPERPLASIA

Test: 17-Hydroxyprogesterone (17-OHP)

Background

The adrenal steroid 17-hydroxyprogesterone is converted to 11-desoxycortisol by the enzyme 21-hydroxylase. Impaired conversion results in congenital adrenal hyperplasia, which is caused by 21-hydroxylase deficiency. When this enzyme is absent or present in decreased amounts, 17-hydroxyprogesterone accumulates and cortisol is not produced effectively. As in other causes of congenital adrenal hyperplasia, the symptoms that occur originate from persistently elevated hormones produced as a consequence of the enzymatic block and the absence of steroids beyond the block. The consequence of lack of negative feedback of cortisol on corticotropin causes elevated corticotropin levels. Depending on the severity of the enzymatic block, other precursors accumulate and are metabolized to the androgens, dehydroepiandrosterone and androstenedione. Androstenedione then is converted peripherally to testosterone. In approximately two-thirds of cases, salt wasting occurs because of a deficiency in aldosterone biosynthesis. If left untreated, aldosterone deficits result in shock and death usually within the first 2 weeks of life. Hyperpigmentation may occur from increased levels of peptides from the ACTH precursor POMC, and bilateral cryptorchidism and hypospadias may occur in genetic females from excessive androgens.

Some patients are born without apparent abnormalities, but acquire signs and symptoms of androgen ex-

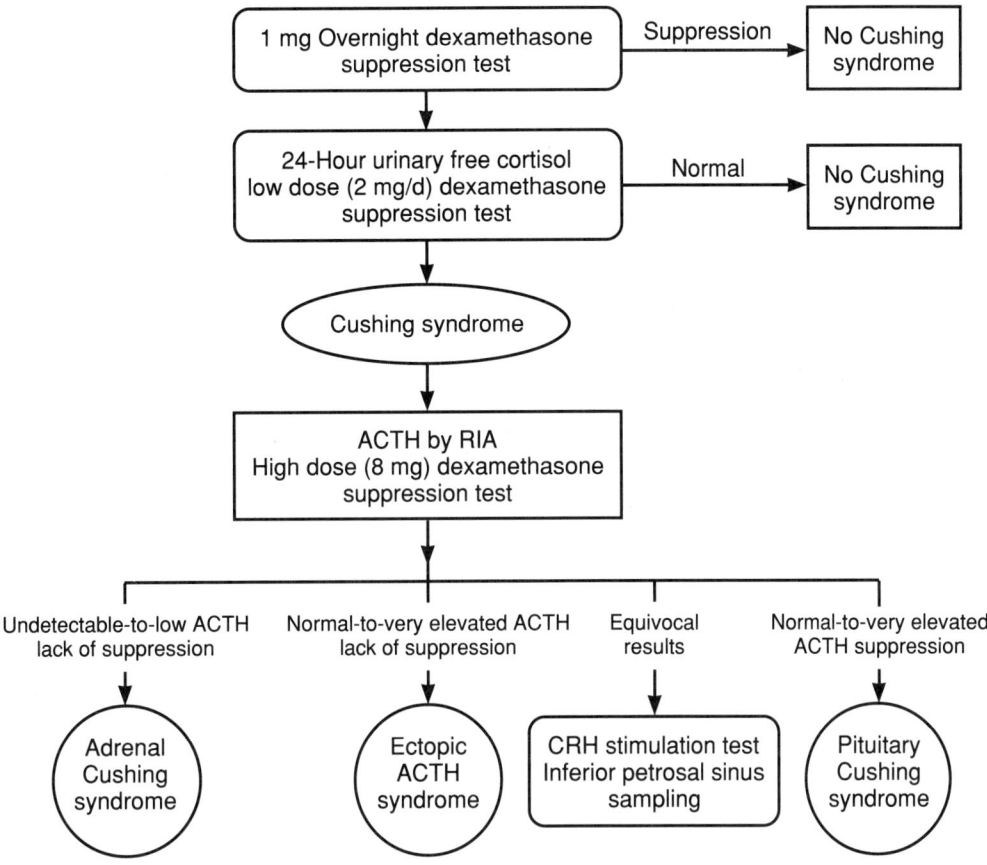

Fig. 11-11. Laboratory evaluation of Cushing syndrome.

cess during childhood, puberty, or later in life. Females may present with irregular menses from elevated progesterone levels that interfere with the ability of estradiol to stimulate the luteinizing hormone (LH) surge. In contrast, males may be infertile because elevated androgens suppress LH, thereby lowering testicular testosterone, resulting in poor spermatogenesis. Because manifestations are variable in severity and time of onset, the disorder has been called acquired adrenal hyperplasia, late-onset 21-hydroxylase deficiency, or cryptic disease when it occurs after the newborn period.

Selection

17-Hydroxyprogesterone serum levels are useful in identifying individuals with 21-hydroxylase deficiency, in identifying heterozygotes following ACTH stimulation of baseline 17-hydroxyprogesterone, and in neonatal screening. In addition, 17-hydroxyprogesterone is used in following adequacy of glucocorticoid replacement therapy in patients with 21-hydroxylase deficiency. Amniotic fluid 17-hydroxycorticosteroid measurements are useful in the diagnosis of prenatal 21-hydroxylase deficiencies.[78]

Logistics

The measurement of 17-hydroxyprogesterone can be performed using serum specimens obtained at about 0800 hours. For ACTH testing, a baseline and a specimen obtained 1 hour after administration of an intravenous bolus of cosyntropin are required. For neonatal diagnoses, screening at least 3 and preferable 5 days after birth is performed with 17-hydroxyprogesterone measurements using blood spots collected on filter paper. Amniotic fluid specimens are collected during the early second trimester.

17-Hydroxyprogesterone is measured by immunoassay; however, 17-hydroxypregnenolone has major cross-reactivity in some assays. Other steroids such as 11-desoxycortisol and corticosterone also cross-react, giving spuriously high results. Studies from several neonatal screening programs have shown interferences with 17-hydroxyprogesterone measurements following dilution of some specimens from filter paper. Most of the interfering water-soluble substances can be eliminated by an ether extraction step, followed by repeat assay.

Interpretation

The usual reference interval for serum 17-hydroxyprogesterone is approximately 20–100 ng/dL (~0.64–3.2 nmol/L). During pregnancy, 17-hydroxyprogesterone levels increase in maternal and fetal blood resulting in concentrations in cord serum that are much higher than those of older children and nonpregnant women. After birth, levels decline rapidly to reach those of healthy adults by 2–7 days. Premature and sick, full term infants between days 2 and 6 after birth have two to threefold higher results than healthy babies of the same age. In these infants, increased 17-hydroxyprogesterone is probably stress-related, and the magnitude of the increase probably depends on the severity of the illness.

Persons who are homozygotes for 21-hydroxylase deficiency have 17-hydroxyprogesterone results in the range of 10,000–100,000 ng/dL (320–3200 nmol/L), whereas heterozygotes usually have results of 100–1000 ng/dL (3.2–32 nmol/L). A nomogram with 17-hydroxyprogesterone levels before and after ACTH stimulation has been developed to describe patients in various diagnostic categories (Fig. 11-9). When following treatment of individuals with 21-hydroxylase deficiency, 17-hydroxyprogesterone results are considered appropriate when they are within the reference interval.

Amniotic fluid 17-hydroxyprogesterone values during the second trimester are in the range of 60–360 ng/dL (1.9–11.5 nmol/L), and with the salt-losing form of the disorder, these values may range up to 1900 ng/dL (≤60.8 nmol/L). Unfortunately, nonclassical cases have values that cannot be distinguished from unaffected homozygotes.[79]

Test: 11-Desoxycortisol and Desoxycorticosterone

In 11-hydroxylase deficiency, 11-desoxycortisol is not converted to cortisol and desoxycorticosterone is not converted to corticosterone. The subsequent deficiency of cortisol results in findings similar to those seen in 21-hydroxylase deficiency. Because desoxycorticosterone accumulates and has mineralocorticoid activity, elevated levels cause hypertension and hypokalemia. A number of variants exist with variable penetrance. Diagnosis is made by finding elevated 11-desoxycortisol (reference range 50–250 ng/dL [1.4–6.9 nmol/L]) and desoxycorticosterone (reference range 2–13 ng/dL [50–360 pmol/L]) in serum, and tetrahydro metabolites in urine several hundred-fold more than the usual trace concentrations seen in healthy individuals.

A number of rare causes of congenital adrenal hyperplasia are summarized in Table 11-11. Patients with lipoid adrenal hyperplasia (desmolase deficiency) usually die soon after birth because all adrenal and gonadal steroidogenesis is inhibited. Patients with 17-hydroxylase deficiency cannot synthesize cortisol and sex steroids: males develop incomplete masculinization and females primary amenorrhea. Frequently patients are hypertensive. Deficiency of 3-β hydroxysteroid dehydrogenase affects all classes of steroids causing slight virilization in female patients and incomplete masculinization in males with variable hypospadias. Frequently salt wasting is found, and 17-hydroxyprogesterone and dehydroepiandrosterone are elevated.[80]

INTRODUCTION: THE ALDOSTERONE-RENIN-ANGIOTENSIN SYSTEM

Aldosterone is secreted by the zona glomerulosa of the renal cortex and increases resorption of sodium in the distal convoluted tubule of the kidney. Aldosterone biosynthesis is controlled directly by ACTH, angiotensin II, and potassium. Other factors such as sodium depletion indirectly effect aldosterone by increasing adrenal responsiveness to angiotensin II.

Renin is a proteolytic enzyme synthesized and stored by specialized cells in the afferent arteriole wall of the renal glomerulus. The release of renin activates a cascade in which renin cleaves angiotensin, an α_2-globulin produced by the liver, to a decapeptide angiotensin I. Angiotensin converting enzyme (ACE), which is found in the highest concentration in the lung, but also is found in the kidney and a systemic vasculature, cleaves angiotensin I to angiotensin II. Because angiotensin II is a potent vasoconstrictor, it elevates blood pressure. It also directly stimulates aldosterone secretion leading to sodium retention and potassium loss. A seven amino acid peptide, angiotensin III, formed by proteolytic cleavage from angiotensin II, also stimulates aldosterone secretion and acts as a vasoconstrictor.

Renin is released in response to decreased kidney perfusion pressure such as occurs in hemorrhage, hypotension, or a reduction in extracellular fluid volume after sodium depletion. Catecholamines also directly stimulate renin secretion. Conversely, hyperkalemia, angiotensin II, and antidiuretic hormone can all inhibit renin secretion.

Table 11-11. Clinical and Biochemical Features of Congenital Adrenal Hyperplasia

Enzyme Deficient	Adrenal Hyperplasia	Virilization	Adrenocortical Insufficiency (Salt Losers)	Hypertension	Anomalous Sexual Development	Aldosterone Production	Laboratory Findings Increased	Laboratory Findings Decreased
21-Hydroxylase	Present	Present	Present in less than one-third	Absent	Female virilized	Deficient (salt losers)	Serum 17-OH progesterone	Cortisol, aldosterone
11-Hydroxylase	Present	Present	Absent	Present in majority	Female virilized	Normal	Plasma 11-desoxycortisol desoxycorticosterone	Cortisol, aldosterone
20,22-desmolase	Present	Absent	Present	Absent	Lack of masculinization	Deficient	None	All urine and plasma steroids
3-β-hydroxysteroid dehydrogenase	Present	Slight (in female)	Present	Absent	Female normal or slight virilization	Deficient	Dehydroepiandrosterone; 17-ketosteroids	
17-Hydroxylase	Present	Absent	Absent	Present	Absent secondary sex characteristics	Deficient	Metabolites of corticosterone and 11-desoxycorticosterone	
18-Hydroxylase and 18-hydroxysteroid dehydrogenase	Absent	Absent	Present	Absent	Normal	Absent	Metabolites of corticosterone and 11-desoxycorticosterone; 17-hydroxycorticosteroids increased in 18-dehydrogenase defect	

Abbreviation: 17-OH, 17-hydroxycorticosteroid.

Table 11-12. Secondary Causes of Hypertension

Renal Hypertension
    Renovascular
    Renal parenchymatous disease
    Primary reninism
Primary hyperaldosteronism
    Unilateral adrenal adenoma
    Bilateral idiopathic hyperaldosteronism
    Glucocorticoid-suppressible hyperaldosteronism
    Aldosterone-producing adrenocorticoid carcinoma
Rare causes of hypertension
    Pheochromocytoma
    Cushing syndrome
    Coarctation of the aorta

A large number of secondary causes of hypertension have been described, of which the most common are endocrine and relate to the aldosterone-renin-angiotensin system. Hypertension is one of the major medical problems of the world affecting up to 15% of the population in western countries. Lowering the blood pressure has been shown to reduce the incidence of stroke, renal failure, and coronary artery disease. In almost 80% of patients, the cause of hypertension cannot be identified, and these patients are defined as having primary or essential hypertension. Table 11-12 shows the causes of secondary hypertension.

BASIC TESTS

Test: Aldosterone

Background

Aldosterone is the major mineralocorticoid in humans and is produced exclusively in the zona glomerulosa of the adrenal cortex. Although weakly bound to albumin, almost all aldosterone circulates as free or unbound hormone with action occurring following binding to mineralocorticoid receptors in the kidney. In the distal renal tubule, aldosterone enhances the reabsorption of sodium and promotes the excretion of potassium and hydrogen ions. Aldosterone is metabolized rapidly by the liver and excreted as tetrahydro aldosterone; it also is metabolized by the kidney and excreted as aldosterone glucuronide.

Although the clinical syndrome was described over 40 years ago, the diagnostic approach for evaluation of patients with primary aldosterone still is controversial. The distinctive syndrome of hypertension, hypokalemia, low plasma renin activity (PRA), and increased aldosterone is easily recognizable, but the underlying cause is difficult to determine. At least four distinct entities occur: (1) a unilateral aldosterone-producing adenoma, (2) bilateral idiopathic hyperaldosteronism, (3) glucocorticoid-suppressible hyperaldosteronism, and (4) aldosterone-producing adrenocorticoid carcinoma. Not only are aldosterone-producing adenomas the most common cause, but the associated symptoms can be cured by unilateral adrenalectomy. However, bilateral idiopathic aldosteronism is frequently confused with an adenoma, and for this condition, unilateral adrenalectomy is not curative. Together, unilateral adenomas and bilateral idiopathic hyperaldosteronism account for over 95% of the causes of primary aldosteronism. Secondary aldosteronism is a group of disorders in which elevated aldosterone occurs in response to excessive renin secretion.

Selection

Aldosterone measurements are used to distinguish primary aldosteronism from other causes of hypertension and to separate unilateral aldosterone-producing adenomas from idiopathic hyperaldosteronism. Several potential screening tests have been used to aid in this identification. Because only patients with adrenal adenomas predictably respond to surgical treatment, accurate diagnosis is imperative. Adrenovenous sampling and subsequent aldosterone measurement is reserved for cases with conflicting screening results.

Logistics

Aldosterone estimations require serum specimens and are made by immunoassay. When adrenovenous sampling is used, a simultaneous specimen for aldosterone determination is obtained from a peripheral vein to aid interpretation. In healthy subjects, a low salt diet (less than 2 g per day), stress, an upright posture, and diuretics all increase plasma aldosterone; whereas a high salt diet, angiotensin converting enzyme inhibitors such as captopril, and lying in the supine position decrease aldosterone secretion. Combinations of those maneuvers that suppress aldosterone are used in the diagnosis of excessive secretion. Demonstration of the relative autonomy of aldosterone secretion frequently is accomplished in two different ways, administration of saline or a synthetic mineralocorticoid such as fludrocortisone. Even when time of sampling, posture, drug ingestion, dietary sodium, and potassium are controlled, it is difficult to discriminate with certainty between primary aldosteronism and other forms of hypertension using serum aldosterone measurements. It follows that

Table 11-13. Some Screening Laboratory Tests for Primary Aldosteronism

Test	Protocol	Comments
Plasma K^+	Supine, no exercise, rapid separation	Improved sensitivity if high sodium intake; normal K^+ unusual in adenomas
Urinary K^+	At least 5 days off diuretics; potassium intake should be known and >60 mmol/d	Only useful if hypokalemic; excretion >30 mmol/d abnormal and confirms urinary loss
Basal serum aldosterone	0800–1000 h; at least 1 h recumbent; should be on sodium intake >100 mmol/d, ideally fixed	Reference values must be age-matched; may only be high-normal in proven aldosteronism
Basal PRA	0800–1000 h; at least 1 h recumbent; should be on sodium intake >100 mmol/d, ideally fixed	Reference values must be age-matched; often overlaps with normal and LREH range
Saline suppression	Supine, infusion 2 L saline (154 mmol/L) between 0900-1300 h; aldosterone specimens at 0900, 1300 h	Healthy subjects and EH patients suppress 139 aldosterone to <5 ng/dL (139 pmol/L); avoid if evidence of heart failure
Fludrocortisone suppression	Fludrocortisone 0.6 mg/d for 3 d	Healthy subjects and EH patients suppress aldosterone to <4.0 ng/dL (111 pmol/L); avoid if evidence of heart failure
Stimulated PRA	Low sodium diet (<20 mmol/d) for 3 d or diet 1 d with furosemide 40 mg at 1000, 1400 and 1800 h; sample after 4 h standing 1300 h next d	Reference values must be age-matched; considerable overlap with LREH
Captopril suppression	Measure serum aldosterone while sitting, before and 2–3 h after captopril 25 mg orally	Healthy subjects and EH patients suppress aldosterone to <10.1 ng/dL (280 pmol/L); limited data, but no overlap of adenomas and LREH/normal subjects
Aldosterone/PRA		Ratios of <200 in EH and >400 in adenomas

Abbreviations: PRA, plasma renin activity; LREH, low renin essential hypertension; EH, essential hypertension.

random serum aldosterone sampling is useless for diagnostic purposes. Some procedures used for the diagnosis of primary aldosteronism are shown in Table 11-13.

To separate aldosterone-producing adenomas from idiopathic hyperaldosteronism, patients with primary aldosteronism are placed on a high salt diet and following overnight recumbency stand for 4 hours. Aldosterone, along with the immediate precursor of aldosterone, 18-hydroxycorticosterone, and cortisol measurements are made using baseline 0800- and 1200-hour specimens.

Urine aldosterone measurements have been used in the past with some reports indicating high discriminatory value after sodium loading. However, generally urine measurements have been replaced by serum measurements.

Interpretation

After 1 hour in the upright position, aldosterone levels usually are not increased to more than 5 ng/dL (>139 pmol/L) in patients with Addison's disease. However, aldosterone measurements for diagnosis of adrenal insufficiency are of little value.

When healthy subjects are placed on a high salt diet and lie supine, they suppress their plasma aldosterone levels to less than 10 ng/dL (<278 pmol/L). In this screening test, nonsuppression is defined as values higher than this cutoff. With administration of large amounts of sodium chloride (in one procedure, 2 L of isotonic saline infused over a 4-hour period), a reference population and those individuals with hypertension not caused by primary aldosteronism suppress their plasma aldosterone to below 5 ng/dL (<139 pmol/L). In contrast, those patients with primary aldosteronism have values above 8.5 ng/dL (>236 pmol/L). This test has been found to be the single best screening technique for outpatients, but it has a false positive rate of over 40%. When four screening tests for primary aldosteronism — (1) serum potassium less than 3.5 mEq/L (<3.5 mmol/L), (2) plasma aldosterone concentration after saline infusion, (3) lack of a depressed response following the administration of the angiotensin II analogue saralasin, and (4) stimulated PRA — are combined, the diagnostic yield is enhanced substantially.[81]

An alternate diagnostic maneuver is the administration of 200 ng of synthetic mineralocorticoid and fludrocortisone, three times a day for 3 days, and demonstration of a nonsuppressibility of serum aldosterone. A reference population suppresses serum aldosterone to less than 4 ng/dL (<111 pmol/L). An important, and often ignored, factor in the interpretation of aldosterone measurements is the pronounced fall in levels in adults with increasing age. Reference ranges appropriate for age must thus be used. Listed in Table 11-14 are some of the screening tests commonly used for primary aldosteronism.

In patients with primary aldosteronism, distinguishing patients with aldosterone-producing adenomas from those with idiopathic hyperaldosteronism, who usually are managed medically, remains a major diagnostic challenge. To separate patients with aldosterone-producing adenomas from idiopathic hyperaldosteronism, the criteria of aldosterone concentrations increasing by greater than 33% over baseline in patients standing for 4 hours are found with idiopathic hyperaldosteronism, whereas absence of an increase of this magnitude supports a diagnosis of an aldosterone-producing adenoma. Healthy persons and those with essential hypertension show a two- to fourfold increase in aldosterone levels over baseline. If the circadian rhythm of ACTH is not substantiated by a decrease in the 1200 hour cortisol value over baseline, the test is invalid. Patients

Table 11-14. Summary of Methods for Differentiation Between Adrenal Adenoma and Idiopathic Hyperaldosteronism

	Adrenal Adenomas	Idiopathic Hyperaldosteronism	Discriminatory Value
Plasma potassium	Very low to normal	Low normal	K^+ <2.5 mmol/L uncommon with IHA
Basal serum aldosterone	High/very high	High/high normal	Poor
Basal PRA	Low	Low/low normal	Poor
Aldosterone response to upright posture	Fall in 70–90%	Rise (90%+)	Fall is good predictor of adenoma
18-OH corticosterone levels	High	Normal/slightly high	Good
Aldosterone response to A II infusion	Suppressed	Increased	Good
CT scanning	Tumor, usually only if >10 mm	Normal/slightly enlarged	Good for adenoma: not for IHA
Scintiscanning	Unilateral uptake	Bilateral uptake	Good with new techniques (90%)
Ultrasonography	Tumor, usually only if >15–20 mm	Indistinguishable from normal	Poor unless large adenoma
Adrenal venograms	Tumor	Enlarged bilaterally	Fair (50–80%)
Adrenal venous sampling for aldosterone	Unilateral increase contralateral suppression	Bilateral aldosterone production	Excellent (80–95%)

Abbreviations: IHA, idiopathic hyperaldosteronism; 18-OH, 18-hydroxycorticosteroid; A II, angiotensin II; CT, computed topography.

with aldosterone-producing adenomas have recumbent 18-hydroxycorticosterone levels of more than 100 ng/dL (>2800 pg/L), whereas patients with idiopathic hyperaldosteronism have results less than this cutoff value.[82] Radiologic scanning procedures are helpful in this differential.

Adrenovenous sampling occasionally is used, but is recommended only when screening procedures and computed tomographic (CT) scanning give conflicting results. A specimen should be obtained simultaneously from a peripheral vein to account for variations in the serum levels. Simultaneous sampling and expression of aldosterone and cortisol as a ratio improve accuracy; cortisol measurements are used to determine correct catheter placement.

Reasons for unexpected aldosterone findings include use of immunoassays that cross-react with steroids in higher concentration than aldosterone such as 11-desoxycortisol, inadequate control of conditions of sampling, and injection of drugs such as aldosterone. In critically ill patients, aldosterone concentrations may be inappropriately low, especially when expressed as PRA/aldosterone ratios. Similarly, low levels and dissociation of renin and aldosterone occur during hypoxemia and during heparin therapy.

Test: Renin (Plasma Renin Activity, Plasma Renin Concentration)

Background and Selection

Plasma renin measurements are used in screening hypertensives, whereas renal vein renin measurements are used to predict the likelihood of surgical cure in patients with renovascular hypertension. A renin measurement made on a random specimen offers no useful information. When used to diagnose primary aldosteronism, a suppressed value is unreliable.

Terminology

Renin measurements are of two types, renin activity and renin concentration. For the measurement of PRA, a plasma specimen containing renin is allowed to react with its substrate, angiotensin I. Then, after a specified period, the reaction is terminated and measurement of generated angiotensin I (or II) is made. For the measurement of plasma renin concentration, the effect of endogenous substrate is eliminated and highly active ovine substrate is added. Because the substrate is in excess, angiotensin I generation occurs linearly with increasing renin concentration. An international reference standard developed for this method, which is expressed in Goldblatt U/dL (GU/dL), allows result comparisons among laboratories. Assays of PRA and plasma renin concentration provide similar information except in a few clinical situations. With oral contraceptive administration, plasma renin concentration remains within the reference interval, whereas PRA increases owing to the increase in substrate. Other procedures such as freezing and thawing have been found to convert prorenin to renin and thereby increase values in plasma renin concentration assays.

Logistics

Because renin release is controlled by many physiologic variables, it is extremely important to know the conditions under which the specimen was obtained. Such conditions as upright posture, the administration of diuretics, or low sodium diets help stimulate renin release, and should be adequately controlled before measurement of plasma renin. Renin also appears to be extremely labile so that the variables involved in specimen processing should be vigorously controlled. Blood should be drawn into iced tubes containing chelating agents for inactivation of enzymes (angiotensinases), centrifuged in the cold, and plasma frozen to avoid substantial loss of angiotensinase activity: with this technique the specimen is stable for several months at $-20°C$.

Comparison of results for PRA measurements among laboratories is an impossibility because of procedural differences such as variations of pH, ionic strength, the length of the assay, the angiotensinase inhibitor, lack of a specific reference preparation, and the conditions under which the specimen was obtained. In addition, renin assays raise confusion regarding units of measurement used, even when an attempt is made to express the many arbitrary units in the same terms (angiotensin liberated/mL/h). There are wide ranges reported for human PRA in reference populations.

One of the simplest procedures requiring PRA measurements is that described by Kaplan et al.[83] Plasma renin activity is determined in fasting subjects after 30 minutes in an upright position after intravenous infusion of 40 mg of furosemide (Lasix). This test does not require hospitalization, special diet, or prolonged standing. Plasma renin also can be interpreted relative to a simultaneous 24-hour urine sodium excretion after several days on stable sodium intake and off diuretics.

Interpretation

Plasma renin measurements are useful in screening hypertensives because an elevated level may suggest renovascular hypertension and a very low level makes renovascular hypertension unlikely. For the procedure requiring a fast upright posture and the infusion of furosemide, a reference population of whites and blacks had plasma renin activity more than 1.0 and 0.5 ng/mL/h, respectively, whereas low renin hypertensive patients were not able to respond as well. When plasma renin is plotted relative to the simultaneous 24-hour urine excretion, an inverse relationship between plasma renin and urine sodium is found, allowing the identification of low, medium, and high plasma renin groups from a nomogram. Listed in Tables 11-15 and 11-16 are causes of hypertension associated with low and high levels of renin. A renin measurement made using a random specimen offers no useful information. A variety of other procedures for renin categorization have been developed using various stimuli for renin release (Table 11-17).

Bravo et al.[84] reported that PRA in patients with aldosteronism is suppressed in approximately 75% of patients and either increased or within the reference interval in others. He concluded PRA, therefore, is not a reliable screening test for primary aldosteronism.

Several series have concluded that elevated PRA is highly suggestive of renal hypertension, but a result within the reference interval by no means excludes the diagnosis. A variety of possible explanations for the relatively low sensitivity and specificity for renin measurement include false negative results from (1) dilution of elevated renin from the affected side by suppressed value on the contralateral side to give a nonelevated plasma value; (2) lack of attention to conditions of collection such as sodium excretion, upright posture, or both; (3) segmental lesions not demonstrating an increased PRA because of dilutional effect of blood draining nonischemic areas of the kidney; and (4) lack of attention to circadian rhythm, which allows better discrimination from the reference population in the evening hours. False positive results can occur in hypertensive conditions such as malignant hypertension, hypertension treated with diuretics or vasodilators, congestive heart failure, or essential hypertension.

Some investigators advocate renin measurements made with blood obtained simultaneously from both

Table 11-16. Some Causes of Hypertension Associated With High Levels of Plasma Renin

Renin-secreting tumor
Malignant accelerated hypertension
Renovascular hypertension
    Major arterial lesions
    Segmental lesions
Chronic renal failure
    End-stage
    Transplant rejection
Cushing syndrome
Iatrogenic
    Volume depleting agents
    Vasodilating agents
    Glucocorticoids
    Estrogens

Table 11-15. Some Causes of Hypertension Associated With Low Levels of Plasma Renin

"Primary" excess of mineralocorticoids
    Primary aldosteronism
    Pseudoprimary (idiopathic) aldosteronism
    Glucocorticoid suppressible aldosteronism
    11-Desoxycorticosterone excess
        18-Hydroxy-11-desoxycorticosterone excess
        Adrenal carcinoma (mineralocorticoid excess)
"Secondary" excess of mineralocorticoids
    Licorice ingestion
    Excess unsupervised sodium intake
    Low renin, low aldosterone syndrome

Table 11-17. Renal Vein Renin Ratios: Pathophysiologic and Technical Causes for False Negative and False Positive Results

Pathophysiologic Causes	Technical Causes
Equivalent bilateral disease	Catheter malposition with admixture
Segmental lesions	Vigorous aspiration of blood causing admixture
Renin suppression by volume, posture, or antihypertensive drugs	Multiple renal veins
Extensive collateral circulation	Valsalva maneuver
Nonrenin-mediated renovascular hypertension	Contrast media interference with renin assay
	Heparin interference with renin assay
	Nonsimultaneous sampling
	Errors in renin assay
	Reduction in renal blood flow without increased renin secretion
	Inadequate surgical repair

renal veins. With unilateral renovascular hypertension, the affected side demonstrates elevated renin measurements and the contralateral side suppressed values. Various cutoff ratios have been advocated, with higher ratios (2:1) yielding better diagnostic sensitivity and poorer specificity whereas lower ratios (1.5:1) offer poorer diagnostic sensitivity and better specificity. Others have recommended expression of renal vein renin results in terms of arterial values (i.e., renal vein renin minus arterial renin/arterial renin). For estimation of arterial renin, specimens are obtained from the inferior vena cava. In healthy persons an increment of renin in the renal veins relative to the renal arteries is 0.24 or 24%; when one kidney is ischemic, its renin secretion is 0.48 or 48% on the ischemic side and it approaches zero on the contralateral side. In a study of comparing the two methods of expressing renin measurements, the incremental method was found diagnostically superior to expressing renin from both renal veins as a ratio.[85] Some argue that renal vein renin measurements are a poor indicator of surgical outcome. Imprecision of renin assays, especially at low values, is responsible for false positive and false negative results. Elevated ratios are obtained frequently in patients with essential hypertension and insignificant renal artery stenosis. Additionally, hypersecretion of renin occasionally is not a factor in causing renovascular hypertension. Listed in Table 11-17 are some causes of false negative and false positive renal vein renin results.

Test: Angiotensin Converting Enzyme (ACE)

Angiotensin converting enzyme is a protease that converts the decapeptide angiotensin I to the octapeptide angiotensin II and also activates bradykinin. By altering concentrations of angiotensin, it plays a central role in the control of blood pressure.

Angiotensin converting enzyme is useful in monitoring patients with sarcoid and to measure compliance of sarcoid patients for treatment with steroids. Angiotensin converting enzyme is of limited value in the diagnosis of sarcoid because only two-thirds of patients have elevated values and patients with a number of other granulomatous diseases such as tuberculosis, alcoholic hepatitis, and hyperthyroidism have elevated values as well. In patients with sarcoid, ACE is elevated due to activation of the monocyte macrophage system involved in developing granulomas. Serum is a specimen of choice for measurement and serum ACE is surprisingly stable during storage. No loss of activity occurs for weeks when specimens are stored at room temperature, or in the cold, or frozen for months. A number of different assays are used including chemical and immunologic methods, but little effort to date has been made toward correlating results between assays.[86]

ADRENAL MEDULLA

INTRODUCTION

The catecholamines and their metabolites are used mainly in confirming the diagnosis of pheochromocytoma and in the diagnosis and follow-up of patients with neuroblastoma.

Biochemistry

Norepinephrine is synthesized in the brain, adrenal medulla, and sympathetic nerve endings (Fig. 11-12). In the adrenal medulla, epinephrine is formed from norepinephrine. Both epinephrine and norepinephrine, which together are known as the catecholamines, are secreted from the adrenal medulla in response to various physiologic stimuli. Small amounts of the catecholamines are excreted in the urine unchanged, but most are metabolized by monoamine oxidase and catechol *O*-methyltransferase. These enzymes are responsible for inactivating circulating catecholamines and probably play a role in disposing of the excess catecholamine stores. When catecholamines are released from the sympathetic nerve endings, they are retaken up by nerve endings by an active transport mechanism and converted to 3,4 dihydroxyphenyglycol (DHPG).

The major end products of epinephrine and norepinephrine metabolism are vanillylmandelic acid (VMA), metanephrine, and normetanephrine. Other metabolites may appear in the urine as well, for example, 3-methoxy-4-hydroxyphenylacetic acid (homovanillic acid [HVA]), the final product of dopamine metabolism. A dopamine metabolite, 3-methoxy-4-hydroxyphenylglycol (MHPG), is thought to be produced by brain catecholamine metabolism.

Specimens

Most commonly, 24-hour urine (acidified) collections are used for VMA, metanephrines, and free catecholamines. Urine is acidified to improve stability of the

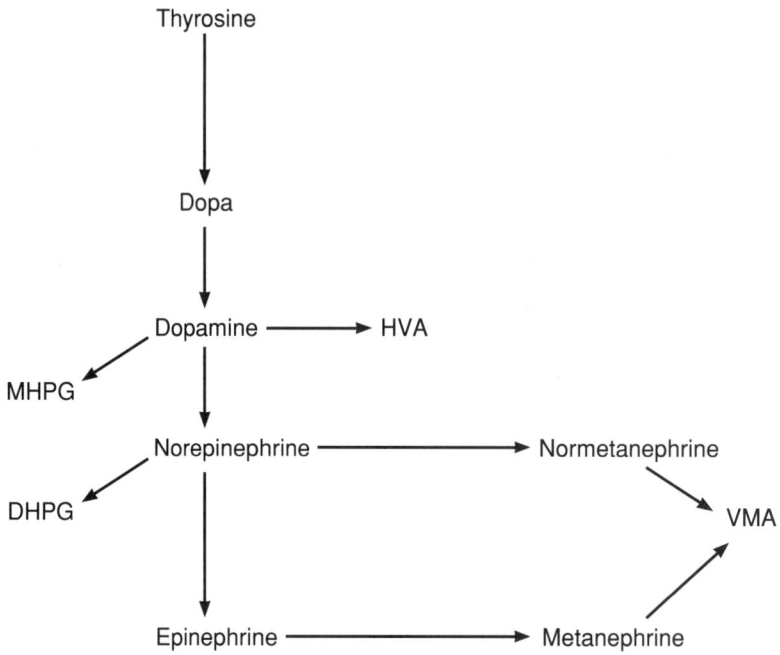

Fig. 11-12. Outline of catecholamine synthesis and metabolism. HVA, homovanillic acid; MHPG, 3-methoxy-4-hydroxyphenylglycol; DHPG, 3,4 dihydroxyphenyglycol; VMA, vanillylmandelic acid.

catecholamines, but this is not strictly necessary for VMA and metanephrines.[87] With the currently used methods, dietary restrictions are not necessary for these analytes. Ideally, specimens should be collected when the patient is drug-free, is medically stable, and is not under stress. Many drugs influence catecholamine metabolism (Table 11-18) and thus can interfere with these measurements. Method dependent interferences also occur especially with the spectrophotometric and fluorimetric assays.

Pheochromocytoma

Pheochromocytomas are catecholamine-producing tumors that are usually benign. Although pheochromocytomas are associated with 1% or less of hypertension cases, proper diagnosis of these patients is important because of the curable nature of the hypertension produced. It is especially important to test patients with signs or symptoms suggestive of pheochromocytoma (e.g., the combination of headaches, palpitations, and excessive sweating) and those with certain clinical characteristics (e.g., malignant hypertension in a young patient). Pheochromocytomas are components of the multiple endocrine neoplasia syndromes, types IIA and B, and can be associated with neuroectodermal disorders such as neurofibromatosis. Urinary catecholamines or their metabolites traditionally are used as the initial screening tests with other tests usually reserved for cases where the diagnosis is not clear.

In the urine of healthy persons, VMA predominates (Fig. 11-13). In contrast, there is a greater proportional increase in urinary-free catecholamines than in VMA in most pheochromocytoma patients.

Neuroblastoma

Neuroblastoma is a relatively common childhood malignant tumor, usually occurring before the age of 6. Symptoms relate primarily to tumor mass rather than to hypertension, which is often mild or absent. About 90% of tumors are associated with elevated catecholamine results. Urinary HVA and VMA traditionally are used to follow neuroblastoma patients, but a variety of other catecholamine metabolites hold promise. Spot urines can be used because they alleviate collection problems in small children. Plasma measurements, especially of dopa, also appear to hold promise. In addition to the catecholamines or their metabolites, other markers are used. Elevated plasma levels of neuropeptide Y have been reported with neuroblastomas, but also occur in pheochromocytoma as well.[89] Plasma levels of GD_2 gangliosides are increased in neuroblastoma patients and appear to correlate disease activity.[90] The N-*myc* oncogene, which is amplified in some neuro-

Table 11-18.	Influences of Catecholamines (Examples)

Increases
    Endogenous stimulation (emotional and physical stress)
    Exogenous catecholamines (nose drops, appetite suppressants)
    Drugs
        Indirect acting sympathomimetic (amphetamines)
        Vasodilators (nitrates, hydralazine, phenothiazines)
        α-Adrenergic antagonist (prazosin, phentolamine)
        Diuretics in doses sufficient to produce sodium depletion
        Miscellaneous (cigarette and marijuana smoking, caffeine ingestion)
        β-adrenergic antagonists
        Tricyclics (increase norepinephrine)
Decreases
    Drugs
        Clonidine
        α-Methyl-para-tyrosine
        Bromocriptine
        Dexamethasone
        Monoamine oxidase inhibitors

(Modified from Cryer,[87] with permission.)

blastoma patients, is used as a prognostic indicator: amplification of N-*myc* is highly correlated with tumor progression.[91]

TESTS TO DIAGNOSE PHEOCHROMOCYTOMA

Test: Vanillylmandelic Acid (3-Methoxy-4-Hydroxymandelic Acid)

Background and Selection

Urinary VMA measurements are commonly used to screen for pheochromocytoma, but they are considered less sensitive, although more specific, than urinary metanephrine measurements. Urinary VMA also is used to follow patients with neuroblastoma.

Logistics

The usual specimen is a 24-hour urine specimen (acidified), but random urine specimens have been used for neuroblastoma patients.[92] Dietary VMA causes inter-

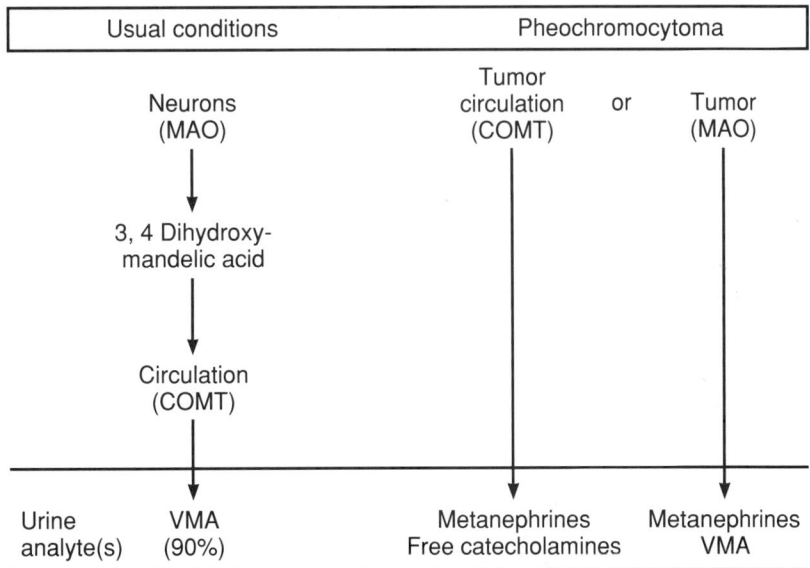

Fig. 11-13. Catecholamine metabolism. (Modified from Benowitz,[88] with permission.)

ference with p-nitroaniline screening methods. The so-called VMA diet, which is free of coffee, vanilla, and certain fruits and vegetables, is not necessary because the p-nitroaniline methods are no longer in use. Dietary phenolic acids do not interfere with the commonly used Pisano technique or chromatographic procedures. Catecholamine-containing or -stimulating drugs (Table 11-18), and other drugs interfering with the VMA method used, should be discontinued approximately 2 weeks before specimen collection if possible.

Interpretation

The reference range for urinary VMA in adults is approximately 7.0 mg/24 h (~35.3 µmol/d). Results for VMA also can be expressed in terms of urinary creatinine. In children, at least up to the age of about 15 years, urinary VMA levels tend to be higher (per milligram of creatinine) and more variable than in adults.[92] In pheochromocytoma patients, there is usually a greater proportional increase in metanephrine and free catecholamines than VMA. Some tumors, however, contain large amounts of monoamine oxidase and in these patients, VMA and metanephrines predominate in the urine. False negative VMA results occur in 10–30% or more of patients. Reliability of urinary VMA results is influenced by completeness in collecting a 24-hour urine specimen, the patient's renal function, and tumors that may secrete catecholamines only intermittently. Drugs that influence catecholamine metabolism can cause increased, decreased, or variable test results and many method dependent interferences occur.

In patients with neuroblastomas, almost 75% have increased urinary VMA levels at the time of diagnosis.[93] Urinary VMA along with urinary HVA traditionally are used to follow neuroblastoma patients. Plasma VMA levels have been used for neuroblastoma patients, but assays are not widely available.

Test: Metanephrine

Background and Selection

Urinary total metanephrine (metanephrine and normetanephrine) measurement is considered the most sensitive urine screening test for pheochromocytoma. Many investigators consider urinary metanephrine the single most reliable test for pheochromocytoma because it has the fewest false negative results.

Logistics

Usually 24-hour urine collections (acidified) are used for total metanephrine determinations, although random 1-hour urine specimens with results expressed per unit of creatinine give comparable results.[94] A variety of methods including colorimetric, fluorimetric, high performance liquid chromatography (HPLC), and immunoassay can be used to measure total metanephrine.

Normetanephrine and metanephrine can be measured separately with some techniques. Catecholamine-containing drugs or those that effect catecholamine metabolism can cause interference (Table 11-18). Especially with the chemical methods, drugs (e.g., methyldopa) or urine pigments can cause assay interference, usually giving rise to small increases in metanephrine results.

Interpretation

For adults, the reference range for urinary metanephrines is less than about 1.0–1.5 mg/24 h (<5.5–7.3 µmol/d) with the exact reference range depending on the method used. In children until about 15 years of age, urinary metanephrine results tend to be higher and more variable than in adults. Metanephrines are markedly elevated in most pheochromocytoma patients. Regardless of their blood pressure patterns, patients with pheochromocytomas tend to have markedly elevated metanephrine results (greater than about 1000 mg/24 h [>5000 µmol/d]).[94] False negative results occur in only about 1–2% of patients,[95] although higher percentages of false negative results have been reported in other studies. Elevated results can occur in patients subject to severe stress such as sepsis, shock, or metastatic disease and small increases can be caused by assay interferences (see above). Urinary metanephrines also can be elevated in neuroblastoma patients, but are not a sensitive measure of residual tumor.

Test: Catecholamines, Urinary (Free)

Background and Selection

Urinary catecholamines (free) are used to screen for pheochromocytoma. Fractionated urinary catecholamines may be helpful in some specific clinical circumstances (see below).

Logistics

A 24-hour urine (acidified) collection is the preferred specimen. Preferably the specimen should be kept cold, because catecholamines are more stable under these conditions. If possible, the patient should be medically stable and not taking any medications. As with urinary VMA and metanephrines, catecholamines and catecholamine-stimulating drugs interfere with results. Method dependent interferences also occur especially with the older fluorimetric method. Urinary-free (unconjugated) catecholamines are measured because total urinary catecholamines (unconjugated plus conjugated forms) include interfering dietary catecholamines. When specific analysis of individual, free (unconjugated) urinary catecholamines is performed, for example by HPLC, this is called fractionation.

Interpretation

The usual reference range for urinary-free catecholamines is up to about 100 µg/24 h (591 nmol/d). Reference ranges for fractionated catecholamines are epinephrine, up to about 20 µg/24 h (110 mmol/d); norepinephrine, up to about 80 µg/24 h (473 nmol/d); and dopamine, up to about 400 µg/24 h (2610 µmol/d). Over 95% of pheochromocytomas cause elevated urinary epinephrine or norepinephrine or both. A few cases of pure dopa or dopamine-producing tumors have been reported. Urinary catecholamines are increased during stress and after ingestion of catecholamine-containing medication. Urinary catecholamines have been used in screening for pheochromocytoma and may be helpful for patients with intermittently secreting tumors. They also have been used in diagnostically difficult cases. Urinary epinephrine levels have been used to screen for pheochromocytoma in patients with multiple endocrine neoplasia (MEA), in which there is a good correlation between elevated urinary epinephrine levels and pheochromocytoma.[95] Fractionation of urinary catecholamine levels into norepinephrine and epinephrine components is used to assist in localization of the tumor, with increased epinephrine levels indicating an adrenal location. However, the most useful procedure for localization of pheochromocytomas is meta-iodobenzyl-guanidine (MIBG) scintigraphy.[96]

OTHER CATECHOLAMINE TESTS

Test: Catecholamines, Plasma

Background and Selection

Plasma catecholamines generally are used only in diagnostically difficult cases of suspected pheochromocytoma and often in conjunction with clonidine. Patients undergo screening with urinary tests, usually metanephrines, often along with catecholamines or VMA. If the diagnosis remains unclear, tests such as fractionated urinary catecholamines or plasma catecholamines are then undertaken.

Logistics

Blood Collection

If possible, patients should be studied when medically stable and when not taking any medications. Strict precautions must be taken in obtaining specimens for plasma catecholamines. The patient should be in the fasting state and should rest in a supine position for 30 minutes before the test and during the testing period. Blood should be drawn via a venous catheter that has been placed long enough in advance to avoid elevations in catecholamines because of apprehension or pain.[97] Noise, stress, discomfort, and body position, as well as caffeine, nicotine, or food may profoundly affect plasma catecholamine results.[95] Catecholamines deteriorate in whole blood specimens at a rate of about 30% per hour at room temperature. Therefore, blood specimens should be drawn into iced tubes preferably with an anticoagulant and antioxidant. Plasma should be promptly separated in a refrigerated centrifuge and frozen. Catecholamines deteriorate at about 5% a month at $-20°C$, but are stable at $-70°C$ for at least 1 year.[87]

Assays

Because conjugated catecholamines have a half-life of 30 minutes to several hours, total catecholamine results remain high, even following clonidine. Radioimmunoassays that measure total catecholamines (free and conjugated) thus give false positive results with the clonidine suppression test (see below). Radioenzymatic assays with catechol O-methyltransferase, which measure free catecholamines, are recommended for use with clonidine suppression.

Interpretation

The reference range for plasma catecholamines is about 150–650 ng/L (~0.89–3.84 nmol/L) for the radioenzymatic method. There appears to be a diurnal variation of catecholamine secretion as well as increases with age. Stress, physical and mental, can cause dramatic elevation in plasma catecholamines. Plasma catecholamine results are increased with change in posture from reclining to standing, exertion, emotional or physical stress, and in patients taking a variety of drugs. They are elevated in acute as well as chronic illnesses and moderate elevations appear in some patients who presumably have essential hypertension.

Plasma catecholamine results are difficult to interpret because of the many physiologic and pharmacologic causes of increased levels. In general, plasma catecholamine results of 1000 ng/L (5.9 nmol/L) or less exclude the diagnosis pheochromocytoma, whereas values of 1000–2000 ng/L (5.9–11.8 nmol/L) are considered equivocal. Plasma catecholamine results greater than 2000 ng/L (11.8 nmol/L) indicate that the patient has a pheochromocytoma.[97] Low plasma catecholamines can occur in patients with pheochromocytoma because the tumor is not secreting during the time the specimen is obtained or because the tumor produces mainly pharmacologically inactive metabolites. Elevation of plasma epinephrine alone may be significant, because rare tumors secrete only epinephrine.

Elevated catecholamine levels also occur in patients with essential hypertension. Other tests including the ratio of DHPG to norepinephrine and the clonidine suppression test have been used to distinguish patients with pheochromocytoma from those with essential hypertension. The ratio of DHPG to norepinephrine in plasma has been used to differentiate pheochromocytoma patients and those with essential hypertension. The ratio of plasma DHPG to norepinephrine is less than 0.5 in pheochromocytoma patients as compared with greater than 2 in essential hypertensives[95] (see Test: 3,4 Dihydroxyphenylglycol).

Clonidine Suppression Test

Clonidine suppression tests usually are reserved for patients with borderline elevations in plasma catecholamines and consist of plasma-free catecholamine measurements before and after oral clonidine administration. The clonidine suppression test was developed to eliminate the sympathetic nervous system contribution to plasma catecholamine levels. Clonidine is a centrally active α-adenergic agonist that suppresses neurogenic catecholamine release. In hypertensive patients with equivocal plasma catecholamines results, a clonidine suppression test is used to distinguish patients with pheochromocytoma from others. Normal clonidine suppression consists of a fall in plasma-free catecholamines to less than 500 ng/L 2–3 hours after clonidine administration.[97] Plasma-free catecholamine results are suppressed in patients with essential hypertension, but are not suppressed in patients with pheochromocytoma.[98]

Other Tests

False negative and false positive clonidine suppression test results occur and appropriate plasma catecholamine assays may not be readily available.[99] Thus other attempts have been made to approach difficult diagnostic cases. Overnight clonidine suppression (measurement of urinary norepinephrine and epinephrine following sleep and clonidine) has been used. Sleep alone suppresses urinary norepinephrine and epinephrine in patients without pheochromocytoma, but greater suppression is obtained with sleep and clonidine combined. After sleep and clonidine, urinary norepinephrine and epinephrine collected overnight are normally suppressed to less than 60 and 20 nmol/mmol creatinine, respectively.[100]

Test: 3,4 Dihydroxyphenyglycol (DHPG)

Background and Selection

Urinary norepinephrine determination is a sensitive diagnostic test for pheochromocytoma, but may be elevated owing to increased sympathetic nervous system activity. Measurement of DHPG has been suggested to improve the specificity of norepinephrine measurements in patients with suspected pheochromocytoma. Norepinephrine released from sympathetic neurons is subject to reuptake and conversion to DHPG by monoamine oxidase. Sympathetic stimulation causes rises in both DHPG and norepinephrine of similar magnitude, whereas norepinephrine infusion causes a large rise in free norepinephrine as compared with DHPG. In patients with pheochromocytoma, norepinephrine appears to be metabolized similar to the infusion model; that is, the DHPG level is low in comparison to norepinephrine. However, DHPG measurements are not considered routine at this time.[101]

Interpretation

The reference range for DHPG in hypertensive patients without pheochromocytoma is about 152–169 mg/24 h (~90–1000 nmol/d). Analysis of 24-hour urine collections for DHPG in addition to free norepinephrine may improve the specificity of urinary catecholamine measurements in confirming the diagnosis of pheochromocytoma. The ratio of DHPG to norepinephrine or norepinephrine to DHPG is used. A comparison of norepinephrine and DHPG levels appears to allow differentiation of sympathetic activity versus pheochromocytoma. Sympathetic stimulation causes rises of similar magnitude in both DHPG and norepinephrine. In contrast, in patients with pheochromocytoma substantial rises in free norepinephrine occur with only modest increases in DHPG.[101] Thus the ratio of DHPG to norepinephrine in plasma is low (less than 0.5) in patients with pheochromocytoma compared with patients with essential hypertension (greater than

2.0). Some patients with pheochromocytoma, however, excrete large amounts of DHPG.

Test: 3,4 Dihydroxyphenylalanine (Dopa)

Patients with neuroblastoma consistently have high plasma dopa levels. In most patients, plasma dopa measurements correlate with the course of the disease and appear more reliable than traditional urinary catocholamine determinations.[102] Patients with benign pheochromocytoma have results within the reference range, but about 60% of patients with malignant pheochromocytomas have been reported to have elevated plasma dopa results.[103]

Test: Dopamine

In patients with dopamine-secreting pheochromocytomas, free dopamine may only be slightly elevated, whereas conjugated levels are markedly increased. Because free plasma dopamine usually is measured, diagnostic difficulties may ensue. Urinary dopamine assays may be a more sensitive test for dopamine-secreting tumors.[88] Elevated dopamine levels also occur in patients with neuroblastoma and in some patients with carcinoids.

Test: Homovanillic Acid

Urinary HVA is used in the diagnosis and monitoring of patients with neuroblastoma. Although 24-hour urine specimens have been used, random urine specimens are suitable for testing and have obvious advantages especially in the pediatric population.[92] Plasma HVA results have been used for the diagnosis and follow-up of neuroblastoma patients,[104] but assays are not widely available. In pediatric patients, the reference range for urinary VMA varies with age with the highest results, expressed as μg/mg creatinine, occurring in the youngest patients. Values decrease with age reaching adult levels by about 15–18 years of age.[92] At the time of diagnosis, about 90% of neuroblastoma patients have elevated urinary HVA results.[93] Urinary HVA also is increased in familial dysautonomia (Riley-Day syndrome) and some pheochromocytoma patients.

Test: 3-Methoxy-4-Hydroxyphenylglycol

Both the central nervous system and the sympathetic nervous system contribute to plasma MHPG, a metabolite of norepinephrine. Measurement of MHPG is used in assessing norepinephrine function in the central nervous system. Plasma, which contains free and conjugated MHPG, is often used, but MHPG also is measured in the cerebrospinal fluid and urine. The concentration of free MHPG in plasma is in the range of 1.5–5.5 μg/L (8.9–32.6 nmol/L). 3-Methoxy-4-hydroxyphenylglycol is a possible marker of depression and has been proposed as a diagnostic tool in the study of anxiety disorders. It also has been studied as a predictor of response to the tricyclic antidepressants and as a monitor for effectiveness in monoamine oxidase inhibitors.[105] It also is increased in patients with pheochromocytoma.

SEX HORMONES

INTRODUCTION

The gonadotropins, lutropin (luteotropic hormone) and follitropin (follicle stimulating hormone), are glycoproteins with a molecular mass of approximately 30,000 da composed of an α- and β-subunit. The gonadotropins have structural similarities not only to each other, but to the other pituitary glycoprotein hormones, TSH and human chorionic gonadotropin (hCG). The α-subunits of these four hormones are nearly identical, with the specificity of each hormone conferred by a different β-subunit. In contrast to apparent cell type specificity for most pituitary hormones, some pituitary cells appear to synthesize both LH and FSH, but cells containing only LH or FSH also are present. In men, LH appears to act on Leydig or interstitial cells of the testes to cause the increased synthesis of testosterone. In women, LH acts on the interstitial cells of the ovary resulting in synthesis of androgens, estrogens, and progestins depending on other local factors. Luteinizing hormone binds to specific hormone receptors on the cell membrane and acts by a mechanism involving activation of adenylate cyclase and induction of AMP. Follicle stimulating hormone appears to control gametogenesis in both men and women. The specific target cell for FSH in the male appears to be the Sertoli cell, which has a supportive function for the developing spermatozoa. In the female, the target cell for FSH is the granulosa cell of the ovarian follicle. Follicle stimulating hormone also is believed to act synergistically with estrogen and LH to cause follicular growth and maturation.

Regulation of gonadotropin secretion still is not understood fully. The hypothalamus synthesizes gonadotropin releasing hormone (GnRH), which stimulates LH and FSH synthesis and release. The gonadal hormones stimulated by LH and FSH, estrogen in females and testosterone in males, in turn feedback on the pituitary and hypothalamus. Puberty occurs as a result of a decreased sensitivity of the hypothalamus and pituitary to feedback inhibition of lower levels of gonadal steroids, resulting in increased pulsatile secretion of GnRH. The gonadotropins are secreted in pulsatile fashion in response to release of GnRH. For example, in women during the follicular phase pulses occur at 1–2 per hour, but during the luteal phase, the frequency is up to every 8 hours. In men, testosterone appears to suppress LH synthesis, whereas inhibin, a peptide usually derived from the testes, is thought to suppress FSH. Inhibin is not well studied, but it is produced by the Sertoli cells in the male and the granulosa cells of graafian follicles in the female.

In women, the regulation of the menstrual cycle is more complex (Fig. 11-14). The differential inhibitory and stimulatory effects of ovarian steroids on the hypothalamus and pituitary appear to be critical. A surge of ovarian estrogen at the end of the follicular phase of the cycle ultimately causes the release of LH and FSH, presumably through GnRH release in the hypothalamus. Inhibin may be important in women as well as in men.

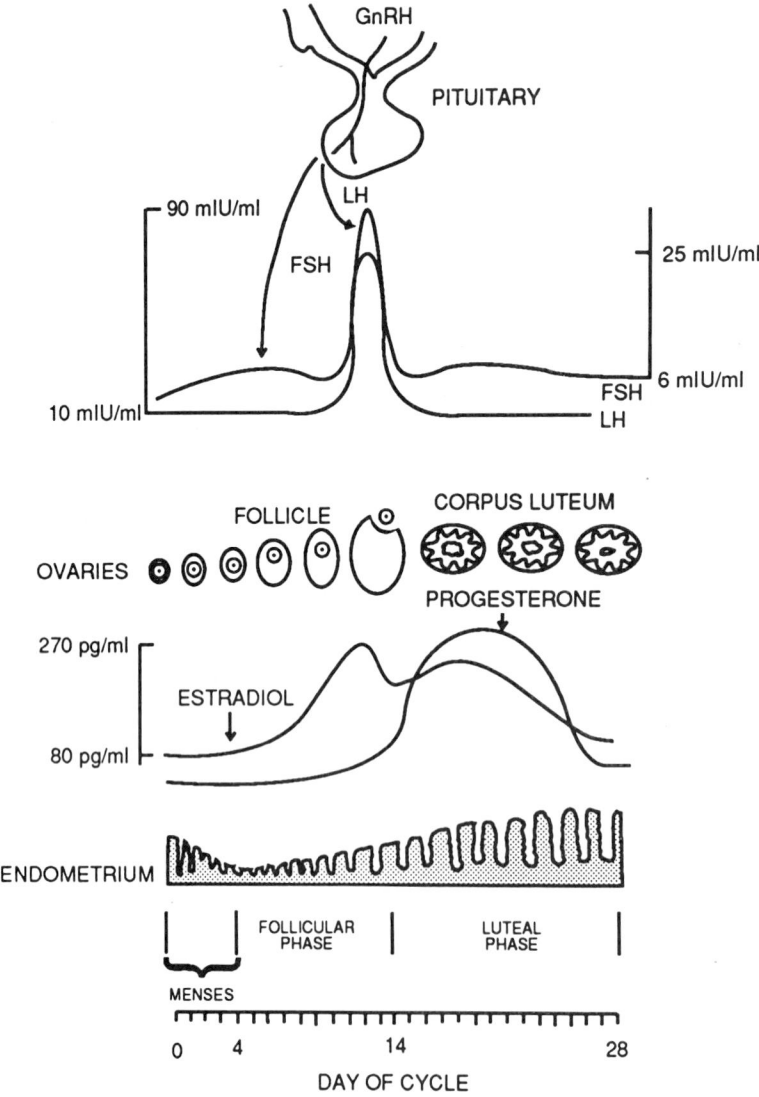

Fig. 11-14. Secretory events of the menstrual cycle. GnRH, gonadotropin releasing hormone; LH, luteinizing hormone; FSH, follicle stimulating hormone.

Test: Gonadotropins (Lutropin [LH, Luteotropic Hormone, Luteinizing Hormone] and Follitropin [FSH, Follicle Stimulating Hormone])

Background

Gonadotropin levels vary with gender and age. The menstrual cycle is characterized by repetitive changes in the hypothalamic-pituitary-ovarian hormone secretion, which regulate development and release of mature ovum and coordinate preparation of the endometrium for fertilization and implantation. If pregnancy does not ensue, each cycle culminates in menses, which designates the beginning of the next menstrual cycle. During menses, a slight rise in FSH occurs, stimulating the growth of follicles and their ability to synthesize estradiol. As the number of growing follicles is reduced, the capacity of the dominant follicle to secrete estradiol increases, thereby gradually increasing estradiol during the follicular phase. When serum estradiol remains at approximately 150 pg/mL (~520 pmol/L) for a 36-hour period, a surge of LH and FSH is triggered. This gonadotropin surge induces ovulation and subsequently promotes transformation of the ovulatory follicle into a corpus luteum. The corpus luteum becomes functional and secretes large amounts of progesterone within 2 days of the gonadotropin surge. Estradiol also is secreted from the corpus luteum, but at approximately one-half the rate of the preovulatory follicle. If the follicle is not fertilized, the corpus luteum degenerates within 14 days as indicated by decreasing serum progesterone and estradiol concentrations. With decline of steroid levels, uterine endometrium is not maintained and menses ensues. As a woman approaches menopause, menstrual cycles become irregular and ultimately terminate as the woman enters menopause. Postmenopausal women have serum estradiol levels below 20 pg/mL (<69.3 mmol/L) and increased LH and FSH levels which, when compared with the follicular phase, are up to 5-fold and 15-fold higher, respectively.

Men older than 50 years of age have age-related increases in both basal LH and FSH levels. Serum LH and FSH levels in some very elderly men can be as high as values found in men with primary testicular failure or in postmenopausal women. Increased basal serum LH levels in older men result from a mild degree of Leydig cell failure or from a decrease in sensitivity to feedback regulation of androgens. Basal elevations in serum FSH in men usually exceed those of LH, may occur without an increase in LH levels, and are generally proportional to the degree of seminiferous tubular atrophy. By contrast in postmenopausal women, gonadotropin levels decrease with age.[106]

Selection

Gonadotropin levels are useful in the diagnosis of infertility in males and females, amenorrhea and hirsutism in females, in response to a number of diagnostic agents such as GnRH, clomiphene, and human menopausal gonadotropin, and in diagnosis of certain tumors. Until recently, low levels of gonadotropin were unmeasurable by assays used, thus diagnosis of gonadotropin deficiency could not be made reliably with basal gonadotropin measurements alone. The gonadotropins LH and FSH are usually measured simultaneously along with testosterone in the male and estradiol in the female (see below).

Logistics

Serum FSH and LH levels vary according to age and sex and in females marked changes occur during the menstrual cycle and menopause. during the first week of life in both sexes, values are similar to adult values.

The specimen of choice for measurement is serum although urine has been used frequently in the past. Generally, LH and FSH both are measured using a single specimen usually obtained at a standard time of day. However, some authors recommend collection of multiple specimens (usually three) at 20-minute intervals, and pooling equal aliquots from each time point for measurement. The additional time for specimen collection and processing is balanced by obtaining a more integrated measure of hormone secretion because secretion of FSH and LH is intermittent. Assays have been standardized with a variety of reference preparations making comparisons between assays difficult.

Interpretation

Reference intervals are given in Table 11-19. In both men and women, primary hypogonadism results in at least a twofold elevation of basal LH and FSH serum levels. If both values are high (LH being more than 25 mIU/mL [>25 IU/L] and FSH being more than 40 mIU/mL [>40 IU/L]) the diagnosis of hypergonadotropic (primary) hypogonadism is established. Although LH levels are increased in hypergonadotropic hypogonadism, these elevated levels can be confused with the ovulatory peak of LH in healthy women. However, nonelevated FSH levels in healthy women along with low concentrations of sex hormones found in hypo-

Table 11-19. Luteinizing Hormone and Follicle Stimulating Hormone Reference Intervals[a]

	Follicle Stimulating Hormone mIU/mL	Luteinizing Hormone mIU/mL
Males		
Prepubertal	2–10	2–12
Adult	4–15	5–25
Females		
Prepubertal	3–7	2–12
Follicular phase	4–15	5–30
Midcycle	15–25	79–90
Luteal phase	4–15	5–40
Postmenopausal	30–200	30–200

[a] Conventional units are mIU/mL; SI units are IU/L; the numerical result remains the same.

gonadism are useful in discrimination of these patients. In patients with oligomenorrhea or amenorrhea with primary hypergonadotropic hypogonadism, FSH levels are similar to those seen in menopausal women. When LH and FSH are low or within the reference interval, the most likely diagnosis is a hypothalamic-pituitary defect or an abnormality of the feedback process. Clinically, those females who have adequate estrogen are identified by a progesterone challenge test, and are candidates for clomiphene or hCG (see below). Individuals with pituitary disease are identified by pituitary stimulation tests.

The combination of serum LH above the reference interval (greater than 15 mIU/mL [> 15 IU/L]) and non-elevated FSH suggest the diagnosis of polycystic ovary disease. These patients frequently are hirsute and have large ovaries as shown by ultrasound scanning. Some investigators have used the relationship of LH to FSH to confirm the diagnosis; patients with polycystic ovary syndrome typically have ratios greater than 2.5:1. However, approximately 25% of patients with polycystic ovary syndrome have LH values that are within the reference interval.

In the male, elevated FSH and LH indicate damage to both testicular interstitial and tubular components. When only FSH is increased, only tubular function is impaired, and measurement of testosterone is essential. When gonadotropins are low or within the reference interval, a hypothalamic or pituitary lesion is suspected. Elevated FSH with LH within the reference interval occurs in patients with gonadotropin-secreting tumors (see below). Some degree of primary hypogonadism manifested by elevated LH levels has been found in men with AIDS, uremia, malignancies, and malnutrition.[107]

Stimulatory Testing

Follicle stimulating hormone and LH can be monitored following stimulatory testing. During clomiphene testing, LH and FSH normally increase by 70% and 45%, respectively (and testosterone by 40%).

Gonadotropin Cell Tumor

A number of patients have been identified with gonadotropin cell adenomas of the pituitary. Most of these are men and most are beyond the age of 40. Frequently, FSH is elevated, which is often accompanied by a hypersecretion of FSH β- and α-subunits, and less often by hypersecretion of β-LH and intact LH. In a few patients intact LH is elevated, and these patients commonly have elevated testosterone. However, most patients with gonadotropin cell tumors have decreased testosterone with decreased LH concentrations because these pituitary tumors are compressing the normal gonadotropin cells and impairing LH secretion.[108]

Test: Gonadotropin Releasing Hormone (GnRH, LRH, LHRH, Luteinizing Releasing Hormone) Stimulation

Gonadotropin releasing hormone, a decapeptide produced by the hypothalamus, acts on the pituitary causing synthesis and release of the gonadotropins LH and FSH. Because it releases mainly LH, GnRH is frequently called luteinizing releasing hormone (LRH).

Gonadotropin releasing hormone has a half-life of approximately 4 minutes.

For the GnRH stimulation test, the releasing hormone usually is administered as a single dose (usually 100 μg) or as part of a multiple dose (usually much lower doses of 1–10 μg/dose) priming test with measurement of LH. Follicle stimulating hormone usually is not measured as the response is of lower magnitude and less reproducible. Healthy persons have baseline LH levels of less than 20 mIU/mL (<20 IU/L) and responses in LH of approximately 60 mIU/mL (~60 IU/L) (range 25–110 mIU/mL [25–110 IU/L]) at 20 or 30 minutes. By 3 hours gonadotropin levels return to baseline. Individuals with hypothalamic or pituitary disease have low baseline values and no response to the infusion, whereas individuals with primary hypogonadism have elevated baseline levels, exaggerated responses, and a delay in results returning to baseline. Peak responses of LH to the single GnRH dose are proportional to basal prevailing LH levels, thus the GnRH test offers only marginal advantages over baseline measurements.[109]

The multiple dose GnRH stimulation test is based on the principle of priming the pituitary gonadotropes by repeated low dose stimulation to simulate normal physiology. The multiple dose GnRH test is useful for separating low or absent LH responses to the single dose test, which occurs in both pituitary and hypothalamic disease. Patients with hypothalamic disease have a brisk response after multiple priming doses are given, whereas little or no response occurs in patients with pituitary disease. The priming test is limited to investigational use only. Gonadotropin releasing hormone also is used therapeutically for the treatment of hypothalamic infertility, induction of ovulation, and cryptorchidism.

Test: Testosterone

Background

The major synthetic pathway of testosterone originates from cholesterol (Fig. 11-15). Testosterone circulates in the serum bound to proteins, predominantly (75%) as sex hormone-binding globulin (SHBG) and albumin (20%). Changes in the concentrations of these binding proteins affect serum testosterone values by changing the amount of testosterone binding. The serum concentration of SHBG, which is synthesized in the liver, also is controlled in part by concentrations of circulating sex hormones. At elevated circulating estrogen concentrations, such as occur during pregnancy, a several-fold increase in SHBG levels occurs, whereas elevated testosterone concentrations may cause up to a 50% increase in this protein as well. Other factors that may increase SHBG concentrations are thyroid hormone excess and cirrhosis.

Only 1–3% of testosterone remains unbound, and this unbound fraction is biologically active. A large propor-

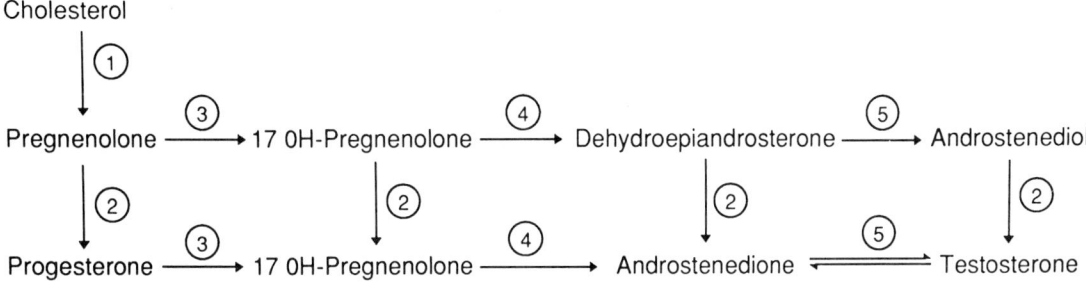

Biosynthesis of testosterone ① =20,22-lyase (desmolase); ② = 3 β-hydroxysteroid dehydrogenase-isomerase; ③ = 17 hydroxylase; ④ = 17,20 lyase (desmolase); ⑤ = 17 β-hydroxysteroid dehydrogenase.

Fig. 11-15. Synthesis of testosterone.

tion (55%) of the albumin bound testosterone is biologically available. Testosterone exerts androgen-like action in tissues where binding occurs to specific cytoplasmic receptors either directly or after conversion to 5 α-dihydrotestosterone by the enzyme 5 α-reductase. The steroid complex travels to the nucleus and then affects gene transcription. At the hypothalamic-pituitary level, feedback occurs either from 5 α-reduction or aromatization of testosterone to estradiol and subsequent binding to specific receptors.

In healthy men, most of the circulating testosterone is derived from direct secretion by the testes (more than 90%). Testosterone concentrations in the male reflect androgen status, because other androgens present in comparable or even greater concentrations are biologically less active. In women, the circulating testosterone concentrations are about one-tenth that of men. Of this, 15% is derived from ovarian secretion and 25% from the adrenal cortex, and peripheral conversion from other androgens, especially androstenedione, accounts for up to 50% of the total. The differential diagnosis of conditions responsible for androgen excess is seen in Table 11-20.

Testosterone is metabolized in the liver to a group of compounds called 17-oxosteroids. Because most of the 17-oxosteroids in men and women are derived from other androgens, they are of no value in assessing testosterone production in either sex.

Table 11-20. Etiology of Hyperandrogenism

Ovarian dysfunction
    Polycystic ovary disease
    Acanthosis nigricans
        Hyperthecosis
        Tumors
            Arrhenoblastoma
            Hilar cell adenoma
            Lipoid cell tumor
Adrenal dysfunction
    Congenital adrenal hyperplasia
        21-Hydroxylase deficiency
        11-β-hydroxylase deficiency
        3-β-Hydroxysteroid dehydrogenase deficiency
    Tumors
        Adenoma
        Carcinoma
    Cushing syndrome
    Metabolic causes
        Hyperthyroidism
Exogenous medications
    Androgens or "anabolic steroids"

Selection

Measurement of serum testosterone in the male is used predominantly for investigating infertility and for monitoring testosterone replacement therapy. It also is used in the investigation of precocious puberty and for monitoring testicular response to hCG stimulation. In women, plasma testosterone is used for investigating hyperandrogenization and has been found to be of most use in cases of hirsutism of recent onset. At birth and during infancy, testosterone measurements are used mainly for patients with cryptorchidism and ambiguous genitalia. Other useful tests are free testosterone or bioavailable testosterone (see below).

Logistics

Serum is the specimen of choice. Because testosterone increases in specimens in which serum and red blood cells are in contact, measurements should not be made using blood that was left unseparated for longer than 6 hours. Immunoassays give variable results depending on the extraction step, the label used, and the cross-reactivity of the reagent antibodies. Dihydrotestosterone has reactivity in most immunoassays. Recently, the concentrations of SHBG has been shown to influence testosterone results in some assays with underestimation at high SHBG levels and overestimation at low SHBG values.[110]

Interpretation

Reference Intervals

Serum testosterone results vary with age and gender (Table 11-21). In male infants, plasma testosterone levels increase in the first day of life owing to decreased clearance and may even reach levels in the low adult range. By the end of the first week, testosterone levels have fallen and are similar to those of females. During the second week of life and continuing to about 3 months of age in males, testosterone levels increase and then decline to prepubertal levels, which are reached at about 6 months of age. This neonatal increase in testosterone does not occur in female infants. At the onset of puberty, testosterone levels in boys follow a pattern dependent upon LH stimulation of the testes, first with pulses at night, then with frequent pulses during the day as well. The major increases in serum testosterone occur usually between 12 and 14 years of age at which time boys enter pubertal stages 3 and 4. In girls, testosterone concentrations increase throughout puberty.

Table 11-21. Serum Testosterone Levels

Age	Mean of Reference Intervals for Testosterone Males ng/mL (nmol/L)	Females ng/mL (nmol/L)
1 d	1.99 (6.9)	0.46 (1.6)
1 wk	0.25 (0.9)	0.14 (0.5)
1–4 mo	1.79 (6.2)	0.06 (.02)
4–48 mo	0.06 (0.2)	0.06 (0.2)
Pubertal (stage 1)	0.12 (0.4)	0.12 (0.4)
Pubertal (stage 2)	0.17 (0.6)	0.20 (0.7)
Pubertal (stage 3)	0.52 (1.8)	0.29 (1.0)
Pubertal (stage 4)	1.70 (5.9)	0.49 (1.7)
Pubertal (stage 5)	3.49 (12.1)	0.37 (1.3)
Adults	5.62 (19.5)	0.46 (1.6)

In men, testosterone secretion is episodic and therefore serum levels are variable. There is also a circadian rhythm with highest levels in early morning and the lowest in the evening. Morning levels in young men are only approximately 20–40% higher than those in the evening, but with age these differences are less. In normal menstruating females, serum testosterone levels fluctuate throughout the cycle with highest levels at midcycle. Serum testosterone decreases temporarily in response to many severely stressful situations such as surgery, respiratory failure, and severe unaccustomed exercise. In well conditioned runners, testosterone levels increase about twofold during exercise and return to baseline about 2 hours after cessation of a race.

Infertility

Levels of testosterone (and LH) usually are decreased in infertile men with primary or secondary hypogonadism. Even though symptoms usually are a more sensitive indicator of gonadal hypofunction than testosterone measurements, some patients with secondary hypogonadism may lack symptoms despite markedly decreased testosterone levels. Markedly elevated serum testosterone (1.0 ng/mL [3.5 nmol/L]) suggests occult hyperthyroidism or insensitivity of peripheral tissues to androgens (both of these conditions are associated with increased LH). An example of resistance to testosterone action occurs in some patients with celiac disease, where elevated testosterone, SHBG, and LH concentrations are found. In some common causes of infertility such as cryptorchidism, azospermia, oligospermia, and varicocele, testosterone results usually are within the reference interval. In Table 11-22 are listed some characteristic laboratory findings when testosterone and gonadotropin levels are used to evaluate infertility. Testosterone measurements sometimes are used to monitor replacement therapy in hypogonadal men. For treatment, a number of different testosterone preparations are used with varying routes of delivery, thus both testosterone and testosterone esters may circulate. Because immunoassays show varying reactivity with testosterone esters, testosterone results are specific to the preparation and immunoassay used.[112]

Human Chorionic Gonadotropin Stimulation Test

This test is used to assess Leydig cell function (hypogonadism) and requires the administration of hCG and subsequent measurement of testosterone and other steroids. Many different protocols are used with variations in the dose, route, and timing of the hCG administration. Generally if infertility or impotence is evaluated, a single dose is used, whereas if anorchia is suspected, multiple doses are given 3–4 days apart. Testosterone measurements are made at baseline and at 72 hours after the injection. In healthy prepubertal boys, in early puberty, and in adults the maximal testosterone increase is about 70-fold, 6-fold, or 2- to 4-fold over baseline, respectively. If expressed as an absolute rise, the increase from baseline is 35–120 ng/mL (10–35 nmol/L). This test has little or no value in assessing ovarian steroid production in women.[112]

Hirsutism

Hirsutism, excessive growth of androgen dependent sexual hair in a male pattern, occurs in women with marked elevation of testosterone. However, elevated testosterone levels are seen in only 50–75% of cases of hirsute women despite obvious clinical signs of hyper-

Table 11-22. Charactic Laboratory Findings in Hypothalamic-Pituitary-Gonadal Axis in Males

Diagnosis	Luteinizing Hormone	Follicle Stimulating Hormone	Testosterone
Gonadal (hypergonadotropic)			
Primary testicular failure	↑	↑	↓
Anorchia	↑	↑	↓
Cryptorchidism	RI	RI or ↑	RI
Azoospermia and oligospermia	RI or ↑	RI or ↑	RI
Varicocele	RI	RI	RI
Klinefelter syndrome	↑ or RI	↑	↓ or RI
Hypothalamus and pituitary (hypogonadotropic)			
Hypopituitarism	↓ or RI	↓ or RI	↓ or RI
Pituitary sarcoid	↓ or RI	↓ or RI	↓ or RI
Kallmann syndrome	↓ or RI	↓ or RI	↓ or RI
Isolated gonadotropin deficiency	↓ or RI	↓ or RI	↓ or RI
Simple delayed puberty	↓ or RI	↓ or RI	↓ or RI
Other			
Complete testicular feminization syndrome	↑	↑ or RI	↑ or RI
Precocious puberty			
Idopathic or CNS lesion	↑	↑	↑
Adrenal tumors or congenital adrenal hyperplasia	↓	↓	↑

Abbreviations: RI, within reference interval; ↑, increase; ↓, decrease; CNS, central nervous system.
(Modified from Marshall,[111] with permission.)

androgenism. In women, testosterone results twice the upper reference interval or greater usually are caused by an androgen-producing tumor. In contrast, in women with Cushing syndrome, polycystic ovary disease, or congenital adrenal hyperplasia, testosterone results are normal to slightly increased. Approximately 50% of women with polycystic ovary syndrome have elevated testosterone levels, but almost all elevations are less than twice the upper reference interval.

Androgenic Tumors

Androgenic tumors arise more frequently from the ovary than the adrenal. In women, testosterone results greater than 1.5 ng/mL (>5 nmol/L) are likely to occur from ovarian tumors, whereas levels less than 1.5 ng/mL (<5 nmol/L) are more likely to occur from adrenal carcinomas. If markedly elevated adrenal androgens such as dehydroepiandrosterone sulfate also occur, the likelihood of an adrenal adenoma is increased. In contrast, ovarian tumors usually are associated with adrenal androgens, which are only slightly increased or not increased at all. Unfortunately, there are many exceptions to these general rules.

In men with testicular tumors, testosterone levels are low or within the reference range with normal or slightly raised gonadotropin levels. Androgen-secreting tumors are one of the causes of precocious puberty.

Test: Free Testosterone

Clinical evidence indicates that the concentration of free testosterone in serum correlates better with biologic activity than does total testosterone concentration. Free testosterone is usually measured following the tedious technique of equilibrium dialysis, although recently direct immunoassays have been introduced. Other methods to estimate free testosterone levels include free androgen index (a measure of testosterone corrected for abnormalities of sex hormone binding) and salivary testosterone.[113] Free testosterone levels are not widely available.

Test: Bioavailable Testosterone

In the past, free testosterone was thought to be the only bioavailable moiety, but recent studies suggest that bioavailable testosterone includes circulating free testosterone and a large proportion (55%) of albumin-bound testosterone. Testosterone bound to SHBG appears to dissociate too slowly to be biologically active. Biologically active testosterone is measured following precipitation of SHBG-bound testosterone by 50% ammonium sulfate. Bioavailable testosterone levels are about 2.5 ng/dL (~8.7 mmol/L) in young men and 1.6 ng/dL (5.5 mmol/L) in elderly men, with lower results occurring in infertile and hyperthyroid men. In women, results are higher in hirsute patients (0.08 ng/mL [0.24 nmol/L]) and lower during pregnancy (0.03 ng/mL [0.09 nmol/L]) than in normal women during the follicular phase of the menstrual cycle. Bioavailable testosterone levels correlate better than other measurements with physiologic androgen activity.[114]

Test: Dehydroepiandrosterone Sulfate (DHEA-S)

Background

Dehydroepiandrosterone sulfate is the most abundant steroid in the circulation, arising primarily by secretion from the adrenal cortex or peripheral sulfation of the dehydroepiandrosterone secreted by the adrenal cortex. Because of a long half-life and little diurnal or menstrual cycle variation, it provides a specific and stable marker of adrenal androgen production. DHEA-S is not adrogenic but exerts its androgenic activity after conversion to testosterone and its metabolites.

Selection

Serum DHEA-S is more reliable than the time honored determination of urinary 17-ketosteroids and should replace it for the assessment of adrenal androgen output.

Logistics

DHEA-S is measured by immunoassay with widely discrepant results occurring by differences in reagent antibodies. Although results from many assays compare well when serum from healthy individuals is used, serum from patients with a variety of diseases yield widely discrepant results between assays.

Interpretation

DHEA-S, which is elevated in neonates, decreases markedly within the first few months of life and remains low until about 7 years of age. During adrenarche, levels peak usually between the ages of 15 and 25 years and then decrease steadily after the third decade. Males generally have higher levels than females at almost all ages (Table 11-23). In conditions of low androgen production, the measurement of choice is testosterone, not DHEA-S. However, DHEA-S levels in patients with secondary adrenal insufficiency are usually moderately decreased.[115] Phenytoin and carbamazepine cause

Table 11-23. Reference Ranges for Serum Dehydroepiandrosterone Sulfate

Age (yr)	Range μg/dL [μmol/L]
Children	
Newborns	30–970 (0.8–26.4)
1–5	0– 20 (0–0.5)
8–12	75–150 (2.0–4.1)
12–15	100–175 (2.7–4.8)
Men	
15–39	150–550 (4.1–14.9)
40–49	100–400 (2.7–10.9)
50–59	60–300 (1.6–8.2)
≥60	30–200 (0.8–5.4)
Women	
15–29	100–500 (2.7–13.6)
30–39	60–350 (1.6–9.5)
40–49	40–250 (1.1–6.8)
≥50	20–150 (0.5–4.1)

DHEA-S levels to decrease, although the mechanism of this decrease is unknown.

In Cushing's disease, DHEA-S levels are usually within the reference interval or moderately elevated, although there are a group of these patients with markedly elevated values (800 μg/dL [21.7 μmol/L]).

In contrast, patients with Cushing syndrome caused by adrenal adenomas have decreased DHEA-S levels (less than 40 μg/dL [<1.1 nmol/L]). In adrenal carcinoma, DHEA-S levels are almost always elevated, but a few patients have adrenal tumors in which testosterone is the only elevated androgen. Usually patients with adrenal carcinoma have serum DHEA-S levels greater than 800 μg/dL (>21.7 μmol/L). By contrast, in patients with ovarian tumors, DHEA-S levels are usually within the reference interval. Patients with congenital adrenal hyperplasia of 21-hydroxylase deficiency type have elevated results with the severity of elevation directly related to the severity of elevation of 17-hydroxyprogesterone results. Usually, however, serum DHEA-S is less than 500 μg/dL (<13.6 μmol/L) in these patients.

Serum DHEA-S levels are moderately elevated in 30% of patients with oligomenorrhea and in about 60% of hirsute females. These elevations are usually less than 600 μg/dL (<16.3 μmol/L). About 50% of patients with polycystic ovary syndrome have moderately elevated levels are well. Patients who exercise strenuously such as running in marathons have elevated levels immediately upon completion, which exist for up to 36 hours. With some immunoassays, cross-reaction with 16-α-hydroxy DHEA-S and other steroid sulfates has been identified as a cause of increased results. An approach to patients with hirsutism has been suggested; it requires measurement of DHEA-S, cortisol, and free testosterone before and after 5 days of dexamethasone, and a subsequent ACTH stimulation test for patients who do not show suppression.[116]

Test: Estradiol (E$_2$)

Background

Estradiol, the most potent estrogen, is found in both males and females. Although over 20 estrogens have been identified, only estradiol, estrone, and estriol have any clinical importance. However, the biologic activity of estrone may depend on its conversion to estradiol. Estriol is useful as an index of fetoplacental function during pregnancy. In the female, estradiol stimulates growth of female sex organs and development of secondary sexual characteristics, influences secretion of gonadotropins by the anterior pituitary, and is involved in bone homeostasis. In the male, the role of estradiol is not well defined, although it is thought to play a role along with testosterone in regulation of gonadotropin secretion. Estradiol is produced by five tissues: the ovaries, testes, adrenal cortex, peripheral tissues, and fetoplacental unit in pregnancy. The pathway for estrogen synthesis is seen in Figure 11-16. In a premenopausal woman, estradiol is the main estrogen secreted by the ovary; however, 10–30% of the estradiol is formed in peripheral tissues from androgen precursors, with adipose tissue being the major site for this conversion. In postmenopausal women, the major source of estradiol is from steroids secreted from the adrenals and ovaries. Throughout a woman's reproductive life, the preovulatory follicle of the ovary is the main source of estradiol.

Only 1–3% of estradiol in plasma is nonprotein bound. About 40% in the female and 20% in the male is bound to SHBG, the transport protein for testosterone as well as estradiol. The remainder is bound with low affinity to albumin. Recently, it has been suggested that estradiol bound to albumin may dissociate rapidly, and this fraction as well as the unbound hormone can cross cell membranes and interact with nuclear receptors. Major pathways for elimination of estradiol is interconversion with estrone and conjugation to glucuronides or sulphates in the liver to form water-soluble metabolites, which are secreted in the bile.

In premenopausal women, changes in secretion of estradiol during the normal menstrual cycle are dependent on the release of gonadotropins from the pituitary. Estradiol in turn exerts negative feedback on the release of gonadotropins at the hypothalamic and pituitary level by controlling the release of GnRH and gonadotropins, respectively. In the late follicular phase, a

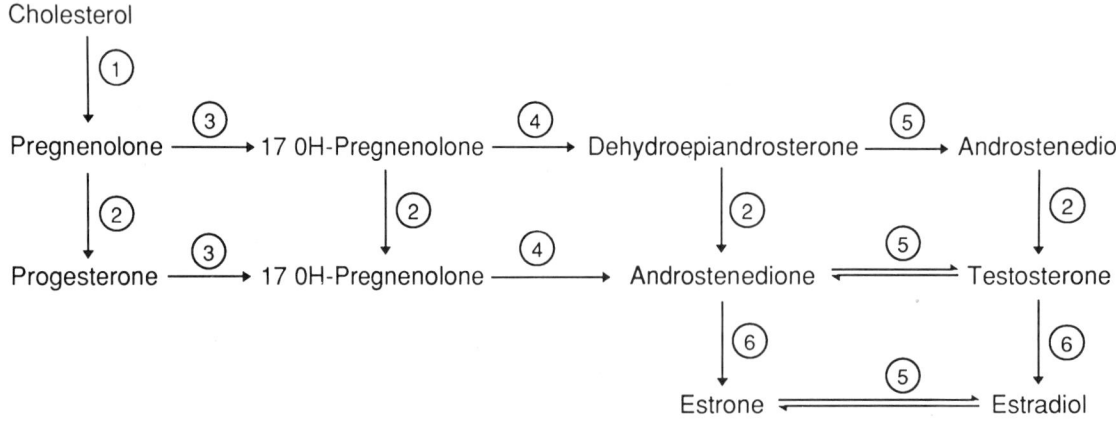

Fig. 11-16. Synthesis of estrogen.

sustained increase in estradiol secretion by a maturing graafian follicle exerts a positive feedback effect resulting in a surge of LH that initiates ovulation. In men, the major proportion of estradiol is derived by peripheral aromatization of androgen secreted by the testes and adrenals. About 20% of serum estradiol is secreted by Leydig cells of the testes: a smaller amount is secreted from the adrenals. Testicular secretion of estradiol is dependent on LH.

Selection

Measurement of estradiol alone is seldom useful, except when monitoring follicular growth or identifying an estrogen-secreting tumor. In other circumstances, concomitant LH and occasionally FSH measurements also are required in order to interpret results properly.[117]

Logistics

Estradiol is measured by immunoassay, with serum being the specimen of choice. Unfortunately, some direct assays exhibit interference by SHBG, giving overestimation of estrogen concentrations at low SHBG levels and underestimation at high levels. A number of synthetic estrogen preparations cause elevated results because of assay cross-reactivity. Although secretion is episodic, fluctuations in the serum estradiol concentrations are not significant except in the preovulatory period, when within 30 minutes, fluctuations of up to 50% occur. These rapid changes necessitate daily measurements during the preovulatory period and when following follicular growth.

Interpretation

Reference ranges for serum estradiol vary with age and gender. During infancy and childhood, serum estradiol levels are generally less than 16 pg/mL (<60 pmol/L) in both sexes, although levels approximately fivefold higher have been reported in female infants between age 4 and 12 months. In the female, levels begin to rise at about 11 years of age, increasing progressively throughout puberty reflecting the onset of cyclic ovarian activity. Estradiol also increases in the male during puberty largely reflecting peripheral conversion of testosterone. During the normal ovulatory cycle, there is a biphasic pattern of estradiol secretion with midcycle peaks at about 270 pg/mL (~1000 pmol/L). In the postmenopausal woman, estradiol concentrations are generally less than 27 pg/mL (<100 pmol/L). In men, estradiol concentrations are in the range of 20–71 pg/mL (75–260 pmol/L).

In ovarian dysfunction and infertility, estradiol is useful for investigating amenorrhea and oligomenorrhea and for identifying hypoestrogenic states. In primary hypogonadism, or failure of follicular development from absent or unresponsive follicular tissue, estradiol is low in the postmenopausal range, and FSH is elevated because of lack of feedback. In secondary hypogonadism from a wide range of conditions, serum estradiol is also in the postmenopausal range. Basal gonadotropins may be low or within the reference interval and show an impaired response to GnRH. In ovulatory dysfunction, such as in polycystic ovary syndrome, estradiol is of limited diagnostic use when ovulation is infrequent or absent, because estradiol and go-

Table 11-24. Characteristic Laboratory Findings in Hypoestrogenic Disorders in the Female

	FSH and LH	Estradiol	Additional Testing
Primary hypogonadism			
Menopause	↑	↓	
Gonadal dysgenesis (Turner syndrome)	↑	↓	Karyotype
Premature ovarian failure	↑	↓	Ovarian biopsy
Ovarian resistance syndrome	↑	↓	Ovarian biopsy
Secondary hypogonadism			
Hyperprolactinemia	RI or ↓	↓	TSH, prolactin
Weight loss amenorrhea	↓	↓	
Exercise amenorrhea	↓	↓	
Anorexia nervosa	↓	↓	
Kallman syndrome	↓	↓	Anosmia testing
Pituitary failure (Sheehan syndrome, Ahumada-del Castillo syndrome)	↓	↓	GH, TSH, ACTH, ITT

Abbreviations: FSH, follicle stimulating hormone; LH, luteinizing hormone; RI, reference interval; TSH, thyrotropin stimulating hormone; ACTH, adrenocorticotropic hormone; ITT, insulin tolerance test.

nadotropin levels are erratic or asynchronous. Table 11-24 shows some disorders in which estradiol and gonadotropin measurements may be useful in the female.

When used to monitor follicular growth for prediction of day of ovulation, serum estradiol measurements are extremely valuable. Serum estradiol rises steadily during the second half of the follicular phase reaching a mean peak concentration of approximately 270 pg/mL (~1000 pmol/L), 1–2 days before ovulation. If the induction of ovulation is monitored following clomiphene or human menopausal gonadotropin, estradiol is measured daily along with ultrasonography to assess development of follicles. Serum estradiol results above approximately 550 pg/mL (~2000 pmol/L) indicate an excessive response and are an indication for withholding hCG to avoid multiple ovulation and the risk of multiple pregnancies.

Serum estradiol measurements may be valuable for diagnosing the cause of precocious puberty (puberty before the age of 8). Although in the majority of cases no etiology is found, estradiol measurements are essential for those patients with estrogen- or hCG-secreting tumors. In both sexes, tumors most frequently occur in the gonads arising from interstitial cells in the testes, or granulosa or theca cells in the ovaries. Rarely do estrogen (estradiol)-secreting tumors arise in the adrenal. In males, estrogen (estradiol)-secreting tumors are commonly associated with gynecomastia and hypogonadism, whereas precocious puberty, amenorrhea, and postmenopausal bleeding are common findings in females.

Test: Sperm Penetration Assay (Hamster Test, Humster Test, Heterologous Ovum Penetration Test, Hamster Zona-Free Ovum Test)

This procedure is a bioassay used to assess human sperm fertilizing ability. Human sperm are evaluated for their ability to penetrate zona-free hamster eggs (human sperm, hamster eggs, hence *humster*). The percentage of eggs penetrated are expressed in terms of a fertile and infertile range.[118]

Test: Inhibin

Inhibin is a glycoprotein produced by the ovary and testicular Sertoli cells in response to FSH and LH. It blocks the action of GnRH at the pituitary and inhibits release of FSH and LH as well. The diagnostic role of inhibin has not yet been established.

POSTERIOR PITUITARY

INTRODUCTION

The posterior pituitary secretes vasopressin (antidiuretic hormone [ADH]) and oxytocin, neither of which are measured in the clinical laboratory. The laboratory diagnoses of the disorders of water metabolism usually are carried out using osmolality measurements. In selected cases, however, ADH measurements are warranted; oxytocin is occasionally used as a tumor marker.

BASIC TESTS

Test: Antidiuretic Hormone (ADH, Arginine Vasopressin)

Background

The posterior pituitary produces an octopeptide, vasopressin (antidiuretic hormone or ADH), in the nerve bodies of the supraoptic and paraventricular nuclei. Antidiuretic hormone is thought to split off from a large precursor, propressophysin, which also gives rise to neurophysin, its binding protein for transport and storage. After synthesis, the vasopressin-neurophysin complexes are packaged as large granules within the cell body, move down the axon, and then are released into the circulation by an endocytic process in response to hypertonicity and volume depletion. Vasopressin is bound to receptors on the basolateral cell membrane of cortical and medullary collecting ducts of the kidney. After a series of events, the luminal cell membrane is transformed with a striking increase in the permeability to water, urea, sodium, and many other solutes.

Selection

When obtained during a dehydration test, ADH levels can separate individuals with nephrogenic and central nervous system causes of diabetes insipidus. Antidiuretic hormone results are useful to document the syndrome of inappropriate ADH (SIADH).

Logistics

Measurements are made using immunoassay, requiring a plasma specimen collected in a chilled tube with EDTA. The specimen should be transported while in an icy slurry and the plasma immediately separated in the cold.

Interpretation

Under usual states of hydration, results are in the range of 1–2 pg/mL (1–2 ng/L). Plasma vasopressin levels are highly dependent on plasma osmolality. Above levels of about 280 mOsm/kg (~280 nmol/kg), plasma vasopressin increases linearly with increasing tonicity. Below 280 mOsm/kg (280 nmol/kg), vasopressin is suppressed to less than 1 pg/mL (<1 ng/L), and at this level diuresis of 10–12 L/d can occur.

Patients who have neurogenic (central) diabetes insipidus have undetectable levels, whereas patients with nephrogenic diabetes insipidus have elevated levels. In patients who have been deprived of water for 8–24 hours, plasma ADH results are usually greater than 2 pg/mL (>2 ng/L). In patients with inappropriate ADH, the hormone concentration is inappropriately high for a given plasma osmolality. A number of other conditions have been reported when ADH levels are inappropriately high for plasma osmolality including congestive heart failure, acute respiratory failure, cirrhosis, renal and adrenal insufficiency, and hypopituitarism.[119]

Test: Water Loading Test

This test is used for the diagnosis of inappropriate ADH excess (SIADH). The syndrome is characterized by hypo-osmolality of serum, urine osmolality less than 300 mOsm/kg (<300 nmol/kg), urine sodium less than 20 mEq/L (<20 mmol/L), and low serum urea nitrogen concentrations.

An oral water load of 20 mL/kg body weight is ingested over 15–20 minutes while the patient is recumbent. Healthy persons excrete over 80% of the water load in 4–5 hours whereas persons with inappropriate ADH concentrations (SIADH) excrete less than 40% in that same time. The test only should be performed in patients without symptoms of hyponatremia and serum sodium values above 125 mEq/L (>125 mmol/L). Measurements of ADH are a more direct way of making this diagnosis. Some common causes of the syndrome are seen in Table 11-25.

Table 11-25. Some Disorders Associated With Inappropriate Antidiuretic Hormone

Malignant tumors
    Lung, duodenum, pancreas
Disorders of central nervous system
    Meningitis, head trauma, brain tumors
Diseases of lung
    Pneumonia, tuberculosis, emphysema
Drugs
    Chlorpropamide, vincristine
Acute psychosis
Postoperative period
Endocrine causes
    Adrenal, pituitary insufficiency
Idiopathic

Test: Water Deprivation (Dehydration Test)

The water deprivation test is used for the diagnosis of diabetes insipidus, a syndrome that usually presents with clinical manifestations of polyuria, thirst, and dehydration. Following fluid deprivation for 16 hours

Table 11-26. Water Deprivation Test

Condition	Serum Osmolality[a] (mOsm/kg) At Plateau	Urine Osmolality At Plateau	After Vasopressin
Healthy individuals	<300	>Serum	<5% ↑
Primary polydipsia	<300	>Serum	<5% ↑
Severe diabetes insipidus	>300	<Serum	>50% ↑
Nephrogenic diabetes insipidus	>300	<Serum	<50% ↑
Partial diabetes insipidus	<300	>Serum	>9% ↑

[a] Conventional units are mOsm/kg; SI units are nmol/kg; the numerical result remains the same.

and constant urine osmolality for 2 hours (difference of two specimens less than 30 mOsm/kg [<30 nmol/kg]), 5 U of aqueous vasopressin are injected and urine osmolality measured. Potential responses are seen in Table 11-26. Although exogenous vasopressin was initially used, aqueous pitressin given subcutaneously or the synthetic vasopressin analogue DDAVP given intranasally (20 μg) or intravenously (2 μg) can be used as an alternative.

Central diabetes insipidus is caused by brain tumors, trauma such as basal skull fractures, neurosurgical procedures, sarcoid, or is idiopathic (Table 11-26). Nephrogenic diabetes insipidus can be caused by renal disease, an X-linked dominant disorder, chronic sickle cell disease, and drugs such as tetracycline. When the accuracy of the water deprivation test was compared with ADH levels, ADH measurements were found superior for diagnosis.[120]

CALCIUM METABOLISM

INTRODUCTION

The concentration of calcium in serum is controlled by parathyroid hormone, calcitonin, and vitamin D and its metabolites (Table 11-27) through a complex feedback loop depending on those hormones as well as other factors such as serum phosphate levels.

The most potent stimulus of parathyroid hormone (PTH) secretion is ionized calcium, with hypocalcemia inducing PTH secretion and hypercalcemia causing inhibition. Although small, rapid decreases in serum magnesium can stimulate PTH secretion, prolonged hypomagnesemia and hypermagnesemia both cause inhibition of PTH release. Parathyroid hormone inhibits phosphate reabsorption by the kidney and low serum phosphate stimulates 1-hydroxylase leading to formation of 1,25-dihydroxyvitamin D.

BASIC TESTS

Test: Calcium, Total

Background

Calcium exists in three states: about one-half protein-bound (mainly to albumin), about 10–15% weakly bound (to phosphates and other anions), and the remainder unbound (or free). The physiologically active form is free calcium, also called ionized calcium.

Selection

Total serum calcium is commonly used in the diagnosis and monitoring of a wide variety of clinical disorders (Table 11-28). Even though total serum calcium is usually measured, ionized calcium is the preferred measurement in many clinical situations.

Logistics

Serum total calcium can be measured by atomic absorption spectroscopy as well as with chromogenic reagents. Serum or heparinized plasma can be used, but specimens anticoagulated with agents that chelate calcium (i.e., EDTA or citrate) cannot be used. For approximately every gram of change in serum albumin, total calcium changes roughly 0.7 mg/dL (0.2 mmol/L), although the ionized calcium may remain constant. Albumin adjustments to serum calcium are not ideal, but in the absence of ionized calcium measurements, they appear to reflect the patient's true calcium status better than adjusted results.

Acidosis increases ionized calcium, generally leading to reduction in total serum calcium. Venous occlusion and upright posture produce hemoconcentration with in-

Table 11-27. Calcium Regulation

	Gastrointestinal Tract	Kidney	Bone
1,25 OH$_2$ D	Increases calcium absorption	Promotes calcium reabsorption	Increased osteoclast activity
PTH	—	Promotes calcium reabsorption	Increased number of osteoclasts
Calcitonin	—	Inhibits calcium reabsorption	Inhibits osteoclastic bone reabsorption

Abbreviations: 1,25 OH$_2$ D, 1,25-dihydroxyvitamin D; PTH, parathyroid hormone.

Table 11-28. Disorders of Calcium Metabolism
Causes of hypocalcemia
Hypoparathyroidism
Pseudohypoparathyroidism
Phosphate overload
Renal insufficiency
Causes of hypercalcemia
Malignancy
Lytic bone metastases
Humoral factors
Endocrine disorders
Hyperparathyroidism
Other: hyperthyroidism, pheochromocytoma, VIPoma
Vitamin D
Toxicity
Granulomatous disease
Lymphoma
Other
Drug-induced (e.g., thiazides, lithium)
Familial benign (hypocalciuric) hypercalcemia
Immobilization
Parenteral nutrition

Abbreviation: VIP, vasoactive intestinal peptide.

creases in total protein, leading to increases in serum total calcium results. These effects can change total calcium results by as much as 10%. Therefore, phlebotomy procedures should be standardized when obtaining specimens for total serum calcium.

Interpretation

The serum concentration of calcium in adults is approximately 8.4–10.2 mg/dL (~2.10–2.55 mmol/L), but the upper limit of the reference range has been reported as considerably higher, especially in the older literature. It is imperative that hypercalcemia be confirmed on at least two separate occasions before the patient is evaluated further. A patient with mild hypercalcemia on one occasion may be shown to have serum total calcium results within the reference interval on subsequent measurements. In over 60% of patients who have mildly elevated results, serum total calcium will be within the reference range on repeat measurement.[121] Other tests useful in delineating the cause of disorders of calcium metabolism include serum phosphate, urine calcium, and serum alkaline phosphatase.

Decreases

Hypocalcemia has a variety of causes including as a complication of thyroid and parathyroid surgery (Table 11-28). Most of the causes of hypocalcemia are related to the production, metabolism, or response to PTH, or vitamin D, or both. Although tetany is its hallmark, hypocalcemia can produce many other signs and symptoms including psychiatric and gastrointestinal symptoms.

Increases

Serum calcium results greater than about 12.8 mg/dL (~3.19 mmol/L) are associated with arrhythmias, coma, and death. Although hypercalcemia can be associated with a number of disorders (Table 11-28), the most common causes of hypercalcemia are neoplasia and hyperparathyroidism. Patients with hyperparathyroidism generally have serum calcium levels in the range of 10.2–12.0 mg/dL (2.55–2.99 mmol/L). Malignant tumors causing osteolytic lesions can cause severe hypercalcemia and malignancies also can produce hypercalcemia via humoral factors, perhaps the most important of which is the elaboration of PTH-like substance (see Ch. 12, Tumor Markers, Test: Parathyroid-Like Substance). In patients with primary hyperparathyroidism, typically serum phosphate tends to be decreased, chloride increased, and urine calcium and phosphate also increased. If bone disease occurs, serum alkaline phosphatase activity and osteocalcin increase along with urinary hydroxyproline. Measurement of PTH is used in making the diagnosis of primary hyperparathyroidism.

The hypercalcemia of familial benign (hypocalciuric) hypercalcemia (FBH) is characterized by nonprogressive hypercalcemia. The disorder has an autosomal dominant pattern of transmission and occurs with PTH results that are usually within the reference range. The most consistent distinction between FBH and primary hyperparathyroidism are the urine calcium results. In patients with FBH, urine calcium excretion is low with a low ratio of calcium clearance to creatinine clearance. However, to diagnose FBH, family studies also are required. The hypercalcemia associated with sarcoidosis and other granulomatous diseases appears to be caused by excess conversion of 25-hydroxyvitamin D to 1,25-dihydroxyvitamin D by activated macrophages.

Test: Calcium, Ionized (Free)

Background and Selection

Measurements of serum or whole blood ionized calcium are important in clinical situations where total serum calcium does not adequately reflect ionized calcium levels. Ionized calcium, which makes up almost one-half of the total circulating calcium, is the biologically active portion. The remainder of calcium is bound mainly to albumin, but about 15% is complexed with various anions. In healthy persons in whom levels of albumin, bicarbonate, phosphate, citrate, and lactate remain relatively constant, concentrations of ionized and total calcium are directly correlated. In clinical situations when this is not the case, ionized calcium measurements can be useful, and additionally ionized calcium may be more reliable than total calcium in patients with disorders of calcium metabolism, especially in those with only mild abnormalities. Expressing PTH results in terms of ionized calcium has been used in delineating mild hyperparathyroidism from healthy persons.

Logistics

Either serum or whole blood, anticoagulated with heparin, specimens are suitable for ionized calcium measurements with ion selective electrodes. The pH of the specimen must remain stable, thus care should be taken to avoid venous stasis and the specimen must be maintained anaerobically. Anticoagulants including citrate, EDTA, and oxalate must not be used because of low results caused by chelation. Heparin should be carefully checked before use and generally if its concentration is kept at 15 U/mL or less, its effect on ionized calcium is minor. Anaerobic specimens are stable at room temperature for up to 2 hours and at 4°C for up to 24 hours. Calculation of ionized calcium from total calcium and albumin or protein results is an unsatisfactory indicator of true ionized calcium.[122]

Interpretation

Various reference ranges have been reported for ionized calcium in the adult, but generally they are in the range of about 4.6–5.3 mg/dL (~1.15–1.33 mmol/L). The reference range tends to be higher in newborns. In critically ill individuals, many factors give rise to changes in total and ionized calcium. For example, these patients commonly have decreased levels of serum albumin as well as acid-base disturbances. Monitoring ionized calcium is indicated in patients who are given rapid transfusions and during liver transplantation. Blood for transfusion is collected with citrate as the anticoagulant; with rapid transfusion, changes in ionized calcium can occur. Blood products administered during liver transplant surgery can cause marked increases in circulating citrate levels because hepatic clearance of citrate is diminished. Decreases in ionized calcium can be a particular problem, especially during the anhepatic phase of the surgery.[123]

Test: Calcium (Urine)

Background and Selection

Urine calcium measurements are important in the diagnosis of certain causes of hypercalcemia and may prove important in studying patients with renal stones.

Logistics

To avoid precipitation, urine specimens should be collected with acid or, if collected without acid, should be adjusted to pH 3–4 before assay or storage.

Interpretation

Urine calcium measurements usually are expressed as 24 hour excretion rate, but also can be expressed as a ratio to creatinine or to creatinine clearance. Generally, males excrete less than 300 mg (<7.5 mmol) of calcium and females less than about 250 mg/24 h (<6.25 mmol/d). The normal ratio of calcium to creatinine is less than 0.14 (when measured in mg/dL) or less than 0.40 (when measured in mmol/L).

In most patients with hypercalcemia, urine calcium results are increased. Urine calcium measurements can be important in the diagnosis of FBH. In patients with FBH or in those taking drugs such as lithium or thiazides, urinary calcium results are decreased. In addition, urine calcium measurements appear to be important in studying patients with renal stones. Between 40% and 75% of patients with calcium-containing renal stones have hypercalciuria, even though their serum calcium results are within the reference range. Idiopathic hypercalciuria is a common disorder that has been attributed to an inherited defect in calcium transport.[124]

Test: Phosphate (Serum)

Background

The phosphorus content of the body consists of phosphate in two main forms: organic (mainly as lipids) and inorganic, important for high energy transfer reactions. Parathyroid hormone controls phosphate levels by blocking its reabsorption in the kidney. Phosphate in turn regulates vitamin D activity with high levels suppressing 1-hydroxylation and low levels increasing enzyme activity.

Selection

Traditionally, serum phosphate is measured along with serum calcium to delineate disorders of calcium metabolism. A wide variety of disorders are associated with changes in serum phosphate levels (Table 11-28). Ordinarily, urine phosphate measurements are reserved for tubular reabsorption of phosphate (TRP) studies used in the study of calcium metabolism.

Terminology

Standard methods measure the inorganic phosphate fraction; however, traditionally results are expressed as phosphorus. Thus the term *phosphorus* is frequently used even though *phosphate* is correct on physiologic grounds.

Logistics

Phosphate is commonly measured using the phosphomolybdate method: potential interference occurs from compounds that complex to molybdate including citrate, oxalate, tartrate, and mannitol. Hemolysis can cause increases in serum phosphate if released erythrocyte phosphate esters are hydrolyzed to phosphate. Results with serum are higher than with heparinized plasma, probably because of release of labile phosphate esters during clotting. For routine use, serum is the preferred specimen because changes on storage are less than with plasma. Phosphate in serum removed from cells is stable for at least several days at 4°C or below.[125] There are several physiologic effects on serum phosphate, for example, vigorous exercise can increase results. Because of influence of the sleep cycle, serum phosphate is 10–30% higher at night than in the morning. The TRP is calculated from serum and urine phosphate. The tubular maximum for phosphate reabsorption also is depressed in hyperparathyroidism.

Interpretation

The reference interval for serum phosphate is about 2.5–5.0 mg/dL (~0.8–1.60 mmol/L) with higher values seen in children, especially during the first 6 months of life. Phosphate depletion of prolonged duration can lead to a variety of clinical problems such as metabolic acidosis and impaired leukocyte and platelet function. The basis of these effects appears related to impaired tissue oxygenation caused by 2,3 DPG deficiency along with reduced energy stores caused by adenosine triphosphate (ATP) depletion.[125]

A large number of factors increase or decrease serum phosphate (Table 11-29). Decreases in gastrointestinal absorption and malnutrition are two important causes of hypophosphatemia. Generally, reciprocal changes in serum calcium and phosphate occur in parathyroid disorders, thus serum phosphate results decrease in hyperparathyroidism and increase in hypoparathyroidism. With vitamin D toxicity and deficiency, serum calcium and phosphate rise and fall together. Phosphate is retained with progressive renal insufficiency, but increased serum phosphate results rarely develop before renal function decreases to about 25% of normal.

Table 11-29. Causes of Serum Phosphate Abnormalities

Decreases
- Alcohol withdrawal
- Diabetic ketoacidosis, treated
- Hyperparathyroidism
- Malabsorption
- Malnutrition
- Sepsis
- Renal tubular defects

Increases
- Hypoparathyroidism
- Hemolysis
- Muscle damage
- Renal insufficiency

Tubular Reabsorption of Phosphate

The TRP used in the study of patients with hypercalcemia is calculated from serum and urine creatinine and phosphate measured on the same specimen.

$$\text{TRP} = 1 - \frac{\text{urinary phosphate} \times \text{serum creatinine}}{\text{serum phosphate} \times \text{urinary creatinine}}$$

In patients with hyperparathyroidism, serum phosphate results are low and urinary levels high yielding decreased TRP. With the introduction of more sensitive and specific methods for PTH measurement, interest in TRP measurements has waned. The set point for serum phosphate concentration is determined by the tubular maximum for phosphate divided by the glomerular filtration rate, TmP/GFR (for calculation see Mallette[127]).

Test: Magnesium

Background and Selection

Magnesium has a mainly intracellular physiologic role, for example, acting as a cofactor for many important enzyme reactions. Only about 1% of the total body magnesium occurs in the serum and interstitial body fluid.

In serum, about one-third of magnesium is protein bound; about 20% is complexed to phosphate, citrate, and other compounds; and the remainder is free.[126] The kidney is the major organ that controls magnesium concentration in serum, but PTH may effect or be effected by magnesium homeostasis. Serum magnesium levels should be monitored when electrolyte testing is required, especially in patients taking diuretic drugs or digitalis.

Logistics

Magnesium can be determined by several different methods including atomic absorption. Magnesium has been measured in serum, urine, red blood cells, and mononuclear blood cells. Serum is generally preferred to plasma, because of potential interference by anticoagulants. The concentration of magnesium in red blood cells is about three times that of serum, thus hemolysis will spuriously increase serum results. Although not routinely available, studies indicate mononuclear blood cell magnesium content may better reflect tissue magnesium content than serum or red blood cell magnesium measurements.[126] A 24-hour urine collection is used for urinary magnesium, because of a circadian rhythm in excretion. The urine should be collected with an acidifying agent to prevent magnesium precipitation at high pH.

Interpretation

The reference range for serum magnesium is about 1.3–2.1 mEq/L (~0.7–1.1 mmol/L). Table 11-30 lists some of the causes of hypomagnesemia. Hypomagnesemia has been reported to cause a variety of clinical manifestations including convulsions and cardiac arrhythmias. Because diuretics promote concurrent potassium and magnesium deficiency contributing to the problem of refractory potassium repletion, assessment of patients taking diuretics is particularly important. Although intracellular magnesium depletion can occur in the presence of normal serum magnesium results, for practical purposes, low serum magnesium values are used as the indicator of magnesium depletion. Even though the magnesium concentration in serum apparently fails to correlate with tissue magnesium, measurement of serum magnesium appears to be of value for assessing acute changes in magnesium status.[126] Hypermagnesemia has a number of clinical manifestations including muscle weakness, hypotension, sedation, and confusion. Most cases of hypermagnesemia are associated with renal disease.

CALCIUM HORMONE TESTS

Test: Parathyroid Hormone

Background

Parathyroid hormone is degraded in the peripheral tissues to form biologically active amino-(N) terminal, biologically inactive carboxyl(C)-terminal, and midregion fragments. In the circulation, the main forms of PTH are the whole molecule, called intact PTH, and the following fragments: carboxyl-terminal, midmolecule, and amino-terminal PTH. The half-life of circulating intact PTH and amino-terminal fragments is normally about 5 minutes, whereas the half-life of the carboxyl-terminal fragments is in the range of 30–40 minutes or more. Usually, less than 25% of the total immunoreactive PTH in the circulation is intact hormone and most of the remainder is inactive carboxyl fragments. Fragments of PTH are cleared by glomerular filtration and thus accumulate in renal failure.

Selection

The main use of serum PTH assays is to separate hyperparathyroid patients from those with other causes of hypercalcemia, especially malignancy. Measurement of PTH is important in the renal failure patient to identify those patients with hyperparathyroid bone disease. Additionally, serum PTH measurements are used to localize PTH-producing adenomas and some assays are suitable for delineation of hypoparathyroidism.

Logistics

Metabolism of PTH within the parathyroid glands and peripheral tissues leads to complications in measurement of serum PTH concentrations. In addition, PTH

Table 11-30. Common Causes of Hypomagnesemia

Acute tubular necrosis
Alcoholism
Cyclosporine treatment
Diabetic ketoacidosis
Diarrhea
Diuretics
Hypercalcemia
Malabsorption
Malnutrition

Table 11-31. Parathyroid Hormone

Assay Type	Amino Acid	Approximate Half-Life	Biologic Activity	Moiety Measured
Intact hormone	1–84	5 min	Active	Intact hormone
Carboxy(C)-terminal fragments	35–84 (or less)	30–40 min	Inactive	Carboxy-terminal fragments Intact hormone
Midmolecule (midregion)	44–68	1 h	Inactive	Midmolecule Carboxy-terminal fragments Intact hormone
Amino(N)-terminal fragments	1–34	5 min	Active	Amino-terminal fragments Intact hormone

results appear to have a diurnal variation and are affected by meals and the season. Age-related increases also have been described. Parathyroid hormone assay antibodies react with intact PTH and, depending on the specificity of the assay, with some PTH fragments. Thus most immunoassays measure biologically active as well as inactive PTH. Immunoassays for PTH are categorized, depending on the specificity of the antibody, into intact PTH, C-terminal, midmolecule (midregion), or N-terminal assays (Table 11-31). Recently, immunometric assays for intact PTH have been developed using two separate antibodies that recognize different antigenic sites on the PTH molecule. Proper specimen collection and handling, especially for the intact assays, is necessary to avoid spurious results. Fasting morning specimens should be processed in a refrigerated centrifuge and the separated serum frozen immediately.

Interpretation

The reference interval and interpretation of PTH results depend on the PTH assay used. Among various PTH assays of the same theoretic specificity, large differences in predictive value occur. Thus, even though a particular midregion or N-terminal assay is useful in distinguishing hyperparathyroids from normals, this does not mean all midregion or N-terminal assays have the same capabilities. Although theoretically it may be best to measure intact PTH, at least in most clinical circumstances, until recently immunoassays proved to be either not sufficiently sensitive to measure the intact hormone or not sufficiently specific to avoid detection of circulating PTH fragments. Some intact PTH assays are now available that are suitable for delineating hypoparathyroidism as well as hyperparathyroidism. The reference range for intact PTH is about 10–65 pg/mL (10–65 ng/L).

Decreases

Some of the newer assays for intact PTH are suitable for detection of hypoparathyroidism. In patients with hypoparathyroidism, PTH is lacking in contrast to patients with pseudohypoparathyroid (PHP) who lack the ability to respond to PTH resulting in hypocalcemia and a secondary rise in PTH. Idiopathic hypoparathyroidism is distinguished from pseudohypoparathyroidism on the basis of clinical evaluation and PTH measurements, but the differentiation of type I and type II PHP depends on renal response to exogenous PTH. The response of urinary cAMP and phosphate to synthetic PTH 1–34 fragment is used to distinguish between the two types.[127]

Increases

Measurement of PTH is important in determining the etiology of hypercalcemia. Often hypercalcemia is found as an unexpected result on biochemical screening, with most of these patients having primary hyperparathyroidism. Typically, patients with primary hyperparathyroidism have hypercalcemia, hypercalciuria, hypophosphatemia, hyperphosphaturia, and elevated 1,25-dihydroxyvitamin D levels. They also tend to have high or high normal serum chloride levels. Intact PTH accounts for a large portion of the circulating immunoreactive PTH in patients with primary hyperparathyroidism. Development of a sensitive immunometric assay for intact PTH has led to improvement in the diagnosis of hypercalcemic patients. About 90% of patients with primary hyperparathyroidism have elevations in intact PTH and the remainder have PTH results inappropriate for their serum ionized calcium. Immunometric assays of intact PTH have their greatest value in separating hyperparathyroid patients from those patients with hypercalcemia of malignancy. Although patients with hypercalcemia of malignancy usually have suppressed intact PTH, about 5% of these patients have results in the low normal range. In a few cases, PTH production in association with malignancy has been reported.

C-Terminal, Midmolecule, and N-Terminal Assays

Because serum concentrations of intact (and N-terminal) PTH are low, C-terminal and midmolecule assays were used until recently when more sensitive assays were developed. Even though biologically inactive, the longer high life and increased serum concentrations of these fragments conferred an assay advantage. Increased results for C-terminal or midmolecule PTH generally correlate well with the diagnosis of hyperparathyroidism, except in patients with renal insufficiency. In patients with chronic renal failure, C-terminal and midmolecule PTH fragments and the ratio of these fragments to intact PTH increases. Thus results for C-terminal and midmolecule assays must be interpreted with caution in renal failure patients. In renal failure patients without evidence of hyperparathyroidism, results for midregion and C-terminal assays can be 10–30 times the upper limit of normal.[128] For unknown reasons, but possibly because of decreased renal clearance, not all patients with hypercalcemia of malignancy have suppressed PTH results as measured by these assays. In contrast, PTH results in patients of hypercalcemia of malignancy are suppressed when measured with intact or some N-terminal assays. The N-terminal assays have been used for catheterization studies to localize PTH-producing adenomas; however, intact PTH assays also are suitable for this use.

Test: Calcitonin

Background and Selection

Serum calcitonin measurements are mainly used to exclude medullary carcinoma of the thyroid, an often familial malignancy of the thyroid C cells. Calcitonin is elevated in a number of other conditions.

Logistics

To screen for medullary thyroid carcinoma, serum calcitonin measurements sometimes are made following stimulation with calcium (by infusion), pentagastrin, or both with the exact protocol depending on the laboratory in which screening is carried out.[129] Stimulation tests allow early detection of medullary thyroid carcinoma before metastatic disease occurs.

Interpretation

The reference range for serum calcitonin may be up to 100 pg/mL (100 ng/L), but the range is variable depending on the assay used. The reference range is higher in children and in pregnant women. Medullary thyroid carcinoma is associated with multiple endocrine neoplasia (MEA) type IIa and IIb, but can occur sporadically as well as in a familial form not associated with MEA. Some patients present with signs and symptoms of MEA such as pheochromocytoma or hyperparathyroidism. In addition, MEA patients can present with signs and symptoms of ACTH or vasoactive intestinal peptide excess.[129] Many patients with familial medullary thyroid carcinoma have basal serum calcitonin results within the reference range. To identify these patients with early disease, provocative tests of calcitonin secretion are performed. Primary relatives of medullary thyroid carcinoma patients should be screened and testing should be repeated periodically in high risk individuals who are negative on the initial screen. The chance of cure is correlated with the calcitonin levels following stimulation. For example, in patients with preoperative stimulated calcitonin results of 1000–5000 pg/mL (1000–5000 ng/L), surgery is curative in about 90%.[130]

Other causes of increased calcitonin results are malignancy, especially lung and breast, renal failure, pernicious anemia, Zollinger-Ellison syndrome, and pancreatitis. Increases in serum calcitonin also are associated with thyroiditis and pheochromocytoma. Acute increases in serum calcitonin occur with calcium infusion, but the effects of chronic hypercalcemia are controversial. Basal calcitonin results apparently are within the reference interval in patients with primary hyperparathyroidism (see also Ch. 12, Tumor Markers, Test: Calcitonin).

Test: Osteocalcin (Bone γ-Carboxyglutamic Acid, GLA)

Osteocalcin is a vitamin K-dependent noncollagenous bone protein. Osteocalcin, which is synthesized by osteoblasts, is incorporated in the bone matrix where it constitutes 1–2% of the total protein. The concentration of osteocalcin in serum reflects the rate of bone formation. Serum and 24-hour urine measurements appear promising in the diagnosis and management of high turnover metabolic bone disease.[131] Serum shows a diurnal pattern with results peaking during the late night and early morning. Serum immunoassay results correlate linearly with age in both women and men, but are generally less than about 8 ng/mL (8 µg/L) in healthy adults.[132]

REFERENCES

1. Sukegawa I, Hizuka N, Takano K et al: Urinary growth hormone (GH) measurements are useful for evaluating endogenous GH secretion. J Clin Endocrinol Metab 1988;66:1119–1123.
2. Baumann G: Acromegaly. Endocrinol Metab Clin North Am 1987;16:685–703.
3. Barkan AL: Acromegaly. Diagnosis and therapy. Endocrinol Metab Clin North Am 1989;18:277–310.
4. Rose SR, Ross JL, Uriarte M et al: The advantage of measuring stimulated as compared with spontaneous growth hormone levels in the diagnosis of growth hormone deficiency. N Engl J Med 1988;319:201–207.
5. Celniker AC, Chen AB, Wert RM et al: Variability in the quantitation of circulating growth hormone using commercial immunoassays. J Clin Endocrinol Metab 1989;68:469–476.
6. Frasier SD, Lippe BM: Clinical Review 11: the national use of growth hormone during childhood. J Clin Endocrinol Metab 1990;71:269–273.
7. Bercu BB, Shulman D, Root AW et al: Growth hormone (GH) provocative testing frequently does not reflect endogenous GH secretion. J Clin Endocrinol Metab 1986;63:709–716.
8. Abboud CF, Laws ER: Diagnosis of pituitary tumors. Endocrinol Metab Clin North Am 1988;17:242–280.
9. Daughaday WH, Hall K, Salmon WD et al: Letter to the Editor: on the nomenclature of the somatomedins and insulin-like growth factors. J Clin Endocrinol Metab 1987;65:1075–1076.
10. Clemmons DR, Underwood LE: Somatomedin-C/insulin-like growth factor I in acromegaly. J Clin Endocrinol Metab 1986;15:629–653.
11. Hammerman MR: Insulin-like growth factors and aging. Endocrinol Metab Clin North Am 1987;16:995–1011.
12. Albertsson-Wikland K, Hall K: Growth hormone treatment in short children: relationship between growth and serum insulin-like growth factor I and II levels. J Clin Endocrinol Metab 1987;65:671–678.
13. Barkan AL, Beitins IZ, Kelch RP: Plasma insulin-like growth factor-I/somatomedin-C in acromegaly: correlation with the degree of growth hormone hypersecretion. J Clin Endocrinol Metab 1988;67:69–73.
14. Unterman TG, Vazquez RM, Slas AJ et al: Nutrition and somatomedin. XIII. Usefulness of somatomedin-C in nutritional assessment. Am J Med 1985;78:228–234.
15. Editorial: Hyperprolactinaemia: when is a prolactinoma not a prolactinoma? Lancet 1987;2:1002–1004.
16. Melmed S, Braunstein GD, Chang J et al: Pituitary tumors secreting growth hormone and prolactin. Ann Intern Med 1986;105:238–253.
17. Kleinberg DL, Noel GL, Frantz AG: Galactorrhea: a study of 235 cases, including 48 with pituitary tumors. N Engl J Med 1977;296:589–600.
18. Jackson RD, Wortsman J, Malarkey MB: Persistence of large molecular weight prolactin secretion during pregnancy in women with macroprolactinemia and its presence in fetal cord blood. J Clin Endocrinol Metab 1989;68:1046–1050.
19. Robinson AG: Prolactinomas in women: current therapies. Ann Intern Med 1983;99:115–118.
20. Fisher DA, Klein AH: Thyroid development and disorders of thyroid function in the newborn. N Engl J Med 1981;304:702–712.
21. Allen DB, Hendricks A, Sieger J et al: Screening programs for congenital hypothyroidism. Am J Dis Child 1988;142:232–236.
22. Editorial: Outcome of screening for congenital hypothyroidism. Lancet 1986;1:1130–1131.
23. Sakata S, Nakamura S, Miura K: Autoantibodies against thyroid hormones or trilodothyronine. Ann Intern Med 1985;103:579–589.
24. Waite KV, Maberly GF, Eastman CJ: Storage conditions and stability of thyrotropin and thyroid hormones on filter paper. Clin Chem 1987;33:853–855.
25. Brent GA, Hershman JM, Braunstein GD: Patients with severe nonthyroidal illness and serum thyrotropin concentrations in the hypothyroid range. Am J Med 1986;81:463–466.
26. Borst GC, Eil C, Burman KD: Euthyroid hyperthyroxinemia. Ann Intern Med 1983;98:366–378.
27. Kennedy L, Griffiths H, Gray TA: Amiodarone and the thyroid. Clin Chem 1989;35:1882–1887.
28. Utiger R: Serum triiodothyronine in man. Annu Rev Med 1974;25:289–302.
29. Bigos RT, Ridgeway EC, Kourides IA et al: Spectrum of pituitary alterations with mild and severe thyroid impairment. J Clin Endocrinol Metab 1978;46:317.
30. Utiger R: Decreased extrathyroidal triiodothyronine production in nonthyroidal illness: benefit or harm? Am J Med 1980;69:807–810.
31. Thonnart B, Messian O, Linhart NC et al: Ten highly sensitive thyrotropin assays compared by receiver-operating characteristic curves analysis: results of a prospective multicenter study. Clin Chem 1988;34:691–695.
32. Berry DJ, Clark PMS, Price CP: A laboratory and clinical evaluation of an immunochemiluminometric assay of thyrotropin in serum. Clin Chem 1988;34:2087–2090.
33. Hershman JM, Pekary AE, Smith V et al: Evaluation of five high-sensitivity American thyrotropin assays. Mayo Clin Proc 1988;63:1133–1139.
34. Nicoloff JT, Spencer CA: Clinical review 12: the use and misuse of the sensitive thyrotropin assay. J Clin Endocrinol Metab 1990;71:553–558.
35. Bartalena L, Martino E, Falcone M et al: Evaluation of the nocturnal serum thyrotropin (TSH) surge, as assessed by TSH ultrasensitive assay, in patients receiving long term L-thyroxine suppression therapy and in patients with various thyroid disorders. J Clin Endocrinol Metab 1987;65:1265–1271.
36. White GH, Gericke L: Diagnostic performance of a commercial assay for thyrotropin, when used as the initial test of thyroid function. Clin Chem 1985;31:1914–1916.
37. Smals AGH, Ross AH, Kloppenborg PWC: Dichotomy between serum free triiodothyronine and free thyroxine concentrations in familial thyroxine-binding globulin deficiency. J Clin Endocrinol Metab 1981;53:917–922.
38. Surks MI, Hupart KH, Pan C et al: Normal free thyroxine in critical nonthyroidal illnesses measured by ultra-

filtration of undiluted serum and equilibrium dialysis. J Clin Endocrinol Metab 1988;67:1031–1039.
39. Hay ID, Klee GG: Thyroid dysfunction. Endocrinol Metab Clin North Am 1988;17:473–509.
40. Wilke TJ: Estimation of free thyroid hormone concentrations in the clinical laboratory. Clin Chem 1986;32:585–592.
41. Nelson JC, Tamel RT: Dependence of the thyroxin/thyroxin-binding globulin (TBG) ratio and the free thyroxin index on TBG concentrations. Clin Chem 1989;35:541–544.
42. Acland JD: The interpretation of the serum protein-bound iodine: a review. J Clin Pathol 1971;24:187–218.
43. Chopra IJ, Solomon DH, Hepner GW et al: Misleadingly low free thyroxine index and usefulness of reverse triiodothyronine measurement in nonthyroidal illnesses. Ann Intern Med 1979;90:905–912.
44. Refetoff S, Lever EG: The value of serum thyroglobulin measurement in clinical practice. JAMA 1983;250:2352–2357.
45. Mariotti S, Martino E, Cupini C et al: Low serum thyroglobulin as a clue to the diagnosis of thyrotoxicosis factitia. N Engl J Med 1982;307:410–412.
46. Chopra IJ, Boado RJ, Geffner DL et al: A radioimmunoassay for measurement of thyronine and its acetic acid analog in urine. J Clin Endocrinol Metab 1988;67:480–487.
47. Editorial: Extrathyroidal actions of TRH. Lancet 1984;2:560–561.
48. Kolesnick RN, Gershengorn MC: Thyrotropin-releasing hormone and the pituitary. Am J Med 1985;79:729–739.
49. Klee GG, Hay ID: Assessment of sensitive thyrotropin assays for an expanded role in thyroid function testing: proposed criteria for analytic performance and clinical utility. J Clin Endocrinol Metab 1987;64:461–471.
50. Takamatsu J, Ando M, Weinberg M et al: Isoelectric focusing of variant thyroxine-binding globulin in American blacks: increased heat lability and reduced serum concentration. J Clin Endocrinol Metab 1986;63:80–87.
51. Smith BR, McLachlan SM, Furmaniak J: Autoantibodies to the thyrotropin receptor. Endocr Rev 1988;9:106–121.
52. Akamizu T, Ishii H, Mori T et al: Abnormal thyrotropin-binding immunoglobulins in two patients with Graves' disease. J Clin Endocrinol Metab 1984;59:240–245.
53. Takaichi Y, Tamai H, Honda K et al: The significance of anti-thyroglobulin and antithyroidal microsomal antibodies in patients with hyperthyroidism due to Graves' disease treated with antithyroidal drugs. J Clin Endocrinol Metab 1989;68:1097–1100.
54. Tamai H, Kasagi K, Takaichi Y et al: Development of spontaneous hypothyroidism in patients with Graves' disease treated with antithyroidal drugs: clinical, immunological, and histological findings in 26 patients. J Clin Endocrinol Metab 1989;69:49–53.
55. Editorial: Autoimmune thyroid disease and thyroid antibodies. Lancet 1988;1:1261–1262.
56. Hamada N, Jaeduck N, Portmann L et al: Antibodies against denatured and reduced thyroid microsomal antigen in autoimmune thyroid disease. J Clin Endocrinol Metab 1987;64:230–238.
57. Larsen PR, Alexander NM, Chopra IJ et al: Revised nomenclature for tests of thyroid hormones and thyroid-related proteins in serum. Arch Pathol Lab Med 1987;111:1141–1145.
58. McKenzie JM, Zakarija M: Clinical Review 3: the clinical use of thyrotropin receptor antibody measurements. J. Clin Endocrinol Metab 1989;69:1093–1096.
59. Speiser PW, Laforgia RI, Kato K et al: First trimester prenatal treatment and molecular genetic diagnosis of congenital adrenal hyperplasia (21-hydroxylase deficiency). J Clin Endocrinol Metab 1990;70:838–848.
60. May ME, Carey RM: Rapid adrenocorticotropic hormone test in practice. Am J Med 1985;79:679–684.
61. Clayton RNI: Diagnosis of adrenal insufficiency. Br Med J 1989;298:271–272.
62. Stewart PM, Corrie J, Seckle JR, Edwards CRW: A rational approach for assessing the hypothalamo-pituitary-adrenal axis. Lancet 1988;1:1208–1210.
63. New MI, Lorenzen F, Lerner AJ et al: Genotyping steroid 21-hydroxylase deficiency: hormonal reference data. J Clin Endocrinol Metab 1983;57:320–326.
64. Wand GS, Niey RL: Disorders of the hypothalamic-pituitary-adrenal axis. J Clin Endocrinol Metab 1985;14:33–53.
65. Gold EM: The Cushing syndromes: changing views of diagnosis and treatment. Ann Intern Med 1979;90:829–844.
66. Finlay WE, McKee JI: Serum cortisol levels in severely stressed patients. Lancet 1982;1:1414–1415.
67. Orbach O, Schussler GC: Increased serum cortisol binding in chronic active hepatitis. Am J Med 1989;86:39–42.
68. Bertrand PV, Rudd BT, Weller PH, Day AJ: Free cortisol and creatinine in urine of healthy children. Clin Chem 1987;33:2047–2051.
69. Raff H, Findling JW: A new immunoradiometric assay for corticotropin evaluated in normal subjects and patients with Cushing's syndrome. Clin Chem 1989;35:596–600.
70. Carpenter PC: Diagnostic evaluation of Cushing's syndrome. J Clin Endocrinol Metab 1988;17:445–472.
71. Nieman LK, Loriaux DL: Corticotropin-releasing hormone: clinical applications. Ann Rev Med 1989;40:331–339.
72. Kaye TB, Crapo L: The Cushing syndrome: an update on diagnostic tests. Ann Intern Med 1990;112:434–444.
73. Ashcraft MW, Van Herle AJ, Vener SL, Geffner DL: Serum cortisol levels in Cushing's syndrome after low- and high-dose dexamethasone suppression. Ann Intern Med 1982;97:21–26.
74. Tyrrell JB, Findling JW, Aron DC et al: An overnight high-dose dexamethasone suppression test for rapid differential diagnosis of Cushing's syndrome. Ann Intern Med 1986;104:180–186.
75. Arana GW, Mossman D: The dexamethasone suppression test and depression. Approaches to the use of a laboratory test in psychiatry. J Clin Endocrinol Metab 1988;17:21–39.
76. Sindler BH, Griffing GT, Melby JC: The superiority of the metyrapone test versus the high-dose dexamethasone test in the differential diagnosis of Cushing's syndrome. Am J Med 1983;74:657–662.
77. Howanitz JH, Howanitz PJ: Evaluation of endocrine function. pp. 299–345. In Henry JB (ed): Clinical Diagnosis and Management by Laboratory Methods. 17th Ed. Philadelphia, WB Saunders, 1984.
78. Gueux B, Fiet J, Couillin P et al: Prenatal diagnosis of

78. *(continued)* 21-hydroxylase deficiency congenital adrenal hyperplasia by simultaneous radioimmunoassay of 21-deoxycortisol and 17-hydroxyprogesterone in amniotic fluid. J Clin Endocrinol Metab 1988;66:534–537.
79. Pang S, Pollack MS, Loo M et al: Pitfalls of prenatal diagnosis of 21-hydroxylase deficiency congenital adrenal hyperplasia. J Clin Endocrinol Metab 1985;61:89–97.
80. White PC, Niew MI, Dupont B: Congenital adrenal hyperplasia. N Engl J Med 1987;316:1580–1586.
81. Streeten DHP, Tomycz N, Anderson GH: Reliability of screening methods for the diagnosis of primary aldosteronism. Am J Med 1979;67:403–412.
82. Young WF, Klee GG: Primary aldosteronism, diagnostic evaluation. J Clin Endocrinol Metab 1988;17:367–395.
83. Kaplan NM, Kem DC, Holand OB et al: Intravenous furosemide test: a simple way to evaluate renin responsiveness. Ann Intern Med 1976;84:639–643.
84. Bravo EL, Tarazi RC, Dustan HP et al: The changing clinical spectrum of primary aldosteronism. Am J Med 1983;74:641–651.
85. Pickering TG, Sos TA, Vaughan ED et al: Predictive value and changes in renin secretion in hypertensive patients with unilateral renovascular disease undergoing successful renal angioplasty. Am J Med 1984;76:398–404.
86. Lieberman J: Enzymes in sarcoidosis. Angiotensin-converting enzyme (ACE). Clin Lab Med 1989;9:745–755.
87. Cryer PE: Phaeochromocytoma. J Clin Endocrinol Metab 1985;14:203–219.
88. Benowitz NL: Pheochromocytoma—recent advances in diagnosis and treatment. West J Med 1988;148:561–567.
89. Grouzmann E, Comoy E, Bohuon C: Plasma neuropeptide Y concentrations in patients with neuroendocrine tumors. J Clin Endocrinol Metab 1989;68:808–813.
90. Ladisch S, Wu ZL, Feig S et al: Shedding of G_{D2} ganglioside by human neuroblastoma. Int J Cancer 1987;39:73–76.
91. Brodeur GM: Clinical significance of genetic rearrangements in human neuroblastomas. Clin Chem 1989;35:B38–B41.
92. Tuchman M, Morris CL, Ramnaraine ML et al: Value of random urinary homovanillic acid and vanillylmandelic acid levels in the diagnosis and management of patients with neuroblastoma: comparison with 24-hour urine collections. Pediatrics 1985;75:324–328.
93. Tuchman M, Ramnaraine MLR, Woods WG et al: Three years of experience with random urinary homovanillic and vanillylmandelic acid levels in the diagnosis of neuroblastoma. Pediatrics 1987;79:203–205.
94. Oishi S, Sasaki M, Ohno M et al: Urinary normetanephrine and metanephrine measured by radioimmunoassay for the diagnosis of pheochromocytoma: utility of 24-hour and random 1-hour urine determinations. J Clin Endocrinol Metab 1988;67:614–618.
95. Sheps SG, Jiang N, Klee GG: Diagnostic evaluation of pheochromocytoma. Endocrinol Metab Clin North Am 1988;17:397–411.
96. Samaan NA, Hickey RC: Pheochromocytoma. Semin Oncol 1987;14:297–305.
97. Bravo EL, Gifford RW: Pheochromocytoma: diagnosis, localization and management. N Engl J Med 1984;311:1298–1303.
98. Bravo EL, Tarazi RC, Fouad FM et al: Clonidine-suppression test: a useful aid in the diagnosis of pheochromocytoma. N Engl J Med 1981;305:623–626.
99. Taylor HC, Mayes D, Anton AH: Clonidine suppression test for pheochromocytoma: examples of misleading results. J Clin Endocrinol Metab 1986;63:238–242.
100. MacDougall IC, Isles CG, Stewart H et al: Overnight clonidine suppression test in the diagnosis and exclusion of pheochromocytoma. Am J Med 1988;84:993–999.
101. Duncan MW, Campton P, Lazarus L et al: Measurement of norepinephrine and 3,4-dihydroxyphenylglycol in urine and plasma for the diagnosis of pheochromocytoma. N Engl J Med 1988;319:136–142.
102. Alvarado CS, Faraj BA, Kim TH: Plasma dopa and catecholamines in the diagnosis and follow-up of children with neuroblastoma. Am J Pediatr Hematol Oncol 1985;7:221–227.
103. Goldstein DS, Stull R, Eisenhofer G et al: Plasma 3,4-dihydroxyphenylalanine (Dopa) and catecholamines in neuroblastoma or pheochromocytoma. Ann Intern Med 1986;105:388.
104. Gahr M, Hunneman DH: The value of determination of homovanillic and vanillylmandelic acids in plasma for the diagnosis and follow-up of neuroblastoma in children. Eur J Pediatr 1987;146:489–493.
105. Harlharan M, VanNoord T, Cameron OG et al: Free 3-methoxy-4-hydroxyphenylglycol determined in plasma by liquid chromatography with coulometric detection. Clin Chem 1989;35:202–205.
106. Kwekkeboom DJ, de Jong FH, van Hemert AM et al: Serum gonadotropins and α-subunit decline in aging normal postmenopausal women. J Clin Endocrinol Metab 1990;70:944–950.
107. Croxson TS, Chapman WE, Miller LK et al: Changes in the hypothalamic-gonadal axis in human immunodeficiency virus-infected homosexual men. J Clin Endocrinol Metab 1989;68:317–321.
108. Snyder PJ: Gonadotroph cell pituitary adenomas. Endocrinol Metab Clin North Am 1987;16:755–764.
109. Harman SM, Tsitouras PD, Paul T et al: Evaluation of pituitary gonadotropic function in men: value of luteinizing hormone-releasing hormone response versus basal luteinizing hormone level for discrimination of diagnosis. J Clin Endocrinol Metab 1982;54:196–200.
110. Slaats EH, Kennedy JC, Kruijswijk H: Interference of sex-hormone binding globulin in the "coat-a-count" testosterone no-extraction radioimmunoassay. Clin Chem 1987;33:300–302.
111. Marshall JC: Investigative procedures. Endocrinol Metab Clin North Am 1975;4:545–567.
112. Ismail AAA, Astley P, Burr WA et al: The role of testosterone measurement in the investigation of androgen disorders. Clin Biochem 1986;23:113–134.
113. Carlström K, Gershagen S, Rannevik G: Free testosterone and testosterone/SHBG index in hirsute women: a comparison of diagnostic accuracy. Gynecol Obstet Invest 1987;24:256–261.
114. Nankin HR, Calkins JH: Decreased bioavailable testosterone in aging normal and impotent men. J Clin Endocrinol Metab 1986;63:1418–1420.
115. Yamaji T, Ishibashi M, Takaku F et al: Serum dehydroepiandrosterone sulfate concentrations in secondary adrenal insufficiency. J Clin Endocrinol Metab 1987;65:448–451.

116. Ehrmann DA, Rosenfield RL: Clinical review 10. An endocrinologic approach to the patient with hirsutism. J Clin Endocrinol Metab 1990;71:1–4.
117. Ratcliffe WA, Carter GD, Dowsett M et al: Oestradiol assays: applications and guidelines for the provision of a clinical biochemistry service. Ann Clin Biochem 1988;25:466–483.
118. Rogers BJ: The sperm penetration assay: its usefulness reevaluated. Fertil Steril 1985;43:821–840.
119. Gross PA, Pehrisch H, Rascher W et al: Pathogenesis of clinical hyponatremia: observations of vasopressin and fluid intake in 100 hyponotremic medical patients. Eur J Clin Invest 1987;17:123–129.
120. Zerbe RL, Robertson GL: A comparison of plasma vasopressin measurements with a standard indirect test in the differential diagnosis of polyuria. N Engl J Med 1981;305:1539–1546.
121. Marcus R: Laboratory diagnosis of primary hyperparathyroidism. Endocrinol Metab Clin North Am 1989;18:339–414.
122. Toffaletti J: Ionized calcium: part 1. Clin Chem News 1989; July:10–11.
123. Gray TA, Buckley BM, Sealey MM et al: Plasma ionized calcium monitoring during liver transplantation. Transplantation 1986;41:335–339.
124. Bianchi G, Vezzoli G, Cusi D et al: Abnormal red-cell calcium pump in patients with idiopathic hypercalciuria. N Engl J Med 1988;319:897–901.
125. Ladenson J: Inorganic phosphorus: review of methods. Am Soc Clin Pathol Check Sample CORE Chemistry No. 89-3, 1989.
126. Elin R: Assessment of magnesium status. Clin Chem 1987;33:1965–1970.
127. Mallette LE: Synthetic human parathyroid hormone 1-34 fragment for diagnostic testing. Ann Intern Med 1988;109:800–804.
128. Endres DB, Villaneuva R, Sharp C et al: Measurement of parathyroid hormone. Endocrinol Metab Clin North Am 1989;18:611–629.
129. Sizemore GW: Medullary carcinoma of the thyroid gland. Semin Oncol 1987;14:306–314.
130. Wells SA, Dilley WG, Farndon JA et al: Early diagnosis and treatment of medullary thyroid carcinoma. Arch Intern Med 1985;145:1248–1252.
131. Taylor AK, Linkhart S, Mohan S et al: Multiple osteocalcin fragments in human urine and serum as detected by a midmolecule osteocalcin radioimmunoassay. J Clin Endocrinol Metab 1990;70:467–471.
132. Pastoureau P, Delmas PD: Measurement of serum bone gla-protein (BGP) in humans with an ovine BGP-based radioimmunoassay. Clin Chem 1990;36:620–1624.

12 Serum Tumor Markers

Joan H. Howanitz
Peter J. Howanitz

INTRODUCTION

Most, if not all, human tumors release a variety of products, some of which may lead to signs and symptoms as indicated in Table 12-1. In common usage, those products appearing in blood or other body fluids are called tumor markers, meaning biochemical indicators associated with the presence of malignancy. Because of their unchecked growth, it is logical to assume malignant cells are different from other cells and, therefore, might produce a component not present in healthy cells. Thus, theoretically at least, a unique biochemical component could occur as a result of malignant transformation. To date, the differences in biochemical components between normal and malignant cells appear to be quantitative. Another theoretic possibility is that biochemical components appear briefly at some early stage of embryogenesis, but are never normally expressed again. Although it is a hypothetical possibility that some components are only expressed in malignant transformation, this does not seem to be the case. For example, the Tennessee antigen has been found not only in association with malignancy, but also in a variety of other illnesses. The so-called tumor markers thus are found in patients with malignancies, in those with benign disease or infection, in fetal tissue, and, indeed, in the serum and tissues of healthy individuals. It is clear the tumor markers that have been described to date are neither specific for a particular type of malignancy nor specific for malignancy itself. One approach to improve sensitivity and specificity is to use one or more tumor markers.

Use of Tumor Markers

An ideal tumor marker fills a number of criteria (Table 12-2), but most of the known markers fall far short of these ideal goals.[1] Tumor markers have been used to screen patients for malignancy, diagnose a specific type of malignancy, determine prognosis, and follow the course of disease in patients with malignancies. Because tumor markers are not specific for a particular malignancy or even malignancy itself, they generally have not found a significant role in screening and diagnosing malignancy. Use of markers in screening, however, has been successful in certain high risk groups. For example, in susceptible families, calcitonin measurements have been used successfully to identify individuals who harbor medullary carcinoma of the thyroid. Tumor markers can be a useful adjunct to the diagnostic process even though nonspecificity of tumor markers is a problem in determining the site of origin of the malignancy with perhaps only a few exceptions. For example, although carcinoembryonic antigen (CEA) is associated with gastrointestinal tract malignancy, increased CEA levels may occur in association with a number of malignant conditions, including breast carcinoma, as well as a variety of nonmalignant conditions, for example, smoking and acute infections. However, CEA levels that are at least 20 times greater than the reference range are usually associated with gastrointestinal malignancy.

Tumor markers are used for determining prognosis and for staging various malignant disorders but, to date, the

Table 12-1. Humoral Syndromes of Cancer

Paraneoplastic syndromes of the nervous system
    Cerebellar syndromes
        Cortical cerebellar degeneration
        Myoclonic encephalopathy
    Encephalomyelitis
    Multifocal leukoencephalopathy
    Peripheral neuropathy
        Sensory
        Sensorimotor
    Skeletal muscle syndromes
        Polymyositis-dematomyositis
        Carcinomatous neuromyopathy
    Myathenic syndromes (e.g., Eaton-Lambert syndrome)
Miscellaneous syndromes
    Digital clubbing and arthropathies
    Enzyme production (e.g., AP)
    Fetal protein production (e.g., AFP, CEA)
    Fever
    Hematologic syndromes (e.g., aplastic anemia, red blood cell aplasia)
    Glomerular kidney disease

Abbreviations: AFP, α-fetoprotein; AP, alkaline phosphatase; CEA, carcinoembryonic antigen.

Table 12-2. Characteristics of an Ideal Tumor Marker

Specific for a particular type of tumor
Released only by, or in response to, the tumor
Results are proportional to the state of differentiation and mass of tumor cells
Quantitatively reflects therapeutic response
Elevations occur in patients with low tumor burden

Table 12-3. Tumor Markers

Enzymes
    Alkaline phosphatase
    Creatine kinase
    Lactate dehydrogenase
    Neuron specific enolase
    Prostate acid phosphatase
    Prostate specific antigen
    Sialytransferase
Glycoproteins[a]
    α-fetoprotein
    Cancer antigen (CA) 15-3
    CA 19-9
    CA 50
    CA 125
    CA 195
    CA 549
    Carcinoembryonic antigen
    Sialic acid/lipid-associated sialic acid
    Tennessee antigen
    Tumor associated glycoprotein
Hormones and hormone-like substances
    Antidiuretic hormone
    Calcitonin
    Corticotropin
    Homovanillic acid
    Human chorionic gonadotropin (B-hCG)
    Parathyroid hormone-like factor
    Tumor necrosis factor (cachectin)
    Vasoactive intestinal peptide
Hormone receptors
    Androgen
    Estrogen
    Progesterone
Oncogenes and oncogene products
    erb
    myc
    ras
    src
Miscellaneous
    $β_2$-Microglobulin
    Immunoglobulins
    Polyamines

[a] With the development of monoclonal antibody technology, it became possible to make antibodies to various glycoprotein markers using cancer cell lines or material from surgical specimens. Many of the antibodies have been developed commercially and are often named for the antigen from which they have been derived or for the antibody that was developed. Currently, a number of commercially developed markers are available in kit form, but many are for investigative use only.

most important use of tumor markers is assessing patient response to therapy. Unfortunately, quantification of serum tumor markers often does not reflect tumor burden accurately. Reasons for this may include relationship of tumor to venous drainage, heterogeneity of tumors as well as varying rates of marker production and metabolism.[2] Production rate of tumor markers varies not only between patients with the same type of tumor but also in the same patients over the course of their disease. Production rates of tumor markers can change as the cell population changes, and varying amounts of a marker may reach the circulation depending on such factors as anatomic location of the tumor or degree of tumor necrosis. Most commonly, relatively specific tumor-derived markers, such as prostate-specific antigen (PSA), are used for predicting prognosis and therapy of patients, but markers made in response to tumor presence also have been used especially in following the course of malignant disease. For example, markers indicating cell turnover or growth are potentially useful for monitoring response to therapy.

Tumor markers also can be used for the location of a metastases in vivo (e.g., by the use of radiolabeled markers) and in therapy, in which radioactivity or drugs are conjugated with an antibody to a given marker. Administration of antibodies to markers can be expected to cause assay interferences. For example, this has already been reported in a patient where radioimmunodetection was performed with anti-CA 125 antibodies.[3]

Classification of Tumor Markers

Tumor markers can be placed into two broad categories, namely (1) tumor-derived markers (molecules produced by the neoplastic cells) and (2) tumor associated markers (metabolic and immunologic products produced by response to the tumor). The tumor markers also can be categorized by their biochemical nature and function (Table 12-3). Many tumor markers have been proposed, but considerable experience in clinical trials is necessary to delineate their value. This chapter includes only some of the more well studied markers.

ENZYMES AS TUMOR MARKERS

Serum enzyme activity often is increased in the presence of malignancy. Increases occur because of increased production by, or leakage from, the tumor or in response to tumor presence. There are many reports of nonspecific changes in malignancy, for example, serum enzyme activity occurring in association with liver metastases[4] (Table 12-4). In addition, more specific changes, such as elevations of PSA in association with prostatic carcinoma, have been reported. Only a few common examples of enzyme activity changes associated with malignancy are covered in this chapter, but it is important to recognize that there have been numerous reports of other enzyme changes; for example, amylase production by lung and ovarian cancers has been reported. Production by, or secondary to, malignancy has been reported with all the commonly measured serum enzymes and many of less commonly ordered ones as well. For details regarding changes reported in association with specific tumors, an excellent source of information is *Effect of Disease on Clinical Laboratory Tests*.[5]

Table 12-4. Serum Enzyme Activity in Patients With Metastatic Liver Disease

Increases
    Alkaline phosphatase
    Arylsulfatase
    Aspartate aminotransferase
    γ-Glutamyl transpepidase
    Glycoprotein galactosyl transferase
    Lactate dehydrogenase
    5' Nucleotidase
Decreases
    Pseudocholinesterase

(From Stefanini,[4] with permission.)

Test: Alkaline Phosphatase (AP) (See Ch. 4)

Background and Selection

Alkaline phosphate occurs in many tissues including the intestine, liver, kidney, bone, and placenta. Elevations in AP activity may be caused by liver and bone metastases or by tumor production of the enzyme. In patients with malignancy, it is often important to identify the source of an elevated AP, although until recently this has been technically difficult. Additionally, specific assays for the placental form of the AP are useful for following patients with certain malignancies (see below).

Terminology

At least three genes encode for AP isoenzyme forms: (1) tissue nonspecific; (2) intestinal (adult); and (3) placental. Other forms such as fetal intestinal and testicular may correspond to other isoenzymes. The tissue nonspecific gene is widely expressed in such tissues as bone, liver, and kidney; thus the isoenzyme sometimes is designated the liver/bone form. The Commission on Biochemical Nomenclature discourages labeling of isoenzymes on the basis of tissue distribution, because confusion may arise owing to species variation. Although labeling based on electrophoretic mobility is recommended, numerous electrophoretic techniques exist, giving rise to differences in relative mobility of the isoenzyme forms. Thus, common practice in the medical literature is to name the isoenzymes depending on the tissue from which they are derived.

In addition to the AP isoenzymes, there are AP forms that occur with differences in carbohydrate composition. The various carbohydrate-containing forms, which probably arise by post-translational modification of the enzyme, should not be classified as isoenzymes, even though in practice all of the enzyme forms are called *alkaline phosphatase isoenzymes*. Isoenzymes associated with malignancy also are named (e.g., the Regan isoenzyme for the placental form, although some differences between this and the placental form may occur; Nagao for a placental-like form; and Kasahara for a relatively heat sensitive, fetal intestinal form).

Logistics

Because separating the AP isoenzymes (especially the bone and liver fractions) is both difficult and important, many techniques have been developed. These include rates of hydrolysis of various substrates and response to inhibitors. Probably the most commonly used method in clinical laboratories, at least until recently, is heat stability.

Heat Stability

There is gradation in heat stability from placental AP, which is stable at 56°C, to bone, which has a half-life of roughly 2 minutes at 56°C. At 56°C the liver fraction has a half-life of approximately 8 minutes. These times, however, are variable depending on the particular serum tested. Small temperature variations affect inactivation rates enough to obscure the relatively small difference in liver and bone AP fractions.

Other Methods

The AP isoenzymes can be separated on the basis of their electrophoretic mobility, with varying degrees of resolution of normal and abnormally occurring forms depending on the media used. Both the liver and bone forms appear to be derived from the same gene locus (see above); thus, it is not surprising that with electrophoresis, the bone and liver bands are resolved incompletely. Recently, isoelectric focusing and high performance liquid chromatography (HPLC) methods have been developed.

Immunoassays

Immunoassays are available for quantitation of placental alkaline phosphatase (PLAP).

Interpretation

Liver and bone metastases can cause increases in serum AP activity. In addition, elevation of serum AP activity caused by tumor production of the enzyme is associated with a variety of malignancies including breast, lung, ovarian, and gastrointestinal malignancies. It appears that some tumors express an enzyme identical to PLAP (as determined by monoclonal antibodies).[6] Usually, however, the APs expressed by malignancies are only similar to, but not identical with, the placental (heat-stable) form. In addition, other AP isoenzyme forms have been described in association with malignancy, for example, a heat-sensitive form reported in Hodgkin's disease.[7] The fetal intestinal form is associated with hepatomas and gastrointestinal tract malignancies.

Placental Alkaline Phosphatase

The reference range of PLAP, as measured by immunoassay, is less than about 0.1 μ/L in males and nonpregnant females. Mean values, however, are roughly five times as high in smokers as compared with nonsmokers, and some smokers have results as high as 10-fold above the upper reference for nonsmokers.[8] Immunoassay of PLAP has been used for following patients with malignancy, especially ovarian and testicular carcinomas. About 45% of patients with ovarian carcinoma have elevated results for PLAP, whereas about 60% of testicular carcinoma patients have elevated results. Results are increased in over 70% of seminoma patients and about 35% of patients with nonseminomas. Only a small portion of patients with breast, lung, or bronchial carcinoma have elevated PLAP results.

Test: Creatine Kinase (CK) (See Ch. 2)

There is at least one report of increased CK-MB in association with a colonic carcinoma, but carcinoma is more commonly associated with macromolecular CK forms or with CK-BB.[9]

Macro CK, type 1 (macromolecular form of BB produced by binding CK-BB to immunoglobulin) and macro CK, type 2 (probably representing a mitochondrial MM) have been reported in patients with malignancy, but neither are specific for malignancy (Fig. 12-1). Macro CK, type 2 has been reported, especially in association with colonic carcinoma, but enzyme activity lacks correlation with stage of disease.[10]

Although not specific for malignancy, the BB isoenzyme of creatine kinase is increased in patients with a variety of malignancies including small cell carcinoma of the lung, lymphomas, and gastrointestinal and head and neck carcinomas. The BB isoenzyme also is increased in patients with carcinomas of the breast, uterus, cervix, prostate, testes, and bladder. Although CK-BB is commonly increased in gastric and prostatic carcinoma patients, the percentage of patients with

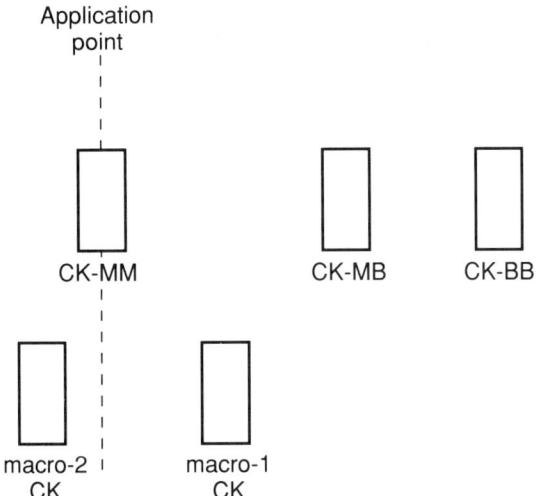

Fig. 12-1. Schematic diagram of agarose gel electrophoresis of the CK isoenzymes and macro-1 and macro-2 CK forms. The position of the macro forms is not constant from patient to patient.

other types of tumors who have increased serum CK-BB activity is relatively low.[11]

Test: Lactate Dehydrogenase (LD) (See Ch. 2)

Increases in serum LD activity are found in some hematologic malignancies (e.g., leukemia and lymphomas), in association with a variety of primary solid tissue tumors (e.g., colorectal carcinoma), and in metastatic disease. Almost one-half the patients with metastatic carcinoma have increases in LD 2, 3, 4 with or without increases in LD 5. In addition to increases in LD 2, 3, 4 (midzone increases), other patterns of increased LD activity have been identified in patients with malignancy including relative increase in all five isoenzymes (isomorphic pattern); increases in LD 4, 5, or LD 5 only, increases in LD 1 and LD 2, and an extra band.

The isomorphic pattern is seen frequently in leukemia and lymphoma patients. In patients with metastatic liver disease, the isomorphic pattern occurs in patients with the highest LD results, perhaps reflecting substantial metastases outside the liver. In contrast, usually only LD 5 is increased in patients with liver metastases, when LD is within the reference range or only slightly elevated.[12] Patients with seminomas or dysgerminomas have elevated serum LD activity, mainly associated with increases in LD 1 and LD 2. Extra bands of LD have been reported in various positions associated with a variety of conditions. Some of these bands are tumor products, but others are genetic variants, complexes with immunoglobulins, and recombinations of monomers; they also may result from a crossreacting enzyme in the LD assay. There have been numerous reports of an extra LD isoenzyme in the serum of patients with hepatic malignancies, but the presence of an extra LD isoenzyme also is associated with a variety of other malignancies.[13]

Test: Acid Phosphatase (Prostatic Acid Phosphatase [PAP], Male PAP Test)

Background

Besides digital examination of the prostate, the oldest and the most widely used diagnostic aid for prostatic carcinoma is the measurement of PAP. Measurement of this enzyme has certain drawbacks, including choice of inhibitor, substrate, or technique used to discriminate among the acid phosphatases from sources other than the prostate. Over 50 years ago, it was established that acid phosphatase was found in the prostate, and its activity was increased in cases of metastatic prostatic carcinoma. When these observations were extended to correlate with disease progression and response to hormonal treatment, a new field of biologic markers for following manifestations of carcinoma was initiated. Because this enzyme has an isoelectric point (pI) between 4.4 and 5.5, the term acid phosphatase was coined. The function of acid phosphatase in semen has been accepted as hydrolyzing phosphate esters with the release of important metabolites for sexual function.

Selection

The major use of PAP has been the evaluation and management of patients with prostatic carcinoma. Enzymatic determinations performed with sera indicate that elevated acid phosphatase determinations are rarely associated with disease localized to the gland. Generally elevated levels indicate carcinoma has extended outside the gland and with progression of disease, values increase. However, even in patients with widely metastatic disease, the percent of patients with elevated values has been reported as only 75–90%. Table 12-5 shows the nonprostatic diseases reported to give elevated acid phosphatase results, but many are from reports using nonspecific substrates. With thymolphthalein monophosphate, elevated values have been reported in growing children, presumably from the contribution of bone, as well as in patients with Gaucher's disease and some leukemias. Elevated values result from a variety of prostatic diseases and trauma, such as prostatic infarction, benign prostatic hypertrophy, prostatic biopsy, massage during the rectal examination, transurethral prostatic resection, and prostatic radiation. Interpretation of immunoassay results

Table 12-5. Some Conditions in Which Acid Phosphatase is Elevated

Bone disease
Gaucher's disease
Manipulation (rectal or surgical) of benign prostatic tissue
Paget's disease
Nonprostatic carcinoma with bone or hepatic metastases
Multiple myeloma
Osteoporosis
Renal osteopathy
Osteogenesis imperfecta
Niemann-Pick disease
Hepatitis
Cirrhosis
Extrahepatic biliary obstruction
Pulmonary embolus and other thromboembolic phenomena
Myocardial infarct
Acute and chronic leukemias
Polycythemia vera
Primary thrombocythemia
Other myeloproliferative disease
Macroacid phosphatase

is similar to enzymatic assays except that antibody specificity has resulted in elimination of reactivity from nonprostatic fractions; however, a number of benign conditions still are cause for elevated results for the prostatic fraction of acid phosphatase. Markedly elevated results have been reported with macroacid phosphatase. In this condition, acid phosphatase is complexed with IgG and measured by both enzymatic and immunologic methods.[14]

Prostate specific antigen, because of its improved sensitivity and specificity, has begun to replace acid phosphatase measurements (see Test: Prostate Specific Antigen). When used as a screening test for prostatic carcinoma in the general population, acid phosphatase is considered useless.

Acid phosphatase activity in vaginal specimens has been used to substantiate the allegation of rape.

Terminology

Serum acid phosphatases are a group of enzymes capable of hydrolyzing phosphate esters in an acid environment. Over 20 isoenzyme bands have been found in human sera, however, isoenzyme 2 originates from the prostate. When this isoenzyme was measured by radioimmunoassay in sera of males suspected of having prostatic carcinoma, it was advertised as the male PAP test.

Logistics

Specimen Requirements

Plasma from healthy individuals contains tartrate resistant isoenzyme 5 but no demonstrable isoenzymes from red blood cells (RBC) or the prostate. Comparable serum contains an additional isoenzyme 3, which is tartrate sensitive and is released from platelets during blood clotting. In a variety of diseases, other isoenzymes may appear in plasma; the most important example is metastatic prostatic carcinoma with which isoenzyme 2 appears.

Acid phosphatase enzymatic activity is unstable if stored at room temperature, or at physiologic pH. Storage at 23°C for a few hours, acidification to pH 5.5, or the addition of citrate preserves enzymatic activity. The immunologic reactivity of acid phosphatase also shows similar sensitivity to heat and neutral and alkaline pH, with some reports even indicating increased degradation as compared with enzymatic estimations. Enzymatic phosphatase measurements should be made within 2 hours after specimen collection. Although a

Table 12-6. Differences in Serum Acid Phosphatases

Occurrence/Properties	Erythrocytes	Hairy Cells, Gaucher Cells, Osteoclasts	Lysosomes, Lymphocytes, Platelets	Prostate, Granulocytes, Pancreas
Electrophoresis	Not detected	Band 5a, 5b	Band 3	Band 2a, b, 4
Molecular size (da)	20,000	30,000	100,000	100,000
Tartrate inhibition	Resistant	Resistant	Sensitive	Sensitive
Substrates Reactivity				
p-Nitrophenyl phosphate	Reactive	Reactive	Reactive	Reactive
Thymolphthalein monophosphate	Reactive	Reactive	Reactive	Reactive
2-Naphthylphosphate	Reactive	Reactive	Reactive	Reactive
1-Naphthylphosphate	Inactive	Reactive	Reactive	Reactive
Glycerolphosphate	Inactive	Inactive	Reactive	Reactive

diurnal pattern similar to cortisol, showing highest values in the early morning and lowest at night, had been described, this has not been validated. However, a wide within-day biologic variation has been shown, with changes frequently up to twofold seen in healthy individuals.

Methods

Enzymatic methods for measurement have used a variety of substrates some of which are listed in Table 12-6. The large number of substrates reflect attempts to devise methods that are simple and specific for PAP with the exclusion of other isoenzymes of nonprostatic sources. Also shown in Table 12-6 are some of the major isoenzymes found in sera in various diseases and their tissue source. Of the various substrates, thymolphthalein monophosphate has been found to provide superior analytic specificity for the prostatic isoenzyme. Other approaches to increase the specificity have included use of organ-specific acid phosphatase inhibitors. L-tartrate, the most commonly used of these, inhibits almost all of the PAP activity while exhibiting little effect on erythrocyte acid phosphatase. However, acid phosphatases from spleen, liver, platelets, and kidney also are inhibited. Many reports have documented elevation of acid phosphatase when nonspecific substrates have been used (Table 12-5). These conditions can be significant when nonspecific methods are used.

The use of immunologic techniques held out the promise of improving specificity and eliminating the problems related to the lack of stability but, to date, this has not been achieved. A list of potential tumor markers from prostatic carcinoma is seen in Table 12-7.

Interpretation

When enzymatic methods using thymolphthalein monophosphate as the substrate and stringent specimen handling conditions are used, typical reference intervals are 0–0.8 IU/L for males and females. Reference values in young children are higher than in adults until puberty, and old men have elevated values as well.

Table 12-7. Prostatic Tumor Markers

Acid phosphatase (enzymatic)
Acid phosphatase (RIA)
Prostate-specific antigen
Creatine kinase, isoenzyme BB
γ-Seminoprotein
Placental alkaline phosphatase
Alkaline phosphatase
Bone alkaline phosphatase

The cause of the elevations is lack of specificity and cross-reaction with osteoclast acid phosphatase in the young, and the presence of prostatic disease in the aged. Other substrates or methods generally yield higher results caused by nonspecificity, and the results are not interchangeable between methods because methodologies are not standardized against each other. When immunoassay is used, the reference interval generally extends from nondetectable up to approximately 10 ng/mL, depending on the assay used.

Test: Prostate Specific Antigen

Background and Selection

Prostate-specific antigen, a glycoprotein enzyme found in the cytoplasm of prostatic duct cells and within the lumina of prostatic ducts, is excreted in urine and seminal plasma. It is a protease showing homology with the kallakrein proteases and has a mass of approximately 33,000 da. The natural substrate for PSA has been identified as seminal coagulum, the prominent protein in seminal vesicle secretion. Stains of prostatic tissue from children demonstrate high PSA concentrations during the first few months of life, which then decrease but reappear after 10 years of age, thereby suggesting a hormonal dependence. Because the half-life of PSA is 2.2 days, it is useful for detecting residual disease shortly after surgical resection. Concentrations of PSA in the serum correlate well with the stage of prostatic disease and the response of patients with prostatic carcinoma. Prostate-specific antigen measurements have a better sensitivity for diagnosing and monitoring disease activity than serum acid phosphatase as well as showing less biologic variation.[15] Consequently, PSA has begun to replace acid phosphatase measurements.

In peripheral blood, PSA is a sensitive marker for prostatic cancer, but the lack of specificity precludes its use as a routine screening test in the general population. Repetitive measurements are extremely valuable for evaluating the response of prostatic cancer to treatment.

Logistics

Measurements are made by immunoassay with monoclonal or polyclonal reagent antibodies. Unexpected low values have been reported as a result of the "high dose hook effect," an analytic artifact when extremely high values yield a factitiously low result. Upon dilution of these patient specimens, values increase, thereby demonstrating assay conditions as a cause of these spurious results.

Interpretation

A typical reference interval for a monoclonal assay is 0–2 µg/L, whereas polyclonal assays give results approximately 50% higher. Women have barely detectable PSA results, with the probable source being the periurethral glands.

Prostate-specific antigen results have been reported as being elevated in up to one-half of patients with benign prostatic hyperplasia, prostatitis, or urinary retention, although prostatic carcinoma had not been excluded in these patients. When patients with urinary tract obstruction were studied, approximately one-third were found to have previously unidentified prostatic carcinoma, suggesting that a large percent of patients with prostatic symptoms also may have cancer. Because of the overlap in patients who have elevated levels and do not have identifiable prostatic carcinoma, PSA is not sufficiently reliable to select patients for radical prostatectomy. However, raised levels of PSA in patients with abnormal prostates or in elderly men with a high risk of prostatic cancer should be an indication for ultrasound or biopsy of any suspicious areas. Following digital rectal examination, some workers have reported elevated PSA levels, whereas others have detected no increase in values. More traumatic procedures, such as cystoscopy or prostatic needle biopsy, cause PSA levels to increase. Slightly elevated results also have been reported in patients with pulmonary, renal, mammary, gastrointestinal, and genital urinary tumors, but are found in less than 10% of cases.

Serum levels also relate to the degree of extraprostatic extension and disease activity, especially when combined with acid phosphatase. Prostate-specific antigen levels may precede development of clinically detectable metastasis by as much as 6–12 months. Following radical prostatectomy, any patient with detectable levels 3 weeks later is considered to have residual cancer and thus is a candidate for further immediate therapy. For following patients treated with radical prostatectomy, Stamey et al.[16] recommend measurement 3 weeks after prostatectomy, every 3 months during the first year, every 4 months during the second year, and every 6 months thereafter if values remain within the reference interval. When compared with PAP for monitoring patients treated for prostatic carcinoma, PSA is superior with up to 50% of patients with elevated PSA results having acid phosphatase values within the reference interval.

Bone marrow PSA measurements do not provide an advantage over serum measurements in the early detection of metastatic prostatic carcinoma and should be discouraged.

GLYCOPROTEINS AS TUMOR MARKERS

Test: α-Fetoprotein (AFP) (See Ch. 15)

Background and Selection

α-Fetoprotein was first found in cord blood almost 40 years ago, and then subsequently identified in sera of patients with hepatocellular carcinomas. It is a glycoprotein with a mass of about 70,000 da containing approximately 4% carbohydrate. As a glycoprotein, AFP shows heterogeneity as demonstrated by chromatography on lectins. The function of AFP is not known, but because it is the primary dominant serum protein during most stages of fetal life and serves functions similar to albumin in the adult, speculation is that it provides for osmotic regulation and is a carrier protein.

Logistics

A diurnal pattern in serum, with changes approximately 10% of mean values, has been described with peak levels found at 1100 hours and a nocturnal dip occurring at 2300 hours. Although a different diurnal pattern of AFP also occurs in patients with cancer, this difference has not found clinical use.

In the human embryo, AFP is produced first by the yolk sac and liver, and after the yolk sac has involuted at the end of the first trimester, by the liver alone. Trace amounts also are produced by the gastrointestinal tract. α-Fetoprotein levels exceed those of albumin until about 8 weeks of gestation, at which time both proteins are present in approximately equal concentrations. The concentration of serum AFP peaks during the 14th week of gestation at approximately 2–3 g/L and thereafter decreases to 5–100 mg/L at birth. Levels then fall rapidly so that by 1 year of age adult values of 4–25 µg/L are reached.

The measurement of AFP levels is useful for monitoring individuals with hepatocellular carcinoma, nonseminomatous germ cell tumors of the testis, and germ cell tumors of the ovary. The measurement is also useful for prenatal diagnosis of neural tube defects (see Ch. 15).

Interpretation

The typical reference interval for AFP is less than 10 µg/L, but pregnant women commonly have serum values up to 500 µg/L. Spuriously elevated results have been seen with sera containing an IgG reactive with AFP assay reagent immunoglobulins.

Liver Disease

Approximately 75% of individuals with hepatocellular carcinoma have elevated levels, however, concentrations vary from within the reference interval up to several grams per liter. Most cases of symptomatic hepatocellular carcinoma have values over 1000 µg/L, whereas the majority of patients with small asymptomatic tumors have AFP levels of less than 200 µg/L. In one study no hepatocellular carcinomas less than 1 cm in size were accompanied by abnormal AFP levels.

Elevated AFP levels commonly are associated with benign diseases of the liver such as hepatitis, cirrhosis, tyrosinemia, and ataxia telangiectasia. Usually in these situations, the elevation is only slight to moderate (less than 50 µg/L). Levels higher than 500 µg/L usually are associated with hepatocellular carcinoma and almost never occur with benign liver diseases. However, no absolute value can be used to distinguish between these two sets of conditions, and at least one case of benign liver disease has been reported to have a level over 3000 µg/L.[17] In general, normalizing or fluctuating values suggest a benign origin, while stabilizing or rising levels are characteristic of malignancy. Because an increase in AFP levels correlate with an increase in tumor size, increased AFP has been used to monitor disease. Spontaneous falls in AFP may occur in spite of a discernible increase in tumor growth, probably owing to tumor necrosis.

In acute hepatitis, AFP levels are elevated in the late phase when serum transaminase levels are decreasing and recovery is ongoing. In these situations elevated levels seem to reflect ongoing liver regeneration rather than malignant change. If AFP levels fail to rise in acute hepatitis, this carries a bad prognosis and indicates impending liver failure. In chronic hepatitis, AFP levels are elevated as well.

It was recently reported that the percentage of lectin reactive AFP is higher in patients with hepatocellular carcinoma than in those with benign liver disease.[18] The usefulness of this difference expressed as the fucosylation index remains to be clarified.

Approximately 10% of patients with metastatic liver carcinoma show elevated AFP levels. These are usually metastatic tumors of embryonal foregut origin such as stomach, pancreas, and gall bladder. Colon tumors with liver metastasis frequently secrete carcinoembryonic antigen (CEA), but rarely AFP. Some authors have recommended characterization of serum AFP by concanavalin A (conA) chromatography to differentiate between primary and metastatic tumor of the liver. Patients with primary hepatocellular carcinoma have reactivity that is higher than that by metastatic tumors. Of the other liver cancers, hepatoblastomas are invariably associated with elevated AFP levels. Elevated AFP levels also have been reported in patients with carcinoma of the bile duct.

Germ Cell Tumor

Elevated levels of AFP are found in approximately 60% of patients with germ cell tumors of the ovary and testis. The AFP synthesis by these germ cell tumors correlates with the occurrence of endodermal sinus elements analogous to the AFP producing yolk sac in early embryogenesis. Other germ cell tumors, such as seminomas, dysgerminomas, choriocarcinomas, and mature teratomas, are not associated with AFP synthesis. Elevated levels of both AFP and human chorionic gonadotropin (hCG) are often observed in patients with germ cell tumors, therefore, both markers should be used in follow-up of these patients (Table 12-8) (see Test: Human Choriogonadotropin).

The usual half-life of AFP is 4–6 days after complete surgical removal of germ cell tumor, with a slower decay after operation suggesting residual tumor tissue. Renewed elevation of serum AFP is an indication of tumor reoccurrence. Experience has indicated that rising levels of AFP and/or hCG precede a clinical confirmation of tumor relapse by 4–8 weeks.

Table 12-8. Immunohistochemical Classification of Testicular Tumors

Tumor Type	AFP	hCG
Pure seminoma	−	−
Seminoma with syncytiotrophoblastic giant cells	−	+
Embryonal carcinoma	+	+
Endodermal sinus tumor	+	−
Choriocarcinoma	−	+
Teratoma	−	−

Abbreviations: AFP, α-fetoprotein; hCG, human chorionic gonadotropin.

Test: Cancer Antigen 15-3 (CA 15-3)

Background and Selection

Serum levels of CA 15-3, a mammary tumor associated antigen, has been used in the evaluation of patients with breast cancer and may be of use in monitoring patients with other malignancies.

Logistics

The antigen designated CA 15-3 has two determinants recognized by the monoclonal antibodies 115D8 (designated MAM 6) and DF3. These antibodies recognize antigens of human milk fat globulin membranes and breast cancer associated antigen, respectively.

Interpretation

The reference range for CA 15-3 is up to about 25 U/mL.[19] Monitoring of serum CA 15-3 appears clinically useful in breast carcinoma patients, with levels correlating with the extent of disease. In breast carcinoma patients, CA 15-3 results correlate well with disease progression, regression, and stability. In patients with metastatic breast cancer, CA 15-3 is a more sensitive indicator than CEA, but both antigens tend to be elevated in patients with hepatic metastases. Over 90% of patients with progressive disease have increases greater than 25% and almost one-half these patients have increases by a factor of two or more. In contrast, CA 15-3 decreases 50% or more in 90% of breast carcinoma patients with disease regression.[20]

Serum 15-3 also can be increased in patients with other tumors including ovarian, uterine, pancreatic, and lung cancers and may prove useful for monitoring patients with these malignancies although the positivity rate is low. A small percentage of patients with nonmalignant disease, such as benign breast or liver disease, also may have increased CA 15-3 results.

Test: Cancer Antigen 19-9 (CA 19-9) (Gastrointestinal Cancer Associated Antigen [GICA])

Background and Selection

Cancer antigen 19-9 has been studied as a marker for patients with gastrointestinal malignancies, especially pancreatic carcinoma. Although the assay originally was developed using a colon cancer derived cell line, CA 19-9 has better sensitivity for pancreatic carcinoma than colon cancer.

Logistics

Cancer antigen 19-9 is a sialylated lacto-N-fucopentaose II, an oligosaccharide similar in structure to the Lewis blood group antigen. Approximately 4–7% of the U.S. population do not have the ability to synthesize the Lewis antigen and are said to be Lewis A negative, Lewis B negative. These individuals lack the transferase responsible for adding a fucose residue to the Lewis antigen at the α-1-4 linkage. There is speculation that Lewis A, Lewis B negative individuals may not test positive for this antigen even in the face of pancreatic carcinoma.[21] In addition, patients with Lewis A negativity and B positivity produce suboptimal levels of the sialylated Lewis A antigen.

Interpretation

Although results up to about 37 U/mL have been considered normal, recently reference ranges up to about 70–75 U/mL have been used. Higher limits allow better separation of patients with pancreatic carcinoma and appropriate controls.[21,22] Of the numerous serum markers (see Table 12-18) that can be associated with pancreatic carcinoma, CA 19-9 appears to be one of the most (see Summary of Tumor Marker Use, Pancreatic Carcinoma). Over 80–90% of patients with pancreatic carcinoma have an elevated CA 19-9 as compared with about 50–60% who have an elevated CEA. Pancreatic cancer patients with results within the reference range tend to have poorly differentiated carcinomas, but some Lewis A negative, Lewis B negative patients may have low results for this antigen. In patients with moderately elevated CA 19-9, that is, not above 120 U/mL, the ratio of CA 19-9 to total protein in pancreatic juice may be helpful in distinguishing patients with localized pancreatic carcinoma from those with chronic pancreatitis.[23]

Additionally, CA 19-9 is elevated in patients with other malignancies of the gastrointestinal tract including adenocarcinoma of the stomach, hepatobiliary tree, and colon. It also may be elevated with other tumors, for example, ovarian carcinoma. Serum CA 19-9 is increased in 45% or more of patients with recurrent colorectal cancer. Because CEA and CA 19-9 do not always rise in parallel, CA 19-9 is an additional marker useful in the follow-up of colorectal cancers.[24] Serum CA 19-9 levels also are elevated in patients with a number of benign diseases (e.g., acute pancreatitis, alcoholic liver disease, and renal failure). In patients with acute cholecystitis, markedly increased (greater than 2000 U/mL) CA 19-9 results have been reported.[21]

Test: Cancer Antigen 50 (CA 50)

Background and Selection

Serum CA 50 has been studied as a marker of gastrointestinal cancer, especially pancreatic carcinoma. The CA 50 antigen is similar to, but not identical with, CA 19-9.

Logistics

The CA 50, like CA 19-9, has a sialylated Lewis A determinant. Additionally, it has at least one other carbohydrate structure, sialosyl-lactotetraose, which lacks the fucose residue present in the sialylated Lewis A structure.

Interpretation

The upper limit of the reference range for serum CA 50 is about 17 U/mL. Over 70% of patients with pancreatic carcinomas have increased serum CA 50, with high levels found especially in those with advanced disease.[25] While CA 19-9 is rarely increased in patients with malignancy outside the gastrointestinal tract, CA 50 is elevated in patients with renal, prostatic, ovarian, breast, and lung cancer. Increased results also have been reported in patients with benign pancreatic, biliary, and hepatic disease.[26]

Test: Cancer Antigen 125 (CA 125)

Background and Selection

The tumor marker CA 125 is a mucin-like glycoprotein that can be identified using monoclonal antibody raised against an ovarian carcinoma line (OVCA 433). Serum CA 125 results are elevated in patients with a variety of malignancies including breast, lung, and gastrointestinal tract, but the marker has been used mainly to follow women with ovarian carcinoma.

Interpretation

The reference range for serum CA 125 is up to about 35 U/mL (~35 kU/L). Only 1% or less of healthy individuals have serum CA 125 concentrations greater than 35 U/mL (>35 kU/L), but elevated levels occur in about 20% of patients in the first trimester of pregnancy. Markedly elevated serum CA 125 levels sometimes occur in healthy subjects, as evidenced by the report of an individual with a CA 125 result greater than 300 U/mL (>300 kU/L) that coincided with the onset of her menstrual period. Results for CA 125 fell into the reference range by the end of her menstrual cycle.[27] Because over one-half of the patients with severe endometriosis have increased CA 125 results, this antigen has been used as an indicator of endometriosis. Serum CA 125 can be elevated in patients with other nonmalignant disorders, for example, cirrhosis, peritonitis, and pancreatitis.

Over 80% of patients with nonmucinous epithelial ovarian carcinoma have CA 125 results greater than 35 U/mL (>3.5 kU/L).[28] In 80–95% of these patients, steady increases or decreases of serum CA 125 correspond with progression or regression of disease. In patients with nonmucinous ovarian carcinoma, elevation of CA 125 precedes clinical disease recurrence by a mean of about 3 months. Although residual tumor nodules can occur in patients who have CA 125 values within the reference range, elevated serum CA 125 mediate against so-called second look surgery for ovarian carcinoma. That is, an elevated serum CA 125 result in a patient who has had surgery and a course of chemotherapy indicates the patient may have disease persistence obviating the usual second laparotomy to stage the disease.[29]

Among different tumor types, the most marked elevations in CA 125 are observed in patients with epithelial ovarian carcinoma, but elevated serum CA 125 is not specific for nonmucinous, epithelial ovarian carcinoma. For example, CA 125 is elevated in gynecologic malignancies besides ovarian carcinoma. About 60% of patients with pancreatic carcinoma also have increases in serum CA 125. Abnormal results occur in a small percentage of patients with other malignancies, such as those of lung, breast, and the gastrointestinal tract. Simultaneous measurement of independent markers, such as CA 15-3 or tumor associated glycoprotein (TAG) 72 may be helpful in patients suspected of having ovarian carcinoma. These antigens are elevated in only about 5% of patients with falsely elevated CA 125, whereas in over 80% of ovarian cancer patients simultaneous increases occur in CA 125 and TAG 72 or CA 15-3. Although CA 125 can be elevated in peritoneal fluid from patients with benign conditions, results usually are less than 200 U/mL (<200 kU/L). In contrast, more than 80% of ovarian cancer patients have ascites values of greater than 200 U/ml (>200 kU/L).[28]

Test: Cancer Antigen 195 (CA 195)

Like CA 19-9 and CA 50, CA 195 is related to Lewis A expression. The antigen, which has determinates of Lewis A and its sialylated form, is elevated in patients with colorectal carcinomas. Depending on the stage of clinical disease, about 30–70% of patients have elevated results.[30]

Test: Cancer Antigen 549 (CA 549)

Background and Selection

Measurement of serum CA 549 holds promise for following patients with breast carcinoma.

Logistics

Serum CA 549 is measured using two monoclonal antibodies, one to a breast cancer cell line (T-417) and the other to antigens of human milk fat globule membrane.

Interpretation

The reference range for serum CA 549 is up to about 11 U/mL. In general, the level of CA 549 correlates with tumor burden in breast carcinoma patients. The marker is rarely elevated in benign breast disorders or pregnancy. Elevated values are reported in nonmalignant disease, especially liver disease, and also occur in patients with metastatic cancer originating from a variety of sites including ovaries, prostate, lungs, and colon. Metastatic cancer from these various sites may give rise to elevated results in up to 50% of patients, but levels are less than 120 U/mL.[31] In contrast, about 30% of patients with metastatic breast carcinoma have results greater than 120 U/mL. In breast carcinoma patients with progression, 70% have a significant increase in CA 549 as compared with about 50% with changes in CEA. In breast cancer patients with tumor regression, CA 549 is significantly decreased.[31] In preliminary studies, CA 549 appears to be more sensitive than CA 15-3 for metastatic breast cancer.[30]

Test: Carcinoembryonic Antigen (Monoclonal CEA)

Background and Selection

Carcinoembryonic antigen is a cell surface-derived glycoprotein with a mass of approximately 200,000 da that has been used as a tumor associated antigen in cases of digestive tract cancers and other malignancies.

Carcinoembryonic antigen is used to monitor postoperative therapy in patients with colorectal, breast, or lung cancer. When used alone, it is not useful for identifying asymptomatic cancers, nor does it provide enough diagnostic certainty to confirm or rule out suspected cancer. Following surgery, CEA values are measured at 3-month intervals beginning at least 4 weeks postoperatively.

Logistics

Carcinoembryonic antigen is the most studied of the oncofetal antigens; however, a number of antigens in sera have CEA reactivity (Fig. 12-2). It has been measured in sera by immunoassay using polyclonal antibodies. Because cross-reacting antigens from spleen, lung granulocytes, and bile are sometimes found in sera, monoclonal CEA assays are currently used, obviating in part this cross-reactivity and thereby providing the best diagnostic performance.

In healthy individuals, CEA values demonstrated a diurnal pattern with values highest at 1600 hours and lowest at 0400 hours with excursions of almost 70% around mean values. Because of differences in assay calibration and reagent antibody specificities, results from one assay system cannot be directly related to another.

Interpretation

Immunoassay reference range is widely dependent upon immunoassay reagents used, with values of 2.5 and 5.0 µg/mL commonly used as cutoff points for dis-

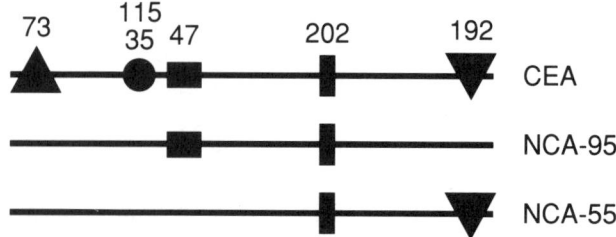

Fig. 12-2. Monoclonal antibody reactivity. Five different antigenic determinants of carcinoembryonic antigen are recognized by six monoclonal antibodies. The site at which each numbered monoclonal antibody reacts is represented. NCA-95 and NCA-55 are two nonspecific cross-reacting antigens with a mass of 95 kd and 55 kd, respectively. (From Buchegger et al.,[32] with permission.)

tinguishing abnormal values. Extreme elevations of CEA levels are unusual in apparently healthy persons, but results in the range of 2.5–10 µg/mL can occur. CEA concentrations are, on the average, somewhat higher in smokers than nonsmokers and higher in men than in women. Concentrations tend to be slightly higher in older persons.

For screening, absolute CEA values of 4.0, 5.0, 7.5, 10.0, and 20.0 µg/mL have been called significant in various studies. The higher the level chosen, the greater the specificity, whereas the lower the level, the greater the sensitivity.[33] Even with optimum cutoff levels, CEA is useful neither for colorectal cancer screening in asymptomatic patients nor in the initial diagnosis of colorectal cancer if used alone nor as an indicator of prognosis. Increasing CEA levels are associated with progressive Dukes stages of colon carcinoma, and larger carcinomas tend to be associated with higher levels.

Carcinoembryonic antigen has great usefulness for monitoring patient response to treatment. Some reports have demonstrated that CEA is of value in detecting recurrence of colorectal cancer after surgery and the basis for "second look" surgery. Included in the literature are various guidelines for predicting tumor recurrence based on postoperative CEA monitoring. These include CEA values exceeding cutoff levels (such as, 5.0, 10, 20 µg/mL) and progressively rising CEA levels exceeding a specific rate of change. However there is no consensus on guidelines that yield adequate sensitivity and specificity for colonic cancer identification. Some workers recommend bimonthly CEA determinations following surgery after primary curative resection, then every 3 months for the next year, then yearly.[34] Clinically important differences occur when assay systems are used interchangeably for the same patient. Carcinoembryonic antigen values are used with a variety of other laboratory tumor markers including CA 19-9 for colon carcinoma.

A preoperatively elevated CEA level should fall to baseline in 6 weeks after curative surgery. If the level fails to fall, or rises, it is highly suggestive of persistent disease. If the level falls to baseline, then sustains a persistent elevation, recurrent disease is assumed until proven otherwise.

Measurement of CEA is even less useful in the management of cancer at various other sites including the gastrointestinal tract, breast, and lung. The major role of CEA measurement in breast cancer is in following patients with advanced disease, especially those with widespread metastases.

Individuals with various types of liver disease may have elevated CEA values. Occasionally these elevated values occur because of impaired CEA clearance by the liver. Individuals with renal failure, fibrocystic breast disease, and other types of inflammatory bowel disease frequently have been reported to have mildly elevated values, and there are case reports of CEA elevations in hundreds of other conditions, some examples of which are shown in Table 12-9.

Body Fluid

Carcinoembryonic antigens have been measured in pleural and other body fluids to aid in the diagnosis of malignancy. Carcinoembryonic antigen is higher in pleural effusion secondary to malignant disease than in that secondary to nonmalignant disease. A large study showed that in benign disease CEA levels were below 40 ng/mL, whereas the majority of patients with metastatic disease had values above this cutoff level.[35]

Test: Tumor Associated Glycoprotein (Cancer Antigen 72 [CA 72])

Tumor associated glycoprotein (CA 72), which is distinct from CEA, CA 125, and CA 19-9, is increased in patients with a variety of malignancies. TAG-72, which has an upper limit of the reference range of about 10

Table 12-9. Causes of an Elevated CEA Level

Benign Conditions	Malignant Conditions
Crohn's disease	Cancer of
Ulcerative colitis	Pancreas
Hepatitis	Lung
Cirrhosis of the liver	Stomach
Collagen vascular disease	Esophagus
	Bladder
Chronic lung disease	Head or neck
Smoking	Female reproductive tract
Pancreatitis	
Polyps	Breast
Transfusion with CEA rich blood	Neuroblastoma
Diverticulitis	
Peptic ulcer disease	
Renal failure	
Fibrocystic breast disease	

Abbreviation: CEA, carcinoembryonic antigen.

U/mL, is increased in more than 85% of patients with colorectal carcinoma. Elevated TAG-72 also occurs in the majority of patients with pancreatic and ovarian cancer and in a significant portion of those with stomach cancer.[36]

HORMONES AND HORMONE-LIKE SUBSTANCES AS TUMOR MARKERS

During the past 20 years, the widespread availability of specific and sensitive immunoassays has resulted in the discovery that virtually all peptide hormones may be produced "ectopically." An ectopic hormone is one secreted by a tissue not normally engaged in the production of this hormone, and in almost all cases, the cells of origin are malignant or potentially malignant. To date, all ectopic hormones described have been polypeptides, thereby excluding steroids, catecholamines, and thyroid hormones from this association. This is not surprising, as the synthesis of steroids, catecholamines, and thyroid hormones would require the ectopic production of all enzymes needed for their synthesis, a highly unlikely situation. A few years ago, we considered the presence of a humoral syndrome caused by cancer rare or unusual; now we believe such manifestations common, and if sought, easily detectable. Current data demonstrate that most or all nonendocrine tissues produce small amounts of a variety of peptide hormones and hormone precursors.

The secretion of most ectopic hormones is identified by the signs and symptoms seen in patients. However, diagnostic certainty of their existence is always difficult, as confusion exists between these syndromes and those caused by eutopic tumors, or tumors of the gland usually responsible for the production of hormone. Generally, the following should be fulfilled if the tumor is to be considered ectopic: (1) demonstration of the hormone is sera quantitatively or qualitatively different from the reference population; (2) disappearance of the endocrine syndrome after tumor removal; (3) demonstration of the hormone tumor tissue in higher concentrations in surrounding tissues; (4) an arterial/venous gradient across the tumor bed; and (5) hormone production by tumor cells in tissue culture. Recently, many workers have used the measurement of the mRNA specific for the ectopic hormone in question as evidence of its occurrence. Table 12-10 shows some of the most commonly produced ectopic hormones. None of these tumor markers alone are useful in screening for disease.

TESTS FOR ECTOPIC HORMONES AND HORMONE-LIKE SUBSTANCES AS TUMOR MARKERS

Test: Antidiuretic Hormone (ADH), (Vasopressin) (See Ch. 11)

Antidiuretic hormone is synthesized in the hypothalamus as propressophysin consisting of the hormone and its carrier, neurophysin. Ectopic production of ADH has been reported in association with a variety of tumors including colon and lung carcinomas (small cell, squamous), and thymomas. Not all patients with excess ADH secretion have symptoms of inappropriate ADH secretion, as demonstrated in cases of hyponatremia. The number of individuals with the ectopic inappropriate ADH syndrome also have alterations in set point of receptors to ADH action. Propressophysin circulates in some patients with oat cell carcinoma of the lung.

Test: Calcitonin (CT) (Thyrocalcitonin [TCT]) (See Ch. 11)

Calcitonin is a peptide hormone with a mass of about 3400 da secreted by the C cells of a thyroid gland and is

Table 12-10. Hormones and Hormone-Like Substances Reported to be Produced by Cancers

Calcitonin
Corticotropin and proopiomelanocortin
Corticotropin-releasing hormone
Eosinophilopoietin
Epidermal growth factor
Erythropoietin
Gastrin
Gastrin-releasing peptide (and bombesin)
Growth hormone
Growth hormone-releasing hormone
Glucagon
Human chorionic gonadotropin and its subunits
Hypophosphatemia-producing factor
Insulin-like growth factor
Osteoclast activating factor
Renin and prorenin
Secretin
Somatostatin
Vasoactive intestinal peptide
Vasopressin

(Modified from Odell,[37] with permission.)

involved in calcium metabolism. Elevated levels frequently are found in serum of patients with tumors of the lung (small cell), liver, breast, as well as carcinoid tumors, and those associated with Zollinger-Ellison syndrome. Some benign diseases such as Paget's disease, hyperparathyroidism, and pancreatitis also cause elevated levels, thereby making interpretation difficult. The CT found in sera from some tumor patients has a mass larger than native CT and is presumably a precursor form. However, not all "big" CT fractions are measured by CT antibodies used in immunoassays. The appearance of high levels of calcitonin with two or more tumor markers frequently occurs throughout the spectrum of lung carcinoma and reflects the amine precursor uptake decarboxylation (APUD) theory. In malignant diseases in which ectopic production of CT occurs, levels of CT are not accurate in predicting reoccurrence of tumor nor response to chemotherapy.

Elevations of serum CT are observed in patients with medullary carcinoma of the thyroid. The primary clinical application of serum measurements is for detection of patients with the familial autosomal dominant condition. Diagnostic tests such as pentagastrin stimulation and calcium infusion with subsequent CT measurements have greatly increased the sensitivity of detection for this condition. Serial measurements of levels of CT in monitoring therapy in patients with medullary carcinoma of thyroid with persistent or recurrent elevations after thyroidectomy indicate residual or recurrent disease.

Test: Corticotropin (Adrenocorticotropin, [ACTH]) (See Ch. 11)

The first and one of the most frequently occurring paraendocrine syndromes is the association of Cushing syndrome with ectopic production of ACTH by small cell carcinoma of the lung. Subsequently, other causative neoplasms including carcinoid tumors, thymomas, pancreatic islet cell tumors, and pheochromocytomas have been identified. Because of the rapidity with which symptoms such as weight loss, muscle wasting, hypertension, hyperpigmentation, and especially severe hypokalemic alkolosis occur, the patient often presents before many of the classic signs of Cushing syndrome have developed. Some patients with minimal symptoms of Cushing syndrome have in their circulation a peptide called *big ACTH*. Big ACTH has a mass of 20,000 da in contrast to 4500 da of bioactive ACTH and approximately 4% of the biologic activity of ACTH. Big ACTH has been subsequently identified as pro-opiomelanocortin (POMC), the precursor of ACTH. Other hormones, such as β endorphin, β lipotrophic hormones, and β and γ melanocyte stimulating hormones, are formed from POMC and found in the circulation, but measurements have little diagnostic utility at this time.

Patients with a variety of other conditions including chronic obstructive pulmonary disease, pulmonary infarction, and pulmonary inflammation may have elevated ACTH levels. This and other data suggest that POMC is synthesized in small amounts by all nonendocrine tissues.

Ectopic secretion of ACTH can be identified by the dexamethasone suppression test. Failure to suppress serum cortisol levels with high dose dexamethasone suggests ectopic secretion of ACTH. However, discrepant responses to dexamethasone suppression test occur, perhaps by episodic release of corticotropin. This complicates the evaluation of the cause of Cushing syndrome in these patients (see Ch. 11).

Measurements of ACTH have no value in screening for carcinoma. Pretreatment levels demonstrate no correlation to patient survival or the stage of the disease. The usefulness of the serial measurements of ACTH to monitor the response of the tumor to therapy remains controversial. For further information see Odell.[37]

Test: Human Choriogonadotropin (hCG) (Human Chorionic Gonadotropin, β-hCG) (See Ch. 15)

Background

Prior to 1970, hCG was believed to be a hormone produced exclusively by the trophoblastic cells during pregnancy and by rare neoplasms derived from trophoblastic cells. Subsequently, a substance with hCG immunoreactivity was isolated from virtually all human tissues and almost all human cancers.

Human chorionic gonadotropin is a glycoprotein composed of two dissimilar subunits, α and β, joined covalently. The α-subunit of the glycoprotein of hCG, follitropin (FSH), lutropin (LH), and thyrotropin (TSH) is coded by a single gene, translated by a single mRNA, and shares almost complete homology among the four different glycoprotein hormones. Immunologically, the α-chain of hCG is virtually indistinguishable from the α-chain of LH, FSH, and TSH despite some differences in carbohydrate moieties. The β-subunit of each glycoprotein hormone is different and confers the hormone's biologic specificity and bioactivity. Approximately 80% of the β-chains of LH and hCG have structural homology with unique structure of 30 amino acids found at the carboxyl terminus of hCG. Free β-hCG reportedly has immunoreactivity similar to hCG, but lacks the bioactivity of hCG. In contrast to the single gene that codes for α-subunits, the β-subunits of hCG are encoded by at least six genes. Because α-hCG and β-hCG are synthesized separately and production appears to be regulated separately, an imbalanced secretion with an excess of one of the chains frequently is found during pregnancy and malignancy. When free β-hCG is measured in serum after the first trimester of pregnancy, it is not detected. Therefore, the synthesis of β-hCG may be the rate-limiting step controlling hCG production during this time. In contrast, α-hCG is rate limiting in early pregnancy and malignancy, because free β-hCG levels are elevated.

The metabolic half-life of the intact hormone is approximately 36 hours, that of the α-subunit approximately 20 minutes, and that of the β-subunit approximately 45 minutes.

Variable quantities of free serum β-hCG have been found in patients with gestational trophoblastic diseases. These diseases occur with a frequency of 1/2000 pregnancies in the United States, but are 10 times more frequent in women in developing countries. Hydatidiform moles and choriocarcinoma have approximately 10 and 20% of hCG as free β-chains, respectively.[38] This suggests that in trophoblastic disease, the production of free β-hCG increases with the immaturity of the trophoblastic cell.

Human chorionic gonadotropin undergoes extensive glycosylation with about 30% of the mass as carbohydrate. The α- and β-subunits each contain two complex carbohydrate units and, in addition, the 30 amino acid COOH terminal sequence of β-hCG contains four smaller disaccharides with O-glycosidic linkages. Recent evidence indicates that free α-subunit of pituitary or placental origin also contains a unique O-glycosidically linked carbohydrate whose presence prevents association with the corresponding β-chain. This additional carbohydrate accounts for the occurrence of a subunit with a larger mass than the native subunit. The nature of the four O-glycosidic linkages is uncertain, with some reports describing identical hexasaccharides and others reporting a variety of heterogenous sugars attached randomly. Approximately 10% of the mass of hCG is N-acetylneuraminic acid (sialic acid), which occupies terminal positions in the carbohydrate chain. The sialic acid residues of hCG influence biologic activity by promoting retention of hCG in the circulation. Removal of sialic acid results in increased metabolic clearance of the asialic molecule by the liver. Changes in carbohydrate content, such as desialated forms, have been described, but changes in structure have not yet been correlated with disease. Desialated hCG has a half-life of about 4 minutes.

Selection

Along with AFP, hCG is used to monitor patients with nonseminomatous germ cell tumors of the testis. In patients with trophoblastic disease of the placenta, levels of hCG correlate with tumor burden, progression, and response to therapy.

Logistics

Assay Specificity and Sensitivity

Human choriogonadotropin is a placental hormone composed of polypeptide chains α and β (see above). Some immunoassays measure intact hCG, others have specificity to the β-chain (β-hCG), whereas others react with both the free β-chain and the intact molecule. The designation β-subunit assay is misleading, because both hCG and β-hCG usually are detected by these assays.

Assays for hCG formerly required urine, but with improvements in assay sensitivity, serum determinations are now the measurement of choice. Sensitivity of pregnancy tests are not sufficient to detect hCG in most tumor patients (Table 12-11). Without assays using monoclonal antibodies, it has been difficult to measure serum free β-hCG accurately, because antibodies generated against the β-subunit of hCG usually recognize intact hCG as well. Also, serum-free β-hCG levels are sometimes too low for detection by some current assays. Because free β-subunit is rapidly cleared from the circulation, the predominant molecular species measured in most circumstances is intact hCG, and not the free β-subunit.

Discordant Results

Two different hCG reference preparations are in use, thereby making comparisons of results between assays difficult. Because discordance between immunoassays

Table 12-11. Comparison of hCG Assays

Type	Sensitivity (mIU/L)	Reactivity	Use
Immunoassay	1–5	hCG	Tumor marker
Immunoassay	1–5	β-hCG	Tumor marker
Radioreceptor assay	1–5	7–10 Days after ovulation	Pregnancy test
Tube hemagglutination inhibition	200–2000	18–30 Days after ovulation	Pregnancy test
Slide test	500–4000	28–35 Days after ovulation	Pregnancy test
Bioassay	400–2000	28–35 Days after ovulation	Pregnancy test

Abbreviations: hCG, human chorionic gonadotropin.

occurs, occasionally patients are seen with widely discrepant results. Because of nearly identical α-chains and similar β-chains, LH frequently cross-reacts, thereby giving spuriously high hCG values. Table 12-12 lists reasons for discrepant results based on immunoassay specificities for altered forms of hCG.[39] Discrepancies are suggested when specimens with elevated values are diluted and demonstrate inconsistencies in values derived from dilutions. The role of specific subunit measurements continues to be debated. Although there is evidence suggesting clinical value for both α- and β-subunit measurements, the data are too limited and conflicting to permit definitive conclusions.

Test Interpretation

Normally hCG is secreted by the placenta, with highest levels (100,000 mIU/mL) occurring in the mother at 60 days of gestation. In nonpregnant women, hCG levels range up to 2 mIU/mL. A large number of tumors have been found to produce hCG ectopically, the most common of which are those of the testis, ovary, pancreas, liver, colon, and kidneys. Significant elevations always occur throughout normal pregnancies, frequently occur in patients with trophoblastic neoplasms and nonseminomatous testicular tumors, and rarely occur with other tumors. A number of conditions with slightly elevated hCG levels easily can be confused with those tumors (Table 12-13). Levels as high as in pregnancy are found in patients with gastric adenocarcinoma and trophoblastic tumors.

In some cases, the amount of hCG secreted by a tumor corresponds to the high concentrations observed during the first trimester of pregnancy, but still no clinical signs or symptoms may be apparent. Most patients with hCG-secreting tumors, however, have hCG concentrations in serum between 5 and 20 mIU/mL. Because of elevated levels, some men present with gynecomastia and some women present with dysfunctional uterine bleeding. Estrogen determinations frequently are elevated in men with gynecomastia.

Because approximately 60% of patients with these nonseminomatous germ cell tumors have elevated levels, it

Table 12-12. Serum hCG Heterogeneity

Altered Forms of hCG	Biologic Source (Human)
Free α- or β-subunits (in addition to complete hCG)	Many (tumors, pregnancy)
Free β-hCG (in absence of hCG)	Testicular cancer serum
Fragment of hCG or β hCG	Pregnancy, many cancers, subjects injected with β-hCG
Heterogeneous forms of α- and β-hCG	Pregnancy, crude hCG preparations; placental extracts; choriocarcinoma and testicular cancer
Large hCG	Placental extracts
Large free α	Pregnancy, many cancers, placental extracts
Asialo-hCG	Choriocarcinoma
Asialo carboxyl terminal fragment of β-hCG	Choriocarcinoma
Altered sugar chains on hCG	Choriocarcinoma
Altered oligosaccharides on hCG-like material	Extracts of normal tissues and tumors
Hyperglycosylated α and/or β	Pregnancy, lung carcinoma, gastric carcinoid, and gastric carcinoma; carcinoma cell lines (choriocarcinoma, cervical carcinoma)
β-hCG minus the carboxyl terminal fragment	Cervical carcinoma cell lines
Multiple genes for β-hCG	Fetal liver, fibroblast cell lines

Abbreviation: hCG, human chorionic gonadotropin.

Table 12-13. Clinical Conditions Associated With Slightly Elevated Levels of hCG

Early Pregnancy (3 weeks since last menstrual period)
Ectopic pregnancy
Undiagnosed (subclinical) abortion
Spontaneous abortion
Blighted ovum
Persistent trophoblastic disease
Follow-up of gestational trophoblastic disease
Regional enteritis
Ulcerative colitis
Cirrhosis
Ulcer disease
Nontrophoblastic malignancies

---

is recommended that AFP and hCG be used together to monitor therapy. In this situation, 90% of patients have an elevation of one or both markers. In contrast, approximately 5% of patients with seminomas have elevated hCG levels. Although the giant tumor cell occasionally found in a seminoma is capable of secreting hCG, one should always consider elements of the nonseminomatous germ cell tumors, choriocarcinoma or embryonal cell carcinoma, when hCG levels are elevated. Those cases with a tentative diagnosis of seminoma and elevated levels of hCG frequently lack serial sectioning or cellular localization of human chorionic gonadotropin production. Accurate diagnosis of the tumor is essential, because the therapeutic approach depends on tumor type.

Although not an example of ectopic production, essentially all patients with trophoblastic tumors have elevated hCG levels. Numerous investigators have demonstrated that elevated levels of hCG correlate with tumor burden and patient prognosis. Also, hCG is an excellent marker for monitoring the response of trophoblastic disease to therapy. During therapy, if elevated levels occur, chemotherapy must be continued until after hCG levels are undetectable. When treatment has reduced hCG to consistently undetectable levels, a decrease in progression is observed. Conversely, when hCG values increase progressively, either with or without treatment, death invariably occurs from choriocarcinoma.

Upon evacuation of a molar pregnancy, hCG titer falls rapidly at first in all patients, but thereafter the pattern is more variable. In some patients, the titer continues to decrease rapidly until the hCG becomes undetectable by about 3 weeks after evacuation. More frequently, values decline more gradually, plateau, or even rise temporarily before falling again, and may ultimately remain detectable for as long as 15 weeks before becoming undetectable. Chemotherapy is instituted when values plateau or rise. Following evacuation of a molar pregnancy, hCG levels should be monitored every 1–2 weeks until undetectable for 3 consecutive weeks and then monthly until 6–12 months after evacuation. When initial hCG levels are in the range of 1000 to 10,000 mIU/mL, the fatality rate is less than 5%, whereas when levels exceed 1,000,000 mIU/mL the fatality rate is over 50%. Patients whose levels exceed 40,000 mIU/mL are usually categorized as having a poor prognosis. Although hCG does not cross the blood brain barrier, cerebrospinal fluid (CSF) hCG, expressed as the ratio of serum to CSF values, can be used as a useful diagnostic test for metastases. A ratio of less than 60 indicates metastases; for further information see Pattillo and Hussa.[40]

Test: Parathyroid Hormone (PTH) (Parathyrin) (See Ch. 11, Test: PTH)

The most common laboratory finding in patients with malignancy is hypercalcemia. Initially, it was thought that hypercalcemia occurred only in patients with bone metastasis, but then it was recognized that a variety of tumors secrete a hormonal substance, presumably PTH, which elevates serum calcium concentrations in the absence of bone metastasis. The true incidence of ectopic PTH production in hypercalcemic patients with cancer remains controversial; more recent studies have attributed hypercalcemia to a variety of causative agents (Table 12-14). Some older reports indicate an incidence of ectopic PTH production as high as 95% of tumors studied. These data remain conflicting owing to heterogeneous population of circulating PTH fragments, poor correlation between PTH levels measured by different assays, and the assumption that detectable PTH immunoreactivity in patients with malignancy was definitive evidence for ectopic PTH secretion.

Table 12-14. Mechanisms of Hypercalcemia in Malignancy

Parathyroid hormone (PTH)
PTH-like peptide
Prostaglandin
Osteoclast-activating factor
Coincidental primary hyperparathyroidism
Direct bone invasion by metastases

Recently, in an investigation of PTH mRNA in a series of human tumors, no mRNA was detected, thereby offering convincing evidence for the lack of PTH secretion by these tumors. Subsequently, evaluation of patients with cancer and hypercalcemia by Broadus et al.[41] indicated that a protein with PTH-like biologic activity, but without PTH immunoreactivity, was responsible for hypercalcemia in a large percentage of their study population. This substance has been characterized as having a mass of 1600 da and a similarity in the 15 amino acids on the N terminal end to that of the 9600 da PTH molecule. This information casts doubt on a high incidence of ectopic PTH previously reported and draws attention to a needed reappraisal of the true incidence of ectopic PTH production. Tumors commonly reported to have ectopic PTH immunoreactivity include those of the lung (squamous, large cell), kidney, pancreas, and ovary.

Test: Parathyroid Hormone-Like Peptide (Protein)

Background and Selection

Parathyroid hormone-like peptide, larger than PTH and similar to PTH only in the amino terminal region, is expressed in normal tissue. Although PTH-like peptide stimulates nephrogenous cyclic AMP (cAMP), inhibits phosphate reabsorption in the proximal tubule, and stimulates osteoclastic bone reabsorption, its activity differs from PTH in other ways. For example, PTH-like peptide has limited capacity to stimulate 1-hydroxylase activity.[41] Recently PTH-like peptide has been linked with humoral hypercalcemia associated with malignancy. Patients with humoral hypercalcemia have marked hypercalcinuria and low circulating levels of 1,25 dihydroxy vitamin D as compared with patients with hyperparathyroidism. Potentially, PTH-like peptide may be useful for assessing patients with hypercalcemia associated with malignancy.

Logistics

Recently, the structure of PTH-like peptide has been elucidated and specific immunoassays developed. Previously, humoral hypercalcemia associated with malignancy was identified by measuring the increase in nephrogenous cAMP excretion.[42] Plasma and urinary cAMP are measured and nephrogenous cAMP calculated as described by Stewart et al.[42] The nephrogenous component of urinary cAMP also is increased in patients with primary hyperparathyroidism.

In many malignancy patients with hypercalcemia, PTH immunoassays do not show suppression of PTH levels appropriate for their degree of hypercalcemia; thus, it has been speculated that PTH assays cross-react with the PTH-like peptide. With the identification of PTH-like peptide, it is now clear that the amino terminal region is similar to PTH. Although the reason is unclear for the relative increases in PTH results in patients with hypercalcemia associated with malignancy, the nonsuppressed PTH levels apparently are not caused by cross-reactivity with PTH antibodies.

Interpretation

Humoral hypercalcemia, when present with malignancy, is associated with osteoclastic bone reabsorption mediated by factors secreted by the malignant cells and is typically associated with squamous, renal, bladder, and ovarian carcinomas. A number of substances, including growth factors and lymphokines, have been implicated as the cause of humoral hypercalcemia associated with malignancy. Currently, humoral hypercalcemia in cancer patients is usually identified by nephrogenous cAMP measurements (see above), but immunoassays for PTH-like peptide are becoming available. In about 70% of hypercalcemic patients with solid tumors, immunoreactive PTH-like peptide is increased. In contrast, patients with parathyroid adenomas appear to have results in the range of those seen in healthy individuals, that is, less than about 4 pmol equivalents/L.[43]

Test: Tumor Necrosis Factor-α (TNF-α) (Cachectin)

Background and Selection

Tumor necrosis factor-α named for its cytolytic affect on certain tumors, is a cytokine produced mainly by macrophages. Tumor necrosis factor-α regulates cellular metabolism and response to inflammation mediating many of the beneficial and adverse effects of endotoxin.[44] Measurements of TNF-α are of potential use in patients with chronic infectious and neoplastic diseases where TNF-α, also known as cachectin, is thought to induce anorexia, fatigability, and wasting.

Interpretation

Preliminary data show that TNF-α levels in healthy subjects are as high as about 35–40 pg/mL.[45] In a large percentage of patients with infections and neoplastic disease, serum TNF-α is increased. Slightly increased

TNF-α levels also occur in patients with rheumatoid arthritis.

TESTS FOR OTHER HORMONE SYNDROMES

Almost every known protein hormone or protein hormone precursor has been reported to have been produced by malignant tumors (Table 12-10). Recently, a number of syndromes have been described in which releasing hormones are produced ectopically. Among these are acromegaly caused by secretion of growth hormone and Cushing syndrome associated with corticotropin-releasing hormone. These cases are easily confused with the ectopic production of pituitary hormones.

Perhaps the best known hematologic abnormality produced by tumors is the erythrocytosis or polycythemia produced by the glycoprotein erythropoietin. The most frequently identified tumors are renal carcinoma and cerebellar hemangioblastomas.

Hypoglycemia occasionally is found with large mesenchymal tumors, as well as hepatic and adrenal carcinomas. None of these tumors have been found to produce insulin. Although mechanisms of this hypoglycemia have not been proven definitively, the current commonly accepted mechanism is the production of a labile protein that possesses insulin-like growth factor properties. In addition, a few metastatic colon carcinomas have been described as producing an increase in insulin receptors in a variety of tissues, thereby causing hypoglycemia.

TESTS FOR HORMONE RECEPTORS

Test: Estrogen Receptors

Background and Selection

Measurements of estrogen receptors in tumor tissue have been used to determine treatment and prognosis in patients with breast carcinoma. Although estrogen receptor assays are currently regarded as an important part of managing patients with breast carcinoma and as prognostic factor, changes in treatment and the development of other tests that predict prognosis probably will change the role of the estrogen receptor measurements. Methods by which estrogen receptors are measured also are changing. Because very small lesions can now be detected, often there is insufficient material to use for the steroid binding methods. Estrogen receptors also have been measured in tumors other than those found in the breast, most notably those of the female genital tract.

Logistics

Specimen Requirement

Estrogen receptors are unstable; tissue specimens must be kept cold and rapidly frozen (at $-70\,°C$) to preserve the receptors. Various compounds, for example, molybdate, are used to retard receptor degradation. In tumors where estrogen receptor binding function is inactivated, it appears antigenic sites necessary for immunoassay also are altered. Precautions must be taken in selecting and handling the specimen; it should come from an area of tumor tissue without necrosis and the specimen should be trimmed of fat and normal tissue. The standard method for measuring estrogen receptors is to use a crude tissue preparation of tumor cytoplasm (cytosol), made by centrifugation of a tissue homogenate.

Method

There are two basic types of methods used to quantitate tissue estrogen receptors: (1) binding assays in which receptor binds to labeled estrogen and (2) immunoassays using antibodies to the estrogen receptor. The methods apparently correlate well, but the immunoassays have the advantage of requiring only a small amount of cytosol. Additionally, antibodies have been used to estimate estrogen receptors directly in tissue preparations.

Steroid Binding Assays. The so-called dextran-coated charcoal technique has been widely used to quantitate estrogen receptors, but requires approximately 1 g of tissue. Tritated estradiol is added to various aliquots of a cytosol preparation. The amount of bound and free radioactive material is separated by dextran-coated charcoal and counted. After bound and free fractions are separated, the results are plotted on a Scatchard plot. The final result, expressed in terms of protein content of the specimen, is a measure of unoccupied cystolic estrogen receptors.

Immunoassays. Cytosol preparations also have been used in immunoassays for the estrogen receptor. Recently, immunoradiometric assays using monoclonal antibodies to the estrogen receptor have been developed. These assays measure total (bound and unbound) cytosolic estrogen receptors.

Histologic Techniques. Using antibody to estrogen receptors, these assays measure occupied and unoccupied receptor, with results obtained by various methods including scoring reactivity. Some of the methods are qualitative at best, but evaluation by computer-assisted image analysis appears effective in objectively quantifying receptors. Histologic techniques have the advantage of identifying tumor heterogeneity, because cells that are receptor positive and receptor negative can be distinguished. In addition, the techniques can be used with very small specimens, even those obtained by fine needle aspiration (FNA). It should be noted that some of the earlier histologic techniques detected lower affinity (types II and III) binding sites in addition to high affinity type I binding sites detected by the biochemical assays.

Interpretation

With the steroid binding assays for cytosol estrogen receptor, usually estrogen receptor positivity is defined as greater than 3 fmol/mg protein. Classically, estrogen receptor status has been used to select which breast carcinoma patient would receive endocrine treatment. The level of estrogen receptor also has been used as an important prognostic factor.

About two-thirds of patients with estrogen receptor positive tumors respond to endocrine treatment regimens, whereas the response rate in estrogen poor tumors is 10% or less. Additionally, estrogen receptor status is reported to be an important prognostic factor with respect to disease-free interval and overall survival.[46] With changes in treatment, the role of estrogen receptors in management of early and advanced breast cancer is changing. For example, both tamoxifen, a relatively nontoxic antiestrogen, and chemotherapy have been found effective in certain patient subgroups regardless of the estrogen receptor status of their tumors.[47] Estrogen receptors, however, continue to have an important role in evaluating new therapeutic agents and interpreting results of clinical trials. Not all patients with estrogen receptor positive tumors respond to endocrine treatment. Many reasons have been proposed to explain this problem including error in the definition of positivity and tumor heterogenity, but receptor defects may help account for the problem. Patients with estrogen receptor positive/progesterone receptor negative tumors have a poor prognosis, perhaps because of an estrogen receptor defect.[48]

A very important problem is predicting eventual metastatic disease in patients with node negative breast carcinoma. About 30% of these patients, if not treated, will eventually develop metastases. If these individuals could be identified reliably, therapy could be better tailored. At least in some patient groups, progesterone receptor appears to be a better prognostic marker than the estrogen receptor, perhaps because an intact estrogen receptor binding and transport system is necessary for production of progesterone receptors. Other markers, for example, the HER-2/neu oncogene, also appear to hold promise for identifying patients who are at risk of developing metastatic disease.

Test: Progesterone Receptors

Background and Selection

Progesterone receptors in tumor tissue have been used to determine treatment and prognosis in patients with breast carcinoma. Because intact estrogen receptors ordinarily are necessary for progesterone receptor production, progesterone receptor measurements are helpful in interpretation of estrogen receptor results (see Test: Estrogen Receptors).

Logistics

Tissue handling and assay of progesterone receptors is analogous to estrogen receptors, but progesterone receptors appear to be even more labile than estrogen receptors. Immunoassays for progesterone receptors correlate well with the dextran-coated charcoal method.

Interpretation

Patients whose tumors contain both estrogen and progesterone receptors have a response rate of 75% or more to endocrine therapy. Patients with estrogen receptor positive/progesterone receptor negative tumors show a response rate of only about 30% to endocrine therapy, in contrast to patients with estrogen receptor negative/progesterone receptor negative tumors, who have a response rate of less than 10%. At least for certain patient groups, progesterone receptor status is a better prognostic marker than estrogen receptor status.[46] Patients with progesterone receptor positive ovarian carcinoma appear to have a better prognosis than those with progesterone receptor negative tumors.

ONCOGENES AND ONCOGENE PRODUCTS AS TUMOR MARKERS

Oncogenes are those genes capable of inducing or maintaining transformation of cells.[49] The rapidly transforming retroviruses carry specific genes directly responsible for retroviral oncogenic potential. Homologs to these so-called oncogenes are found in normal human DNA and are known as proto-oncogenes. Proto-oncogenes from which viral oncogenes arise are authentic cellular genes normally lacking any oncogenic activity. Several proto-oncogenes are known to produce gene products that are related to growth factors or growth factor receptors, thus they appear to be important in normal cellular proliferation or differentiation. When proto-oncogenes become altered or overexpressed, they are called oncogenes. Alterations occur by mutation, amplification (multiple gene copies), or translocation. The oncogenes encode oncoproteins that lack important regulatory control of their activity. The exact mechanisms by which these changes cause malignant transformation are being studied.[49]

Measurement of oncogenes or oncogene products appears to hold future promise in the diagnosis, prognosis, and follow-up of patients with malignancies. Table 12-15 shows some of the oncogenes that have been identified in association with malignant tumors. Additionally, there is a growing recognition of the importance of suppressor genes, also known as anti-oncogenes or recessive oncogenes. For at least some malignancies, genetic susceptibility appears determined by inherited lesions affecting tumor suppressor genes.[50] Inactivation or loss of these genes presumably allows a cell to escape normal growth controls. Although deletions have been found frequently in some tumors (e.g., 13q in retinoblastomas) these genetic alterations appear to be just one component in the complex process of tumor generation.[51]

SUMMARY OF TUMOR MARKER USE

Breast Cancer

Tissue Markers

Measurements of estrogen and progesterone receptors have been used routinely as parameters for determining therapy and prognosis in breast cancer patients. Although receptors are measured as a standard practice, the method by which they are measured is changing as well as their role in determining prognosis and treatment. Receptors have been used in combination with other markers; for example, patients with tumors positive for haptoglobulin-related protein and negative for progesterone receptors have a greater than 90% incidence of reoccurrence.[52] Other hormone receptors including growth hormone and epidermal growth factor have been studied as well as other substances, especially proteolytic enzymes and oncogenes. For example, cathepsin D, an estrogen-induced lysosomal protease, is mitogenic for breast carcinoma cells and may facilitate cancer spread via its protease action on the extracellular matrix.[53] Oncogene and DNA content measurements also appear to hold promise for determining prognosis. The HER-2/neu (c-erb B2) gene appears to encode for a protein with properties similar to the epidermal growth factor receptor.[46] Amplification of HER-2/neu oncogene occurs in 20–30% of primary breast cancers and appears to be highly correlated with prognosis. Patients with tumors having multiple copies of the HER-2/neu gene have a shorter time to relapse. In tumors with amplification of HER-2/neu, estrogen and progesterone receptors tend to be absent, whereas the DNA content is tetraploid or near tetraploid.[54] Some investigators, however, conclude ploidy is not a useful prognostic factor.[53] Other changes associated with aggressive breast cancer include changes in c-myc and c-myb oncogenes as well as loss of alleles at the H-ras locus.

Serum

Serum markers, most notably CEA, have been used in the management of breast cancer. Many other markers have been studied (Table 12-16) and recently, CA 15-3 and CA 549 have been introduced. Both CA 15-3 and CA 549 use two monoclonal antibodies one of which is an antibody to antigen of milk fat globule membranes.

Table 12-15. Examples of Oncogenes Associate With Malignancy

Malignancy	Oncogene[a]
Burkitt's lymphoma	c-myc (translocation)
Breast carcinoma	HER-2/neu (C-erb B-2) (amplification)
Colon cancer	c-K-ras (mutation)
Neutroblastoma	N-myc (amplification)
Small cell lung cancer	c-myc, N-myc, or L-myc (amplification)

[a] Oncogenes are designated by three lowercase letters indicating the tumor and/or species in which they were initially identified (e.g., myc from myelocytomatosis, ras from rat sarcoma). For similarly designated oncogenes, preceding letters are used as a modifier to distinguish between different oncogenes in the same group.

Table 12-16. Elevation in Circulating Antigens Associated With Breast Cancer

α-Lactalbumin
Cancer antigen (CA) 15-3
CA 549
Casein
Carcinoembryonic antigen
Ceruloplasmin
CK-BB
Glycolipids
Gross cystic disease protein
MAM 6
Phospholipids
Procathepsin D
Sialytransferase
Tissue polypeptide antigen

In each case, the second antibody is to a human breast cancer antigen. Both CA 15-3 and CA 549 appear to have better sensitivity and specificity than CEA in breast carcinoma patients (see Test: Carcinoembryonic Antigen).

Ovarian Carcinoma

The diagnosis of ovarian carcinoma is often not made until the late stages of the disease. Measurement of tumor markers has been tried to improve early diagnosis but, as with other tumors, sensitivity and specificity of markers have been inadequate. Many of the markers shown in Table 12-17 have been studied for use in diagnosis and follow-up of ovarian carcinoma patients. Of the available markers, CA 125 is found to be increased in about 80% of nonmucinous, epithelial ovarian carcinoma patients.[28] If CA 125 is increased, its concentration correlates with disease course in up to 95% of patients. Elevation of CA 125 also occurs in benign disease (e.g., endometriosis) and in nongynecologic cancer, especially pancreatic carcinoma. In patients with mucinous ovarian carcinoma, CA 125 is not as useful. In contrast, CEA is increased in about 50% of ovarian cancer patients, but except for a few cases of mucinous ovarian carcinoma, CEA has not been a proven monitor in ovarian carcinoma.[55] The addition of CEA does not appear to improve results obtained with CA 125 in patients with nonmucinous ovarian carcinoma, but monitoring of TAG-72 or CA 15-3 in addition to CA 125 may be helpful.

Pancreatic Carcinoma

Pancreatic carcinoma usually gives rise to nonspecific symptoms and thus only about 10% of patients are diagnosed at an early stage. Measurement of tumor markers has been evaluated in efforts to improve early diagnosis, but the sensitivity and specificity of markers have not proven adequate for screening. Measurement of tumor markers, especially combinations of markers, may be a useful adjunct in diagnosis of pancreatic carcinoma, but must be used with caution because the markers are not specific for the disorder. Many markers, including those shown in Table 12-18, have been studied for use in diagnosis and follow-up of pancreatic carcinoma patients. Of the available markers, CA 19-9 and CA 50 have better diagnostic accuracy than many other markers including DU-PAN-2. Both CA 19-9 and CA 50 also appear useful in monitoring the

Table 12-17. Serum Tumor Marker Elevation in Ovarian Carcinoma

Cancer antigen (CA) 15-3
CA 19-9
CA 125
Carcinoembryonic antigen
Galactosyltransferase
Human chorionic gonadotropin
Human milk fat globule antigen
Human placental lactogen
MOV$_2$
NB 70k
Ovarian carcinoma antigen
Ovarian cystadenocarcinoma antigen
Placental alkaline phosphatase
Procollagen (N-terminal propeptide of type III)
Tumor associated trypsin inhibitor

Table 12-18. Serum Tumor Marker Elevation in Pancreatic Carcinoma

α-Fetoprotein
Cancer antigen (CA) 50
CA 19-9
CA 125
Carcinoembryonic antigen
DU-PAN-2
Galactosyltransferase isoenzyme II
Human chorionic gonadotropin (β-hCG)
Tumor-associated trypsin inhibitor
Pancreatic oncofetal antigen
Pancreatic ribonuclease

postoperative course of pancreatic carcinoma patients. The markers, which are closely related, usually, but not always, are elevated in the same patients.[26] Although up to 20–30% of patients have CA 19-9 and CA 50 results within the reference range, only marginal benefit is achieved by using these markers in combination with each other or with other markers. Although they have the higher sensitivity for the disease, the specificity of CA 19-9 and CA 50 for pancreatic carcinoma are similar to CA 125 and CEA. Increased CA 19-9 and CA 50 are seen in some patients with benign pancreatic disease, more commonly in acute than chronic pancreatitis.[26]

REFERENCES

1. Virji MA, Mercer DW, Herberman RB: Tumor markers in cancer diagnosis and prognosis: CA-A. Cancer J Clin 1988;38:104–126.
2. Neville AM: Tumour markers—an overview. pp. 1–14. In Griffiths K, Neville AM, Pierepoint CG (eds): Tumour Markers. Baltimore, University Park Press, 1977.
3. Reinsberg J, Heydweiller A, Wagner U et al: Evidence for interaction of human anti-idiotypic antibodies with CA 125 determination in a patient after radioimmunodetection. Clin Chem 1990;36:164–167.
4. Stefanini M: Enzymes, isoenzymes, and enzyme variants in the diagnosis of cancer. Cancer 1985;55:1931–1936.
5. Friedman RB, Young DS: Effects of Disease on Clinical Laboratory Tests. 2nd Ed. Washington, DC, AACC Press, 1989.
6. Loose JH, Damjanov I, Harris H: Identity of the neoplastic alkaline phosphatase as revealed with monoclonal antibodies to the placental form of the enzyme. Am J Clin Pathol 1984;82:173–177.
7. Beilby JP, Garcia-Webb P, Bhagat CI et al: Atypical alkaline phosphatase isoenzyme in serum from a patient with Hodgkin's disease. Clin Chem 1984;30:800–802.
8. Muensch HA, Maslow WC, Azama F et al: Placental-like alkaline phosphatase. Cancer 1986;58:1689–1694.
9. Annesley TM, McKenna BJ: Ectopic creatine kinase MB production in metastatic cancer. Am J Clin Pathol 1983;79:255–259.
10. Rogalsky VY, Koven IH, Miller DR et al: Electrophorectic characteristics of macro creatine kinase type 2 in serum. Clin Chem 1986;32:13–21.
11. Hirata RDC, Hirata MH, Strufaldi B et al: Creatine kinase and lactate dehydrogenase isoenzymes in serum and tissues of patients with stomach adenocarcinoma. Clin Chem 1989;35:1385–1389.
12. Rotenberg Z, Weinberger I, Davidson E et al: Lactate dehydrogenase isoenzyme patterns in serum of patients with metastatic liver disease. Clin Chem 1989;35:871–873.
13. Kalpaxis DL, Giannoulaki EE: Partial characterization of an abnormal lactate dehydrogenase isoenzyme, LDH-1ex, in serum from a patient with hepatocellular carcinoma. Clin Chem 1989;35:844–848.
14. Schifferli JA, Roth P, Steiger G et al: Macroprostatic acid phosphatase in a patient's serum. Clin Chem 1988;34:2172–2174.
15. Schifman RB, Ahmann FR, Elvick A et al: Analytical and physiological characteristics of prostate-specific antigen and prostatic acid phosphatase in serum compared. Clin Chem 1987;33:2086–2088.
16. Stamey TA, Yang N, Hay A et al: Prostate-specific antigen as a serum marker for adenocarcinoma of the prostate. N Engl J Med 1987;317:909–916.
17. Aoyagi Y, Suzuki Y, Isemura M et al: The fucosylation index of alphafetoprotein and its usefulness in the early diagnosis of hepatocellular carcinoma. Cancer 1988;61:769–773.
18. Aoyagi Y, Isemura M, Yosizawa Z et al: Fucosylation of serum alpha fetoprotein in patients with primary hepatocellular carcinoma. Biochem Biophys Acta 1985;830:217–223.
19. Pons-Anicet DMF, Krebs BP, Mira R et al: Value of CA 15:3 in the follow-up of breast cancer patients. Br J Cancer 1987;55:567–569.
20. Hayes DF, Zurawski VR, Kufe DW: Comparison of circulating CA 15-3 and carcinoembryonic antigen levels in patients with breast cancer. J Clin Oncol 1986;4:1542–1550.
21. Steinberg WM, Gelfand R, Anderson KK et al: Comparison of the sensitivity and specificity of the CA 19-9 and carcinoembryonic antigen assays in detecting cancer of the pancreas. Gastroenterology 1986;90:343–349.
22. Pleskow DK, Berger HF, Gyves J et al: Evaluation of a serologic marker, CA 19-9, in the diagnosis of pancreatic cancer. Ann Intern Med 1989;110:704–709.
23. Malesci A, Tommasini M, Bonato C et al: Determination of CA 19-9 antigen in serum and pancreatic juice for differential diagnosis of pancreatic adenocarcinoma from chronic pancreatitis. Gastroenterology 1987;92:60–67.
24. Kuusela P, Jalanko H, Roberts P et al: Comparison of CA 19-9 and carcinoembryonic antigen (CEA) levels in the serum of patients with colorectal diseases. Br J Cancer 1984;49:135–139.
25. Kuusela P, Haglund C, Roberts PJ et al: Comparison of CA-50, a new tumour marker, with carcinoembryonic antigen (CEA) and alpha-fetoprotein (AFP) in patients with gastrointestinal diseases. Br J Cancer 1987;55:673–676.
26. Haglund C, Kuusela P, Roberts PJ: Tumour markers in pancreatic cancer. Ann Chir Gynaecol 1989;78:41–53.
27. Mastropaolo W, Fernandez Z, Miller EL: Pronounced increases in the concentration of an ovarian tumor marker, CA-125, in serum of a healthy subject during menstruation. Clin Chem 1986;32:2110–2111.
28. Bast RC, Hunter V, Knapp RC: Pros and cons of gynecologic tumor markers. Cancer 1987;60:1984–1992.
29. Ryder KW, Oei TO, Hull MT et al: An enzyme immunoassay procedure for cancer antigen 125 evaluated. Clin Chem 1988;34:2513–2516.
30. Virji MA, Mercer DW, Herberman RB: New immunologic markers for monitoring of cancer. Ann Chir Gynaecol 1989;78:13–26.
31. Beveridge RA, Chan DW, Bruzek D et al: A new biomarker in monitoring breast cancer: CA 549. J Clin Oncol 1988;6:1815–1820.
32. Buchegger F, Schreyer M, Carrel S, Mach JP: Monoclonal antibodies identify a CEA crossreacting antigen of 95 kD (NCA-95) distinct in antigenicity and tissue distribution from the previously described NCA of 55 kD. Int J Cancer 1984;33:643–649.

33. Fletcher RH: Carcinoembryonic antigen. Ann Intern Med 1986;104:66–73.
34. Minton J, Chevinsky AH: CEA directed second-look surgery for colon and rectal cancer. Ann Chir Gynaecol 1989;78:32–37.
35. Faravelli B, D'Amore E, Nosenzo M et al: Carcinoembryonic antigen in pleural effusions. Diagnostic value in malignant mesothelioma. Cancer 1984;53:1194–1197.
36. Klug TL, Sattler MA, Colcher D et al: Monoclonal antibody immunoradiometric assay for an antigenic determinant (CA 72) on a novel pancarcinoma antigen (TAG-72). Int J Cancer 1986;38:661–669.
37. Odell WD: Paraendocrine syndromes of cancer. Adv Intern Med 1989;34:325–352.
38. Fan C, Goto S, Furuhashi Y et al: Radioimmunoassay of the serum free B-subunit of human chorionic gonadotropin in trophoblastic disease. J Clin Endocrinol Metab 1987;64:313–318.
39. Hussa RO, Rinke ML, Schweitzer PG: Discordant human chorionic gonadotropin results: causes and solutions. Obstet Gynecol 1985;65:211–219.
40. Pattillo RA, Hussa RO: The hCG assay in the treatment of trophoblastic disease. J Reprod Med 1984;29:802–812.
41. Broadus AE, Mangin M, Ikeda K et al: Hymoral hypercalcemia of cancer. Identification of a novel parathyroid hormone-like peptide. N Engl J Med 1988;319:556–563.
42. Stewart AF, Horst R, Deftos LJ et al: Biochemical evaluation of patients with cancer-associated hypercalcemia. N Engl J Med 1980;303:1377–1383.
43. Budayr AA, Nissenson RA, Klein RF et al: Increased serum levels of a parathyroid hormone-like protein in malignancy-associated hypercalcemia. Ann Intern Med 1989;111:807–812.
44. Beutler B, Cerami A: Cachectin (tumor necrosis factor): a macrophage hormone governing cellular metabolism and inflammatory response. Endocrine Rev 1988;9:57–66.
45. Michie HR, Manogue KR, Spriggs DR et al: Detection of circulating tumor necrosis factor after endotoxin administration. N Engl J Med 1988;318:1481–1486.
46. Duffy MJ: Biochemical markers as prognostic indices in breast cancer. Clin Chem 1990;36:188–191.
47. Barnes DM, Millis RR, Fentiman IS et al: Who needs steroid receptor assays? Lancet 1989;1:1126–1127.
48. Brocklehurst D, Wilde CE, Finbow JAH et al: Relative importance of estrogen and progesterone receptor assays as prognostic indicators in primary breast cancer: a short-term study. Clin Chem 1989;35:238–240.
49. Druker BJ, Mamon HJ, Roberts TM: Oncogenes, growth factors, and signal transduction. N Engl J Med 1989;321:1383–1390.
50. Mackay J, Steel CM, Elder PA et al: Allele loss on short arm of chromosome 17 in breast cancers. Lancet 1988;2:1384–1385.
51. Vogelstein B, Fearon ER, Kern SE et al: Allelotype of colorectal carcinomas. Science 1989;244:207–211.
52. Kuhajda FP, Piantadosi S, Pasternack GR: Haptoglobin-related protein (Hpr) epitopes in breast cancer as a predictor of recurrence of the disease. N Engl J Med 1989;321:636–641.
53. Ingle JN: Assessing the risk of recurrence in breast cancer. N Engl J Med 1990;322:329–331.
54. Heintz NH, Leslie KO, Rogers LA et al: Amplification of the c-erb B-2 oncogene and prognosis of breast adenocarcinoma. Arch Pathol Lab Med 1990;114:160–169.
55. Halila H, Alfthan H, Stenman UH: Clinical use of gynaecologic tumour markers. Ann Chir Gynaecol 1989;78:65–70.

13 Therapeutic Drug Monitoring

Bruce Ackerman
Alex A. Pappas

INTRODUCTION

Because individuals vary in their response to a prescribed drug dose as a result of a variety of factors, individualization of drug dosage is desirable to ensure therapeutic effectiveness without undue toxicity. Ideally, pharmacologic response can be quantified accurately, but in many cases it is not possible to use clinical means to assess a drug's effects. For some drugs, the intensity of pharmacologic action and the severity of side effects correlate better with the steady-state concentration of the drug in blood than with daily dosage. Measurement of serum drug concentrations, therefore, may be helpful, but generally only for drugs for which the dosage should be individualized or the therapeutic and toxic action cannot be quantified adequately by other means. In this chapter, major drugs that are monitored are covered; however, psychotropic agents, namely lithium, phenothiazines, and tricyclic antidepressants, are discussed in Chapter 14.

For a drug to be therapeutically effective, it must reach the site of its intended pharmacologic activity within the body at a sufficient rate and in sufficient amounts to yield an effective concentration. Although the dose of a drug is the major determinant for the resulting serum level, the relationship of dose to serum level is not always directly proportional. Marked intraindividual and interindividual variability in serum drug levels can occur after administration of the same dose. Factors important in attaining drug concentrations in serum and eventually at the site of drug action include (1) dosage and route of administration, (2) compliance, (3) bioavailability, (4) drug pharmacokinetics (absorption, binding distribution, biotransformation, and elimination), (5) physiologic factors, (6) genetic factors, (7) intercurrent disease, and (8) drug interactions.

Bioavailability of Drugs

Bioavailability is the amount of drug that enters the systemic circulation in active form and depends on the drug's absorption from the gut lumen, its ability to bypass inactivating enzymes, or its ability to be metabolized to active drug by liver and blood enzymes.[1] Although bioavailability is most often used to describe oral and intramuscular doses of drug, the intravenous drugs clindamycin phosphate and chloramphenicol hemisuccinate represent intravenous "prodrugs" that need to be metabolized to less water-soluble active forms. For some patients (especially pediatric patients), renal elimination of the "prodrug" can reduce the bioavailability of the intravenous dose during an infusion.

Pharmacokinetics

Protein Binding of Drugs

For many drugs, a total serum concentration represents both unbound (pharmacologically active) drug and drug bound to proteins.[2] Under usual circumstances, drug displacement from protein binding sites is only significant if a drug is greater than 95% bound to serum proteins.[3] Protein binding changes as serum protein concentration changes. For example, in hypoalbuminemic patients treated with phenytoin, total

Table 13-1. Serum Concentrations and Distribution Volumes for Monitored Drugs

Drug	Therapeutic Range	Analytic Sensitivity	Panic Values	Distribution Volume
Acetaminophen	10–20 µg/mL (66–132 µmol/L)	10 µg/mL (66 µmol/L)	20 µg/mL (132 µmol/L)	
Amikacin				0.2 L/kg
Trough	0–5 µg/mL (0–8.6 µmol/mL)	0.6 µg/mL (1.0 µmol/L)	>8 µg/mL (>13.7 µmol/L)	
Peak	25–32 µg/mL (42.8–54.8 µmol/L)			
Amiodarone	1–2.5 µg/mL (1.6–3.9 µmol/L)	0.2 µg/mL (0.3 µmol/L)	>2.5 µg/mL (>3.9 µmol/L)	15–40 L/kg
Amitriptyline	120–250 ng/mL (430–900 nmol/L)[a]	10 ng/mL (36.1 nmol/L)	>250 ng/mL (>900 nmol/L)	
Amoxapine	200–400 ng/ml (638–1276 nmol/L)	10 ng/mL (32 nmol/L)	>400 ng/mL (>1276 nmol/L)	
Caffeine	3–15 µg/mL (15.5–77.3 µmol/L)	1 µg/mL (5.2 µmol/L)	>15 µg/mL (>77.3 µmol/L)	0.4–0.7 L/kg
Carbamazepine	4–12 µg/mL (16.9–50.8 µmol/L)	2 µg/mL (8.5 µmol/L)	>12 µg/mL (>50.8 µmol/L)	0.8–1.8 L/kg
Chloraphenicol				
Trough	0–5 µg/mL (0–15.5 µmol/L)			
Peak	15–25 µg/mL (46.4–77.4 µmol/L)			
Clonazepam	20–70 ng/mL (63.3–222 nmol/L)	10 ng/mL (31.7 nmol/L)	>25 ng/mL (>77.8 µmol/L)	1.0 L/kg
Cyclosporin-A			>70 ng/mL (>222 nmol/L)	
HPLC (whole blood)	50–200 ng/mL (41.5–166 nmol/L)	5 ng/mL (4.2 nmol/L)	>200 ng/mL (>166 nmol/L)	10 L/kg
RIA (plasma)	50–300 ng/mL (41.5–249 nmol/L)[a]	5 ng/mL (4.2 nmol/L)	>300 ng/mL (>249 nmol/L)	
Desipramine	75–160 ng/mL (280–600 nmol/L)	5 ng/mL (18.8 nmol/L)	>160 ng/mL (>600 nmol/L)	7.1 L/kg
Digoxin	0.5–2.0 ng/mL (0.7–2.6 nmol/L)	0.2 ng/mL (0.25 nmol/L)	>2.0 ng/mL (>2.6 nmol/L)	0.81 L/kg
Disopyramide	2–5 µg/mL (5.9–14.7 µmol/L)	0.04 µg/mL (0.12 µmol/L)	>5.0 µg/mL (>14.7 µmol/L)	
Doxepin	110–250 ng/mL (394–895 nmol/L)	5 ng/mL (17.9 nmol/L)	>150 ng/mL (>537 nmol/L)	
Ethosuximide	40–100 µg/mL (283–708 µmol/L)	10 µg/mL (70.1 µmol/L)	>100 µg/mL (>708 nmol/L)	
Free phenytoin	1–3 µg/mL (3.96–11.9 µmol/L)	<0.2 µg/mL (<0.79 µmol/L)	>3 µg/mL (>11.9 µmol/L)	
Flecainide	100–1000 ng/mL (241–2410 nmol/L)	25 ng/mL (60.3 nmol/L)	>1000 ng/mL (>2410 nmol/L)	
Gentamicin				0.2 L/kg
Trough	0–2 µg/mL (0–4.0 µmol/L)	<0.2 µg/mL (<0.40 µg/L)	>2.5 µg/mL (>5.0 µmol/L)	
Peak	5–12 µg/mL (9.9–23.9 µmol/L)		>12 µg/mL (>23.9 µmol/L)	
Imipramine	125–250 ng/mL (446–892 nmol/L)[a]	10 ng/mL (35.7 nmol/L)	>250 ng/mL (>892 nmol/L)	
Lidocaine	0.5–5 µg/mL (2.1–21.4 µmol/L)	1 µg/mL (4.3 µg/L)	>5 µg/mL (>21.4 µmol/L)	0.5–1.0 L/kg
Lithium	0.8–1.2 mEq/L (0.8–1.2 mmol/L)	0.1 mEq/L (0.1 mmol/L)	>1.5 mEq/L (>1.5 mmol/L)	
Methotrexate	0.91 µg/mL (2 µmol/L)	4.5 ng/mL (0.01 µmol/L)	>0.9 µg/mL (>2 µmol/L)	
N-acetyl Procainamide	10–25 µg/mL (37.7–94.3 µmol/L)	1 µg/mL (3.8 µmol/L)	>30 ng/mL (>113 µmol/L)	
Nortriptyline	50–150 ng/mL (170–570 nmol/L)	5 ng/mL (19.0 nmol/L)	>150 ng/mL (>570 nmol/L)	0.7 L/kg
Phenobarbital	15–40 µg/mL (65–172 µmol/L)	0.5 µg/mL (2.2 µmol/L)	>40 µg/mL (>172 µmol/L)	0.75 L/kg
Phenytoin	10–20 µg/mL (39.6–79.2 µmol/L)	0.5 µg/mL (19.8 µmol/L)	>25 µg/mL (>99 µmol/L)	
Primadone	5–10 µg/mL (22.9–45.8 µmol/L)	2.5 µg/mL (11.5 µmol/L)	>10 µg/mL (>45.8 µmol/L)	
Procainamide	4–8 µg/mL (17.0–34.0 µmol/L)	1 µg/mL (4.2 µmol/L)	>8 µg/mL (>34 µmol/L)	1.8 L/kg
Protriptyline	70–250 ng/mL (266–950 nmol/L)	5 ng/mL (19.0 nmol/L)	>250 ng/mL (>950 ng/L)	
Quinidine	2–5 µg/mL (6.2–15.4 µmol/L)	0.5 µg/mL (1.5 µmol/L)	>5 µg/mL (>15.4 µg/L)	2.0 L/kg
Salicylate	15–30 mg/dL (1.1–2.2 mmol/L)	2.8 µg/mL (2.0 µmol/L)	>30 mg/dL (>2.2 mmol/L)	
Theophylline	6–20 µg/mL (33.3–111 µmol/L)	2.0 µg/mL (11.1 µmol/L)	>25 µg/mL (>139 µmol/L)	0.45 L/kg
Tobramycin				0.2 L/kg
Trough	0–2 µg/mL (0–4.3 µmol/L)	0.18 µg/mL (0.38 µmol/L)	>2.5 µg/mL (>5.3 µmol/L)	
Peak	5–12 µg/mL (10.7–25.7 µmol/L)		>12 µg/mL (>25.7 µmol/L)	
Valproic acid	100–150 µg/mL (693–1040 µmol/L)	10 µg/mL (69 µmol/L)	>150 µg/mL (>1040 µmol/L)	
Vancomycin				0.6–0.9 L/kg
Trough	8–20 µg/mL (5.5–13.8 µmol/L)	0.6 µg/mL (0.41 µmol/L)	>25 µg/mL (>17.3 µmol/L)	
Peak	30–40 µg/mL (20.7–27.6 µmol/L)		>45 µg/mL (>31.1 µmol/L)	

[a] Sum of parent compound and active metabolites.
Abbreviations: HPLC, high performance liquid chromatography; RIA, radioimmunoassay.

phenytoin serum concentrations are reduced (phenytoin is 90% bound to albumin), whereas unbound phenytoin concentrations may actually be in the toxic range.[4] Patients with cancer, myocardial infarctions, and other disease states may have elevated α_1-acid glycoprotein concentrations that lead to increased binding of basic drugs and decreased unbound concentrations. In this situation, pharmacologic effects of drugs are decreased, but total serum concentrations remain in the therapeutic range.[5]

Distribution Volumes and Total Body Clearance

Clearance represents the portion of the total distribution volume that is returned to the body free of drug from an eliminating organ over a unit of time.[6] The distribution volume is a theoretic volume of water in which a known dose of drug would have to be dissolved in order to achieve the observed serum concentrations.[7] For some drugs, the distribution volume approximates a compartment of body water, but for others, the distribution greatly exceeds the total body water and can be explained by binding to tissue proteins or intracellular drug accumulation.[8] For some drugs, disease states such as congestive heart failure either increase or decrease the size of the distribution volume depending on the extent of tissue binding and decreased hepatic perfusion. Liter per kilogram distribution volumes for commonly used drugs are listed in Table 13-1.

For some commonly used drugs, there is little variation in the distribution volume, but considerable variation in clearance.[9] Thus, patients receive essentially the

Table 13-2. Factors Altering Theophylline Clearance Means ± Standard Deviations (Age, Exposures, and Underlying Disease)

Age/Factor	Mean Age	Mean Clearance (mL/kg/min)	Mean Half-Life (h)
Neonates (apnea)	7.5 ± 4.4 d	0.29 ± 0.1	30 ± 6.5
Infants	41 ± 12 d	0.64 ± 0.3	20 ± 5.3
Infants	18 ± 2 wk	0.8 ± 0.1	6.9 ± 1
6–11 mo	34 ± 7 wk	2.0 ± 0.5	4.6 ± 1.2
1–4 yr	2.5 ± 0.9 yr	1.7 ± 0.6	3.4 ± 1.1
Older children			
4–12 yr	9.4 ± 3 yr	1.5 ± 0.4	?
13–15 yr	14 ± 0.8 yr	0.8 ± 0.2	?
6–17 yr	10.7 ± 2.6 yr	1.4 ± 0.6	3.7 ± 1.1
Adults			
Nonsmoking asthma patients	31 ± 10 yr	0.65 ± 0.19	8.7 ± 2.2
Nonsmoking volunteers	22–35 yr	0.86 ± 0.35	8.1 ± 2.4
Elderly			
Nonsmoking healthy patients	67 ± 5.7 yr	0.59 ± 0.07	7.4 ± 1.1
Abnormal physiology			
Cor pulmonale	64 yr	0.48 ± 0.2	?
Acute pulmonary edema	71 ± 10 yr	0.33 (range, 0.067–2.35)	19 (3.1–82)
Hepatic cirrhosis	52 ± 8.2 yr	0.43 (0.13–3.3)	14.1 (7.1–59.1)
Smoking	56 ± 4 yr	0.21 (0.1–0.6)	32 (10.4–4.56)
Marijuana	20–25 yr	1.2 ± 0.5	4.3 ± 1.2
Marijuana and cigarettes	19–27 yr	1.5 ± 0.4	4.3 ± 1.0
Heavy cigarette use	22–31 yr	1.05 ± 0.32	5.4 ± 1.0
Ex-cigarette smokers (>2 yr)	22–39 yr	0.85 ± 0.2	6.4 ± 1.0
Concurrent drug therapy			
Patient baseline	23 ± 2.2 yr	0.82 ± 0.17	6.7 ± 0.2
Erythromycin exposure	23 ± 2.2 yr	0.60 ± 0.11	8.3 ± 1.8
Patient baseline	23–32 yr	0.75 ± 0.35	?
Phenobarbital exposure	23–32 yr	1.0 ± 0.5	?
Cimetidine exposure		Decreases clearance by 50%	

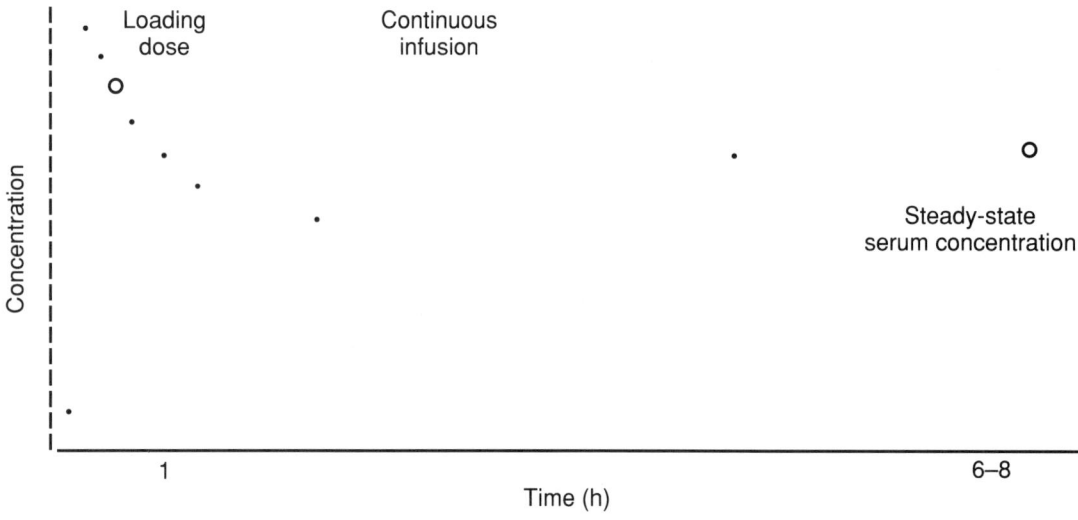

Fig. 13-1. Following loading doses of quinidine and lidocaine, redistribution of the drug occurs. As the continuous infusion of either drug is begun steady-state is reached when the drug has distributed to the peripheral compartment.

same loading dose, but they have considerable differences in required maintenance doses. Theophylline and many cardiovascular drugs demonstrate greater variance in clearance than in distribution volume (Table 13-2), permitting accurate prediction of serum concentrations following loading doses. For these drugs, estimates of clearance are necessary for determining a maintenance dose.

The continuous infusion of a drug is calculated from an estimated clearance and may result in elevated, expected, or subtherapeutic drug concentrations depending on prediction accuracy. As can be seen in Figure 13-1, a loading dose followed by a continuous infusion of drug may result in toxic, expected, or subtherapeutic concentrations.

Elimination Half-Life

The observed fall in serum concentration following the administration of a drug reflects drug metabolism, distribution to peripheral tissues, and renal elimination of parent drug and its metabolites.[6] The half-life may be defined as the time required for the serum concentration of a drug to fall to 50% of the initially observed serum concentration. The half-life is dependent on total body clearance of the drug and its distribution volume as can be seen with equation 3 in Table 13-3.[10]

Table 13-3. Helpful Pharmacokinetic Equations

Ideal body weight (IBW) = 2.3 kg/in in height over 5 feet + (50 kg for males or 45.5 kg for females)	(1)
Creatinine clearance = $\dfrac{(140 - \text{patient age}) \times \text{patient IBW (kg)}}{72 \times \text{patient serum creatinine}}$	(2)
Half-life = $\dfrac{0.693 \times \text{distribution volume}}{\text{total body clearance}}$	(3)
Renal failure half-life = $\dfrac{\text{normal half-life}}{\text{fraction excreted} \times (\text{patient creatinine clearance}/100 - 1) + 1}$	(4)
Maintenance dose (MD) equation MD renal = MD Normal × [fraction excreted × (patient creatinine clearance/100 − 1) + 1]	(5)
Accumulation ratio (AR) equation AR = $\dfrac{1}{1 - e^{-k_e(t_{1/2} \times n)}}$, where n = number of half-lives and $t_{1/2}$ = half-life[a]	(6)

[a] Ke is the elimination rate constant for particular drugs.

One or both of these parameters can vary considerably in ill patients, therefore a wide range in half-lives is observed within a patient population.[10-12]

The half-life indicates when steady-state will occur and provides a rough measure for estimating the dosing interval. Steady-state, a time dependent process taking greater than five half-lives,[13] occurs when there is an equilibrium between the amount of drug administered and the amount of drug eliminated during a dosing interval. At steady-state, serum concentrations drawn at exactly the same time interval will be equal provided no change in pharmacokinetic parameters has occurred. Table 13-4 describes the relationship between the percentage of steady-state and the number of half-lives since initiation of drug therapy. As the number of half-lives approaches five, serum concentrations approach 100% of steady-state.

Figure 13-2 graphically describes the half-life of a drug with a serum concentration of 40 mg/L at 1 hour after administration of a dose. At 4 hours, the concentration has fallen to 20 mg/L and at 7 hours to 10 mg/L. The apparent half-life for this drug is 3 hours and the patient will not have steady-state peak and trough concentrations for at least 15 hours after initiating drug therapy. Figure 13-3 demonstrates that it often takes several doses of a drug for a patient to achieve steady-state serum concentrations. Figure 13-4 demonstrates that the levels drawn from serum concentration monitoring are not the true peak and trough (the highest and lowest serum concentrations during the dosing interval) and these need to be calculated for the serum concentrations at 30 minutes before and 30 minutes after the infusion following the one compartment model. The points marked with (o) are the extrapolated true peak and trough needed to calculate pharmacokinetic

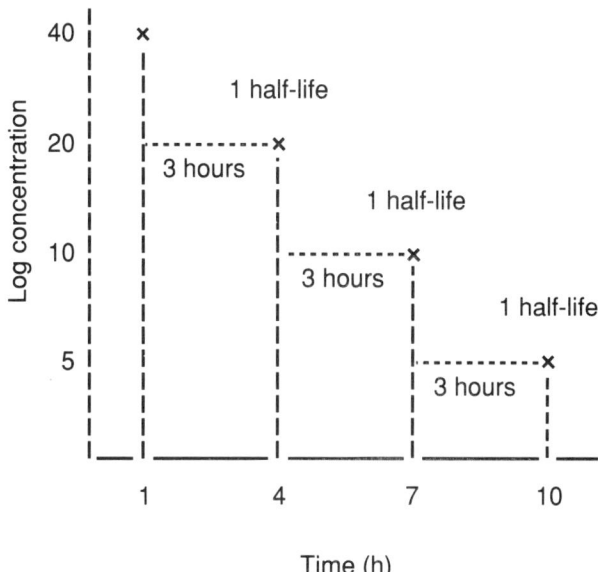

Fig. 13-2. Half-life of a linear drug in the body. The half-life represents the time required for the serum concentration of a drug to decrease by 50% from the initial measured serum concentration, here a 3-hour period.

parameters from a peak-trough check. With a short half-life this difference can be quite marked, and conversely, with renal impairment this difference is insignificant.

Pharmacokinetics

One Compartment Models

Drugs with linear one compartment models are said to have first order or first order appearing drug elimination. That is, for a given period of time, a consistent percent of the drug will be eliminated during the entire dosing interval. A linear one compartment open model in clinical pharmacokinetics is applied to a number of drugs that actually are two compartment open model drugs. For example, the aminoglycosides, quinidine and theophylline, are technically multicompartmental drugs with very small distribution phases. A one compartment model can be used to characterize the disposition of these drugs, because the distribution phase following an infusion of the drug contributes less than 5% to the area under the concentration time curve (AUC). Thus the use of a one compartment model estimate of the distribution volume can be based on greater than 95% of the AUC, an estimate close enough for clinical use in dose calculation.

Table 13-4. Number of Half-Lives and Percentage of Steady-State Serum Concentrations

Half-Lives	% Steady-State
0.5	29
1	50
2	75
3	87
4	94
5	97
6	98

338 • Laboratory Medicine

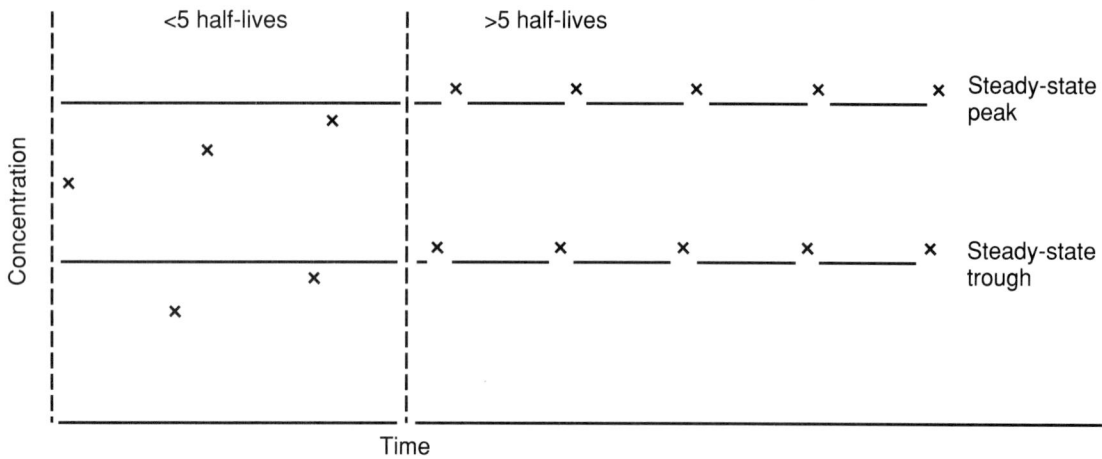

Fig. 13-3. Approaching steady-state peak and trough concentrations. As steady-state is approached, trough concentrations accumulate to a maximum serum concentration at which point the amount of drug entering the body during the dosing interval is equal to the amount of drug leaving the body during the same interval.

Two Compartment Models

For drugs clearly demonstrating a biphasic serum concentration decline, at least when greater than 5% of the AUC is contributed by the distribution phase, major errors may occur with dose adjustments based on a one compartment model as demonstrated in Figure 13-5. By ignoring the "alpha" distribution phase, resulting AUCs are such that the distribution volume and clearance are overestimated. The formulas for drugs demonstrating two compartment models are much more complex and accurate prediction of serum concentrations requires more serum samples than needed for drugs adjusted with one compartment model programs.

Non-Linear Pharmacokinetics

Almost all drugs used in therapeutic doses will demonstrate linear pharmacokinetics. This means that there is a proportional change in serum concentrations with increasing and decreasing doses of a given drug. With nonlinear pharmacokinetics, this proportional relationship is lost and serum concentrations either geo-

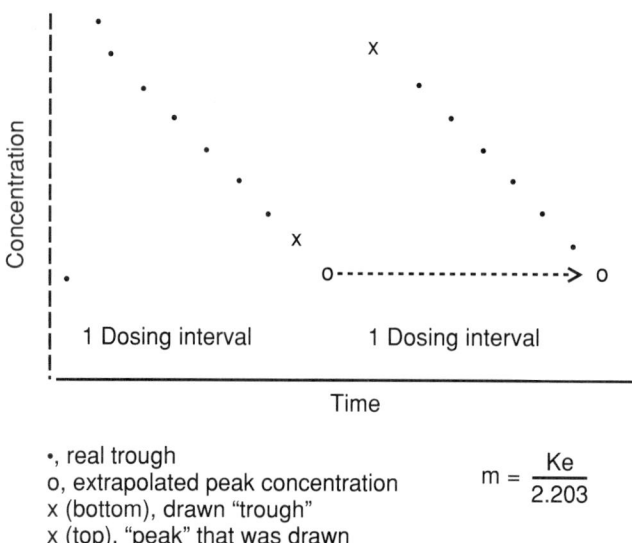

•, real trough
o, extrapolated peak concentration
x (bottom), drawn "trough"
x (top), "peak" that was drawn

$$m = \frac{Ke}{2.203}$$

Fig. 13-4. Graphic depiction of how a peak-trough check can be used to calculate pharmacokinetic parameters for dose adjustment. The trough and peak must be extrapolated to immediately preinfusion and postinfusion levels (----) to the end of the second dose in order to calculate the Ke.

Therapeutic Drug Monitoring • 339

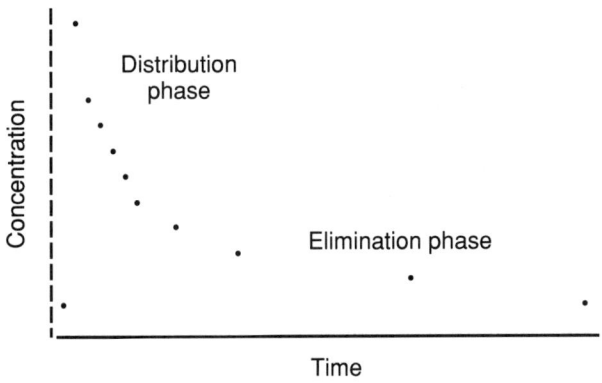

Fig. 13-5. Serum concentration time curve for a drug described by a two compartment model. The serum concentration time curve for a two-compartment drug that is best described by the $Cp_t = Ae^{-at} + Be^{-bt}$ where A and B are intercepts for the hybrid constants "a" and "b." For any given postinfusion time (t) a serum concentration Cp_t can be calculated.

linear pharmacokinetic models using Michaelis-Menten equations. The two parameters that remain constant in a nonlinear system are the V_{max} and Km, which represent, respectively, the maximum enzymatic biotransformation and affinity of a subtrate (drug) for hepatic enzymes. For drugs demonstrating saturable pharmacokinetics, these two parameters (Km and V_{max}) alone are constant, whereas the half-life and other more commonly known pharmacokinetic parameters change as serum concentrations rise or fall.[14]

Accumulation of Drug in the Body

For drugs that are not given as continuous infusions, a steady-state peak and trough concentration also are achieved. For drugs that are given as intermittent boluses or as oral doses, a certain percentage of the previous dose remains at the time of the administration of the next dose; the percentage is dependent on the half-life of the drug. When the dosing interval is set at two half-lives then significant drug accumulation begins (72% accumulation) and at one half-life the drug will accumulate in the body to 144% of the administered dose (Table 13-3, equation 6). For drugs with a narrow therapeutic range, such as antiarrhythmics and theophylline, this drug accumulation can be exploited to keep serum concentrations within the therapeutic range between doses. Development of new drugs with greater potential for toxicity has motivated development of methods of pharmacokinetic dose adjustment to assure therapeutic drug concentrations while minimizing the risk of toxicity.[15] Pharmacokinetic models

metrically increase or decrease with changes in doses. Figure 13-6 demonstrates graphically the difference between drugs demonstrating linear and nonlinear (saturable) kinetics after administration of equal doses of drug. In addition, many of the pharmacokinetic parameters discussed previously, such as half-life and clearance, change with rises and falls in serum concentrations and thus cannot be used for dose adjustment. The disposition of alcohol, phenytoin, theophylline in children, and overdoses of tricyclic antidepressants and a few other drugs can be best described with non-

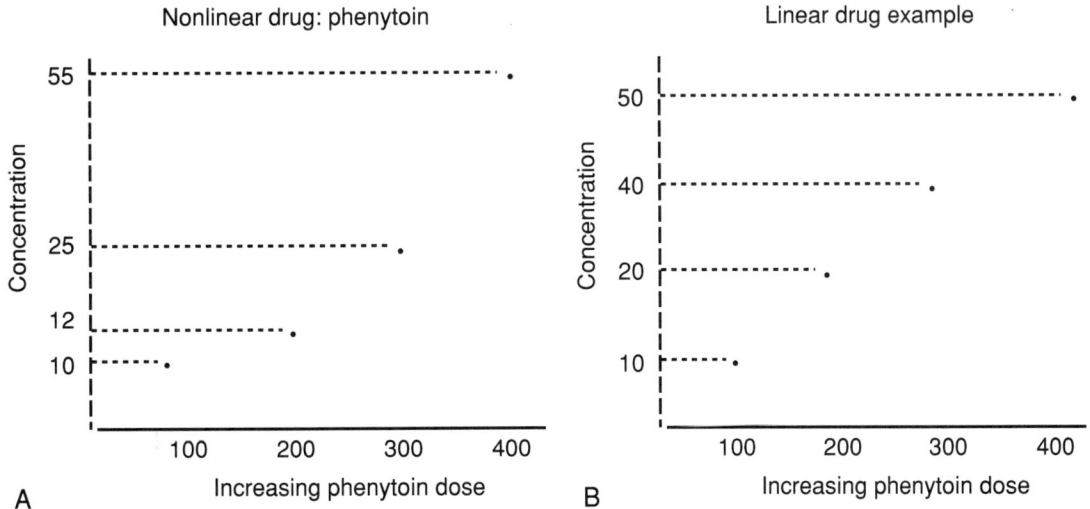

Fig. 13-6. Two graphs demonstrating the difference in serum concentrations as doses of (**A**) nonlinear drug (phenytoin) and (**B**) linear are increased by 100-mg increments.

are applied in therapeutic drug monitoring to make appropriate dose adjustments.

Monitoring Serum Concentration

Specimens for serum drug levels should be drawn when steady-state is reached. With oral medications serum specimens are usually obtained during steady-state just before the administered drug dose. For drugs that are continuously infused, serum specimens should be obtained at approximately one half-life after the beginning of the continuous infusion or when patients demonstrate manifestations of toxic or subtherapeutic concentrations. If there have been changes in the dose, five half-lives must pass after the dose change before steady-state serum concentrations are achieved and peak and trough data can be used. For the sustained release products, absorption can be prolonged, therefore no real "peak" occurs during the dosing interval. Likewise the trough concentration will be higher, as demonstrated in Figure 13-7. Release of drug from sustained release products is assumed to be analogous to a continuous infusion and dose adjustments are made to either attain a mid-interval specific concentration or a specific trough concentration as demonstrated in Figure 13-7.[16]

There are a number of points to remember before ordering and evaluating serum levels: (1) is the patient at steady-state (more than five half-lives from any dose change); (2) have there been any missed or late doses recently; (3) are the infusion periods and dosing intervals essentially unchanged; (4) at what time has the specimen been obtained in relationship to dose, and (5) has there been a significant change recently in renal or hepatic function (is the half-life changing)?

ANTICONVULSANT DRUGS

Test: Carbamazepine

Background and Selection

Carbamazepine, which is structurally related to the tricyclic antidepressants, is indicated for the treatment of generalized and partial complex seizures. Carbamazepine is considered as effective as phenobarbital, phenytoin, or primadone, and is often used as an alternative agent for patients with serious adverse effects to phenytoin. Carbamazepine also is used to treat trigeminal neuralgia and investigationally for treatment of lithium resistant manic depression, diabetes insipidus, and migraine headaches.[17] The side effects that occur in up to 25% of treated patients include diplopia, drowsiness, and blurred vision. The most serious side effects are the rare bone marrow and hepatic toxicity. Paradoxic intoxication with low serum concentrations of carbamazepine has been noted and is an indication for obtaining an unbound carbamazepine serum concentration. The pharmacokinetic parameters of carbamazepine and the other commonly used anticonvulsants are listed in Table 13-5. The apparent half-life is affected by the persistent absorption phase and must be

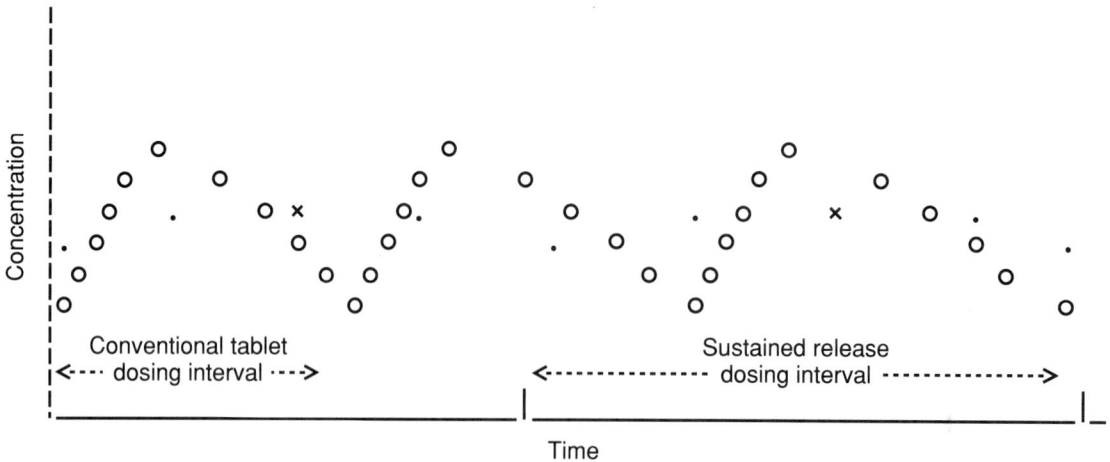

Fig. 13-7. The greater fluctuation in serum concentrations are more frequent with conventional tablets, while sustained release tablets produce less fluctuations. Sustained release products are indicated for short half-lives or peak-related toxicities.

Table 13-5. Pharmacokinetic Properties of the Anticonvulsant Drugs

	Phenytoin	Phenobarbital	Primadone	Carbamazepine	Valproate
Absorption	70–100%	80–90%	Unknown	70–80%	85–100%
Protein binding	80–95%	50%	10%	65–85%	90–95%
Distribution volume (L/kg)	0.75	0.7–1.0	0.6	0.8–1.9	0.13–0.4
Metabolism	95%	65%	15–25%	98%	
Half-life					
Adults (h)	24–48	50–120	10–12	9–24	8–15
Children (h)	12–22	40–70			8–15

interpreted with caution. Serum carbamazepine concentrations cannot be predicted from administered doses and therapy is complicated by carbamazepine's induction of its own metabolism. Thus, increasing doses of carbamazepine are required over the first 6 to 8 weeks following initiation of therapy to maintain therapeutic serum concentrations.

Logistics

Carbamazepine induces the metabolism of other anticonvulsants, warfarin, oral contraceptives, and doxycycline thus reducing their pharmacologic effects. Erythromycin and propoxyphene have been reported to interfere with carbamazepine's metabolism with accumulation of carbamazepine to toxic serum concentrations. Table 13-6 lists common drug interactions for the anticonvulsant drugs as a group.

Interpretation

The therapeutic concentration range for serum carbamazepine is from 6–12 µg/mL (25.4–50.8 µmol/L), but therapeutic effects are seen with serum concentrations as low as 4 µm/mL (16.9 µmol/L). It is difficult to interpret carbamazepine serum concentrations because of its complex absorption characteristics and protein binding as well as displacement of carbamazepine from serum proteins by its own metabolites. Although toxicity can occur with concentrations greater than 12 µg/mL (> 50.8 µmol/L),[17] toxic serum concentrations have been reported as high as 23–60 µg/mL (97.4–254 µmol/L). Table 13-7 lists routine laboratory tests for monitoring patients over the first 3 months of therapy: these tests and carbamazepine concentration should be repeated at least annually.

Test: Free Carbamazepine

Background and Selection

As with the other anticonvulsants, there has been a significant interest in developing methods for monitoring unbound concentrations in serum and attempting to correlate these to seizure control. Like valproic acid and phenytoin, carbamazepine is extensively bound to serum proteins with variable and unpredictable un-

Table 13-6. Major Drug-Drug Interactions With Anticonvulsant Drugs

Oral anticoagulants (warfarin)	Induction of metabolism—increase dose and monitor patient with all anticonvulsant dose changes
Corticosteroids and oral contraceptives:	Induction of metabolism—increased risk pregnancy
Isoniazid (INH)	Inhibits primadone conversion to active metabolites
Quinidine	Induction of metabolism—draw quinidine levels after initiating phenobarbital or primadone therapy
Antidepressants	Induction of metabolism
Monoamine oxidase inhibitors	Inhibit phenobarbital metabolism—reduce maintenance dose
Tetracycline	Induction of metabolism
Valproic acid	Inhibits metabolism?

Table 13-7. Routine Laboratory Tests for Carbamazepine Toxicity Monitoring
Complete blood count with platelets
Serum iron—before and after 3 weeks of therapy
Blood urea nitrogen
Urinalysis
Liver function tests as a baseline and following initiation of therapy
Serum carbamazepine trough concentrations

bound carbamazepine serum concentrations. Free concentrations in serum range from 19.6–34.7% of the total serum concentration, indicating problems in predicting seizure control from total serum concentrations. One problem with interpretation of unbound carbamazepine concentrations has been the displacement of the parent compound from protein binding sites by the 10,11-epoxide metabolite. Recently, the protein binding of carbamazepine and the 10,11-epoxide metabolite were characterized as 81% and 62% bound, respectively, with considerable greater variance in metabolite binding. Thus, ultrafiltrates will contain higher metabolite concentrations when compared with total serum concentrations. In addition, most immunoassays overestimate the unbound concentration of carbamazepine by approximately 34% because of filtration of the metabolite and its being read as carbamazepine when the enzyme-multiplied immunoassay technique (EMIT) assay was compared with a high performance liquid chromatography (HPLC) assay.[18] The use of gas liquid chromatography (GLC) appears to reduce this to only a 14–16% overestimation of carbamazepine when compared with the EMIT assay. Prediction of the percent 10,11-epoxide metabolite is also difficult due to the considerable variance in its formation.

Baruzzi et al[19] noted an inverse correlation between the unbound concentration of carbamazepine and α_1-acid glycoprotein. This has implications on the management of seizure patients following myocardial infarction, with renal disease, cancer and burns.

Logistics

Drug Interactions

The major drug interactions involve other anticonvulsant drugs that are known to induce carbamazepine metabolism and 10,11-epoxide metabolite formation.

Assay

After ultrafiltration, the sample is assayed by HPLC, GLC, EMIT, or fluorescence polarization immunoassay (FPIA) methods. Assay interference occurs with immunoassay methods due to the measurement of the active metabolite, 10,11-epoxide carbamazepine.

Interpretation

Therapeutic unbound concentrations for carbamazepine have not been fully defined but appear to range somewhere near 1.3 ± 0.5 µg/mL (5.5 ± 2.1 µmol/L) and the metabolite concentration approximates 0.5 ± 0.3 µg/mL (2.1 ± 1.3 µmol/L).[20] Variance in α_1-acid glycoprotein and induced metabolite formation by other anticonvulsants complicates unbound carbamazepine concentration interpretation. Further definition of the unbound concentration therapeutic range has yet to be fully determined.

Test: Ethosuximide

Background and Selection

Ethosuximide is a hydantoin anticonvulsant indicated for the management of absence seizures. The drug is readily absorbed over a period of 3 hours with little biotransformation by the liver before entering the systemic circulation. The drug distributes in the total body water and is not extensively bound to serum or tissue proteins. Serum concentrations approximate cerebrospinal fluid concentrations and the drug will distribute to breast milk to concentrations equaling those in plasma. Metabolism is mainly directed toward hydroxylation of the ethyl side chain followed by glucuronidation and accounts for 40–50% of the ingested dose. Hydroxylation of the hydantoin ring followed by glucuronidation also occurs and represents a minor metabolite. Approximately 20% of ethosuximide is excreted unchanged in the urine. The hepatic clearance is rather small for the drug representing 7.5 mL/min/m² reflected as a half-life of 40–60 hours in patients with normal renal and hepatic function. Initial therapy in children is 15–20 mg/kg in children under age 10. This should provide serum concentrations in excess of 40 µg/mL (280 µmol/L) but such large doses in adolescents and adults are likely to approach serum concentrations of 60–80 µg/mL (430–570 µmol/L). Because of gastric upset, ethosuximide is often given in divided doses rather than once a day.

Ethosuximide is a hydantoin anticonvulsant analogous to phenytoin and sharing many of the side effects in common with hydantoin drugs. The most common side effects of the drug involve the gastrointestinal tract and include anorexia, gastric upset, cramps, abdominal pain, and diarrhea. Central nervous system toxicity includes headache, drowsiness, fatigue, dizziness, ataxia, and lethargy or hyperactivity. Sleep disturbance and night terrors have also been described for ethosuximide. The most serious side effects are blood dyscrasias that limit the use of this drug in preference for valproic acid and benzodiazepines. Leukopenia, eosinophilia, agranulocytosis, pancytopenia, and aplastic anemia have been described, some cases of which have been fatal. Rarely, Stevens-Johnson syndrome has been reported in treated children. Gum hypertrophy and hirsuitism similar to that of phenytoin have also been described. As with other anticonvulsants, liver function tests, complete blood count, and urinalysis should be obtained before and during initial treatment with ethosuximide with annual or semiannual monitoring.

Logistics

Drug Interactions

Combination therapy with other anticonvulsants is likely to augment the pharmacokinetic parameters and the serum concentrations of all other concomitant anticonvulsants included in a treatment regimen. With the addition or subtraction of anticonvulsants, serum concentration monitoring of all remaining anticonvulsants with dose adjustment is almost always required.

Analysis

Ethosuximide serum concentrations may be determined by HPLC, gas chromatography (GC), GLC, or by one of several immunoassays.

Interpretation

Seizure frequency has been demonstrated to be suppressed by 75% or more by maintaining serum concentrations of ethosuximide in excess of 40 μg/mL (280 μmol/L) and currently this is thought to be the minimum trough concentration for the management of absence seizures. There is little data correlating toxicity with specific serum concentrations, but an upper limit of 100 μg/mL (710 μmol/L) has been suggested as the maximal therapeutic concentration of ethosuximide. Decision to decrease or increase doses should be predicted on seizure control and toxicity rather than serum concentrations as a less clear relationship exists between seizure control and specific trough concentrations.

Test: Phenobarbital

Background

Phenobarbital was first used clinically to treat seizure disorders in 1912 when it was used as an alternative to the sedating and very toxic bromides. Phenobarbital was the first safe and effective drug for the treatment of epilepsy, but all seizure patients do not respond to phenobarbital. Phenobarbital is indicated for the management of generalized tonic-clonic seizures and complex partial seizures. It also is used for the management of febrile seizures in the pediatric age group and in patients with status epilepticus who are unresponsive to parenteral phenytoin. Rash and allergic manifestations occur in about 2% of patients treated with phenobarbital and these lesions may progress to life-threatening exfoliative dermatitis.[21] Pharmacokinetic parameters for phenobarbital, which has a half-life ranging from 50–120 hours, are listed in Table 13-5.[21]

Phenobarbital exerts its pharmacologic activity by preventing synaptic transmission through elevation of the enuronal cell threshold. This rise in threshold causes generalized slowing of the central nervous system characterized by drowsiness and sedation and, in children, irritability. Patients often become tolerant to the sedative effects of phenobarbital, but no tolerance to disinhibition and other behavioral changes occurs.

Selection

Variance in response can occur with empiric doses; thus, routine serum concentration monitoring should be done within several months of initiating empiric therapy. Patients complaining of lethargy, diplopia, ataxia, or dizziness should have a phenobarbital serum concentration obtained to rule out drug toxicity. Monitoring of serum anticonvulsant concentrations in children is complicated by changes in hepatic clearance that occur with increasing age. As children enter puberty, serum concentrations should be obtained about every 3–4 months. Doses for children with substantial weight gain or loss likewise should be reevaluated based on serum concentration data. For trauma-induced and temporal lobe epilepsy, several anticonvulsants are prescribed in combination to manage seizure activity. As a result, predictable and unpredictable changes in the serum concentrations of one or more of these anticonvulsants may occur, and therefore it is important to monitor serum concentrations of all anticonvulsants with the addition or removal of any others.

Logistics

Barbiturates induce hepatic microsomal enzymes increasing the hepatic clearance of other drugs (see Table 13-6). Alcohol and central nervous system depressants potentate the sedative and disinhibitory effects of barbiturates. Warfarin, oral contraceptives, digoxin, antiarrhythmics, and doxycycline may have reduced effectiveness due to their increased hepatic clearance in the presence of phenobarbital. Patients taking these drugs concomitantly with phenobarbital should be carefully monitored and have drug doses appropriately adjusted to ensure appropriate therapy.

Interpretation

The therapeutic range for phenobarbital is 15–40 μg/mL, but most patients require serum concentrations less than 30 μg/mL for adequate therapeutic effects. Many patients taking phenobarbital chronically can tolerate serum concentrations of phenobarbital as high as 50 μg/mL with no apparent toxicity, but frank coma occurs when serum concentrations exceed 90 μg/mL.

Test: Phenytoin

Background and Selection

Phenytoin is used in the treatment of generalized tonic-clonic seizures, status epilepticus, and complex partial seizures. Drowsiness and disinhibition are much less marked with phenytoin than phenobarbital, thus it is often chosen for initial therapy. Patients with reduced albumin binding or reduced albumin concentration may demonstrate ataxia and intoxication from "therapeutic" total phenytoin serum concentrations. Phenytoin is used 60–80% of the time for generalized tonic-clonic seizures, although use of carbamazepine for this indication is increasing. Even though phenytoin is a structural analogue of phenobarbital, there are pharmacologic differences between phenytoin and phenobarbital. Phenobarbital increases the seizure threshold with global pharmacologic action, whereas phenytoin does not suppress a seizure focus but prevents its spread to a generalized seizure.[22] Treatment of epilepsy with phenytoin is complicated by nonlinear pharmacokinetics in which changes in dose do not correlate with changes in serum concentrations (Fig. 13-6). Therapeutic doses of phenytoin saturate hepatic enzymes, thus the liver is capable of metabolizing only a limited amount of phenytoin per day. The disposition of phenytoin is further complicated by slow and variable drug absorption, interference of absorption with some drugs, and variable protein binding especially with hypoalbuminemic patients. All of the metabolites of phenytoin are inactive.

Logistics

Concomitant administration of barbiturates, alcohol, or other central nervous system depressants may potentiate the sedation caused by phenytoin. In addition, phenytoin induces the metabolism of some drugs thus lowering their serum concentrations and their pharmacologic effects (Tables 13-6 and 13-8). These include warfarin, levodopa, doxycycline, chloramphenicol, isoniazid, sulfonylureas, propranolol, lidocaine, and oral contraceptives. In addition, the absorption of phenytoin may be inhibited by antacids and folic acid. Valproic acid displaces phenytoin thus lowering serum concentrations, whereas disulfram impairs the hepatic metabolism of phenytoin.

Interpretation

The therapeutic range of phenytoin is 10–20 μg/mL (70–140 μmol/L), but Lund[23] and Troupin and Friel[24] noted that many patients may require serum concen-

Table 13-8. Specific Drug-Drug Interactions That Occur With Phenytoin

Metabolism is increased with
    Phenobarbital
    Primadone
    Carbamazepine
    Alcohol

Protein binding displacement occurs with
    Valproic acid
    Salicylates
    Sulfonylureas
    Uremia
    Hyperlipidemia and nephrotic syndrome

Metabolism is decreased with
    Barbiturates
    Chloramphenicol
    Disulfiram
    Isoniazid
    Benzodiazepines
    Warfarin
    Phenylbutazone
    Estrogens
    Propoxyphene
    Ethosuximide
    Liver disease

Table 13-9.	Common Side Effects of Phenytoin

Dose related
  Nystagmus, blurred vision, ataxia, dysarthria, drowsiness: Css < 30, 15%; Css > 30, 50%
Nondose related
  Hirsutism and acne
  Gingival hyperplasia
  Facial coarsening
  Hypocalcemia and osteomalacia
  Rashes and exfoliative dermatitis
  Pseudolymphoma, blood dyscrasias, IgA deficiency, and eosinophilia
  Anicteric hepatitis with 38% mortality

Abbreviation: Css, trough concentration of phenytoin at steady-state.

trations as high as 25 μg/mL (180 μmol/L) for single agent seizure control. Lund[23] and Troupin and Friel[24] demonstrated a clear correlation between serum phenytoin concentrations and clinical efficacy. Likewise, many of the adverse effects of phenytoin also have been correlated with elevated serum concentrations (Table 13-9).

Wide variations in phenytoin serum concentrations occur whether dosing is done empirically or based on body weight. Although there are limitations to using average patient data, phenytoin doses can be predicted from average V_{max} and Km data using the equations in Table 13-10. The only pharmocokinetic dose adjustment method that can be used with a single serum concentration: dose pair for prediction of V_{Max} and Km

Table 13-10.	Michaelis-Menten Equations

$$V = \frac{V_{max} \times [S]}{Km \times [S]} \quad (1)$$

Vozeh nomogram formulas

$$\text{Dose} = \frac{\text{Y-intercept mg/kg/d} \times \text{IBW Css desired}}{\text{X-intercept mg/L} + \text{Css desired}} \quad (2)$$

Note: equations [2] and [3] are identical

$$\text{Dose} = \frac{V_{max}/F \times \text{desired serum concentration}}{Km + \text{desired serum concentration}} \quad (3)$$

$$\text{Css} = \frac{\text{dose} \times Km}{V_{max} - \text{dose}} \quad (4)$$

Abbreviations: V, enzyme velocity at specific substrate concentrations; V_{max}, maximum enzyme velocity; [S], substrate concentration; Km, reciprocal of substrate affinity for the enzyme; IBW, ideal body weight; Css, steady-state concentration; F, percentage of dose absorbed.

is the Vozeh et al.[25] nomogram method. Other methods described by Mullen[26] (Fig. 13-8) and Ludden et al.[27] require a minimum of two sets of phenytoin serum concentrations obtained from two different doses.

Antiarrhythmic Indications for Phenytoin

The mechanism of action of phenytoin remains controversial, but certainly the "calcium channel blocking" effect of the drug at teliodendria of nerves contributes considerably to the anticonvulsant effect of the drug. Likewise, a selective calcium channel blockade by phenytoin has been proposed to reverse the drug-induced arrhythmias observed in digoxin overdoses. The clinical use of phenytoin for the general management of arrhythmias has been disappointing as it is generally less effective than quinidine, procainamide, and lidocaine. Phenytoin currently is specifically indicated for the management of paroxysmal atrial tachycardia and digoxin-induced atrial tachycardias. Therapeutic concentrations for arrhythmia suppression are less clearly defined. Serum concentrations for management of arrhythmias do not differ from those required for management of epilepsy. The limited clinical use of phenytoin has not afforded study as to the therapeutic unbound concentration range for arrhythmia management.

Test: Free Phenytoin

Background and Selection

Usually about 10% of the total phenytoin in serum is the free (unbound) form. Patients with hypoalbuminemic nutritional deficiencies, renal insufficiency, patients demonstrating severe toxicity with therapeutic phenytoin concentrations, and pregnant patients should be monitored with free phenytoin serum concentrations to assure adequate seizure control without unnecessary toxicity.[28]

Logistics

Drug Interactions

Valproic acid displaces phenytoin from its albumin binding sites, but the effects of other drugs are unknown. For poorly controlled diabetics, nonspecific glycation of albumin occurs with altered phenytoin protein binding.

Analysis

Following ultrafiltration, the specimen is analyzed for free phenytoin by assays that provide an accurate assay at low concentrations of phenytoin. Nomograms and formulas have been developed to estimate the free

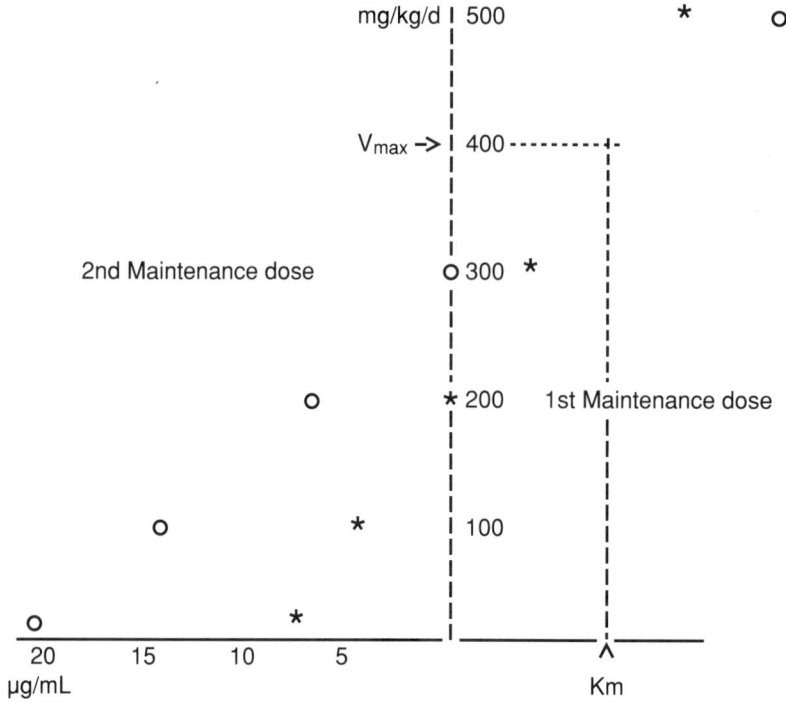

Fig. 13-8. A Mullen plot for determining the V_{max} and Km following two phenytoin dose changes is demonstrated. At the intersection of two dose:steady-state serum concentration lines, perpendicular lines to the X and Y axes may be drawn. The perpendicular intercept to the Y axis estimates the V_{max} and the perpendicular intercept to the X axis estimates the Km.

phenytoin concentrations from serum albumin results, but these methods often fall short of the actual free phenytoin concentration and are not recommended.

Interpretation

The therapeutic range for free (unbound) phenytoin is 1.5–3 μg/mL (5.9–11.9 μmol/L).[4,5] No method is currently available for predicting dose adjustment in patients with hypoalbuminemia, thus empiric dose adjustment with repeated measurement of free phenytoin concentrations is required.

Test: Primadone

Background and Selection

Primadone is a complex drug because the parent compound as well as its principal metabolite phenobarbital have anticonvulsant properties. For patients treated with primadone, both phenobarbital and primadone serum concentration monitoring is required. Primadone is used to treat generalized tonic-clonic and psychomoter seizures by empiric dose adjustment.[29] Following the addition or subtraction of any anticonvulsant, serum concentrations of all the anticonvulsants used in the management of the patient's seizures should be obtained.

Logistics

When primadone is taken with phenytoin, there is an increased conversion of primadone to its active metabolite, phenobarbital. Therefore, therapeutic drug monitoring of phenytoin, primadone, and phenobarbital is important after initiation of therapy and at steady-state.

Interpretation

The therapeutic range for primadone is 5–12 μg/mL (22.9–55.0 μmol/L) and side effects (diplopia, dizziness, ataxia) are commonly associated with serum primadone concentrations in excess of 15 μg/mL (68.7 μmol/L). The major metabolite of primadone is phenylethylmalonamide (PEMA), but it is considered to have little anticonvulsant activity. Phenobarbital is the other primadone metabolite that accumulates to therapeutic concentrations.

Test: Valproic Acid

Background and Selection

The pharmacologic action of valproic acid is controversial. Valproic acid (dipropylacetate), a short chain fatty acid, is thought to increase γ-aminobutyric acid (GABA) concentrations in the brain by inhibiting GABA transaminase and succinic semialdehyde dehydrogenase activity. Although some investigators have demonstrated a rise in GABA following valproic acid therapy, others have not. Some workers have proposed that valproic acid exerts its pharmacologic effects by inhibiting the pharmacologic effects of aspartate and other excitatory neurotransmitter amino acids.

The disposition of valproic acid varies considerably among patients with considerable variance occurring in half-life, total body clearance, rate of absorption, and bioavailability. Valproic acid also is metabolized to several active metabolites that may contribute significantly to the therapeutic effect of valproic acid. Several of these metabolites have been noted to accumulate in the brain, but their seizure suppressing potentials have not been characterized. Bauer et al.[30] demonstrated diurnal variance in the clearance of valproic acid noting decreased clearance in the evening in 10 volunteers. These authors noted that both clearance and protein binding demonstrated diurnal variation with decreased clearance and free fraction in the evening. Bowdle et al.[31] noted a decline in total body clearance with increasing doses of valproic acid indicating that valproic acid may, like phenytoin, demonstrate saturable pharmacokinetics in high therapeutic doses. With valproic acid, there is less central nervous system toxicity than other anticonvulsants, but a greater risk for hepatotoxicity. Other acute side effects are rare with valproic acid, but bizzare behavior and hallucinations may occur in up to about 20% of treated patients. Weight gain, which occurs in over 40% of treated patients, may affect the disposition of valproic acid and other concomitantly used anticonvulsants. Tremors, hair loss, drowsiness, and hyperactivity occur in about 3% of treated patients.

Marty et al.[32] demonstrated changes in protein binding between doses of valproic acid indicating nonlinear protein binding and, more importantly, changes in the free fraction of the drug with changes in dose. Patel and Levy[33] have suggested that the variance in valproic acid protein binding may reflect competitive binding of valproic acid and free fatty acids for albumin and other serum proteins. Although total serum valproic acid measurements fail to demonstrate a clear relationship of serum concentration to therapeutic effect, total serum valproic acid concentrations are monitored. In early fetal development teratogenicity combined with higher than maternal unbound valproic acid serum concentrations is an additional concern. Unbound valproic acid serum concentrations have been suggested for monitoring patients, but therapeutic unbound concentrations have not been defined.

Logistics

Alcohol, tricyclic antidepressants, and monoamine oxidase inhibitors all add to the sedative effects of valproic acid. Valproic acid also displaces aspirin and warfarin from their binding sites on albumin increasing the risk of bleeding. Phenobarbital, primadone, and phenytoin also are displaced by valproic acid; thus total serum concentrations of these drugs decrease with concomitant valproic acid therapy.

Interpretation

The therapeutic range for valproic acid has been reported to range from 50–100 μg/mL, but a clear correlation between serum concentration and suppression of seizures is lacking. Variance in free (unbound) serum concentrations and the diurnal variations in protein binding and clearance add to the complexity of interpreting valproic acid serum concentrations. In spite of an increase in the free fraction of valproic acid with increasing doses, total serum concentrations of valproic acid continue to rise inferring that valproic acid either autoinhibits its metabolism or demonstrates saturable pharmacokinetics. There are increases in valproic acid free fractions among patients with renal disease, hypoalbuminemia, liver disease, burns, and in pregnancy. Likewise, elderly patients and patients with hyperlipidemia have increased free valproic acid concentrations. Because of the many changes, free concentration monitoring of valproic acid has been suggested; however, the therapeutic range for free valproic acid has not been defined (see below).

Test: Free Valproic Acid

Background and Selection

The protein binding of valproic acid averages 88.7% throughout the dosing interval. As such, the unbound or free concentration of valproic acid should warrant serum concentration monitoring.[34] Data from several sources indicate that the free fraction or unbound concentration ratio is not constant throughout the dosing interval and thus diurnal variation in unbound concentrations of valproic acid occurs as reported by Riva et al.[35] These authors noted considerable changes in the fluctuation in free concentrations over a 10-hour period form 08:00 to 18:00. Drug interaction with phenobarbital was proposed to explain the wide fluctuations noted in three of the patients, and free fatty acid concentration changes throughout the day were proposed for the other observed changes. Roman et al.[36] demonstrated a rather poor correlation between total and unbound valproic acid concentrations from blood samples obtained from 30 epileptic patients. Data demonstrated a wide scatter of points with a correlation coefficient of 0.68 and evidence suggestive for nonlinear protein binding. These authors demonstrated no predictable relationship between free and total valproic acid concentrations and thus recommended monitoring free rather than total valproic acid concentrations. Rene Levy[37] is one of the strongest advocates of free valproic acid serum concentration monitoring. The nonlinearity of valproic acid binding, its displacement by free fatty acids, and its low extraction ratio suggest that free concentration monitoring should be done. Rapeport et al.[38] demonstrated a close correlation of 0.934 between unbound valproic acid concentrations in serum and cerebrospinal fluid concentrations. The best arguments for unbound valproic acid serum concentration monitoring come from Haidukewych and Rodin,[39] Cramer et al.,[40] and Patel and Levy[41] who argue that drug and free fatty acid displacement of valproic acid warrants unbound concentration monitoring for patients managed with multiple anticonvulsants. Bauer et al.[42] and Riva et al.[43] affirm that in both the elderly and among pregnant patients, higher unbound concentrations occur with greater potential for adverse effects of the drug. Current monitoring of total valproic acid concentrations demonstrate wide therapeutic and toxic serum concentration ranges as well as wide ranges in serum concentrations with standard milligram per kilogram doses as discussed by Chadwick.[44]

Logistics

Drug Interactions

The principal drug interactions with valproic acid unbound serum concentration determinations involve displacement of valproic acid by anticonvulsants, aspirin, and potentially other drugs. In addition, disease states known to augment α_1-acid glycoprotein, or albumin binding are likely to disturb the protein binding and thus the unbound concentration of valproic acid. Uncontrolled or poorly managed diabetes mellitus and uremia will alter the valproic acid binding to albumin and hypoalbuminemic states, as occur with cirrhosis, pregnancy, and nephritis, will also affect free concentrations.

Analysis

Following ultrafiltration, the specimen is analyzed for free valproic acid concentrations using either GLC or by FPIA as described by Bauer et al.[42]

Interpretation

Definition of the unbound concentration therapeutic range for valproic acid remains controversial. Froscher et al.[45] studied 101 patients treated with valproic acid and were able to correlate seizure control and side effects. Others have not been able to demonstrate such a close correlation with free concentrations or to demonstrate predictable cerebrospinal fluid (CSF) concentrations from unbound concentrations. Data indicate that although unbound concentrations correlated with CSF concentrations, the CSF concentrations were substantially lower than unbound concentrations. The relationship between unbound concentrations and CSF concentrations appears to be the least perfect of the anticonvulsants. Therapeutic unbound serum valproic acid concentration ranges between 7 and 23 μg/mL (48.5 and 159.5 μmol/L) have been reported by Cramer et al.[40] with tremor occurring at unbound concentrations of 11–24 μg/mL (76.3–166.4 μmol/L) obtained 2 hours after estimated peak concentrations. The utility of unbound valproic acid serum concentration determination is likely to be limited to evaluation of potential fetal toxicity in pregnant patients and for the evaluation of tremor or other toxicity among patients with decreased serum albumin or a disease-induced decrease in valproic acid binding.

ANTIARRHYTHMIC DRUGS

Test: Disopyramide

Background and Selection

Disopyramide is a quinidine-like type 1a antiarrhythmic agent indicated for the treatment of atrial and ventricular arrhythmias. Disopyramide depresses myocardial responsiveness, slows automaticity, and raises the cardiac tissue threshold prolonging the effective refractory period.[46,47] Disopyramide prolongs cardiac conduction and also may cause "quinidine syncope." The n-dealkylated metabolite of disopyramide possesses

Table 13-11. Pharmacokinetic Parameters for the Cardiovascular Drugs

	Digoxin	Quinidine	Procainamide	Disopyramide
% Protein binding	20–40	70–95	15	10–65
Therapeutic concentrations	1.0–2.0 ng/mL	2.3–5.0 µg/mL	4.0–10.0 µg/mL	2.0–5.0 µg/mL
Toxic concentrations	>2.0 ng/mL	>6.0 µg/mL	>12.0 µg/mL	>5.0 µg/mL
Distribution volume (L/kg)	7.0	2.3	2.0	1.3
Distribution volume in congestive heart failure	5.0	1.8	1.6	0.85
Bioavailability	60–70%	60–90%	85%	95%
Half-life	1.6 d	4–7 h	3–4 h	4.5–9 h

anticholonergic activity and causes most of the reported side effects including the negative inotropic effect.[46] Accumulation of this metabolite in patients with renal failure (creatinine clearance less than 20–25 mL/min) precipitates congestive heart failure.[48] Dose adjustment for decreased renal function should not be accomplished using the Tozer equation (Table 13-3, equations 4 and 5) because patients have demonstrated considerable variance in apparent distribution volume and clearance. Pharmacokinetic parameters for disopyramide are listed in Table 13-11.

In general, dose adjustment based on total disopyramide serum concentrations is difficult.[49] Use of simple linear pharmacokinetic formulas such as cp 1/dose 1 = cp 2/dose 2 cannot be used for disopyramide dose adjustment (Table 13-12, equations 5 and 6) because this formula leads to underestimation of the desired dose. There has been considerable controversy concerning the distribution volume of disopyramide and in particular, the distribution volume in congestive heart failure. Because disopyramide protein binding is nonlinear (Fig. 13-9), the renal clearance and the fraction of the drug excreted unchanged in the urine decrease over the dosing interval as protein binding increases. The free (unbound) concentration therapeutic range of disopyramide has not been determined, but dosing methods using pharmacokinetic parameters derived from unbound serum concentration time data have been investigated. Sustained release disopyramide is available permitting less frequent dosing. The impact of such a product on the apparent total body clearance, distribution volume, and half-life remains to be investigated.[49,50]

Logistics

Drug interactions have been noted particularly with concomitant therapy with lidocaine, procainamide, propranolol and other β-blockers, quinidine, and verapamil. Disopyramide also appears to enhance effects of warfarin and oral antihyperglycemic agents. Metabolism of disopyramide is increased with concomitant treatment with phenobarbital, phenytoin, and rifampin.

Interpretation

Although serum concentrations of 2–4 µg/mL (5.9–11.8 µmol/L) are reported as the therapeutic range, higher serum concentrations (more than 6 µg/mL [>17.7 µmol/L]) are necessary to suppress ventricular

Table 13-12. Oral Dose Pharmacokinetic Formulas

Distribution volume = L/kg value × ideal body weight   (1)

$$\text{Steady-state peak} = \frac{(\text{bioavailability}) \times (\text{dose})}{(\text{distribution volume}) \times (1 - e^{-ke \times \text{dosing interval}})} \quad (2)$$

Trough = peak × $e^{-ke \times \text{dosing interval}}$ (3)

Dose = peak × distribution volume × 1 − $e^{-ke \times \text{dosing interval}}$ × bioavailability   (4)

$$\frac{\text{Trough 1}}{\text{Dose 1}} = X = \frac{\text{trough 2}}{\text{dose 2}} \quad (5)$$

$$\text{Desired dose} = \frac{\text{steady-state trough}}{\text{present dose} \times \text{desired trough}} \quad (6)$$

Abbreviations: e, base for natural log; ke, elimination rate constant.

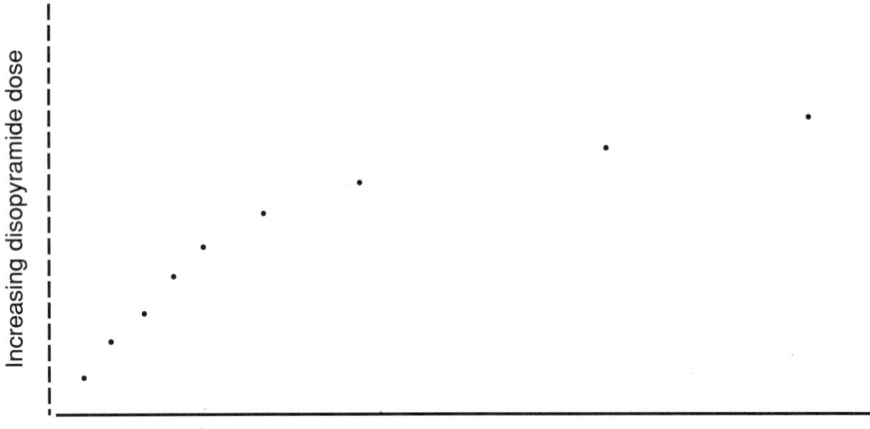

Fig. 13-9. Saturable protein binding occurring with increasing total serum concentrations of disopyramide. As total serum concentrations of disopyramide rise, the free fraction (the pharmacologically active form) of the drug increases.

arrhythmias.[46] Disopyramide therapeutic drug monitoring is complicated by nonlinear (saturable) protein binding within the therapeutic range (protein binding from 35–95%).[49,51] Considerable changes in free (unbound) disopyramide concentrations thus occur over a dosing interval as is shown in Figure 13-9. As the free (unbound) concentrations increase, the metabolism of disopyramide is increased, thus disopyramide pharmacokinetic parameters are difficult to determine and are not constant over a dosing interval.

Test: Encainide

Background and Selection

Encainide, an antiarrhythmic drug of the Ic class, is highly effective for refractory arrhythmias not responding to conventional 1a and 1b antiarrhythmic agents. Encainide is most effective for ventricular arrhythmias and less effective for supraventricular arrhythmias. It is ineffective for the management of atrial fibrillation. Like other members of the class 1 antiarrhythmic agents, encainide prolongs the QRS complex, the QT interval, and has negative inotropic effects. It differs from other members of its class; it is more effective on the PR and QT intervals than on the QRS complex and has less of a negative inotropic effect. Encainide shortens the action potential duration, slows sodium influx via slow and fast channels, and lengthens the effective refractory period.[52,53] Encainide has a half-life of approximately 21 hours. Encainide undergoes extensive hepatic biotransformation of o-demethyl encainide, 3 methyoxy-o-demethyl encainide, and n-desmethyl encainide. The major metabolite ODE has a half-life of 8 hours and is a more potent antiarrhythmic than the parent compound. The most common side effects from encainide are tremors, blurred vision, and dizziness with the incidence of side effects correlating with doses greater than 100 mg/24 h.

Electrophysiology studies have demonstrated that encainide and flecainide have the potential to induce as well as suppress arrhythmias due to their unique activity on sodium channels. Among the potential drug-induced arrhythmias were sudden death arrhythmias, and recently both encainide and flecainide were demonstrated to have a significantly higher risk of drug-induced arrhythmias. As a result, the indications for the use of both encainide and flecainide have been restricted to serious life-threatening arrhythmias.

Logistics

An HPLC assay that is capable of measuring encainide serum concentrations and its metabolites has been published; ODE, MODE, and NDE.

Interpretation

Some authors have noted a nonlinear relationship between resulting serum concentrations and increasing doses of encainide. Therapeutic concentrations of ODE range form 100–300 mg/mL (300–900 nmol/L) and for MODE from 60–280 ng/mL (165–760 nmol/L). With acute therapy, ODE, a metabolite with greater potency than encainide, is noted to rise in serum concentrations. MODE and NDE are about as potent as encainide and for patients with efficient encainide metabolism, both ODE and MODE exceed the encainide serum concentrations.

Test: Flecainide

Background and Selection

Flecainide is a class Ic antiarrhythmic agent that produces a concentration dependent inhibition of sodium influx in a manner similar to other members of the class and like lidocaine, appears to affect calcium entry in the conducting tissues as well. Flecainide's principal pharmacologic effect is the slowing of impulse conduction with less effect on refractoriness, repolarization time, and action potential duration. Conduction of impulses though the His-Purkinje system is markedly affected by the presence of flecainide giving rise to prolongation of the PR interval, QRS complex, and QT interval. Flecainide exhibits mild negative inotropic effects and should be used with caution in patients with coronary artery disease, recent myocardial infarction, and congestive heart failure.[52,54]

Flecainide, like encainide, is a benzanilide antiarrhythmic agent with slowed binding to the sodium channels of cardiac tissue. As a result of this pharmacodynamic activity at sodium channels, there is a potential for drug-induced arrhythmias including sudden death arrhythmias. A recent study of antiarrhythmic agents noted an increased risk of sudden death arrhythmias among patients treated with encainide or flecainide. As a result, the widespread use of these agents for arrhythmias has been curtailed and the drugs have been limited to the treatment of serious life-threatening arrhythmias.

Flecainide is rapidly and almost completely absorbed from the gastrointestinal tract with peak concentrations occurring 2–3 hours after an oral dose. Early disposition studies with flecainide indicate possible mixed order pharmacokinetics with both linear and nonlinear processes occurring simultaneously. The distribution volume for flecainide ranges from 5.5–8.7 L/kg indicating substantial tissue binding and sequestration. Serum protein binding, which is primarily to α_1-acid glycoprotein, ranges from 40–50%. The half-life of flecainide ranges from 7–25 hours in healthy adults.

Approximately 25–40% of the total clearance of flecainide occurs through the kidney. Adjustment of doses for renal impairment with formulas such as the Tozer equation (Table 13-3, equation 5) inadequately predicts changes in clearance and half-life.[52,54] Adverse effects of flecainide include dizziness, headaches, paresthesias, and visual disturbances (including diplopia and blurred vision). Cardiac effects include induction of arrhythmias, first degree heart block, and torsades de pointes. About 10% of treated patients show gastrointestinal side effects, whereas malaise, rash, and fever occur in 1–3% of patients.

Logistics

Combinations of antiarrhythmic agents can give rise to arrhythmogenicity, additive effects, synergism, and antagonism. The combination of flecainide and amiodarone appears to permit lowering of amiodarone doses by 30–50%, thus reducing the risk of amiodarone toxicity. Flecainide interferes with the disposition of digoxin increasing serum concentrations by 15–25%. Concomitant flecainide and propranolol therapy increases the serum concentrations of both drugs and the risk for synergistic negative inotropic effects. Verapamil should not be used in patients receiving flecainide, because of the combined effects of these two drugs on the atrioventricular node. Cimetidine appears to reduce hepatic biotransformation and active renal tubular secretion of flecainide, thus flecainide doses should be reduced.

Interpretation

Therapeutic serum concentrations of flecainide are from 0.2–0.6 µg/mL (0.5–1.4 µmol/L). The therapeutic effects of flecainide correlate with serum concentrations, but changes in PR, QRS, and QT intervals do not correlate with increasing serum concentrations. Toxicity appears to correlate with serum concentrations in excess of 1.0 µg/mL (2.4 µmol/L). Changes in serum digoxin concentrations do not appear to be clinically significant, but patients receiving concomitant digoxin therapy should be monitored carefully for digoxin toxicity.

Test: Lidocaine

Background and Selection

Lidocaine is a class Ib antiarrhythmic agent indicated for the prophylactic management of immediately post myocardial infarction patients. Lidocaine differs from other class 1b antiarrhythmic agents in that it is rapidly cleared by hepatic biotransformation and thus is used clinically as a continuous infusion. As with other antiarrhythmic agents, variance in protein binding, distribution volume, and hepatic clearance complicate therapeutic dose prediction and thus therapeutic drug monitoring is required. Standard doses of lidocaine result in serum concentrations outside the therapeutic range in almost 40% of treated patients with toxicity reported in 15%.[55]

The half-life for lidocaine is thought to range from 1–2 hours with a prolongation in half-life following myocardial infarction, congestive heart failure, and liver disease. Lidocaine is principally metabolized by n-dealkylation to monoethyl-glycinexylidide (MEGX) and glycinexylidide (GX). These two metabolites are further metabolized to xylidine and hydroxyxylidine, which are the principal urinary metabolites. For patients with renal impairment, MEGX accumulates from 20 to over 60% lidocaine serum concentration with a greater free fraction in serum than does lidocaine. Because MEGX has about 80% of the potency of lidocaine, it may contribute to the pharmacologic effects of lidocaine particularly in acute myocardial infarction complicated by renal impairment. MEGX is not measured as lidocaine with the current immunoassays. The activity of this metabolite and its potential toxicity remain controversial. Measurement of MEGX by FPIA is in development and may be beneficial in evaluating possible lidocaine toxicity. As compared with MEGX, GX is less protein bound but has a much longer half-life. For most patients with renal impairment, MEGX and GX do not accumulate to toxic serum concentrations, thus early discontinuation of lidocaine in all renal patients may not be justifiable.[56] Aging appears to reduce both the clearance and the distribution of lidocaine.

Logistics

Drug Interactions

Propranolol and other β-blockers decrease hepatic perfusion thus affecting the hepatic clearance of lidocaine. Cimetidine reduces hepatic clearance by competing for cytochrome P_{450} thus decreasing lidocaine biotransformation. Phenytoin and phenobarbital induce cytochrome P_{450} thus increasing its hepatic biotransformation.

Specimen Collection

With serum separator tubes lower than actual serum lidocaine concentrations may be reported.

Interpretation

The therapeutic range for lidocaine is 1.5–5 μg/mL (6.4–21.4 μmol/L) when α_1-acid glycoprotein levels are less than 100 mg/dL (1000 μg/L). Lidocaine is used in acute management of intensive care patients: in these patients frequently α_1-acid glycoprotein (orsomucoid) synthesis has been induced. Because of the extensive binding of lidocaine and other antiarrhythmics to this serum protein, the total serum concentrations of lidocaine will appear to rise acutely while the patient response declines. Studies of free (unbound) lidocaine concentrations among these patients have demonstrated a marked decrease in unbound (pharmacologically active) lidocaine due to increased serum protein binding with decreased tissue distribution.

Test: Mexiletine

Background and Selection

Mexiletine is a class Ib antiarrhythmic agent with a pharmacologic profile similar to lidocaine. The drug demonstrates anesthetic, antiarrhythmic, and anticonvulsant properties by altering fast sodium channel activity. Mexiletine shortens the action potential duration and decreases the effective refractory period. Mexiletine appears to be rapidly absorbed within 1.5 hours of ingestion and serum concentration time data indicate the drug demonstrates a two compartment open model (Fig. 13-5). The half-life for mexiletine ranges from 8–14 hours.[52] Renal impairment (greater than 10 mL/min creatinine clearance) and congestive heart failure appear to have little impact on the disposition of mexiletine, but the half-life is markedly prolonged in patients with hepatic failure. The protein binding of mexiletine is about 75%, the drug is well absorbed from the gut, and is extensively metabolized by the liver. Like other antiarrhythmic agents, mexiletine is actively secreted in the urine and this pathway of elimination appears to be pH dependent.

Logistics

Drug Interactions

Antacids and cimetidine therapy have been reported to affect the disposition of mexiletine. Narcotic analgesia may cause a partial ileus thus affecting the absorption of the drug and treatment with metoclopramide reverses this decreased absorption. Enzyme inducers such as the anticonvulsants effect the disposition of mexiletine resulting in a decrease in total serum concentrations.

Assay

Mexiletine is measured by HPLC using a fluorescence detector with precolumn derivitization as described by McErlane et al.[57] Assays using GLC have also been published. Currently no immunoassay has been developed or marketed for mexiletine or tocainide.

Interpretation

Mexiletine has a narrow therapeutic range of 0.75–2.0 µg/mL and most of the toxic effects of the drug are serum concentration related.[52] Side effects reported for mexiletine include tremor, diplopia, nausea, and vomiting in up to 70% of treated patients. These effects appear to be serum concentration dependent and patients often respond to dose reduction.

Test: N-Acetyl Procainamide (NAPA)

See Test: Procainamide/NAPA below.

Test: Procainamide/NAPA

Background and Selection

Procainamide is a class Ia antiarrhythmic agent that decreases automaticity and the action potential thus prolonging the effective refractory period and action potential duration by interfering with potassium fluxes. Like quinidine, procainamide prolongs the QRS complex, the PR interval, and the QT_c by approximately 10–25%.[58] Procainamide is an extremely potent antiarrhythmic agent indicated for atrial and ventricular arrhythmias. Intravenous procainamide is used to treat lidocaine refractory ventricular arrhythmias. Procainamide is metabolized to NAPA, which is then hydroxylated, deacetylated, de-ethylated, and metabolized to yet undetermined metabolites.[59] Although NAPA formation depends on patient fast or slow acetylator status, this does not predict differences in procainamide disposition.[60,61] Side effects of procainamide include skin rashes and itching that usually occur in patients with allergies, local anesthetics, thrombocytopenia, leukopenia, and hemolytic anemia and fevers. Nausea, vomiting, and anorexia are serum concentration-related side effects of procainamide and NAPA warranting serum concentration determination. Procainamide induces a systemic lupus-like disease possibly by the production of an epoxide metabolite.[62] Patients with drug-induced systemic lupus erythematosus usually complain of fever and joint pain and most often do not have a rash or renal disease.

Logistics

Drug Interactions

Procainamide in combination with other antiarrhythmic agents may aggravate arrhythmias in patients; thus, the addition of other antiarrhythmic agents must be carefully evaluated. Procainamide may increase and prolong the neuromuscular blockade induced by curariform drugs. Equation 5 in Table 13-12 provides a simple method for dose adjustment using steady-state serum concentrations. Absorption of procainamide may be significantly delayed; Figure 13-10 demonstrates this delayed absorption and the complications in interpreting single trough concentrations.

Blood Collection and Analysis

After initiation of continuous infusion therapy, blood samples for procainamide should not be obtained for at least 2 hours and NAPA concentrations should not be obtained until after 12–24 hours. Various dosage forms including sustained release procainamide products are available and differing blood sampling strategies for sustained release products are needed (Fig. 13-7). Blood samples for sustained release procainamide products are collected at 4 hours after dose administration or drawn just before the next dose. Either method will provide information that can be used for pharmacokinetic dose adjustment using the continuous infusion equation (Table 13-13, equation 1). The HPLC method permits the simultaneous determination of both procainamide and NAPA concentrations and may have an advantage when monitoring patients with renal impairment.

Interpretation

Therapeutic serum concentrations range from 4–10 µg/mL (17–42.5 µmol/L) and the pharmacokinetics of procainamide are complex enough to make dose prediction difficult.[63] Recent electrophysiologic study data indicate that procainamide concentrations in excess of 10 µg/mL (42.5 µmol/L) may be required for particularly aggressive arrhythmias. Procainamide and NAPA serum concentrations should be added and this sum should not exceed 25–30 µg/mL (106–128 µmol/L).[63,64] Toxicity does not commonly occur until serum concentrations of 12 µg/mL (51 µmol/L) are exceeded at which point "quinidine syncope" occurs complicated with hypotension, conduction disturbances, and ventricular tachycardia, which can progress to cardiac arrest.[63] Electrophysiologic studies using procainamide have demonstrated that many refractory arrhythmias require serum concentrations above 8 µg/mL (>34

354 • Laboratory Medicine

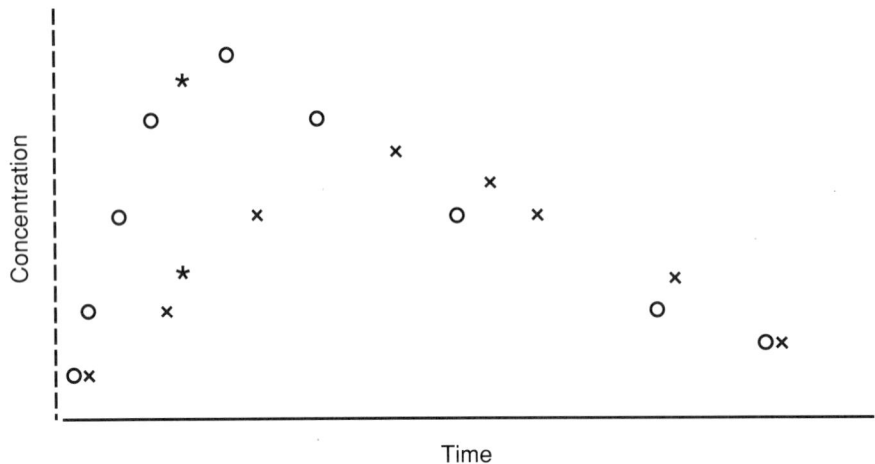

Fig. 13-10. Variance in the absorption of procainamide. Serum concentration time data are presented for a patient with normal (o) and a patient with delayed (x) drug absorption. At 1 hour after ingestion, the patient with delayed absorption (bottom asterisk) appears subtherapeutic although trough concentrations for both patients are very close and are more predictable.

μmol/L).[63] Procainamide will induce heart block at serum concentrations greater than 20 μg/mL (>85 μmol/L) or at NAPA plus procainamide sums in excess of 30 μg/mL (>128 μmol/L).[65]

Test: Propranolol

Background and Selection

Propranolol is a β-blocker used for the treatment of hypertension, angina pectoris, and for the acute management of arrhythmias of atrial and ventricular origin. Propranolol is structurally related to the local anesthetics and shares many of the characteristics of this class of drugs as well as its β-receptor activity. Propranolol is a class II antiarrhythmic agent with quinidine-like activity. Propranolol is mainly used for its suppression of conduction of impulses through the atrioventricular node especially in patients with atrial fi-

Table 13-13. Continuous Infusion Formulas

$$C_{ss} = \frac{K_o}{TBC} \quad (1)$$

$$TBC = \frac{K_o}{C_{ss}} \quad (2)$$

$$K_o \text{ desired} = TBC \times \text{desired } C_{ss} \quad (3)$$

Abbreviations: Css, steady-state concentration; Ko, rate of infusion; TBC, total body clearance.

brillation and symptomatic supraventricular tachycardias. The major manifestation of overdose is atrioventricular dissociation progressing to cardiac arrest. Treatment of propranolol overdoses is accomplished by the administration of glucagon that has innate inotropic effects acting independently of the β-receptors.

Unlike other antiarrhythmic agents, the relationship between serum concentrations and the desired therapeutic effects has not been demonstrated. Variance in β-receptors may explain this variance in the serum concentration-response relationship. The introduction of esmolol (an ultrashort acting β-blocker with a 6-minute half-life) has just about eliminated the need for continuous propranolol infusions for tachycardias, but continuous propranolol infusions may be necessary in patients not responding to esmolol.

Propranolol's disposition is complicated by an extensive first pass effect and apparent nonlinear pharmacokinetics within the therapeutic range.[66] Therapeutic drug monitoring in propranolol treated patients is most helpful in evaluating treatment failure with large oral or parenteral doses. Propranolol is extensively protein bound (85–95%) with an exceedingly large distribution volume averaging 200–300 L indicating extensive tissue binding. α_1-Acid glycoprotein accounts for most of the serum binding of propranolol and acute changes in this protein will have major effects on the pharmacologic response. A minor metabolite of propranolol, 4-hydroxypropranolol, is produced only with oral doses of propranolol. The enzyme biotransforming propranolol is saturated at therapeutic doses; thus, with chronic doses, the ratio of propranolol to its active metabolite 4-hydroxypropranolol increases.

Logistics

Drug Interactions

Indomethacin antagonizes the antihypertensive effects of propranolol. Cimetidine reduces hepatic biotransformation of propranolol. Synergistic toxicity at the atrioventricular node occurs when calcium entry blockers or digoxin are used concomitantly with propranolol.

Assay

Propranolol serum concentrations have been assayed by published methods using HPLC, GLC, radioimmunoassay (RIA), and thin-layer chromatography (TLC). Several HPLC methods have been published that are superior to the other methods. All current methods are designed to measure total propranolol concentrations. Free concentration monitoring has been done investigationally and data indicate similar problems with interpretation of total serum concentrations noted with valproic acid (see Test: Free Valproic Acid).

Interpretation

The therapeutic range for serum propranolol is from 25–100 ng/mL (96–386 nmol/L) with serum concentrations in excess of 100 ng/mL (386 nmol/L) necessary for maintaining complete β-blockage of the heart.[67] Evaluation serum of propranolol concentrations is difficult because there is no close correlation between serum concentrations and desired pharmacologic effects. For propranolol overdoses, serum concentrations do not reliably predict the rate of propranolol elimination or provide meaningful pharmacokinetic data. Monitoring of 4-hydroxypropranolol is considered unnecessary because its formation is rate limited.

Test: Quinidine

Background and Selection

Quinidine is a type 1a antiarrhythmic agent with direct and indirect effects on cardiac tissue, thus affecting automaticity, conduction velocity, and membrane potential of cardiac tissue.[58,68,69] These effects result in the prolongation of the effective refractory period and widening of the QRS complex. Quinidine has antimuscarinic effects that blunt vagal regulation and also is an α-adrenergic blocker.[58] Quinidine was first used in France to treat atrial fibrillation in 1749 and still is used to treat atrial fibrillation and flutter, premature atrial contractions, paroxysmal supraventricular tachycardia, premature ventricular contractions, ventricular tachycardias, and as prophylaxis against ventricular fibrillation.[58]

Quinidine sulfate is usually 70–80% absorbed, whereas quinidine gluconate bioavailability ranges from 60–70%. Quinidine has been reported to cause drug fevers, thrombocytopenia, hemolytic anemias, hepatitis, asthma, and respiratory depression as well as rashes, urticaria, psoriasis-like lesions, and exfoliation of the skin.[58] Patients with glucose 6-phosphate dehydrogenase deficiency also may develop hemolytic anemia.

Drug absorption may range from 40–80% and varies with the sulfate and the gluconate salts. Quinidine is extensively metabolized by liver enzymes with only 20% excreted unchanged in the urine.[58] Quinidine is eliminated mainly by hydroxylation of the quinidine molecule to active and inactive metabolites that are conjugated with glucuronic acid and excreted in the bile or urine. Between 60 and 80% of a dose of quinidine is metabolized and at least two have antiarrhythmic activity.[70,71] Thus, the liver plays a principal role in the elimination of quinidine and any change in this metabolizing capacity effects disposition of the drug causing a smaller required loading dose and maintenance dose of quinidine.

For patients with right-sided heart failure and hepatic congestion, hepatic metabolism of quinidine is likely to be decreased as is the distribution volume.[2,72] Observed changes in the distribution volume with congestive heart may actually reflect changes in tissue perfusion and differences in acute versus stable congestive heart failure. Quinidine metabolites accumulate in renal failure and are not substantially removed by peritoneal dialysis. Serum concentration monitoring is particularly important for patients with hypokalemia, congestive heart failure, acute or chronic renal failure, and liver disease. Certain types of patients should be monitored very carefully with therapeutic drug monitoring of serum concentration. These include patients with myocardial infarction, those treated concomitantly with cimetidine or anticonvulsants, and patients with unusual cardiac rhythms.

Logistics

Drug Interactions

Quinidine in combination with other antiarrhythmic agents or with reserpine may induce serious arrhythmias. Quinidine also has additive effects on the anticoagulant effects of warfarin, thus doses of warfarin need to be reduced and prothrombin time monitored closely. Quinidine competes with digoxin for uptake into cardiac and muscle tissue resulting in greater central nervous system digoxin toxicity. Phenytoin, phenobarbital, and rifampin induce hepatic metabolism of quinidine with resulting reduction in serum concentrations.

Specimen Collection and Assay

Quinidine trough concentrations are usually collected just prior to ingestion of the next oral dose of the drug. Blood should be obtained from an evacuated glass tube with a rubber stopper (red top tube) containing no anticoagulant. Harvested sera may be assayed by several methods including an HPLC method using acid back extraction and a fluorescence detection as described by Patel et al. and others. Hemolyzed, hyperbilirubin, or lipemic samples may not be read correctly by the EMIT assay, but do not appear to be a problem with the FPIA method. The quinidine metabolites 3-hydroxyquinidine, 2'-quinidinone, o-desmethylquinidine, and dihydroquinidine are measured as quinidine with fluorometry and some immunoassays.

Interpretation

The therapeutic range for quinidine is 2–5 µg/mL (6.2–15.4 µmol/L), but varies with the assay used. Serum quinidine concentrations in excess of 6 µg/mL (18.5 µmol/L) are considered toxic. Serum concentrations of quinidine correlate with its pharmacologic effects, but Ha et al.[73] also have noted that free quinidine concentrations may better predict the desired pharmacologic effects of quinidine.[72]

Test: Tocainide

Background and Selection

Tocainide is a class Ic antiarrhythmic with similar structure to lidocaine and mexiletine and is classified as an "oral lidocaine." Tocainide suppresses all refractory periods when used in electrophysiologic studies in patients with severe ventricular arrhythmias.[52] Like lidocaine, the QRS complex is minimally effected by the drug and the QT_c is decreased or unchanged in the presence of the drug. Minimal changes that most resemble the effects of lidocaine also occur in the AH and HV intervals in the presence of tocainide.

The bioavailability of tocainide is about 90%, and at steady-state about 40% of the drug is excreted unchanged in the urine. Tocainide is extensively metabolized to lactoxylidide (LX) and tocainide carbamoyl glucuronide (TG). The half-life of tocainide ranges from 11–15 hours, whereas that of LX averages 29 hours and of TG is 13 hours.[74] Monitoring of the metabolites of tocainide is not as important as with other antiarrhythmic agents, because these metabolites appear to have no pharmacologic activity.

The distribution volume for tocainide ranges from 1.6–2.9 L/kg in healthy volunteers and from 1.4–3.2 L/kg in patients with myocardial infarction. Renal clearance of tocainide appears to be pH dependent as has been observed with other antiarrhythmic agents. For patients with congestive heart failure, limited data indicate that the distribution volume is contracted to an average of 1.36 L/kg. No change in distribution of volume was noted with renal failure, but with hepatic failure the average distribution volume was 3.8 L/kg with a half-life of 27 hours.

Suppression of the number of premature ventricular contractions is correlated with serum tocainide concentrations, although a clear relationship between therapeutic concentrations and therapeutic effect has not been demonstrated. Patients treated with tocainide have been reported to have central nervous system toxicity characterized by hallucinations, severe confusion, and paranoid behavior. Other reported side effects include anorexia, nausea and vomiting, lightheadedness, tremor, sweating, pathesthesias, and altered vision and hearing. Pulmonary infiltrates with symptoms of pneumonitis also have been described.

Logistics

Drug Interactions

Anticonvulsants are likely to induce the metabolism of tocainide. Combinations of antiarrhythmic agents are more likely to induce arrhythmias; therefore, combinations of tocainide with other antiarrhythmic agents should be monitored carefully.

Assay

Serum tocainide concentrations may be determined by several methods including several published HPLC and GLC methods. Currently no immunoassay methods are available and the toxicity profile of the drug may have reduced interest in developing immunoassays for the drug.

Interpretation

Electrophysiologic studies have demonstrated a therapeutic range for tocainide of 4–10 µg/mL (20.8–52.0 µ/mol/L), but for serious ventricular arrhythmias serum concentrations tocainide in excess of 6 μg/mL (31.2 μmol/L) may be necessary to suppress ectopy. For some arrhythmias, serum concentrations in excess of 10 μg/mL (52 μmol/L) may be necessary, but often serum concentrations in excess of this will result in a high incidence of unwanted side effects.[52]

CARDIAC GLYCOSIDES

Test: Digoxin

Background and Selection

Digoxin remains a controversial drug for the treatment of congestive heart failure with about one-third of the treated patients benefiting from chronic digoxin therapy.[75,76] Digoxin is a plant steroid conjugated with amino sugars that affect the activity of adenosinetriphosphatase (ATPase). The half-life for digoxin ranges from 1.8–5.6 days, and it takes approximately 2–4 weeks for a patient to reach steady-state. The distribution volume of digoxin varies little; however, this is not the case with digoxin clearance. Thus, clearance changes have considerable impact on individual patient digoxin half-lives. Seventy percent of the total body clearance of digoxin is renal clearance, thus changes in renal function will have major impact on digoxin clearance. Pharmacokinetic parameters for digoxin may be found in Table 13-11.

The distribution volume of digoxin can be calculated by multiplying the ideal body weight times the 7.3 L/kg distribution volume, but 6.0 L/kg should be used for congestive heart failure and 5.0 L/kg for renal or hepatic failure. Estimates of clearance can be used to adjust doses of digoxin. The Tozer equation can be used to estimate the half-life due to renal impairment or to calculate a maintenance dose reduction (see Table 13-3, equation 4 or 5).[11] The Tozer equation adjusts for the contribution of renal clearance to total body clearance by a factor designated as "kidney function." *Kidney function* is defined as the ratio of the patient's creatinine clearance and the creatinine clearance for normal renal function (100 mL/min). The equations for this dosing method can be found in Table 13-3 as well. For this formula, the maintenance dose or the half-life for patients with normal renal function can be obtained from reference sources such as *The American Hospital Formulary Service, Clinical Use of Drugs in Patients with Kidney and Liver Disease*, or *Clinical Drug Data*. However, subtle changes in renal and hepatic function may not be fully corrected, and careful patient monitoring will be required.

The distribution volume is decreased in patients with renal impairment and immunoassay methods measure digoxin, some of its metabolites, and digoxin-like substances in serum and urine particularly among end-stage renal disease patients. Digoxin is metabolized by removing amino sugars from the digoxigenin (steroid) nucleus. All amino sugar conjugates are pharmacologically active, but all dihydro metabolites and sulfated conjugates are pharmacologically inactive. The metabolized drug and the parent compound are eliminated (60–80%) by glomerular filtration. In renal impairment, hepatic biotransformation may account for 75% of the elimination of digoxin by formation of dihydrogenin conjugates.

Logistics

Drug Interactions

Verapamil has been reported to reduce the hepatic clearance of digoxin, whereas anticonvulsants have been reported to increase its hepatic clearance. Cimetidine effects the renal tubular secretion of several drugs, but its effects on digoxin clearance have not been described. Serum digoxin concentrations should be obtained at 2–3 days after the start of quinidine therapy. For some patients, a significant rise in serum digoxin concentrations occurs, with such rises being as great as 2.5 times the stable digoxin serum concentrations.[77–79] Quinidine's effect on digoxin tubular secretion has been described in hypoakalemic and hyponatremic patients, where digoxin accumulates in the brain causing extensive central nervous system side effects without cardiac toxicity.[73–75] The same mechanism preventing active secretion also prevents the uptake of digoxin in peripheral tissues leading to accumulation of digoxin in the brain.

Analysis

Currently, digoxin serum concentrations are determined using RIA, EMIT, and FPIA methods. RIA methods are accurate but require prolonged incubation time and disposal of radioactive waste. Assay problems emerge with the use of hemolyzed or hyperbilirubinemic serum with the EMIT assay. Digoxin-like reactive species in serum also will affect digoxin serum concentration determinations in infants, patients with hypertension and renal and hepatic failure, and third trimester pregnancy females. For pediatric monitoring, dilution of both the antiserum and iodine labeled digoxin prior to addition to the serum samples combined with a longer incubation period appears to resolve the problem. For immunoassays, the digoxin-like immunoreactive substance can be removed by ultrafiltration of the serum sample and then assaying the ultrafiltrate.

For patients treated with digoxin binding Fab globulins, measurement of serum digoxin concentrations are complicated by the appearance of measured Fab fragment bound digoxin along with the unbound drug. This can be resolved by ultrafiltration of plasma samples that will leave the Fab bound drug behind the filter permitting a determination of the active digoxin in the serum.

Interpretation

The therapeutic index for digoxin is very narrow, and over 75% of patients in the high therapeutic range (1.5–2 ng/mL [1.9–2.6 nmol/L]) will have side effects. It is important to not overreact to elevated digoxin levels before carefully determining the time of dose administration, the time of sampling, and the serum creatinine.[80] Often early sampling is the cause of apparent elevated digoxin serum concentrations. The bioavailability of the various dosage forms of digoxin also affects serum concentrations particularly if the oral microgram dose of digoxin is administered as the elixir or parenterally (Table 13-14). Lower serum concentrations may occur in hospitalized patients due to generic digoxin usage, diarrhea, high fiber diets, and untreated hyperthyroidism. Food and gastric resection do not impair digoxin absorption.

Digoxin toxicity is a serious complication of digoxin therapy in the elderly and in the management of symptomatic atrial fibrillation, often resulting in empiric and overly aggressive digoxin loading. For patients with serum concentrations in excess of 6 ng/mL (>7.7 nmol/L) serious toxicity is likely with resulting bradycardia and atrioventricular nodal block. In addition to the management of the arrhythmias with phenytoin, a recent antibody fragment product has been marketed for the management of digoxin overdoses. As with charcoal hemoperfusion discussed in Chapter 14, the use of antibody products to reduce the toxicity of drug overdoses may result in variable responses in some tissues. Digoxin has an extremely large distribution volume and therefore the Fab fragments must greatly increase the hepatic and renal clearance of digoxin in order to have a substantial effect in preventing the full range of digoxin toxicity. Arguments against such methods note that little drug is actually removed from the patient by either digibind or charcoal hemoperfusion of drugs with large distribution volumes. Others argue that the patient's symptoms in some organ systems are improved with "adsorption" of the drug from the systemic circulation. Clearly the cardiovascular symptoms at the atrioventricular node will be most affected by the digoxin binding Fab product; thus, patients demonstrating digoxin-induced arrhythmias will most benefit, and patients demonstrating gastrointestinal or central nervous system toxicity from digoxin are likely to have more variable responses.

Test: Digitoxin

Background and Selection

Digitoxin differs from digoxin in that it has a longer half-life and smaller distribution volume. The half-life averages 7.6 days and the distribution volume is 0.73 L/kg. Only 25% of the drug is excreted unchanged in the urine, and one of its metabolites is digoxin. Approximately 70% of an oral dose is absorbed and between 30 and 50% of a dose is metabolized by the liver. Digitoxin is greater than 90% protein bound; thus, the distribution volume of digitoxin is considerably smaller than digoxin.

Logistics

Diuretics and glucocorticoids waste potassium and thus aggravate cardiac glycoside toxicity. Antacids and kaolin suspensions indicated for the treatment of diar-

Table 13-14. Digoxin Dosing Formulas

Digoxin clearance = 1.0 × Clcr + 40 mL/min nonrenal clearance   (1)

$$\text{Maintenance dose} = \frac{\text{digoxin TBC} \times \text{C ave ss} \times \text{24-h dosing interval}}{\text{bioavailability}} \quad (2)$$

    Intravenous dose bioavailability is 1.0
    Oral tablet bioavailability is 0.6
    Lanoxicap and lanoxin elixir bioavailability is 0.8

$$\text{Daily dose (mg/d)} = \frac{(3.56 \times \text{Clcr}) + 93}{1000} \quad (3)$$

Abbreviations: Clcr, creatinine clearance; TBC, total body clearance; C ave ss, average steady-state concentration.

rhea and bile acid resins affect cardiac glycoside absorption. Sympathomimetics add to the pharmacologic effects of cardiac glycosides. Barbiturates and anticonvulsants are well known inducers of hepatic biotransformation that reduce digitoxin serum concentrations. Quinidine causes accumulation of digoxin in the brain.

Interpretation

The therapeutic range for digitoxin is 15–30 ng/mL (19.2–38.5 nmol/L) and digitoxin toxicity with symptoms similar to those described for digoxin occurs at serum concentrations about 35 ng/mL (44.8 nmol/L).

PSYCHOTROPIC AGENTS (SEE CH. 14)

Desipramine

Background and Selection

Desipramine is the active secondary amine metabolite of the tricyclic antidepressant, imipramine. Like other secondary amine metabolites of antidepressants, desipramine causes greater norepinephrine than serotonin turnover in contrast to imipramine, which has more marked effects of serotonin turnover. Catecholamine turnover effects though are short-lived following initiation of therapy, and tricyclic antidepressants may exert their pharmacologic effects by altering receptor expression in the synaptic cleft rather than by preventing the reuptake of catecholamines in the synaptic cleft. All of the tricyclic antidepressants have an approximately 70% response rate and patients may respond to one agent while failing therapy with others. Desipramine has anticholinergic effects that account for most of the drug's side effects including blurred vision, urinary retention, dry mouth, and arrhythmias following toxic ingestions.

Logistics

There is a relative contraindication for administering both monoamine oxidase inhibitors and tricyclic antidepressants together and their concomitant use should be carefully monitored in treated patients.

Interpretation

Less information is available concerning the therapeutic range of desipramine than the other tricyclic antidepressants. Serum concentrations of about 145 ng/mL have been reported to be effective for the management of depression, but lower serum concentrations have resulted in the desired therapeutic effects as well. For all of the tricyclic antidepressants, serum concentrations in excess of 1700 ng/mL are associated with a high incidence of cardiac arrhythmias and permanent cardiac damage.

Test: Imipramine

Background and Selection

Imipramine is a tertiary amine tricyclic antidepressant with moderate sedating side effects due to initial increased serotonin turnover in treated patients. Imipramine is indicated for the management of endogenous depression with an approximately 70% of patients responding to therapy. Similar to other tricyclic antidepressants, imipramine demonstrates anticholinergic side effects such as blurred vision, urinary retention, and dry mouth. Like amitriptyline, imipramine is metabolized to desipramine and thus the pharmacologic effect of the drug may be due to concentrations of imipramine and desipramine. Imipramine and the other tricyclic antidepressants were noted to affect catecholamine turnover and this was proposed as their mechanism of action and pharmacologic effect. Recent studies have demonstrated that this effect is short-lived and that there must be other mechanisms for their pharmacologic action. Recent research indicates that chronic therapy with tricyclic antidepressants may induce changes in the relative concentrations of receptors in the synaptic clefts of nerves and that alterations in mood may reflect these receptor concentration changes.

Logistics

There is a relative contraindication for the coadministration of monoamine oxidase inhibitors and tricyclic antidepressants; thus, patients treated with this combination should be monitored carefully. Alcohol and other central nervous system depressants may add to the sedative effects of imipramine and anticonvulsants may reduce serum concentrations. Centrally acting antihypertensives such as clonidine, guanabenz, and alphamethyldopa also may add to the sedative effects of this drug.

Interpretation

Therapeutic response is correlated with serum concentrations greater than 180 ng/mL. Although a therapeutic window has been demonstrated for other tricyclic agents, this is not the case for imipramine.

Test: Lithium

Background and Selection

Lithium is used for the management of manic depression, and migraine and cluster headaches. The mood stabilizing effects of lithium are thought to relate to decreased catecholamine release due to disturbed sodium-potassium exchange or due to decreased cyclic adenosine monophosphate (cAMP) synthesis or increased degradation. For vascular headaches, the mechanism of action has not been characterized, but likely also involves the decreased concentrations of cAMP in vascular smooth muscle. Altered release of histamine and serotonin caused by lithium also may alter the course of cluster headaches. The half-life of lithium is reported to range from 18–24 hours in adults and may be as long as 36 hours in elderly patients. Lithium demonstrates a biphasic serum concentration decline with a distribution phase lasting 5–6 hours followed by an elimination phase (Fig. 13-5). Lithium is almost completely eliminated in the urine with extensive renal tubular reabsorption. Toxicity from lithium therapy may be characterized by clumsiness, muscle weakness, tremulousness, and slurred speech. Patients also may have confusion, dizziness, loss of appetite, or symptoms consistent with hypothyroidism. Alternate therapy to lithium should be initiated in pregnant patients.

Logistics

Theophylline and caffeine may increase the toxicity or the elimination of lithium; thus, patients treated for asthma and manic depression should be carefully monitored. Lithium has been demonstrated to reduce the gastrointestinal absorption of chlorpromazine by 40% and concomitant use of phenothiazines and lithium may be associated with an increased risk of neuroleptic malignant syndrome, although this association is controversial. Increased toxicity also has been noted in patients treated with haloperidol and lithium. Lithium aggravates the neuromuscular blocking effects of succinylcholine and pancuronium prolonging neuromuscular blockade. Thiazide diuretics and potassium sparing diuretics may decrease lithium secretion resulting in elevation of serum lithium concentrations. Furosemide and other loop diuretics cause variable and unpredictable changes in lithium serum concentration and thus patients treated with these drugs require careful monitoring. Indomethacin is associated with decreased renal perfusion with accumulation of lithium in treated patients.

Interpretation

During acute management of manic episodes, lithium serum concentrations are in the range of 1.0–1.5 mEq/L (1.0–1.5 mmol/L), whereas for patient management the therapeutic range is thought to be 0.6–1.2 mEq/L (0.6–1.2 mmol/L). As with most other drugs, serum concentration monitoring is directed at maintaining trough concentrations in the therapeutic range and peak concentrations should not be obtained unless apparent peak related toxicity is noted. Interpretation of peak concentrations is complicated by variable rates of absorption and the prolonged distribution phase. In addition to lithium levels, routine monitoring of lithium treated patients should include a complete blood count, serum creatinine, blood urea nitrogen, and thyroid function tests. Sodium intake by patients should be carefully monitored.

Test: Nortriptyline

Background and Selection

Nortriptyline is a secondary amine tricyclic antidepressant increasing the turnover of norepinephrine to a greater extent than serotonin upon initiation of therapy. The catecholamine turnover hypothesis has been questioned for nortriptyline as well as the other tricyclic antidepressants, and it is hypothesized that either nortriptyline or its metabolites alters receptor expression in the synaptic cleft. Catecholamine turnover lasts only about 5 weeks and appears to decrease in significance at the point when the full therapeutic effects of the drug are seen.

Nortriptyline is less sedating than amitriptyline but more sedating than desipramine. Nortriptyline is also more potent than most other tricyclic antidepressants and has a longer half-life ranging from 18–83 hours. Therapeutic response varies from 50–80% of patients and may reflect the serum concentration dependent response observed by Kragh-Sorensen and others.

Nortriptyline, which has a bioavailability ranging from about 50–70%, is highly protein bound. There is considerable variance in hepatic biotransformation and clearance of nortriptyline. Because of the extensive tissue and serum protein binding of nortriptyline, it has a large apparent volume of distribution greater than 90%. Less than 5% of nortriptyline is excreted unchanged in the urine with 2-hydroxy-nortriptyline and its glucuronide being the most common urinary metabolites indicating extensive metabolism via the cytochrome P_{450} enzyme complex. The 2-hydroxy-nortriptyline metabolite appears also to be an active metabolite, as well as 10-hydroxy-nortriptyline, which accumulates in the central nervous system.

Logistics

Barbiturates, smoking, and chloral hydrate all induce the metabolism of nortriptyline via increased cytochrome P_{450} enzyme complex induction. Trihexyphenidyl reduces the absorption of nortriptyline thus decreasing serum concentrations. Serum concentrations of nortriptyline are increased as a result of competition for biotransforming enzymes when methylphenidate, chloramphenicol, haloperidol and phenothiazines, or cimetidine is given concomitantly.

Interpretation

Nortriptyline has been demonstrated to have a "therapeutic window" between 50 and 150 ng/mL (190 and 570 nmol/L) within which approximately 70% of endogenously depressed patients respond. Patients with serum concentrations below or in excess of this therapeutic window are less assured to have the desired drug effects.[81,82]

XANTHINES

Test: Caffeine

Background and Selection

The therapeutic use of caffeine is limited to the treatment of neonates and infants with apnea and bradycardia syndrome. Either caffeine or theophylline is used for their brain stem stimulating effects to prevent sudden apnea and bradycardia. The half-life of caffeine can exceed 100–160 hours in neonates, but can substantially decrease over the first few months of life to a half-life of 2.5–4.5 hours, which is the normal half-life range in adults. During the first months of life, theophylline is methylated to caffeine, a less toxic, but longer half-life xanthine. Both theophylline and caffeine exert similar pharmacologic effects in the brain stem. As the infant matures, the half-life of theophylline and caffeine approach those of adults and older children, and thus caffeine will have a shorter half-life than theophylline. At this time, children treated with caffeine may be switched to theophylline. Caffeine is also an active ingredient in prescription drugs, in some over-the-counter diet products, and in "street speed" capsules made to look like real amphetamine capsules.

Overdoses of caffeine can be fatal and are characterized by cardiac arrest or life-threatening arrhythmias.

Logistics

Fatal arrhythmias have been noted in patients receiving β-agonists and theophylline as well as "street speed" that contains caffeine and ephedrine. Management of bronchopulmonary dysplasia and early infant asthma with theophylline and β-agonists should be initiated with caution.

Interpretation

The therapeutic range for caffeine in neonates is 40–100 μg/mL (206–515 μmol/L). For adults there is a wide range in therapeutic serum concentrations, but fatal caffeine serum concentrations have been as low as 121 μg/mL (623 μmol/L).

Test: Theophylline

Background and Selection

Theophylline has been used to treat asthma for over 50 years.[83] It is also used clinically for apnea and bradycardia syndrome in neonates, as a diaphragmatic stimulant in intubated patients, in nonreversible chronic obstructive airways disease, and rarely as a cardiac stimulant and diuretic.[84] The phosphodiesterase inhibitor mechanism for theophylline has been questioned since 1956 and it appears theophylline may effect prostaglandins and calcium metabolism in smooth muscle cells.[85,86] Theophylline is eliminated from the blood by metabolism through hepatic biotransformation to inactive xanthine metabolites.[84] For patients treated with theophylline, alteration in hepatic metabolism due to liver impairment or induction of metabolizing enzymes by some drugs and not impaired renal function will affect maintenance dose estimations. The distribution volume is dependent on serum proteins. Pharmacokinetic parameters for theophylline are listed in Table 13-15. The clearance of theophylline shows considerable variance and therefore maintenance doses must be selected based on expected theophylline clearance.[87,88] Over 90% of theophylline clearance is due to hepatic metabolism of theophylline to inactive metabolites, thus changes in renal function do not significantly affect the clearance of theophylline.[84] For intensive care unit and postoperative patients, the half-life of theophylline may be prolonged and thus an adjustment in theophylline infusion rate may be necessary before steady-state is reached.[84,89] In these patients, daily

Table 13-15. Pharmacokinetic Parameters for Theophylline

Therapeutic range: 10–20 μg/mL
Toxic range: >30 μg/mL (75% of patients are symptomatic at 25 μg/mL)
Protein binding: 55–65% in patients with normal serum albumin
Hepatic clearance: >90%, averaging 0.68 mL/kg/min
Half-life: 3–8 hours in normal patients, half-life may be prolonged in intensive care patients
Distribution volume: 0.45–0.5 L/kg

monitoring of theophylline serum concentrations may be necessary until steady-state is reached.

Metabolism of Theophylline in Infants

Most biotransformation pathways for drugs result in compounds with increased polarity and a decrease in half-life and distribution volume. Several metabolic pathways in the adult result in the formation of less polar and less soluble enzyme products of which uric acid is a prime example. For neonates, n-demethylase activity in the liver is impaired and for theophylline the expected formation of methyluric acid metabolites does not occur but rather the biotransformation of theophylline to caffeine due to hepatic n-methylase activity. From birth the infant slowly develops n-demethylase activity characterizing a decreased formation of caffeine usually by 4–6 months of age, thus indicating the need to use caffeine rather than theophylline for management of apnea and bradycardia because of its longer half-life in older infants. Thus, management of infants treated with theophylline requires caffeine therapeutic monitoring and likewise the management of apnea and bradycardia patients with caffeine requires theophylline serum concentration monitoring as well. Therapeutic serum concentrations for caffeine range from 40–100 μg/mL while theophylline serum concentrations in infants range from 5–10 μg/mL.

Metabolism of Theophylline in Adults

Hepatic metabolism cannot be predicted by liver function tests or other commonly available clinical laboratory tests; tables of diseases, age, and drug exposures are used to provide mean patient pharmacokinetic parameters.[90] Table 13-2 contains a list of mean theophylline clearances in mL/kg/min and half-lives for patients of differing ages, concomitant drug use, and underlying diseases. When the patient is at steady-state, the rate of infusion and steady-state theophylline concentration can be used to calculate total body clearance, which can be normalized and compared with the mean clearances found in Table 13-2.

Logistics

Changing a Patient From a Continuous Infusion to Oral Theophylline

It is most important to remember that aminophylline is not the same as theophylline. Aminophylline is an ethylene diamine salt of theophylline that is more soluble in water than is theophylline. The dose of theophylline calculated following a continuous infusion of aminophylline will be less than the aminophylline dose, because aminophylline is 80% theophylline. Thus, the theophylline content in aminophylline can be calculated by multiplying the aminophylline dose by 0.80 and an aminophylline dose can be calculated by dividing a theophylline dose by 0.80.[84]

Drug exposures such as smoking and antiepileptic drugs may increase theophylline clearance.[90,91,94,95]

Specimen Collection

Following a loading dose of theophylline, a 5-mL peak concentration should be obtained followed by initiating a continuous infusion of aminophylline based on the estimated mean theophylline clearance. For patients taking antiepileptic drugs and young patients, a second serum theophylline concentration should be obtained about 6 hours after the start of the maintenance infusion as shown in Figure 13-11.[91] For patients with drugs inhibiting theophylline metabolism or suspected of having a long theophylline half-life, a serum concentration should be obtained 12 hours after initiating the maintenance infusion.

Interpretation

The therapeutic range of theophylline is 10–20 mg/L (55.5–111 μmol/L), but some pharmacologic benefit is often seen as serum concentrations exceed 5 mg/L. At serum theophylline concentrations of 15–20 mg/L (83.3–111 μmol/L), ~2.5% of the patients experience adverse effects. As the serum concentrations exceed 20 mg/L (>111 μmol/L), the incidence of adverse effects of theophylline increase dramatically to greater than 25% of those exposed.[84] Nausea, cramps, insomnia, and headaches are common as serum concentrations of theophylline approach and exceed 20 mg/L (>111 μmol/L).[83,84] Acid stomach occurs as the serum theophylline concentrations rise from 15 mg/L–35 mg/L (83.3–194 μmol/L).

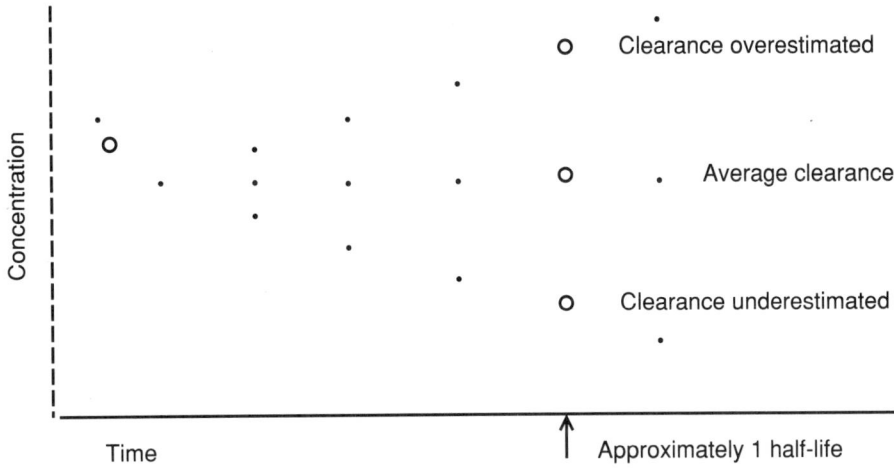

Fig. 13-11. Continuous infusion serum concentration monitoring. Graph depicting the administration of a loading dose of a drug followed immediately by a continuous infusion of the same drug to maintain a constant steady-state concentration. Average clearance estimates may result in the desired steady-state concentration, less than the estimate, or greater than the desired concentration. The resulting circle (○) on the graph represents the range in serum concentrations for patients with less than expected, as expected, and more than expected drug clearance, respectively.

Patients with low serum albumin will have a decreased total theophylline concentration, but an increased therapeutically active unbound theophylline concentration. For these patients, a therapeutic response may occur at total serum concentrations below 10 mg/L (<55.5 μmol/L) and toxicity may occur at serum concentrations as low as 15 mg/L (83.3 μmol/L). As serum concentrations in adults exceed 35 mg/L (>194 μmol/L), the risk of a theophylline-induced seizure increases.[83,89] Children tend to be more tolerant of elevated theophylline concentrations and may not seize until the serum concentrations approach 70 mg/L (389 μmol/L).[96]

MISCELLANEOUS DRUGS

Test: Cimetidine

Background and Selection

Cimetidine is an antihistamine blocking the pharmacologic activity of histamine on histamine-2 receptors that are found in parietal cells, large blood vessels, helper thymocytes, and the brain. Cimetidine is indicated for the treatment of peptic ulcers and has been used investigationally as an immunostimulant for chronic candidiasis, melanomas, and renal cell cancers. Schentag et al.[97] reported a correlation between creatinine clearance and cimetidine clearance indicating that the drug is actively secreted by the kidney tubules.[97] Cimitidine serum concentrations are not routinely monitored, but dose adjustment may be necessary to renal impairment as 45–75% of the drug is eliminated unchanged in the urine.

Logistics

Drug Interactions

Cimetidine is a potent inhibitor of the cytochrome P_{450} enzyme complex that metabolizes most drugs and foreign substances introduced into the body. The most significant drug-drug interactions involving cimetidine include warfarin, theophylline, lidocaine, and phenytoin.

Assay

Several HPLC assays for the quantitation of cimetidine have been published in the *Journal of Chromatography* and other sources. A method permitting the quantitation of both ranitidine and cimetidine has also been published.

Interpretation

No therapeutic range for serum cimetidine concentrations has been determined. Therapy in intensive care is often monitored by following the pH of stomach aspirates with dose adjustment to a desired gastric pH. For patients with Zollinger-Ellison syndrome, larger and more frequent doses of cimetidine and other histamine-2 blockers may be required to control gastric acid secretion.

Test: Cyclosporine

Background and Selection

Cyclosporin A (cyclosporine) is a peptide derived from the fungus *Tolypocladium inflatum*. The immunosuppressive effect of the drug is due to the suppression of interleukin-2 production. Suppression of interleukin-2 favors suppressor T-cell proliferation and induces a more specific immunosuppression when compared with azathioprine and prednisone therapy. The drug is reported to have inherent nephrotoxicity and hepatotoxicity and therefore needs to be carefully monitored to assure that effective immunosuppressive concentrations are maintained while potentially toxic serum concentrations are avoided. Serum concentration time data from parenteral doses of the drug have been described by multicompartment pharmacokinetic models involving five or more exponents. Oral absorption is variable and incomplete with only 36% of the dose is absorbed.[98]

Logistics

Drug Interactions

Cyclosporine serum concentrations have been reported to rise with concomitant treatment with amphotericin B and ketoconazole. Treatment of fungal infections in patients treated with cyclosporine needs to be initiated slowly and with caution as these drugs may increase the risk of nephrotoxicity.

Specimen Collection

Either anticoagulated whole blood or clotted blood can be used for the two available assay methods. Either total blood cyclosporine concentrations or serum cyclosporine concentrations are determined and institutions should not report results from both methods as there are considerable differences and conversion factors to convert from one method to the other are inaccurate. For the whole blood assay, a time consuming process of preparing the specimen is required. For whole blood cyclosporine measurements by HPLC, the specimen is lysed and digested. Specimen preparation requires approximately 24 hours including double extraction, and resulting whole blood concentrations are more than twice those obtained from serum due to the compartmentalization of cyclosporine into red blood cells. The immunoassay for cyclosporine is more difficult to interpret, because of the lack of antibody specificity between the parent compound and its active and inactive metabolites. In addition, cyclosporine concentrations in serum decreased by as much as 40% if the blood is centrifuged at room temperature rather than at body temperature.

Interpretation

Whole blood cyclosporine concentrations range from 150–300 ng/mL, whereas serum cyclosporine concentrations range from 100–150 ng/mL (83–125 nmol/L) when the immunoassay method is used. Dose adjustment for cyclosporine is accomplished using a clearance model for the drug where a single serum trough concentration is used to characterize cyclosporine clearance assuming a constant distribution volume and absorption rate. Because trough related toxicity reflects the serum AUC, it is important to remember that therapeutic concentrations may still be toxic if there is rapid clearance, but a small distribution volume.

Test: Gold

Background and Selection

Gold salts are used for the management of rheumatoid arthritis with accompanying joint destruction and deformity. Gold salts suppress further joint destruction thus further suppressing joint degeneration, but they do not reverse pre-existing joint damage. Parenteral gold has been used for over 50 years to treat rheumatoid arthritis, but the mechanism for this suppression remains controversial. Some have proposed that gold salts displace copper from the liver, whereas others have proposed that gold interferes with sulfhydryl-containing enzymes in macrophages and joint tissue. Others, noting the accumulation of gold in macrophages, have postulated that accumulation of gold in these cells prevents phagocytosis and degranulation thus sparing the joint tissue. Finally, gold has been demonstrated to affect both collagen and prostaglandin synthesis and thus may exert its pharmacologic effects through this mechanism. Gold is extensively bound to serum and tissue proteins and the half-life for gold is reported to be 5.5 days in patients with normal renal function. Gold is primarily excreted by the kidney, with fecal elimination and colonic exfoliation being two minor routes of elimination. Skin rash, itching, and mouth sores may occur in treated patients as well as gold-induced glomerulonephritis and colitis. With prolonged use, neurotoxicity, skin discoloration, and fever may suddenly appear.

Logistics

Clotted blood with no preservatives or anticoagulants should be used because EDTA may chelate gold. Gold distributes extensively in red blood cells thus hemolysed blood will show factitiously high serum gold concentrations. Urine collection also is used for monitoring gold therapy and only polyethylene containers prepared by washing in nitric acid should be used for urine collection. Patients with hematuria will have factitiously elevated urine gold concentrations.

Interpretations

Peak serum gold concentrations drawn at 2–6 hours after injection should range between 6 and 8 μg/mL (30.5 and 40.6 μmol/L) and therapeutic benefit seems to correlate with serum concentrations in excess of 3 μg/mL (5.2 μmol/L). Urinary excretion for gold treated patients should range between 1 and 5 mg/L/24 h (50 and 25.4 μmol/d). Routine monitoring of patients receiving gold salts also should include a complete blood count with differential, liver function tests, urinalysis for urine protein, ophthalmologic examination, as well as assessment of therapeutic benefit.

Test: Methotrexate

Background and Selection

Methotrexate is a folic acid antiagonist used extensively in the treatment of various solid tumors and hematologic cancers, psoriasis, and now indicated for rheumatoid arthritis refractory to other treatment. Therapeutic drug monitoring of methotrexate is particularly indicated for high dose methotrexate therapy with leucovorin rescue. The disposition of methotrexate following high dose protocols is complicated by subtle changes in renal and hepatic function, toxicity of concomitant chemotherapy, and sequestration of methotrexate conjugates in cells. Methotrexate impairs pyrimidine synthesis by preventing formation of n-formidyl tetrahydrofolate (leucovorin), which is necessary for DNA and RNA synthesis. Methotrexate competitively binds to dihydrofolate reductase preventing cellular leucovorin synthesis. Total inhibition of this enzyme is necessary for the desired therapeutic effect in high dose regimens as partial inhibition does not inhibit DNA synthesis. Common toxicities with high dose therapy include myelosuppression, gastric ulcerations, renal toxicity, and hepatitis progressing to frank cirrhosis. Therapeutic drug monitoring has substantially reduced patient morbidity and mortality as demonstrated by Evans et al.[99] Methotrexate, like phenytoin, demonstrates nonlinear increases in time to peak absorption with increasing doses with a bioavailability of 50–70%.[99]

The volume of the central compartment for methotrexate approximates the extracellular volume, but the steady-state distribution volume is 0.75–0.8 L/kg indicating intracellular sequestration as methotrexate is 50% protein bound. Penetration of methotrexate into the peripheral compartment and intracellularly appears to follow Michaelis-Menten nonlinear disposition with a saturable carrier system and an affinity constant at low doses, but others have noted a mixed order process with high dose therapy. Methotrexate penetrates poorly into the brain except when patients have sustained massive intracranial irradiation where they are then at risk of methotrexate associated leukoencephalopathy.

Methotrexate is metabolized to weakly active metabolites by gut flora and hepatic enzymes. Methotrexate is actively secreted into forming urine, and few drugs other than probenicid clinically inhibit this excretion route. Methotrexate demonstrates a biexponential serum concentration decline with an α-phase half-life (Fig. 13-5).[99] Major errors may occur if serum concentration time data are analyzed using completer programs fitting data to a one compartment model as clearance and the elimination rate constant will be overestimated. Toxicity to methotrexate appears to be both serum concentration and exposure duration dependent; therefore, urinary alkalinization, leucovorin administration, and aggressive hydration are often added to patient management for patients with prolonged β-phase half-lives. Methotrexate serum concentration monitoring is particularly indicated for patients treated with high dose methotrexate who have in addition renal or hepatic impairment.

With the increased aggressive management of leukemia patients and the central nervous system prophylaxis for lymphomas with intrathecal methotrexate, concerns have emerged concerning the potential toxicity of such therapy. Neurotoxicity, particularly leukoencephalopathy is a concern particularly among renally impaired patients requiring methotrexate therapy. Recently Glascoe et al.[100] published a report on the use of a commercial FPIA method for monitoring cerebrospinal fluid methotrexate concentrations.

Logistics

Drug Interactions

Alcohol, hepatotoxic medications, cytarabine, nonsteroidal anti-inflammatory agents such as phenylbutazone or salicylates, as well as sulfonamides, phenytoin, chloramphenicol, and probenicid displace methotrexate from its serum and tissue protein binding sites.

Specimen Collection

Serum or cerebrospinal fluid should be obtained no later than 48 hours after administration of the drug. For immunoassays, serum samples obtained more than 24 hours following high dose methotrexate generally show a high rate of crossreactivity with metabolites.

Interpretation

The toxicity of methotrexate reflects the size of the serum AUC that reflects resulting serum concentrations and the duration of tissue exposure. Thus, serum concentrations obtained 24–48 hours after the administration of methotrexate reflect the extent of methotrexate clearance and resulting serum concentrations. Although serum concentrations do not necessarily predict tissue toxicity, they indicate how much leucovorin will be needed. The dose-response relationship between methotrexate and drug toxicity is complex and serum concentrations of methotrexate in excess of (>0.1 mmol/L) at 72 hours correlate with tissue toxicity.

REFERENCES

1. Gibaldi M, Perrier D: Absorption kinetics and bioavailability. pp. 145–198. In Gibaldi M, Perrier D (eds): Pharmacokinetics: Drugs and the Pharmaceutical Sciences. 2nd Ed. Vol. 15, New York, Marcel Dekker, 1982.
2. Taylor EH, Ackerman BH: Free drug monitoring by liquid chromatography and implications for therapeutic drug monitoring. J Liquid Chromatogr 1987;10:323–343.
3. MacKichan JJ: Pharmacokinetic consequences of drug displacement from blood and tissue proteins. Clin Pharmacokinet 1984;9:suppl.1, 32–41.
4. Eadie MJ: Plasma level monitoring of anticonvulsants. Clin Pharmacokinet 1976;1:52–66.
5. Levy RH, Schmidt D: Utility of free level monitoring of antiepileptic drugs. Epilepsia 1985;26:199–205.
6. Rowland M, Tozer TN: Hepatic clearance and elimination. In Clinical Pharmacokinetics; Concepts and Applications. Philadelphia, Lea & Febiger, 1980.
7. Gibaldi M, Levy G; Pharmacokinetics in clinical practice: 1. Concepts. JAMA 1976;235:1864–1867.
8. Greenblatt DJ, Koch-Weser J: Clinical pharmacokinetics (in two parts). N Engl J Med 1975;293:702–705, 964–970.
9. Rowland M, Tozer TN: Variability in drug response. In Clinical Pharmacokinetics: Concepts and Applications. Philadelphia, Lea & Febiger, 1980.
10. Rowland M, Tozer TN: Intravenous dose. In Clinical Pharmacokinetics: Concepts and Applications. Philadelphia, Lea & Febiger, 1980.
11. Rowland M, Tozer TN: Clearance and renal excretion. In Clinical Pharmacokinetics: Concepts and Applications. Philadelphia, Lea & Febiger, 1980.
12. Burton ME, Vasko MR, Brater DC: Comparison of drug dosing methods. Clin Pharmacokinet 1985;10:1–37.
13. Gibaldi M, Levy G: Pharmacokinetics in clinical practice: 2. Applications. JAMA 1976;235:1987–1992.
14. Gibaldi M, Perrier D: Nonlinear pharmacokinetics. pp. 271–318. In Gibaldi M, Perrier D (eds): Pharmacokinetics: Drugs and the Pharmaceutical Sciences. 2nd Ed. Vol. 15. New York, Marcel Dekker, 1982.
15. Roland M, Tozer TN: Why clinical pharmacokinetics? In Clinical Pharmacokinetics: Concepts and Applications. Philadelphia, Lea & Febiger, 1980.
16. Rowland M, Tozer TN: Dosage regimens. In Clinical Pharmacokinetics: Concepts and Applications. Philadelphia, Lea & Febiger, 1980.
17. Riva R, Albani F, Ambrosetto G et al: Diurnal functuations in free and total steady-state plasma levels of carbamazepine and correlation with intermittent side effects. Epilepsia 1984;25:476–481.
18. Contin M, Riva R, Albani F et al: Determination of total and free plasma carbamazepine concentrations by enzyme multiplied immunoassay: Interference with the 10,11-epoxide metabolite. Ther Drug Monit 1985;7:46–50.
19. Baruzzi A, Contin M, Perucca E et al: Altered serum protein binding of carbamazepine in disease states associated with an increased alpha 1-acid glycoprotein concentration. Eur J Clin Pharmacol 1986;31:85–89.
20. Agbato OA, Elyas AA, Patsalos PN et al: Total and free serum concentrations of carbamazepine and carbamazepine 10,11-epoxide in children with epilepsy. Arch Neurol 1986;43:1111–1116.
21. Rall TW, Scheifer LS: Drugs effective in the therapy of the epilepsies. pp. 446–472. In Goodman LS, Gilman AG (eds): The Pharmacological Basis of Therapeutics. 6th Ed. New York, Macmillan, 1985.
22. Louis S, Kutt H, McDowell F: Intravenous diphenylhydantoin in experimental seizures. II. Effect on penicillin-induced seizures in the cat. Arch Neurol 1968;18:472–477.
23. Lund L: Anticonvulsant effect of diphenylhydantoin relative to plasma levels. A prospective three-year study in ambulant patients with generalized epileptic seizures. Arch Neurol 1974;31:289–294.
24. Troupin AS, Friel P: Anticonvulsant levels in saliva, serum and cerebrospinal fluid. Epilepsia 1975;16:223–227.
25. Vozeh S, Koelz A, Martin E et al: Predictability of phenytoin serum levels by nomograms and clinicians. Eur Neurol 1980;19:345–352.
26. Mullen PW: Optimal phenytoin therapy: A new technique for individualizing dosage. Clin Pharmacol Ther 1978;23:228–232.
27. Ludden TM, Hawkins DW, Allen JP, Hofman SF: Op-

timum phenytoin dosage regimens. Lancet 1976;1:307–309.
28. Levi RH, Schmidt G: Utility of free level monitoring of antiepileptic drugs. Epilepsia 1985;26:199–205.
29. Primadone: Drug Information for the Health Care Provider. USPDI, 5th Ed. Rockville, MD, United States Pharmacopeial Convention, 1985.
30. Bauer LA, Davis R, Wilensky A et al: Diurnal variation in valproic acid clearance. Clin Pharmacol Ther 1984;35:505–509.
31. Bowdle TA, Patel IH, Levy RH, Wilensky AJ: Valproic acid dosage and plasma protein binding and clearance. Clin Pharmacol Ther 1980;28:486–492.
32. Marty JJ, Kilpatrick CJ, Mounds RF: Intra dose variation in plasma protein binding of sodium valproate in epileptic patients. Br J Clin Pharmacol 1982;14:399–404.
33. Patel IH, Levy RH: Valproic acid binding to human serum albumin and determination of free fraction in the presence of anticonvulsants and free fatty acids. Epilepsia 1979;20:85–90.
34. Klotz U, Antonin KH: Pharmacokinetics and bioavailability of sodium, valproate. Clin Pharmacol Ther 1977;21:736–743.
35. Riva R, Albani F, Cortelli P et al: Diurnal fluctuations in free and total plasma concentrations of valproic acid at steady state in epileptic patients. Ther Drug Monit 1983;5:191–196.
36. Roman EJ, Ponniah P, Lambert JB, Buchanan N: Free sodium valproate monitoring [letter]. Br J Clin Pharmacol 1982;13:452–454.
37. Levy RH: Monitoring of free valproic acid levels [commentary]? Ther Drug Monit 1980;2:199–201.
38. Rapeport WG, Mendelow AD, French G et al: Plasma protein-binding and CSF concentrations of valproic acid in man following acute oral dosing. Br J Clin Pharmacol 1983;16:365–369.
39. Haidukewych D, Rodin EA: Monitoring free valproic acid in epilepsy patients medicated with anticonvulsants. Ther Drug Monit 1982;4:209–212.
40. Cramer JA, Mattson RH, Bennett DM, Swick CT: Variable free and total valproic acid concentrations in sole- and multi-drug therapy. Ther Drug Monit 1986;8:411–415.
41. Patel IH, Levy RH: Valproic acid binding to human serum albumin and determination of free fraction in the presence of anticonvulsants and free fatty acids. Epilepsia 1979;20:85–90.
42. Bauer LA, Davis R, Wilensky A et al: Valproic acid clearance: Unbound fraction and diurnal variation in young and elderly adults. Clin Pharmacol Ther 1985;37:697–700.
43. Riva R, Albani F, Contin M et al: Mechanism of altered drug binding to serum proteins in pregnant women studies with valproic acid. Ther Drug Monit 1984;6:25–30.
44. Chadwick DW: Concentration-effect relationships of valproic acid. Clin Pharmacokinet 1985;10:155–163.
45. Froscher W, Burr W, Penin H et al: Free level monitoring of carbamazepine and valproic acid: Clinical significance. Clin Neuropharmacol 1985;8:362–371.
46. Morady F, Scheinman MM, Desai J: Disopyramide. Ann Intern Med 1982;96:337–343.
47. Meltzer RS, Robert EW, McMorrow M et al: Atypical ventricular tachycardia as a manifestation of disopyramide toxicity. Am J Cardiol 1978;42:1049–1053.
48. Siddoway LA, Woosely RL: Clinical pharmacokinetics of disopyramide. Clin Pharmacokinet 1986;11:214–222.
49. Taylor EH, Pappas AA: Disopyramide: Clinical indications, pharmacokinetics, and laboratory assessment. Ann Clin Lab Sci 1986;16:289–295.
50. Ekelund LG, Nilsson E, Walldius G: Efficacy of and adverse effects of disopyramide: Comparison of capsules, controlled release tablets, and placebo in patients with chronic ventricular arrhythmias. Eur J Clin Pharmacol 1986;29:673–677.
51. Shaw LM, Doherty JU, Waxman HL et al: The pharmacokinetic and pharmacodynamic effects of varying the free fraction of disopyramide. Angiology 1987;38:192–197.
52. Gillis AM, Kates RE: Clinical pharmacokinetics of the newer antiarrhythmic agents. Clin Pharmacokinet 1984;9:375–403.
53. Winkle RA, Peters F, Kates RE et al: Clinical pharmacology and antiarrhythmic efficacy of encainide in patients with chronic ventricular arrhythmias. Circulation 1981;64:290–296.
54. Anderson JL, Stewart JR, Perry BA et al: Oral fecainide acetate for the treatment of ventricular arrhythmias. N Engl J Med 1981;305:473–477.
55. Lie KI, Wellens HJ, van Capelle FJ, Durrer D: Lidocaine in the prevention of primary ventricular fibrillation: A double blind, randomized study of 212 consecutive patients. N Engl J Med 1975;291:1324–1326.
56. Collingsworth KA, Strong JM, Atkinson AJ Jr: Pharmacokinetics and metabolism of lidocaine in patients with renal failure. Clin Pharmacol Ther 1975;18:59–64.
57. McErlane KM, Igwemezie L, Kerr CR: Stereoselective analysis of the enantiomers of mexilitine by high performance liquid chromatography using fluorescence detection and study of their stereoselective disposition in man. J Chromatogr 1987;415:335–346.
58. Bigger JT, Hoffman BF: Antiarrhythmic agents. In Gilman AG, Goodman LS, Rall TW, Murad F (eds): The Pharmacologic Basis of Therapeutics. 7th Ed. New York, Macmillan, 1985.
59. Rou TI, Morita Y, Atkinson AJ et al: Identification of desethy procainamide in patients: A new metabolite of procainamide. J Pharmacol Exp Ther 1981;216:357–362.
60. Tilstone WJ, Lawson DH: Capacity-limited elimination of procainamide in man. Res Commun Chem Pathol Pharmacol 1978;21:343–346.
61. McKinney TD: Heterogeneity of organic base secretion by proximal tubules. Am J Physiol 1982;243:F404–F407.
62. Freeman RW, Woosley RL, Oates JA et al: Evidence of the biotransformation of procainamide to a reactive metabolite. Toxicol Appl Pharmacol 1979;50:9–16.
63. Karlsson E: Clinical pharmacokinetics of procainamide. Clin Pharmacokinet 1978;3:97–107.
64. Gibson TP, Atkinson AJ, Matusik E et al: Kinetics of procainamide and N-acetylprocainamide in renal failure. Kidney Int 1977;12:422–429.
65. Connolly SJ, Kates RE: Clinical pharmacokinetics of N-acetylprocainamide. Clin Pharmacokinet 1982;7:206–220.
66. McAnish J, Gay MA: Theoretical Michaelis-Menten elimination model for propranolol. Eur J Drug Metab Pharmacokinet 1985;10:241–245.
67. Duff HJ, Mitchell LB, Wyse DG: Antiarrhythmic effi-

cacy of propranolol; comparison of low and high serum concentrations. J Am Coll Cardiol 1986;8:959–965.
68. Duff HJ, Wyse G, Manyari D et al: Intravenous quinidine: Relations among concentration, tachyarrhythmia suppression, and electrophysiologic actions with inducible sustained ventricular tachycardia. Am J Cardiol 1985;55:92–97.
69. Torres V, Flowers D, Miura D et al: Intravenous quinidine by intermittent bolus for electrophysiologic studies in patients with ventricular tachycardia. Am Heart J 1984;106:1437–1442.
70. Bowers LD, Nelson KM, Connor R et al: Evidence supporting 3(S)-3-hydroxyquinidine-associated cardiotoxicity. Ther Drug Monit 1985;7:308–312.
71. Vozeh S, Bindschedler M, Ha HR: Pharmacodynamics of 3-hydroxyquinidine alone and in combination with quinidine in healthy persons. Am J Cardiol 1987;59:681–684.
72. Woosley RL, Echt DS, Roden DM: Effects of congestive heart failure on the pharmacokinetics and pharmacodynamics of antiarrhythmic agents. Am J Cardiol 1986;57:25B–33B.
73. Ha HR, Vozeh S, Follath F: Evaluation of a rapid ultrafiltration technique for determination of quinidine protein binding and comparison with equilibrium dialysis. Ther Drug Monit 1986;8:331–335.
74. Ronfeld RA, Wolshin EM, Block AJ: On the kinetics and dynamics of tocainide and its metabolites. Clin Pharmacol Ther 1982;31:384–392.
75. Lee DC-S, Johnson RA, Bingham JB et al: Heart failure in outpatients, a randomized trial of digoxin versus placebo. N Engl J Med 1982;306:699–705.
76. Mulrow CD, Feussner JR, Velez R: Reevaluation of digitalis efficacy: New light on an old leaf. Ann Intern Med 1984;101:113–117.
77. Mungall DR, Robichaux RR, Perry W et al: Effects of quinidine on serum digoxin concentration: A prospective study. Ann Intern Med 1980;93:689–693.
78. Leahey EB, Reiffel JA, Elsa-Grace VG et al: The effect of quinidine and other oral antiarrhythmic drugs on serum digoxin. Ann Intern Med 1980;92:605–608.
79. Burkle WS, Matzke GR: Effect of quinidine on serum digoxin concentrations. Am J Hosp Pharm 1979;36:968–971.
80. Reuning RH, Sams RA, Notari RE: Role of pharmacokinetics in drug dosage adjustment. I. Pharmacologic effect, kinetics, and apparent volume of distribution of digoxin. J Clin Pharmacol 1973;13:127–141.
81. Preskorn SH: Tricyclic antidepressant plasma level monitoring: An improvement over the dose-response approach. J Clin Psychiatry 1986;47:suppl. 1, 21–30.
82. Orsulak PV: Therapeutic monitoring of antidepressant drugs: Current methodology and applications: J Clin Psychiatry 1986;47:suppl. 1, 39–52.
83. Bukowskyj M, Nakatsu K, Munt PW: Theophylline reassessed. Ann Intern Med 1984;101:63–73.
84. Hendeles L, Weinberger M: Theophylline: A "state of the art" review. Pharmacotherapy 1983;3:2–44.
85. Bergstrand H: Phosphodiesterase inhibition and theophylline. Eur J Respir Dis 1980;61:suppl. 109, 37–44.
86. Horrobin DF, Manku MS, Franks DJ et al: Methyl xanthine phosphodiesterase inhibitors behave as prostaglandin antagonists in a perfused rat mesenteric artery preparation. Prostaglandins 1977;13:33–40.
87. Uden DL, Smith GD: Asthma. pp. 381–405. In Katcher BS, Young LY, Koda-Kimble MA (eds): Applied Therapeutics: The Clinical Use of Drugs. 3rd Ed. San Francisco, Applied Therapeutics, 1983.
88. Anderson G, Koup J, Slaughter R et al: Evaluation of two methods for estimating theophylline clearance prior to achieving steady-state. Ther Drug Monit 1981;3:325–332.
89. Massey KL, Gotz VP, Russell WL: Dose-dependent kinetics of theophylline in adults with pulmonary diseases. Ther Drug Monit 1984;6:284–289.
90. Postelnick MJ, Lesher CA, Steiner VI et al: Rapid adjustment of theophylline: A kinetic model. Drug Intell Clin Pharmacol 1984;18:519–522.
91. Reed WE Jr, Cooper MW: Sustained release procainamide: Use of serum concentrations to determine dosage. South Med J 1985;78:1190–1193.
92. Powell JR, Thiercelin J, Vozeh S et al: The influence of cigarette smoking and sex on theophylline disposition. Am Rev Respir Dis 1977;116:17–23.
93. Hunt SN, Jusko WJ, Yurchak AM: Effect of smoking on theophylline disposition. Clin Pharmacol Ther 1976;19:546–551.
94. Reitberg DP, Bernhard H, Schentag JJ: Alteration of theophylline clearance and half-life by cimetidine. Ann Intern Med 1981;95:582–585.
95. Green JA, Clementi WA: Decrease in theophylline clearance after the administration of erythromycin to a patient with obstructive lung disease. Drug Intell Clin Pharmacol 1983;17:370–372.
96. Baker MD: Theophylline toxicity in children. J Pediatr 1986;109:538–542.
97. Schentag JJ, Cerra FB, Calleri GM et al: Age, disease, and cimetidine disposition in healthy subjects and chronically ill patients. Clin Pharmacol Ther 1981;29:737–743.
98. Cohen DJ, Loertscher R, Rubin MF et al: Cyclosporine: A new immunosuppressive agent for organ transplantation. Ann Intern Med 1984;101:667–682.
99. Evans WE, Pratt CB, Taylor RH et al: Pharmacokinetic monitoring of high-dose methotrexate: Early recognition of high-risk patients. Cancer Chemother Pharmacol 1979;3:161–166.
100. Glascoe GB, Taylor EH, Chadduck WM, Pappas AA: Analysis of methotrexate in cerebrospinal fluid by fluorescence polarization immunoassay. Drug Intell Clin Pharmacol 1988;22:912–913.

14 Toxicology and Drugs of Abuse

Alex A. Pappas
E. Howard Taylor
Bruce Ackerman

INTRODUCTION

Clinical toxicology can be defined as the measurement of drugs or toxins in human physiologic fluids for the purpose of meeting patient management needs. To meet these needs it is necessary that an integrated approach be made (1) to establish a close working relationship between the laboratory and the attending physician, (2) to develop analytic services and test ordering guidelines to meet local needs, (3) to correlate the analytic results with the clinical history and findings (e.g., a formal written interpretation), and (4) to establish ongoing continuing education.[1]

The epidemiologic spectrum of clinical toxicology is indeed broad, and no one laboratory can screen for all potential drugs or substances that can cause patient morbidity or death. Intentional ingestions of drugs or toxins may be seen in suicide attempts, substance abuse, with recreational use, or as a result of accidental exposure (Table 14-1). The data from the Drug Abuse Warning Network (DAWN) were collected from a nonrandom sampling of emergency rooms and medical examiners' cases. The "mentions" compiled by DAWN may be circumstantial in many cases; however, the data are supported by previous retrospective and prospective studies using confirmatory laboratory methods.[2,3] The 10 drugs in Table 14-1 constituted 80% of the drugs seen in emergency room patients. An additional 20% of drugs encountered by these patients include amitriptyline, propoxyphene, phenytoin, methadone, flurazepam, over-the-counter sleep aids, phenobarbital, ibuprofen, diphenhydramine, and chlordiazepoxide. These data do not include pediatric patients. Table 14-2 is a compilation of pediatric exposures and reveals a high frequency of involvement with substances that may or may not cause significant toxicity. The representation of these substances reflects their ready availability. It is important to know if the laboratory is capable of providing support for substance analysis. Intentional poisoning in the elderly is an emerging problem that is increasing as the population ages. The more common ingestions in this age group include sedative/hypnotics, cardiovascular drugs, analgesics, and antidepressants.[4]

A request for a toxicologic examination, even when the toxin or substance is known, may require a multitude of complex analytic procedures. As with any laboratory examination, the request must be accompanied by an adequate clinical history and properly collected specimens. There need to be readily available consultative services to guide the clinician through the myriad of specimen collection protocols, test methods, and results. A formal interpretive report, delivered in a timely fashion and correlating the clinical and laboratory findings, assists in current and future patient management. Any clinical specimen or result may very quickly become entangled with legal intricacies in which a formal interpretive report would be most helpful.

Table 14-1. Drug Categories Most Frequently Encountered by Emergency Room Patients According to Motive by the Drug Abuse Warning Network

Drug	Number (% of Total)	Motive Psychic (%)	Dependence (%)	Suicide (%)
Alcohol (alone or in combination)	21,100 (20)	33	22	34
Heroin or morphine	14,700 (14)	18	73	3
Cocaine	13,500 (13)	40	45	6
Diazepam	8300 (8)	17	17	60
Acetaminophen	5800 (5)	12	1	76
Phencyclidine (PCP)	5700 (5)	29	26	5
Aspirin	5300 (5)	11	1	76
Marijuana	5300 (5)	63	22	6
Alprazolam	2700 (3)	16	5	65
Codeine	2600 (2)	23	25	34

(Data from National Institute on Drug Abuse.[61])

Comprehensive laboratory testing should focus on meeting patient care needs, which are dictated by local drug prevalence or patterns of abuse. The dilemma of deciding the tests that should and can be offered, and the availability of these tests, are decisions that must be made with full consultation of the technical and clinical staff involved. Because physicians have difficulty in predicting the substances that have been ingested, a broad comprehensive approach will be of greater value in determining the nature and extent of drug exposure in a given patient. Screening panels have been developed to assist in the triage of the patient presenting with an acute toxic emergency when the history, clinical signs, and symptoms are not particularly helpful (Table 14-3). If the drug or substance ingested is known or highly suspected, a quantitative or a semiquantitative analysis of a particular drug or drug class is preferred. An example of a suggested single item "menu" of toxicologic tests is given in Table 14-4. The qualitative screens using thin-layer chromatography (TLC) can be advantageous in detecting a wider range of drugs or substances.

The therapeutic, toxic, and lethal ranges presented in this chapter are representative of those found in the literature and are not a substitution for the proper evaluation and management of the patient.

Analytic Methods in Toxicology

Immunoassays

In clinical laboratories, the two most common immunoassays for toxicology are the enzyme multiplied immunoassay technique (EMIT, Syva, Palo Alto, CA) and fluorescence polarization immunoassay (FPIA,

Table 14-2. Pediatric (<6 Years Old) Toxic Exposures in 630,000 Cases (% of Total)

Nonpharmaceutical Exposures (%)	Pharmaceutical Exposures (%)
Plants (11)	Analgesics (8), mostly acetaminophen
Cosmetics/personal care (11)	Cold/cough preparations (6)
Cleaning substance (10)	Topical medications (5)
Foreign bodies (5)	Vitamins/minerals (4)
Insecticide/pesticides (4)	Antibiotics (3)
Hydrocarbons (4)	Antacids/laxatives (2)
Solvents (2)	Hormones (2)
Art/office supplies (2)	Electrolyte preparations (1.5)
Alcohols (2)	Sedative/hypnotic (1)
Chemicals (2)	Stimulants and street drugs (1)

(Data from Litovitz et al.[62])

Table 14-3. Toxicology Panels Based on Acute Patient Presentation

Presenting History or Symptoms	Drug Panel
Lethargic or comatose	Ethanol, tricyclic antidepressants barbiturates, benzodiazepines, opiates
Agitated or combative	Amphetamines, cocaine, Phencyclidine (PCP)
Hallucinating or delusional	Marijuana, PCP
Motor vehicle accident or trauma	Amphetamine, cocaine, ethanol, marijuana, PCP

Abbott Laboratories, North Chicago, IL). In general, these techniques are rapid, nonisotopic, automated, and are easily performed. There are numerous drug assays available that lend themselves well to a clinical laboratory (Table 14-5).

Immunoassays detect very low drug concentrations and are well suited for therapeutic drug monitoring (TDM) and screening techniques for drugs of abuse; however, interferences can occur. For example, structurally similar drugs, such as over-the-counter decongestants, phenylpropanolamine, pseudoephedrine, or phenteramine, can interfere in the assay for amphetamine.[5] In TDM, some interferences may also be present, such as the theophylline metabolite 1,3-dimethyluric acid present in increased concentrations in the serum of patients with renal impairment, and may cause a problem in the theophylline assay. Interferences can arise from endogenous sources such as a digoxin-like immunoreactive substance, which has been found to be a naturetic hormone produced in neonates that can cause a falsely elevated immunoassay result for digoxin.[6] With EMIT, the indicator drug is labeled with the enzyme glucose 6-phosphate dehydrogenase (G-6-PD) (Fig. 14-1). As enzyme labeled drug binds to a drug-specific antibody, enzyme activity is inhibited. The drug present in the patient's serum will compete with the enzyme labeled drug for the available antibody binding sites. At greater drug concentrations, there is greater enzyme activity, which may be conveniently monitored on a spectrophotometer by measuring the increase with time in the absorbance of reduced nicotinamide-adenine dinucleotide (NADH) at 340 nm.

In FPIA, the drug of interest is labeled with a fluorescent tracer, fluorescein. This fluorescein labeled drug competes with the drug present in the patient's serum for antibody binding sites. The labeled drug, which is bound to the large antibody molecule, will emit largely

Table 14-4. Availability of Clinical Toxicologic Testing

Quantitative (7 d/wk, 1-h turnaround)	Semiquantitative (7 d/wk, 1-h turnaround)	Qualitative (7 d/wk, 3-h turnaround)
Acetaminophen	Amphetamine class	Antihistamines
Carboxyhemoglobin	Barbiturates	Carbamazepine
Iron and iron binding	Benzodiazepines	Cocaine
Lithium	Cannabinoids	Cyclobenzaprine
Methemoglobin	Cocaine metabolite	Ethchlorvynol
Phenobarbital	Opiates	Glutethimide
Phenytoin	PCP	Haloperidol
Pseudocholinesterase	Tricyclics	Hydroxyzine
Salicylate		Ibuprofen
		MDA/MDMA
		Meprobamate
		Methaqualone
		Narcotics
		Phenothiazines
		Propoxyphene
		Pentazocine
		Quinidine
		Sympathomimetic amines
		Strychnine

Abbreviations: PCP, phencyclidine; MDA, methelynedioxamphetamine; MDMA,
(Modified from Pappas et al.,[63] with permission.)

Table 14-5. Drugs and/or Metabolites Detected by Immunoassay

Acetaminophen
Amikacin
Amphetamine/methamphetamine
Antidepressant (class)
Barbiturate (class)
Benzodiazepine (class)
Cannabinoids (THC)
Carbamazepine
Cocaine
Cyclosporine
Digoxin
Disopyramide
Ethosuximide
Flecainide
Gentamicin
Lidocaine
Methotrexate
N-acetyl procainamide
Opiates (class)
Phencyclidine (PCP)
Phenobarbital
Phenytoin
Primidone
Procainamide
Quinidine
Salicylate
Theophylline
Tobramycin
Valproic acid
Vancomycin

polarized light when excited with a polarized incident beam. Due to their slower rotational rates, large molecules undergo only a few degrees of rotation, and coupled with limited Brownian motion during the same time interval the emitted light remains largely polarized in the same plane with the incident polarized light. The unbound fluorescein labeled drug is small and therefore emits light that is depolarized. These small molecules become randomly oriented during the inter-val between excitation and emission and thus emit randomly oriented (depolarized) light when excited by a polarized incident beam. As the serum concentration of the drug increases, the ratio of unbound labeled drug to antibody bound indicator drug increases, and thus the degree of fluorescence polarization diminishes. At low patient drug concentrations, a large proportion of the labeled drug is bound by antibody, and this will show a high amount of fluorescent polarization. The relationship of concentration to fluorescence depolarization is therefore inversely related.

Thin-Layer Chromatography

Drugs are extracted from the urine or gastric contents with an organic solvent (e.g., methylene chloride), evaporated to near dryness, and then spotted onto a stationary phase, either a silica-coated glass plate or silica impregnated paper. The plate or paper is then placed in a covered tank with a small volume of organic solvent; this is the mobile phase. By capillary action (Fig. 14-2) the drugs migrate up the plate to a point determined by the compound's polarity. Nonpolar compounds are more soluble in the mobile phase than on the more polar silica plate and migrate a greater distance. Identification is based on relative migration distance (R_f). The solvent front and origin are assigned the values 1.0 and 0.0, respectively. The R_f is defined as migration distance from application point/migration distance of solvent front. The plates are then stained with developing solutions such as sulfuric acid, followed by Dragendorf's reagent (iodide). Drugs are identified by R_f and color development and then compared with a set of standards. An excellent commercial system (Toxi-Lab, Marion Laboratories, Inc.) is available.

With TLC a large number of drugs can be detected; however, some drugs are metabolized rapidly to more water soluble forms and are difficult to extract with organic solvents without pretreatment. Morphine is metabolized to the more water soluble morphine 3-glucuronide, and cocaine is metabolized rapidly to benzoylecgonine and ecgonine. Because these compounds are more water soluble than the parent drug, they are more difficult to extract and detect at lower concentrations. Also, compounds with similar structures will comigrate and may be difficult to resolve. With TLC approximately 0.5–1.0 μg/mL of the drug can be detected. Such drugs as phencyclidine (PCP or angel dust) and lysurgic acid diethylamide (LSD) are present at very low concentrations and are better detected by an immunoassay. Combinations of immunoassays and TLC provide a very comprehensive means of drug detection in a hospital clinical toxicology laboratory.

$$\text{Drug} + \text{drug–E} \xrightleftharpoons{\text{antibody}} \text{Ab–drug} + \text{Ab–drug–E}$$
$$\text{(active)} \qquad\qquad\qquad \text{(inactive)}$$

Fig. 14-1. Principle of the enzyme multiplied immunoassay technique (EMIT). Drug present in patient serum will compete with the enzyme labeled drug (drug-E) for available antibody binding sites (Ab). Drug competes with the enzyme, glucose 6-phosphate dehydrogenase tagged drug for the specific antibody. When the substrate, glucose 6-phosphate, is added, the enzyme converts NAD$^+$ to NADH. The active site of the enzyme is not available to react when drug is bound to antibody (Ab-drug-E) and produces no reaction.

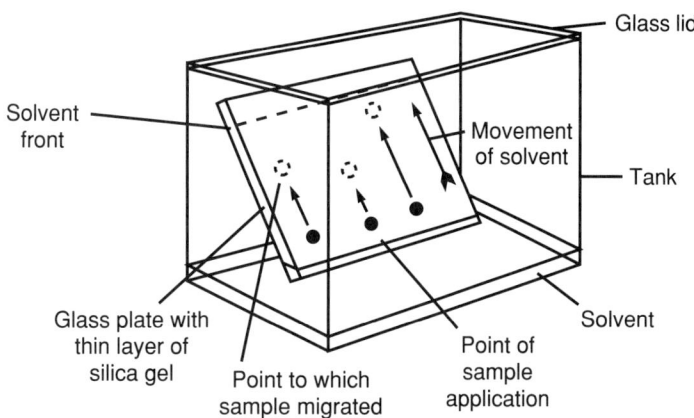

Fig. 14-2. Illustration of the principle of thin layer chromatography (TLC). (Modified from Bennett,[71] with permission.)

High Performance Liquid Chromatography (HPLC)

High performance liquid chromatography (Fig. 14-3) is a powerful technique used when it is desirable to measure a drug and its pharmacologically active metabolite, particularly if no immunoassay technique is available. With this technique, a drug is extracted from the serum or urine and concentrated. The sample is then injected onto a chromatographic column (usually a nonpolar stationary phase such as C18). By using a mobile phase specific for elution of the particular class of drugs, many different members of a specific drug class (e.g., antidepressants or benzodiazepines), can be analyzed simultaneously. The chromatographic separation depends on pH, ionic strength, and organic solvent composition of the mobile phase. On a C18 reverse phase column, most polar drugs elute first, while fewer polar drugs are late eluting due to the hydrophobic nature of the compound and interaction with the column. Detection is usually by absorbance at an optimal wavelength for a particular drug class. Fluorescence or electrochemical detection also is available but is usually reserved for compounds that have poor ultraviolet absorbance spectra. Quantitation is achieved by evaluating peak heights or areas and comparing unknown peak heights or areas with a known set of calibration standards that are extracted in the same manner as the unknown samples.

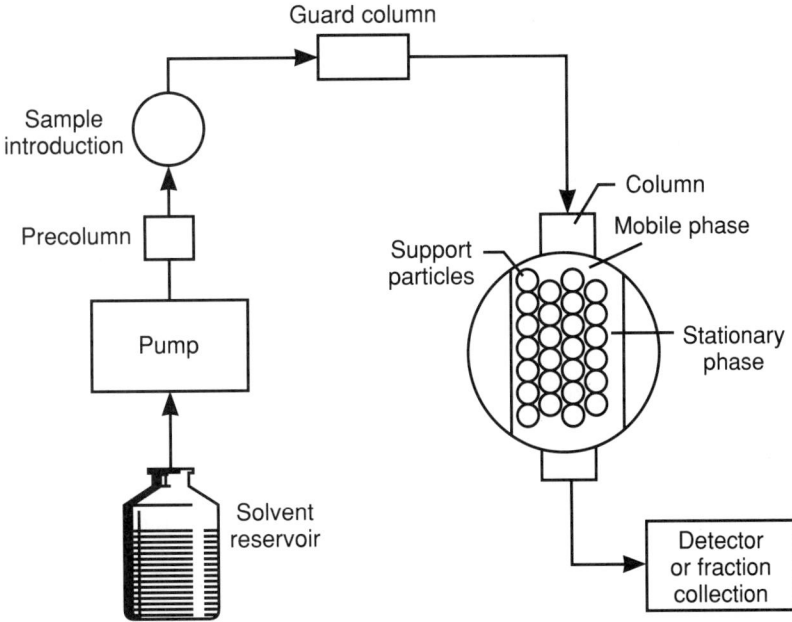

Fig. 14-3. Diagram of components of a high performance liquid chromatograph. (From Bowers and Carr,[72] with permission.)

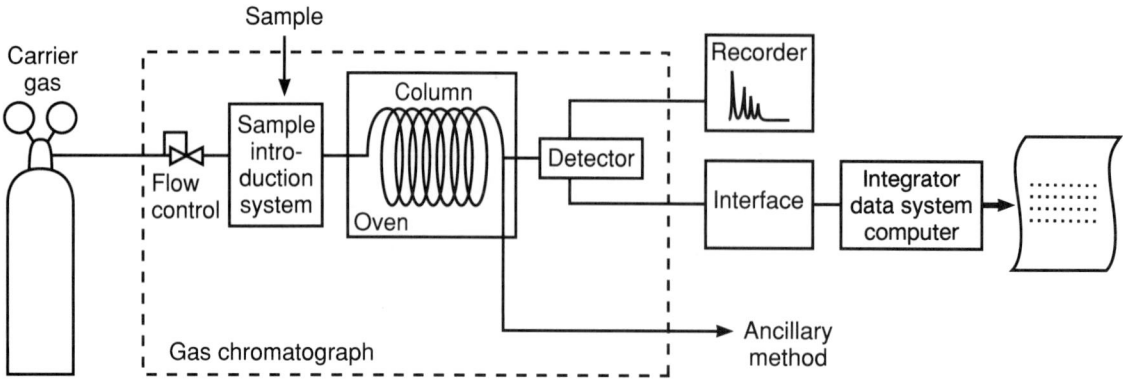

Fig. 14-4. Components of a gas chromatograph. (From Ettre,[73] with permission.)

Gas Chromatography (GC)

In gas liquid chromatography (GLC) (Fig. 14-4) a mixture of drugs is extracted from the serum or urine, injected in a volatilized form carried by the mobile phase (a gas, usually helium) into a chromatographic column (stationary phase), and eluted from the column following a rise in oven temperature. The degree of interaction of the drug with the relatively polar stationary phase determines the elution time. Just as in HPLC, identification of an unknown is based on column retention time and compared with internal and known standards for quantitation (Table 14-6). For drugs, approximately 1 μL of liquid is injected into the column; however, for volatiles such as alcohols, a gas phase can be injected into the column (Fig. 14-5).

GC provides a variety of drug detectors. The most common are flame ionization (FID), nitrogen-phosphorus (NP), and mass spectrometry (MS). Compounds that contain carbon can be detected with FID, and compounds containing nitrogen (most drugs) or phosphorus can be detected with NP. These detectors are widely used; however, as in any of the above techniques, the possibility exists for a false positive result if only retention times are used to identify analytes. In GC/MS, each GC peak is bombarded by a stream of electrons (electron impact ionization), which breaks the drug into many different mass fragments. Each drug fragmentation spectrum is unique and is analogous to a fingerprint pattern. Qualitative identification is usually the result of mass spectral identification with GC/MS. By preselecting certain mass fragments in the selected-ion monitoring (SIM) mode, quantitative analysis of very low (ng/mL) drug concentrations can be performed. Because of the specificity of the technique, GC/MS is the method of choice for confirmation of immunoassay results for forensic drugs of abuse testing.

THE ALCOHOLS

Alcohol (ethanol) is the most commonly encountered drug ingestion observed in the clinical setting. It may be seen as an acute intoxication or its complications (e.g., pancreatitis and aspiration pneumonia), as syn-

Table 14-6. Comparison of Analytic Techniques Used in Clinical Toxicology

Technique	Pretreatment of Sample	Major Instrumentation	Sensitivity (μg/mL)	Personnel Experience
TLC	Yes	No (<$1000)	0.5–1.0	Moderate
EMIT/FPIA	No	Yes ($25–50,000)	2.5–5.0	Moderate
HPLC	Yes	Yes ($25–50,000)	0.02–10	High
GC	Yes	Yes ($25–50,000)	0.01–10	Moderate
GC/MS	Yes	Yes ($75–125,000)	0.001–5	High

Abbreviations: TLC, thin-layer chromatography; EMIT, enzyme multiplied immunoassay technique; FPIA, fluorescence polarization immunoassay; HPLC, high performance liquid chromatography; GC, gas chromatography; MS, mass spectrometry.
(Modified from Council on Scientific Affairs of the American Medical Association,[64] with permission.)

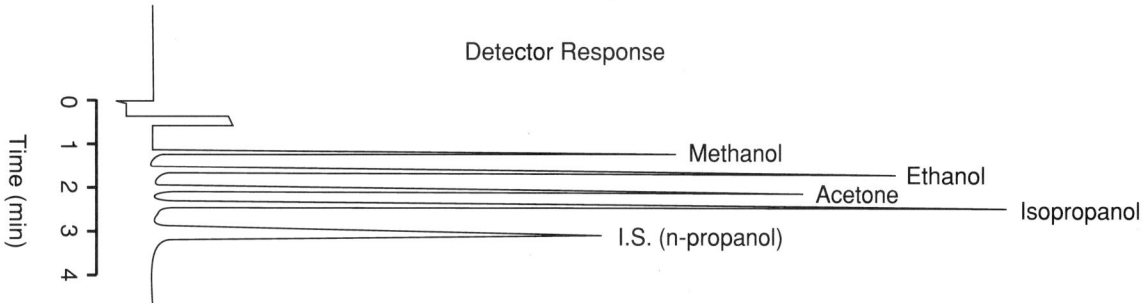

Fig. 14-5. Chromatogram from a head-space gas chromatograph showing separation of volatiles.

ergistic effects in combination with other drugs, or in connection with accusations of operating a motor vehicle while intoxicated ("driving under the influence," [DUI] or "driving while intoxicated," [DWI]).[7,8]

Although ethanol is the most frequently encountered "alcohol" or low molecular weight volatile, other toxic volatiles such as methanol, isopropanol, and ethylene glycol may be seen clinically and share similar chemical, metabolic, and toxicity characteristics (Table 14-7). Ethanol is absorbed rapidly from the gastrointestinal tract with peak levels observed within 30–60 minutes after ingestion. Ethanol is metabolized primarily (80%) by liver alcohol dehydrogenase (ADH) to acetaldehyde, by catalase to acetic acid, and then ultimately to carbon dioxide and water. The ADH reaction causes the generation of NADH with the depletion of NAD. A minor oxidative microsomal (cytochrome P_{450}) pathway exists. It is the cytochrome P_{450} mediated metabolism that explains the alcohol's interaction with other drugs or toxins. Over 90% of ingested ethanol is metabolized via ADH leaving less than 10% to be excreted unchanged, primarily in urine and in the breath. Ethanol, as well as the other low molecular weight volatiles, is distributed throughout body water having a profound effect on serum osmolality and can significantly alter the patient's metabolic status.[9]

Test: Ethanol (Alcohol, Ethyl Alcohol, Grain Alcohol)

Background and Selection

Alcohol measurements most often are ordered to establish whether a patient's altered mental status or appearance of intoxication is due to alcohol (ethanol) ingestion or to establish whether an individual was under the influence of ethanol while operating a motor vehicle (DUI or DWI). Serious ethanol poisoning occurs most often in children as a consequence of ingesting liquor, wine, cough medicine, or nonpotable sources of ethanol such as perfumes, mouthwashes, or antiseptics.

Logistics

Specimen Requirements

To determine the presence of alcohol, blood is the specimen of choice for either the living or the dead. When blood is not available, other specimens such as urine, spinal fluid, blood clot, and tissues may be used. Special attention must be paid to specimen collection; it is *not* acceptable to use preparatory wipes containing *ethanol*

Table 14-7. Comparative Properties of the Low Molecular Weight (M_r) Volatiles

Volatile	Structure	M_r	D-Osm at 100 mg/dL in Serum	Anion Gap Metabolic Acidosis	Acetonemia or Acetonuria
Methanol	CH3OH	32	31.3	Yes	No
Ethanol	CH3CH2OH	46	21.7	No[a]	No[a]
Isopropanol	CH3CHCH3 OH	60	16.7	No	Yes
Ethylene glycol	CH2=CH2 OH OH	62	16.1	Yes	No

[a] Not present unless alcoholic ketoacidosis supervenes.

Table 14-8. Comparison of Analytic Methods for Alcohol Analysis

Method	Sample and Treatment	Sensitivity and Specificity	Equipment
Enzymatic alcohol dehydrogenase	Serum or plasma (deproteinize blood)	Most sensitive for ethanol; insensitive for other volatiles	Spectrophotometer
Gas chromatography	Headspace equilibration	Detects all alcohols	Gas chromatograph
Osmometry	Serum or plasma	Detects total volatiles	Freezing point osmometer

(Modified from Dubowski,[65] with permission.)

to clean the arm before drawing blood. In these circumstances hexachlorophene or iodine alcohol-free antiseptics should be used. For medicolegal purposes, whole blood is the specimen of choice, with fluoride added as a preservative. In the clinical setting, serum or plasma may be used with oxalate, citrate, or heparin added as an anticoagulant. Specimens should be tightly sealed to avoid loss of the volatile and may be stored at room temperature (25°C) for 1 year, refrigerated (2-8°C) for 3 years, or frozen (−20°C) indefinitely.[10]

Analysis

Ethanol is most frequently measured in clinical situations using an enzymatic method employing alcohol dehydrogenase (ADH), and for medicolegal or forensic purposes using head-space GC (Fig. 14-5). The GC is the method of choice for ethanol and other low molecular weight volatile analyses, but may not be practical in meeting urgent clinical needs (Table 14-8). The ADH method is very sensitive for ethanol, but will not detect the other low molecular weight volatiles. With the ADH ethanol method, interferences from other volatiles occur only if they are present in extremely high concentrations. Freezing point osmometry can be used clinically to reasonably estimate ethanol and is useful in combination with the readily available ADH methods to screen for other low molecular weight volatiles (Fig. 14-6). Breath analysis (Breathalyzer) using a differential dichromate reduction is used in some states as a convenient and portable method for ethanol detection.

Interpretation

Ethanol exerts its pharmacologic effects in the same way that a general anesthetic does. There are generalized cumulative clinical effects of ethanol at increasing concentrations; however, these effects may vary with tolerance and drinking experience (Table 14-9). A blood content or breath ethanol equivalent of 100 mg/dL or 0.100 g%-wt/vol (21.7 mmol/L) is per se legal evidence of DUI or DWI.[11] There is evidence of a signifi-

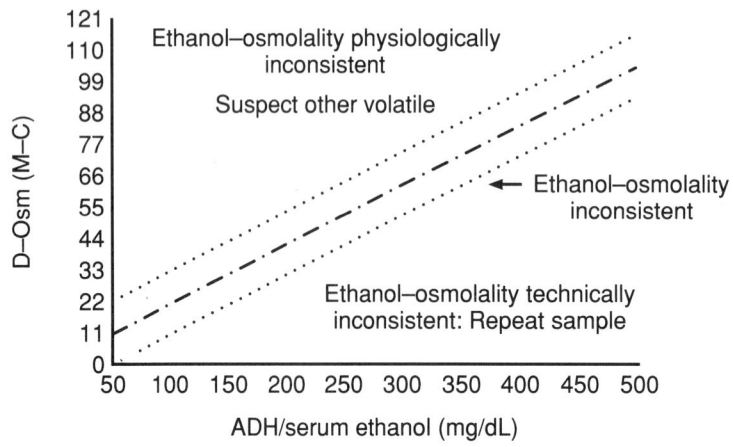

Fig. 14-6. Comparison of ethanol concentrations by ADH and D-Osm values, indicating areas of discrepancy and laboratory action. ADH, alcohol dehydrogenase; D-Osm, delta-osmolality; M−C, measured−calculated.

Table 14-9. Ethanol Concentrations and Clinical Symptoms

Concentration mg/dL (mmol/L)	Clinical Symptoms
<50 (<10.9)	None to limited euphoria
50–100 (10.9–21.7)	Incoordination, sensory impairment, impaired driving
100 (21.7)	Per se legally intoxicated
100–150 (21.7–32.6)	Personality and mood changes, slurred speech
150–200 (32.6–43.4)	Poor coordination and reaction time, thought processes impaired
200–300 (43.4–65.1)	Ataxia, visual disturbances, nausea and vomiting
300–400 (65.1–86.8)	Stuporous, hypothermia
500–700 (108.5–130.2)	Unconscious, respiratory failure, death

(Modified from Dubowski,[65] with permission.)

cant reduction in reaction response time attributable to ethanol ingestion even with lower blood ethanol concentration. It has been recommended that the presumptive blood alcohol concentrations (BAC) be reduced to 50 mg/dL (10.8 mmol/L) for defining legal intoxication.[12] Concentrations in excess of 50 mg/dL or 0.05 g%-wt/vol (10.8 mmol/L) but less than 100 mg/dL or 0.100 g%-wt/vol (21.7 mmol/L) are not currently considered presumptive evidence that the individual is DWI or DUI. However, ethanol concentrations in this range can be used to substantiate other evidence of apparent intoxication (e.g., roadside coordination testing). Ethanol is distributed throughout the body water, and its respective concentration in plasma or serum is 10–20% higher than in whole blood.[12] Most hospital clinical laboratories routinely use serum for ethanol determinations. Although there is some difference between whole blood and serum levels, it is not clinically significant. In forensic cases, however, this distinction may be critical. Ethanol is metabolized at a rate of 15–18 mg/dL/h (3.3–4.0 mmol/L/h) in the adult. This rate can be increased twofold in the tolerant individual owing to enzyme induction. The lethal range can vary from 180–600 mg/dL (39–130 mmol/L), and conversely only moderate central nervous system depression, albeit uncommon, can be observed with concentrations of 520–780 mg/dL (113–170 mmol/L). Survival has been observed with ethanol concentrations of up to 1130 mg/dL (245 mmol/L).[13] Results obtained from specimens other than blood can be of diagnostic help. The use of tissue/blood ratios to convert to a "calculated" BAC is not acceptable.[10]

Test: Methanol (Methyl Alcohol, Wood Alcohol)

Background

Methanol is used widely in windshield washer fluids, in paint removers, and sometimes, intentionally or unintentionally, in bootlegged whiskey (moonshine). Methanol intoxication often occurs accidentally by oral ingestion, but can also occur through skin absorption or inhalation. Methanol intoxication can occur in an epidemic fashion and may indeed present as a forensic emergency.[14] Methanol is metabolized to formaldehyde by ADH at a rate of one-tenth that of ethanol and then oxidized to its toxic metabolite, formic acid. Formic acid produces a severe anion gap metabolic acidosis and is directly toxic to the optic nerve. There is a consistent decrease in the serum bicarbonate, which is reciprocal to the accumulation of formate.

Selection

Methanol measurements are indicated in patients suspected of methanol ingestion and serve as a guide to therapy. Initially the patient with methanol intoxication may present with mild central nervous system depression similar to ethanol poisoning (the latent period). After 12–36 hours, an anion gap, metabolic acidosis with visual disturbances, and possible blindness develop. There may be further central nervous system deterioration leading to coma and death.

Logistics

Blood should be collected as for ethanol. Electrolyte measurements should also be performed and the patient's acid-base status assessed. Most clinical laboratories do not have GC readily available to perform methanol quantitations. Clinicians should clearly request a test for methanol levels, because a request for "alcohol quantitation" will be interpreted to mean ethanol. If GC is not available in a timely fashion, the performance of the serum osmolality and the presence of an anion gap with a metabolic acidosis will help establish the diagnosis.

Interpretation

Toxicity does not correlate well with the amount of methanol ingested or with blood methanol concentrations. Blood methanol concentrations are not good prognostic indicators in regards to the clinical course. As little as 10 mL of methanol ingested is considered toxic, and ingestions of 100–200 mL are usually fatal. In the untreated patient, blood concentrations in excess of 50 mg/dL (16 mmol/L) are potentially fatal. Concentrations below 50 mg/dL (<16 mmol/L) are adequately treated with ethanol blockade therapy and should be initiated during the latent phase. Specific therapy is achieved by slowing the metabolic degradation of methanol by administering a 5% ethanol infusion to maintain a blood ethanol level of 100 mg/dL (21.7 mmol/L). Dialysis is indicated for patients with a blood methanol concentration above 50 mg/dL (>16 mmol/L).[15] The accompanying metabolic acidosis must be corrected and attention paid to the possibility of a supervening acute pancreatitis.

Test: Isopropanol (Isopropyl Alcohol, Rubbing Alcohol)

Background and Selection

Isopropanol is readily available as a 70% solution known as rubbing alcohol and is the major ingredient in numerous cosmetics such as skin lotions and hair tonics. Ingestion is usually accidental in children and deliberate in the alcoholic because it is cheaper than ethanol and provides a slightly different intoxication. Inhalation of isopropanol vapors or dermal absorption can cause toxicity and even coma. Isopropanol is metabolized (80%) to acetone by ADH with an accompanying acetonemia and acetonuria usually without acidosis, although at a much slower rate than ethanol. Isopropanol is a potent central nervous system depressant with two to three times the intoxicating effect of ethanol. Gastrointestinal symptoms are caused by isopropanol's direct irritating effects, which are more frequently observed with isopropanol than with ethanol. Lethal ingestion is estimated to about 250 mL (8 oz) but is variable. Treatment is usually supportive.[16]

Logistics

Specimen collection and stability requirements for whole blood are the same for isopropanol as for ethanol. Gas chromatographic techniques (Fig. 14-5) are the best methods for detection and quantitation. The analyst should report any isopropanol and acetone detected. A urine specimen will show acetonuria (ketonuria) in the absence of hyperglycemia. In urgent clinical situations where GC is not available, an estimation of the isopropanol level can be made using the serum delta osmolality (D-Osm) value and supported by detecting the presence of acetone in either the blood or urine.

Interpretation

Blood levels of isopropanol should be interpreted in conjunction with its primary metabolite, acetone. In fact, only acetone in the blood or urine may be detected with late ingestion. Toxicity can be observed in children beginning at 50 mg/dL (8.3 mmol/L) with fatalities reported at 150 mg/dL (25 mmol/L). In adults, concentrations in excess of 400 mg/dL (65 mmol/L) can occur in nonfatal cases. Acetone levels accumulate in the blood and urine, persisting for 24 hours or more as isopropanol levels decline.[17]

Test: Ethylene Glycol (Antifreeze, Radiator Fluid)

Background and Selection

Ethylene glycol is an odorless, sweet-tasting solvent most commonly used in antifreeze and coolants. It has soporific effects similar to ethanol and has been used as a beverage by those unfamiliar with its toxicity, as a suicidal agent, or ingested accidentally by children (or household pets). Ethylene glycol itself is only mildly toxic, but is metabolized by ADH to its major toxic metabolite, glycolic acid, which causes a profound anion gap with a metabolic acidosis and central nervous system depression. Glycolic acid is further metabolized to several organic acids, including oxalate, which may in turn cause hypocalcemia and oxalate deposition in the kidneys. Oxalate crystals are found in urine relatively late after ingestion, but can be a helpful confirmatory finding.

The half-life of ethylene glycol is approximately 3 hours. The onset of acidosis usually occurs within 4–8 hours after ingestion as glycolic acid accumulates. The resulting acidosis is one of the most severe and treatment refractory found in clinical practice. Patients surviving this initial toxic period almost invariably develop renal failure. Treatment consists of correction of the profound metabolic acidosis, ethanol blockade of ADH, and possibly charcoal or hemoperfusion.[15]

Logistics

Specimen collection and stability requirements are the same for blood ethylene glycol levels as for ethanol. Assessment of the patient's acid-base status should be made. The GC techniques are the best methods for detection and quantitation for ethylene glycol. It may be helpful to perform blood oxalate and glycolic acid levels, if available. Urine should be examined for oxalate crystals. In urgent clinical situations where specific GC methods are not readily available, an estimation of the ethylene glycol level can be made using the serum D-Osm or osmol gap. The D-Osm discrepancy may not be sensitive enough to pick up the relatively low toxic levels of ethylene glycol; however, the profound metabolic acidosis and other metabolic derangements will give rise to an unexplainable hyperosmolality associated with ethylene glycol ingestion.

Interpretation

The presence of any ethylene glycol or its metabolites in blood or urine confirms the diagnosis. Because concentrations drop precipitously with time, ethylene glycol may not be detectable if time has elapsed since ingestion.

Examination of the urine for oxalate crystals is helpful in these late circumstances. Refractory metabolic acidosis with an unexplainable hyperosmolality and an increased anion gap suggest the diagnosis. The blood concentrations associated with death have ranged from 30–430 mg/dL (4.8–69.3 mmol/L).[18]

Test: Delta Osmolality (Osmol Gap)

Background

The presence of any of the aforementioned alcohols causes a linear increase in measured serum osmolality (M-Osm), which is proportional to its respective concentration and inversely proportional to its respective molecular weight (Table 14-7). The M-Osm must be performed using a freezing point osmometry. The M-Osm can be calculated (C-Osm) using the following formula[19]:

$$C\text{-}Osm = 2 \times Na + \frac{Glucose}{20} + \frac{BUN}{3}$$

where BUN is blood urea nitrogen and Na is sodium.

The difference between the M-Osm and the C-Osm is known as the D-Osm or osmol gap. The concentration of the respective volatile can be reasonably estimated from the patient's D-Osm (Fig. 14-6 and Table 14-10) or from the formula: concentration mg/dL = D-Osm $\times$ M_r/10.

The use of the D-Osm and the simultaneous measurement of ethanol by ADH is valuable in rapidly evaluating the acutely intoxicated patient when facilities are not available to identify and quantify the specific alcohols by GC on an emergency basis (Fig. 14-6).[2] This method gives the physician a rapid and reasonable estimation of the concentration of the intoxicant and can help differentiate between low molecular weight solvent ingestion versus other causes of metabolic acidosis.

Logistics

Blood collection is handled in the same manner as for ethanol analysis. Osmolality must be measured using the freezing point depression method. Care must be taken that specimens are not drawn into containers with anticoagulants (including sodium oxalate) because these substances are osmotically active, and the resultant M-Osm will be spuriously high leading to an unexplained D-Osm. The administration of physiologically active volume expanders such as dextran also

Table 14-10. Estimated Volatile Concentration (mg/dL) From D-Osm (mOsm/kg H_2O)[a]

D-Osm	Ethanol	Methanol	Acetone	Isopropanol	Ethylene Glycol
5[b]					
10	46	32	58	60	62
12	55	38	70	72	75
14	64	45	81	84	87
15	69	48	87	90	93
20	92	64	116	120	124
30	138	96	174	180	186
35	161	112	203	210	217
40	184	128	233	240	248

[a] The SI equivalent for the conventional concentration is equal to the D-Osm value.
[b] D-Osm values below 10 are within potential physiologic variation.
(Modified from Bell et al.,[66] with permission.)

causes a spuriously high M-Osm and resultant D-Osm. The use of the D-Osm to estimate volatile concentration is not valid in postmortem specimens because the method requires a homeostatically intact individual. A urine sample also should be collected to detect acetone and oxalate and a follow-up drug screen should be taken, if indicated.

Interpretation

The reference range for the D-Osm is 0 ± 10 mOsm/kg (0 ± 10 mmol/kg) H_2O. The variability in the D-Osm of ± 10 mOsm/kg (± 10 mmol/kg) H_2O reflects the presence of unmeasured electrolytes and proteins not considered in the C-Osm formula as well as analytic imprecision. Metabolic disorders such as hyperglycemia, uremia, or dehydration increase both the M-Osm and C-Osm and usually do not cause a D-Osm greater than 10 mOsm/kg (10 mmol/kg) H_2O. The D-Osm can be very helpful in ruling out the presence of ethanol and other volatiles and can be used to presumptively estimate the quantity of the suspected volatile (Table 14-9). The potential limitations of this method are its sensitivity in detecting ethylene glycol or methanol. For instance, an ethylene glycol concentration of 50 mg/dL theoretically results in a D-Osm of 8 (8 mmol/kg), a result within the reference range. Similarly, methanol concentrations as low as 23–30 mg/dL (7.2–9.4 mmol/L) have been observed in serious or fatal cases of methanol poisoning, but would result in D-Osm of approximately 7–9 mg/dL (7.2–9.4 mmol/L), again within the reference range. Caution should be exercised in evaluating a D-Osm value within the reference range in the patient with the history and clinical signs and symptoms of ethylene glycol, isopropanol, or methanol ingestion.[20]

A significant negative D-Osm (C-Osm greater than M-Osm) is usually indicative of an error in the calculation of D-Osm or C-Osm, or the analysis of serum M-Osm, glucose, urea nitrogen, or sodium.

NON-NARCOTIC ANALGESICS

Salicylate (aspirin) and acetaminophen, both non-narcotic analgesics, are the most widely used drugs in the world. Both drugs have equal antipyretic and analgesic effects. Acetaminophen does not have the anti-inflammatory effect of aspirin, but is virtually free of side effects in therapeutic doses. In contrast, aspirin even at low doses is associated with hypersensitivity reactions especially in asthmatic patients, as well as bleeding disorders and gastrointestinal distress. These drugs are available in so many different formulations, in combination with other prescriptions, and over-the-counter preparations that patients may not even be aware that they are ingesting the drug(s).[21,22] In addition, confusion can occur about proper dosages and timing, particularly in pediatric or geriatric populations. Wide variance in metabolism and excretion of these drugs also occurs in these two patient populations. Both of these drugs account for a significant number of reported poisonings whether intentional or unintentional.

Both drugs are rapidly absorbed from the gastrointestinal tract with an onset of action within 30 minutes, peak absorption in 1–2 hours, and a duration of action of approximately 4 hours. The metabolism and toxic manifestations, however, differ considerably.

Test: Salicylate (Aspirin, Acetylsalicylic Acid [ASA])

Background

Accidental acute ingestion of salicylate accounts for the majority of poisonings seen in the pediatric age group. Unrecognized toxicity can occur in adults on chronic therapy for diseases such as osteoarthritis, rheumatoid arthritis, or collagen vascular disorders. In adults, the half-life for the usual doses of 650 mg is 2–3 hours, whereas with larger doses, such as those used in rheumatoid disorders, the half-life increases to 15–30 hours.

The pharmacokinetics and toxicokinetics of aspirin have been described using nonlinear models like those used for phenytoin and barbiturates where the half-life increases as serum concentration increases. Salicylic acid and ASA (aspirin) are highly protein bound (80%) (to albumin) and are metabolized primarily to salicyluric acid. Both agents as well as salicyluric acid occupy cyclo-oxygenase active sites, which account for almost all of the pharmacologic activity. Renal excretion of salicylic acid and its metabolites is very sensitive to urine pH. An alkaline urine favors a more rapid excretion of salicylate and conversely an acidic environment favors drug reabsorption from the urine as well as hinders elimination. Displacement of salicylic acid from albumin by other drugs (e.g., probenecid and other nonsteroidal anti-inflammatory agents) and saturation of the metabolic pathways even at relatively low therapeutic levels can lead to accumulation and intoxication. Withdrawal of corticosteroids in patients concomitantly treated with high doses of salicylate results in salicylism if aspirin doses are not reduced.

Severe salicylate intoxication has four primary effects on the body: (1) hyperventilation with respiratory alkalosis caused by increasing the sensitivity of the respiratory centers to carbon dioxide and oxygen tension, (2) increasing the metabolic rate by uncoupling oxidative phosphorylation (which can result in fever and tachycardia), (3) production of an anion gap with ketoacidosis by inhibiting lipid and carbohydrate metabolism, and (4) interference with coagulation by inhibiting platelet aggregation or by decreasing coagulation factors. If seen, central nervous system depression is preceded by agitation and restlessness. Most patients with significant poisoning initially complain of tinnitus and some hearing loss caused by the direct ototoxic effects of salicylates. The broad spectrum of toxic effects can cause a perplexing diagnostic problem if salicylate toxicity is not suspected.

Selection

Salicylate is monitored in rheumatoid arthritis and other inflammatory diseases to achieve effective blood concentrations. In chronic high dose therapy with resulting serum levels of 30–40 mg/dL (2.2–2.9 mmol/L), aspirin demonstrates dose dependent or saturable kinetics. The dose required to reach the upper therapeutic range nearly approximates that producing toxic concentrations, frequently causing patients an insidious toxicity. Salicylate levels should be measured periodically in patients on high dose regimens or in suspected cases of salicylate intoxication.

Logistics

For therapeutic monitoring, the specimen is collected just prior to the next dose. In acute overdoses, the specimen should be collected as soon as possible. Because of impaired dispersion, absorption, and distribution, a second level should be determined 4–6 hours after the suspected ingestion to detect peak levels, that are used to predict the seriousness of the toxicity (Fig. 14-7). After initial levels are drawn and determined, serial monitoring every 2–4 hours should be done to assess if there is continued absorption of salicylate from the gut. With liquid salicylate ingestions (e.g., Oil of Wintergreen), levels should be measured within 1–2 hours after ingestion because these salicylate preparations

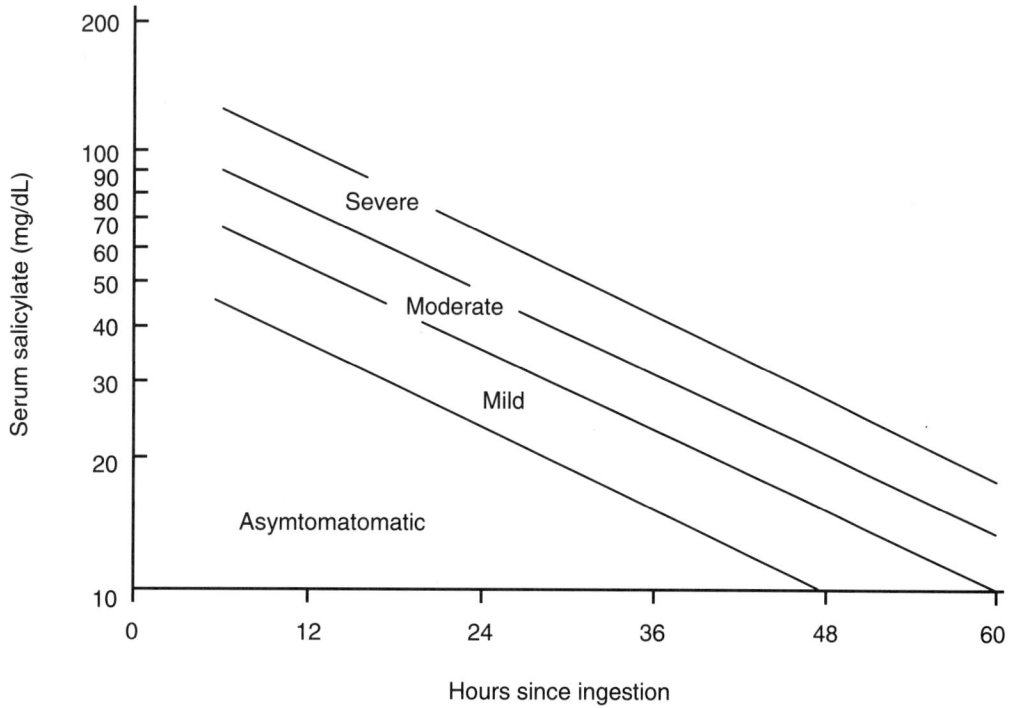

Fig. 14-7. Salicylate poisoning. Nomogram relating serum salicylate level to severity of intoxication at time intervals postingestion of single doses of aspirin. (Modified from Done,[74] with permission.)

are absorbed rapidly. The analytic method for quantifying serum salicylate is a colorimetric assay using the Trinder reaction and is readily available as a stat procedure in most laboratories.

Interpretation

The usual dose of two tablets of aspirin (650 mg) results in serum concentrations of less than 6 mg/dL (<0.4 mmol/L). Although analgesia occurs with salicylate concentrations less than 10 mg/dL (<0.72 mmol/L), levels of 15–30 mg/dL (1.1–2.2 mmol/L) are necessary for patients with osteoarthritis or rheumatologic disorders.

Patients with excess salicylate ingestion who present with tinnitus or a serum concentration in excess of 40–50 mg/dL (>2.9–3.6 mmol/L) should be hospitalized. At levels above 40 mg/dL (>2.9 mmol/L), respiratory alkalosis is common and may be complicated by a compensatory metabolic acidosis. At levels above 500 mg/dL (>36 mmol/L), there is significant mortality. A nomogram relating potential toxicity to peak serum concentrations can be used in acute overdoses (Fig. 14-7). The predictive nomogram for salicylate toxicity is not appropriate to use in cases of chronic salicylate therapy, because severe salicylate toxicity can occur at much lower concentrations.[23]

Test: Acetaminophen

Background

Acetaminophen is rapidly absorbed orally with peak concentrations observed 2 hours after ingestion. The half-life is approximately 4 hours. Acetaminophen is metabolized primarily by glucuronic acid conjugation and by a minor oxidative pathway (cytochrome P_{450}). The postulated toxic, oxidative metabolite, N-acetyl-imidoquinone, is detoxified by conjugation with limited amounts of hepatic glutathione and subsequent renal excretion. This postulated toxic metabolite is highly reactive, and in toxic ingestions its rate of formation increases as other metabolic pathways are saturated. Glutathione becomes rapidly depleted with toxic ingestions forcing N-acetyl-imidoquinone to covalently bind to hepatic macromolecules causing the observed hepatic necrosis.[24] Cytochrome P_{450} inducers such as ethanol increase the concentration of the toxic, oxidative metabolite.

N-acetylcysteine (NAC) (Mucomist) provides an analogue of glutathione and can be used as a direct antidote (sequestering agent) for acetaminophen toxicity. To be effective, NAC must be given within 24 hours after a toxic ingestion. An acute ingestion of 10–15 g of acetaminophen is toxic and if untreated results in hepatic necrosis. Doses of 25 g are potentially fatal. Toxicity occurs in four distinct phases. In contrast to many other analgesics, it is important to note that central nervous system depression does not occur until late when hepatic encephalopathy supervenes (Table 14-11).

Selection

Acetaminophen is not routinely monitored because poor correlation exists between analgesic relief and serum concentrations. Acetaminophen levels are principally determined to predict potential toxicity and to institute NAC therapy.[25] If acetaminophen quantitations are not readily available, it is prudent to treat the

Table 14-11. Stages of Acetaminophen Toxicity and Associated Findings

Stage/Time	Clinical Symptoms	Laboratory Findings
I/12–24 h	Nausea, vomiting, anorexia, diaphoresis	None except serum toxic level for acetaminophen
II/24–48 h	Clinical improvement	Increase in liver enzymes, prothombin time begins to increase
III/72–96 h	Hepatic failure and encephalopathy	Marked elevation of liver enzymes, coagulopathy, and renal failure
IV/7–8 d	Recovery or Death	Resolution Persistence of abnormally high liver enzymes

(Modified from Rumack et al.,[26] with permission.)

patient with NAC on the basis of the clinical history. Chronic hepatotoxicity with chronic acetaminophen ingestion can occur among alcoholics and patients taking known inducers of cytochrome P_{450}.[26]

Logistics

Serum levels most accurately predict toxicity when blood samples are drawn at least 4 hours after ingestion. If the analysis cannot be performed in a timely manner, treatment should begin with NAC and be terminated only if the initial serum concentration is below the toxic threshold for the appropriate postingestion time (Fig. 14-8). Baseline liver function tests (aspartate transaminase [AST], alanine transaminase [ALT], lactate dehydrogenase [LD], bilirubin) and coagulation studies (prothrombin time [PT], partial thromboplastin time [PTT]) should be ordered concomitantly and are useful in follow-up care.

Interpretation

The therapeutic range of acetaminophen associated with analgesia is 5–20 µg/mL (31–124 mmol/L). In suspected overdoses, *only* the initial or presenting concentration of acetaminophen is valid for predicting toxicity. Concentrations of 150 µg/mL (930 mmol/L) at 4 hours, 75 µg/mL (465 mmol/L) at 8 hours, and 37 µg/mL (237 mmol/L) or greater at 12 hours postingestion are indications to begin immediate treatment with NAC. Because the toxic metabolite represents only 4% of the total biotransformation of acetaminophen, it is inappropriate to extrapolate subsequent acetaminophen concentrations to a presumptive initial concentration to predict toxicity. Subsequent acetaminophen levels that fall below the toxic threshold line are not an indication to discontinue NAC treatment, nor are they indicative of the efficacy of treatment.[26]

BENZODIAZEPINES

The benzodiazepines are used primarily for the relief of anxiety, insomnia, muscle spasm, and for the control of epilepsy. Although benzodiazepines are the most frequently prescribed drugs in the United States and are chosen principally for their low incidence of addiction, psychological dependence or toxicity has been reported.[27] They are rarely the sole cause of death.[28] They are rapidly absorbed following ingestion and may be metabolized to active metabolites with varying half-lives (Table 14-12). Virtually all the therapeutic effects of the benzodiazepines involve modulation of γ-aminobutyric acid (GABA) (an inhibitory neurotransmitter) with resulting increases in GABA activity.

Test: Benzodiazepine (Table 14-12)

Background and Selection

Therapeutic monitoring of benzodiazepines is not performed routinely; however, plasma levels are obtained for the assessment of toxicity. The most common side effects of benzodiazepines are sedation, somnolence, ataxia, and intellectual impairment. With toxic reactions, the probability that benzodiazepines are the sole cause is rare, and other causes of toxicity should be sought.

Logistics

No special specimen or patient preparation is necessary. Semiquantitative identification can be made by immunoassays and definitive quantitations by GC or HPLC. Immunoassays may show significant crossreactivity, and it is necessary to know the specificity and limitations of the respective immunoassay method used in a laboratory.

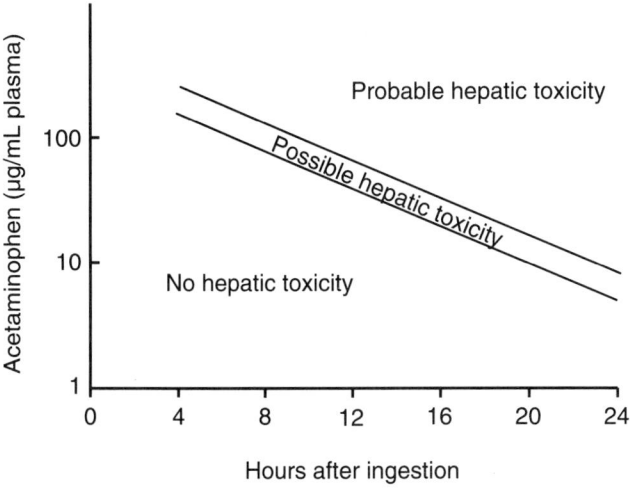

Fig. 14-8. Acetaminophen toxicity. Nomogram relating serum acetaminophen level to the potential hepatotoxicity at time intervals postingestion of single doses of acetaminophen. (Modified from Rumack and Matthew,[75] with permission.)

Table 14-12. Benzodiazepines, Comparison of Half-Life, Therapeutic and Toxic Concentrations

Indication Drug Active Metabolite(s)	Half-life (h)	Serum Concentration Therapeutic µg/mL (µmol/L)	Toxic µg/mL (µmol/L)
Anxiolytic			
Alprazolam	12–19	0.011–0.018 (0.036–0.058)	—
Hydroxy-alprazolam			
Chlordiazepoxide	7–14	0.5–1.0 (1.67–3.34)	>5 (>16.7)
Demoxepam	14–95	0.5–0.74 (1.74–1.86)	
Oxazepam	4–18	0.2–1.4 (0.7–4.9)	
Chlorzepate	30–97	0.12–1.0 (0.36–3.0)	>5 (>15.6)
Desmethyldiazepam			
Diazepam	21–37	0.5–2.5 (1.76–8.78)	>5 (>17.6)
Desmethyldiazepam			
Oxazepam	4–18	0.2–1.4 (0.7–4.9)	—
Temazepam	3–38	0.3–0.75 (1–2.5)	—
Halazepam	7		
Desmethyldiazepam			
Lorazepam	10–20	0.05–0.24 (0.16–0.75)	—
Oxazepam	4–18	0.2–1.4 (0.70–4.9)	—
Prazepam	36–200	0.8 (2.46)	—
Hypnotic			
Flurazepam	<2	<0.004 (<0.01)	—
Desalkylflurazepam			
Temazepam	10	0.017–0.13 (0.057–0.44)	—
Oxazepam			
Anticonvulsant			
Clonazepam	20–60	0.015–0.06 (0.048–0.19)	—
Diazepam	21–37	0.5–2.5 (1.76–8.78)	>5 (>17.6)

(Data from Moffat[39] and Tietz.[67])

Interpretation

The therapeutic ranges should be interpreted cautiously in conjunction with the patient's hepatic and renal status. The coingestion of other drugs such as phenobarbital or cimetidine may alter metabolism and prolong or decrease the effects of benzodiazepines, respectively. Serum determinations correlate poorly with the observable clinical effects caused by the extensive protein binding with variances in central nervous system penetration. In cases of suspected benzodiazepine toxicity with more than mild central nervous system depression, other drugs such as alcohol, barbiturates, or tricyclic antidepressants should be suspected. In only 2 of over 1200 deaths associated with diazepam ingestion was the cause of death solely related to diazepam. Toxic (5–20 µg/mL [17.6–70.2 µmol/L]) and lethal (720 µg/mL [2527 µmol/L]) ranges have been defined, but they rely on single case reports or small series of patients, reflecting the overall safety of the benzodiazepines.[29]

BARBITURATES

The barbiturates are chemically similar drugs with hypnotic, anticonvulsant, and sedative properties. The barbiturates are usually classified according to their duration of action (Table 14-13). Phenobarbital and mephobarbital are long-acting barbiturates used primarily to control seizure disorders. The barbiturates decrease the excitability of neurons by increasing intracellular sodium, thus increasing the threshold for seizures and inhibiting the spread of discharges through the cerebral cortex. The shorter-acting barbiturates, namely, amobarbital, pentobarbital, and secobarbital, are used primarily as hypnotics or sedatives. Their popularity is waning as other drugs with greater efficacy and safety, such as the benzodiazepines, are being prescribed as anxiolytics or hypnotics. These changes have resulted in a 50% reduction in barbiturate associated deaths. It is the shorter-acting barbiturates that have the highest abuse potential. The ultra-short-acting barbiturates such as thiopental are used

Table 14-13. Comparative Data on the More Commonly Used Barbiturates

Class (Duration of Action) Generic Name	Dose (mg)	Half-life (h)	Serum Concentration Therapeutic µg/mL (mmol/L)	Toxic µg/mL (mmol/L)
Long-acting (>6 h)				
Mephobarbital	200–600	48–52	0.5–1.7 (2–6.9)	—
Phenobarbital	50–100	50–100	15–40 (65–172)	>40 (172)
Intermediate (3–6 h)				
Amobarbital	60–200	15–4	1–5 (4–22)	>10 (44)
Butabarbital	100–200	35–40	1–10 (5–47)	>10 (>50)
Short-acting (<3 h)				
Pentobarbital	50–100	20–30	1–5 (4–22) 20–40 (80–160)	>10 (>44) Therapeutic coma
Secobarbital	50–100	15–40	1–2 (4.2–8.4)	>5 (>21)
Ultrashort-acting (10 min)				
Thiopental	50–70 IV	6–46	1–5 (4.1–20.7) 7–130 (29–537) 30–100 (124–414)	Hypnotic Anesthesia Therapeutic coma

intravenously for induction of general anesthesia and do not present with clinical toxicity except on rare occasions.

Phenobarbital is the most widely prescribed barbiturate and has the greatest margin of safety; however, chemical dependence can occur as with any of the barbiturates. Sudden cessation of chronic phenobarbital maintenance can precipitate generalized tonic-clonic seizures. The barbiturates cause clinically observable depression of the central nervous system that may range from mild sedation to deep coma accompanied by a corresponding respiratory depression. The degree of central nervous system depression is dependent on the particular barbiturate, the route of administration, and the cumulative dose. In general, the shorter acting the barbiturate, the more potent its depressive effects on the central nervous system and respiratory system. Potential lethal ingestions produce apnea with cardiac arrest. If the patient survives, the clinical course may be complicated with pulmonary edema, circulatory failure, and pneumonia.[30] Ethanol potentiates the depressant effects of the barbiturates and other central nervous system depressants. The long-acting barbiturates are metabolized by hepatic biotransformation with dose dependent pharmacokinetics and serum concentration dependent half-lives.

Test: Barbiturates (Amobarbital, Butabarbital, Butalbital, Mephobarbital, Pentobarbital, Phenobarbital, Secobarbital, Thiopental, Goof Balls, Sleeping Pills)

Background and Selection

Phenobarbital, mephobarbital, and a closely related compound primidone are used primarily for treating various seizure disorders. Mephobarbital is converted to phenobarbital by oxidative demethylation, which accounts for its anticonvulsant effects. Primidone has anticonvulsant properties of its own and is also converted to phenobarbital and phenylethylmalonamide (PEMA), which have anticonvulsant properties. The therapeutic ranges for these drugs as anticonvulsants have been established; however, adverse reactions can occur at lower than expected levels, and tolerance can occur because the barbiturates are inducers of the cytochrome P_{450} system of the liver.

Phenobarbital, mephobarbital, and primidone are monitored to optimize dosage in individual patients. Although therapeutic ranges have been established, toxic reactions can occur at subtherapeutic ranges, and conversely, control of seizures may not be achieved until nominally "toxic" ranges have been achieved. Monitoring of levels is indicated anytime there are changes in the dosage regimen, suspected toxicity, addition or deletion of concomitant anticonvulsants, or drug interaction. Barbiturate poisoning is most often due either to the ingestion of phenobarbital, phentobarbital, or secobarbital, one of the more common causes of drug-induced coma. Reduction of intracranial pressure with pentobarbital in patients with closed head injury also requires careful monitoring.[31]

Logistics

In interpreting results, it is important to know the analytic methods that have been used to determine levels of phenobarbital and the other barbiturates. Methods specific for phenobarbital may not detect the other barbiturates and conversely there may be crossreactivity in analytic methods for the other barbiturates with phenobarbital. The barbiturates can be measured using immunoassays, differential ultraviolet spectrophotometry, GLC, or HPLC. Immunoassays are the most frequent clinical methods used to determine levels of phenobarbital and total barbiturates. The barbiturate class immunoassays primarily detect secobarbital, whereas TLC can classify the barbiturates as short, intermediate, or long-acting.

Interpretation

Serum levels should complement clinical findings and can be correlated with clinical findings if the patient is not a habitual user of the drug. In addicted individuals, tolerance can develop and apparently toxic concentrations may be associated with few clinical findings of toxicity. Most barbiturate overdoses arise from attempted suicide typically with a short-acting barbiturate along with alcohol. The more potent short acting barbiturates have greater toxicity at lower concentrations (Table 14-13).

The correlation of clinical state and blood concentration of short-acting barbiturates in nonaddicted individuals is found in Table 14-14. Associated lethal blood levels by duration of action are short-acting barbiturates, 30–40 µg/mL (16.3–21.7 µmol/L); intermediate-acting barbiturates, greater than 30 µg/mL (>16.3 µmol/L); long-acting barbiturates, greater than 80–150 µg/mL (>34.4–64.6 µmol/L).

DRUGS OF ABUSE

Drug abuse is an increasing public health problem. Drug screening programs have been instituted in the workplace (for pre-employment, random testing, or job-related incidents), at drug rehabilitation centers, and by the criminal justice system to monitor compliance with abstinence programs. Drug abuse can be broadly defined as the use of a drug for purposes other than for which it is legitimately prescribed (drug class II-VI) or as possession or use of class I substance (e.g., heroin, psilocybin, or the methylenedioxyamphetamine compounds, methelynedioxamphetamine [MDA] and methoxymethylenedioxyamphetamine [MMDA]). The laboratory testing for drugs of abuse has been controversial, and a final resolution as to the limits of its applications in specific cases is yet to be resolved.[33] The drugs of abuse over the years have changed; however, marijuana, cocaine, opiates, amphetamines, and PCP are currently screened as recommended by the National Institute of Drug Abuse (NIDA) (Table 14-15). Other drugs, such as LSD, certainly have a high abuse potential; however, these are not discussed because they are not routinely measured by the clinical laboratory, and the treatment is symptom management.

Amphetamines are central nervous system stimulants for which there are few legitimate uses. (Legitimate uses include documented adult narcolepsy and childhood attention deficit disorders.) With the exception of methamphetamine, which is taken intravenously, the rest are taken orally. Clinical toxicity from amphetamines can be classified as mild (restlessness, insomnia, combativeness), moderate (panic reaction, vomiting, diffuse diaphoresis), and severe (hyperpyrexia, convulsions).[34] Deaths are infrequent and are usually associated with violent actions or cardiovascular complications. Cocaine is currently one of the most widely abused members of the class I drugs and is the most potent naturally occurring stimulant with psychologically addictive properties; with chronic, habitual use it

Table 14-14. Effect of Short-Acting Barbiturates in Nonaddicted Individuals

Clinical State	Blood Concentration µg/mL (µmol/L)
Alert	<6 (<3.3)
Drowsiness	6–10 (3.3–5.4)
Stuporus	11–17 (5.9–9.2)
Coma I	16–20 (6.8–10.8)
Coma II	20–24 (10.8–13.0)
Coma III	24–28 (13.0–15.2)
Coma IV	28–34 (15.2–18.5)

(Data from McCarron et al.[32])

Table 14-15. Positive Decision Levels for Screening and Confirmation of Selected Drugs of Abuse in Urine

Drug	Screening Test, ng/mL (µmol/L)	Confirmatory Test, ng/mL (µmol/L)	Duration of Detection
Marijuana			3 days to month depending on chronicity
Metabolites	100[a]	—	
9-Carboxy-THC	—	15 (0.042)	
Cocaine			
Metabolites	300[a]	—	
Benzoylecgonine	—	150 (1.04)	2–3 d
Opiates			
Metabolites	300[a]	—	
Morphine	—	300 (3.51)	2–3 d
Phencyclidine	25 (0.103)	25 (0.103)	2–3 d
Amphetamines	1000[a]	—	2–3 d
Amphetamine	—	500 (3.70)	
Methamphetamine	—	500 (3.70)	

[a] Cumulative total for metabolites or structurally related compounds.
(Modified from the Federal Register,[68] with permission.)

induces paranoia. It is estimated that over 20 million individuals in the United States have used cocaine, with approximately 10% becoming addicted. Cocaine's only medical use is for mucous membrane anesthesia and vasoconstriction. The drug does not cause the classic addiction patterns seen with the opiates but does lead to compulsive drug-oriented behavior. The street drug invariably contains various adulterants (e.g., quinine, strychnine, and lactose) or substitutes for cocaine (e.g., ephedrine, phenylpropanolamine [PPA], and lidocaine). Adverse reactions to "cocaine" may indeed be reactions to these compounds.

The most common form of cocaine administration is by insufflation, "snorting." The free base form of cocaine ("crack") is sublimed by heating chunks of cocaine, and the resulting fumes are inhaled and rapidly absorbed systemically in a manner similar to cigarette smoking. Cocaine toxicity can be divided into three sequential phases: early (euphoria, bruxism, mild circulatory changes with increased respirations), late (convulsions, cyanosis, cardiovascular instability, respiratory failure), and depressive (paralysis, coma, and death).[35] Phencyclidine, similar to the anesthetic ketamine, was used as an animal anesthetic and is currently abused by humans as a hallucinogen. Patients with PCP intoxication may be categorized into two classes: minor (stupor, violent, or bizarre behavior) and major (toxic psychosis, catatonia, or coma). Patients with PCP symptoms belonging to the major group should be hospitalized.[36] Marijuana is a natural product containing several psychoactive compounds of which δ-9-tetrahydrocannabinol (THC) is the most abundant. After smoking, THC is rapidly absorbed through the oral mucous membranes and pulmonary alveoli. Because it is extremely lipophilic, THC is readily sequestered into adipose tissue and slowly released back into the circulation with prolonged disappearance of metabolites. The primary metabolite measured in drug testing is 11-nor-δ-9-THC carboxylic acid (9-carboxy-THC), which has a half-life of days to weeks. The clinical features of acute marijuana intoxication may be so subtle that it should be suspected in patients having difficulty with cognitive functions, such as thinking and speaking.

Test: Drug Screen (Drug of Abuse Panel, Pre-Employment Drug Screen)

Background and Selection

The performance of any laboratory test for drugs of abuse serves to document prior use, but neither blood nor urine levels correlate with clinical findings. Management is based on the patient's clinical initial presentation and course.

Logistics

The specimen for drug abuse screening usually is urine. There must be rigorous specimen handling to assure that there is no adulteration of the specimen, that

Table 14-16. Comparative Data on Selected Drugs of Abuse

Drug Street Name	Clinical Effects	Duration (h)	Half-life (h)	Blood Concentrations Toxic ng/mL (µmol/L)	Blood Concentrations Lethal ng/mL (µmol/L)
Amphetamines Speed, uppers, pep pills	Insomnia, anorexia, arrhythmias, paranoia	2–4	7–24	200 (1.48)	>500 (>3.7)
Cocaine Coke, snow, flake, nose	Euphoria, confusion, cardiac arrhythmia	1–2	2–5	250 (0.82)	>1000 (>3.30)
Marijuana Grass, weed, Mary Jane	Altered perception, disorientation	2–4	14–38	—	—
Opiates Junk, skag, dope	Euphoria, drowsiness	3–6	10–18	Heroin 10 (30) Morphine 200 (0.7)	3000 (8.1) 5000 (17.5)
Phenycyclidine PCP, hog, angel dust	Bizarre behavior, acute brain syndrome	2–4	8–16	>100 (>0.4)	>300 (>1.2)

proper legal chain of custody is maintained, and that security of the specimen handling and the facility is adequate to assure that unauthorized individuals do not have access to the specimens or results. Generally, drugs are screened for by a sensitive immunoassay and confirmed by GC/MS. The immunoassays used for detecting amphetamines crossreact with many similar but legal substances such as phenteramine, PPA, or pseudoephedrine.[37] Confirmation is mandatory for absolute identification of a presumptively positive immunoassay screen. The primary metabolite of cocaine, benzylecgonine, is readily detectable in urine using immunoassays. The primary metabolite of the opiates and opioids, morphine, is readily detected using an immunoassay. The immunoassays do not have sufficient crossreactivity to detect synthetic narcotics such as propoxyphene. Determination of PCP by TLC procedures may lack sufficient sensitivity; therefore, suspected PCP ingestion should be tested using immunoassay techniques. Immunoassays for marijuana detect total cannabinoids, and because confirmatory testing by GC/MS is generally directed against 9-carboxy-THC, quantitative GC/MS levels are lower than those detected by immunoassay screening.

Interpretation

Positive urine tests indicate probable prior use and cannot be correlated with impairment. The negative threshold cutoffs for an immunoassay screen and the follow-up quantitative positive threshold levels using GC/MS are given in Table 14-15. The duration of detectability in urine must take into account variables such as route, frequency of ingestion, metabolism, state of hydration, and the individual's overall physical condition. In general, there is poor correlation between blood concentrations and toxic effect or even impairment. Wide ranges in concentrations have been reported for toxic or fatal cases (Table 14-16).[38,39]

Test: Opiates and Opioids

Background

This class of drug includes drugs actually contained in the poppy itself (opiates), drugs derived from morphine (semisynthetics or opioids), and the synthetic narcotics (Table 14-17). These drugs are most often prescribed for the relief of pain. Opiate intoxication presents classically with coma, respiratory depression, and constricted pupils. The most common cause of death is respiratory depression, which is potentiated by the presence of other drugs such as alcohol. In the adult, poisoning is most commonly seen after intravenous heroin or oral methadone ingestion by addicts or nontolerant individuals. Propoxyphene (a cogener of methadone) is often taken in suicides. Children may accidentally ingest methadone, propoxyphene, or diphenoxylate. Neonates of mothers who are heroin addicts or on methadone maintenance often show signs of withdrawal within hours of birth. Iatrogenic opiate

Table 14-17. Comparative Characteristics of the Opiates and Opioids

Subclass Drug	Half-life (h)	Blood Concentrations Therapeutic μg/mL (mmol/L)	Toxic μg/mL (mmol/L)
Opiates			
Codeine	2.0–3.0	0.010–0.100 (0.033–0.334)	>0.2 (>0.67)
Morphine	1.3–6.7	0.065–0.08 (0.185–0.228)	>0.2 (>0.7)
Semisynthetic opioids			
Heroin	1–1.5	—	>0.01 (>0.03)
Hydromorphone	1.5–3.8	0.001–0.03 (0.003–0.105)	>0.1 (>0.35)
Oxycodone	—	0.01–0.1 (0.032–0.317)	>0.2 (>0.63)
Synthetic opioids			
Anileridine	1–3	—	—
Butorphanol	2–4	0.0003–0.003 (0.0009–0.009)	—
Dextromethorphan	2–4	0.001–0.008 (0.0036–0.0295)	—
Diphenoxylate	~2	—	—
Fentanyl	1–6	—	—
Levorphanol	~13	—	—
Meperidine	2–5	0.7–0.5 (0.28–2.0)	>1.0 (>4.04)
Methadone	15–55	0.1–0.4 (0.32–1.29)	>2.0 (>6.46)
Pentazocine	2.1–3.5	0.05–0.2 (0.17–0.70)	>1.0 (>3.5)
Propoxyphene	8–24	0.1–0.4 (0.3–1.2)	>0.5 (>1.5)

(Data from Lancet [Editorial].[40])

overdoses are seen in association with meperidine, morphine, and pentazocine overadministration.

The opiates are well absorbed from the gastrointestinal tract and other routes of administration such as intramuscularly, intravenously, or subcutaneously. The opiates are metabolized in the liver and then conjugated with glucuronide or sulfate for enhanced renal excretion. The drugs are excreted in the urine in the unchanged form or as metabolites.

Selection

The opiates are rarely monitored for clinical purposes, and analysis is usually limited to toxicologic and forensic purposes. Whenever an opiate overdose is suspected, administration of a narcotic antagonist (naloxone) will promptly reverse the coma, respiratory depression, and hypotension of morphine, codeine, and almost all semisynthetic opioids.[41,42] Administration of naloxone thus provides a useful clinical test for the presence of toxic levels of opioids.

Logistics

Urine is the specimen of choice in documenting the presence of an opiate or opioid. The immunoassays are more sensitive than TLC and are primarily directed against morphine, the primary metabolite of these drugs. Thus, codeine ingestion may give a result that cannot be distinguished from morphine or some other compound in this class. Screening methods need to be confirmed by definitive GC/MS methods if the results are being used to monitor patients for abstinence. Quantitative methods using blood are technically difficult and do not usually help in the acute assessment of the patient for opiate or opioid intoxication. The quantitative methods include GC, GC/MS, and HPLC methods.

Interpretation

The precise dosage and hence blood concentration that is considered toxic or lethal cannot be determined due to individual variation in tolerance and sensitivity (Table 14-17). In general, the shorter the onset and duration of action of the opiate the greater the rapidity of symptom onset and intensity (e.g., heroin is less intense than morphine, which is less intense than propoxyphene, which is less intense than methadone). All positive screening tests need to be confirmed by definitive methods since crossreactivity can occur and because of the serious consequences of inadvertently labeling a patient as having a history of opiate abuse.

METALS

> **Test:** Arsenic (As, Arsenic Triioxide, Cacodylic Acid), Cadmium (Cd, Cigarettes), Iron (Fe, Ferrous Sulfate, Ferrous Gluconate, Feosol), Lead (Pb, Antiknock Gasoline, Paint), Mercury (Hg, Electronics, Pesticides, Explosives)

Background

There are approximately 40 elements that are classified as metals, the toxicity of which is variable as is the means of exposure (Table 14-18). The precise mechanism of toxicity is different for each metal; toxicity results from the metals binding to metabolically active functional groups on enzymes and structural proteins within selected organs. Most exposures are industrial (aerosols), with occasional episodes of intentional or accidental ingestion (primarily iron in children). A few but notable instances of poisoning have occurred when metals (mercury or cadmium) have been introduced into the ecosystem because of industrial pollution. With the exception of iron, none of these metals is needed for human homeostasis. The signs and symptoms of metal toxicity are so nonspecific and variable that a good medical history is essential as is a high index of suspicion.

Selection

Metal poisoning may be acute or chronic. With potential industrial exposure (As, Cd, Pb, Hg), an initial pre-employment baseline urine level should be determined. After individual baseline urine levels have been established for the respective metal, the employee should be monitored for exposure with quantitative levels taken every 3-6 months.

Logistics

Specimen Requirements

In industrial monitoring or in cases of chronic toxicity, a 24-hour urine collection is the preferred specimen. The urine containers used for metal analysis need to be "acid washed" by soaking them in nitric acid and rinsing them several times with distilled or deionized water of the highest purity. In cases of suspected acute iron poisoning, serum is analyzed for iron and total iron binding capacity (TIBC). Iron levels must be taken within 3-5 hours after ingestion because iron is cleared so rapidly, thus serum levels after this period of time may be misleadingly low. In cases of acute toxicity involving the heavy metals, whole blood samples are the initial specimens of choice; gastric contents may be helpful and subsequent 24-hour urine collections are useful to monitor the rate of excretion particularly if a chelator (e.g., British anti-Lewisite (BAL), desferoxamine, or EDTA) is used to promote excretion.[43]

Hair analysis has been used for diagnosing chronic arsenic poisoning, because arsenic binds to sulfhydryl groups, but meticulous attention must be paid to collection and analysis.[44] The use of hair analysis for metal analysis other than arsenic is controversial and not recommended.[45] Even if urine or blood levels are not elevated in suspected cases of chronic metal toxicity, a provocative trial with a chelating (mobilization) agent (e.g., BAL or EDTA) may be helpful for mobilizing the metal from tissue stores helping to confirm the diagnosis, particularly in chronic lead poisoning.[43] A 24-hour urine collection to measure the efficacy of this procedure is warranted. In acute cases, it is useful to test blood and gastric contents, followed by 24-hour urine collection to monitor the rate of excretion. When collecting whole blood, it is best to use silicon-coated heparinized syringes *except* for iron, which requires only a routine vacutainer without anticoagulant. The

Table 14-18. Types and Examples of Exposures to Various Metals

Metal	Type of Exposure	Example
Arsenic	Occupational	Dust from smelting (copper, lead, zinc), chemicals (pesticides, herbicides)
	Ecosystem	Seafood, water
Cadmium	Occupational	Dust from refining of metals (zinc, lead), plastics, pigments, tires, nuclear reactor rods
	Ecosystem	Contamination of irrigation water
Iron	Ingestions	Accidental or intentional overingestions
Lead	Occupational	Dust from smelters, refining, welding
	Ingestions	Paint, illicit alcohol, ceramics
Mercury	Occupational	Mining, metal production, manufacturing
	Ecosystem	Seafood, water

use of any chelating anticoagulant (e.g., EDTA or oxalate) causes falsely low results in blood.

Analysis

The method for analyzing all of these metals is atomic absorption spectroscopy (AAS), again with the exception of iron, which may be measured colorimetrically. Measurement of these metals by AAS may not be a routine clinical procedure in many laboratories, and specimens may have to be referred to regional or specialized industrial laboratories. Iron is measured routinely using serum, and in cases of acute toxicity, measuring the iron binding capacity is useful. Because an acute iron overdose is a serious situation, especially in children, measurement of serum iron should be available 24 hours a day, 7 days a week in timely fashion for hospitals offering emergency services. If a child is symptomatic from iron ingestion or has ingested more than 40 mg of elemental iron, treatment is indicated.[46] If the patient is being treated with desferoximine, it is useful to monitor the efficacy of iron excretion. It will be necessary to pretreat the urine with thioglycolic acid and 10% trichloroacetic acid if the iron concentration is being measured chromogenically. Serum in this case must be measured by AAS to avoid falsely low urine iron results.

Table 14-19. Toxicity Levels for Iron

Level µg/dL (µmol/L)	Toxicity Risk
<100 (<19.90)	Normal for children
100–350 (17.90–62.65)	Poisoned, ? toxicity
350–500 (62.65–89.50)	Possible serious toxicity
500–1000 (89.50–179.0)	Definite serious toxicity
>1000 (>179.0)	Potentially fatal

(Data from Tong and Banner.[47])

Interpretation

In suspected acute iron overdose, patients are at risk for toxicity if the free iron exceeds the TIBC. Correlation of serum iron with probable toxicity is seen in Table 14-19.[47]

Representative toxic ranges for acute and chronic heavy metal toxicity are given in Table 14-20. The levels for exposure to male industrial workers are given in Table 14-21. Chronic lead toxicity in children is particularly insidious, leading to learning disorders, mental

Table 14-20. Symptoms and Concentrations Associated With Acute and Chronic Metal Toxicity

Metal	Symptoms Acute	Symptoms Chronic	Toxic Concentrations Blood µg/dL (mmol/L)	Toxic Concentrations Urine µg/dL (mmol/L)
Arsenic	Bloody diarrhea, abdominal pain, cardiac failure	Neuropathy, palmar keratosis, mental changes	Acute: >60 (7.98) Chronic: >10–50 (>1.33–6.65)	>100 (>13.3) 5–50 (0.67–6.65)
Cadmium	Diarrhea, renal failure, hepatic failure	Renal disease, pulmonary fibrosis, testicular atrophy	>1.0 (>0.89)	—
Iron			>280 (50.1)	—
Early (2–6 h)	Diarrhea, vomiting			
Latent (~12 h)	None			
Recurrent (12–48 h)	Shock, coma, hepatorenal failure			
Late (4–6 wk)		Gastrointestinal obstruction		
Lead	Gastrointestinal symptoms, convulsions, coma	Abdominal pain, anemia, neuropathy, nephropathy	>60 (>2.90), adult male	See text
Mercury	Vomiting, dehydration, coma, death	Central nervous system damage, impaired sensation, paralysis, coma	>5.0 (>0.25)	>15 (>0.75)

Table 14-21. Recommendations for Monitoring Occupational Exposure to Metals

Metal	Urine (µg/g Creatinine)	Blood µg/dL (µmol/L)
Arsenic (inorganic)		
Normal	<10	—
T-MPV	<220	
Cadmium		
Normal	<2	<0.5 (<0.4)
T-MPV	<10	<1.0 (<0.9)
Lead (male workers)		
Normal	<50	<35 (<101.5)
T-MPV	<150	
Delta-aminolevulinic acid		
Normal	<4.5	
T-MPV	<10	
Zinc protoporphyrin		
Normal		<2.5/g Hgb (<0.04/g Hgb)
T-MPV		<12.5/g Hgb (<0.23/g Hgb)
Mercury (inorganic)		
Normal	<5	<2 (<100)
T-MPV	<50	<3 (<1000)

Abbreviations: T-MPV, tentative maximum permissible value; Hgb, hemoglobulin.
(Modified from Lauwerys RR,[69] with permission.)

retardation, and neuropathy.[48] Lead impairs heme biosynthesis, and this inhibition leads to elevation of free erythrocyte protoporphyrin (FEP), which can be used as a sensitive screen for chronic lead poisoning. The Centers for Disease Control recommends that an FEP be used to screen children at risk between the ages of 6, 9, 12, and 18 months, and 2, 3, 4, 5, and 6 years of age. If the FEP is greater than 35 µg/dL (>0.63 µmol/L), a whole blood lead quantitation is indicated. Childhood lead poisoning has been defined as blood lead greater than 25 µg/dL in association with an FEP of 35 µg/dL (0.63 µmol/L) or greater.[49] Obvious clinical symptoms may not occur in children until lead blood levels of 60 µg/dL (2.90 µmol/L) and in adults until 80 µg/dL (3.96 µmol/L) is reached. Chelation is indicated in symptomatic children or adults. Chelation therapy is indicated in asymptomatic children when the blood lead is greater than 55 µg/dL (>2.64 µmol/L) or less than 55 µg/dL (<2.64 µmol/L) if the EDTA provocation test is positive.[50] Chelation therapy in asymptomatic adults is indicated when the blood lead level is in excess of 100 µg/dL (>4.83 µmol/L) or in the range of 80–100 µg/dL (3.96–4.83 µmol/L) with a positive BAL or EDTA provocation test.

These thresholds are periodically evaluated as we gain more knowledge about the real and potential toxicity of these metals. As a rule, the thresholds are being revised downward. The usually associated ranges for acute and chronic toxicity are given in Table 14-20. With arsenic and mercury, transient elevations can be observed with recent ingestion of contaminated seafood. Associated laboratory findings, which reflect end organ damage (e.g., with lead toxicity, anemia, erythrocyte basophilic stippling, or renal insufficiency), are corroborative of metal intoxication but are not particularly sensitive or specific within themselves.

PSYCHOTROPIC DRUGS

Test: Lithium

Background

Lithium is a light metal that is handled physiologically in a manner very similar to sodium. It is used specifically in the treatment and prophylaxis of bipolar depression or manic-depressive disorders and has found additional use in migraine headache therapy. The efficacy of lithium in other psychiatric disorders has not been established. The exact mechanism for its mood stabilizing effect is not known; however, there appears to be altered cell membrane transport of ions, inhibition of norepinephrine and dopamine release, and altered production of cyclic adenosine monophosphate (cAMP). A psychotropic effect is not seen in healthy individuals who are given the drug. Because lithium can reduce hypothyroidism, thyroid function should be monitored, particularly in those patients with a history of thyroid dysfunction. Renal dysfunction also can occur, thus baseline renal function should be established and then monitored periodically. Lithium also impairs the ability to concentrate urine and may complicate management of patient fluid status with toxic ingestions.[51]

Selection

Lithium is monitored because the therapeutic index is narrow and toxicity can occur with nominally therapeutic doses and ranges (Table 14-22). It is administered orally in doses of 300–600 mg two to three times per day. Peak absorption occurs after 1–3 hours followed by a long distributional half-life of about 4 hours. Lithium is not metabolized and elimination is entirely renal with the blood half-life of 24–40 hours. Elimination of the drug is complicated by renal tubular reabsorption and coingested drugs such as thiazide diuretics, which may increase reabsorption. Conditions associated with sodium loss (e.g., with diuretic therapy or gastrointestinal disease) may lead to toxicity even at maintenance doses. For proper interpretation, specimens must be drawn 8–12 hours after the last dose. Specimens drawn before this period of time may give falsely high levels, conversely specimens drawn after this time period may give falsely low levels. The full therapeutic effects of lithium are not seen until 7–10 days after the initiation of therapy.

Logistics

Blood specimens for monitoring therapeutic use of lithium should be collected 5–7 days after the initiation of therapy to allow for the establishment of a steady-state condition. After steady-state has been achieved, on the next consecutive 3 days, 12-hour postadministration samples should be analyzed daily. The dosage should be adjusted to establish a mean serum concentration between 0.4 and 1.30 mmol/L. When the therapeutic level has been reached, a standardized 12-hour postadministration specimen should be drawn weekly for 4 weeks and thereafter every other month. The patient must be monitored for renal and cardiac function.

The analyzed blood specimen should be separated into serum/plasma within 4 hours. Lithium is most commonly measured by either flame emission photometry, AAS, or by ion-specific electrode (ISE). The expected trough therapeutic range is 0.40–1.30 mEq/L (0.40–1.30 mmol/L) assuming steady-state conditions and that the last dose was taken 12 hours previously.

Interpretation

A 12-hour postadministration lithium level of 1.50 mEq/L (1.50 mmol/L) or greater must be regarded as potentially toxic. Most cases of lithium intoxication occur during chronic maintenance.[52] Toxicity usually arises from several predisposing factors that cause a general imbalance in sodium and water such as dehydration, diarrhea, or diuretic therapy. If the patient on chronic lithium maintenance inadvertently takes lithium on the day of testing (less than 12 hours), an inappropriately high result may be obtained.

Table 14-22. Lithium Serum Concentrations and Associated Toxic Manifestations

Serum Concentration[a] (mEq/L)	Clinical Stage	Severity of Symptoms
0.4–1.3	0	Therapeutic range
1.5–2.5	I	Drowsiness, vomiting, nystagmus
2.5–3.5	II	Toxic psychosis, fasciculations, & blurred vision
>3.5	III	Convulsions, stupor, coma, & death

[a] Conventional units are mEq/L; SI units are mmol/L; the conversion factor is 1.
(Data from Hansen and Amdisen.[70])

When lithium toxicity is suspected, the patient should be admitted to the hospital. Toxic symptoms may progress slowly or precipitously and may become life-threatening. The drug, as well as any diuretics that may have been prescribed, should be withdrawn immediately. Saline diuresis may have an equivocal response in lowering serum lithium levels, and use of theophylline to induce lithium diuresis is no longer recommended. Fluid and electrolyte balance should be maintained. It may take as long as 5–7 days before serum lithium levels fall within the desired therapeutic range. In severe lithium intoxication, dialysis is the treatment of choice.[53]

Test: Phenothiazines

Background

The phenothiazines are a class of drugs (neuroleptics) used for managing acute and chronic psychotic behavior. They also are useful as antiemetics and can be used to potentiate analgesia and general anesthesia. Chlorpromazine, thioridazine, and their derivatives are the most commonly used phenothiazines. Multiple metabolites of the phenothiazines have been identified with varying degrees of pharmacologic activity. Therapeutic drug monitoring is not routinely feasible because of the rapid formation of metabolites and wide therapeutic indices for these agents.[54] Serum concentration monitoring is directed toward determination of inactive sulfoxide metabolites as an indication of potential treatment failure. Side effects, although uncommon, can occur.

The acute toxic effects of phenothiazines are primarily extrapyramidal (Parkinson-like syndrome) and cardiac (arrhythmias and hypotension). Individuals who are chronically taking phenothiazines are at greater risk for developing spontaneous hypothermia or hyperthermia.[55] Peak blood levels are reached 3 hours from deep compartments after oral administration. Most phenothiazines are excreted slowly and can be detected in urine up to 18 months after the end of therapy and thus may limit the usefulness of urine screening.

Selection

In cases of acute toxicity, a urine screen using ferric chloride will give a pink-purple color reaction. The test is nonspecific and may crossreact with other substances (e.g., salicylate, acetoacetate).[56]

Logistics

Phenothiazines can be detected and quantitated with difficulty by a variety of techniques including ultraviolet spectrophotometry, GC/MS, and HPLC. For rapid detection in cases of suspected toxicity, TLC or a spot urine test using ferric chloride (Phenistix-Ames) may be helpful. For therapeutic monitoring, serum should be obtained just before the next dose. There is a wide variability in gastrointestinal absorption and drug inactivation from gut wall enzymes. Food or antacids can cause a significant decrease in orally absorbed chlorpromazine. The serum sample should be determined as soon as practical because the phenothiazines undergo extensive degradation with storage.

Interpretation

The presence of a phenothiazine as detected by a qualitative test (TLC or ferric chloride) will help confirm the clinical diagnosis of phenothiazine ingestion. Treatment is based on the clinical signs and symptoms. Quantitative levels show wide variability and clinical correlation is needed (Table 14-23).

Table 14-23. Comparative Data on the More Commonly Used Phenothiazines

Generic (Trade Name)	Half-life (h)	Serum Concentrations µg/mL (mmol/L) Therapeutic	Toxic
Chlorpromazine (Thorazine)	18–30	0.01–0.12 (0.03–0.37)	>0.5 (>1.5)
Promethazine (Phenergan)	4–7	0.002–0.018 (0.007–0.06)	—
Prochlorperazine (Compazine)	—	0.0008 (—)	
Trifluoperazine (Stelazine)	7–18	0.001–0.028 (.0024–.068)	
Thioridazine (Mellaril)	26–36	0.4–2.0 (1.1–5.5)	>2 (>5.5)
Fluphenazine (Prolixin)	1–12 days	0.0002–0.0004 (0.0004–0.0008)	
Haloperidol (Haldol)	10–40	<0.05 (<0.139)	—

Test: Tricyclic Antidepressants (See Ch. 13)

Background

Tricyclic antidepressants (amitriptyline, amoxapine, clomipramine, desipramine, doxepin, imipramine, maprotiline, nortriptyline, and protriptyline) are the treatment of choice for endogenous depression. The tricyclic antidepressants (TCAs) consist of a seven-membered central ring surrounded by two benzene rings. The various formulations are made by differing the radicals attached to the central ring or by modifying the central ring itself. Maprotiline, trazadone, alprazolam, and amoxapine have been advertised as "tetracyclics," but are similar pharmacologically to the secondary amine tricyclics.[57] Cyclobenzaprine (Flexeril), a skeletal muscle relaxant, and carbamazepine (Tegretol), an anticonvulsant, are chemically related to the TCAs and present similar toxicities in overdoses and are difficult to differentiate analytically from the TCAs.

The TCAs block the reuptake of the biogenic amines norepinephrine and serotonin at the presynaptic neuron ("amine pump"). Accumulation of biogenic amines at the receptor site occurs, thus alleviating depression. Long-term therapy with these drugs alters the expression of presynaptic and postsynaptic receptors, thus reversing depression. The TCAs also are sedatives, exert an anticholinergic effect, and can produce cardiac arrhythmias by a direct quinidine-like effect. The therapeutic index for these drugs is narrow, and these side effects can be seen in varying degrees depending on the TCA ingested (Table 14-24). The most common side effects are caused by anticholinergic effects such as dry mouth and urinary retention. In the United States, TCAs are among the most widely prescribed drugs and represent the singularly most lethal drug class presenting in drug overdose. Most overdoses are suicidal ingestions with legitimate prescriptions.[58]

The TCAs are rapidly absorbed from the gastrointestinal tract with a high degree of protein binding (80–95%). Distribution occurs from blood to tissues, especially the myocardium. Most of the TCAs demonstrate a therapeutic window, thus dose adjustment based on serum concentrations is warranted. The drug is metabolized by the liver by N-demethylation. The tertiary amines (amitriptyline, doxepin, imipramine) are metabolized to pharmacologically active secondary amines (nortriptyline, desmethyldoxepin, desipramine), which accumulate to concentrations approximately equal to the parent drug. It is thus important to measure not only the parent drug but its metabolite (e.g., amitriptyline plus nortriptyline or doxepin plus desmethyldoxepin).

Selection

The individual variation in response to the various TCAs makes monitoring quite useful in individualizing therapy, particularly in the elderly, children, pregnant women, and in patients with renal or hepatic disease. The administration of other drugs that alter binding or absorption makes monitoring essential. Levels should be obtained when patients do not show the anticipated therapeutic response (to monitor compliance) or before switching drug regimens. Patients on early maintenance therapy should have levels performed biweekly or monthly. For long-term therapy, levels determined every 3–4 months are usually sufficient. In any suspected cases of toxicity, serum levels can help confirm the diagnosis of TCA toxicity, but may be misleading even in true cases of toxicity. In managing TCA overdose, the patient's clinical status should dictate the appropriate treatment regime. Patients with TCA overdose often present as "mixed" and other drugs such as alcohol may be present.

Logistics

The TCAs can be detected qualitatively using TLC, semiquantitated for presumptive toxic levels using immunoassay, and quantitated definitively for parent drug and metabolite using HPLC or GC. The immunoassay methods, although readily available clinically, lack specificity because the antisera crossreact with both tertiary and secondary amines and with chemically similar drugs such as cyclobenzaprine or thioridizine.[59,60] The immunoassay is positive when the individual or the cumulative concentrations of the TCA exceed a pre-established threshold. A negative result implies that the limits of detection have not been exceeded and not necessarily that TCAs are absent. All presumptively positive results should be quantitated using a definitive method as soon as practical. For therapeutic monitoring, levels should be obtained after a steady-state has been attained. This will vary for each particular drug. Sampling should be performed during the elimination phase of the drug, which is usually 8 hours after the last dose. For possible toxicity, levels may be obtained at any time.

Interpretation

For therapeutic monitoring, ranges have been established, but therapy must be individualized. Toxicity with any of the TCAs is associated with a serum con-

Table 14-24. Tricyclic Antidepressant Therapeutic Ranges and Associated Toxicities

Group Name Drug	Therapeutic Range ng/mL (µmol/L)	Half-life (h)	Anticholinergic	Associated Toxicity Central Nervous System	Cardiac
Tertiary Amines					
Amitriptyline	120–250 (0.433–0.903)[a]	31–46	+++	+++	+++
Imipramine	125–250 (0.466–0.893)	9–24	+++	+++	+++
Doxepin	30–150 (0.107–0.537)	8–24	+++	+++	++
Trimipramine	10–240 (0.3–0.816)	16–40	+++	+++	
Secondary Amines					
Nortriptyline	50–150 (0.190–0.570)	18–93	++	+++	+++
Desipramine	75–160 (0.281–0.600)	14–62	+	+++	+++
Protriptyline	70–250 (0.266–0.950)	54–198	++	+++	++
Polycyclics					
Amoxapine	200–500 (0.637–1.59)[a]	6–10	+	+++	++
Maprotiline	—	30–50	+	+	++
Trazodone	~700 (1.88)	4–7	+	+	+

[a] Sum of parent drug and metabolite.
(Data from Moffat[39] and Tietz.[67])

centration in excess of 500 ng/mL (1800 nmol/L) cumulatively for the parent drug and metabolite or for combinations of TCA. Toxicity is associated with seizures, central nervous system depression, and cardiac abnormalities as evidenced by sinus tachycardia, increased QT interval, and alteration of the QRS vector. The high negative predictive value of a normal electrocardiogram suggests that a patient is not likely to have ingested a TCA in significant amounts.[58] Combined antidepressant concentrations in excess of 1000 ng/mL are associated with significant morbidity and possibly death. Prolonged in-hospital observation may be necessary until the patient is arrhythmia-free and serum levels consistently fall within the range.

REFERENCES

1. Helper BR, Sutheimer CA, Sunshine I: The role of the toxicology laboratory in emergency medicine II: An integrated approach. Clin Toxicol 1985;22:503.
2. Pappas AA, Gadsden RH, Taylor EH: Serum osmolality in acute intoxication. Am J Clin Pathol 1985;84:74.
3. Bailey DN: The role of the laboratory in treatment of the poisoned patient: laboratory perspective. J Toxicol Clin Toxicol 1984;7:136.
4. Dean BS, Krenzelok, EP: Poisoning in the elderly an increasing problem for health care providers. J Toxicol Clin Toxicol 1987;25:411.
5. Baselt RC: Urine drug screening by immunoassay. p. 81. In Baselt RC (ed): Advances in Analytical Toxicology. Forest City, CA, Biomedical Publications, 1984.
6. Valdes R: Endogenous digoxin immunoreactive factors: impact on digoxin measurements and potential physiologic implications. Clin Chem 1985;31:1525.
7. Holder HD, Blose JO: Alcoholism treatment and total health care utilization and costs. JAMA 1986;256:1456.
8. Weston J: Alcohol's impact on man's activities. Am J Clin Pathol 1980;74:755.
9. Gennari JF: Serum osmolality, uses and limitation. N Engl J Med 1984;310:102.
10. Kaye S: The collection and handling of blood alcohol specimen. Am J Clin Pathol 1980;74:743.
11. Uniform vehicle code and model traffic ordinance. p. 65. Revised 1987. National Committee on Uniform Traffic Laws and Ordinances, Evanston, IL, 1987.
12. Council on Scientific Affairs Report: Alcohol and the driver. JAMA 1986;255:522.
13. Baselt RC: Ethanol. p. 299. In Baselt RC (ed): Disposition of Toxic Drugs and Chemicals in Man. 2nd Ed. Davis, CA, Biomedical Publications, 1982.
14. Bennet IL, Freeman CH, Mitchell GL, Cooper MN: Acute methyl alcohol poisoning: A review based on experiences in an outbreak of 323 cases. Medicine 1953;32:431.
15. Jacobsen D, McMartin KE: Methanol and ethylene glycol poisonings. Mechanism of toxicity, clinical course, diagnosis, and treatment. Med Toxicol 1986, 1:309.
16. Skoutakis VA, Koumbourlis AC, Carter CA: Isopropyl alcohol intoxication. Clin Toxicol 1983;5:88.
17. Daniel DR, McAnalley BH, Garriott JC: Isopropyl alcohol metabolism after acute intoxication in humans. J Anal Toxicol 1981;5:110.
18. Baselt RC: Ethylene glycol. p. 316. In Baselt RC (ed): Disposition of Toxic Drugs and Chemicals in Man. 2nd Ed. Davis, CA, Biomedical Publications, 1982.
19. Weisberg HF: Osmolality calculated, "delta," and more formulas. Clin Chem 1975;21:1182.
20. Pappas AA, Gadsden RH, Porter WH, Mullins RH: Osmolality of serum for evaluating the acutely intoxicated patient. p. 85. In Frings CS, Faulkner WR (eds): Selected Methods of Emergency Toxicology. Vol. 11. American Association for Clinical Chemistry Press, Washington, DC, 1986.
21. Billups NF, Billups SM (eds): American Drug Index. 28th Ed. Philadelphia, JB Lippincott, 1984.
22. Beaver WT: Aspirin and acetaminophen as constituents of analgesic combinations. Arch Intern Med 1981;141:293.
23. Temple AR: Acute and chronic salicylate intoxication. Arch Intern Med 1981;141:364.
24. Gillette JR: An integrated approach to the study of chemically reactive metabolites of acetaminophen. Arch Intern Med 1981;141:375.
25. Smilkstein MJ, Knapp GL, Kulig KW, Rumack BH: Efficacy of oral N-Acetylcysteine in the treatment of acetaminophen overdose. Analysis of the National Multicenter Study (1976 to 1985). N Engl J Med 1988;319:1157.
26. Rumack BH, Peterson RC, Koch GG, Amara IA: Acetaminophen overdose: 662 cases with evaluation of oral acetylcysteine treatment. Arch Intern Med 1981;141:380.
27. Woods JH, Katz JL, Winger G: Use and abuse of benzodiazepines. JAMA 1988;260:3476.
28. Finkle BS, McCloskey KL, Goodman LS: Diazepam and drug-associated death. JAMA 1979;242:249.
29. Jatlow P, Dobular K, Bailey D: Serum diazepam concentrates in overdose, their significance. Am J Clin Pathol 1979;72:571.
30. Goodman JM, Bischel MD, Wagers DW et al: Barbiturate poisoning. West J Med 1976;124:179.
31. Marshall LF, Smith RW, Shapiro HM: The outcome with aggressive treatment in severe head injuries. J Neurosurg 1979;50:26.
32. McCarron MM, Schulze BB, Walbert CB et al: Short acting barbiturate overdose correlation of intoxication score with serum barbiturate concentration. JAMA 1982;248:55.
33. Lundberg GD: Mandatory unindicated urine drug screening: still chemical McCarthyism. JAMA 1986;256:3003.
34. Espelin DE, Done AK: Amphetamine poisoning. N Engl J Med 1986;278:1361.
35. Gay GR: Clinical management of acute and chronic cocaine poisoning. Ann Emerg Med 1982;11:567.
36. McCarron MM, Schulze BW, Thompson GA et al: Acute phencyclidine intoxication: clinical patterns, complications and treatment. Ann Emerg Med 1981;10:290.
37. Budd RD: Amphetamine EMIT—structure versus reactivity. Clin Toxicol 1981;18:91.
38. Baselt RC: Disposition of Toxic Drugs and Chemicals in Man. 2nd Ed. Davis, CA, Biomedical Publications, 1983.
39. Moffat AS: Clarke's Isolation and Identification of Drugs. 2nd Ed. London, Pharmaceutical Press, 1986.
40. Opiates or Opioids? (Editorial.) Lancet 1983;1:687.

41. Goldfrank LR: The several uses of naloxone. Emerg Med 1984;16:105.
42. Baselt RC: Codeine. p. 198. In Baselt RC (ed): Disposition of Toxic Drugs and Chemicals in Man. 2nd Ed. Davis, CA, Biomedical Publications, 1982.
43. Chisolm JJ: Treatment of lead intoxication—choice of chelating agents and supportive therapeutic measures. Clin Toxicol 1970;3:527.
44. Baselt RC: Arsenic in disposition of toxic drugs and chemicals in man. p. 59. In Baselt RC (ed): Disposition of Toxic Drugs and Chemicals in Man. 2nd Ed. Davis, CA, Biomedical Publications, 1982.
45. Barrett S: Commercial hair analysis. Science or scam? JAMA 1985;254:1041.
46. Lacouture PG, Wason S, Temple AR et al: Emergency assessment of severity in iron overdose by clinical and laboratory methods. J Pediatr 1981;99:89.
47. Banner W Jr, Tong TG: Iron poisoning. Pediatr Clin North Am 1986;33:393.
48. Marecek J, Shapiro IM, Burke A et al: Low level lead exposure in childhood influences neuropsychological performance. Arch Environ Health 1983;38:355.
49. CDC: Preventing lead poisoning in young children. A statement by the Centers for Disease Control, USDHEW, PHS, Bureau of State Services, Environment of Health Services, Atlanta, GA, January 1985.
50. Piomelli S, Rosen JF, Chisolm JJ et al: Management of childhood lead poisoning. J Pediatr 1984;105:527.
51. Singer I: Lithium and the kidney. Kidney Int 1981;19:374.
52. Lewis DA: Unrecognized chronic lithium neurotoxic reactions. JAMA 1983;250:2029.
53. Jacobsen D, Aa G, Frederichsen P, Eiseng AB: Lithium intoxication: pharmacokinetics during and after terminated hemodialysis in acute intoxications. Clin Toxicol 1987;25:81.
54. Sakalis G, Curry SH, Mould GP et al: Physiologic and clinical effects of chlorpromazine and their relationship to plasma levels. Clin Pharmacol Ther 1972;13:931.
55. Caroff S, Rosenburg H, Gerber JC: Neuroleptic malignant hyperthermia and malignant hyperthermia (letter). Lancet 1983;1:244.
56. Forrest FM, Forrest IS, Mason AS: Review of rapid urine tests for phenothiazines and related drugs. Am J Psychiatry 1961;118:300–307.
57. Orsulak PJ: Therapeutic monitoring of antidepressant drugs: current methodology and applications. J Clin Psychiatry 1986;47:39.
58. Flomenbaum N, Price D: Recognition and management of antidepressant overdoses: Tricyclics and trazadone. Neuropsychobiology 1986;15, suppl 1:46.
59. Ryder KW, Glick MR: The effect of thioridazine on the automatic clinical analyzer serum tricyclic anti-depressant screen. Am J Clin Pathol 1986;86:248.
60. Schroeder TJ, Tassed JJ, Otten EJ, Hedges JR: Evaluation of Syra EMIT Toxicological serum tricyclic antidepressant assay. J Anal Toxicol 1986;10:221.
61. National Institute on Drug Abuse (DHHS 86-1469): Annual Data from the Drug Abuse Warning Network. Series I 1985;5:24.
62. Litovitz TL, Martin TG, Schnitz B: 1986 Annual Report of the American Association of Poison Control Center's national data collection system. Am J Emerg Med 1987;5:405.
63. Pappas AA, Taylor EH, Shifman MA: Manual of Clinical Pathology Services. 1st Ed. Little Rock, University of Arkansas for Medical Sciences, 1986.
64. Council on Scientific Affairs of the American Medical Association: Scientific issues in drug testing. JAMA 1987;257:3110.
65. Dubowski KM: Alcohol determination in the clinical laboratory. Am J Clin Pathol 1980;74:747.
66. Bell R, Pappas AA, Taylor EH: The use of osmolality in detecting alcohols. p. 37. In Sunderman FW (ed): Manual of Proceedings for Clinical and Analytical Toxicology. Philadelphia, Institute for Clinical Science, 1987.
67. Tietz NW: Clinical Guide to Laboratory Tests. Philadelphia, WB Saunders, 1983.
68. Federal Register 53:11983, April 11, 1988. US Government Printing Office, Washington, DC.
69. Lauwerys RR: Summary of recommendations. p. 133. In Lauwerys RR (ed): Industrial Chemical Exposure. Davis, CA, Biomedical Publications, 1983.
70. Hansen HE, Amdisen A: Lithium intoxication. QJ Med 1978;47:123.
71. Bennett TB: Graphic Biochemistry. Chemistry of Biological Molecules. Vol. 1. New York, Macmillan, 1968.
72. Bowers LD, Carr PW: Quantitative Aspects of HPLC Workshop. Minneapolis, 1983.
73. Ettre LS: Practical Gas Chromatography. Norwalk, CT, Perkin Elmer Corp., 1973.
74. Done AK: Aspirin overdosage: incidence, diagnosis, and management. Pediatrics 1978;62:suppl, 895.
75. Rumack BH, Matthew H: Acetaminophen poisoning. Pediatrics 1975;55:871.

15 Pregnancy and Genetics

Wayne W. Grody
Peter J. Howanitz
Alan I. Lipsey

INTRODUCTION

In pregnant patients, many changes occur in results for routine laboratory tests. For example, serum total thyroxine increases because of increases in thyroxine-binding globulin caused by rises in estrogens. For these and other changes associated with pregnancy, refer to the specific analyte in question. Tests related to laboratory confirmation of pregnancy and monitoring the pregnant patient are reviewed in this chapter.

The perinatal period includes a period of time before and after birth. During this period, the well-being of the fetus can be evaluated in a number of ways. In recent years, techniques such as ultrasonography have enhanced the obstetrician's ability to evaluate the fetus. When potential problems are detected by history, physician examination, or ultrasound, laboratory tests often are indicated. These tests may be placed into several categories, namely, fetal well-being or maturity, congenital malformations, and genetic abnormalities. For fetal monitoring, amniotic fluid is obtained by amniocentesis, usually performed at 15–16 weeks' gestation. Amniotic fluid contains fetal somatic cells that will grow in culture and can be used to identify certain cytogenetic and biochemical abnormalities. Indicators for amniocentesis include maternal age older than 35, a fetus at risk for a chromosomal abnormality, or an inborn error of metabolism. For details on indications for amniocentesis and overview of amniotic fluid assessment, see Smith.[1]

During the birth process, monitoring of adequate oxygenation is a major concern. During a difficult delivery, fetal pH can be monitored as an indicator of distress or jeopardy. As birth occurs, concern shifts from placental and fetal circulation to initiation of respiration and the fetal functional lung capacity. In the postnatal period, biochemical tests play an important role in the detection of inherited metabolic disorders. Many states have implemented mandatory screening programs for the more commonly inherited disorders. In the postnatal period, malformations may be discovered requiring genetic study. This is especially true for infants of young and elderly mothers as well as of those who did not receive appropriate prenatal care.

PREGNANCY TESTING

Test: Chorionic Gonadotropin (hCG, Pregnancy Test) (See Ch. 12)

Background

Although frequently called pregnancy tests, these procedures measure high concentrations of human chorionic gonadotropin (hCG), the hormone the placenta begins to produce in increasing amounts about 10 days after fertilization (Fig. 15-1). In the past, tests for pregnancy were used after the first missed menstrual period, but with increased analytic sensitivity, hCG now

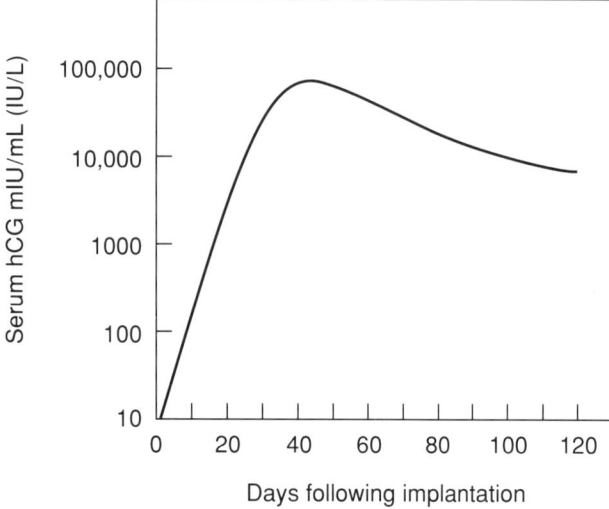

Fig. 15-1. Serum human chorionic gonadotropin levels during a normal pregnancy. (Modified from Stephenson,[2] with permission.)

is first measurable in maternal serum approximately 10 days after conception, that is, 48–72 hours after implantation. On the basis of production rates, hCG doubles every 2 days within the first 30 days. Unfortunately, hCG is not specific for pregnancy as many tissues including the pituitary secrete hCG and are responsible for the low levels found in sera from males and nonpregnant women.

In normal pregnancy, fertilization takes place in the distal third of the Fallopian tube and the blastocyst implants in the endometrium lining of the uterus. By contrast, occasionally implantation occurs at other sites and implantation at any of these sites is considered ectopic. Almost all ectopic pregnancies occur in the Fallopian tube. In the United States, ectopic pregnancy is the leading cause of maternal death, and its incidence has tripled in the past 20 years with over 1.5% of pregnancies now ectopic.

The hCG molecule is composed of an α- and β-chain with variable amounts of carbohydrate attached (see p. 316). The β-chain gives hCG immunologic and biologic specificity, distinguishing it from the other glycoprotein hormones of similar structure, thyrotropin (TSH), lutropin (LH), and follitropin (FSH). In sera, the free β subunit is found as well, but usually in much lower concentrations than intact hCG. Although some procedures are called β-hCG pregnancy tests because they measure the free β subunit of hCG, they react with the β subunit of the intact hormone as well.

Selection

Measurements of hCG are used to diagnose or rule out early pregnancy, identify an ectopic or failing pregnancy, a missed abortion, or as a confirmation test for molar disease. Frequently, serial measurements are used. Measurement of hCG also is used as a tumor marker (see Ch. 12).

Logistics

For the diagnosis of pregnancy, hCG reagent kits that have an analytic sensitivity of 25 mIU/mL (25 IU/L) are currently used. For information on analytic sensitivity of these assays see p. 401. The assays used are quantitative, semiquantitative, or qualitative. For diagnosis of pregnancy, qualitative or semiquantitative urine or serum measurements are recommended. By contrast, quantitative measurements are used for substantiating ectopic pregnancy, missed abortion, hydatidiform moles, or choriocarcinoma. Urine measurements are usually qualitative or semiquantitative although with home-use kits, results are qualitative. Qualitative assays can be used to provide semiquantitative results by diluting specimens with elevated values and interpreting results in relation to results from control specimens. For measurements made in clinical laboratories, serum is now the specimen of choice for quantitative assays, although in the past urine measurements were widely used. The major reason for using serum for semiquantitative determinations of hCG is that its concentration is not subject to the wide variation of hCG concentrations found in urine owing to changes in the specific gravity. Most reagent kits that are used for both serum or urine show better analytic sensitivity with serum than urine specimens.

The measurement of choice is immunoassay, with reagent specificity for either intact hCG alone, or both the free β-chain of hCG and the β-chain of intact hCG. Generally, assays that measure only intact hCG are more specific. hCG assays have been calibrated against either the World Health Organization (WHO) Second International Reference Preparation or more recently, against the WHO First International Reference Preparation. Both preparations give equivalent bioassay results. The First Reference Preparation is more pure and when calibrated by that standard, usually immunoassay results are approximately twice as high as those using the Second International Reference Preparation. In this chapter, all results are expressed using the First International Reference Preparation.

Interpretation

Males and nonmenstruating and postmenopausal females have serum hCG results of approximately 0.1 mIU/mL (0.1 IU/L). During the LH surge in menstruating women, serum hCG may increase up to sevenfold from this baseline, then rapidly decline. At 48–72 hours after implantation, hCG results are greater than 25 mIU/mL (> 25 IU/L), the value usually used to confirm pregnancy. One week postimplantation, the serum levels are 70–100 mIU/mL (70–100 IU/L), and by 2 weeks they exceed 250 mIU/mL (250 IU/L). Concentrations continue to increase approaching 10,000 mIU/mL (10,000 IU/L) after the first 6 weeks and reach a peak of about 100,000 mIU/mL (100,000 IU/L) during the third gestational month. When pregnancy is suspected but the test is negative, the test should be repeated in 48–72 hours or a test with an analytic sensitivity of 5 mIU/mL (5 IU/L) should be used.[3] Several conditions are associated with low hCG values, such as ectopic pregnancy, abortion, blighted ovum, or "ruling out" early pregnancy.

Ectopic pregnancy is effectively ruled out if hCG values are less than 5 mIU/mL (< 5 IU/L). Moreover, positivity at this level cannot be used as an indication of pregnancy, as many nonpregnant persons have been reported with hCG values this high.[3] Depending on the hCG level, transabdominal ultrasonography can be used to substantiate the diagnosis of an ectopic pregnancy. Failure to detect a gestational sac at a preset level of hCG indicates the likely occurrence of an ectopic pregnancy. Some workers recommend setting this level at about 6500 mIU/mL (6500 IU/L). The absence of a gestational sac when the serum hCG concentration is above this level is associated with ectopic gestations in almost 90% of cases. Others use 3600 mIU/mL (3600 IU/L) as the level at which transabdominal ultrasound can be used to identify a gestational sac.[4] Similarly, cutoff levels of 1000 mIU/mL (1000 IU/L) have been used when vaginal ultrasonography is used.

Declining hormone levels indicate a failing pregnancy. Low or declining levels do not differentiate between intrauterine and ectopic pregnancies. Because repeat measurements are usually performed, many workers recommend evaluating serial hCG levels in response to standards they have developed. For example Kadar et al.[5] have established usual serum hCG increases with intrauterine pregnancy. If values are less than this percentage increase, a healthy intrauterine pregnancy is unlikely (Table 15-1).

Table 15-1. Lower Limits of Serum Human Chorionic Gonadotropin Expressed as a Percentage of the Initial Result Over Time

Sampling Interval (days)	Lower Limits of Percentage Increase
1	29
2	66
3	114
4	175
5	255

Because there is overlap between hCG levels of normal pregnancies and hydatidiform moles, the determination of hCG alone is of limited value. When hCG is combined with ultrasonography, an hCG level below 25,000 mIU/mL (< 25,000 IU/L) coupled with a normal intrauterine sac makes the diagnosis of molar disease unlikely. Values of hCG between 25,000 and 85,000 mIU/mL (25,000 and 85,000 IU/L) with the presence of an intrauterine sac may be associated with normal or abnormal pregnancies. Above 82,350 mIU/mL (> 82,350 IU/L), the failure to observe a pulsating heart by ultrasound permits the identification of patients at risk for gestational trophoblastic disease in the first trimester.[6]

False Results

False negative results are seen when "prozoning" occurs, that is, exceedingly high hCG concentrations that are nonreactive. False negative results occur with some reagents when blood is in the specimen. With home pregnancy test kits, false negative results occur in up to 40% of cases, because of failure to comply with reagent kit directions.[7] Because of these errors, women should repeat a negative test within 1 week to avoid delays in seeking prenatal care.

Some reports indicate that hCG levels of 10–50 mIU/mL (10–50 IU/L) may occur in nonpregnant women, causing false positive results. In some assays, false positive test results occur with postmenopausal sera. Injections of human menopausal gonadotropins cause false positive test results. Urine specimens that are turbid or have high protein concentrations have been reported to produce false positive pregnancy test results. Psychotropic drugs have been reported to cause false positive results with some assays, but improved assay reagents appear to have eliminated this problem.

MONITORING THE PREGNANT PATIENT

Test: α-Fetoprotein (AFP) (See Ch. 12)

Background

α-Fetoprotein, a glycoprotein of 70,000 da, is the major globulin in fetal serum, synthesized first in the yolk sac and later in the fetal liver. It attains peak levels of about 300 mg/dL (3 g/L) during week 13 of gestation and then begins to decline, finally reaching normal adult levels (less than 1.0 mg/dL [<10 mg/L]) by about 8 months of age. AFP appears in the amniotic fluid, probably via fetal urination, and also crosses the placental barrier to enter the maternal circulation. Levels in amniotic fluid peak at about 5.3 mg/dL (53 mg/L) at weeks' 15–17 gestation, while the concentration in maternal serum continues to rise throughout pregnancy, exceeding 10 mg/dL (100 mg/L) by 25 weeks.

Open neural tube defects (NTD), such as anencephaly and spina bifida, result in direct leakage and transudation of AFP from the fetal serum into the amniotic fluid at the site of the defect, increasing its concentration both within that compartment and in the maternal serum. Hence, elevation of AFP level can be used as a convenient prenatal screening marker for these devastating birth defects. Conversely, an association with decreased AFP levels has been found in certain fetal chromosomal anomalies, most consistently in trisomy 21 (Down syndrome).

The incident of Down syndrome increases so dramatically at maternal ages above 35 that these women are routinely offered amniocentesis with fetal karyotype analysis to identify affected pregnancies and provide the option for termination. Even though the risk in younger women is too low to justify such an invasive screening procedure as amniocentesis, with its low but definite fetal loss rate, the overall population of younger women becoming pregnant is so much larger than the over-35 group that the majority of Down syndrome babies will be born to younger mothers. The ability to ascertain low AFP levels in the maternal serum makes mass screening possible for Down syndrome (and the other trisomies) even in the low risk population, with no risk of harm to the fetus.

To some extent, a similar rationale holds true for NTD, where the majority of affected children are born to couples with a negative family history and who would therefore be considered of having too low a risk to justify amniocentesis. However, in contrast to Down syndrome, neural tube defects are detectable by fetal ultrasound, a procedure currently performed routinely in virtually all pregnancies.

Selection

These tests are performed for the detection of specific fetal anomalies early enough in pregnancy so that the option for termination can be offered if the fetus is found to be affected. In general, amniotic fluid AFP (AF-AFP) is offered to pregnant women with some increased a priori risk (positive family history [e.g., previously affected fetus or relative] for NTD, or advanced maternal age for Down syndrome). In contrast, maternal serum AFP (MS-AFP), with its absence of iatrogenic risk to the fetus, is more amenable to mass population screening of low risk pregnancies. Because these tests are not in themselves diagnostic of fetal defects, but merely suggest the likelihood of a problem, they must be followed up by more definitive procedures: fetal ultrasound for an NTD, and fetal karyotype analysis for Down syndrome. In addition, AF-AFP is often performed after detecting an elevated MS-AFP. At that time, amniotic fluid acetylcholinesterase (AChE) may also be measured; it leaks from the fetal cerebrospinal fluid at the site of an NTD and thus provides an additional level of confirmation (see Test: Acetylcholinesterase).

Logistics

α-Fetoprotein levels in body fluids can be measured by immunoelectrodiffusion, radial immunodiffusion, radioimmunoassay, or enzyme immunoassay. The extreme sensitivity of the latter two methods is required for measurement of MS-AFP, whereas the first two are adequate for AF-AFP. Because AFP levels vary markedly at different stages of pregnancy, accurate knowledge of gestational age at the time the specimen is collected is essential. The specimen should be free of blood contamination, because the presence of fetal blood will cause a false elevation. Screening usually takes place during weeks 16–18 of gestation.

Interpretation

Because of significant variations in AFP measurement between laboratories, it has been recommended that levels be expressed as multiples of the median (MoM) of each laboratory's values obtained in normal pregnancies of the same gestational age as the patient specimen. Thus, most cases of open NTD show MS-AFP levels of higher than 2.5 MoM; and AF-AFP levels are even higher, up to 4.0 MoM, depending on gestational age.

Maternal race, weight, and insulin-dependent diabetes have been reported to influence MS-AFP levels. Black women have values that average 10% higher at each week of gestation than other women. Therefore for black women, the MoM must be decreased by 10%. Because insulin-dependent diabetics exhibit 20–40% lower MS-AFP levels than do nondiabetic mothers, the MoM can be corrected by dividing it by 0.7. For maternal weight corrections of the MoM, a more complex formula is used.

Data indicate that if amniocentesis and chromosomal analysis are offered to all women with serum AFP levels below a specified maternal age-dependent cutoff level (1.0 MoM or less at 37 years, 0.9 or less at 36 years, 0.8 or less at 35 years, 0.7 or less at 34 years, 0.6 or less at 32–33 years, 0.5 or less at 25–31 years), 40% of all pregnancies with Down syndrome and 6–8% of unaffected pregnancies would be selected.[8] The concentration of AFP in maternal serum and amniotic fluid in early pregnancy is shown in Figure 15-2.

False elevations of AF-AFP (i.e., not caused by an NTD) may result from (1) fetal blood contamination, (2) underestimation of gestational age, (3) multiple pregnancy (e.g., twins), (4) threatened abortion, (5) fetal death, (6) congenital nephrosis, (7) duodenal atresia, (8) Turner syndrome, and (9) body wall defects such as omphalocele. False elevation of MS-AFP may additionally be caused by (1) maternal malignancies such as hepatoma, (2) hepatitis, (3) cirrhosis, and (4) ataxia-telangiectasia. False depression of MS-AFP may occur in maternal insulin-dependent diabetes and with obesity.

Test: Acetylcholinesterase

Background

Cholinesterases are a family of enzymes that hydrolyze choline esters and are found in almost all tissues, including red blood cells. Neural tissue is rich in AChE where it has an important role in neurotransmission. Neural tissue is the source of amniotic fluid AChE until day 28 of fetal development (6 weeks' gestation), at which time the neural tube closes. However, amniotic fluid AChE normally persists until about the 11th week of fetal development. The persistence of amniotic fluid AChE throughout pregnancy indicates that the neural tube is not closed.

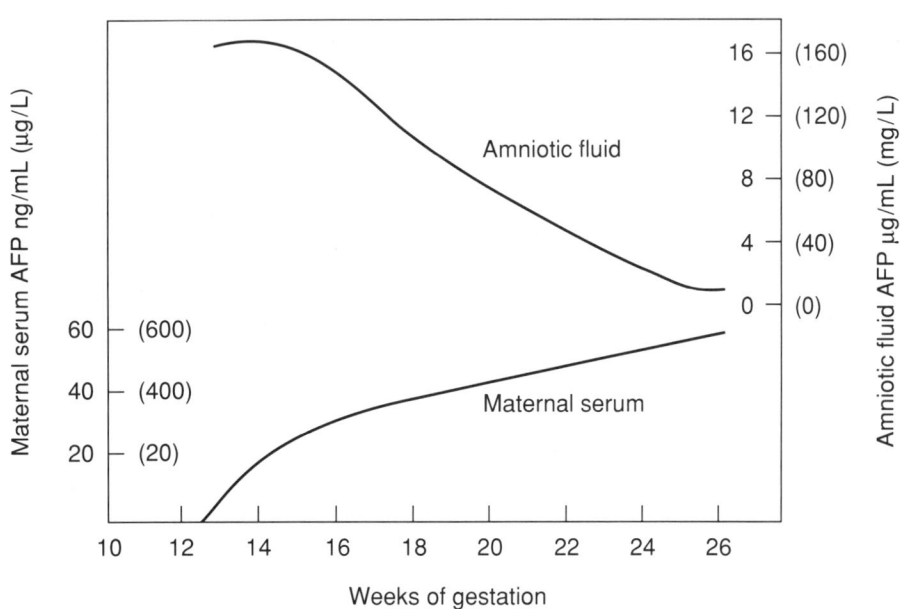

Fig. 15-2. Maternal serum and amniotic fluid concentrations in normal pregnancy during midgestation. (Modified from Burton,[9] with permission.)

Selection

Amniotic fluid AChE is used to confirm the presence of an NTD. It is usually measured when MS-AFP and AF-AFP measurements are elevated, or when a mother has had a previous pregnancy with an NTD (Table 15-2). Some investigators recommend measuring AChE in all amniotic fluids obtained because of high MS-AFP concentrations.

Logistics

Because the measurement of amniotic fluid AChE is a much more labor intensive test than AF-AFP, it has not had widespread use in screening. For measurement, amniotic fluid obtained between weeks 13 and 24 of gestation is subjected to electrophoresis. In a normal pregnancy, only one band representing pseudocholinesterase occurs, but with an NTD a second, faster migrating band (AChE) also is found. Specific inhibitors of either AChE or pseudocholinesterase are used for confirmation. A ratio of AChE-to-pseudocholinesterase can be used to separate open spina bifida from ventral wall defects such as gastroschisis and omphalocele.

Interpretation

The presence of amniotic fluid AChE and AF-AFP is powerful evidence of a fetal NTD (Table 15-3). The use of specific inhibitors of AChE or pseudocholinesterase improves test accuracy.[11] Further evidence that the defect is a ventral wall defect in contrast to an open spina bifida can be made by determining the ratio of AChE-to-pseudocholinesterase. Typically, the ratio is below 0.10 in ventral wall defects and greater than 0.15 in open spina bifida.

A common cause of a false positive result is the contamination of amniotic fluid with blood. Fetal calf serum has high concentrations of AChE and is used as a culture medium for determining the fetal karyotype of amniotic cells. A number of instances have been reported where fetal calf serum has contaminated amniotic fluids awaiting AChE measurements, thereby causing false positive results.

AChE is used mainly for the confirmation of AFP results. However, the major difference between the two tests is in congenital nephrosis where AChE bands are not observed and AFP values are markedly elevated.

Test: Bilirubin Pigments in Amniotic Fluid (Liley scan, Delta OD [Optical Density] 450)

Background and Selection

As part of prenatal care, pregnant women are screened for antibodies to red blood cell antigens.[12] Before the introduction of Rhesus (Rh) immunoglobulin, maternal alloimmunization to red blood cell antigens and subsequent severe hemolytic disease in the child most often was caused by antibodies against the Rh antigen. Irregular antibodies of the IgG type that occur in maternal serum now are seen relatively more frequently as a cause of this problem. Once maternal isoimmunization has been identified, management includes amniotic fluid analysis for bilirubin to predict severity of fetal anemia caused by the incompatibility.

Logistics

Specimen Requirements

To ensure bilirubin stability, the amniotic fluid specimen must be protected from light and the test performed as soon as possible. The specimen is centrifuged to remove debris. Contamination of the amniotic fluid with blood or meconium causes interference lasting for approximately 3 weeks. Error in sampling the amniotic fluid also can occur, most commonly by aspiration of the maternal urinary bladder. Several tests can be used

---

Table 15-2. Step-Wise Laboratory Testing to Detect Neural Tube Defects

Step	Laboratory Test	Test Purpose
1	Maternal serum α-fetoprotein	Screening for neural tube defects
2	Repeat maternal serum α-fetoprotein	Confirm elevated test result
3	Diagnostic ultrasound examination	Confirm gestational age and singleton fetus
4	Amniotic fluid α-fetoprotein	Confirm abnormal screening test
5	Amniotic fluid	Confirm abnormal amniotic fluid α-fetoprotein
6	Other testing	Define defect

(Modified from Knight and Wu,[10] with permission.)

Table 15-3. Odds of Having a Fetus With Open Spina Bifida Given Positive Amniotic Fluid Results for Different Policies According to Reason for Amniocentesis

Policy	Amniocentesis for Raised Maternal Serum α-Fetoprotein — Specimen not Bloodstained	Amniocentesis for Raised Maternal Serum α-Fetoprotein — Specimen Bloodstained	Amniocentesis for a Previous Neural Tube Defect Pregnancy — Specimen not Bloodstained	Amniocentesis for a Previous Neural Tube Defect Pregnancy — Specimen Bloodstained
α-Fetoprotein ≥ Specified cut-offs[a]	7:1	2:1	30:1	3:1
Acetylcholinesterase positive and α-fetoprotein				
≥ 1.0 MoM	36:1	3:1	14:1	2:1
≥ 2.0 MoM	40:1	4:1	59:1	4:1
≥ 3.0 MoM	42:1	5:1	86:1	5:1

[a] Cut-offs were 2.5 MoM at 13–15 weeks, 3.0 MoM at 16–18 weeks, 3.5 MoM at 19–21 weeks, and 4.0 MoM at 22–24 weeks. (Modified from Wald et al.,[11] with permission.)

to distinguish maternal urine from amniotic fluid, including pH, urea nitrogen, and creatinine. Amniotic fluid creatinine is in the range of 2–3 mg/dL (180–270 μmol/L) as compared with urine creatinine, which is several-fold higher in concentration.

Analysis

The test is based on the qualitative measurement of the maximum absorption peak of bilirubin (OD at 450 nm) using a narrow band pass scanning spectrometer. Normally the absorption curve descends linearly from 365–550 nm; the amount of bilirubin present is proportional to the degree to which there is deviation from the expected absorbance at 450 nm. The change in OD is plotted versus gestational age giving a so-called Liley curve (Fig. 15-3).

Interpretation

In amniotic fluid, normally there is only a small amount of bilirubin, which decreases with gestational age in association with fetal kidney maturation. Increases in bilirubin, as determined by the OD at 450 nm, is an indicator of hemolysis in the fetus. Because the amount of bilirubin varies with gestational age, accurate dating of gestation is necessary for proper interpretation of results. Additionally, sequential studies are often needed to document the increase in bilirubin pigment over time.

Results falling within the upper zone of the Liley chart indicate the fetus is at risk for intrauterine or neonatal death. Results falling within the lower zone of the chart indicate the fetus is at little or no risk of untoward effect of isoimmunization. For results falling in the midzone, prognosis of the fetus depends on the magnitude and trend in the delta OD. Because it may be necessary to provide obstetric intervention, tests for fetal lung maturity often are ordered as well. Maternal jaundice or hemolysis can lead to problems in interpretation of results, but otherwise the Liley method has proven reliable in the third trimester. Four possible patterns of results are shown in Figure 15-4. The ability of the method to predict the severity of anemia during the second trimester, however, is limited and therefore direct measurement of fetal hemoglobulin (Hgb) has been advocated. Other methods such as ultrasonography also may be valuable in certain of these patients.[13]

Test: Estriol (E$_3$) Unconjugated (Free)

Background

Estriol, the principal estrogen of pregnancy, has been used as a biochemical test of fetal well-being. Both the placenta and the fetus must be intact to produce estriol, and if either becomes compromised, decreased production of the hormone occurs. In the nonpregnant state estriol is the major metabolite of estradiol, whereas in pregnancy, almost all maternal estriol originates from 16 α-hydroxydehydroepiandrosterone sulfate (DHEA-S) synthesized in the fetal adrenal and subsequently converted to estriol by the placenta (Fig. 15-5). Almost all estriol is conjugated with either sulfate or glucuronide and then excreted by the kidneys. Approximately

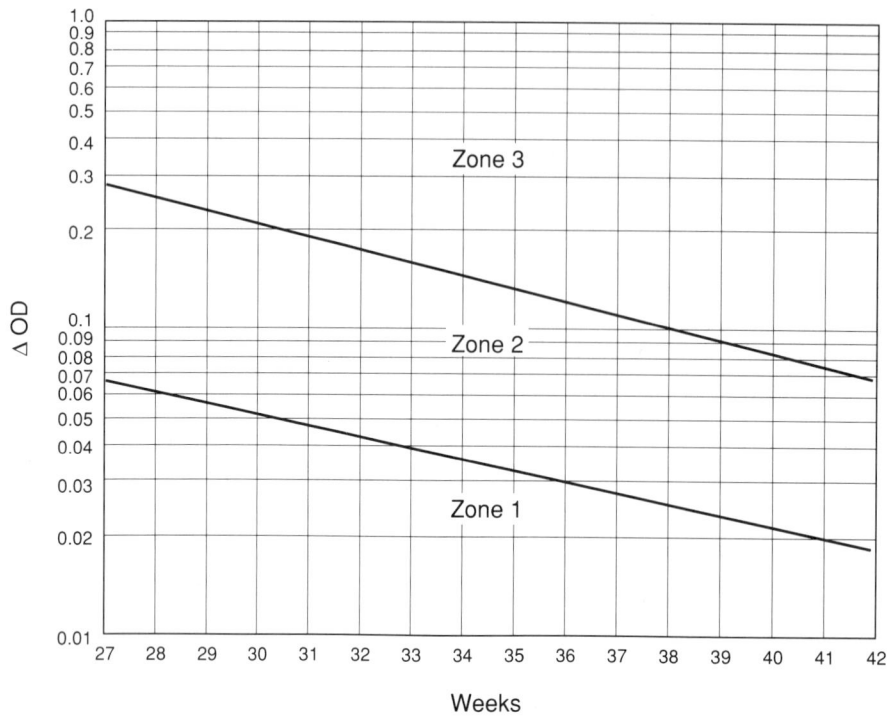

Fig. 15-3. Liley graph used to depict degrees of sensitization. (From American College of Obstetricians and Gynecologists,[12] with permission.)

9% is unconjugated (free) and it is this fraction that is measured.

Total urinary estrogens have been measured; estriol is the largest contributor to the measurement of total estrogens. As compared with total urinary estrogens, ease of serum specimen collection, increased analytic specificity, and more rapid laboratory turn-around time are reasons for abandonment of urinary estrogen measurements in favor of serum unconjugated estriol. In addition, the short half-life of serum estriol allows identification of fetal changes earlier, and measurements are valid in renal or hepatic failure. Salivary estriol measurements have been used in a research setting as an alternative to serum unconjugated estriol.

Selection

Unconjugated serum estriol results are valuable in managing past date pregnancies. Although earlier work indicated that unconjugated estriol values were useful in managing pregnancies complicated by diabetes mellitus, recent work has indicated that the measurement provides little useful information. Unconjugated serum estriol has been used in other high risk conditions such as multiple gestations, intrauterine growth retardation, hypertensive disorders, and Rh sensitization, but little evidence substantiates its value.[14] Although unconjugated serum estriol levels in the second trimester are low in the presence of fetal Down syndrome, controversy exists about the value of these measurements for screening because of the overlap in results with healthy fetuses.[15] Clinical patterns indicate that modern obstetric management is moving away from unconjugated estriol and other biochemical tests toward biophysical antenatal tests of well-being.

Logistics

Maternal serum is the specimen of choice but many still use plasma, although plasma values are approximately 7% lower. It has been the practice to obtain serum specimens at the same time of day to minimize circadian variation; however, a recent report indicates that there is no diurnal pattern in late pregnancy.[16] For past date pregnancies, recommendations are to measure estriol twice weekly. In the management of diabetic pregnancies daily measurements are required. Measurement of unconjugated estriol levels requires a modification of assays when used in the second trimes-

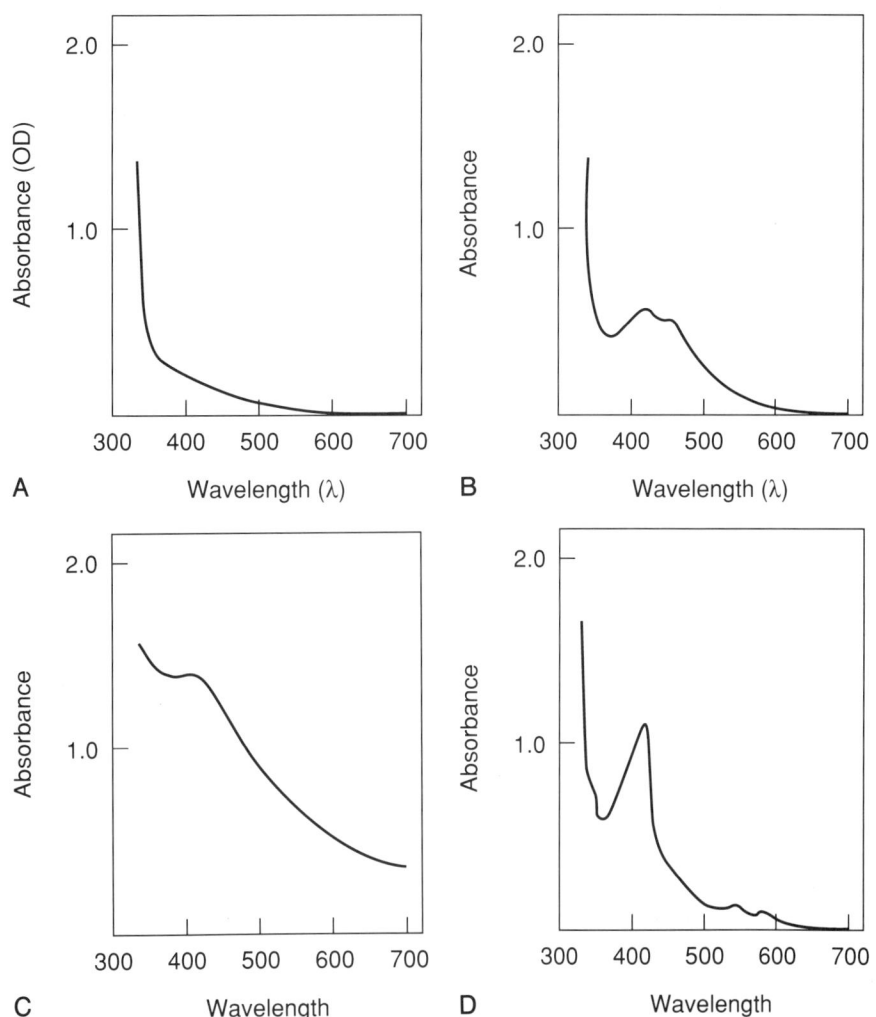

Fig. 15-4. Amniotic fluid scans. **(A)** Normal scan. **(B)** Moderately jaundiced fluid indicative of hemolytic disease. **(C)** Slight to moderate meconium staining. **(D)** Blood amniocentesis without jaundice.

ter, because values are about one-tenth those in the third trimester. Immunoassay is the measurement of choice because estradiol, estrone, progesterone, glucuronide, and sulfate conjugates of estriol have minimal cross-reactivity (less than 2%) in current assays.

Interpretation

The reference range for serum estriol during the third trimester is 3–40 ng/mL (10.4–138.7 nmol/L) and increases as delivery approaches (Fig. 15-6). Values in the second trimester are about 0.5–5.0 ng/mL (1.7–17.3 nmol/L). With frequent measurements, either a trend or an absolute value is followed. For past date pregnancies, a significant decrease is 35% or 40% of the mean of the three previous values, or three consecutive values: this is usually interpreted to mean fetal jeopardy, even though the result may be within the reference range. Values below 12 ng/mL (<41.6 nmol/L) predict intrapartum distress and perinatal death.

Estriol results may be decreased with pre-eclampsia or when the fetus has intrauterine growth retardation, but overlap with ostensibly healthy fetuses is large. In patients with Rh sensitization, estriol values are within the reference range. Estriol results may be increased secondary to increased fetal and placental mass such as with multiple fetuses. In diabetic pregnancies, maternal estriol concentrations are elevated in relation to control subjects.

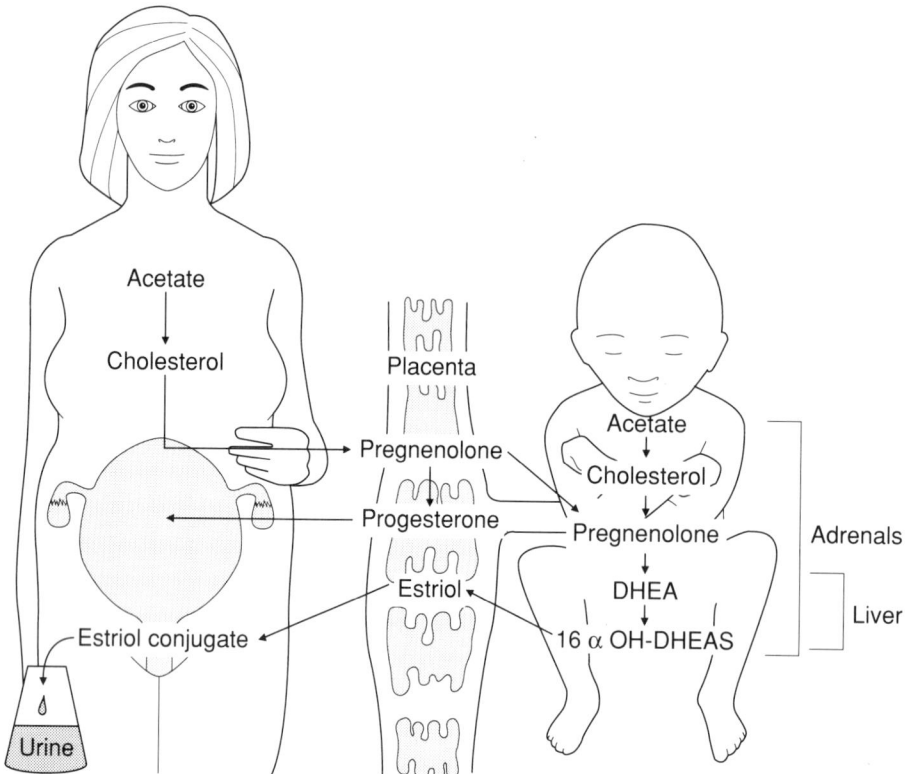

Fig. 15-5. Synthesis of estriol requiring an intact placental and fetal unit. DHEA, dehydroepiandrosterone; 16 α-OH-DHEA-S, 16 α-hydroxydehydroepiandrosterone sulfate.

Test: Human Placental Lactogen (HPL) (Human Chorionic Somatomammotropin [HCS])

Human placental lactogen, a polypeptide hormone produced by the trophoblast, is used to evaluate placental function. Normally, maternal serum HPL increases throughout pregnancy, but there is a wide range of values, especially during the second half of pregnancy. Because of this variability, serial specimens obtained over several days usually are used for assay. Results for HPL in the period 36 weeks to term generally are in the range of 5 to over 8 µg/mL (232 to over 450 mmol/L).

Measurements of HPL have been suggested as a routine determination to complement ultrasonic scanning in the assessment of length of gestation.[17] Measurement of HPL has been advocated in a variety of other clinical circumstances, but its main use is in the management of high risk pregnancies. For example, HPL monitoring in severely hypertensive women shows low results in most cases before fetal death. Because decreased results precede abortion, HPL measurements have been used to assess patients with vaginal bleeding during pregnancy. The finding of a low HPL in combination with an elevated hCG is indicative of molar disease. High HPL results may occur in association with large placentas such as seen in diabetic women and in a patient with a multiple pregnancy.

Test: Lecithin-to-Sphingomyelin (L/S) Ratio

Background and Selection

Phospholipids in amniotic fluid are predictors of fetal lung maturity because they reflect fetal surfactant levels. Surfactant is necessary to keep the air spaces open when the infant is born; in the absence of adequate pulmonary surfactant, respiratory distress syndrome (RDS) occurs. Amniotic fluid contains phospholipids including lecithin (phosphatidylcholine), sphingomyelin, phosphatidylglycerol, acidic phospholipids, lamellar bodies, and specific apoproteins. Lamel-

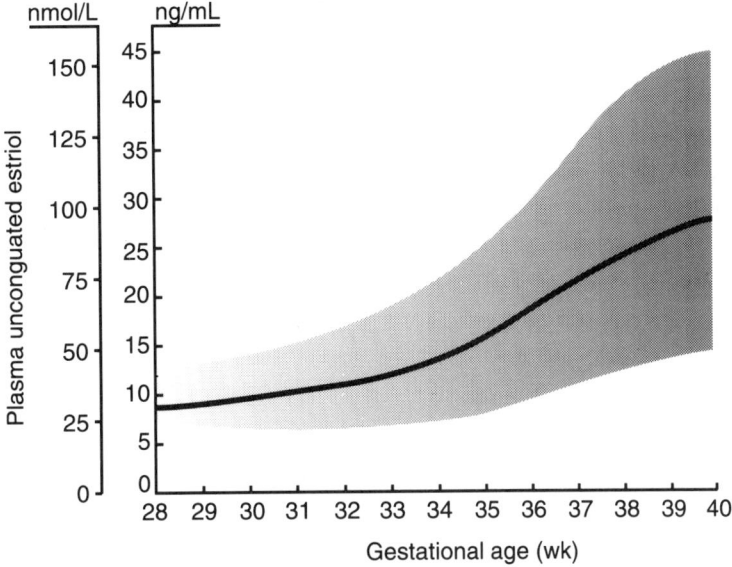

Fig. 15-6. Confidence limits for unconjugated estriol in plasma during the third trimester of pregnancy. Mean indicated by solid line.

lar bodies (Fig. 15-7) are the actual packages of surfactant in amniotic fluid. The L/S ratio is the usual test performed, but a variety of other indicators of fetal lung maturity have been used.

Logistics

Amniotic fluid is collected in a sterile tube, protected from light, centrifuged to remove cells and cellular debris, and frozen if the analysis cannot be performed immediately. Excessive centrifugation must be avoided because it removes lamellar bodies leading to alteration in measurements. Prolonged storage of the specimen at room temperature before assay decreases the L/S ratio. Most investigators suggest the specimen should be stored at 4°C for no more than 24 hours.[18]

Throughout gestation, sphingomyelin concentrations remain relatively constant as compared with the increases in lecithin, which occur starting around week 35. Thus, sphingomyelin concentration provides a corrective factor for amniotic fluid volume. The phospholipids usually are determined by thin-layer chromatography (TLC). Because of its high lipid content, blood gives an elevated L/S ratio, with the degree of interference depending on the method used. Meconium can interfere with the analysis by a number of mechanisms, but these are assay dependent. For assay details, see Spillman and Cotton.[19]

Interpretation

Generally, an L/S ratio of 2 or greater indicates fetal lung maturity and a neglible risk of RDS. Although an L/S ratio less than 1.5 is indicative of fetal lung immaturity, RDS will not develop in a large percentage of these cases. Additionally, an unacceptable level of false predictions of maturity (1–15%) also occurs, especially in pregnancies complicated by diabetes mellitus. The poor predictive value of the L/S ratio has led to the introduction of other tests including phosphatidylglycerol. The presence of phosphatidylglycerol makes it very unlikely the infant will develop RDS. In the presence of meconium or blood pigment staining, only phosphatidylglycerol methods are considered accurate.[20] Even though phosphatidylglycerol is not found in blood or meconium, some assay dependent problems still may occur.[19]

Other Tests of Lung Maturity

Many other tests of fetal lung maturity have been introduced, including the shake test (stable ring formation in the presence of ethanol), assessment of microvis-

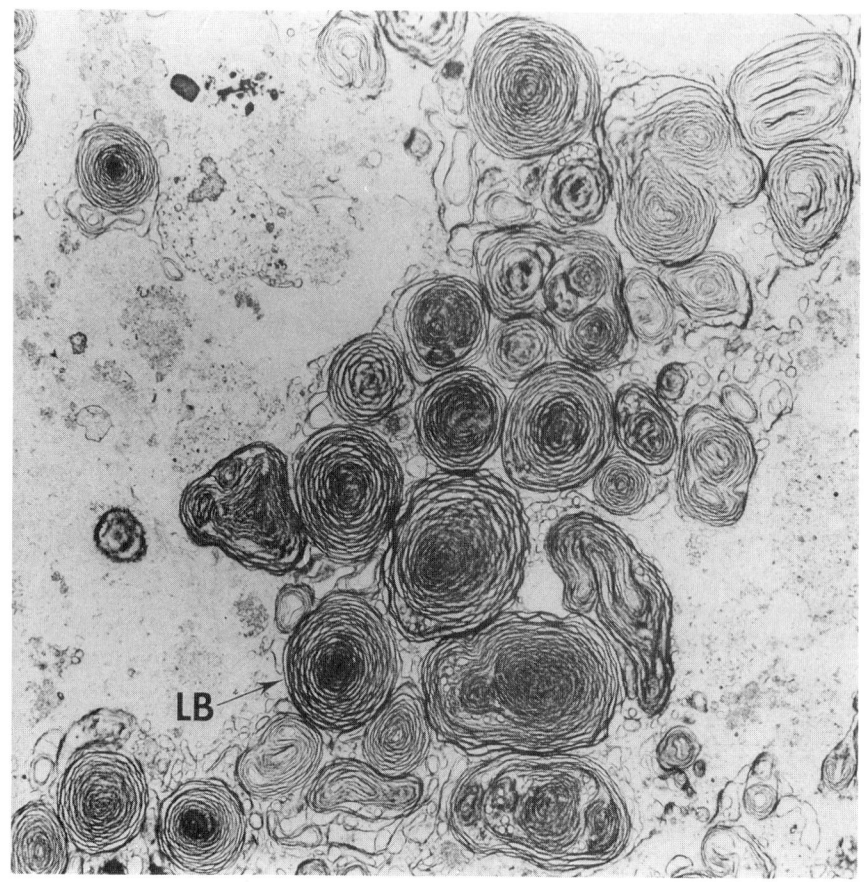

Fig. 15-7. Lamellar bodies (LB) in amniotic fluid from a woman near term. The specimen was centrifuged and viewed using an electron microscope.

cosity by fluorescence polarization, and determination of lamellar bodies (measured by absorbance at 650 nm or use of electronic particle detectors) (Table 15-4). Some of these tests (e.g., the shake test) have the advantages of speed, low cost, and simplicity. In general, if test results indicate maturity, the predictive value is good. By contrast, if the results indicate immaturity, they are relatively poor at predicting the occurrence of RDS. This has led some investigators to suggest using rapid screening tests, then proceeding to the standard L/S by TLC if the screening tests fail to predict maturity.[20] Other assays including immunoassay of apoprotein A, palmitic acid, and saturated phosphatidylcholine assays hold promise for the future.

Table 15-4. Biochemical and Biophysical Assays for Evaluation of Fetal Lung Maturity

Biochemical
    Lecithin-sphingomyelin (L/S) ratio
    Lung profile (L/S ratio, % saturated lecithin, phosphatidylglycerol, phosphatidylinositol)
    Lamellar body phospholipid
    Surfactant associated apoproteins
Biophysical
    Foam stability
    Surface tension
    Fluorescence polarization
    Optical density, 650 nm

SCREENING THE NEWBORN

Test: Routine Biochemical Screening (Genetic Screen, Neonatal Screen)

Background

To be applicable and cost-effective for screening of newborns on a mass population scale, a genetic disease must meet several criteria. It must be relatively common in the population screened, it must be detectable by an inexpensive, automated method, and its natural history must be such that early diagnosis and treatment is essential to prevent severe illness or mental retardation. The prototype disorder in this group is phenylketonuria (PKU), and screening of all newborns for this disease is now mandatory in most states and many countries. In addition, the newborn screening programs of many states include such other disorders as galactosemia, hypothyroidism, maple syrup urine disease, and biotinidase deficiency.

Selection

These tests are used to diagnose unsuspected, preclinical genetic disease as early in life as practical, to institute therapy before the onset of postnatal damage. Depending on state law, tests for PKU and certain of the other disorders may be mandatory before discharge of the newborn from the hospital.

Logistics

For PKU, galactosemia, and some other metabolic disorders, accumulation of the involved metabolite will not be evident before the onset of regular milk feedings. Current recommendations, mindful of the increasing trend toward early discharge of healthy neonates, call for testing at least 24 hours after the start of milk feeding and as close to discharge as possible. For mass screening purposes, most of these tests use a few drops of whole blood applied to a spot of filter paper. The PKU screen, for example, uses the Guthrie bacterial inhibition assay, in which elevated phenylalanine or its metabolites in the blood spot circumvent growth inhibition of a strain of *Bacillus subtilis*. A false negative clear zone around the blood spot can occur if the infant was receiving antibiotics at the time of specimen collection. Fluorimetric and chromatographic assays are also available for PKU and the other screens. A false positive fluorescent assay for phenylalanine can result from interference by ampicillin.[21] The thyroxine (T_4) screen is usually done by radioimmunoassay. A urine specimen spotted on galactose-specific test paper can be used to screen for galactosemia, using a galactose oxidase assay. Such specimens should be refrigerated or frozen to prevent bacterial breakdown of galactose. Additionally, high levels of ascorbic acid in the urine can inhibit the test reaction. Some normal newborns, especially those on a high milk diet, may have galactosuria.

Interpretation

The legal reference range limits are less than 4 mg/dL (<0.24 mmol/L) for phenylalanine and more than 7.0 µg/dL (>90 mmol/L) for thyroxine. In general, a result of more than 10 mg/dL (>0.6 mmol/L) galactose in the urine is considered positive. Abnormal results on such newborn screening tests usually require further workup and/or therapeutic trials (e.g., to classify the type of galactosemia, to rule out transient or benign hyperphenylalaninemia, etc.). (See also Ch. 8, Test: Phenylalanine; Ch. 11, Test: Thyroxine; and Test: Galactosemia below.)

Test: Molecular Genetic Analysis (DNA Hybridization, Southern Blot Analysis, Restriction Fragment Length Polymorphism [RFLP], Polymerase Chain Reaction [PCR])

Background

With continuing advances in recombinant DNA technology and further extensive mapping of the human genome, an increasing number of single gene defects are becoming amenable to diagnosis and screening at the molecular level using DNA probes. This technology utilizes the principle of nucleotide base pairing between two complementary strands of DNA, otherwise known as hybridization, to elucidate information about gene structure in a patient or fetus. Hybridization is performed on fragmented patient DNA that has been cleaved at discrete recognition sequences by restriction endonucleases, electrophoresed through an agarose gel, and blotted onto a filter membrane; this is the so-called Southern blot technique (Fig. 15-8). Based on the presence or absence of hybridization with a DNA probe specific for the disease gene or a sequence close to it, as well as the sizes of the hybridizing target fragments, it is possible to ascertain the presence of point mutations and deletions in the patient's DNA. It is also possible to generate large amounts of particular patient DNA fragments for further analysis via the recently developed PCR.

Selection

These tests are indicated when clinical, preclinical, or prenatal screening is required to ascertain the presence of a heritable genetic disorder or carrier state for purposes of family planning, pregnancy termination, or definitive clinical diagnosis. At present, only Mendelian single gene disorders, for which a locus-specific or closely linked DNA probe is readily available, are amenable to this type of diagnosis. Examples of applicable disorders include sickle cell anemia, thalassemia, PKU, hemophilia A, Duchenne muscular dystrophy, adult onset polycystic kidney disease, Huntington's disease, and cystic fibrosis.

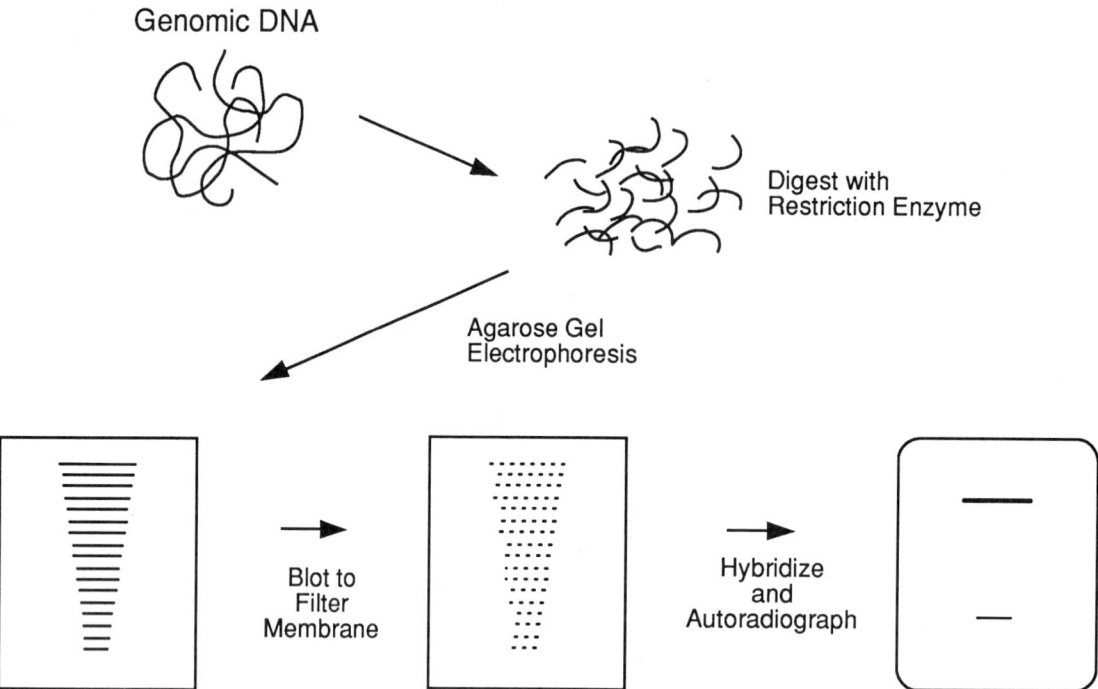

Fig. 15-8. Southern blot technique.

DNA-based tests for genetic disease fall generally within two major categories. When the gene for a disease is already known and its normal homologue cloned, the clone can be used as a probe to directly hybridize Southern blots of the patient's DNA to search for signs of deletions or internal mutations that would be seen as alterations in band pattern on the blot. For diseases in which the actual site of mutation at the individual base pair level is known, such as sickle cell anemia, hybridization can be performed with short oligonucleotide probes for the region of the mutation (called allele-specific oligonucleotides). If the probes are short enough (about 10 base pairs), then even a single base mismatch with the target DNA, as would be caused by a point mutation, will prevent hybridization of probe under sufficiently stringent conditions. Conversely, an oligonucleotide probe containing the point mutation will hybridize only to the mutant DNA and not to normal DNA.

On the other hand, a genetic disease can still be screened for even if the causative gene or its protein product has not yet been identified. All that is required is a DNA probe that maps close enough to the actual disease locus so that the chance of spontaneous recombination between the two loci, disrupting their linkage, is rare. The probe itself does not even have to be a real gene, but may be just a piece of anonymous DNA cloned from an area near the disease locus and suitably linked to it as determined by family studies. The probe is used to detect differences in DNA fragment sizes, presumably containing the disease gene, which are generated by benign polymorphisms between people in certain restriction enzyme recognition sites. These benign variations in DNA restriction fragment sizes between people are called restriction fragment length polymorphisms. In family studies it may be found that a particular restriction site, or its absence, always cosegregates with a disease gene, even though it does not lie within the gene itself. Thus, this site, and the particular DNA fragment size it generates on a Southern blot, can be used as a marker of the disease gene, even though the precise nature of the latter may not be known. This technique has been used for prenatal diagnosis and carrier detection of Mendelian diseases for which the gene is not yet precisely identified, such as Huntington's disease.

Logistics

The genomic DNA required for Southern blot analysis may be obtained from white blood cells, amniocytes, or chorionic villus sampling (CVS). Sufficient DNA can be extracted from 5–10 mL of whole blood, stored at 4°C for up to 48 hours, or from a standard CVS specimen. Amniotic fluid cells, on the other hand, frequently need to be placed in culture for 1–2 weeks to obtain enough material with which to work. In certain circumstances, however, a miniscule amount of patient material can be used by first amplifying the target DNA sequences using the PCR. For prenatal diagnosis, the usual parameters for minimum gestational age apply (17–18 weeks for amniocentesis, 8–9 weeks for CVS), with the caveat that specimens should be obtained as early as possible to allow time for completion of the rather lengthy (2–4 weeks) Southern blot procedure while termination of the pregnancy is still an option. For tests using the cloned disease gene or its normal homologue as probe, the patient's or fetus' DNA alone is sufficient for screening. For those tests using a linked RFLP, DNA from multiple family members, including a previously affected individual, must be analyzed alongside that of the patient or fetus to determine the informativeness of the segregation pattern in that particular family. Because the DNA probe used in such cases is linked but not identical to the disease gene, there is always a chance, however slight, of a recombination event between the two loci, leading to the possibility of misdiagnosis. The magnitude of this uncertainty factor is inversely proportional to the proximity of linkage between the two markers, and family members must always be advised of this when they receive genetic counseling based on the results of RFLP analysis.

Interpretation

Performance and interpretation of diagnostic Southern blots require considerable expertise in molecular biology, and the relevant parameters will vary depending on the type of DNA probe used, the size and structure of the target locus (e.g., the huge dystrophin gene involved in Duchenne muscular dystrophy may require a battery of individual subclones as probes), the proximity of linkage in RFLP analysis, and the mode of inheritance of the disease in question. Results tend to be faster and more straightforward for those diseases in which allele-specific probes can be used, as opposed to those diseases relying solely on RFLPs. Because the information obtained through this technology often engenders a considerable emotional burden, as in the elective termination of a pregnancy or the diagnosis of inevitable Huntington's disease in an at risk adult, ancillary genetic and psychological counseling is mandatory in presenting these results to patients.

TESTS FOR GENETIC DISORDERS

Test: α_1-Antitrypsin (AAT) (See Ch. 8)

Background

α_1-antitrypsin, a glycoprotein with a molecular weight of 25,000, is the primary protease inhibitor found in serum and the major inhibitor of neutrophil elastase within the lungs. In the absence or diminution of AAT, and particularly in settings of chronic inflammation and/or cigarette smoking, the unchecked activity of leukocyte elastase can lead to lung damage in the form of emphysema. α_1-Antitrypsin is synthesized in the liver and secreted continually to maintain adequate serum levels. Over 30 electrophoretic variants of the protein have been described; these are inherited in an autosomal condominant manner and classified under the protease inhibitor (Pi) system of nomenclature. The most common type is M and 95% of the population is homozygous PiMM. Genotype PiZZ, arising from a point mutation in the AAT structural gene, results in defective glycosylation of the molecule and diminished secretion from the hepatocyte. These patients have low circulating levels of AAT (10–15% of normal) and massive accumulation of AAT polypeptide, leading to both emphysema and cirrhosis. PiMZ heterozygotes exhibit serum levels about one-half of normal and some degree of AAT accumulation in the liver, whereas Pi$^-$ homozygotes, carrying a null mutation or deletion of the AAT locus, show no detectable AAT in either the serum or liver.

Selection

Evaluation of AAT status is indicated in the workup of otherwise unexplained neonatal hepatitis, cryptogenic cirrhosis in adults, and patients with chronic obstructive pulmonary disease, especially if they are smokers. Whether asymptomatic smokers should be screened on a large scale is currently being debated.

Logistics

The various AAT variants are separated and quantitated by acid-starch gel electrophoresis. About 2 mL of serum is sufficient for this test. α_1-Antitrypsin accounts for the major portion of the α_1-globulin fraction on standard serum protein electrophoresis.

Interpretation

The reference range for AAT in serum is 85–225 mg/dL (850–2250 mg/L). Many of the rare variants of AAT seen on acid-starch gel electrophoresis are of no clinical significance. Detection of homozygous or heterozygous Z protein is useful for the understanding and further workup of lung and/or liver disease and for providing a rational basis for urging affected smokers to quit. Inspissated AAT can be observed on liver biopsy by immunohistochemistry or diastase resistant periodic acid-Schiff (PAS) positivity. PiZ$^-$ heterozygotes cannot be reliably distinguished from PiZZ homozygotes by electrophoresis alone, but must be confirmed by pedigree analysis of the family. α_1-Antitrypsin is an acute-phase reactant and can be elevated in conditions of stress, malignancy, pregnancy, and infection.

Test: Amino Acid Screen (Metabolic Screen) (See Ch. 8)

Background

Patients with inborn errors of amino acid metabolism exhibit elevated plasma or urine levels for one or more biochemical intermediates proximal to the enzymatic defect. These can include not only the 20 common amino acids found as structural components of protein, but many intermediary metabolites of the amino acid family, such as citrulline and argininosuccinic acid in the urea cycle, isovaleric acid in the leucine metabolic pathway, and so forth.

Selection

This screening test should be performed to confirm or rule out an inborn error of amino acid metabolism. Often it is performed on newborns presenting with unexplained metabolic acidosis, hyperammonemia, or failure to thrive, but it is also requested for older children or adults with unexplained mental retardation, seizures, or other persistent symptoms. An unusual odor to the urine also may suggest one of these disorders. The qualitative test is usually requested first as a quicker and less expensive screening method.

Logistics

Urine must be refrigerated or frozen to prevent breakdown of analytes by contaminating bacteria. For qualitative amino acid screen by two dimensional paper chromatography, using one of several equally good methods, a random urine specimen of approximately 15 mL is sufficient. Quantitative methods using high performance liquid chromatography (HPLC), or a standard amino acid analyzer, require the same type of specimen. A number of medications and foodstuffs, if ingested within 3 days before collection, can produce falsely elevated levels of particular amino acids. The most common offenders and their affected analytes are valproic acid (glycine), penicillin derivatives (alanine), and benzoic acid preservatives (glycine).

Interpretation

The interpretation of plasma and urine amino acid profiles is complex, requiring a specialized laboratory for performance of the procedures and a skilled metabolic disease expert well versed in the subtle and complex interplay between the various metabolites in the many known specific disorders. Reference ranges are generally established by the individual laboratory (see Ch. 8). The various disorders are far too numerous to list here; some of the more common findings include elevated methionine and homocysteine in homocystinuria, increased phenylalanine and phenylacetic acid in PKU (more often diagnosed by a simpler newborn screening test), increased branched-chain amino acids in maple syrup urine disease, and elevated tyrosine and methionine in tyrosinemia. The urine screen will also pick up disorders in amino acid transport, such as cystinuria and Hartnup's disease. Note that an abnormal plasma amino acid profile may not always be reflected in the urine, depending on the kidney's reabsorptive capacity for the particular metabolites involved.

In many cases the qualitative or quantitative amino acid screen will be sufficient to clinch the diagnosis. In other instances further tests, such as liver biopsy with specific enzymatic studies, may be required for confirmation. Because a few disorders may be mimicked by benign or transient elevations of particular amino acids in the newborn period (e.g., hyperphenylalaninemia, transient neonatal hypertyrosinemia), serial measurements are often necessary. Sometimes assay or trial administration of known cofactors for the enzyme in question is helpful in further pinpointing the molecular defect involved (e.g., tetrahydrobiopterin deficiency as a rare cause of PKU).

Test: Carnitine

Background

Carnitine (β-hydroxy-γ-N-trimethylammonium butyrate) is a cofactor involved in the transport of fatty acids and acyl CoA compounds across the mitochondrial membrane. In this capacity it also assists in the detoxification and excretion of these compounds. Two types of primary carnitine deficiency have been described: a systemic form characterized by encephalopathy, hepatic abnormalities, and cardiomyopathy; and a myopathic form localized to skeletal muscle.[22] In addition, a secondary deficiency can arise because of consumption of carnitine by the toxic levels of acyl compounds that accumulate in the organic acidemias.[23]

Exogenous administration of carnitine is often of direct or ancillary benefit in these conditions.

Selection

These tests are ordered to diagnose primary or secondary carnitine deficiency, and to monitor achievement of adequate levels during carnitine administration.

Logistics

Carnitine circulates in plasma in both a free and esterified form. Both should be measured when assessing carnitine levels. The assay is performed on plasma, which should be frozen during transport, using a radiometric method.

Interpretation

The reference range for free plasma carnitine is 5.7–8.9 µg/mL (35–55 µmol/L), although values will vary somewhat among individual laboratories. Total plasma carnitine is reported to be in the same range. Additional laboratory tests, along with the clinical picture, are required to determine whether the carnitine deficiency is primary or secondary. A muscle biopsy may be necessary to confirm a diagnosis of the primary myopathic deficiency, and empiric carnitine supplementation is also often revealing. When carnitine is administered to patients with organic acidemias to promote excretion of organic acids such as carnitine esters, both free and esterified carnitine should be measured periodically to assure that effective blood levels are maintained.

Test: Copper and Ceruloplasmin (See Chs. 8 and 10)

Background

Copper is an essential micronutrient, serving as the integral divalent cation of a number of important enzymes of intermediary metabolism. It is also a very toxic ion when increased above homeostatic levels. Normally this homeostasis is maintained by a balance between intestinal absorption of copper and processing by the liver both into an unabsorbable form excreted in the bile and into a complex with ceruloplasmin, a copper-containing enzyme of the oxygen reductase class that may also serve as a copper transport protein in the plasma.

Two hereditary defects of copper metabolism are known. In Wilson's disease, the rate of biliary excretion of copper and the rate of its incorporation into ceruloplasmin are both decreased. The net effect is a progressive accumulation of copper stores in the liver, leading eventually to cirrhosis, with spillover deposition and damage in the brain, cornea (producing Kayser-Fleischer rings), and other tissues. In Menkes disease, by contrast, there is a net deficiency of copper resulting from defective absorption of the ion from intestinal mucosal cells and into other tissues. The disease is fatal in early childhood, with symptoms of hypothermia, neuronal and arterial degeneration, and brittle hair. For neither of these disorders has the precise molecular defect been identified.

Selection

These tests are ordered to confirm a diagnosis of one of the disorders of copper metabolism discussed above. Ceruloplasmin is also an acute-phase reactant.

Logistics

Copper can be measured in serum (5 mL) or urine (24-hour collection preserved with 30 mL of 6 N HCl). For definitive diagnosis of Wilson's disease, especially when a biopsy is already being performed for histologic classification of chronic liver disease, the copper content per gram dry weight of liver tissue can be measured. The techniques used are atomic absorption spectroscopy and quantitative spectrophotometry of copper reactive chromogens. Serum copper levels are about 10% higher in blacks than in whites and may be double the normal adult value in women who are pregnant or taking oral contraceptives.

Ceruloplasmin is measured in serum by immunochemical, enzymatic, and colorimetric methods. On plasma protein electrophoresis, it is found in the α_2-globulin fraction. As an acute-phase reactant, it can be increased up to double the reference value in conditions of stress, infection, pregnancy, and oral contraceptive use. It also tends to be higher in young children than in adults.

Interpretation

The reference range for serum copper is 10–155 µg/dL (1.6–24.4 µmol/L) and for urine copper it is 15–50 µg/24 h (0.24–0.79 µmol/d). Liver copper content is normally about 30–40 µg/g (0.48–0.65 µmol/g) dry weight and judged to be significantly increased when more than 300 µg/g (>4.8 µmol/g). Reference ranges for ceruloplasmin are 20–40 mg/dL (200–400 mg/L) in infants and adults, and 30–50 mg/dL (300–500 mg/L) in young children. The classic findings in Wilson's disease are low serum ceruloplasmin concentration and increased free serum copper, urinary copper excretion, and liver copper content. It should be kept in mind that elevated copper levels may also be the result of such other conditions as copper poisoning and enhanced retention secondary to other liver and biliary diseases. In Menkes disease, low levels of both serum copper and ceruloplasmin are the hallmarks. However, as these values are low in normal newborns as well, diagnosis is difficult in the first 2 weeks of life. The diagnosis can be further confirmed by finding increased copper content in the mucosal cells of a jejunal biopsy, and microscopic examination of the kinky, steely hair (pili torti) is also helpful.

Test: Galactosemia Screening (Galactose-1-Phosphate Uridyl Transferase Assay, Galactokinase Assay)

Background

A clinical defect in galactose metabolism can result from deficiency of either galactose-1-phosphate uridyl transferase or galactokinase. Both types are inherited in an autosomal recessive fashion. The clinical features result from toxicity of galactose and its metabolites, and include cataracts associated with galactokinase deficiency and failure to thrive, mental retardation, and liver failure associated with the more severe transferase deficiency. The transferase defect is more common (1 in 80,000 births) and has justified the institution of widespread newborn screening programs.

Selection

The diagnosis is suspected when nonglucose reducing substances are found in the urine, and elevated levels of galactose and/or galactose-1-phosphate are found in the plasma. In many cases such patients will come to attention through newborn screening tests using a bacterial assay of dried blood spots on filter paper. In all cases the diagnosis and definitive subtyping of galactosemia should be confirmed by the specific enzyme assays.

Logistics

Both disorders can be ascertained by assay of the relevant enzyme activities in erythrocytes. The galactose-1-phosphate uridyl transferase assay indirectly measures uridine diphosphate (UDP)-glucose remaining after incubation with the patient's red blood cell hemolysate and galactose-1-phosphate. Patients with galactokinase deficiency have normal red blood cell transferase activity, but an inability to oxidize radiolabeled galactose to radiolabeled CO_2. Galactosuria may be intermittent or absent in those patients with poor feeding or absent intake of milk products. Newborns who are receiving third generation cephalosporins have false positive antimicrobial assays because the *Escherichia coli* strains are inhibited in their growth by antibiotics. False negative transferase results are found when affected individual specimens are collected using citrate rather than ethylenediaminetetraacetic acid (EDTA) as the anticoagulant.

Interpretation

Galactosemic patients show absent red blood cell activity of the particular enzyme involved, whereas heterozygotes demonstrate approximately 50% of normal levels. Rare patients picked up in the newborn screening test have been found to have normal activity of both galactokinase and transferase in the erythrocyte assay. Further investigation showed a deficiency of another enzyme of galactose metabolism, UDP galactose-4-epimerase. This disorder is of no clinical significance, however, and no treatment is required.

Management of the transferase deficiency involves monitoring the level of erythrocyte galactose-1-phosphate. The reference interval is less than 40 µg/g Hgb and levels greater than 110 µg/g of Hgb indicate noncompliance with a diet of galactose restriction.

Test: Mucopolysaccharides

Background

The mucopolysaccharidoses include the Hurler, Hunter, Schie, Sanfilippo A and B, and Morquio syndromes. Among the storage diseases, this group of disorders is particularly amenable to detection by urine screening tests, since the acid mucopolysaccharides are freely dispersed among many tissues and body fluids, obviating the need for specific organ biopsy as is required, for example, in the glycogen storage diseases.

Selection

These tests are used to screen for the presence of accumulated acid mucopolysaccharides excreted in the urine in the mucopolysaccharide storage diseases.[24] Such a diagnosis may be suspected in pediatric patients presenting with coarse facial features, hepatosplenomegaly, skeletal and cardiac abnormalities, and sometimes mental retardation.

Logistics

The cetyltrimethyl-ammonium bromide test or acid albumin turbidity test can be used. Thirty milliliters of urine should be collected and refrigerated, as false negative results can occur from bacterial action. Both of these tests produce turbid precipitates when reagents are added to urine containing mucopolysaccharides. Borderline and other questionable results should be repeated on a fresh urine specimen.

Interpretation

In these disorders, one or more of the following acid mucopolysaccharides accumulate and produce positive screening reactions in the urine: dermatan sulfate, heparan sulfate, keratan sulfate, chondroitin sulfate, and hyaluronic acid. The particular compound(s) present are characteristic of the particular syndromes, but are not distinguished from one another in these screening tests.

Appearance of a white precipitate indicates the presence of accumulated acid mucopolysaccharides and suggests a diagnosis of one of the mucopolysaccharidoses. The diagnosis can be confirmed and subtyped by assay of the specific enzyme deficiency in leukocytes or cultured fibroblasts.[25]

Test: Organic Acids (Organic Acid Screen)

Background

The organic acidurias (also called organic acidemias) are a group of serious inborn errors of metabolism having in common the accumulation and elevated excretion of organic acids other than amino acids. These compounds arise as metabolic intermediates in the catabolic pathways of amino acid metabolism as well as in fatty acid oxidation, glycolysis, and other pathways. As in the analysis of amino acids, the detection and identification of specific organic acids accumulating in the patient's plasma or urine can allow one to deduce the locus of the enzymatic defect.

Selection

These tests are used to diagnose and differentiate the various organic acidemia syndromes, including methylmalonic acidemia, propionic acidemia, isovaleric acidemia, and so forth. As most of these disorders cause catastrophic illness during the newborn period, organic acid analysis should be included in the workup of any infant with otherwise unexplained metabolic acidosis, hyperammonemia, or failure to thrive.

Terminology

The organic acids of clinical relevance are defined as those compounds containing either carboxylic acid groups or phenolic acid groups but no amino groups. The amino acids are thus not included in this class of analytes. The organic acids are further subdivided into volatile, such as propionic acid and isobutyric acid, and nonvolatile, such as isovaleric acid and fatty acids. The latter compounds must first be volatilized by chemical derivatization before they can be analyzed by gas chromatography.

Logistics

Urine is the preferred specimen for initial screening purposes, because the concentrations of these acids are usually higher in urine than in plasma. The specimen should be refrigerated or frozen to prevent bacterial breakdown of the analytes. On the other hand, certain disorders, such as propionic acidemia, show more consistent elevations in plasma, so that a subsequent blood specimen may be necessary to confirm the diagnosis. Levels of the various metabolites can vary widely depending on the clinical condition and dietary intake of the patient, making diagnosis difficult and repeat tests sometimes necessary. The standard method for identification and quantitation is gas chromatography with or without mass spectrophotometry.[26,27]

Interpretation

As in amino acid analysis, the interpretation of the organic acid profile is highly complex, requiring an experienced laboratory and metabolic disease expert for accurate diagnosis. In most of the disorders, the levels of the involved acids, expressed as mEq/mg creatinine, are many times above normal, so that the detection of an abnormality is usually not based on subtle changes. Indeed for many of the acids the concentrations in normal persons are below the level of detection. However, the pattern of elevation of the various intermediates, although usually characteristic of the particular disorders, can be quite complicated, requiring considerable expertise for proper diagnosis. In most clinical settings, quantitative analysis of amino acids should be obtained in tandem with the organic acid profile to complement the diagnostic information and to rule out a primary amino acid or urea cycle disorder that may have a similar presentation. For certain disorders the diagnosis can be confirmed by assay of the defective enzyme in cultured skin fibroblasts or liver biopsy. Detection of elevated organic acids in amniotic fluid can be used for prenatal diagnosis of some of these disorders.

Test: Porphyrins (See Ch. 3)

Background

The porphyrias are a family of disorders caused by specific enzyme defects in the heme biosynthetic pathway, resulting in the accumulation of one or more of the metabolic intermediates, called porphyrins, which are proximal to the defect. Certain of the inherited disorders can also be mimicked by acquired defects secondary to lead poisoning or hexachlorobenzene toxicity.

Selection

These tests are ordered for diagnosis of patients suspected of having an inherited or acquired defect in heme biosynthesis. Six different inherited forms are seen, characterized by skin lesions (photosensitivity) and/or neurologic symptoms manifesting as psychiatric illness, abdominal pain, or peripheral neuropathy.

Logistics

All porphyrins exhibit a red fluorescence when exposed to ultraviolet light (400 nm), and this is the basis for the rapid qualitative screening tests that can be performed on blood, feces, or urine, most commonly the latter (frozen or refrigerated and stored in the dark at neutral pH after collection). Differentiation of urobilinogen and porphobilinogen can be accomplished rapidly by the Watson-Schwartz test, in which porphyrins producing a pink color on reaction with Ehrlich's reagent (p-dimethylamino benzaldehyde in HCl) are differentially extracted into chloroform or butanol. A specific test for porphobilinogen can also be performed by direct reaction of urine with a large amount of Ehrlich's reagent (the Hoesch test). These initial screening tests must always be confirmed by quantitative chromatographic methods, for which a 24-hour urine specimen, stored in the dark at neutral pH, is preferred. These specimens are best collected at the time of an acute clinical attack; porphyrin excretion may not be elevated during remissions.

Interpretation

The expected porphyrin species elevations during an acute attack of the various porphyrias, and the appropriate specimens in which they should be sought, are summarized in Table 15-5. Approximate reference

Table 15-5. Biochemical Profiles of the Porphyrias[a]

Porphyrias	Biochemical Profiles
Acute intermittent porphyria	Urine δ-aminolevulinic acid, porphobilinogen; fecal uroporphyrin
Protoporphyria	Fecal coproporphyrin, protoporphyrin; red blood cell protoporphyrin
Congenital erythropoietic porphyria	Urine uroporphyrin, coproporphyrin
Hereditary coproporphyria	Urine δ-aminolevulinic acid, porphobilinogen; fecal coproporphyrin
Porphyria cutanea tarda	Urine uroporphyrin
Variegate porphyria	Urine δ-aminolevulinic acid, porphobilinogen

[a] Findings listed are for evaluations in acute attacks.

ranges (which vary among laboratories and methods) are 10–30 μg/24 h (15.3–45.9 nmol/d) for urine uroporphyrin, 30–170 μg/24 h (45.9–260 nmol/d) for urine coproporphyrin, less than 1.0 mg/24 h (<4.4 μmol/d) for urine porphobilinogen, 1.5–7.5 mg/24 h (11.4–57.2 μmol/d) for urine δ-aminolevulinic acid, 20–75 μg/dL (0.35–1.33 μmol/L) erythrocytes for red blood cell protoporphyrin, 0.5–2.0 μg/dL (76–305 pmol/L) erythrocytes for red blood cell coproporphyrin, 0–500 μg/24 h (0–764 nmol/d) for fecal coproporphyrin, and 0–600 μg/24 h (0–916 nmol/d) for fecal protoporphyrin. An exposure to potential etiologic toxins (i.e., lead) should be ruled out by history or laboratory measurement before a diagnosis of one of the hereditary porphyrias is made.

Test: Sweat Chloride (See Ch. 5)

Background and Selection

Cystic fibrosis is an inherited defect of the exocrine glands causing abnormally viscid secretions that lead to meconium ileus, chronic obstructive pulmonary disease, exocrine pancreatic insufficiency, and male infertility. A reliable clinical laboratory marker of the disease is elevated sodium or chloride concentration in sweat. The eccrine sweat glands are histologically normal but exhibit a defect in ductal reabsorption of these ions.

Logistics

The sweat abnormality is present in the immediate newborn period and can be detected at any age. Localized sweating is stimulated for collection by pilocarpine iontophoresis and assayed by chloride ion electrode or other acceptable quantitative methods. At least 50 mg of sweat is required, an amount that may be difficult to obtain in newborn infants.

Interpretation

A sweat sodium or chlorine concentration of more than 60 mEq/L (>60 mmol/L) is consistent with a diagnosis of cystic fibrosis. Values in the range of 40–60 mEq/L (40–60 mmol/L) are found in patients with variant or atypical cystic fibrosis; these patients usually exhibit chronic bronchitis of less severe degree and normal pancreatic function. Some normal newborns can have elevated sweat electrolytes, as can patients with adrenal insufficiency, nephrogenic diabetes insipidus, hypothyroidism, ectodermal dysplasia, and certain storage diseases. However, the clinical picture will almost always allow differentiation of cystic fibrosis from these other disorders. Although the sweat electrolyte test remains the only reliable diagnostic clinical marker of the disease, the recent cloning of the cystic fibrosis gene on chromosome 7 makes possible genetic screening and prenatal diagnosis at the molecular level in most families. Such studies will only be applicable in those families with a prior affected member and will not be informative in all cases. Apart from DNA studies, there is no analogue of the sweat test or any other clinical chemistry procedure that can be applied to prenatal diagnosis or carrier detection.

Test: Tay-Sachs Screening (Hexosaminidase A Assay)

Background

Tay-Sachs disease, one of the GM2 gangliosidoses, is caused by a hereditary deficiency of hexosaminidase A (Hex A) and leads to rapidly progressive mental and motor impairment and death at an early age. As there is no effective therapy and the carrier gene frequency is quite high (1 in 27) in Ashkenazi Jews, a mass screening program has been undertaken with considerable success in this population.

Selection

This test is ordered on couples, usually premaritally, who are at risk of carrying the Tay-Sachs gene, primarily those of Ashkenazi Jewish descent. If both members of the couple are found to be carriers, an analogous test of the fetus by amniocentesis in any subsequent pregnancy is indicated.

Logistics

Hexosaminidase A is usually assayed in serum, using any of a number of ganglioside derivatives as substrate. The same assay can be performed on leukocytes, cultured fibroblasts, tears, or amniocytes. The procedure has been automated for use in mass screening programs. Women taking oral contraceptives may show false positive assay values in the heterozygote range.

Interpretation

Reference ranges are established by the individual laboratory. Heterozygotes show values intermediate between those of normal persons and patients with Tay-Sachs disease. If both members of a couple are found to be carriers, the same assay can be performed on cultured amniocytes for prenatal diagnosis. Rare families have been reported who appear deficient for hexosaminidase A in this assay using synthetic substrates, but are nevertheless clinically normal with adequate enzyme activity for the in vivo substrate, GM2 ganglioside.

Test: Very Long Chain Fatty Acids

Background

Recently a number of severe congenital disorders, including neonatal adrenoleukodystrophy, childhood adrenoleukodystrophy, Zellweger syndrome, Refsum's disease, and hyperpipecolatemia, have been localized to defects in the peroxisome, a small, membrane bound cytoplasmic organelle that is especially numerous in hepatocytes. Peroxisomes are involved in the oxidation of fatty acids, shortening them to smaller carbon chains; they also assist in the production of bile acids through cleavage of the cholesterol side chain. Hence, patients with these disorders can now be diagnosed by the finding of increased accumulation of very long chain fatty acids in serum.

Selection

This test is indicated to confirm or rule out a suspected diagnosis of peroxisomal disorder in patients presenting with otherwise unexplainable characteristic symptoms and signs, including hypotonia, demyelination, hepatic fibrosis, adrenal atrophy, or, in the case of Zellweger syndrome, facial dysmorphism.

Terminology

The very long chain fatty acids are classified by a shorthand nomenclature based on the number of carbon atoms in the chain, followed by the number of unsaturated double bonds in the molecule (e.g., C24:0, C26:1, etc.).

Logistics

At present this test is performed in only a few specialized reference and research laboratories. The test is performed on serum, but can also be done on cultured fibroblasts from a skin biopsy and other tissues.

Interpretation

Reference ranges are established by the individual laboratory, using control sera run in tandem with the patient specimen. The degree of elevation will be different for the various fatty acid species, but typically run 10–100 times higher than control values. Conversely, levels of the shorter species, such as C22:0, as well as common bile acids, are often reduced. An elevation of very long chain fatty acids is usually found in each of the peroxisomal disorders listed above. The diagnosis can often be confirmed further by electron microscopic documentation of absent, abnormally small, or unusually shaped peroxisomes on liver biopsy. Specific peroxisomal enzyme assays can also be performed in some research laboratories. Elevation of pipecolic acid, an intermediate in lysine metabolism, is found in hyperpipecolic acidemia and sometimes in Zellweger syndrome, Refsum's disease, and neonatal adrenoleukodystrophy. C27 bile acid intermediates and phytanic acid are especially elevated in Refsum's disease.

GLYCOGEN STORAGE DISEASE TESTS

The glycogen storage diseases are a rare group of diseases inherited in almost all cases as autosomal recessive defects. They are characterized by a deficiency or abnormality in one of the enzymes responsible for the formation or degradation of glycogen.[28] Almost all present early in childhood with a variety of symptoms occurring from hypoglycemia, hepatomegaly, and muscular weakness. Important characteristics of these diseases are summarized in Table 15-6. Many, such as type II (deficient lysosomal 1,4 glucosidase) and type IV (deficient amylo-1, 4-1, 6 transglucosidase), as well as those caused by specific muscle enzyme defects, are not associated with hypoglycemia. In many cases, however, supporting laboratory data involve the use of baseline glucose and lactate measurements followed by the response of these analytes to glucagon (see Ch. 7, p. 131 and below).

Those diseases in which the diagnosis is dependent on the reaction to the IM injection of 0.5 mg glucagon include type I (von Gierke's), type III (Cori-Forbes), and type VI (Hers). These patients have little increase in glucose and large increases in lactate. The normal response is a 60–80 mg/dL (3.3–4.4 mmol/L) rise in glucose with no change in lactate in 10 minutes. Plasma lactate increases by 3–6 mEq/L (3–6 mmol/L) in patients with von Gierke's disease 1 minute after exercising the forearm with a blood pressure cuff inflated.[29] Usually the specific diagnosis is made by measurement of the suspected enzyme deficiency in affected tissues following biopsy.

Test: L-Lactate (Lactate, Lactic Acid)

Background

L(+)-Lactate is the end product of anaerobic metabolism and its levels relate to oxygen availability. When the supply of oxygen is limited, the cytochrome system is unable to function as an intermediate in transfer of hydrogen to molecular oxygen. In this situation reduced nicotinamide adenine dinucleotide (NADH) accumulates and is oxidized by lactate dehydrogenase with the production of L(+)-lactate. Accumulation of L(+)-lactate in blood occurs from physiologic or pathophysiologic mechanisms. Physiologic increases are transient, occurring after extreme exercise, convulsive seizures, or shaking chills and in these circumstances concentrations decline by one-half in 60 minutes or less. In contrast, pathophysiologic increases such as from shock are more protracted and require over 2 hours for L(+)-lactate concentrations to decline by one-half.

Selection

Measurements of lactate are valuable in the diagnosis of glycogen storage diseases, types I (von Gierke's), III (Cori-Forbes), VI (Hers), and V (McArdle's).[28] However, the most common use of lactate measurements is to substantiate metabolic acidosis, a commonly encountered metabolic disorder in critically ill patients, most often caused by tissue hypoperfusion (see Ch. 2). Measurements also are used to identify and quantitate the severity of shock and to assess response to therapy.

Table 15-6. Glycogen Storage Diseases

Type	Major Clinical Features	Plasma Glucose Enzyme Deficiency (Tissue Affected)	Response to IM Glucagon (0.5 mg)
Ia (von Glerke's)	Hepatomegaly, lactic acidosis, hyperlipidemia, severe fasting hypoglycemia, renal disease	Glucose 6-phosphatase (liver, kidney)	No response
Ib	As Ia and pyogenic infections	Glucose 6-translocase (fresh liver)	No response
II (Pompe's)	Cardiomegaly, muscle weakness, death in infancy	$\alpha_{1,4}$-glucosidase (all tissues)	Normal
	Adult	$\alpha_{1,4}$-glucosidase (muscle)	Normal
III (Cori-Forbes)	Variable degrees of hepatomegaly, muscle weakness, fasting hypoglycemia	Debrancher (all tissues)	Normal after food; poor after fasting
IV (Anderson's)	Portal cirrhosis; usually death in infancy	Brancher (all tissues)	Normal
V (McArdle's)	Pain and stiffness after exertion; myoglobinuria in 50% of cases	Phosphorylase (muscle)	Normal
VI (Hers)	Hepatomegaly, mild fasting hypoglycemia	Phosphorylase (liver)	No response fasting or after food
VII (Tarul's)	Pain and stiffness on exertion	Phosphofructokinase muscle (? liver)	Normal
VIII	Spasticity, decerebration, high urinary catecholamines, death in infancy	Adenylate kinase (liver, brain)	Normal
IX	Hepatomegaly, occasional fasting hypoglycemia	Phosphorylase kinase (liver)	Normal, poor
X	Hepatomegaly only	Cyclic AMP dependent kinase (liver, muscle)	Normal

Logistics

For the diagnosis of types I (von Gierke's), III (Cori-Forbes), and VI (Hers) glycogen storage diseases, lactate is measured following the IM injection of 0.5 mg of glucagon. Laboratory diagnosis of type V (McArdle's) disease is made by applying a blood pressure cuff on the exercising forearm of suspected individuals and sampling blood lactate as a baseline and 1 minute after exercise begins.

Although venous blood specimens may yield higher results than arterial specimens, venous specimens often are used for convenience. If before obtaining the specimen the patient remains at complete rest, venous and arterial levels are identical. Venostasis performed in applying a tourniquet has little effect, but such minor movements as hand clenching can raise blood L(+)-lactate significantly. If whole blood is collected, it should be deproteinized immediately by adding the blood to a tube containing perchloric acid. Plasma kept at 25°C is also a satisfactory specimen if tubes containing sodium fluoride in potassium oxalate are used for blood collection and separation of plasma is complete within 15 minutes. Specimens collected and stored in 0.5 g/L iodoacetate at room temperature for up to 2 hours also provide acceptable results. If blood is not collected by these or comparable methods, lactate will increase rapidly from glycolysis by red blood cell enzymes. When the specimen is not collected in a correct tube, lactate increases may be as great as 20% in 3 minutes or 70% within 30 minutes at 25°C.

Interpretation

Following the injection of glucagon in patients with von Gierke's disease, plasma lactate increases by 3–6 mEq/L (3–6 mmol/L) over baseline. Patients who do not have this disorder have no increase in lactate levels. In type III (Cori-Forbes disease) lactate increases following the injection of glucagon in the fasting stage. With feeding and retesting 2 hours later, however, there is no increase in plasma lactate concentrations. The absence of a rise of L(+)-lactate levels following the application of a blood pressure cuff before mild exercise of the forearm is an important criterion for diagnosis of patients with McArdle's disease (type V glycogen storage disease).

Listed in Table 15-7 are the most widely recognized causes of lactic acidosis, with shock being the most frequent. An anion gap in a patient with metabolic acidosis suggests the diagnosis of lactic acidosis. It can be suspected when the sum of anions minus the sum of cations $[(Na^+ + K^+) - (Cl^- - HCO_3^-)]$ exceeds 18 mEq/L (18 mmol/L) in the absence of other causes of an increased anion gap, such as renal failure, salicylate ingestion, methanol poisoning, or significant ketonemia. Plasma L(+)-lactate concentrations have a reference range of 0.6–1.7 mEq/L (0.6–1.7 mmol/L) for venous blood, but even mild exercise will increase lactate levels substantially. Lactic acidosis values exceeding 7–8 mEq/L (7–8 mmol/L) usually are associated with fatal outcomes. When L(+)-lactate increases from 2–8 mEq/L (2–8 mmol/L) and remains at this level for over 2 hours, survival rates decrease from approximately 90% to 10%. Few cases with D(−)-lactic acidosis from abnormal gut flora have been described but D(−)-lactate is not measured by the usual enzymatic procedures for L(+)-lactate.

The findings of elevated L(+)-lactate in cerebrospinal fluid can discriminate between meningitis of bacterial and viral etiology (see Ch. 6). Its measurement can also aid in differentiating septic from other forms of monoarticular arthritis. Recently, it has been demonstrated that infusion of a sodium lactate solution can precipitate panic attack in patients with panic disorders or agoraphobia.

REFERENCES

1. Smith CV: Amniotic fluid assessment. Obstet Gynecol Clin North Am 1990;17:187–200.
2. Stephenson JN: Pregnancy testing and counseling. Pediatr Clin North Am 1989;36:681–696.
3. Bandi ZL, Schoen I, Waters M: An algorithm for testing and reporting serum choriogonadotropin at clinically significant decision levels with use of "pregnancy test" reagents. Clin Chem 1989;35:545–551.
4. Ammerman S, Shafer MA, Snyder D: Medical progress. Ectopic pregnancy in adolescents: a clinical review of pediatricians. J Pediatr 1990;117:677–686.
5. Kadar N, Caldwell BV, Romero R: A method of screening for ectopic pregnancy and its indications. Obstet Gynecol 1981;58:162–165.
6. Romero R, Horgan JG, Kohorn EI et al: New criteria for the diagnosis of gestational trophoblastic disease. Obstet Gynecol 1985;66:553–558.
7. Lee C, Hart LL: Accuracy of home pregnancy tests. DICP Ann Pharmacother 1190;24:712–713.
8. Knight GJ, Palomaki GE, Haddow JE: Use of maternal serum alpha fetoprotein measurements to screen for Down's syndrome. Obstet Gynecol 1988;31:306–327.
9. Burton BK: Elevated maternal serum alpha fetoprotein (MSAFP) Interpretation and follow-up. Clin Obstet Gynecol 1988;31:293–305.
10. Knight JA, Wu JT: α-Fetoprotein: its role in the prenatal diagnosis of congenital anomalies. Lab Med 1988;19:219–224.
11. Wald N, Cuckle H, Nanchahal K: Amniotic fluid acetylcholinesterase measurement in the prenatal diagnosis of open neural tube defects. Prenat Diagn 1989;9:813–829.
12. American College of Obstetricians and Gynecologists: Management of isoimmunization in pregnancy. ACOG Technical Bulletin 148. Washington, DC, ACOG, 1990.
13. Nicolaides KH, Rodeck CH, Mibashan RS, Kemp JR: Have Liley charts outlived their usefulness? Am J Obstet Gynecol 1986;155:90–94.
14. Polin JI, Frangipane WL: Current concepts in management of obstetric problems for pediatricians. Pediatr Clin North Am 1986;33:621–647.
15. Haddow JE, Palomaki GE, Knight GJ et al: Maternal serum unconjugated estriol levels are lower in the presence of fetal Down's syndrome. Am J Obstet Gynecol 1990;162:1372–1373.
16. Bernstein D, Zer J, Zakut H: Diurnal variations in conjugated plasma and total urinary estriol levels in late normal pregnancy. Gynecol Endocrinol 1989;3:99–106.
17. Whittaker PG, Lind T, Lawson JY: A prospective study to compare human placental lactogen and menstrual

Table 15-7. Common Causes of L-Lactic Acidosis

Congenital
    Glucose 6-phosphatase deficiency (type I glycogen storage disease)
    Fructose 1,6-diphosphatase deficiency
Shock
Exercise
Drugs
    Phenformin
    Sorbitol
    Fructose
    Ethanol
    Epinephrine
    Acetaminophen
Seizures
Hepatic disease
Neoplasms
Diabetic ketoacidosis
Idiopathic

dates for determining gestational age. Am J Obstet Gynecol 1987;156:178–182.
18. Cosmi EV, Di Renzo GC: Assessment of foetal lung maturity. Eur Respir J 1989;2:S40–S49.
19. Spillman T, Cotton DB: Current perspectives in assessment of fetal pulmonary surfactant status with amniotic fluid. CRC Crit Rev Lab Sci 1989;4:341–389.
20. Dubin SB: Assessment of fetal lung maturity: in search of the holy grail. Clin Chem 1990;36:1867–1869.
21. Mabry CC, Reid MC, Kuhn RJ: A source of error in phenylketonuria screening. Am J Clin Pathol 1988;90:279–283.
22. Winter SC, Szabo-Aczel S, Curry CJR et al: Plasma carnitine deficiency: clinical observations in 51 pediatric patients. Am J Dis Child 1987;141:660–665.
23. Ohtani Y, Ohyanagi K, Yamamoto S, Matsuda I: Secondary carnitine deficiency in hyperammonemic attacks of ornithine transcarbamylase deficiency. J Pediatr 1988;112:409–414.
24. Denny W, Dutton G: Simple urine test for gargoylism. Br Med J 1962;1:1555–1556.
25. Manley G, Hawksworth J: Diagnosis of Hurler's syndrome in the hospital laboratory and the determination of its genetic type. Arch Dis Child 1966;41:91–96.
26. Goodman SI: An introduction to gas chromatography-mass spectrometry and the inherited organic acidemias. Am J Hum Genet 1980;32:781–792.
27. Sweetman L: Qualitative and quantitative analysis of organic acids in physiologic fluids for diagnosis of the organic acidurias. pp. 419–453. In Nyhan WL (ed): Abnormalities in Amino Acid Metabolism in Clinical Medicine. E. Norwalk, CT, Appleton-Century-Crofts, 1984.
28. Collins JE, Leonard JV: Hepatic glycogen storage disease. Br J Hosp Med 1987;38:168–174.
29. Wakid NW, Bitar JG, Allam CK: Glycogen storage disease type I: laboratory data and diagnosis. Clin Chem 1987;33:2008–2010.

16 Hematopoiesis and Blood Cell Morphology

Bong Hak Hyun
Gene L. Gulati
John K. Ashton

INTRODUCTION

Erythrocytes (red blood cells, RBCs), leukocytes (white blood cells, WBCs), and thrombocytes (platelets) represent the three populations of cells normally present in the blood. Among these, the erythrocytes and thrombocytes form relatively uniform cell populations, whereas the leukocytes are subclassified into three groups, that is, the granulocytes (neutrophils, eosinophils, and basophils), monocytes, and lympocytes. Each of these blood cell populations is bestowed with specific morphologic characteristics and functions essential to normal life. An understanding of the origin, production, kinetics, morphology, and function of these cellular elements of blood is important to the identification and appropriate management of reactive and malignant disease processes of the hematopoietic system.

It is now common knowledge that all blood cells are derived from a common ancestor, frequently referred to as the hematopoietic stem cell (also known as the pluripotent stem cell or multipotent stem cell), which, although morphologically indistinct, has been operationally identified, using the mouse spleen-colony assay of Till and McCullock,[1] as colony forming unit–spleen (CFU-S).[2-7] These stem cells are capable of proliferation, self-renewal, and differentiation into committed stem cells with uni-, bi-, or trilineage specificities (Figs. 16-1 and 16-2). The process by which the blood cells are produced from their ancestor is termed *hematopoiesis*, and the sites or tissues in which it takes place represent the so-called hematopoietic sites or tissues, which in the developing human (intrauterine life) include the yolk sac, liver, spleen, bone marrow, and lymphoid tissues (thymus, lymph nodes, and gut-associated lymphoid structures). Postnatally, hematopoiesis[3,8-10,12,14] normally occurs only in the bone marrow, with lymphoid tissues contributing lymphocytes and plasma cells. The liver and spleen, although normally inactive, maintain the potential for hematopoiesis throughout life.

For 2–3 years after birth, virtually all bone cavities are completely filled with hematopoietic cells (red marrow). With advancing age, however, the red marrow is gradually replaced by yellow marrow (fatty tissue), particularly in the cavities of peripheral bones. In adults, the red marrow is confined essentially to the cavities of centrally located bones of the sternum, ribs, vertebrae, clavicles, scapulae, cranium, and pelvis and to the proximal ends of the femurs and humeri.[8,13] These age-related changes are referenced when defining marrow cellularity (Fig. 16-3). A normocellular marrow consists of normal proportions of red and yellow marrow. A hypocellular marrow represents reduction in red marrow with a corresponding increase in yellow marrow. Similarly, a hypercellular marrow reflects an increase in the red marrow with a corresponding decrease in yellow marrow.

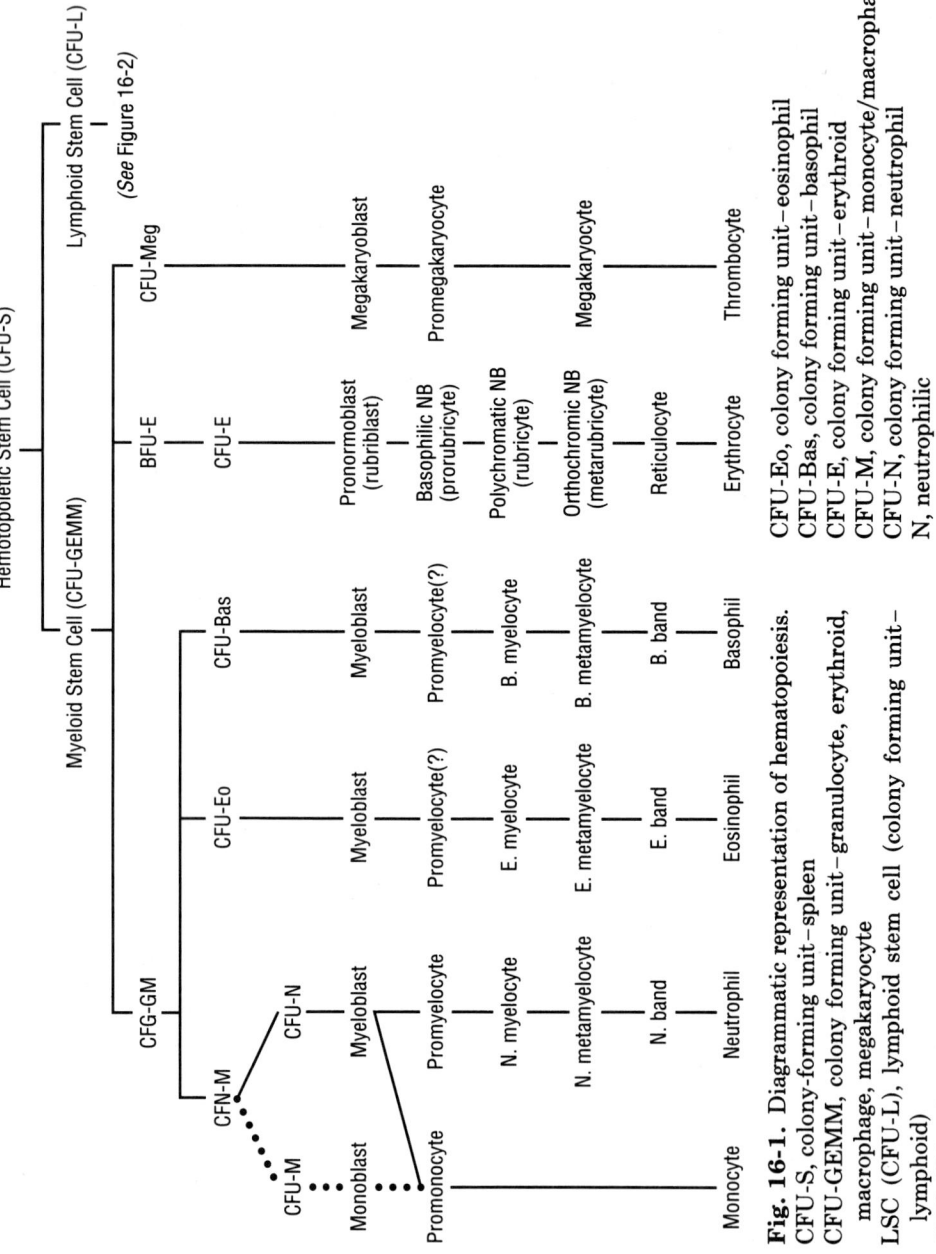

Fig. 16-1. Diagrammatic representation of hematopoiesis.
CFU-S, colony-forming unit–spleen
CFU-GEMM, colony forming unit–granulocyte, erythroid, macrophage, megakaryocyte
LSC (CFU-L), lymphoid stem cell (colony forming unit–lymphoid)
CFU-GM, colony forming unit–granulocyte, monocyte
BFU-E, burst forming unit–erythroid
CFU-Meg, colony forming unit–megakaryocyte
CFU-NM, colony forming unit–neutrophil, monocyte
CFU-Eo, colony forming unit–eosinophil
CFU-Bas, colony forming unit–basophil
CFU-E, colony forming unit–erythroid
CFU-M, colony forming unit–monocyte/macrophage
CFU-N, colony forming unit–neutrophil
N, neutrophilic
E, eosinophilic
B, basophilic
NB, normoblast
(Modified from Gulati et al.,[8] with permission.)

For the purpose of discussion and clear understanding, the process of hematopoiesis is divided into five parts, each representing a pathway for the production of one type of mature blood cell as described below.

ERYTHROCYTES AND ERYTHROPOIESIS[3,4,6,8,10,13,15,16]

The process of erythrocyte production (erythropoiesis) begins in a sequential manner with the differentiation of a pluripotent hematopoietic stem cell, colony forming unit–spleen (CFU-S), through the intermediate stages of colony forming unit–granulocyte, erythrocyte, macrophage, and megakaryocyte (CFU-GEMM), and burst forming unit–erythrocyte (BFU-E), into a unipotent stem cell, colony forming unit–erythrocyte (CFU-E), committed to produce RBCs. None of these stem cells is morphologically recognizable; however, further differentiation of CFU-E gives rise to a progeny that is morphologically identified as a pronormoblast. Each pronormoblast (rubriblast) undergoes a series of heteromorphogenic mitotic divisions, through the stages of early and late basophilic normoblasts (prorubricytes), leading to the production of a total of 16 polychromatophilic normoblasts (rubricytes) (Fig. 16-4). By further maturation without division, each polychromatophilic normoblast yields first an orthochromic normoblast (metarubricyte) and then a reticulocyte. Each mitotic division results in reduction of cell size and nuclear size; progressive differentiation and maturation lead to the disappearance of nucleoli and an increase in density of nuclear chromatin. Ultimately, the nucleus becomes pyknotic and is extruded at the orthochromic normoblast stage. The extruded nucleus is phagocytosed and digested by macrophages.

The synthesis of hemoglobin from the late basophilic normoblast stage onward brings about changes in the staining characteristics of the cytoplasm from blue (because of RNA content) in the pronormoblasts and basophilic normoblasts to varying degrees of pink (because of hemoglobin content) mixed with a bluish tinge in the polychromatophilic normoblasts, orthochromic normoblasts, and reticulocytes. It normally takes 3–5 days for the production of reticulocytes from pronormoblasts. The reticulocytes remain in the marrow for 1–2 days before being released into the circulation, where they lose their cytoplasmic reticulum within 1 or 2 days and become mature RBCs. The normal biconcave mature RBCs circulate for about 120 days, carrying out their function of protecting and transporting hemoglobin, the oxygen-carrying pigment. Over the course of its life span, RBC enzymatic activities diminish, adenosine triphosphate (ATP) content/concentration decreases, and surface area is reduced, resulting in increased density, or increased mean cell hemoglobin concentration (MCHC). The senescent RBCs are degraded by the cells of the reticuloendothelial system. In the degradation process within the macrophages, hemoglobin is broken down into its three components: (1) iron, which is reused in the synthesis of new hemoglobin and other iron-containing compounds; (2) globin, which is further degraded and returned to the amino acid pool of the body; and (3) protoporphyrin, which is converted to bilirubin and ultimately excreted from the body in the form of urobilinogen in feces and urine. In the normal steady-state, the daily loss of about 1% of circulating senescent RBCs is balanced by the production and release of an equivalent number of new RBCs. Although multiple factors, including vitamins (e.g., B_{12} and folate), minerals (e.g., iron, calcium, cobalt, and zinc), hematopoietic microenvironment, hormones (e.g., androgens, triiodothyronine [T_3], and growth hormone), and lymphokines (e.g., interleukin-3), influence the rate of RBC production, the humoral factor, erythropoietin, which is produced by the kidneys, is considered the chief regulator of erythropoiesis.[16–18]

The normal process of RBC production is designated normoblastic erythropoiesis; however, certain vitamin deficiencies, such as B_{12} and/or folate deficiency, are associated with an abnormal process of maturation of erythroid precursors commonly referred to as megaloblastic erythropoiesis. Megaloblastic erythropoiesis proceeds through the same stages of development as normoblastic erythropoiesis but, because of the impaired ability of the cells to synthesize DNA, the cells produced are large and nuclear maturation lags behind cytoplasmic maturation (asynchronous nuclear to cytoplasmic development). The morphologic characteristics of these normal (normoblastic) and abnormal (megaloblastic) RBC precursors as seen on Romanowsky-stained smears are noted below.

Morphology of Normoblastic Erythropoiesis[9,10,14,15,19–21] (Plate 1)

Pronormoblast

The pronormoblast is the largest RBC precursor (14–19 μm), with a large, round, or slightly oval nucleus; fine reticular chromatin; one or two prominent nucleoli; sparse indistinct parachromatin; and basophilic cytoplasm appearing as a thin band around the nucleus. The nuclear to cytoplasmic (N/C) ratio is 8:1.

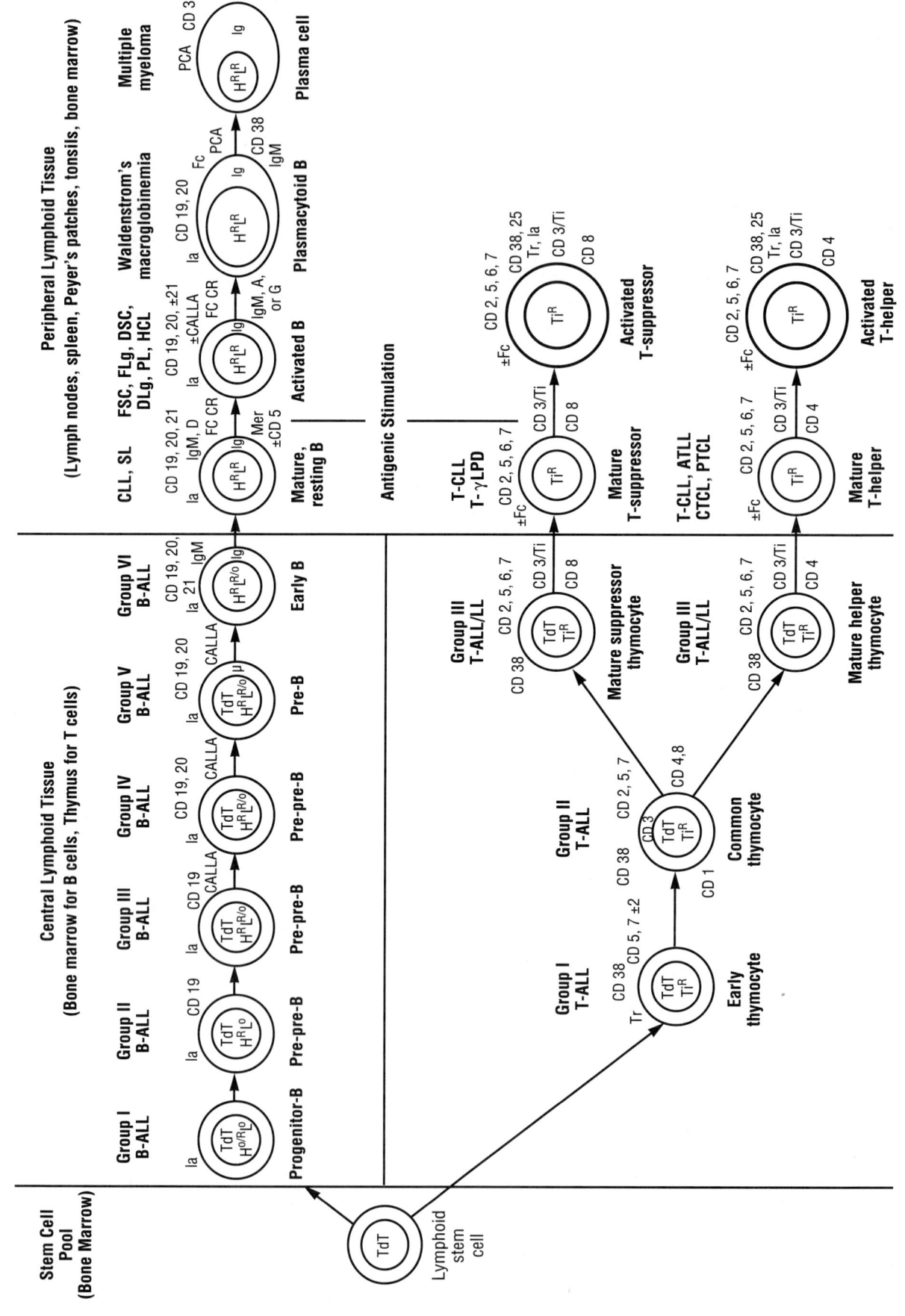

Basophilic Normoblast

The basophilic normoblast is smaller (10–17 μm) than the pronormoblast, with a large, round, or slightly oval nucleus; slightly coarse chromatin; one (in early basophilic normoblast) or no (in late basophilic normoblast) nucleolus; sparse but distinct parachromatin; and a slightly larger amount (than in the pronormoblast) of deeply basophilic cytoplasm. The N/C ratio is 6:1.

Polychromatophilic Normoblast

The polychromatophilic normoblast is slightly smaller (10–15 μm) than the basophilic normoblast, with a round nucleus; deep-staining, coarse, and clumped chromatin; distinct parachromatin; and abundant blue-gray to pink-gray cytoplasm surrounding the nucleus. The N/C ratio is 4:1.

Orthochromic Normoblast

The orthochromic normoblast is smaller (8–12 μm) than the polychromatophilic normoblast, with a small pyknotic nucleus, homogeneously dense chromatin, and more abundant orange-staining cytoplasm. The N/C ratio is 1:2.

Reticulocyte

The reticulocyte is an anucleate cell (7–10 μm) with pinkish gray cytoplasm containing a small amount of fine basophilic reticulum (RNA) and a large amount of

---

Fig. 16-2. Diagrammatic representation of lymphopoiesis.[38,39]
TdT, terminal deoxynucleotidyl transferase
H°, germline configuration for immunoglobulin heavy chain
H^R, rearranged gene for immunoglobulin heavy chain
L°, germline configuration for immunoglobulin light chain
L^R, rearranged gene for immunoglobulin light chain
Ti°, germline configuration for T-cell receptor antigen
Ti^R, rearranged gene for T-cell receptor antigen
Ig, immunoglobulin
μ, μ-heavy chain immunoglobulin
CD10, common acute lymphocytic leukemia antigen (CALLA)
PCA, plasma cell associated antigens
Fc, receptor for Fc portion of immunoglobulin
CR, receptor for complement component
MER, mouse erythrocyte receptor
Ia, HLA-DR associated antigen, appearing on B cells and activated T cells
Tr, transferrin receptor
CD, cluster of differentiation group of leukocyte antigen;
CD19, 20, 21, pan-B antigens present at various stages of B-lymphocyte differentiation
CD2, 5, 6, 7, pan-T antigens present at various stages of T-lymphocyte differentiation—CD2 is the antigen associated with E-rosette formation, while CD5 is the T antigen anomalously present on CLL B cells
CD3, pan-T antigen intimately associated on the surface membrane with Ti, the T-cell receptor antigen
CD1, common thymocyte surface antigen
CD4, T-helper cell surface antigen
CD8, T-suppressor cell surface antigen
CD38, T10, an antigen appearing on early thymocytes and activated mature T and B cells
CD25, IL-2 receptor surface antigen
CLL, chronic lymphocytic leukemia
SL, small cell lymphocytic lymphoma
FSC, follicular center small cleaved cell lymphoma
FLg, follicular center large cell lymphoma
DSC, diffuse small cleaved cell lymphoma
DLg, diffuse large cell lymphoma
PL, prolymphocytic leukemia
HCL, hairy cell leukemia
LL, lymphoblastic lymphoma
T-γ LPD, T-γ lymphoproliferative disease
ATLL, adult T-cell leukemia/lymphoma
CTCL, cutaneous T-cell lymphoma (Sézary syndrome)
PTCL, peripheral T-cell lymphoma
"Activated" cells, may represent several cell divisions with different T and B morphologic forms
(Data from Foon and Tood[38] and McMichael.[39])

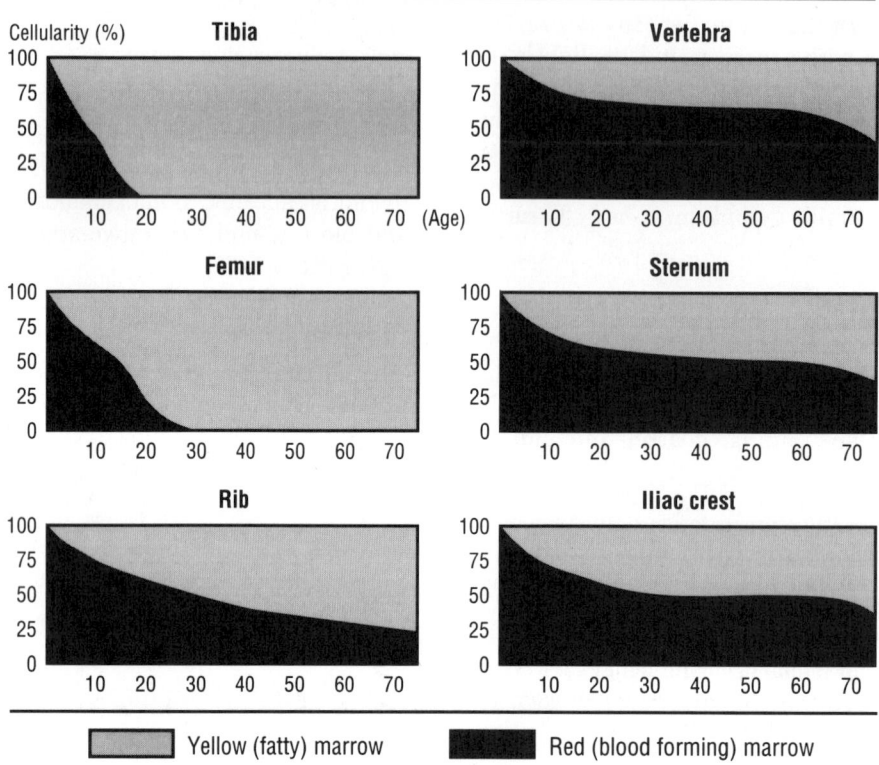

Fig. 16-3. Bone marrow cellularity. (From Hyun et al.,[13] with permission.)

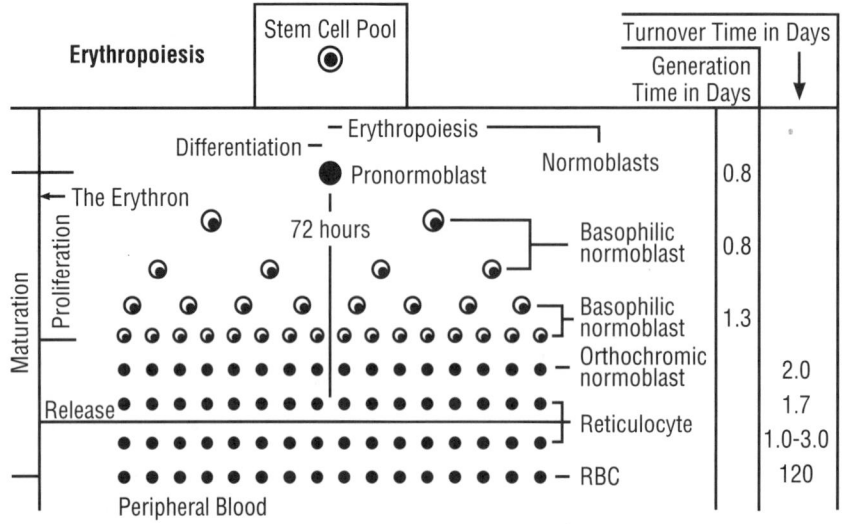

Fig. 16-4. Erythropoiesis. (From Hyun et al.,[13] with permission.)

pink-staining hemoglobin. Fine basophilic stippling is sometimes seen in the reticulocyte.

Erythrocyte

The erythrocyte is a mature RBC, biconcave in shape (6.7–7.8 μm), 0.2-μm thick, that contains but is no longer able to synthesize, pink-staining hemoglobin. A zone of central pallor covering approximately one-third of the cell diameter is devoid of hemoglobin. Normal RBCs are designated normocytic, implying normal size, and normochromic, implying normal hemoglobin content/concentration.

Morphology of Megaloblastic and Dysplastic Erythropoiesis[15,19-21] (Plate 1)

Megaloblastic Nucleated Red Blood Cells (Promegaloblast, Basophilic Megaloblast, Polychromatophilic Megaloblast, Orthochromic Megaloblast)

Megaloblasts are larger than the corresponding normal cells of the erythroid series, with delayed nuclear maturation (asynchronous nuclear to cytoplasmic development). They are classified into similar stages of development as the normal counterpart cells, based on the stage of cytoplasmic development (Plate 7).

Large Reticulocyte

The large reticulocyte is larger (10–13 μm) than the normal reticulocyte, with pink to pink-gray cytoplasm containing a small amount of basophilic reticulum and a large amount of pink hemoglobin.

Macro-ovalocyte

The macro-ovalocyte is a large (9–12 μm) oval shaped RBC containing (but unable to synthesize) pink hemoglobin in the peripheral two-thirds of the cell space.

Macronormoblast (Megaloblastoid Nucleated RBC)

The macronormoblast is a nucleated RBC in transition from normoblastic to megaloblastic development or vice versa, characterized by large (10–20 μm) size, round or slightly oval nucleus, moderately clumped chromatin, and abundant bluish pink (depending on the stage of maturation) cytoplasm; parachromatin spaces may be prominent. The N/C ratio is 1:1–1:2.

Dysplastic Nucleated Red Blood Cells

Morphologic changes in dysplastic nucleated RBCs include nuclear abnormalities, such as lobation, budding, karyorrhexis, and multinuclearity. Cytoplasmic vacuolization or uneven hemoglobinization may be seen. Megaloblastic or megaloblastoid forms commonly occur. Ringed sideroblasts may be seen with Prussian blue stain for iron (Plates 22A and 31B).

Abnormal Red Blood Cell Morphology[13-15,19,20,22] (Plates 4 and 5)

Acanthocytes (Spur Cells, Spiculated Cells)

Acanthocytes are spheroid RBCs (often lacking the zone of central pallor), with multiple (3–10) irregularly distributed spine-like projections of variable length, formed as a result of an increased ratio of cholesterol to lecithin in the membrane often attributable to the deficiency of lecithin/cholesterol acyltransferase (LCAT). Associated conditions include hereditary acanthocytosis accompanying abetalipoproteinemia, liver disease, McLeod phenotype (lack of Kell blood group, Kx), infantile pyknocytosis (vitamin E deficient mother), pyruvate kinase deficiency, and postsplenectomy state.

Anisocytosis

Anisocytosis is a variation in size among RBCs, a common finding in most moderate or severe anemias.

Autoagglutination

Autoagglutination is aggregation/clumping of RBCs, often caused by the presence of an antibody as seen in cold agglutinin disease and other autoimmune hemolytic anemias.

Basophilic Stippling (Punctate Basophilia)

Basophilic stippling is characterized by fine, medium, or coarse blue granules (representing ribosomal RNA precipitated during staining) uniformly distributed throughout the RBC. Fine granulation (stippling) usually represents polychromatophilia (reticulocytes), whereas medium-sized or coarse stippling often reflects impaired erythropoiesis. Associated conditions include heavy metal poisoning (e.g., lead and arsenic), thalassemias, hemoglobinopathies, sideroblastic anemias, and pyrimidine-5′-nucleotidase deficiency.

Blister Cells

Blister cells are RBCs that contain one or more vacuoles or markedly thinned area(s) at the periphery, giving the appearance of a blister. They are often formed as a consequence of the removal of Heinz bodies from the RBCs by reticuloendothelial cells. Rupture of the vacuoles yields what is called a bite cell, a helmet cell, or a schistocyte; they are generally seen during acute hemolytic episodes after exposure to an oxidant in patients with glucose 6-phosphate dehydrogenase (G-6-PD) deficiency.

Burr Cells (Echinocytes, Crenated RBCs, Sea Urchin Cells)

Burr cells are RBCs with short, evenly distributed, blunt (knobby) projections. They may be formed as a result of depletion of ATP, exposure to hypertonic solution, contact with glass surface, or as an artifact during air drying of thick smears or with the use of aged blood. Associated conditions include uremia, cirrhosis of the liver, hepatitis, chronic renal disease, and pyruvate kinase deficiency.

Cabot Rings

Cabot rings are ring, figure-8, or loop-shaped, red, reddish purple, or bluish purple structures representing the remnants of microtubules of the mitotic spindle probably following an anomalous mitosis, within RBCs. They may be seen in nucleated and non-nucleated RBCs and in association with coarse basophilic stippling. Associated conditions include megaloblastic anemia and dyserythropoiesis; they may also be seen, rarely, in other types of severe anemias.

Elliptocytes (Ovalocytes)

Elliptocytes are elliptic (pencil-shaped) or oval (egg-shaped) RBCs with polarization of hemoglobin that may be found in small numbers (usually less than 5%) in normal persons; however, they are most abundant (25–95%) in hereditary elliptocytosis and pyropoikilocytosis, a variant of hereditary elliptocytosis. A moderate degree of elliptocytosis may be seen in other anemias, including iron deficiency, thalassemia minor, megaloblastic anemias, and myelophthisic anemias.

Heinz Bodies

Heinz bodies are round, single or multiple, blue-purple inclusions that represent precipitate(s) of denatured hemoglobin. They are often attached to the inner surface of the RBC membrane and are visualized only by supravital stains (not visible with Wright or Wright-Giemsa stain). Heinz bodies are more readily seen postsplenectomy. Associated conditions include defective RBC glycolytic enzyme system, overdose of oxidant drugs, and unstable hemoglobins.

Hemoglobin C Crystals

Hemoglobin C crystals are tetragonal, rectangular, or rod-shaped, dense-staining, single or multiple crystals of hemoglobin C seen inside RBCs (with a portion of the cell being devoid of hemoglobin), particularly after splenectomy in patients with hemoglobin CC disease or SC disease.

Howell-Jolly Bodies

Howell-Jolly bodies consist of one or more, usually small (mean diameter about 1 μm, but size may vary), round, purple structures or bodies (representing nuclear remnants) within RBCs and sometimes within RBC precursors. They are more readily seen postsplenectomy. Associated conditions include megaloblastic anemia, severe hemolytic process, asplenism, hyposplenism, and myelophthisic anemia.

Hyperchromia

Hyperchromia is characterized by a greater than normal concentration of hemoglobin (MCHC of more than 36 g/dL [360 g/L]) in RBCs, usually associated with moderate or marked spherocytosis, as seen in some patients with hereditary spherocytosis or immune hemolytic anemias. By contrast, a greater than normal amount of hemoglobin, with a mean cell hemoglobin (MCH) above 32 pg is noted in many conditions associated with macrocytosis.

Hypochromia

Hypochromia is characterized by a lower than normal amount (MCH) and concentration (MCHC) of hemoglobin in RBCs, often recognized morphologically by the expansion of the zone of central pallor to more than one-third the diameter of the cell. The most common associated condition is moderate or severe iron deficiency. Slight hypochromia also may be seen in other conditions associated with microcytosis.

Macrocytes

Macrocytes are RBCs that are larger than normal (more than 8.5 μm in diameter, more than 95 fL in volume), formed as a result of impaired DNA synthesis resulting from a lack of vitamin B_{12} or folate, stress erythropoiesis, or excessive surface membrane. Macrocytes are often normochromic, may sometimes be hyperchromic, and may be oval (as in megaloblastic anemias) or round (as in nonmegaloblastic anemias). Associated conditions include vitamin B_{12}/folate deficiency producing oval macrocytes, inherited or acquired conditions (chemotherapy) with impaired DNA synthesis, myeloproliferative disorders, myelodysplastic syndromes, liver disease, obstructive jaundice, alcoholism, and postsplenectomy.

Microcytes

Microcytes are RBCs that are smaller than normal (below 6.5 μm in diameter and/or less than 80 fL in volume) in size, formed as a result of the failure of hemoglobin synthesis because of a lack of iron, defective globin chain(s), imbalance of globin chains or defective porphyrin synthesis. They may or may not be hypochromic. Associated conditions include iron deficiency, thalassemias, anemia of chronic disease, lead poisoning, and sideroblastic anemias.

Pappenheimer bodies

Pappenheimer bodies are one or more, often in clusters of two to five, small (0.3–2.0 μm), bluish black or greenish blue granules (representing nonheme iron particles, as demonstrated by Prussian blue staining) within RBCs (siderocytes) and/or nucleated RBCs (sideroblasts). Associated conditions include postsplenectomy state, hemosiderosis, severe hemolytic anemia, hemoglobinopathies, thalassemias, sideroblastic anemias, defective heme synthesis, and myelodysplastic syndrome.

Poikilocytosis

Poikilocytosis is a variation in shape among RBCs. Although a nonspecific finding, it is usually caused by an irreversible alteration of the membrane and is often associated with active erythroid regeneration and/or extramedullary hematopoiesis. Red blood cells may take many different shapes under various conditions, including a resemblance to teardrop, helmet, bull's eye, and fish mouth. Red blood cell shapes with individual descriptive terms are defined below, whereas those that are not yet defined are simply designated as poikilocytes.

Polychromasia (Polychromatophilia)

Polychromasia is a blue-gray coloration of RBCs that indicates the presence of an admixture of RNA and hemoglobin, as seen in reticulocytes. Normally, about 1% of RBCs in an adult are polychromatophilic, but the percentage rises significantly in severe anemias with increased erythropoietic activity (e.g., hemolytic anemias) and after hematinic therapy in anemic patients.

Rouleaux

Rouleaux is an alignment of RBCs in a linear fashion, appearing as a stack of coins, often caused by increased blood concentration of fibrinogen, globulin, or paraproteins. It must be seen in the thin readable area (next to the feather edge) of the blood smear, as it is commonly encountered as an artifact in the thick area of the blood smear. Associated conditions include acute and chronic inflammatory disorders, Waldenström's macroglobulinemia, and multiple myeloma.

Schistocytes (Helmet Cells, Bite Cells, RBC Fragments, Keratocytes)

Schistocytes are fragments of RBCs, varying in size and shape (e.g., helmet-shaped, triangular), often produced by the arrest of their passage through the circulation by fibrin strands, damaged prosthetic valves, altered vessel walls, or increased shear force. They may also result from the action of macrophages on the defective RBCs. Associated conditions include disseminated intravascular coagulation (DIC), thrombotic thrombocytopenic purpura (TTP), vasculitis, glomerulonephritis, microangiopathic hemolytic anemia, heart valve hemolysis, severe burns, malignant hypertension, and march hemoglobinuria.

Sickle Cells (Drepanocytes)

Sickle cells involve sickling activity related to polymerization/gelation of deoxygenated hemoglobin S, giving the RBCs a crescent shaped, filament shaped appearance with two pointed extremities, in holly leaf form, boat shaped, and/or as envelope cells. The sickled cells usually lack the zone of central pallor. Associated conditions include sickle cell anemia, hemoglobin SC disease, hemoglobin S-β-thalassemia, hemoglobin SD disease, and hemoglobin Memphis/S disease.

Sideroblasts, Ringed

Ringed sideroblasts are nucleated RBCs that contain siderotic granules (nonheme iron particles seen with Prussian blue staining) arranged in a ring form around the nucleus (perinuclear arrangement). Electron microscopy has shown the iron particles to be present in mitochondria. Associated conditions include sideroblastic anemias and dyserythropoietic states (Plate 31B).

Spherocytes

Spherocytes are dense-staining, nondeformable, spherical RBCs with decreased diameter (usually less than 6.5 μm), increased thickness (frequently more than 3 μm), normal cell volume, and little if any central pallor zone. Associated conditions include hereditary spherocytosis and isoimmune and autoimmune hemolytic anemias. Microspherocytes, probably representing rounded-up fragments of RBCs, are common findings in patients with severe burns and in hereditary pyropoikilocytosis.

Stomatocytes

Stomatocytes are RBCs with a central, slit-like or oval pallid zone surrounded by a dense hemoglobinized area giving the appearance of a fish mouth or smiling face. They may occur as an artifact of slow air drying of smears. Associated conditions include hereditary stomatocytosis (an extremely rare disorder), Rh-null disease, acute alcoholism, liver disease, and malignant disease.

Target Cells (Leptocytes, Codocytes)

Target cells are thin, flat RBCs with an excess of surface membrane to volume ratio, showing a peripheral rim of hemoglobin along with a central hemoglobinized area, giving the appearance of a bull's eye or Mexican hat. They may also appear as artifacts of air drying of smears in a humid environment or of smears made from blood specimens anticoagulated with excessive EDTA (e.g., less than 1 mL of blood collected in a vacutainer tube containing EDTA adequate for 5 mL blood). Associated conditions include hemoglobinopathies (e.g., hemoglobin SS, SC, CC, AC, EE, AE disease), thalassemias, liver disease, LCAT deficiency, iron deficiency, and postsplenectomy state.

Teardrop Cells (Dacrocytes)

Teardrop cells are RBCs that have the shape of a teardrop or a pear with a single elongated, often blunted/rounded (rarely pointed) end. They are seen in significant numbers in myelophthisic anemias, particularly myelofibrosis with myeloid metaplasia, and in moderate numbers in pernicious anemia, thalassemias, anemia of renal failure, and other forms of severe anemias.

GRANULOCYTES AND GRANULOPOIESIS[3,6,8,13,23,24]

An orderly production of mature granulocytes (neutrophils, eosinophils, and basophils) begins in the marrow under the influence of the hematopoietic microenvironment and/or some humoral factor(s). Pluripotent hematopoietic stem cells (CFU-S) differentiate through the stages of colony forming unit–granulocyte, erythroid, monocyte/macrophage (CFU-GEMM), colony forming unit–granulocyte, monocyte/macrophage (CFU-GM), and colony forming unit–neutrophil, monocyte (CFU-NM), into three unipotent stem cells — colony forming unit–neutrophil (CFU-N), colony forming unit–eosinophil (CFU-Eo), and colony forming unit–basophil (CFU-Bas), committed to produce neutrophils, eosinophils, and basophils, respectively (Fig. 16-1). Differentiation of each of these unipotent stem cells leads to the production of a morphologically recognizable cell designated a myeloblast. The myeloblast divides (by mitosis) and differentiates into two promyelocytes, each of which undergoes mitosis and differentiation, giving rise to two myelocytes. At this stage, two additional mitotic divisions result in self-replication of myelocytes. The simultaneous development of specific granulation permits classification of myelocytes into three cell lines, neutrophilic, eosinophilic, and basophilic. Ultimately, each myelocyte undergoes progressive maturation without further division, sequentially generating a metamyelocyte, a band, and a segmented cell. Neutrophils, eosinophils, and basophils are the end products of the maturation of neutrophilic, eosinophilic, and basophilic myelocytes, respectively. Each mitotic division from the promyelocyte stage onward progressively reduces the cell size, the nuclear size, and the number of azurophilic (primary) granules. Furthermore, as differentiation and maturation proceed from the myeloblast to the segmented cell stage, there is progressive condensation of nuclear chromatin with the disappearance of nucleoli by the late myelocyte stage, and the cytoplasm gradually loses its basophilia, acquiring pink-staining characteristics. The maturation process from the myelocyte to the mature cell stage is also marked by the development of specific (secondary) granulation (neutrophilic, eosinophilic, and basophilic) and by nuclear shape changes from round or ovoid at the myelocyte stage, to kidney shaped at the metamyelocyte stage, to band or C shaped at the band stage, and ultimately to the segmented or lobulated (two to five) form at the mature cell stage (Plate 2).

It takes about 14 days from the myeloblast stage to the release of mature granulocytes from the marrow into the circulation. On entering the circulation, the granulocytes, particularly the neutrophils, are distributed between two pools of roughly equal size: a marginal granulocyte pool (MGP), representing granulocytes marginated along the walls of capillaries and venules and a circulating granulocyte pool (CGP), consisting of free-floating granulocytes. The circulating granulocyte pool is reflected in the usual total and differential leukocyte counts. However, a free exchange of cells occurs between the two pools continually. Although their total life span (in the blood and tissues) is estimated to be 9-10 days, the granulocytes remain in the blood for only 6-8 hours before migrating to the tissues, where they perform their specific functions.

Granulocytes are attracted (chemotaxis) to the sites of tissue invasion by microorganisms. Neutrophils, and to a lesser degree eosinophils, are capable of phagocytosis, killing, and digesting bacteria and yeast. In addition, eosinophils are involved in certain hypersensitivity reactions and provide defense against parasitic infestations. The function of basophils is less well understood. They are often involved in immediate and delayed hypersensitivity reactions. The regulation of granulocyte production is maintained by certain humoral factors produced by T cells, monocytes, and/or marrow stromal cells, collectively called colony stimulating factors (CSFs) or activities (CSAs) or granulopoietins, and by colony inhibitory activities or factors (CIAs or CIFs) released by mature granulocytes.[25-28]

Morphology of Granulopoiesis[9,10,14, 19-21,29] (Plate 2)

Myeloblast

The myeloblast is a cell of variable size (10-20 μm) with a relatively large, often round or oval (occasionally indented or lobulated) nucleus, very finely reticulated chromatin, sparse but distinct parachromatin, zero to five nucleoli, and usually scanty basophilic cytoplasm devoid of granules or may contain occasional azurophilic granules. The N/C ratio is 5:1-7:1.

Promyelocyte (Progranulocyte)

The promyelocyte is usually slightly larger (12-21 μm) than the myeloblast with a large, round, or oval nucleus, fine chromatin, sparse parachromatin, zero to three nucleoli, and a small amount of pale blue cytoplasm containing a few or many azurophilic granules. These granules represent membrane-bound organelles containing primarily lysosomal enzymes (acid hydrolases and peroxidase) and a small amount of muramidase. The N/C ratio is 5:1.

Myelocyte

The myelocyte is a cell of variable size (10-18 μm), generally smaller than the promyelocyte, with a centrally or eccentrically located, large, round, oval or occasionally slightly indented nucleus, relatively coarse chromatin, no or one nucleolus, sparse parachromatin, and a moderate amount of bluish pink or light pink cytoplasm containing some azurophilic granules and large number of specific granules of either neutrophilic (lilac color), eosinophilic (orange-red), or basophilic (deep blue) type. The N/C ratio is 2:1. The neutrophilic granules also represent membrane-bound organelles and contain muramidase, lactoferrin, peroxidase, collagenase, phagocytin, alkaline phosphatase, and several other enzymes. The eosinophilic granules are similar to the neutrophilic granules in that they are also rich in peroxidase and lysosomal enzymes, with the exception of muramidase. It is unclear whether the basophilic granules contain peroxidase, but they are known to contain histamine, heparin, hyaluronic acid, and minimal amounts of acid and alkaline phosphatases. By electron microscopy, crystalloid protein structures (Charcot-Leyden crystals) have been seen within the granules of eosinophils and after degranulation in the basophils.

Metamyelocyte

The metamyelocyte is slightly smaller (10-16 μm) than the early myelocyte or is same size as the late myelocyte, with a kidney shaped nucleus, dense chromatin, no nucleolus, sparse parachromatin, and abundant pinkish or colorless cytoplasm containing a few azurophilic granules and numerous neutrophilic, eosinophilic, or basophilic granules. The N/C ratio is 5:1.

Band

The band is the same size as the metamyelocyte or is slightly smaller (10-15 μm), with a band or sausage shaped, stab form, or lobulated nucleus, a thick (greater than or equal to one-third the average diameter of lobes) bridge containing dense chromatin connecting the lobes, coarse clumpy chromatin, no nucleolus, very scant, if any, parachromatin, and abundant pinkish or colorless cytoplasm containing numerous neutrophilic, eosinophilic, or basophilic granules and may or may not contain a few azurophilic granules.

Neutrophil

The neutrophil is a mature cell (10–15 μm) with segmented or lobulated (two to five lobes) nucleus, one or more thin (less than one-third the average diameter of lobes) filament(s) connecting the lobes, no nucleolus, coarse and clumped chromatin, and abundant pinkish or colorless cytoplasm containing abundant neutrophilic granules. The N/C ratio is 1:3.

Eosinophil

The eosinophil is a mature cell (10–15 μm), with segmented or lobulated (two or three lobes) nucleus, no nucleolus, coarse and clumped chromatin, and abundant pinkish or colorless cytoplasm containing abundant eosinophilic granules. The N/C ratio is 1:3 (Plate 8B).

Basophil

The basophil is a mature cell (10–15 μm), with a segmented or lobulated (one to three lobes) nucleus, no nucleolus, coarse and clumped chromatin, and abundant pinkish or colorless cytoplasm; several blackish blue granules often spread over the nucleus and in the cytoplasm. The N/C ratio is 1:3 (Plate 8A).

Morphologic Abnormalities Associated with Granulocytes[13,19,21,24]

Alder-Reilly Granules

Alder-Reilly granules are large, purple or purplish black, coarse, azurophilic granules in the cytoplasm of virtually all mature leukocytes and even their precursors. They are a characteristic finding in Alder-Reilly anomaly and are also seen in association with mucopolysaccharidoses.

Auer Bodies (Auer Rods)

Auer bodies are pink or red-staining, round or rod-shaped structures, representing agglomeration of azurophilic granules, seen in the cytoplasm of immature granulocytes and sometimes in precursors of monocytes in acute nonlymphocytic leukemias (Plate 14B).

Chédiak-Higashi Granules

Chédiak-Higashi granules are giant, red, blue, or greenish gray lysosomal granules (reacting positively with peroxidase and Sudan black stains) in the cytoplasm of leukocytes (granulocytes, lumphocytes, and monocytes) and sometimes of RBC precursors, seen in patients with Chédiak-Steinbrinck-Higashi syndrome (Plate 12).

Döhle Bodies

Döhle bodies are variably sized (0.1–2.0 μm), single or multiple, blue or grayish blue cytoplasmic inclusions representing remnants of free ribosomes or rough endoplasmic reticulum. They are seen in the neutrophils of patients with severe infections, burns, and toxic states, frequently in association with toxic granules (Plate 9B).

Dysplastic Granulocytes

Dysplastic granulocytes reveal morphologic changes that include nuclear hyposegmentation and hyperclumping of chromatin with prominent parachromatin spaces (pseudo-Pelger-Huët cells), hypogranulation, and eosinophilic and basophilic granules in the same cells. Nuclear maturation may be delayed, and cells with the cytoplasmic specific granules of a myelocyte, but with fine nuclear chromatin may be seen. Rarely, binucleate granulocytic precursors, or cells with a donut shaped nucleus may be seen (Plate 11B).

Giant Metamyelocyte

The giant (megaloblastic) metamyelocyte has less condensed nuclear chromatin, sometimes seen in the bone marrow in megaloblastic anemias.

Hypersegmentation (Right Shift)

Right shift or hypersegmentation is increased segmentation or lobulation of granulocyte nuclei, most evident in neutrophils, and defined as any neutrophil with six or more lobes, 5% of neutrophils with five or more lobes, or 50% of neutrophils with four lobes. It is a common finding in megaloblastic anemias.

Hyposegmentation (Pelger-Huët Cells)

Hyposegmentation is decreased segmentation or lobulation of granulocyte nuclei, most evident in neutrophils, and defined as single-lobed or bilobed neutrophils. It is seen in Pelger-Huët anomaly and pseudo-Pelger-Huët cells (a distinguishing feature being pyknotic nuclei of psuedo-Pelger-Huët cells), and may be seen in chronic granulocytic leukemia and as an after effect of chemotherapy for malignant disorders (Plate 11A).

Toxic Granules

Toxic granules are large, purple or dark blue azurophilic granules in the cytoplasm of neutrophils, bands, and metamyelocytes. They are seen in severe infections, chemical poisoning, and toxic states (Plate 9A).

Toxic Vacuoles

Toxic vacuoles represent phagocytosis and depletion of granules in the cytoplasm of neutrophils and bands. They are seen frequently in association with toxic granules in septicemia, severe infections, and toxic states (Plate 9A).

MONOCYTES AND MONOCYTOPOIESIS[3,8,10]

Like granulopoiesis, monocytopoiesis begins with the differentiation, under the influence of the hematopoietic microenvironment and/or some humoral factor(s), of the pluripotent hematopoietic stem cell (CFU-S), through the operationally defined stages of CFU-GEMM, CFU-GM, and CFU-NM, into a unipotent stem cell, CFU-M (colony forming unit–monocyte/macrophage). Differentiation of CFU-M generates a morphologically recognizable progenitor designated monoblast. In addition, it is generally believed that the myeloblast—the earliest morphologically recognizable progenitor of granulocytes—is capable of producing monocytes. Whether from monoblast or myeloblast, the production of monocytes proceeds sequentially through the stages of promonocyte and monocyte by way of several (two or more) mitotic divisions. The process of maturation is characterized by progressive, albeit slight to moderate in degree, condensation of nuclear chromatin, disappearance of nucleoli, appearance of nuclear indentations, and changes in staining characteristics of the cytoplasm from blue at the blast stage to blue-gray at the promonocyte stage, to grayish blue or gray at the monocyte stage, along with the appearance of fine azurophilic granules.

On release from the marrow into the circulation, the mature monocytes are also believed to be distributed between a circulating monocyte pool (CMP) and a marginal monocyte pool (MMP), in an approximate ratio of 1:3.5.[30] Monocytes remain in the blood for a short period (16–36 hours) and then migrate to tissues, where they transform into macrophages/histiocytes. The life span of macrophages is perhaps within the range of several months to a few years.

Besides being involved in the disposal of senescent cells, microorganisms, and foreign matter, monocytes/macrophages play an important role in the regulation of hematopoiesis by releasing humoral growth factors and/or inhibitory factors and in the development of the immune response by mechanisms not yet fully elucidated. Regulation of monocyte production is also believed to be under the control of humoral regulators such as colony stimulating factors (e.g., GM-CSF and M-CSF) produced by T cells and marrow stromal cells.[25,28]

Morphology of Monocytopoiesis[14,19,21]

Monoblast

The monoblast is a large cell (12–20 μm) with a large, round, oval or slightly indented nucleus, zero to three nucleoli, fine chromatin, abundant parachromatin, and moderate amount of basophilic, homogeneous and nongranulated cytoplasm. The N/C ratio is 6:1.

Promonocyte

The promonocyte is a large cell (15–20 μm) that may be larger than the monoblast and myeloblast, with a relatively large, indented nucleus with or without nucleoli, slightly clumped chromatin, sparse indistinct parachromatin, and a moderate amount of gray-blue, opaque cytoplasm with or without a few fine, pink granules (containing acid phosphatase, aryl sulfatase, and peroxidase), and vacuoles. The N/C ratio is 5:1.

Monocyte

The monocyte is a large motile cell (12–20 μm) with an indented or folded nucleus, often no visible nucleolus, moderately clumped chromatin, moderate amount of parachromatin, and abundant gray or grayish blue cytoplasm with or without fine pink granules (containing acid phosphatase, aryl sulfatase, diminishing levels of peroxidase, β-glucuronidase, galactosidase), and vacuoles. The N/C ratio is 4:1 (Plate 8A).

Macrophage/Histiocyte

The macrophage/histiocyte is an irregularly shaped, huge tissue cell (15–80 μm) that is motile and phagocytic, often revealing bleb-like or filiform psuedopodia, with a round, oval, or indented nucleus (occasionally more than one nucleus may be present), distinct nuclear membrane, spongy reticular chromatin, and abundant sky blue cytoplasm containing many coarse azurophilic granules and vacuoles. The cytoplasmic vacuoles may appear empty or may contain phagocytosed material (Plate 30A).

LYMPHOCYTES, PLASMA CELLS, AND LYMPHOCYTOPOIESIS[2-4,8,10,14,31-39]

Lymphocytes, the major cell population involved in the development of the immune response, are produced in three groups of tissues designated (1) stem cell pool, located in the bone marrow; (2) primary or central lymphoid tissues consisting of bone marrow (for B lymphocytes) and thymus (for T lymphocytes); and (3) secondary or peripheral lymphoid tissues composed of spleen, lymph nodes, gut-associated lymphoid structures (e.g., Peyer's patches, tonsils), and bone marrow. Lymphoid stem cells, colony forming unit–lymphoid (CFU-L), produced by the differentiation of the pluripotent hematopoietic stem cells (CFU-S) in the yolk sac, migrate to the liver and subsequently to the bone marrow. In the adult, the bone marrow remains the source of primitive precursors for T and B lymphocytes (stem cell pool).

An undefined proportion of the lymphoid stem cells migrate to the thymus, where, under the influence of the thymic microenvironment, hormones, and certain lymphokines, they proliferate and differentiate, ultimately producing immunocompetent T-helper and T-suppressor lymphocytes. As the maturation process within the thymus progresses, the lymphoid stem cells acquire and lose certain membrane antigens (Fig. 16-2), and produce a surface membrane T-cell receptor that can respond to specific foreign antigen determinants and can distinguish between self and nonself histocompatibility antigens.[33-38] From the thymus, the mature thymocytes migrate to the peripheral lymphoid tissues, where the T cells are predominantly localized in the so-called T-cell dependent areas. These include periarteriolar regions of the spleen, paracortical regions of lymph nodes, and interfollicular regions of gut-associated lymphoid tissues. While in the peripheral lymphoid tissues, the T cells recirculate continuously from one lymphoid tissue to another through the lymphatics and/or vascular channels but apparently not back to the thymus.

Some of the lymphoid stem cells that remain in the bone marrow proliferate and differentiate to produce mature B cells (B lymphocytes) within the marrow. The maturation process is marked by development and/or loss of certain surface antigens and production of unique surface immunoglobulin[35,38] (Fig. 16-2). The mature B cells, also sometimes called virgin B cells, are characterized by surface IgM and IgD, and the membrane receptors for Fc and C3. While some immunocompetent B cells remain in the bone marrow, many mature and some immature B cells are released from the marrow into the circulation to be distributed to the so-called B cell-dependent areas of peripheral lymphoid tissues, which include primary follicles and red pulp of the spleen, follicular and medullary regions of lymph nodes, and follicular regions of gut-associated lymphoid tissues.

Both the T-cell development in the thymus and the B-cell development in the marrow are under the control of their respective microenvironment and humoral factors,[26,28] for example, thymosin, interleukins-1 and -2 (IL-1, IL-2), B-cell growth factor, and T-cell replacement factor, being completely independent of systemic antigenic stimulation. By contrast, however, the proliferation of T and B cells in the peripheral lymphoid tissues is dependent on antigenic stimulation. On appropriate stimulation, T cells undergo blastic transformation (immunoblasts) leading to the clone proliferation of committed T cells. Although B-cell stimulation occurs with antigen exposure, it also involves interaction among various cells including macrophages/monocytes and T cells, as well as the presence of certain humoral factors, for example, B-cell growth factor, IL-1, and T-cell replacement factor. Activated B cells also undergo blastic transformation and clonal proliferation to produce plasma cells, which synthesize and secrete immunoglobulins (IgG, IgM, and IgA). Plasma cells are generally characterized by loss of pan-B surface antigens, acquisition of specific plasma cell surface antigens, and by abundant cytoplasmic immunoglobulin (CIg) with very little, if any, surface immunoglobulin (SIg).

Natural killer (NK) cells are a subset of lymphocytes that are capable of cytotoxic activity without antigen specificity or antigen-directed proliferation. This may be accomplished by direct interaction with the target cells or by antibody dependent cell-mediated cytotoxicity (ADCC). Mediation of ADCC occurs through attachment of specific IgG antibody to a surface antigen on the target cell and binding of NK cells to the Fc portion of IgG. Although NK cells are characterized by Fc receptors for IgG, other surface antigens are variable. The heterogeneous NK cells have a combination of NK-associated antigens, myelomonocytic antigens, and/or pan-T and suppressor lymphocyte antigens.[36] Lymphocytes that express the T-suppressor phenotype as well as Fc receptor for IgG are referred to as T-γ lymphocytes. The genesis of NK cells is poorly understood, but they may not require thymic conditioning for maturation.[37] In the adult, NK cells are found primarily in the bone marrow, peripheral blood, and spleen. The activity of NK cells can be modulated by a variety of lymphokines, and the NK cells secrete many lymphokines that can affect other hematopoietic cells. The morphologic equivalent of the NK cell is the large granular lymphocyte (LGL), which contains azurophilic lysosomal granules. Release of these granules appears to be an important mechanism in target cell killing.[36]

Approximately 60–80% of normal blood lymphocytes in an adult are T cells in a helper to suppressor ratio of 2:1, 10–20% are B cells, and less than 10% are non-T, non-B cells (i.e., not revealing either specific T or B antigens). A portion of these null cells express Fc receptors and appear to be NK cells, in contrast to FcR-negative cells that may represent hematopoietic stem cells.[36] Most of the B cells are short-lived with a life span of a few days, whereas the T cells comprise two populations: one short-lived (life span of a few days), and another long-lived (life span of months to years). The functions of T cells include (1) development of cellular immune responses such as graft-versus-host reaction, graft rejection, delayed hypersensitivity, and defense against intracellular organisms (e.g., tubercle bacilli, viruses, and fungi); (2) regulation of humoral immune reactions either by helping (T-helper cell action) or by suppressing (T-suppressor cell action) the activation of B lymphocytes by antigen; and (3) regulation of hematopoiesis by producing various growth factors (e.g., colony stimulating factors). Mainly by way of producing antibodies, B cells and plasma cells are the chief participants in the development of humoral immune responses. The functions of NK cells are not clearly understood but seem to include lysis of virus-infected cells or tumor cells and inhibition of the proliferation of erythroid and granulocytic progenitors.[14,36]

In the past, lymphopoiesis was depicted morphologically as progressing from the lymphoblast, to the prolymphocyte form, and then into the small, mature lymphocyte. Likewise, plasma cell production was thought to arise from a bone marrow plasmablast, dividing or differentiating to a proplasmacyte form, which gave rise to a mature plasma cell. However, availability of monoclonal antibodies to lymphocyte surface antigens has led to better characterization of lymphocyte function and differentiation as described above. Although we know that these traditional morphologic stages of lymphocyte development are no longer valid, the morphologic appearance of many of the "antigenic" stages of development and activation presented in Figure 16-2 are not yet clearly identified. The appearance of these classic stages of lymphopoiesis and plasma cell production is described below, followed by a description of benign and malignant morphologic variants.

Morphology of Lymphocytes, Plasma Cells, and Their Benign and Malignant Variants[9,13,14,19–21,31]

Lymphoblast

The lymphoblast is a round or ovoid cell (10–18 μm), with a round or oval nucleus, definite nuclear membrane, stippled chromatin (less fine compared with that of the myeloblast), zero to three nucleoli, moderately basophilic, and a homogeneous-appearing (sometimes lighter near the nucleus and darker at the periphery) cytoplasm revealing no granules by Romanowsky stain. The N/C ratio is 7:1–5:1. It may represent the lymphoid stem cell or early T or B forms in thymus or bone marrow (Plate 20).

Prolymphocyte

The prolymphocyte is the same size as the lymphoblast or slightly smaller, with a round, ovoid, or slightly indented nucleus, somewhat coarse chromatin (coarser than in the lymphoblast but less dense than that in the lymphocyte), indistinct parachromatin, one nucleolus, and a moderate amount of basophilic, homogeneous-appearing cytoplasm. The N/C ratio is 5:1. It may represent a cell of intermediate differentiation in T or B lineage or activated lymphocyte (Plate 26B).

Lymphocyte

The lymphocyte is a cell of variable size (7–18 μm), frequently round or ovoid, with a round, oval, or indented nucleus, coarse and clumpy chromatin, indistinct sparse parachromatin, no visible nucleolus, and a variable amount of sky blue or moderately basophilic, homogeneous-appearing cytoplasm, which may or may not contain a few azurophilic granules. The N/C ratio is 5:1–2:1. Sometimes lymphocytes are classified on the basis of cell size into three categories: small (7–10 μm), medium (10–12 μm), and large (more than 12 μm). The nucleus of the small lymphocyte is usually the size of a normal mature RBC; the larger the lymphocyte, the greater the amount of cytoplasm, but not necessarily the larger the nucleus. It is thought to represent the mature T-suppressor or T-helper cell, or the mature resting B lymphocyte (Plate 8A).

Plasmablast

The plasmablast is a moderately large cell (15–25 μm) with a round or oval, often eccentric nucleus, fine reticulated chromatin, one or more nucleoli, distinct parachromatin, and moderately to deeply basophilic cytoplasm without granules. The N/C ratio is 1:1–2:1. This immature plasma cell is not found in normal bone marrow but is seen only in rare cases of multiple myeloma.

Proplasmacyte

The proplasmacyte is the same size as the plasmablast or slightly smaller, with a round or oval, often eccentric nucleus, moderately coarse chromatin, one or two nucleoli, and moderately blue cytoplasm with a lighter paranuclear zone and without granules. The N/C ratio is 1:1–2:1. Proplasmacytes are not seen in normal bone marrow or with reactive plasmacytosis; however, they may be a common finding in multiple myeloma (Plate 29B).

Plasmacyte (Plasma Cell)

The plasmacyte is of variable size (10–20 μm), with round or oval, eccentric nucleus, coarse and clumpy chromatin, sparse distinct parachromatin, no nucleolus, a halo (Golgi apparatus) touching the nucleus, and abundant dark blue cytoplasm, which may or may not contain protein globules. The N/C ratio is 1:2 (Plate 29A).

Atypical Lymphocyte (Reactive Lymphocyte, Virocyte)

The atypical lymphocyte is a cell of variable size (10–20 μm) and variable shape (round, ovoid, or irregular), with a central or eccentric, round, oval, indented or lobulated nucleus; fine, medium, or coarse chromatin pattern; zero to one or more nucleoli; and abundant blue cytoplasm, which is often darker at the periphery and lighter near the nucleus, and which may or may not contain a few azurophilic granules and rarely even a few vacuoles. It probably represents an activated form of lymphocyte. The large granular lymphocyte is thought to be an NK cell or activated cytotoxic T-suppressor cell (Plate 10A).

Basket Cell (Smudge Cell)

The basket cell is a squashed, degenerated nucleus in the form of a basket or simply a smudge. It may normally be seen in small numbers as an artifact of the smearing process but is characteristically seen in large numbers in the blood smears from chronic lymphocytic leukemia patients, whose lymphocytes are very fragile and smudge easily upon smearing. Smudging can be eliminated by preparing smears from a mixture of 4 drops of blood and 1 drop of 22% bovine serum albumin (BSA).

Flame Cell

The flame cell is a plasma cell with pinkish red (flame color) cytoplasm that is frequently found, although not specifically, in association with IgA myeloma.

Grape Cell (Mott Cell, Thesaurocyte)

The grape cell is a plasma cell that is variable in size (10–30 μm), often with a small nucleus and abundant cytoplasm containing a few (frequently one to three) large protein globules (Russell bodies, Mott cells) or numerous protein globules, giving the appearance of a bunch of grapes (grape cell) or storage histiocyte (thesaurocyte).

Hairy Cell

The hairy cell is a relatively large cell (12–20 μm) that contains a round, ovoid, or indented nucleus placed centrally or eccentrically, delicate nuclear membrane, fine or slightly coarse chromatin, one or more nucleoli, a moderate amount of pale blue cytoplasm, and fine filamentous (hairy) projections arising from the cell membrane; seen in hairy cell leukemia. It cytochemically reacts positively with tartrate-resistant acid phosphatase (Plate 26A).

Immunoblast

The immunoblast is a large round cell (15–20 μm) with a relatively large nucleus, finely dispersed chromatin, distinct parachromatin, one or more small nucleoli, and moderate amount of basophilic cytoplasm. The N/C ratio is 3:1–2:1. It may resemble a plasmacytoid lymphocyte, but the immature nucleus of the immunoblast is helpful in distinguishing between the two. It probably represents the activated form of T or B lymphocytes.

Lymphoma Cell

The appearance of the lymphoma cell as stained with Wright-Giemsa varies greatly, depending on the type of lymphoma. Large cell lymphoma cells (15–20 μm) have a large, often irregularly shaped nucleus, finely dispersed chromatin, one or more large nucleoli, and a small to moderate amount of basophilic cytoplasm, which may occasionally contain punched-out vacuoles. The N/C ratio is 4:1–3:1 (Plate 27B).

Burkitt's lymphoma cells are 10–20 μm, with a large, round nucleus, finely dispersed chromatin, one or more nucleoli, and small amounts of intensely basophilic cytoplasm; punched-out vacuoles characteristically appear in the cytoplasm and over the nucleus. The N/C ratio is 5:1–3:1 (Plates 21A,B).

Small cell follicular lymphoma cells may be of identical size as small resting lymphocytes, but the N/C ratio is extremely high (more than 7:1), the nuclear chromatin may be hyperchromatic, and some of the nuclei may be very irregular in shape and/or clefted (Plate 28A).

Well differentiated lymphoma or chronic lymphocytic lymphoma will show a uniform population of small to large lymphocytes that cannot be distinguished morphologically from normal lymphocytes. Lymphoblastic lymphoma appears similar to the lymphoblasts described above, except that a more folded or convoluted nuclear shape may be present. Adult T-cell leukemia/lymphoma cells are medium-size lymphocytes with a high N/C ratio. Nuclei have a characteristic lobulated or knobby appearance.

Plasmacytoid Lymphocyte

The plasmacytoid lymphocyte is essentially a round cell of variable size (10–18 μm) with a round, slightly eccentric nucleus, no or very small nucleolus, slightly to moderately coarse "ropy" chromatin, and a moderate amount of deeply basophilic, homogeneous cytoplasm around the nucleus. The N/C ratio is 1:1–3:1. These cells often represent stimulated lymphocytes and hence can be included in the category of atypical or reactive lymphocytes (Plate 10B).

Sézary Cell

The Sézary cell is a round or ovoid cell of variable size (small measuring 8–11 μm, and large measuring 12–20 μm), with a round or oval, cerebriform, convoluted, or grooved nucleus, chromatin of variable density (fine to moderately coarse), zero to one nucleolus, and a relatively narrow rim of blue cytoplasm around the nucleus. It is seen in the Sézary syndrome (Plate 27A).

THROMBOCYTES AND THROMBOCYTOPOIESIS[3,6,8,10,13,40,41]

Platelet production, like other cellular elements of blood, begins with the differentiation of the pluripotent hematopoietic stem cell (CFU-S), through the operationally defined stages of CFU-GEMM and colony forming unit–megakaryocyte (CFU-Meg), into a megakaryoblast, the earliest morphologically recognizable progenitor committed to produce platelets (Fig. 16-1). The megakaryoblast undergoes endomitosis (nuclear endoreduplication, i.e., chromosomal division without cell division) once or twice and matures to become a larger cell with two or four nuclei, the promegakaryocyte. Subsequent endomitotic divisions with continued maturation yield megakaryocytes containing 8, 16, or 32 nuclei. The maturation of megakaryoblast to megakaryocyte, which takes about 5 days, is marked by (1) progressive increase in cell size, cell ploidy (number of nuclei), nuclear chromatin density and cytoplasmic volume; (2) disappearance of nucleoli; and (3) gradual decrease in cytoplasmic basophilia with simultaneous acquisition of increasing amounts of azurophilic granulation and a well developed membrane demarcation system. Ultimately, small membrane-bound cytoplasmic portions break off from mature granular megakaryocytes and are released into the circulation in the form of platelets. The remaining megakaryocyte nuclei are probably phagocytosed and digested by the cells of the reticuloendothelial system. Some of the mature megakaryocytes apparently pass through the marrow sinusoids intact and travel through the bloodstream to the lungs, where they may also shed platelets.

Under normal steady-state conditions, the circulating platelets represent approximately two-thirds of the total platelet mass, the remaining one-third being stored in the spleen. Platelets survive in the circulation for 8–10 days. As with leukopoiesis and erythropoiesis, thrombocytopoiesis is under the control of microenvironmental factors and humoral agents such as megakaryocyte–colony stimulating activity (Meg-CSA) and thrombopoietin; however, their precise source of origin, true nature, and mechanism(s) of action remain poorly understood.[28,42]

On the basis of combined findings by light microscopy, electron microscopy, and cytochemical staining of platelets and megakaryocytes, four groups of cytoplasmic granules have been identified: (1) α-granules containing β-thromboglobulin, platelet factor 4 (PF4), factor VIII-related antigen, fibrinogen, fibronectin, platelet growth factor, albumin, and thrombospondin; (2) δ-granules or dense bodies containing calcium, serotonin, pyrophosphate, and storage pools of adenosine phosphate (ADP) and ATP; (3) γ- or lysosomal granules containing acid phosphatase, β-glucuronidase and aryl sulfatase; and (4) peroxisomes containing catalase.

Platelets play an essential role in primary hemostasis by at least maintaining vascular integrity and forming a platelet plug (platelet aggregation) at sites of injury and in secondary hemostasis by at least providing phospholipids, a major constituent required in blood clot formation.

Morphology of Thrombocytopoiesis[14,19,21,40,43–45] (Plate 3)

Megakaryoblast

The megakaryoblast is the earliest morphologically recognizable nucleated cell in the platelet production pathway, often larger (15–35 μm) than other blast cells in the marrow, but it may sometimes be smaller (micromegakaryoblast, 7–15 μm) resembling immature lymphoid cells, with a round, oval, or indented nucleus, zero to six nucleoli, chromatin of variable density (dense in small and fine in large cells), and a small amount of blue cytoplasm, which sometimes exhibits a few small, round, bud-like projections. The N/C ratio is 8:1–10:1.

Promegakaryocyte

The promegakaryocyte is an intermediate cell in the formation of the megakaryocyte; larger (30–50 μm) than the megakaryoblast, with a two- or four-lobed nucleus, coarse chromatin, zero to two nucleoli, and a moderate amount of bluish cytoplasm containing fine purplish red azurophilic granules. The N/C ratio is 6:1.

Megakaryocyte

The megakaryocyte is the largest nucleated cell (40–100 μm) in the platelet production pathway, often larger than all other hematopoietic cells in the marrow, but it may rarely be smaller (15–30 μm, micromegakaryocyte), with a multilobed (8, 16, or 32) nucleus, no nucleoli, coarse chromatin, and abundant light blue or pink cytoplasm containing numerous purplish red or pink granules frequently clustered in small aggregates. The N/C ratio is 1:1–1:2.

Thrombocyte (Platelet)

The thrombocyte is the smallest cell (2–4 μm) among the normal peripheral blood cells, and is round or ovoid, devoid of nucleus, with a small amount of pale blue or colorless cytoplasm containing several purplish red granules generally aggregated toward the center.

Morphology of Megakaryocyte and Platelet Variants

Dysplastic Megakaryocyte

Dysplastic megakaryocytes may be small, approaching the same size as myeloid precursors. Mononuclear forms, or multinucleate forms with small, separate nuclei, may occur (Plate 22B).

Small Platelets

Small platelets are defined as smaller than normal (less than 2 μm) in size. They are seen in Wiskott-Aldrich syndrome.

Large Platelets

Large platelets are defined as larger than normal (more than 4 μm) in size. They may be seen in small numbers in normal blood smears but are usually seen in large numbers in conditions associated with thrombocytopenia and thrombocytosis (benign and malignant).

Giant Platelets

Giant platelets are of the size of normal RBCs (7–8 μm) or larger, seen in conditions associated with thrombocytopenia and myeloproliferative disorders, including thrombocythemia (Plate 25).

Bizarre Platelets

Bizarre platelets are irregularly shaped platelets that may take any shape other than normal round or ovoid and may show one or more psuedopod projections. They may be seen in myeloproliferative disorders (Plate 25).

Gray Platelets (Agranular Platelets)

Gray platelets are pale blue-staining platelets lacking granules. They are seen in gray platelet syndrome and may also be found occasionally in myelodysplastic and myeloproliferative disorders.

OTHER CELLS IN BONE MARROW[8,12,13,19]

In addition to the cells of the hematopoietic series, a variety of other cell types are encountered in the bone marrow.

Morphology of Miscellaneous Bone Marrow Cells (Plate 6)

Gaucher Cell

The Gaucher cell is a macrophage/histiocyte, variable in size (20–90 μm), ovoid, with a relatively small, round or ovoid nucleus, coarse chromatin, and abundant lipid (glucocerebroside)-laden cytoplasm with reticular, fibrillar, or wrinkled tissue paper appearance. It is found in Gaucher's disease in hematopoietic (i.e., marrow, spleen, liver, thymus, and lymph nodes) and nonhematopoietic (i.e., lungs, kidneys, adrenals, and meninges) tissues. Gaucher-like histiocytes also may be seen in the bone marrow with chronic granulocytic leukemia, formed from the degeneration and digestion of phagocytosed granulocytes (Plate 32A).

Lipocyte (Fat Cell, Adipocyte)

The lipocyte is a large cell (25–75 μm) with an eccentrically located, small, densely staining nucleus and abundant pale-staining empty cytoplasm. It is a normal constituent of yellow marrow (fatty tissue).

Niemann-Pick Cell (Foam Cell)

The Niemann-Pick cell is a histiocyte of variable size (20–90 μm), with one or more nuclei as a consequence of endomitosis, moderately coarse chromatin, and abundant sphingomyelin-laden cytoplasm filled with many relatively uniform droplets or particles giving a foamy or mulberry appearance. It may be distributed throughout the body but is predominant in hematopoietic tissues, particularly the liver and spleen. It is characteristic, but not diagnostic, of Niemann-Pick disease (Plate 32B).

Osteoblast

The osteoblast is a large bone-forming cell (25–50 μm), ellipsoid in shape, with a round or ovoid nucleus, one or more nucleoli, prominent clear zone away from the nucleus, and copious blue-gray cytoplasm. It is often seen in clusters in marrow specimens from growing children and may be seen in small numbers in specimens from adults.

Osteoclast

The osteoclast is a gigantic cell (100 μm) with multiple (usually an even number) uniformly shaped, round or oval nuclei, at least one nucleolus per nucleus, dense chromatin, and abundant smoky cytoplasm containing many fine red granules. It is involved in bone resorption, commonly seen in marrow specimens from young children. Associated clinical conditions include metastatic carcinoma, acute leukemias, myelofibrosis, and secondary osteoporosis.

Reed-Sternberg Cell

The Reed-Sternberg cell is a neoplastic histiocyte, often with two or more nuclei (frequently mirror images in configuration), each containing a large, prominent, round or ovoid nucleolus, and abundant purple-pink cytoplasm. It is considered the hallmark of Hodgkin's disease, commonly seen in lymph nodes, but it may be present in any tissue involved by the disease.

Reticulum Cell (Endothelial Cell, Adventitial Cell)

The reticulum cell is a large (20–30 μm), round, ovoid, or spindle-shaped cell with irregularly shaped nucleus, one to six nucleoli, and abundant pale blue cytoplasm containing vacuoles and a few red or blue-green granules. It may occupy the interstitial space (reticulum cell) or periphery of small vessels (adventitial cell) or may line the inner wall of sinuses (endothelial cell).

Tissue Eosinophil

The tissue eosinophil is a large tissue cell (20–30 μm), often with indistinct cell borders, a round nucleus, fine chromatin without nucleolus, and abundant cytoplasm packed with numerous eosinophilic granules. Its relationship to blood eosinophils or their precursors is unclear.

Tissue Mast Cell

The tissue mast cell is a large (15–30 μm), round or elliptical connective tissue cell with a small, round nucleus and abundant cytoplasm packed with black or bluish black metachromatic granules. Its relationship to circulating basophils or their precursors is unclear. It is seen in large numbers in patients with systemic mastocytosis and in moderate but significant numbers in association with non-Hodgkin's lymphomas and after chemotherapy, irradiation, or other toxic marrow damage.

Tissue Neutrophil (Ferrata Cell)

The tissue neutrophil is a large cell (20–40 μm), often irregular in shape, with a round or oval nucleus, one or more nucleoli, coarsely granular chromatin, and abundant pale cytoplasm with scattered azurophilic granules. It may resemble a reticulum cell, a histiocyte, or a degenerating promyelocyte. Its relationship to blood neutrophils or their precursors is unclear.

ACUTE LEUKEMIAS[3,10,44-51]

Typical morphologic features of predominant cell types in acute nonlymphoid and acute lymphocytic leukemias are illustrated in Table 16-1 and described below.

Morphology of Subclasses of Acute Nonlymphocytic Leukemias

M1: Acute Myeloid Leukemia Without Maturation

Subclass M1 consists of small or large blast cells without (type 1) or with (type 2) a few azurophilic granules and/or one or two Auer bodies. It shows Sudan black and peroxidase and sometimes even specific esterase positivity in 3% or more of the blasts and little differentiation to or beyond the promyelocyte stage (less than 10%) (Plate 13).

M2: Acute Myelocytic Leukemia with Maturation

Subclass M2 has features similar to those of M1, but maturation from promyelocytes to mature polymorphonuclear cells are evident (more than 10%) and a greater number of cells with significant numbers of azurophilic granules with or without occasional Auer bodies reacting positively with Sudan black, peroxidase, and specific esterase stain (Plate 14).

M3: Acute Promyelocytic Leukemia

Subclass M3 consists of many promyelocytes, often containing numerous azurophilic granules and sometimes several Auer rods in the form of a faggot (faggot cell). A microgranular variant may also occasionally occur. It reacts positively with Sudan black, peroxidase, and specific esterase stains (Plate 15).

M4: Acute Myelomonocytic Leukemia

Subclass M4 has many blasts (20–80%) with myeloblastic and/or monocytic features (at least 20% of each form), thereby reacting positively with any or all of the following stains: Sudan black, peroxidase, specific esterase, and nonspecific esterase (Plate 16).

Table 16-1. Acute Nonlymphocytic versus Acute Lymphocytic Leukemias

MORPHOLOGIC FEATURES	Acute Nonlymphocytic Leukemia (Myeloblasts)	Acute Lymphocytic Leukemia (Lymphoblasts)
Romanowsky stain		
Cell size	Variable	Variable
Cell shape	Usually round or ovoid	Usually round or ovoid
Nuclear indentation	May be present	Rare
Nuclear chromatin	Finer	Fine
Nucleoli	0–5	0–2
Cytoplasmic volume	Comparatively more	Relatively less
Granules in cytoplasm	Occasional	Absent
Auer bodies/rods	May be present	Absent
Special stains		
Peroxidase	May be positive	Negative
Sudan black	May be positive	Negative
Chloroacetate esterase (specific esterase)	May be positive	Negative
α-Naphthyl acetate or α-naphthyl butyrate (nonspecific esterase)	May be positive in blasts with monocytic features	Negative
Periodic acid-Schiff	Variable diffuse staining	Often coarse granular positivity
Terminal deoxynucleotidyl transferase	Often negative	Nearly always positive (except L3, Burkitt type)

M5: Acute Monocytic Leukemia

Subclass M5 consists of blasts with predominantly (more than 80%) monocytic features exhibiting positivity primarily with nonspecific esterase reaction (Plate 17).

M6: Acute Erythroleukemia

Subclass M6 consists of a mixed population of erythroblasts (often reacting positively with PAS stain) comprising more than 50% of the marrow nucleated cell population and myeloblasts (some of which stain positively with Sudan black, peroxidase, and specific esterase, and some may contain Auer bodies) representing more than 30% of the nonerythroid cell population. Megaloblastic features may be present. Dyserythropoiesis, characterized by multinucleation, abnormal shaped nuclei, and karyorrhexis, is a frequent finding (Plate 18).

M7: Acute Megakaryoblastic Leukemia

Subclass M7 consists of many (more than 20%) megakaryoblasts, often identified by the morphologic features described earlier and whenever feasible the identification should be confirmed by electron microscopy and cytochemical agents (e.g., platelet peroxidase) and/or immune markers (e.g., antibodies against factor VIII-related antigen and/or against platelet glycoproteins Ib or IIb/IIIa) (Plate 19).

Morphology of Subclasses of Acute Lymphocytic Leukemias

L1: Acute Lymphocytic Leukemia

Subclass L1 is a fairly uniform population of small, often round blast cells, each usually with a round nucleus, rarely with an inconspicuous nucleolus, homogeneous chromatin pattern, and small amount of basophilic cytoplasm with or without a few vacuoles. Some of the blasts exhibit positive staining with terminal deoxynucleotidyl transferase (TdT) and PAS (Plate 20).

L2: Acute Lymphocytic Leukemia

Subclass L2 is a heterogeneous population of blasts of different sizes, each with a round, ovoid, or indented/clefted nucleus, zero to two nucleoli, heterogeneous chromatin pattern, and moderate amount of basophilic cytoplasm with or without a few vacuoles. At least some of the blasts react positively with PAS and TdT.

L3: Acute Lymphocytic Leukemia (Burkitt Type)

Subclass L3 is a homogeneous (monotonous) population of medium or large blasts, each with a round or ovoid nucleus, one or more distinct nucleoli, stippled homogeneous chromatin, and moderate amount of deeply basophilic cytoplasm containing prominent vacuoles. TdT is negative (Plate 21).

REFERENCES

1. Till JE, McCullock EA: A direct measurement of the radiation sensitivity of normal mouse bone marrow cells. Radiat Res 1961;14:213–222.
2. Boggs DR, Winkelstein A: White Cell Manual. 4th Ed. Philadelphia, FA Davis, 1983.
3. Hyun BH, Gulati GL, Ashton JK: Color Atlas of Clinical Hematology. New York, Igaku-Shoin, 1986.
4. Jandl JH: Blood: Textbook of Hematology. Boston, Little Brown, 1987.
5. Kushner JA: Hematopoietic stem cell proliferation. Lab Med 1981;12:279–283.
6. Lipton JM, Nathan DG: The anatomy and physiology of hematopoiesis. pp. 128–158. In Nathan DG, Oski FA (eds): Hematology of Infancy and Childhood. 3rd Ed. Philadelphia, WB Saunders, 1987.
7. Sieff CA: Membrane antigen expression during hemopoietic differentiation. CRC Crit Rev Oncol Hematol 1986;5:1–36.
8. Gulati GL, Ashton JK, Hyun BH: Structure and function of the bone marrow and hematopoiesis. Hematol Oncol Clin North Am, 1988;2:495–511.
9. Lewis SM: The constituents of normal blood and bone marrow. pp. 3–56. In Hardisty RM, Weatherall DJ (eds): Blood and Its Disorders. 2nd Ed. Oxford, Blackwell Scientific, 1982.
10. Nelson DA, Davey FR: Hematopoiesis. pp. 626–651. In Henry JB (ed): Clinical Diagnosis and Management by Laboratory Methods. 7th Ed. Philadelphia, WB Saunders, 1984.
11. Oski FA, Naiman JW: Hematologic Problems in the Newborn. 3rd Ed. Philadelphia, WB Saunders, 1982.
12. Wintrobe MM, Lee GR, Boggs DR, et al: Clinical Hematology. Philadelphia, Lea & Febiger, 1981.
13. Hyun BH, Ashton JK, Dolan K: Practical Hematology. Philadelphia, WB Saunders, 1975.
14. Thorup OA Jr: Fundamentals of Clinical Hematology. 5th Ed. Philadelphia, WB Saunders, 1987.
15. Bessis M, Lessin LS, Beutler E: Morphology of the erythron. pp. 257–279. In Williams WJ, Beutler E, Erslev A, Lichtman MA (eds): Hematology. 3rd Ed. New York, McGraw-Hill, 1983.
16. Hillman RS, Finch CA: Red Cell Manual. 5th Ed. Philadelphia, FA Davis, 1985.
17. Erslev A: Erythropoietin coming of age. N Engl J Med 1987;316:101–103.
18. Spivak JL: The mechanism of action of erythropoietin. Int J Cell Cloning 1986;4:139–166.
19. Bauer JD: Morphology of blood and bone marrow cells. pp. 653–726. In Sonnenwirth AC, Jarett L (eds): Grad-

wohl's Clinical Laboratory Methods and Diagnosis. 8th Ed. St Louis, CV Mosby, 1980.
20. Brown BA: Hematology: Principles and Procedures. 4th Ed. Philadelphia, Lea & Febiger, 1984.
21. Miale JB: Laboratory Medicine-Hematology. 6th Ed. St Louis, CV Mosby, 1982.
22. Kraus JR: Red-cell abnormalities in the blood smear: disease correlations. Lab Management 1985;23:29–35.
23. Cronkite EP, Burlington H, Chanana AD, Joel DD: Regulation of granulopoiesis. Prog Clin Biol Res 1985;184:129–144.
24. Laszlo J, Rundles RW: Morphology of neutrophils. pp. 719–725. In Williams WJ, Beutler E, Erslev A, Lichtman MA (eds): Hematology. 3rd Ed. New York, McGraw-Hill, 1983.
25. Clark SC, Kamen R: The human hematopoietic colony-stimulating factors. Science 1987;236:1229–1237.
26. Dexter TM, Moore M: Growth and development in the hemopoietic system: the role of lymphokines and their possible therapeutic potential in disease and malignancy. Carcinogenesis 1986;7:509–516.
27. Sieff CA: Hematopoietic growth factors. J Clin Invest 1987;79:1549–1557.
28. Zoumbos N, Raefsky E, Young N: Lymphokines and hematopoiesis. Prog Hematol 1986;14:201–227.
29. Wickramasinghe SN (ed): Blood and Bone Marrow. New York, Churchill Livingstone, 1986.
30. Meuret G, Hoffman G: Monocyte kinetic studies in normal and disease states. Br J Haematol 1973;24:275.
31. Hyun BH, Gulati GL: Lymphocytosis and lymphocytopenia. Lab Med 1984;15:319–324.
32. Roitt IM: Essential Immunology. 6th Ed. Boston, Blackwell Scientific, 1988, pp. 134–153.
33. Rapaport SI: Introduction to Hematology. Philadelphia, JB Lippincott, 1987.
34. Denning SM, Haynes BF: Differentiation of human T cells. pp. 1–14. In Davey FR (ed): Classification, Diagnosis, and Molecular Biology of Lymphoproliferative Disorders. Clinics in Laboratory Medicine Vol. 8. Philadelphia, WB Saunders, 1988.
35. Bertoli LF, Burrows PD: Normal B-lineage cells: Their differentiation and identification. pp. 15–30. In Davey FR: Classification, Diagnosis, and Molecular Biology of Lymphoproliferative Disorders. Clinics in Laboratory Medicine Vol. 8. Philadelphia, WB Saunders, 1988.
36. Ferrarini M, Grossi CE: Definition of the cell types within the "null lymphocyte" population of human peripheral blood: an analysis of phenotypes and function. Semin Hematol 1984;21:270–286.
37. Reynolds CW, Foon KA: T-gamma lymphoproliferative disease and related disorders in humans and experimental animals: a review of the clinical, cellular, and functional characteristics. Blood 1984;64:1146–1158.
38. Foon KA, Tood RF: Immunologic classification of leukemia and lymphoma. Blood 1986;68:1–31.
39. McMichael AJ (ed): Leukocyte Typing III, White Cell Differentiation Antigens. New York, Oxford University Press, 1987.
40. Gerwirtz AM: Human megakaryocytopoiesis. Semin Hematol 1986;23:27–42.
41. Mazur EM: Megakaryocytopoiesis and platelet production: a review. Exp Hematol 1987;15:340–350.
42. Evalt BL, Kellor KL, Ramsey RB: Thrombopoietin: past, present and future. Prog Clin Biol Res 1986;215:143–155.
43. White JG: Platelet morphology and function. pp. 1121–1135. In Williams WJ, Beutler E, Erslev A, Lichtman MA (eds): Hematology. 3rd Ed. New York, McGraw-Hill, 1983.
44. Bennett JM, Catovsky D, Daniel MT, et al: Criteria for the diagnosis of acute leukemia of megakaryocyte lineage (M7): a report of the French-American-British Cooperative Group. Ann Intern Med 1985;103:460–462.
45. Sternberg PE: Ultrastructural organization of maturing megakaryocytes. Prog Clin Biol Res 1986;215:373–386.
46. Bennett JM, Catovsky D, Daniel MT, et al: Proposals for the reclassification of the acute leukemias: French-American-British Cooperative Group. Br J Haematol 1976;33:451–458.
47. Bennett JM, Catovsky D, Daniel MT, et al: The French-American-British Cooperative Group: the morphological classification of acute lymphoblastic leukemia: concordance among observers and clinical correlations. Br J Haematol 1981;47:553–561.
48. Bennett JM, Catovsky D, Daniel MT, et al: Proposed revised criteria for the classification of acute myeloid leukemia: a report of the French-American-British Cooperative Group. Ann Intern Med 1985;103:620–625.
49. Catovsky D, DeSalvo CL, O'Brien M, et al: Cytochemical markers of differentiation in acute leukemia. Cancer Res 1981;41:4824–4832.
50. Bloomfield CD, Brunning RD: FAB M7: acute megakaryoblastic leukemia—beyond morphology. Ann Intern Med 1985;103:450–452.
51. Bloomfield CD, Brunning RD: The revised French-American-British classification of acute myeloid leukemia: is new better? Ann Intern Med 1985;103:614–616.

17 Erythrocyte Disorders

James Baker
P. Joanne Cornbleet

INTRODUCTION

Erythrocyte disorders can be divided into those with too few red blood cells (RBCs), *anemia*, and those with too many RBCs, *polycythemia*.

Anemia

Anemia is one of the most frequently encountered medical problems. It is not a diagnosis in itself, but a sign of many hematologic and nonhematologic disorders. Because anemia has a multitude of causes, a careful history and physical examination often provide clues to its etiology and aid in the selection of further laboratory investigation.[1] Inquiry into a prior diagnosis of anemia, family history of anemia, and ethnic background may suggest a hereditary anemia. Dietary history may disclose potential iron or folate deficiency. A careful inquiry into medications is important, because many drugs can lead to anemia through a variety of mechanisms. Exposure to environmental toxins such as lead, benzene, and pesticides can cause anemia. Three nonhematologic disorders—uremia, liver disease, and hypothyroidism—can present with unexplained anemia; specific questioning, as well as physical and laboratory examination, should be directed toward these possibilities. Chronic blood loss, with resultant iron deficiency, may be indicated by symptoms of peptic ulcer or colon carcinoma, a history of excessive menstrual bleeding, or the presence of black stools. Hemolytic anemia may be associated with jaundice and dark urine, whereas neurologic symptoms, such as altered mental state, paresthesias, and unsteady gait, may be clues to pernicious anemia. Splenomegaly on physical examination raises the question of a hematopoietic malignancy. Prominent lymphadenopathy in the anemic patient suggests possible hematopoietic malignancy, metastatic tumor, or an infectious process. Finally, inquiry should be made about prior therapy for anemia, as partial treatment for iron, folate, or vitamin B_{12} deficiency may alter expected laboratory results.

Before extensive investigation of anemia is undertaken, it is important to ensure that anemia is not spurious, because of hemodilution. This may occur in pregnancy, congestive heart failure, hypoalbuminemia, or renal disease.[2] In addition, the hematocrit (Hct) may fall 4–10% in 1 hour after assuming the recumbent position, with an even greater decrease in edematous patients.[2] Occasionally, blood is collected from above the site of intravenous fluid administration, giving erroneously low hemoglobin/hematocrit (Hgb/Hct) results.

The primary laboratory tests designed for the initial classification of anemia include the hemogram, blood smear, and reticulocyte count (Fig. 17-1). This initial laboratory evaluation will document the presence of anemia (considering the patient's age and sex) and will define the severity. Anemias can be classified as microcytic, macrocytic, or normocytic, using the mean cell volume (MCV) from the hemogram. The reticulocyte count is useful in dividing the normocytic anemias into

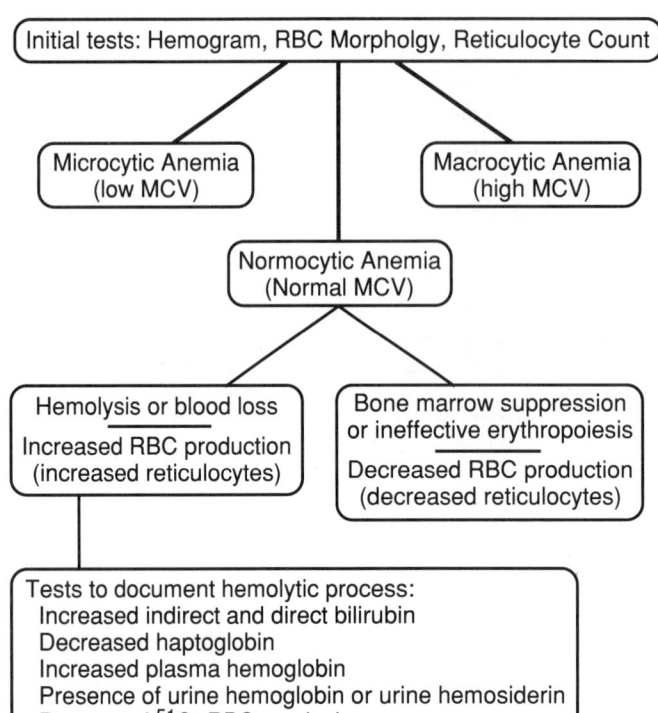

Fig. 17-1. Classification of anemia. ^{51}Cr, chromium 51; MCV, mean cell volume; RBC, red blood cell.

those with decreased production (indicating bone marrow suppression or ineffective erythropoiesis) and those accompanied by increased production (indicating hemolysis or blood loss). Occasionally, abnormalities in RBC morphology are seen on the peripheral blood smear that suggest a specific diagnosis. In addition, as microcytic or macrocytic anemia develops, minor populations of small or large RBCs may be apparent on the blood smear or RBC volume histogram before the MCV becomes abnormal.

Microcytic Anemias

Microcytosis occurs when there is insufficient hemoglobin production in the developing RBCs. This anemia can be produced by several factors[1]:

1. Insufficient iron, following a reduction in total body iron stores (iron deficiency anemia) or impaired release of iron from macrophage stores (anemia of chronic disease)
2. Hereditary hemoglobinopathies with diminished globin synthesis (e.g., thalassemic syndromes, hemoglobin E)
3. Impairment of enzymes involved in heme synthesis (e.g., sideroblastic anemias, lead poisoning, pyridoxine deficiency)

The causes of microcytic anemia, along with helpful laboratory tests in each disorder are presented in Table 17-1. The most common causes of microcytic anemia are iron deficiency, anemia of chronic disease (which more often presents as a normocytic anemia), and thalassemia trait. The differential diagnosis of these disorders is presented in Table 17-2. Thalassemia trait occurs with high frequency in Mediterranean, Asian, Middle Eastern, and African populations (and black Americans) and can be suspected by finding a low normal or mildly decreased hemoglobin, markedly decreased MCV, and an elevated RBC count. Anemia of chronic infectious, inflammatory, or malignant disease may be evident from the patient history. Iron defi-

Table 17-1. Microcytic Anemias

Disorder	Helpful Laboratory Tests
Iron deficiency	Ferritin[a] Serum iron/TIBC/% saturation[a] Erythrocyte protoporphyrin[a] Bone marrow iron stain
Anemia of chronic disease	Ferritin[a] Serum iron/TIBC/% saturation[a] Bone marrow iron stain Erythrocyte sedimentation rate[a]
β-Thalassemia trait, β-∂-thalassemia trait, hereditary persistence of fetal hemoglobin, β-thalassemia intermedia or major	Hemoglobin electrophoresis[a] Hemoglobin A_2[a] Hemoglobin F[a]

α-Thalassemia trait	Often a diagnosis of exclusion for microcytosis:
	  Hemoglobin electrophoresis (normal)[a]
	  Hemoglobin A_2 (normal)[a]
	  Hemoglobin F (normal)[a]
	  Ferritin (normal)[a]
	  Hemoglobin H inclusions (in Asian ethnic groups)[a]
	  Globin chain synthesis studies (research test)

Hemoglobin H disease	Hemoglobin electrophoresis[a] Hemoglobin H inclusions[a]
Other hemoglobins producing thalassemic syndrome (e.g., Hgb E, Lepore, Constant Spring)	Hemoglobin electrophoresis[a]
Double heterozygotes for abnormal hemoglobin and thalassemia trait	Hemoglobin electrophoresis[a]
Hereditary sideroblastic anemia	Serum iron/TIBC/% saturation[a] Ferritin[a] Bone marrow iron stain
Lead poisoning	Serum or urine lead Erythrocyte protoporphyrin[a]

[a] See text for discussion of analytes.

ciency is common, particularly during periods of rapid growth (e.g., in children between the ages of 6 months and 4 years and in adolescents), in pregnancy, and in menstrual-age females. Thus, it is useful to measure serum ferritin as an assessment of iron stores in the initial evaluation of microcytic anemia. Ferritin levels are low in iron deficiency, normal in thalassemia trait, and often elevated in anemia of chronic disease. Difficulty arises when iron deficiency is combined with chronic disease, which may result in a misleading normal ferritin level. In rare cases, a bone marrow examination for stainable iron stores may be necessary for diagnosis. Alternatively, the patient may be given a therapeutic trial of oral iron therapy; a rise in Hgb level of 1–2 g/dL (0.2–0.3 mmol/L) within 4 weeks is expected if iron deficiency is a contributing cause of anemia.[1]

Macrocytic Anemia

Macrocytic RBCs occur when mitotic divisions are skipped during maturation in the bone marrow.[1] This can occur with abnormal nuclear maturation (megaloblastic erythropoiesis) or with erythropoietin stimulation (polychromatophilic macrocytes or reticulocytes). Macrocytic RBCs can also occur with changes in lipid content in the circulating RBC membrane, as seen in liver disease.

Table 17-3 lists disorders associated with macrocytic anemia along with useful laboratory tests. Large increases in MCV (more than 110 fL) may be seen with megaloblastic erythropoiesis caused by vitamin B_{12} or folate deficiency, whereas more modest increases usually occur with other disorders. The finding of oval macrocytes on the blood smear suggests megaloblastic anemia or myelodysplastic syndrome, whereas round macrocytes are seen in most other causes of macrocytosis. However, the distinction between oval and round shape is not always readily apparent from blood smear morphology.

Macrocytic anemia caused by both vitamin B_{12} or folate deficiency and myelodysplasia can be accompanied by pancytopenia; however, dysplastic morphology of the white blood cells (WBCs) and platelets is often present in myelodysplastic syndromes, while hypersegmented neutrophils are typically found in the megaloblastic anemias. (For a description of the specific causes of vitamin B_{12} deficiency, see Fig. 17-6, and of folate deficiency, see Table 17-16.)

Table 17-2. Differential Diagnosis of Common Microcytic Anemias

Laboratory Test	Iron Deficiency	Anemia of Chronic Disease	β-Thalassemia Trait	α-Thalassemia Trait
Hemoglobin	Mild to severe decrease	Usually 9–12 g/dL	Usually >10 g/dL	Usually >10 g/dL
Smear morphology	Mild to severe hypochromia, elliptocytes, variable numbers of other poikilocytes	Mild hypochromia, few poikilocytes	Mild hypochromia; target cells, basophilic stippling, teardrop cells may be seen	Mild hypochromia; target cells, basophilic stippling, teardrop cells may be seen
RBC count	Usually decreased; occasionally normal to increased	Decreased	Normal to increased	Normal to increased
Serum iron	Decreased	Decreased	Normal	Normal
TIBC	Normal to increased	Normal to decreased	Normal	Normal
% saturation	Decreased	Normal to decreased	Normal	Normal
Ferritin	Decreased; may be normal if combined with acute or chronic disease	Normal to increased	Normal	Normal
Marrow iron stores	Decreased	Normal to increased	Normal	Normal
Hgb A_2	Normal to decreased	Normal	Increased	Normal

Abbreviations: Hgb A_2, quantitative hemoglobin A_2; RBC, red blood cell; TIBC, total iron binding concentration.

Macrocytic anemia is seen in more than 50% of patients with liver disease, usually associated with target cells (thin macrocytes).[3] Rarely, in a patient with advanced cirrhosis, a severe hemolytic anemia develops with numerous acanthocytes or spur cells. Mild macrocytosis, with or without anemia, may be seen in alcoholism, resulting from a direct effect of alcohol on erythropoiesis.[1] Alcohol-induced macrocytosis takes 2–4 months to disappear after cessation of alcohol consumption.[1]

Normocytic Anemia

The normocytic anemias comprise the most commonly encountered category. They may be divided into two subcategories by the reticulocyte count: those with decreased RBC production, and those with increased RBC destruction (Fig. 17-1). Although an elevated reticulocyte production index (see Reticulocyte Count) indicates a disorder with shortened RBC life span, such as hemolysis or blood loss, failure to find increased reticulocyte production does not eliminate these entities from consideration. Concurrent chronic disease, bone marrow suppression or infiltration, or folate and iron deficiency may suppress the expected increase in erythropoiesis. In addition, a rise in the reticulocyte production does not occur during the first few days after acute blood loss or with slow chronic blood loss.

The presence of a normal MCV does not exclude an acquired microcytic or macrocytic anemia from consideration. These anemias are normocytic during the early stages of development or may be combined to produce a normal mean RBC size. Either normocytic or macrocytic anemia occurs in primary hematopoietic disorders, such as myelocytic leukemias, myelodysplastic syndromes, myeloproliferative disorders, and aplastic anemia. In addition, although anemias associated with hemolysis or blood loss usually are normocytic, pronounced reticulocytosis may result in a mildly elevated MCV.

Normocytic Anemia with Decreased Red Blood Cell Production

Impaired RBC production may be a sign of many nonhematologic disorders or may be attributable to an intrinsic disease of the bone marrow (Table 17-4). Most patients with chronic infectious or inflammatory disorders or malignancy develop a mild to moderate anemia, with Hgb uncommonly below 9 g/dL. The Hgb typically falls within the first 2 months of illness, then stabilizes, improving only when the underlying dis-

Table 17-3. Macrocytic Anemias

Disorder	Helpful Laboratory Tests
Spurious macrocytosis (cold agglutinins, osmotic effect, e.g., very high glucose)	MCHC (high in cold agglutinins, low with osmotic effect)[a] RBC morphology (no macrocytes present)[a] RBC histogram[a]
Neonate (first few weeks)	
Reticulocytosis (marked)	Reticulocyte count[a] RBC morphology (polychromasia)[a]
Alcoholism	Liver function tests RBC morphology (round macrocytes)[a]
Liver disease	Liver function tests RBC morphology (round macrocytes, target cells)[a]
Myxedema	Thyroid function tests
Drugs (chemotherapeutic agents, drugs that interfere with folate absorption or metabolism)	
Megaloblastic anemia	RBC morphology (oval macrocytes, hypersegmented neutrophils)[a] Serum B_{12}[a] Serum folate[a] RBC folate[a] Schilling test Antibodies to intrinsic factor[a]
Myelodysplastic syndromes (including idiopathic acquired sideroblastic anemia)	RBC morphology (oval macrocytes, dysplastic changes)[a] Bone marrow examination Bone marrow iron Bone marrow cytogenetics
Aplastic anemia	Bone marrow examination
Inherited disorders of DNA synthesis	Organic acids
Congenital dyserythropoietic anemias	Bone marrow examination

[a] See text for discussion of analytes.
Abbreviations: MCHC, mean cell hemoglobin concentration; RBC, red blood cell.

Table 17-4. Normocytic Anemias with Decreased Production

Disorder	Helpful Laboratory Tests
Anemia of chronic disease	Erythrocyte sedimentation rate[a] Serum iron/TIBC/% saturation[a] Ferritin[a] Bone marrow iron stain Urinalysis
Renal failure	Creatinine
Endocrinopathy	T_4 Tests for pituitary function
Bone marrow failure (aplastic anemia, pure RBC aplasia, Fanconi's anemia)	Bone marrow examination
Myelophthisic anemia (marrow infiltration or fibrosis, e.g., carcinoma, hematopoietic malignancy, storage disease)	Bone marrow examination
Combined microcytic and macrocytic anemia	RBC histogram (see hemogram)[a] Tests for each disorder
Early iron or folate deficiency	Tests for each disorder
Recent acute blood loss or chronic blood loss	Stool occult blood Reticulocyte count[a] Ferritin[a]
Bleeding or hemolysis in combination with anemia of chronic disease, renal disease, or marrow suppression or infiltration	Tests for blood loss or hemolysis[a] (see Table 17-5)

[a] See text discussion of analytes.
Abbreviations: RBC, red blood cell; T_4, thyroxine; TIBC, total iron binding capacity.

order improves. In children, a rapid fall in Hgb of 1–2 g/dL (0.1–0.2 mmol/L) may occur with acute inflammatory processes.[4] Occasionally, asymptomatic chronic pyelonephritis may cause anemia of chronic disease; thus, a urinalysis may be useful if the underlying disorder is not apparent. Other characteristic laboratory findings include a low serum iron, total iron binding concentration (TIBC), and percentage saturation of TIBC, elevated ferritin, elevated erythrocyte protoporphyrin, abundant marrow histocytic iron stores, and elevated erythrocyte sedimentation rate (ESR).

Anemia of chronic disease is thought to be caused by a combination of decreased RBC life span (possibly by stimulation of macrophage phagocytic activity)[1] and of decreased RBC production. Possible mechanisms of suppression of erythropoiesis are shown in Figure 17-2. Stimulated macrophages secrete cytokines, such as interleukin-1 (IL-1), that directly suppress erythropoiesis. Neutrophils, which are stimulated by IL-1, release lactoferrin, which tightly binds iron and removes it from transferrin. The lactoferrin-bound iron is phagocytosed by macrophages and is unavailable to the RBC precursors. Thus, the marrow erythroids are iron deficient, even though marrow macrophage storage iron is increased. In addition, there is frequently a suboptimal increase in erythropoietin in response to anemia of chronic disease; early studies indicate that some patients with anemia of chronic disease respond to recombinant erythropoietin injections.[5]

Patients with chronic renal failure develop a severe anemia (Hgb 5-7 g/dL [0.8-1.1 mmol/L]). Marrow erythroid hypoplasia is caused by failure of the kidney to produce sufficient erythropoietin and retention in the plasma of a substance, possibly a polyamine, that inhibits erythropoiesis.[1] In addition, iron deficiency

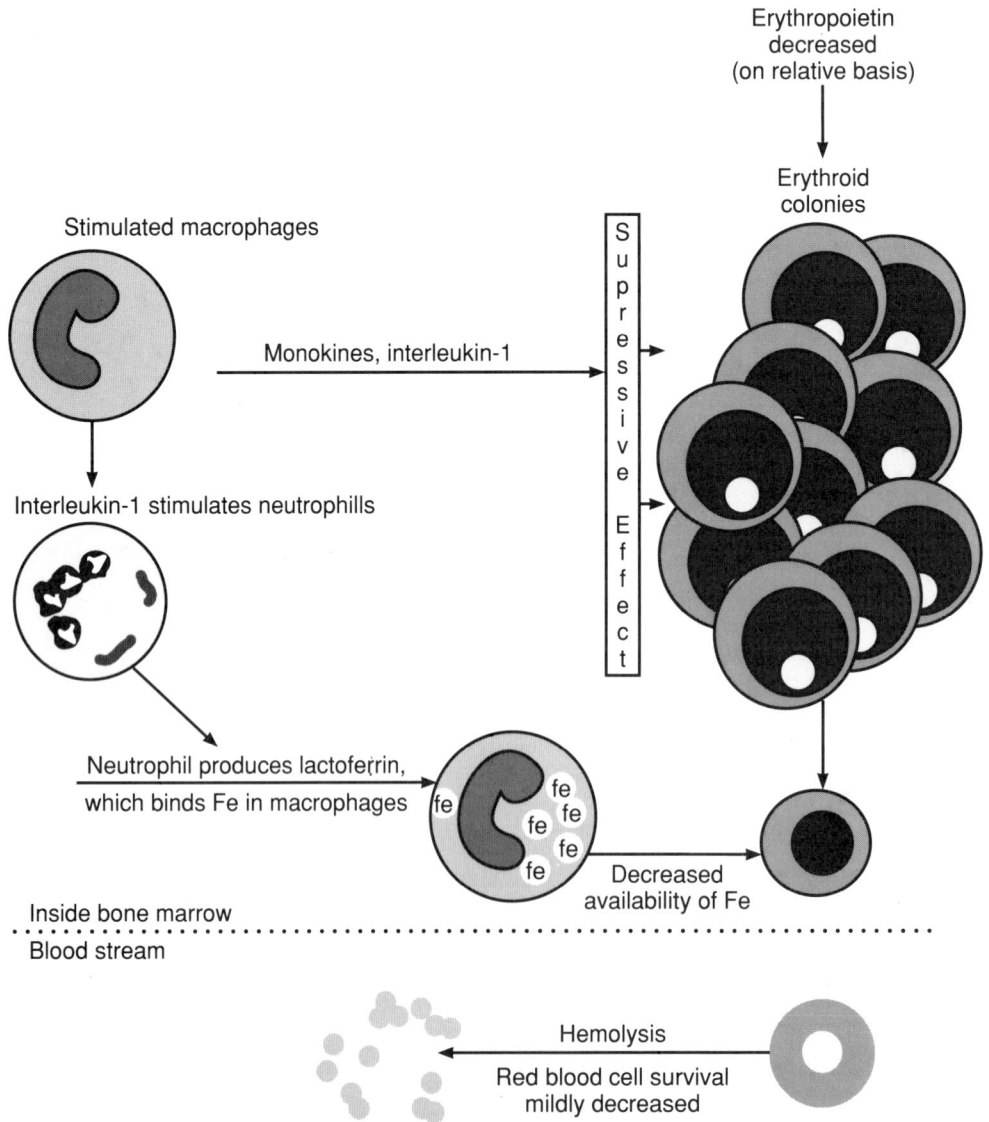

Fig. 17-2. Anemia of chronic disease. Theories of causation. Fe, iron; RBC, red blood cell.

may develop with chronic hemodialysis caused by blood loss. Mild anemia may accompany endocrine disorders such as hypothyroidism and hypopituitarism. Decreased tissue demand for oxygen leads to a need for fewer RBCs to carry oxygen.[6]

Failure of bone marrow erythroid production with hypocellular marrow occurs in combination with impaired granulopoiesis and thrombopoiesis in aplastic anemia or, more rarely, as pure RBC aplasia. Marrow suppression caused by bone marrow infiltration (myelophthisic anemia) may produce a normocytic to macrocytic anemia with characteristic findings in the peripheral blood. Findings include a leukoerythroblastic reaction (nucleated RBCs and immature neutrophils), prominent poikilocytes (especially teardrop cells), and a small number of polychromatophilic RBCs (although the absolute reticulocyte count is not elevated). Larger numbers of immature WBCs may be seen with primary hematopoietic malignancies involving the bone marrow (e.g., leukemias, myeloproliferative disorders, and myelodysplastic syndromes).

Normocytic Anemias with Increased Red Blood Cell Destruction

Anemia with a prominent polychromasia and increased reticulocyte production index (see Reticulocyte Count) is seen with acute blood loss and hemolysis. In addition, replacement of a nutritional deficiency (e.g., iron, folate, or vitamin B_{12}) results in a burst of erythropoiesis, simulating an anemia with increased reticulocytosis. Neither anemia nor reticulocytosis is immediately apparent after acute blood loss. Because both plasma and RBCs are removed, the hemoglobin does not fall for 1–3 days, until tissue fluid moves into the circulation to replenish the lost blood volume. With intravenous fluid therapy to replace the volume loss, a more rapid fall in hemoglobin occurs. The decrease in RBCs perfusing the kidneys increases erythropoietin, which stimulates RBC production in the marrow. However, it takes 3–5 days until reticulocytes appear in the circulation, with a maximum reticulocytosis within 10 days.[6] When blood loss is chronic, the reticulocyte count is usually normal or slightly elevated.[6] Iron deficiency anemia occurs in chronic blood loss after iron stores are depleted.

Hemolytic anemias are characterized by a decrease in the normal 120-day RBC life span. Red blood cell catabolism is thus increased, leading to biochemical changes, as illustrated in Figures 17-1 and 17-3. Normally, 80–90% of senescent RBCs are removed by extravascular mechanisms, within the macrophages of the liver and spleen. Globin is converted to amino acids, and heme is degraded to iron, carbon monoxide, and bilirubin. After conjugation and excretion in the bile, bilirubin is converted to urobilinogen and excreted in the feces; a small amount of urobilinogen is resorbed and excreted in the urine. Approximately 10–20% of normal RBC catabolism occurs intravascularly, with release of free hemoglobin into the plasma. The hemoglobin breaks down into dimers and is rapidly bound to haptoglobin. Hemoglobin-haptoglobin complexes are removed by the liver macrophages and the iron reused. Moderate to severe amounts of extravascular or intravascular hemolysis results in increased indirect and direct serum bilirubin, increased urine urobilinogen, and decreased haptoglobin. If the hemolytic process is mild or obscure, chromium 51 RBC survival studies may be helpful in documenting the decreased RBC half-life and determining the site of RBC destruction.

A small number of hemolytic anemias show primarily intravascular hemolysis (Table 17-5 and Fig. 17-3). With massive acute intravascular hemolysis, the haptoglobin binding capacity is exceeded. In this instance, the oxidized heme portion of the dimer binds to hemopexin and albumin (methemalbumin). Free dimers of hemoglobin also can be excreted in the urine (hemoglobinuria). With chronic intravascular hemolysis, Hgb dimers may be resorbed and broken down within the renal tubular cells, to form hemosiderin. When these renal epithelial cells are shed in the urine, hemosiderinuria can be detected. Thus, an increase in plasma Hgb or the presence of urine Hgb or hemosiderin is indicative of intravascular hemolysis. The presence of serum methemalbumin and decrease in serum hemopexin also occurs with intravascular hemolytic episodes, but these tests are infrequently used.

The hemolytic anemias may be divided into hereditary and acquired disorders. Hereditary disorders are caused by intrinsic defects in the patient's RBCs, whereas acquired disorders are mainly caused by factors extrinsic to the RBCs. Further testing depends on the suspected clinical entities, as listed in Table 17-5. In many of these disorders, RBC morphology may be useful in suggesting the etiology. Other commonly used first-line tests include a direct antiglobulin test and a screen for glucose 6-phosphate dehydrogenase (G-6-PD). A Heinz body stain is useful in acute hemolytic episodes when an oxidant drug or chemical is the suspected etiologic agent. When the cause of hemolysis is obscure, selected tests, depending on clinical presentation, include Hgb electrophoresis, isopropanol screen for unstable hemoglobin, sucrose hemolysis test for paroxysmal nocturnal hemoglobinuria, Donath-Land-

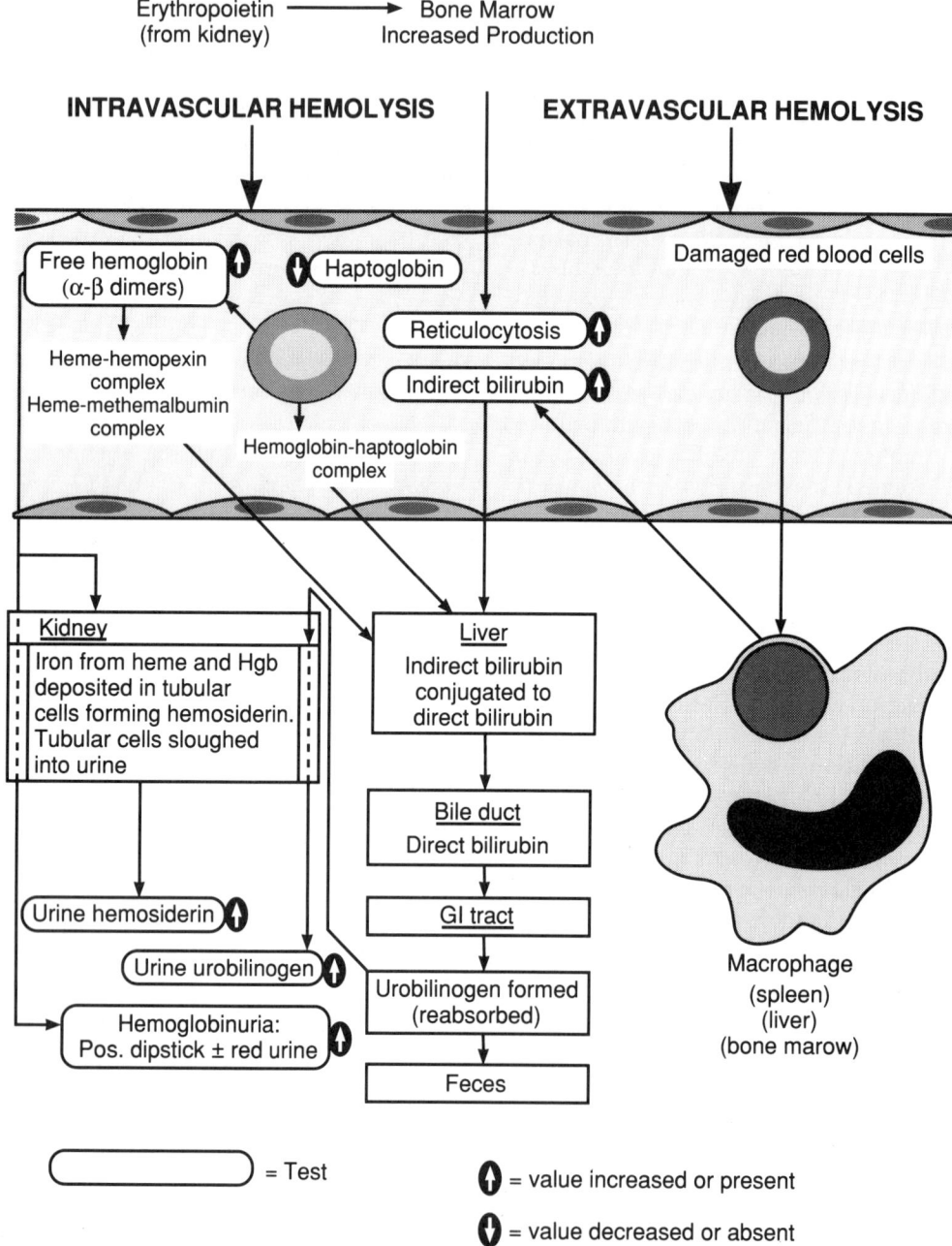

Fig. 17-3. Hemolysis. GI, gastrointestinal; Hgb, hemoglobin; Pos, positive.

Table 17-5. Hemolytic Anemias

Disorder	Helpful Laboratory Tests
Hereditary disorders	
Hemoglobinopathies (homozygous and double heterozygotes for abnormal hemoglobins and thalassemia; unstable hemoglobins)	Red blood cell morphology[a] (target, sickle cells, C crystals; microcytosis in thalassemia) Hemoglobin electrophoresis[a] Hemoglobin A_2[a] Hemoglobin F[a] Hemoglobin H inclusions[a] Heinz bodies[a] Sickle hemoglobin solubility test[a] Unstable hemoglobin screen[a] (isopropanol and heat denaturation)
Enzyme deficiencies (deficiencies in the glycolytic, pentose, or glutathione pathways, see Figs. 17-4 and 17-5)	G-6-PD screen[a] RBC enzymes, quantitative[a] Heinz bodies[a]
Membrane abnormalities (hereditary spherocytosis, elliptocytosis, stomatocytosis, pyropoikilocytosis)	RBC morphology, as described[a] Autohemolysis[a] Osmotic fragility[a]
Acquired disorders	
Antibody mediated[b] (transfusion reaction, hemolytic disease of newborn, cold autoantibody, warm autoantibody, drug-induced antibody, paryoxysmal cold hemoglobinuria)	Red blood cell morphology[a] (spherocytes) Direct antiglobulin Indirect antiglobulin Cold agglutinins Donath-Landsteiner test Antibody screening Antibody screening with drug-treated cells
Mechanical, traumatic[b] (prosthetic values, DIC, hemolytic uremic syndrome, thrombotic thrombocytopenic purpura, thermal injury)	RBC morphology[a] Platelet count APTT, PT Fibrinogen, fibrin-split products
Membrane injury[b] (paroxysmal nocturnal hemoglobinuria)	Acid serum lysis test[a] Sucrose hemolysis test[a]
Altered plasma lipids (severe liver disease, α-β-lipoproteinemia, cachexia)	Red blood cell morphology[a] (acanthocytes) Liver enzymes Lipoprotein analysis
Oxidant drugs[b] (usually in association with enzyme deficiency or unstable hemoglobin)	RBC morphology[a] (bite cells, ghost cells, fragmented cells) Heinz bodies[a]
Infectious agents, toxins[b] (malaria, *Clostridia*, *Bartonella*, babesiosis, snake venom)	RBC morphology[a] (organisms) Cultures
Hypersplenism	White blood cell count, platelet count

[a] See text discussion of analytes.
[b] Primarily intravascular hemolysis.
Abbreviations: APTT, activated partial thromboplastin time; DIC, disseminated intravascular coagulation; PT, prothrombin time; RBC, red blood cell; G-6-PD, glucose 6-phosphate dehydrogenase.

steiner test for paroxysmal cold hemoglobinuria, and a panel of RBC enzymes.

Polycythemia

Technically, polycythemia refers to an increased concentration of erythrocytes that is above normal for age and sex. Generally, microcytic erythrocytosis without a concomitant increase in Hgb or Hct (e.g., in thalassemia trait or some instances of iron deficiency) is not included in this category of disorders. A patient should be investigated for polycythemia if the Hgb is consistently higher than 18 g/dL (2.8 mmol/L) in the adult male and higher than 16 g/dL (2.5 mmol/L) in the adult female.

Absolute polycythemia refers to an increase in the total RBC mass, whereas in relative polycythemia, the RBC mass is normal to slightly elevated, but the plasma volume is decreased. If the Hgb is higher than 20 g/dL or the Hct is greater than 60%, it is safe to assume that the RBC mass is increased.[1] However, if values are moderately elevated, a determination of RBC mass and plasma volume may be necessary. This is a very expensive and time-consuming procedure, often fraught with interpretation problems. Thus, attention first should be directed to clinical findings and other laboratory tests that can establish a cause for polycythemia. Absolute polycythemia may be secondary to an increase in erythropoietin or may be a primary hematologic stem cell disorder, polycythemia vera. Table 17-6 indicates the causes of polycythemia, as well as useful tests.

The use of diuretics or dehydration can cause relative polycythemia. Hemoglobin should be measured when the patient is adequately hydrated. Careful attention should be given to factors that can decrease oxygen saturation, including cardiopulmonary disease, smoking, exposure to carbon monoxide, and high altitude. Chronic hypoxia can be documented by finding a pO_2 of less than 90%. With mild polycythemia in a smoker, an attempt should be made to repeat Hgb and pO_2 measurements after cessation of smoking for several weeks. Rarely, methemoglobinemia caused by RBC enzyme defect, drug effect, or abnormal Hgb M may result in decreased oxygenation or Hgb. Measurement of pO_2 may be normal in polycythemia associated with sleep apnea, because arterial oxygen desaturation occurs only with sleep.[1]

Tissue hypoxia caused by a variant Hgb with a high affinity for oxygen may cause an increase in erythropoi-

Table 17-6. Classification of Polycythemia

Disorder	Helpful Laboratory Tests
I. Relative (pseudopolycythemia)	**RBC mass normal**
Dehydration	**Erythropoietin normal**
Stress erythrocytosis (Gaisböck syndrome)	
II. Absolute polycythemia	**RBC mass increased**
A. Secondary	*Erythropoietin increased (or normal)*
Decreased O₂ saturation	Arterial pO_2 decreased
High altitude	
Pulmonary disease	
Pulmonary AV fistula	
Cyanotic heart disease	
Smoking	Carboxyhemoglobin
Methemoglobin	Methemoglobin
	RBC enzymes[a]
	Hgb M determination
Sleep apnea	
Inappropriate erythropoietin production	
Tumors: renal cell carcinoma, hypernephroma, Wilms tumor, cerebellar hemangioblastoma, hepatoma, leiomyoma, pheochromocytoma	
Local renal hypoxia: renal cysts, hydronephrosis, renal transplant, mass compressing kidney	IVP, kidney ultrasound
High affinity hemoglobin	P_{50}-oxygen saturation curve
	Hemoglobin electrophoresis[a]
Familial polycythemia	
Testosterone administration	Urinary androgens
B. Polycythemia vera	*Erythropoietin decreased (or normal)*
	WBC count and differential
	Platelet count
	Leukocyte alkaline phosphatase
	Serum B_{12}[a]
	Uric acid
	Ferritin[a]
	Bone marrow

[a] See text discussion of analytes.
Abbreviations: AV, arteriovenous; Hgb, hemoglobin; IVP, intravenous pyelogram; RBC, red blood cell; WBC, white blood cell. (Modified from Henry[6] with permission.)

etin and polycythemia. The disorder occurs in the heterozygote, and a family history of erythrocytosis suggests this possibility. The P_{50} (oxygen pressure at which Hgb is 50% saturated) is decreased, and approximately 50% of these variant hemoglobins yield an abnormal alkaline or acid electrophoresis. In addition, rare families with an autosomal recessive inheritance of polycythemia attributable to defective regulation of erythropoietin have been described.[3]

Renal disorders that produce local hypoxia lead to increased erythropoietin production and polycythemia. An intravenous pyelogram (IVP) or ultrasound examination provides evidence for a renal lesion. Autonomous production of an erythropoietin-like hormone has been observed in the tumors listed in Table 17-5.[7] However, polycythemia is uncommon, even in renal carcinoma, the most frequent tumor associated with increased erythropoietin.[6] Finally, iatrogenic testosterone administration has become an increasingly common cause of secondary polycythemia. This may be a particularly elusive etiology, because all diagnostic tests will show normal findings.

Polycythemia vera is a clonal stem cell malignancy that produces a malignant proliferation of granulocytes and megakaryocytes as well as erythrocytes. Autonomous proliferation of the RBCs occurs even with low levels of erythropoietin. Neutrophilia, thrombocytosis, basophilia, and splenomegaly are commonly seen, findings that usually do not occur in secondary polycythemia. Leukocyte alkaline phosphatase, vitamin B_{12}, and uric acid are often elevated. The bone marrow shows hypercellularity with increased megakaryocytes. Iron stores are frequently absent, caused by increased utilization in Hgb synthesis and gastrointestinal blood loss. With prolonged iron deficiency, the Hgb may fall, leaving a microcytic erythrocytosis and normal RBC mass. If polycythemia vera is suspected because of ancillary findings, measurements should be repeated after iron therapy. Further characteristics of polycythemia vera and differentiation from other myeloproliferative disorders are discussed in Chapter 19.

If polycythemia is moderate (Hgb less than 20 g/dL [<3.1 mmol/L]) and no apparent cause can be identified from the above considerations, a RBC mass and plasma volume may be helpful. A normal to borderline RBC mass and decreased plasma volume are often seen in stress erythrocytosis (or Gaisböck syndrome).[1] This disorder of middle-aged men is associated with overweight, stress, fatigue, headache, mild to moderate hypertension, lack of exercise, and smoking. Inhaled carbon monoxide from smoking is thought to be a major cause for reduction in plasma volume in this syndrome. Often the relative polycythemia disappears when the patient stops smoking. Erythropoietin values may be useful in selected cases to differentiate primary polycythemia (low or normal) from secondary polycythemia (normal or elevated), but there is considerable overlap in values between these conditions.

BASIC TESTS

Test: Hemogram (CBC, Complete Blood Count, Blood Count, Blood Cell Profile)[2,6–9]

Background and Selection

The hemogram is the test panel on a multiparameter automated hematology instrument that includes the Hgb, Hct, RBC count, and RBC indices. The Hgb and/or Hct portion of a hemogram validates a presumptive diagnosis of anemia or polycythemia and determine its severity. The MCV is the key RBC index used in the initial classification of anemia. The hemogram is often ordered as a screening test on routine physical examination, in prenatal evaluation, or at admission to the hospital and is usually required before a surgical procedure. It is used after therapy for anemia; after treatment involving chemotherapeutic drugs, many of which are toxic to the bone marrow; in checking for possible idiosyncratic reactions to medications; and in evaluating blood loss from gastrointestinal bleeding, trauma, or surgery.

Terminology

The name of the test for routine blood cell measurements and the number of parameters included vary between laboratories. Automated cell counters are used to measure WBC count, Hgb, Hct, RBC count, MCV, mean cell hemoglobin (MCH), and mean cell hemoglobin concentration (MCHC). With many cell analyzers, a RBC distribution width (most frequently called RDW), which is based on either the coefficient of variation or the standard deviation (SD) of the volume of the RBC population, is also reported. This parameter is a measure of variation in RBC size or anisocytosis. The platelet count can be determined simultaneously with many cell counters. Some laboratories require a separate order for platelet count, because low platelet counts often are verified by additional methods (Ch. 19). The latest generation of hematology analyzers also may produce a screening WBC differential (Ch. 19).

The WBC differential from the blood smear is sometimes included with the cell analyzer results when a hemogram or CBC is ordered, whereas other laboratories require a separate request or perform the slide differential only when certain parameters from the automated counts are abnormal. Likewise, the policy for inclusion of RBC morphology and platelet estimate from the blood smear with the CBC differs between laboratories. In very small laboratories, manual methods may be used and the hemogram components ordered separately.

Logistics

EDTA-anticoagulated blood is the preferred specimen. Blood should be promptly mixed in anticoagulant to prevent clotting. Heparinized blood may be acceptable for some of the hemogram parameters, depending on the type of laboratory instrumentation. Citrate-anticoagulated blood is used occasionally when an EDTA dependent platelet agglutinin is present, and values (except for indices) are multiplied by 1.1 to correct for anticoagulant dilution (see Platelet Count in Ch. 19). Newer instruments use very small sample volumes (e.g., 0.25 mL or less). Thus, capillary blood from neonates or children can be collected directly into EDTA-coated microcollection vials. Alternatively, capillary blood may be diluted directly into a measured amount of saline. The specimen should not be diluted by intravenous fluid or, in the case of capillary blood, obtained by squeezing the finger or heel, which may dilute the specimen with tissue juices.

The ambulatory patient who is placed in bed has an average drop in Hgb 0.5 g/dL (0.1 mmol/L), but the drop may be as great as 1.5 g/dL (0.2 mmol/L). This change is due to a shift of extracellular fluid in the legs into the vascular compartment. Exercise does not normally affect the hemogram unless dehydration occurs. Hydration and dehydration can produce dramatic changes in hemogram parameters; for example, the Hgb can change by more than 3 g/dL.

All RBC parameters are stable for approximately 8 hours at room temperature and for 24 hours when refrigerated. The Hgb value is stable for several days. With time, fluid moves into the RBC, causing MCV to increase (approximately 3% in 8 hours) and the MCHC to fall.

Hematologic measurements are based on particle counts and volumes by electrical impedance or laser light scatter. Cells in a saline solution are drawn through a narrow aperture at a fixed rate. The cells impede the passage of electrical current or scatter light, producing a signal or pulse. The integrated area of the pulse curve or the intensity of light scattered at particular angles is proportional to cell volume. A frequency histogram of RBC volume can be generated for the entire population of RBCs, which is usually gaussian in healthy persons (Fig. 17-4). The mean of this histogram is the MCV, whereas the coefficient of variation (for some instruments, the standard deviation) is the RDW. The shape and Hgb concentration of the RBC may affect the volume measurement, causing a signifi-

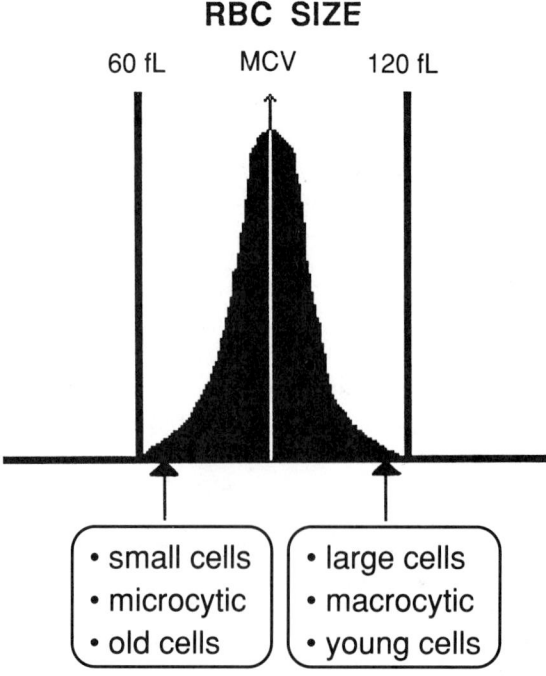

Fig. 17-4. Normal RBC volume histogram. MCV, mean cell volume; RBC, red blood cell.

cant degree of inaccuracy in patients with severe poikilocytosis. A new light scatter instrument induces sphering of the RBCs before analysis, a maneuver that may improve the accuracy of the MCV and that also permits direct measurement of Hgb concentration in individual cells. This instrument produces a frequency histogram of Hgb concentration for the RBC population (Fig. 17-5); the mean of the direct measurement of Hgb concentration in individual RBCs is the Hgb concentration density (HCD), and the standard deviation is the Hgb distribution width (HDW).

The Hct is automatically calculated as the total RBC volume per volume of aspirated blood by multiplying the RBC count by the MCV. In smaller laboratories, the Hct may be obtained by centrifugation in a capillary tube. Spun microhematocrits are higher than electronically determined hematocrits because of plasma trapping, particularly when abnormally shaped or microcytic RBCs are present or when the Hct is elevated. When centrifugation is used, it is important to check periodically the speed at which the centrifuge rotates and the time required for maximal packing of the RBCs.

After lysis of the RBCs, Hgb is converted to cyanmethemoglobin by potassium ferricyanide and potassium cyanide (Drabkin's reagent). The absorbance of the cyanmethemoglobin solution at 540 nm is proportional to Hgb concentration. Because Hgb is measured with greater precision than is the Hct, it is the preferable parameter in evaluating anemia.

The MCH is the average amount of Hgb per RBC, calculated as Hgb/RBC. The MCHC is the average Hgb concentration per RBC, calculated as Hgb/MCV*RBC or Hgb/Hct.

Inspection of histograms of RBC volume and RBC Hgb density may reveal small populations of abnormal cells that do not change the mean or standard deviation of the total population beyond the reference range. Upper and lower boundary "markers" for size and Hgb concentration abnormalities can be set (Figs. 17-4 and 17-5), and the instrument may print a flag for microcytosis, macrocytosis, hypochromia, or hyperchromia, when a significant number of cells exceed these limits.

Multichannel hematology instruments are accurate and precise, with coefficients of variation for most parameters of less than 2%; however, spurious results can sometimes occur (Table 17-7). Many of these situations are identified and corrected by alert laboratory technologists before results are reported.

Interpretation

Table 17-8 indicates adult and pediatric reference ranges for the RBC parameters of the hemogram. After 2 years of age, children maintain a fairly constant Hgb value, with a lower limit of approximately 11.5 g/dL (1.8 mmol/L). The lower reference limit of MCV in

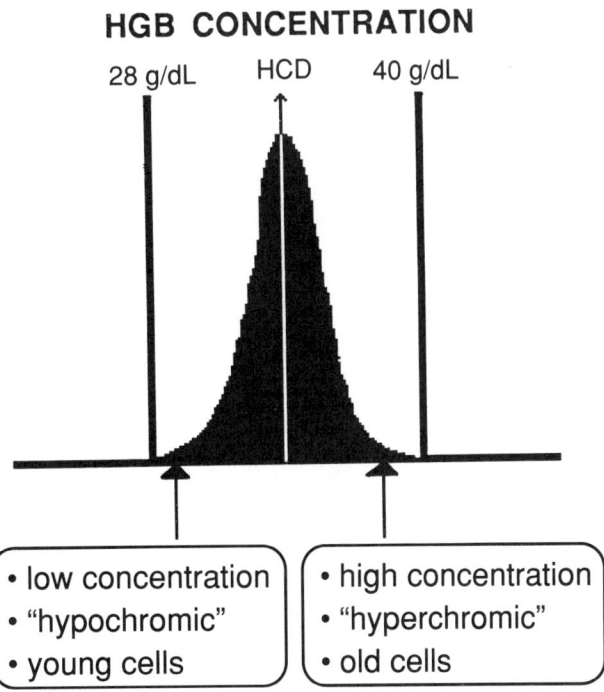

Fig. 17-5. Normal RBC hemoglobin concentration histogram, RBC, red blood cell; HCD, hemoglobin concentration density.

Table 17-7. Spurious Results for Red Blood Cell Parameters

Cause	Parameters Affected	To Obtain Correct Results
RBC autoagglutination	↓ RBC; ↑ MCV; ↓ Hct; ↑ MCH, MCHC, RDW; Hgb correct	Warm blood to 37°C, if cold agglutinin is present
Hyperlipemia (triglyceride >1000 mg/dL)	↑ Hgb, MCH, MCHC; Hct correct	Replace plasma with saline
Hypergammaglobulin on some instruments		
High WBC (>50,000/μL)	↑ RBC, Hgb, Hct, MCV, MCH; spun Hct correct	Centrifuge Hgb before reading; subtract WBC count from RBC count
Clotting	Low values for all counted parameters	Recollect blood
Excess EDTA (tube less than half full)	Low value for spun Hct only; automated counts correct	
Microcytic RBC	Only extreme microcytosis will lead to ↓ Hct, RBC; ↑ MCV, MCH, MCHC; Hgb correct	
Hyperglycemia (>600 mg/dL)	↑ MCV, Hct; ↓ MCHC; spun HCT correct	Dilute blood 1:1 with saline, incubate 5 min, and reassay
Cryoglobulin	↑ Hgb, RBC, Hct; ↓ MCV	Warm blood to 37°C

Abbreviations: ↑ increased; ↓ decreased. Hct, hematocrit; Hgb, hemoglobin; MCH, mean cell hemoglobin; MCHC, mean cell hemoglobin concentration; MCV, mean cell value; RBC, red blood cell, RDW, red blood cell distribution width; WBC, white blood cell.

children above 1 year of age is approximately 70 fL plus the age of the child. At puberty, testosterone increases RBC production; thus, the normal range for Hgb in men is about 2 g/dL (0.3 mmol/L) higher than in women. Placental hormones in pregnancy decrease the Hgb by approximately 1 g/dL (0.2 mmol/L) during the second and third trimesters, although wide swings in fluid volume can result in a more pronounced decline. In the United States, normal Hgb values for blacks are approximately 0.5–1.0 g/dL (0.1–0.2 mmol/L) lower

Table 17-8. Reference Values for RBC Parameters of Hemogram: Mean ±2 SD

	Hgb[a] (g/dL; g/L)[b]	Hct (%; 1)[b]	RBC (×10/μL; ×10/L)[b]	MCV (fL)[b]	MCH (pg)[b]	MCHC (g/dL; g/L)[b]	RDW (%)
Birth-cord[c]	13.5–19.5	42–60	3.9–5.4	98–118	31–37	30–36	—
1–3 days–cap[d]	14.5–22.5	45–67	4.0–6.6	95–121	31–37	29–37	—
1 week	13.5–21.5	42–66	3.9–6.3	88–126	28–40	28–38	—
2 weeks	12.5–20.5	39–63	3.6–6.2	86–124	28–40	28–38	—
1 month	10.0–18.0	31–55	3.0–5.4	85–123	28–40	29–37	—
2 months	9.0–14.0	28–42	2.7–4.9	77–115	26–34	29–37	—
3–6 months	9.5–13.5	29–41	3.1–4.5	74–108	25–35	30–36	—
0.5–2 years	10.5–13.5	33–39	3.7–5.4	70–86	23–31	30–36	—
2–6 years	11.5–13.5	34–40	3.9–5.3	75–87	24–30	31–37	—
6–12 years	11.5–13.5	35–45	4.0–5.2	77–95	25–34	31–37	—
Adult female	11.7–15.7	34.9–46.9	3.8–5.2	80.8–100	26.4–34.0	31.4–35.8	<15
Adult male	13.5–17.5	39.8–52.2	4.4–5.9	80.5–99.7	26.6–33.8	31.5–36.3	<15

[a] Mean Hgb level in blacks of both sexes and all ages may be 0.5–1.0 below the mean for whites.
[b] Values for SI units (second unit in parentheses) are the same as for conventional units, except:
Hgb (g/L) = Hgb (g/dL) × 10
Hct (1) = Hct (%)/100
MCHC (g/L) = MCHC (g/dL) × 10
[c] For premature infants, cord Hgb = 7.016 + 0.243 (gestational age). Hemoglobin values will remain approximately 1.0 g/dL less than those of the full term infant until 1 year of age.
[d] Capillary blood hemoglobin is approximately 2 g/dL higher than venous blood during the first 3 days of life due to seepage of plasma from the capillary bed. However, if the capillary specimen is contaminated by tissue fluid from improper collection, the Hgb level will be lower.
Abbreviations: Cap, capillary; Hct, hematocrit; Hgb, hemoglobin; MCH, mean cell hemoglobin; MCHC, mean cell hemoglobin concentration; MCV, mean cell volume; RBC, red blood cell; RDW, red blood cell distribution width.
(Data from Miller et al.[31] and Rudolph et al.[44])

than those of whites. Prolonged exposure to high altitude increases the Hgb 1 g/dL (0.2 mmol/L) for each 3–4% decrease is arterial oxygen saturation. Taking into account the pertinent variables, a Hgb value persistently below the lower limit of the reference range is termed *anemia*, whereas that above the upper limit is termed polycythemia. With normal RBC indices (normocytic, normochromic RBCs), the RBC count times 3 should approximately equal the Hgb level, and the Hgb value times 3 should approximately equal the Hct.

The RBC count may be useful in differentiating thalassemia trait from iron deficiency in patients with microcytosis. In thalassemia trait, the RBC count is normal to elevated, whereas in iron deficiency, it is often decreased. A number of mathematical discriminant functions have been proposed, based on the observation that the microcytosis in thalassemia trait exceeds that expected from the RBC count; a simple formula uses the MCV divided by the RBC count; a quotient greater than 13 suggests iron deficiency, and a value of less then 13 is seen in thalassemia trait.

The most important of the RBC indices is the MCV, which forms the basis for initial classification of anemia (see Introduction). In iron, folate, and vitamin B_{12} deficiency, the MCV can be abnormal before anemia develops. The MCH is linearly related to MCV and is a redundant parameter; MCHC is also of little diagnostic value. A decrease in MCHC occurs late in the progression of iron deficiency anemia. Occasionally, high values are noted in patients with spherocytosis, but high MCHC values are much more likely to be due to instrument or specimen problems. Before the introduction of automated counting, a low MCHC (Hgb/Hct) was seen more frequently in iron deficiency. This phenomenon was due to the falsely high centrifuged Hct in the patient with microcytic anemia and poikilocytosis caused by plasma trapping in the RBC column.

An increase in RDW or the finding of a small population of large or small RBCs by visual inspection of the histogram may be a more sensitive indicator of changes in cell size than the MCV (Fig. 17-4). In particular, in combined macrocytic and microcytic anemias or sideroblastic anemia, the RDW may be very large, whereas the MCV is normal. A classification for anemias using RDW as well as MCV has been proposed (Table 17-9). However, as discussed in the footnotes for Table 17-9, many exceptions have been noted. RDW may be most clinically useful in detecting early iron deficiency, discriminating thalassemia trait (normal or increased RDW) from iron deficiency (increased RDW), indicating a combined microcytic/macrocytic process, and indicating response to vitamin B_{12}, folate, or iron therapy.

Table 17-9. Classification of Anemia with MCV and RDW[9]

	MCV		
RDW	Low	Normal	High
Normal (≤14.5%) (homogeneous)	Thalassemia trait[a] Transfusion[b] Chemotherapy Malignancy Hemorrhage Hereditary spherocytosis Post-traumatic splenectomy	Normal Chronic disease[d]	Aplastic anemia Liver disease[f]
High (heterogeneous)	Iron deficiency S-β-thalassemia Hgb H RBC fragmentations[c]	Transfusion[b] Early iron, B_{12}, or folate deficiency Homozygous hemoglobinopathy Myelofibrosis Sideroblastic anemia[e]	Folate deficiency B_{12} deficiency Cold agglutinin[g] Hemolytic anemia Chemotherapy

[a] Many cases of thalassemia trait may have an elevated RDW.
[b] Transfusion can elevate the RDW, and use of RDW in anemia classification after transfusion is not valid.
[c] Specimens with a small amount of RBC fragmentation will not present with a low MCV or elevated RDW.
[d] Some cases of chronic disease may have slightly lower MCV and slightly elevated RDW.
[e] "Preleukemia" or myelodysplastic syndrome, with or without sideroblastic RBCs, may have a high MCV and RDW.
[f] Liver disease is not well classified by MCV and RDW; usually, MCV is high normal or macrocytic, and RDW may be slightly elevated.
[g] If agglutinated RBCs are excluded from calculation, samples may show a normal RDW, despite marked elevation of MCHC.

Abbreviations: Hgb, hemoglobin; MCHC, mean cell hemoglobin concentration; MCV, mean cell volume; RBC, red blood cell; RDW, red blood cell distribution width.

(Modified from Bessman et al.,[9] with permission.)

Individual RBCs with decreased Hgb density are seen in iron deficiency, and cells with increased Hgb density are seen with spherocytic or elliptocytic RBCs, or in homozygous CC and SS hemoglobinopathies.

Evaluation of anemia and polycythemia depends on clinical presentation and ancillary laboratory findings (see Introduction). In anemia, classification by MCV, the examination of the peripheral smear, and the reticulocyte count constitute basic tests that can direct subsequent investigation.

Test: Red Blood Cell Morphology (Peripheral Blood Smear Morphology, RBC Morphology)[2,6,7]

Background and Selection

Examination of RBC morphology on the peripheral blood smear can be helpful in evaluating unexplained anemia. Along with the hemogram and reticulocyte count, this initial laboratory test will aid in narrowing the diagnostic possibilities. In addition, abnormalities in the WBCs in the blood smear may be seen when anemia is due to hematopoietic malignancies.

Logistics

An evaluation of RBC morphology is usually made when a slide WBC differential is performed. In some laboratories, this is part of the CBC. In other laboratories, the preparation of a slide may be triggered by the presence of anemia, abnormal RBC indices or RDW, or an abnormal screening differential. Smears may be prepared from either finger or heel puncture capillary blood, or from EDTA-anticoagulated venous blood. If EDTA anticoagulant is used, smears should be prepared within 2 hours, to avoid artifactual changes. A small drop of blood is placed on one end of a slide and spread by means of another slide at a 30-degree angle. The well-made smear has a wedge shape and covers approximately one-half of the slide. No portion of the smear should extend to the edges, and no ridges or holes should be present. In some laboratories, slides are produced with centrifugal devices.

Blood smears are stained with a Romanowsky stain, such as Wright or Wright-Giemsa. These stains contain various combinations of methylene blue, oxidation products of methylene blue, and eosin. A time adjustment in the stain, in a buffer-stain mixture, and in the buffer alone as well as the buffer pH produces the optimal color characteristics. The nuclei of the leukocytes should be purple-blue, whereas the neutrophil cytoplasm should appear tannish (nonspecific neutrophil granules) with violet azurophilic granules (primary or nonspecific granules). Red blood cells should be salmon pink.

Red blood cells are examined in an area of the peripheral smear in which they do not quite overlap. If the thinnest edge of the smear is studied, all the RBCs have a spherocytic or cobblestone appearance. In the thick part of the smear, the RBCs are clumped and cannot be individually evaluated. Information to be gained includes observation of size, Hgb content (hypochromia), variation of size (anisocytosis), presence of abnormally shaped cells (poikilocytosis) or RBC inclusions, and the presence of polychromasia. Abnormalities are reported as an approximate percentage or are graded subjectively as mild, moderate, or marked.

Artifacts in RBC appearance that can be caused by excessive moisture include a donut-hole or cookie-cutter appearance to the RBCs, burr cells, stomatocytes, and even target cells. Prewashing the glass slides with alcohol sometimes can eliminate these problems. In addition, blood films prepared from older blood can have many crenated RBCs (burr cells or echinocytes).

Interpretation

The usual RBC morphology is normocytic, normochromic with minimal numbers of poikilocytes and polychromatophilic cells. The neonate has macrocytic RBCs and may have small numbers of poikilocytes because of their inefficient splenic removal. A description of various RBC poikilocytes and inclusions, along with possible etiology, is given in Chapter 16.

Among the microcytic anemias (Table 17-1), the RBC morphology may be nonspecific, and findings can often overlap between the potential causes. However, coarse basophilic stippling, targets, and occasional teardrops may be seen in thalassemia trait. Target cells are prominent in Hgb E and Hgb H disease, whereas coarse basophilic stippling also occurs in lead poisoning.

When the MCV is elevated (see Table 17-3, for causes), it is useful to confirm the presence of macrocytosis on the blood smear. Spurious macrocytosis may occur with hyperglycemia, which causes transient swelling of the RBCs in isotonic saline, or in vitro RBC agglutination. Macrocytosis caused by pronounced reticulocytosis is evident by the finding of a large number of polychromatophilic RBCs. Oval macrocytes may be seen in megaloblastic anemias, accompanied by occasional teardrop forms, small bizarre-shaped erythrocytes with central pallor (a product of ineffective erythropoiesis), and hypersegmented neutrophils. The high MCV of liver disease is characterized by round macrocytes and target cells. Myelodysplastic syndromes may show similar RBC changes to megaloblastic anemia, but dysplasia of the leukocytes and platelets is usually present.

An estimate of the reticulocyte count can be made by doubling the approximate percentage of polychromatophilic RBCs. The normocytic anemias can then be characterized by increased or decreased production (see Reticulocyte Count). Among the normocytic anemias with decreased production (Table 17-4), the presence of teardrop cells is an important clue to marrow infiltration or fibrosis. In addition, WBC abnormalities can indicate that a leukemic or myeloproliferative disorder is the cause of the normocytic anemia. Evaluation of RBC morphology in normocytic anemia may also indicate combined macrocytic and microcytic anemia, producing a normal MCV.

In hemolytic anemia (Table 17-5), specific RBC poikilocytes may provide an important clue to the diagnosis. Sickle cells and target cells are usually present in hemoglobin S disease or S-C disease. Target cells and rare Hgb C crystals occur in Hgb C disease. Hereditary membrane defects can produce a predominance of spherocytes, elliptocytes, or stomatocytes. Small bizarre poikilocytes are produced with higher temperatures in hereditary pyropoikilocytosis. "Bite" cells or "ghost" cells may be seen with oxidant drug stress in a patient with RBC enzyme deficiencies. Spherocytes are prominent in immune hemolytic anemias. Microangiopathic hemolysis (e.g., in disseminated intravascular coagulation, heart valve hemolysis, vasculitis) is characterized by the presence of schistocytes and spherocytes.

Finally, splenectomy leads to the production of many RBC poikilocytes because of the role of the spleen in remodeling the reticulocyte membrane. Target cells, acanthocytes, and spherocytes may be seen, as well as an occasional Howell-Jolly body and Pappenheimer bodies. Other RBC abnormalities may be accentuated after splenectomy. Tables 17-1 and 17-3 to 17-5 list additional tests useful for the diagnosis of various RBC disorders, many of which can be suggested by peripheral blood smear findings.

Test: Reticulocyte Count[1,6,10–12]

Background and Selection

Once the developing RBC extrudes its nucleus, it is called a reticulocyte. This term is derived from the reticulin-like network of RNA that remains in the cell for the next 3–4 days as Hgb production continues. Normally, the reticulocyte spends 2–3 days in the bone marrow, passes through the bone marrow sinus lining into the peripheral circulation, and matures in the peripheral blood for 1 day. With increased erythropoietin and stimulation of RBC production, reticulocytes are prematurely released from the bone marrow and may circulate for 2–3 days. These stress reticulocytes are less well hemoglobinized and have a bluish or polychromatophilic appearance on the Wright-stained blood smear. Stress reticulocytes are also larger in size than normal reticulocytes, and persistent reticulocytosis can result in an elevated RDW and MCV.

The reticulocyte count is a part of the initial evaluation of any unexplained anemia. It is particularly useful in the normocytic anemias, classifying the anemia as one of increased or decreased production (Fig. 17-1). The reticulocyte count also may be used to follow the response of a nutritional deficiency anemia to replacement therapy.

Logistics

Only a few drops of heparin- or EDTA-anticoagulated blood are required. Blood may be stored for up to 48 hours before reticulocyte determination. Equal amounts of blood are mixed with a supravital stain, usually new methylene blue, and a wedge smear is prepared. The dye complexes and precipitates the RBC RNA, which appears as a blue reticulum network or as two or more blue granules. The number of reticulocytes per 1000 RBCs is enumerated and expressed as a percentage. Care must be taken not to confuse reticulum granules with other RBC inclusions, such as Heinz bodies, Howell-Jolly bodies, or Pappenheimer bodies.

Because a small number of reticulocytes are present, the imprecision in manual reticulocyte counting is large: 95% confidence limits for a 1% count are 0.4–1.6%; for a 5% count, 3.6–6.4%; and for a 10% count, 8.1–11.9%. Recently, methods employing fluorescent dyes for RNA and using flow cytometry have been developed. This technique improves precision by counting larger numbers of reticulocytes but can give spuriously elevated results with DNA inclusions such as Howell-Jolly bodies and nucleated RBCs. In the patient with anemia, the presence of the same absolute number of reticulocytes as in the healthy person will appear as an elevated percentage of reticulocytes because of the reduced RBC count. Thus, absolute reticulocyte counts are frequently calculated by multiplying the percentage of reticulocytes by the RBC count.

Interpretation

A reference range of 0.5–1.5% (0.005–0.015) and 24,000–84,000/μL (24–84 × 10^9/L) is frequently sited for adults, but other studies have shown reticulocytes as high as 2.5% (0.025) and 125,000/μL (.125 × 10^{12}/L) for males and postmenopausal women, and up to 3.5% (0.035) for menstrual-aged females. In the newborn, 2.5–6.5% (0.025–0.065) are observed, with a return to the adult reference range by the end of the second week.

As an alternative to calculating the absolute reticulocyte count, a "corrected" percentage reticulocyte or reticulocyte index can be calculated to normalize the reticulocyte count to the patient's Hgb or Hct:

Reticulocyte index = % reticulocytes
  × (patient Hgb/mean normal Hgb)

A further refinement in estimating the rate of RBC production can be added if the effect of premature reticulocyte release with erythropoietin stimulation is considered. The presence of premature or stress reticulocytes can be confirmed by noting polychromasia on the Wright-stained blood smear. Because these stress reticulocytes reside in the peripheral blood for twice the usual amount of time, the "corrected" reticulocyte count or reticulocyte index should be divided by two:

Reticulocyte production index = reticulocyte index/2

A reticulocyte production index more than two times normal (normal is 1) occurs with blood loss, hemolysis, or correction of a production defect; further laboratory tests that are useful in these disorders are shown in Figure 17-3 and in Table 17-5.

With blood loss, the percentage reticulocyte count doubles during the first 24 hours, caused by the presence of premature or stress reticulocytes from the bone marrow. The reticulocyte production index does not increase until 4–7 days, however, when new RBC precursors have emerged from the maturation sequence. A maximal response of three times basal production should occur within 7–10 days. In chronic hemolysis, with maximal bone marrow RBC hyperplasia, the reticulocyte production index may be more than 6. With correction of a production defect (e.g., replacement of nutritional deficiency), a burst of reticulocyte production in 7–10 days is evidence that the anemia is responding to the particular therapy.

It is important to be aware that low reticulocyte production does not eliminate blood loss or hemolysis from diagnostic consideration. Concurrent iron or folate deficiency and infectious or inflammatory disease can suppress erythropoiesis in these states, and an increase in reticulocytes will not be seen. In particular, folate depletion may frequently occur with chronic hemolysis, and urinary iron loss (hemosiderinuria) in intravascular hemolysis may lead to iron deficiency.

A modest increase in the reticulocyte count without increase in production rate may seen with escape of immature RBCs into the circulation in infiltrative marrow disorders with extramedullary hematopoiesis or with marrow damage caused by radiation or chemotherapy. A marked decrease (less than 0.4%) in reticulocyte count suggests anemia caused by marrow aplasia, marked marrow infiltration, renal disease, or marrow suppression by an infectious agent or drug.

Test: Sedimentation Rate (Erythrocyte Sedimentation Rate, ESR, Sed Rate)[2,6,12–14]

Background and Selection

The ESR measures the distance that RBCs fall in plasma over a period of time. The RBCs first form rouleaux-like stacks, then spherical aggregates, which sediment rapidly. Red blood cells have a net negative charge (ζ [zeta] potential) and normally repel each other. Many plasma proteins are positively charged and can promote RBC aggregation. In particular, an increase in asymmetric acute phase reactant proteins, such as fibrinogen, is an important cause of elevated ESR. In addition, RBC factors, such as shape, size, and concentration, influence the ESR.

Historically, the ESR has been used to detect and monitor acute and chronic inflammatory or infectious conditions. However, it is not a useful test in screening for disease in an asymptomatic patient. Unexplained mild to moderate elevations are usually transitory and are seldom caused by serious disease. Extreme elevations of ESR rarely occur in the absence of apparent disease. In addition, the ESR is often normal in patients with infectious, neoplastic, and inflammatory (connective tissue) diseases, and normal results cannot exclude these conditions in patients with nonspecific complaints. The absolute number of neutrophils is a more sensitive and specific test than the ESR in screening for inflammatory or infectious disorders. Although the ESR is more often normal in viral than bacterial infections, there is significant overlap in ESR values for both types of infections.

The ESR may be useful in the diagnosis and monitoring of temporal arteritis and polymyalgia rheumatica. It is sometimes used in conjunction with other laboratory tests to differentiate noninflammatory arthritis or nonspecific musculoskeletal complaints from rheumatoid arthritis or collagen vascular disease. The ESR may be useful in monitoring therapy in rheumatoid arthritis and Hodgkin's disease. As noted in Figure 17-7, the ESR may be of help in evaluating ferritin levels when diagnosing iron deficiency in the presence of inflammatory disease.

Logistics

EDTA-anticoagulated blood is most often used. Tubes should be at least half full, because high concentrations of EDTA decrease the ESR. Heparin alters the RBC membrane (ζ) potential and cannot be used as an anticoagulant. For the Westergren ESR, blood may be collected in sodium citrate anticoagulant, with a dilution of 4 parts blood to 1 part anticoagulant. Blood should be stored no longer than 2 hours at room temperature, or 6 hours refrigerated before starting the test.

The Wintrobe ESR is performed by pipetting blood into a 100-mm tube and measuring the distance (mm) of fall of the RBCs in 1 hour. The Westergren ESR is similarly measured by placing citrate-diluted blood, or EDTA-anticoagulated blood diluted 4:1 with saline, into a 200-mm tube. For the less frequently performed ζ ESR (ZSR), blood is centrifuged at a low speed in vertically placed capillary tubes, with rotation between four short spins. The distance the RBCs fall is divided by the Hct measured in the same capillary tube and expressed as a percentage.

The Wintrobe ESR is more sensitive to mild elevations, whereas the Westergren is more sensitive to change at higher levels. Both are increased by anemia and decreased by polycythemia. Although a correction for anemia has been proposed for the Wintrobe ESR, the formula was developed using normal blood adjusted to various Hct levels and does not appear to apply to many abnormal blood samples. The ZSR is not affected by anemia but is difficult to perform in a consistent manner; subtle changes in the microcentrifuge can affect the results. All methods of ESR are influenced by changes in RBC size and shape. Significant macrocytosis leads to more rapid sedimentation, whereas extreme microcytosis delays sedimentation. Pronounced poikilocytosis, in particular sickle cells, spherocytes, and acanthocytes, prevent rouleaux formation, resulting in a low ESR.

Interpretation

Reference ranges are age and sex dependent. Typical values for the Westergren sedimendation rate are given in Table 17-10. A useful algorithm for the adult upper limit of normal for the Westergren ESR is to divide the age by 2 for men and to divide the age plus 10 by 2 for women. For the ZSR, 41–54% (0.41–0.54) is normal for both sexes, 55–59% (0.55–0.59) represents a mild elevation, 60–64% (0.60–0.64) is a moderate elevation, and more than 64% (0.64) is a marked elevation.

As indicated under Background and Selection, the ESR is elevated in a somewhat variable fashion in inflammatory, infectious, and neoplastic disorders. Most unexpected elevations in ESR are transitory. Thus, an elevated ESR without explanation after history, physical examination, and routine studies should be repeated in a few weeks. Patients with persistent elevation of ESR most frequently remain undiagnosed or are found to have benign monoclonal gammopathy; rarely, occult carcinoma is discovered. Most patients with a very high ESR (i.e., Westergren greater than 100 mm/h) have obvious malignancy, severe infection, or connective tissue disease. In the patient with malignancy, a very high ESR usually indicates metastasis. If the cause of a very high ESR is not apparent, a protein electrophoresis is indicated because myeloma is a common cause of a very high value.

The ESR is nearly always elevated (usually greater than 50 mm/h) in patients with temporal arteritis and polymyalgia rheumatica. However, if clinical evidence

Table 17-10. Values for Westergren Sedimentation Rate

Age	Male (mm/h)	Age	Female (mm/h)
<25	0–10	<15	0–10
26–35	0–15	15–25	0–15
36–45	0–20	26–35	0–20
46–55	0–25	36–45	0–25
>55	0–30	>55	0–35

is strong, a patient with suspected temporal arteritis should have an artery biopsy or trial of steroids, because a normal ESR has rarely been reported. Although the ESR has been used to monitor disease activity and to adjust steroid dose in temporal arteritis and polymyagia rheumatica, the clinical status of the patient also should be considered. An elevation of ESR is evidence of relapse in Hodgkin's disease if other causes of inflammation or infection have been eliminated from consideration.

TESTS FOR MICROCYTIC ANEMIA

Test: Ferritin[1,7,10,15-19]

Background and Selection

Ferritin consists of a spherical protein shell (apoferritin) filled with an iron complex that contains up to 4000 iron molecules. It provides a form of readily available storage iron. Because free iron is toxic within cells, ferritin is present in all cells to protect against damage from uncomplexed iron. Ferritin is most abundantly present in macrophages of the liver, spleen, and bone marrow and in hepatic parenchymal cells. In healthy persons, serum ferritin concentration reflects the magnitude of body iron stores; 1 µg of ferritin per liter equals approximately 8–10 mg (1.4–1.8 mmol) of total body storage iron. As the iron content of tissue rises, ferritin molecules aggregate to form insoluble hemosiderin.

Serum ferritin is the best single test for the diagnosis of iron deficiency. Thus, it is important in the evaluation of microcytosis or microcytic anemia. It is also an appropriate test in the assessment of any unexplained anemia, because the earlier stages of iron deficiency do not have a low MCV (Table 17-11). The importance of obtaining a ferritin result to confirm possible iron deficiency depends on the clinical situation. Iron deficiency is particularly common during periods of rapid growth (e.g., in children aged 6 months to 4 years), in pregnancy, and in menstrual-age females. In these clinical settings, the physician may elect to follow the patient response to iron therapy. Apart from these groups, it is generally advisable to confirm iron deficiency by low ferritin. The presence of iron deficiency suggests gastrointestinal blood loss, which, in turn, may be an indication for an expensive and lengthy evaluation of the gastrointestinal tract. Serum ferritin testing is useful in renal failure, in which diminished kidney erythropoietin and transfusion lead to increased iron stores, but dialysis and gastrointestinal bleeding may diminish stores.

The role of ferritin in detection of idiopathic hemochromatosis is less well established. The finding of an elevated serum iron and percentage saturation above 60% is a more sensitive test, because serum ferritin may be normal in precirrhotic hemochromatosis. In addition, ferritin may be elevated in acute and chronic inflammation, but this situation produces a low, rather than high serum iron and percentage saturation. Ferritin is probably a sensitive guide to hemosiderosis in transfusion dependent anemias and may be used to

Table 17-11. Sequential Development of Iron Deficiency Anemia

	Iron Depletion	Iron Deficient Erythropoiesis	Iron Deficiency Anemia
Marrow iron stores	Decreased	Absent	Absent
Ferritin	Decreased	Decreased	Decreased
Serum iron	Normal	Decreased	Decreased
TIBC	Normal	Increased	Increased
% saturation	Normal	<15%	<10%
Erythrocyte protoporphyrin	Normal	Increased	Increased
Anemia	None–mild	Mild–moderate	Moderate–marked
Indices	Normal	Increased RDW; low–normal MCV	Increased RDW; decreased MCV; decreased MCHC as progresses
RBC morphology	Normal	Mild microcytosis	Microcytic/hypochromic; poikilocytosis as progresses

MCHC, mean cell hemoglobin concentration; MCV, mean cell volume; RBC, red blood cell; RDW, red blood cell distribution width; TIBC, total iron binding concentration.
(Modified from Sun,[34] with permission.)

monitor progressive iron accumulation in such iron-loading disorders as thalassemia major and sideroblastic anemia and to determine the response to treatment with chelation agents.

Logistics

Serum is required and is stable when refrigerated for 2 days or for longer periods when frozen. Grossly hemolyzed specimens may give erroneous results. Ferritin is measured with an immunoradiometric or immunoenzymatic sandwich assay.

Interpretation

The upper limit for the reference range is approximately 200 ng/mL (200 µg/L) in children, adolescents, and menstruating women and 300 ng/mL (300 µg/L) for men and postmenopausal women. In general, ferritin levels less than 12 ng/mL (12 µg/L) indicate absent iron stores in children, adolescents, and menstruating women, whereas ferritin levels of less than 20 ng/mL (20 µg/L) are seen with absent iron stores in men and postmenopausal women.

Decreases

A low serum ferritin is diagnostic of iron deficiency. Because serum ferritin generally reflects body iron stores, it steadily falls as iron stores are depleted. Thus, ferritin may be diminished before serum iron and percentage transferrin saturation decrease and before anemia is present (Table 17-11). Using ferritin results, the microcytic hypochromic anemias can be differentiated into iron deficiency anemia (low ferritin), anemia of chronic disease (normal to high ferritin), and thalassemia (normal in thalassemia trait, high in thalassemia major), as shown in Table 17-2. Iron therapy rapidly raises ferritin levels, which, in some patients, can re-

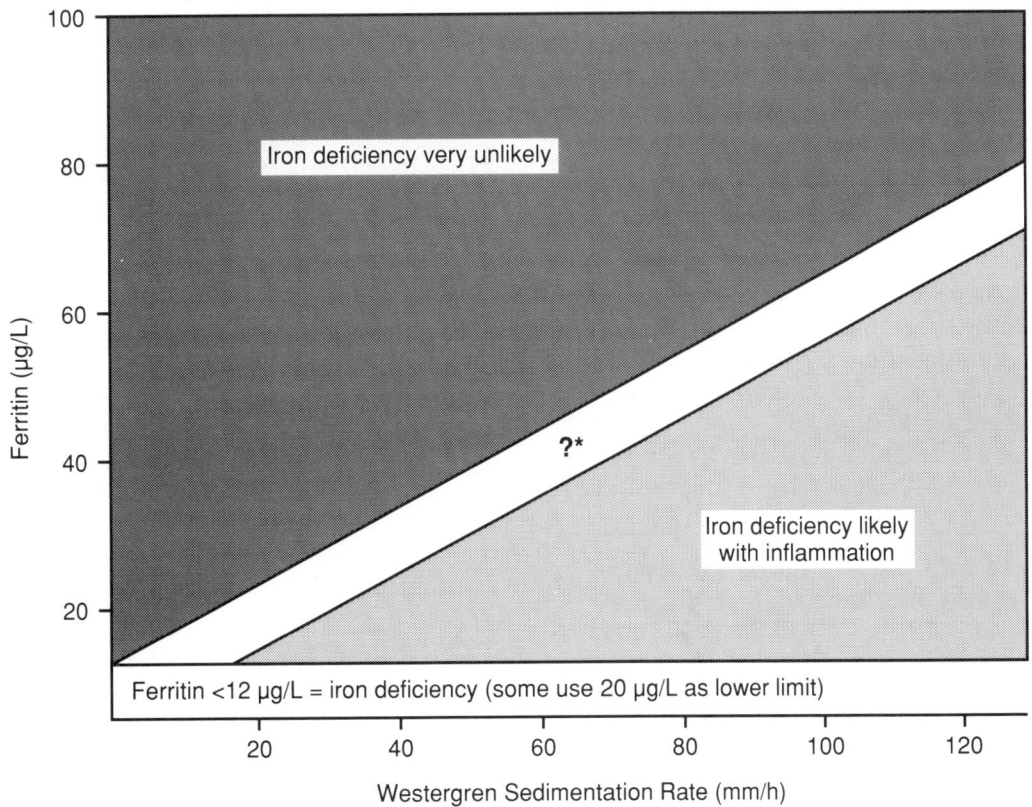

Fig. 17-6. Iron deficiency in inflammatory disorders. ?*, indeterminate—iron deficiency neither established nor excluded. (From Witte et al.,[19] with permission.)

turn to the reference range within 1–3 days. The clinician can monitor the serum ferritin level at intervals of 3–4 weeks; iron therapy should be continued until serum ferritin rises above 50 ng/mL (50 µg/L), a level consistent with body iron stores of about 400–500 mg (72–90 mmol).

Ferritin is an acute phase reactant, rising with infection, inflammation, and some forms of cancer. Increased ferritin synthesis can occur within 2 days and may last several weeks. Inflammatory states serve as a stimulus for continued ferritin synthesis by macrophages and the relationship of serum ferritin levels to stored body iron may be distorted. Likewise, in hepatocellular disease, or certain neoplasms with high levels of ferritin (e.g., leukemia and lymphoma), release from damaged cells can greatly elevate serum ferritin. Thus, in the presence of inflammatory disease, many malignancies, or liver disease, a normal ferritin level does not exclude concomitant iron deficiency. An attempt has been made to use the sedimentation rate to define ferritin levels reflecting iron deficiency for various degrees of inflammatory stimulation, as shown in Figure 17-6. However, many variables affect the sedimentation rate, including age, sex, and the degree of anemia. Such nomograms can only serve as a rough guideline. In addition, studies relating ferritin levels to bone marrow iron content in various chronic inflammatory disorders and renal disease (with the exclusion of liver disease) suggest that ferritin levels may be interpreted as in Table 17-12.

In the situation in which chronic inflammation is present with a high sedimentation rate and the ferritin value is nondiagnostic, iron and total iron binding concentration (TIBC) are rarely helpful. A trial of iron therapy can be initiated, but failure to respond does not exclude iron deficiency. The definitive test is a bone marrow, stained for hemosiderin stores. The importance of establishing the diagnosis needs to be weighed against the pain, risk, and expense of this procedure.

Table 17-12. Ferritin Levels in Chronic Inflammatory Disorders and Renal Disease[1]

Ferritin Levels (ng/mL)[a]	Status of Iron Stores
<30	Depleted
30–50	Probably depleted
50–100	Uncertain
>100	Present

[a] Conventional units are ng/mL, SI units are µg/L; the conversion factor is 1.
(Data from Rapaport.[1])

Iron deficiency in men or postmenopausal women requires further investigation to determine the source of blood loss. External bleeding such as epistaxis, hemorrhoids, or blood donations can be identified by patient history. Occult blood loss from adenocarcinoma of the gastrointestinal tract can be evaluated by performing stool guaiac tests and, if indicated, radiographic and endoscopy examinations. Unusual causes of iron deficiency include malabsorption (sprue or postgastrectomy state), hemosidinuria (intravascular hemolysis), or pulmonary hemosiderosis. In the latter two disorders, hemosiderin may be detected in the renal tubular cells of the urinary sediment or the sputum macrophages with Prussian blue stain.

Increases

Elevated ferritin is associated with acute or chronic infection and inflammatory disease, liver disease, malignancy, hemolytic anemia, anemias with ineffective erythropoiesis (e.g., sideroblastic anemia, megaloblastic anemia, thalassemia major), and iron overload (hemochromatosis, hemosiderosis). Periodic measurement of ferritin is occasionally used to document diminishing iron stores with phlebotomy treatment of iron overload; ferritin levels should be within the reference range with successful iron depletion.

Test: Iron, Total Iron Binding Capacity, and Transferrin (Iron Profile; FE, TIBC, and % Saturation)[1,7,10,15–17,20]

Background and Selection

Transferrin, a β_1-globulin, is the transporting protein for iron in the plasma. Transferrin carries the iron from macrophages, where iron is released after the breakdown of old RBCs, or from the intestines, where iron is absorbed. In the bone marrow, the transferrin-iron complex attaches to a transferrin receptor on the surface of the developing RBC. When this complex enters the cell by endocytosis, the iron is released, and the transferrin is returned to the plasma.

Transferrin is a glycoprotein with a single polypeptide chain synthesized by the liver. It is capable of carrying two iron molecules; 100 mL of plasma contains sufficient transferrin to combine with 300 µg of iron but is normally one-third saturated.

Levels of iron in serum are very labile. The amount of serum iron is regulated by the rate of absorption from the gastrointestinal tract and by the exchange with ferritin or hemosiderin stores in reticuloendothelial cells or hepatocytes. A rapid decrease in iron can occur with leukocyte activation. Release of a leukocyte endogenous mediator, interleukin-1 (IL-1), is thought to lead to retention of iron by the reticuloendothelial cells (Fig. 17-2). In addition, serum iron may decrease transiently when there is a sudden burst of erythropoiesis (e.g., immediately after treatment of a patient with vitamin B_{12} or folate deficiency).

Serum iron, TIBC and/or transferrin, and percentage saturation are generally ordered together. In the past, measurement of serum iron and TIBC have been the most important diagnostic tests for the confirmation of iron deficiency and for distinguishing iron deficiency from anemia of chronic disease. This combination is still widely used and is of value, but the ferritin determination is a better test for this purpose. (See Test: Ferritin, Background and Selection, for further discussion of circumstances in which iron deficiency is suspected.)

Increased iron and percentage saturation by iron of the TIBC are sensitive indicators of hemochromatosis and should be ordered when this disorder is a consideration. Measurement of iron before and after a Schilling test for pernicious anemia may be of value in the untreated patient. A marked drop after administration of vitamin B_{12} in the Schilling test is evidence of enhanced erythropoiesis and supports the diagnosis of B_{12} deficiency. Iron measurements are important in evaluating toxic iron ingestion (see Ch. 10). Transferrin is decreased in protein malnutrition and transferrin levels may be requested as part of a nutrition panel.

Terminology

When transferrin protein is directly measured by immunoassay, the result is expressed in mg/dL transferrin (SI units, g/L). However, in iron studies, transferrin is measured by its iron binding capacity, or TIBC. A TIBC of 300 µg/dL (54 µmol/L) corresponds to transferrin protein concentration of approximately 250 mg/dL (2.5 g/L). The percentage saturation refers to the calculation of the percentage of transferrin iron binding sites occupied with iron.

Logistics

Serum iron concentration shows marked diurnal variation, with morning values approximately 30% higher than values later in the day. References ranges are usually established with fasting morning blood specimens. The patient should not have received therapeutic iron-containing medications for at least 24 hours. Recent blood transfusion is an equivocal contraindication; it may be advisable to delay testing for several days. Blood for iron determination should be the first tube collected, as contamination by any anticoagulant may invalidate the results. The serum should be separated from the RBCs within 1 hour. Serum is stable for at least 1 week in the refrigerator, and for at least 1 month if frozen. Large amounts of RBC hemolysis may elevate serum iron.

Serum iron is disassociated from transferrin and reduced to the ferrous state by an acid solution, then bound to a chromophobe, such as bathophenanthroline, which changes color in the presence of iron. Total iron binding capacity is determined by adding an excess of iron to the patient's serum, completely saturating the transferrin. Excess free ferric ions are removed by a column or chelator. Acid is added to the serum with saturated TIBC, and iron is colorimetrically determined. Alternatively, some methods measure the portion of added iron that is not bound to TIBC and calculate the TIBC by subtraction. Percentage saturation is calculated by dividing the iron by the TIBC.

Interpretation

Typical reference ranges are found in Table 17-13. Serum iron is decreased in iron deficiency (in which body iron stores are depleted) and in acute and chronic infections and inflammatory states (in which release of iron from macrophages is impaired). Typically, in well established iron deficiency, the serum iron is low, the TIBC is elevated, and the percentage saturation is less than 15%. In inflammatory states, both iron and TIBC fall, and the saturation of transferrin may be greater than 15% (Tables 17-2 and 17-11). In actual practice, many cases of both iron deficiency and inflammatory states show low serum iron, normal TIBC, and percentage saturation of less than 15%. Thus iron/TIBC measurements frequently cannot differentiate between iron deficiency and anemia of chronic disease. A serum ferritin may be more helpful in making this differentia-

Table 17-13. Reference Ranges for Iron, TIBC, and Transferrin

	Conventional Units	SI Units
Iron	50–150 µg/dL	(9–27 µmol/L)
TIBC	270–400 µg/dL	(48–72 µmol/L)
Transferrin	200–350 mg/dL	(2–3.5 g/L)
% saturation	20–50%	

Abbreviation: TIBC, total iron binding capacity.

tion. If the ferritin value is inconclusive, a bone marrow stain for iron stores may be worthwhile, depending on the clinical situation. (Causes of iron deficiency and subsequent investigation are discussed in Interpretation, under Test: Ferritin.)

A dramatic and rapid fall in serum iron may be seen with acute inflammation or infection. Within 24 hours, low iron values may be seen after myocardial infarction, extensive surgery, multiple trauma, massive blood loss, and severe systemic infection. This decrease may persist for several weeks. Low iron values also may be seen when there is a sudden burst of erythropoiesis and sudden removal of plasma iron. For example, iron falls dramatically shortly after treatment of vitamin B_{12} deficiency.

Serum TIBC (and transferrin) may be low in protein depletion. This may occur with malnutrition, renal disease, and liver disease. Increased iron and percentage saturation (more than 62% in males, more than 50% in females) is a useful clue to the possibility of idiopathic (primary hereditary) hemochromatosis, which is present in approximately 1% of adult men. However, an increase also may be seen in cirrhosis, hemolytic anemia, with transfusion therapy of chronic anemia, and in anemias with ineffective erythropoiesis (thalassemia major and intermedia, sideroblastic anemia). Secondary hemochromatosis, or deposition of large amounts of iron in tissue parenymal as well as reticuloendothelial cells may occur particularly in patients with anemias of ineffective erythropoiesis with repeated transfusion. In some cases of hemochromatosis, the percentage saturation exceeds 100%, generally within the range of 110% but can be as high as 140%. It has been suggested that this indicates free iron or in vitro dissociation of iron from serum ferritin during the assay. The definitive test for diagnosing hemochromatosis is the liver biopsy with demonstration of stainable iron in hepatic parenchymal cells.

Test: Protoporphyrin, Erythrocyte (Free Erythrocyte Porphyrin, FEP, Zinc Protoporphyrin, ZnPP)[1,7,15,21]

Background and Selection

Iron is added to the protoporphyrin molecule within the mitochondria of the developing RBC to form heme. Ferrochelatase, normally bound to the inner cristae of the mitochondria, catalyzes this reaction and is inhibited with lead toxicity. In the presence of iron deficiency or lead poisoning, erythrocyte protoporphyrin accumulates and remains elevated throughout the 120-day life span of the RBC. The term free erythrocyte protoporphyrin is often incorrectly used for this iron-free protoporphyrin, which is bound to the Hgb molecule in the form of a zinc protoporphyrin.

Erythrocyte protoporphyrin can be measured on a single drop of blood and can provide a rapid screening test in children to detect iron deficiency or lead poisoning. In patients with a low MCV, it can differentiate iron deficiency (high values) from thalassemia (normal values).

Logistics

A single drop of blood is required, which may be placed directly on a coverslip or collected in EDTA. EDTA-anticoagulated blood is stable for 1 day at room temperature and 1 week in a dark refrigerator (light may gradually degrade the protoporphyrin).

Red blood cell zinc protoporphyrin fluoresces and may be determined directly by a portable filter fluorometer with front-face optics (hematofluorometer). A single drop of blood is placed on a coverslip, mixed with a stick to ensure oxygenation, and inserted into the instrument. The instrument incorporates internal standards and performs computerized calculations to provide an instant assay result.

False positive results occur with high serum bilirubin and plasma Hgb. In these situations, the RBCs can be washed, resuspended in saline, and reassayed. Falsely elevated values can also occur with fingerprints on the coverslide and within 24 hours of high doses of riboflavin. Failure to mix the blood thoroughly to reoxygenate an anticoagulated sample can give erroneously low readings.

Interpretation

The reference range is less than 35 μg/dL ($<$350 μg/L) for determinations performed on whole blood. Values in the range of 35–60 μg/dL (350–600 μg/L) are seen in iron deficiency. As a test for iron deficiency, erythrocyte protoporphyrin is not as sensitive or specific as decreased ferritin. As with serum iron and TIBC, it may remain normal in iron deficient erythropoiesis, before microcytosis or anemia is apparent (Table 17-11). Because the protoporphyrin level of RBCs persists throughout their life span, the aggregate erythrocyte protoporphyrin level of whole blood does not rise until iron deficient erythropoiesis has persisted for several weeks, and it does not return to normal for several weeks after iron therapy. Thus, erythrocyte protoporphyrin levels are not subject to dramatic changes with acute inflammatory events, as are iron, TIBC, and ferritin. However, persistent impaired iron availability for reticuloendothelial cells in chronic disease causes elevated erythrocyte protoporphyrin levels. Modest elevations also may be seen in hemolytic anemias, sideroblastic anemias, and secondary polycythemia.

Erythrocyte protoporphyrin is an excellent screening test for chronic lead exposure. It is consistently elevated with blood lead levels above 50 µg/dL (>500 µg/L), with values often in excess of 100 µg/dL (>1000 µg/L) whole blood. Extremely high levels of erythrocyte protoporphyrin can also be found in erythrocyte protoporphyria, a rare congenital disorder with prominent cutaneous photosensitivity.

TESTS FOR MACROCYTIC ANEMIA

Test: B_{12} (Vitamin B_{12}, Cobalamin)[1,6,10,22-26] (See Ch. 10)

Background and Selection

Cobalamins are compounds with a corrin ring group surrounding a cobalt atom and a connected nucleotide (5,6-dimethylbenzimidazole). Vitamin B_{12} is a stable form of cobalamin with cyanide attached to the cobalt atom (cyanocobalamin). In vivo, the active cobalamins are methylcobalamin (methyl group ligand) and adenosylcobalamin (5'-deoxyadenosyl ligand). Methylcobalamin is the coenzyme for methionine synthetase, which, in the presence of N^5-methyl tetrahyrofolate, converts homocysteine to methionine. Adenosylcobalamin is the coenzyme for methyl malonyl CoA mutase, which converts methyl malonyl-coenzyme A to succinyl-coenzyme A.

Lack of cobalamin with blockage of methionine metabolism interferes with cell utilization of folate for reactions involved in DNA synthesis; folate becomes trapped as N^5-methyl tetrahydrofolate and cannot be recycled to N^5,N^{10}-methylene tetrahydrofolate, the form needed to convert deoxyuridilate to thymidylate for use in DNA synthesis. In addition, the methyl group of methionine is not available for formation of the folate derivatives that can be converted from a monoglutamate (the soluble form of folate entering the cell) to a polyglutamate (the insoluble form of folate that can be retained by the cell). Thus, with lack of cobalamin, the cells are depleted of folate.

Humans cannot synthesize cobalamin and obtain it by eating animal protein in meat, poultry, fish, and dairy products. Only small amounts (5 µg/d) are required, and most people store an approximately 5-year supply in the liver. Dietary cobalamin is released from food by peptic acid. Binding to intrinsic factor, a glycoprotein secreted by the gastric parietal cells, is necessary for absorption in the terminal ileum. In addition, saliva, gastric juice, and intestinal fluid contain R proteins, proteins that are similar in structure to intrinsic factor but with more rapid electrophoretic mobility. These R proteins compete for cobalamin in the stomach but, unlike intrinsic factor, liberate bound cobalamin in the intestine when digested by trypsin. Cobalamin stores in the liver are released and transported to tissues or secreted into bile with reabsorption in the small intestine (enterohepatic cycle). With defective absorption in the ileum, liver stores may be more rapidly depleted.

In the plasma, cobalamin is bound by proteins transcobalamin I and transcobalamin II. Transcobalamin II (produced in the liver) is the important carrier for transport into the cells, whereas transcobalamin I (an R protein synthesized by granulocytes) is a passive reservoir. Some individuals may have high plasma concentrations of cobalamin analogues that are metabolically inactive. These analogues bind to transcobalamin I and other R proteins but bind poorly to transcobalamin II or intrinsic factor.

Cobalamin deficiency leads to two major clinical syndromes. Impaired DNA synthesis (through disturbances in folate metabolism) results in defective proliferation of all rapidly dividing cells, including erythrocytes (megaloblastic erythropoiesis). In addition, a variety of neurologic symptoms occur, but it is yet unclear how metabolic reactions involving vitamin B_{12} cause neuropathy.

Serum B_{12} determination is appropriate for patients with an unexplained anemia, primarily when a high MCV or population of macrocytes is present. Neutropenia with hypersegmented neutrophils and thrombocytopenia may also be seen in vitamin B_{12} deficiency, as well as biochemical signs of ineffective erythropoiesis, such as increased indirect bilirubin and increased lactate dehydrogenase (LD). Because similar hematologic findings occur with folate deficiency, vitamin B_{12} and folate levels are often ordered simultaneously. Vitamin B_{12} results may be necessary for appropriate interpretation of RBC folate, because vitamin B_{12} deficiency depletes tissue folate. Although it was previously thought that vitamin B_{12} deficiency first presented with anemia and progressed to a neurologic disorder, many studies have suggested that neurologic damage may often precede hematologic changes. Thus, vitamin B_{12} assay is useful in patients with a variety of neurologic disorders, including paresthesias of hands and feet, loss of proprioception and vibratory sensation, and more subtle disturbances, such as somnambulance and problems with taste, smell, or vision. Severe psychological and mental derangements can occasionally occur as a result of vitamin B_{12} deficiency. The most common cause of vitamin B_{12} deficiency, pernicious anemia, is an autoimmune disorder associated with gastric atrophy and loss of intrinsic factor. The presence of other autoimmune disorders strongly associated with pernicious anemia, such as hypothyroidism and vitiligo, may be an indication for ordering the vitamin B_{12} test. In addition, methionine synthetase may be inhibited by prolonged exposure to the anesthetic gas NO_2, precipitating symptoms in patients with borderline vitamin B_{12} deficiency.

Logistics

A fasting serum specimen is preferred. Blood should be drawn before therapy with vitamin B_{12}, transfusion, or administration of radioactive tracers. Serum should be frozen within 2 hours. Analysis is performed by competitive binding radioimmunoassay (RIA) using cobalt 57-labeled B_{12}. Older assays frequently gave spuriously high results by using R proteins rather than purified intrinsic factor as the binding protein. These R proteins also bound inactive cobalamin analogues present in high concentration in some patient samples.

Interpretation

The reference range may vary with different reagents but is generally 200–800 ng/L (150–590 pmol/L). Results below 100 ng/L (<75 pmol/L) are considered deficient and are generally accompanied by macrocytic anemia and/or neurologic disturbances, whereas 100–200 ng/L (75–150 pmol/L) is considered borderline. Some patients with only neurologic symptoms have been seen with borderline serum vitamin B_{12} values and demonstrated pernicious anemia (by Schilling test or intrinsic factor antibodies). In view of the severe yet preventable consequences of vitamin B_{12} deficiency, further investigation and a trial of therapy in patients with borderline results are recommended.

Interpretation of vitamin B_{12} levels is usually considered in conjunction with serum and RBC folate (Table 17-14). In typical vitamin B_{12} deficiency, serum vitamin B_{12} is decreased, levels of RBC folate are decreased (caused by an inability of tissues to retain folate in an insoluble form in the absence of vitamin B_{12}), and serum folate is normal to increased. If serum folate is also decreased, considerations include combined folate and vitamin B_{12} deficiency (which would occur with malabsorption) or a recent diet deficient in folate. However, for unknown reasons, an occasional patient with folate deficiency also may have a decreased vitamin B_{12} level. In addition, low levels of vitamin B_{12} have been seen in transcobalamin I deficiency, in pregnancy, and in multiple myeloma.

A diagnosis of vitamin B_{12} deficiency may be confirmed by therapeutic trial, using a physiologic replacement dose (10 μg parenterally). Brisk reticulocytosis should begin on the third day and peak by the seventh day. Normoblastic erythropoiesis is seen by 2 days, and hypersegmented neutrophils disappear in 2 weeks.

Table 17-15 shows the causes of vitamin B_{12} deficiency. A Schilling test, with and without intrinsic factor, is the next diagnostic test that should be performed. Pernicious anemia, with gastric atrophy and failure to secrete intrinsic factor, is the most common cause of vitamin B_{12} deficiency. Testing for serum antibodies to intrinsic factor also may be useful in establishing this diagnosis. Concomitant iron deficiency is often masked in patients with vitamin B_{12} deficiency and may particularly become apparent with the brisk erythropoiesis that follows vitamin B_{12} replacement therapy. Increased serum vitamin B_{12} may be seen in any cause of release of transcobalamin I binding protein, including increased granulocytes (myeloproliferative disorders, leukemoid reaction) and liver disease.

Table 17-14. Interpretation of Folate/Vitamin B_{12} Testing

Disorder	Serum Vitamin B_{12}	Serum Folate	RBC Folate
Vitamin B_{12} deficiency	Decreased	Normal to increased	Decreased
Folate deficiency	Usually normal (Occasionally decreased)	Usually decreased (may be normal with recent dietary intake)	Decreased
Combined vitamin B_{12}/folate deficiency	Decreased	Usually decreased (may be normal with recent dietary intake)	Decreased

(Data from Rapaport.[1])

Table 17-15. Vitamin B_{12} Deficiency — Schilling Test

Site of Defect	Causes of Deficiency	Initial	With Intrinsic Factor
Oral intake	Dietary: strict vegetarian	Normal	—
Stomach (source of intrinsic factor)	Pernicious anemia Gastric surgery Extensive carcinoma	Low	Normal
	Inability to "separate" B_{12} from food	Normal	—
Proximal small intestine	Jejunal diverticula Blind loop syndromes (bacteria ingest B_{12})	Low	Low
Mid-small intestine	*Diphyllobothrium latum* (ingests B_{12})	Low	Low

Distal ileum	Regional ileitis
	Surgical resection
	Malabsorption
	    Nontropical sprue
	    Tropical sprue
		Low	Low

Kidney	Failure to excrete absorbed radioactive B_{12}	Low	Low

Test: Folate (Serum and Red Blood Cell Folic Acid)[1,5,10,23,24,26–28]

Background and Selection

Folic acid contains a pteridine double ring attached to paraminobenzoate, with one to nine molecules of glutamic acid. The reduced form, tetrahydrofolate, participates in metabolic reactions involving transfer of single carbon units. One such reaction, the methylation of deoxyuridilate to thymidylate, is essential for DNA synthesis in tissues that rapidly produce new cells. Thus tissue folate deficiency results in defective proliferation of all rapidly dividing cells, including erythrocytes (megaloblastic erythropoiesis).

Folates are found in fresh green vegetables, fruits, beans, nuts (including peanut butter), liver, and kidney. Rapid loss of the vitamin occurs with prolonged cooking or heating for canning. The daily requirement is 50–100 µg but increases in pregnancy to 400 µg. Unlike vitamin B_{12}, body stores in the liver last only a few weeks in patients with very low folate intake.

Folates in food are polyglutamates that are broken down by intestinal mucosal conjugase enzymes to more soluble monoglutamates before absorption. In addition, folate is converted to N^5-methyl tetrahydrofolate as it is transported through the mucosal cell. This form of folate circulates in the plasma free, or loosely bound to albumin, and rapidly enters the tissues. For folate to remain in the tissues, it must be reconverted to the insoluble polyglutamate form, a process that requires the presence of vitamin B_{12}. In addition, vitamin B_{12} is required to obtain N^5,N^{10}-methylene tetrahydrofolate, the form needed to convert deoxyuridilate to thymidylate for use in DNA synthesis.

Utilization of liver stores of folate involves excretion into the bile and reabsorption by the jejunum (enterohepatic circulation). Thus diseases of the small intestine or inhibitory drugs not only decrease absorption of folate from the diet but prevent utilization of body stores. Alcohol intake can impair release of folate from the liver into bile, resulting in a rapid fall in serum folate levels.

Serum and RBC folate determinations are appropriate for patients with an unexplained anemia, primarily when a high MCV or population of macrocytes is present. Neutropenia with hypersegmented neutrophils and thrombocytopenia may also be seen in folate deficiency, as well as biochemical signs of ineffective erythropoiesis (increased indirect bilirubin, increased LD). Changes with progression of folate deficiency are shown in Table 17-16. Because similar hematologic

Table 17-16. Progression of Folate Deficiency

Onset (wk)	Abnormality
2	Low serum folate
10	Hypersegmentation of neutrophils
17	Low RBC folate
18	Macroovalocytes
19	Megaloblastic marrow
20	Anemia
≥20	MCV elevated

Abbreviations: MCV, mean cell volume; RBC, red blood cell. (Data from Herbert.[28])

Table 17-17. Causes of Folate Deficiency

Mechanism	Specific Problem
Inadequate intake (lack of green vegetables, fresh fruit)	Chronic alcoholism
	Elderly
	Infants with diarrhea or infection
	Heavily cooked food (seen in India)
Decreased absorption (occurs in jejunum)	Nontropical sprue
	Tropical sprue (responds dramatically to folate treatment)
	Regional enteritis
	Lymphoma of small bowel
	Whipple's disease
	Amyloidosis
	Diabetes and malabsorption
	Extensive intestinal resection
Increased utilization	Pregnancy
	Chronic hemolysis
	Neoplastic disease
	Severe exfoliative dermatitis
Drugs that impair folate absorption	Dilantin (and other anticonvulsants)
	Sulfasalizine
	Isoniazid, cycloserine
	Oral contraceptives (rarely)
Drugs that interfere with folate metabolism	Methotrexate
	Pyrimethamine (antimalarial)
	Trimethoprim (Bactrim, Septra)
Inborn errors of folate metabolism	Rare cases of congenital enzyme deficiencies that may or may not respond to folate therapy

(Data from Williams et al.[7])

findings occur with vitamin B_{12} deficiency, serum B_{12} and serum and RBC folate levels are usually ordered simultaneously. The vitamin B_{12} value may be necessary for appropriate interpretation of RBC folate, because vitamin B_{12} deficiency will deplete tissue folate. In addition, folate deficiency may be suspected from the appropriate clinical setting (Table 17-17), including pregnancy, hemolytic disorders, malabsorption, deficient diet, and alcoholism.

Terminology

Folate is an inclusive name for folic acid and its derivatives. The reduced form, tetrahydrofolate, is the active coenzyme and can have methyl, methylene, formyl, or forminino groups bound to the N^5 or N^{10} positions. One or more glutamic acid residues may be attached.

Logistics

Folate is measured by ligand assays using milk protein as the binder.

For serum folate a fasting sample is preferred. With hospitalized patients, obtaining the specimen on admission is important, as dietary replenishment can rapidly raise serum folate levels. The patient should not receive transfusion, folate therapy, or radioisotope before specimen collection. Serum for folate should be immediately separated and frozen. Hemolysis and prolonged exposure to light must be avoided.

For the red blood cell folate test the patient should not receive transfusion or radioisotope before sample collection. EDTA-anticoagulated blood is collected and transported on ice and the Hct is determined. A hemolysate of 0.5 mL EDTA blood and 4.5 mL ascorbic acid solution is prepared on receipt into the laboratory and immediately frozen. From the recorded Hct, RBC folate is calculated per mL of RBCs. Correction can be made for serum folate, but this is usually ignored unless the RBC folate is very low and the serum level is high.

Interpretation

The reference range for serum folate is 3–15 μg/L (7–24 mmol/L) and for RBC folate is 200–800 μg/L (400–1800 mmol/L). Serum folate levels must be interpreted with caution. A low serum folate means that the recent supply of folate has been subnormal but does not constitute evidence for tissue folate deficiency. Conversely, tissue folate deficiency may exist, but serum folate can be normal as a result of recent dietary sufficiency.

Low levels of RBC folate provide evidence of tissue folate deficiency. However, vitamin B_{12} deficiency may also lead to low tissue folate levels. Thus, interpretation of vitamin B_{12} levels is often considered in conjunction with serum and RBC folate (Table 17-14), particularly when pernicious anemia is a consideration in older patients. In typical folate deficiency, serum and RBC folate levels are decreased, whereas vitamin B_{12} levels are normal. In folate deficiency with recent dietary intake, serum folate results are within the reference range, RBC folate decreased, and serum vitamin B_{12} within the reference range. In vitamin B_{12} deficiency, serum B_{12} is decreased, levels of RBC folate are decreased (caused by the inability of tissues to retain folate in an insoluble form in the absence of vitamin B_{12}), and serum folate is within the reference range or is increased. If all three laboratory tests are decreased, considerations include combined folate and vitamin B_{12} deficiency (which would occur with malabsorption) or vitamin B_{12} deficiency with a recent diet deficient in folate. However, for unknown reasons, an occasional patient with folate deficiency also may have decreased serum B_{12}. In anemic patients with unclear laboratory results, a diagnosis of folate deficiency may be confirmed by therapeutic trial using a physiologic replacement dose of folic acid (100–200 µg parenterally). Brisk reticulocytosis should begin on the third day and peak by the seventh day. Bone marrow erythropoiesis becomes normoblastic by 2 days, although peripheral blood macrocytes and hypersegmented neutrophils take much longer to disappear. Larger therapeutic doses of folic acid should not be used until the absence of vitamin B_{12} deficiency has been established, because a megaloblastic anemia caused by vitamin B_{12} deficiency will respond to large doses of folic acid, but neurologic damage may still progress.

Table 17-17 shows the causes of folate deficiency. Once folate deficiency is established, the specific cause can generally be suspected on the basis of clinical history. Tropical sprue should be considered in patients from the Caribbean or Southeast Asia; after treatment with folic acid, studies for malabsorption can be performed.

Test: Schilling Test (B_{12} Absorption Test)[1,3,7,24,29] (See Ch. 5)

Background and Selection

The Schilling test, named after its originator, measures the absorption of radioactively labeled vitamin B_{12} with and without intrinsic factor. A Schilling test is indicated in patients with low serum B_{12} (less than 100 ng/L [75 pmol/L]) to determine the cause of deficiency (i.e., pernicious anemia versus intestinal malabsorption). It is also useful in patients with borderline serum B_{12} levels (100–200 ng/L [75–150 pmol/L]), particularly when neurologic symptoms are present. The Schilling test also may be performed in patients with a questionable diagnosis of pernicious anemia who are receiving vitamin B_{12} therapy.

Logistics

The patient should be fasting and should receive no vitamin B_{12} for 3 days before the test. Radioisotopic scans performed before the test should be avoided. The test measures the amount of vitamin B_{12} absorbed by measuring the percentage of an oral dose secreted in a 24-hour urine specimen. A small amount of radiolabeled vitamin B_{12} is given orally, followed 2 hours later by a large parenteral dose of nonradioactive vitamin B_{12}. The cold loading dose saturates the vitamin B_{12} binding proteins in the serum, resulting in the rapid excretion of oral radioactive vitamin B_{12}. The total radioactivity in the 24-hour urine specimen is measured and compared to the total radioactivity of the oral dose of vitamin B_{12}. The ratio is expressed as a percentage.

When the test is abnormal, it may be repeated with porcine intrinsic factor. Because cobalamin deficiency itself may lead to gastrointestinal mucosal dysfunction and malabsorption, the patient should be treated with parenteral vitamin B_{12} for several weeks before performing the Schilling test with intrinsic factor. If bacteria overgrowth is suspected (blind loop syndrome), the patient can be retested after antibiotic therapy. Valid results will not be obtained in patients with renal dysfunction or with incomplete collection of the 24-hour urine specimen.

Interpretation

Usually, more than 7% of the ingested radioactivity is excreted in the urine. When absorption is impaired, less than 3% is recovered. Correction of vitamin B_{12} absorption by addition of intrinsic factor is evidence for pernicious anemia or other gastric abnormalities resulting in lack of intrinsic factor production. Intestinal malabsorption of vitamin B_{12} is not corrected with administration of intrinsic factor (Table 17-15).

Some investigators advocate a modified Schilling test, in which the radioactive B_{12} is administered with food (e.g., eggs). Patients with the gastric atrophy of pernicious anemia may lose the ability to split vitamin B_{12}

from the peptide bonds in food before the complete loss of intrinsic factor. Thus, the food Schilling test may be more sensitive in detecting early development of pernicious anemia. Defective absorption of protein-bound cobalamin, with normal absorption of the unbound cobalamin in the Schilling test, may also be seen after partial gastrectomy or vagotomy, or in patients with gastric ulcer or cimetidine therapy. Testing for serum antibodies to intrinsic factor may also be useful in establishing the diagnosis of pernicious anemia.

Test: Deoxyuridine Suppression[1,6,24]

The deoxyuridine suppression test measures the ability of peripheral blood or bone marrow lymphocytes to use deoxyuridine in DNA synthesis, which is dependent on adequate vitamin B_{12} and folate supply. Lymphocytes are incubated with radioactive thymidine and nonradioactive deoxyuridine. Normally, DNA synthesis uses deoxyuridine. With vitamin B_{12} or folate deficiency, however, deoxyuridine cannot be efficiently converted to thymidine, thus, radioactive thymidine is used and labels the DNA. The test may be repeated in the presence of added folate or vitamin B_{12} to determine which one corrects the abnormally high (greater than 10%) uptake of radioactive thymidine into DNA. The deoxyuridine suppression test is used mainly in research laboratories and is not widely available for clinical testing.

Test: Methylmalonic Acid[6,24,25]

Vitamin B_{12} is necessary for conversion of methylmalonate to succinate, and accumulation of methylmalonic acid is seen with vitamin B_{12} deficiency. Although an increase in urinary methylmalonic acid is thought to be a sensitive test for vitamin B_{12} deficiency, this assay is not generally available in clinical laboratories.

TESTS FOR HEMOLYTIC ANEMIA

Test: Acidified Serum Lysis Test for Paroxysmal Nocturnal Hemoglobinuria (HAM Test, Acid Serum Test for PNH)[6,7,12,30]

Background and Selection

Red blood cells in patients with paroxysmal nocturnal hemoglobinuria have a defect in membrane inactivation of complement leading to susceptibility to complement-mediated hemolysis. Lysis occurs in acidified fresh serum because of the activation of the complement system. The acidified serum lysis test should be performed to confirm a positive sucrose hemolysis test for PNH. It may also be ordered with a strongly suggestive clinical presentation (see Test: Sucrose Hemolysis, Background and Selection) such as chronic hemolytic anemia with hemosiderinuria or pancytopenia. A positive acidified serum lysis test is also seen in type II congenital dyserythropoietic anemia (CDA), a very rare disorder.

Logistics

Washed patient RBCs are obtained from defibrinated whole blood or blood collected in EDTA or acid citrate dextrose anticoagulant. Cells should be promptly separated from serum or plasma and assayed on the day of collection. Serum samples from the patient and normal ABO-compatible or AB serum (fresh or stored properly for preservation of complement) are also required. Patient RBCs are incubated with buffer, normal serum, acidified normal serum, heated acidified normal serum (inactivated complement), and acidified patient serum. The tubes are centrifuged, and the supernatent is assessed for hemolysis. If percentage hemolysis is to be quantitated, an additional aliquot of cells is completely hemolyzed. Careful adjustment of the acidified serum pH to 6.8 ± 0.1 is important for reliable results. For a valid test result, normal control washed RBCs should show no lysis when incubated with the acidified normal serum.

Red blood cells in PNH show hemolysis only in the tubes containing acidified serum with complement. The patient's acidified serum may or may not promote lysis, depending on the complement level. For valid test results, all other tubes should be negative. Lysis may occur with acidified serum in other disorders, such as hereditary spherocytosis, autoimmune hemolysis, aplastic anemia, leukemia, and myeloproliferative syndromes and after transfusion with older units of blood. However, in these conditions, hemolysis occurs in the tube with inactivated complement, whereas hemolysis in PNH is complement dependent.

Interpretation

A carefully performed acidified serum lysis test, with attention to proper control tubes, is highly specific for PNH. If the lysis is quantitated, 10–50% lysis of RBCs is typically obtained in PNH, but lysis may be as low as 5%. Other tests that may be abnormal in PNH include decreased RBC acetylcholinesterase, neutrophil alkaline phosphatase, and sucrose hemolysis.

False negative results may occur if the population of complement-sensitive RBCs is too small to produce detectable hemolysis. This may be seen after transfusions, after severe hemolysis of abnormal cells, or in early stages of the disorder. Because reticulocytes are often more susceptible than older RBCs, the sensitivity of the test may be increased by centrifugation and analysis of the upper reticulocyte-rich cells.

In CDA type II (HEMPAS, hereditary erythroblastic multinuclearity with positive acidified serum test), the RBCs lyse in a proportion (approximately 30%) of acidified normal sera, but no lysis occurs in the patient's acidified serum. Lysis in CDA type II can be caused by the presence of an unusual RBC antigen that reacts with a complement-fixing IgM antibody present in some normal sera. The sucrose hemolysis test is normal in CDA type II. In addition, this disorder does not affect platelets or neutrophils as is often seen in PNH.

Test: Glucose 6-Phosphate Dehydrogenase Screen (G-6-PD Screen)[1,7,30,31]

Background

Glucose 6-phosphate dehydrogenase catalyzes the first step in the hexose monophosphate shunt pathway in the RBC, resulting in the reduction of NADP to NADPH (Figure 17-7). NADPH is a cofactor for the reduction of glutathione, which is important in protecting the RBCs from oxidative damage. The G-6-PD deficient RBC is particularly vulnerable to hemolysis when stressed by oxidant drugs, infection, or acidosis or in the neonatal period. Hemolytic anemia is usually self-limited in most variants, because the younger reticulocytes have relatively normal G-6-PD levels, whereas the sensitive, older RBCs are more easily hemolyzed.

Because the G-6-PD gene is located on the X chromosome, full expression of the deficiency is found in the male hemizygote. Partial expression can occur in the heterozygous female who has a large proportion of deficient RBCs. Deficiency of G-6-PD is the most prevalent congenital RBC enzyme defect, affecting more than 130 million people worldwide. More than 150 variant forms of the enzyme have been identified, with the clinical severity dependent on the degree of activity of the particular variant (the most prevalent variants are listed in Table 17-18). In many variants, the enzyme is unstable with near-normal activity in the reticulocyte but deteriorates more rapidly than normal as the RBC ages. Glucose 6-phosphate dehydrogenase deficiency is particularly concentrated in Africa (G-6-PD A$^-$ variant), the Mediterranean, and the Far East (China, Malaysia, Indochina, the Philippines, and Oceania). The rare cases of severe deficiency, presenting as chronic congenital hemolytic anemia, are primarily from Northern Europe. The African variant occurs in approximately 10% of black males in the United States, but most patients have no hematologic problems unless stressed by oxidant drugs or serious infection.

Selection

Glucose 6-phosphate dehydrogenase deficiency should be suspected when an acute hemolytic episode occurs 1–3 days after administration of an oxidant drug or during infection. Common oxidant drugs that may precipitate hemolysis include nalidixic acid, niridazole, nitrofurantoin, primaquine, sulfacetamide, sulfanilamide, sulfapyridine, sulfamethoxazole, and thiazolsulfone. Occasionally, the peripheral blood smear may show the presence of abnormal RBCs, such as ghosts, bite cells, or fragmented cells. Heinz bodies may be seen early in the hemolytic episode, before removal by the spleen. Before an oxidant drug is given, screening for G-6-PD activity may be useful for a male in a high-incidence ethnic group. In addition, the test may be useful in unexplained neonatal jaundice in susceptible ethnic groups (Table 17-18). Glucose 6-phosphate dehydrogenase measurement is also appropriate in the evaluation of congenital hemolytic anemia. Female heterozygotes may have a range of 20–80% of G-6-PD deficient RBCs and cannot be detected reliably with either screening or quantitative G-6-PD assays. Histochemical demonstration of individual RBC G-6-PD activity may detect heterozygote deficiency, but this test is not widely available.

Logistics

Whole blood anticoagulated with EDTA or heparin is stable at 4°C for at least 1 week; blood anticoagulated with acid citrate dextrose is stable at 4°C for more than 2 weeks. The test should not be performed when the patient has received a recent blood transfusion. Simple screening tests for G-6-PD activity are effective in detecting deficiency in both mildly and severely affected hemizygote males. Blood is added to a mixture of glucose 6-phosphate (G-6-P), NADP, saponin, and buffer. A spot of this mixture is placed on filter paper and observed for fluorescence with ultraviolet light. If G-6-PD is present, fluorescent NADPH is formed. An alternate dye-reduction screening method detects production of NADPH by reduction of a colored dye (dichlorophenol indophenol) to a colorless form. The quantitative G-6-

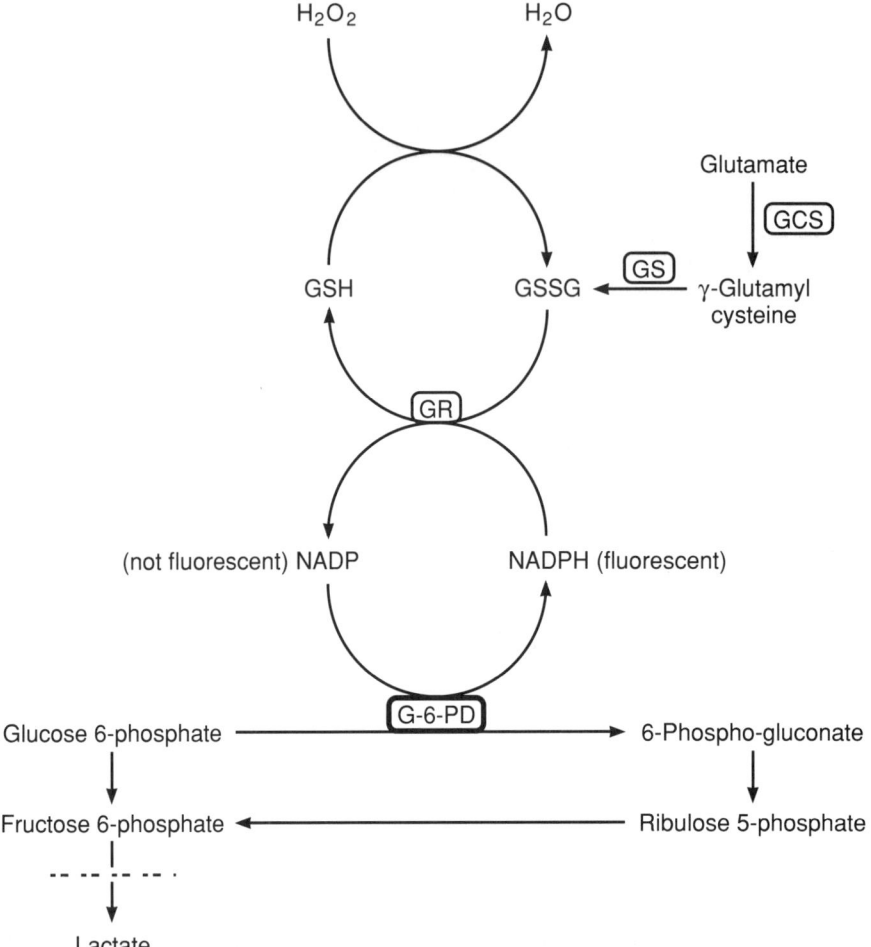

Fig. 17-7. Hexose monophosphate shunt. Enzyme deficiencies associated with hemolytic anemia: G-6-PD, GR, GCS, GS. G-6-PD, glucose 6-phosphate dehydrogenase; GR, glutathione reductase; GCS, γ-glutamyl cysteine synthetase; GS, glutathione synthetase; GSH, reduced glutathione; GSSG, oxidized glutathione; NADP, nicotinamide-adenine dinucleotide phosphate; NADPH, reduced NADP; dashes indicate steps omitted.

PD assay measures the rate of NADPH formation spectrophotometrically in a RBC hemolysate.

Interpretation

The G-6-PD screening test results are reported as normal or deficient. At times, a borderline result is obtained, and G-6-PD enzyme levels in these specimens should be determined quantitatively. A G-6-PD assay or screening test is positive only in G-6-PD deficiency, however, falsely normal results may occur after an acute hemolytic episode, in which the older deficient RBCs have been destroyed and replaced by reticulocytes. The younger reticulocytes contain near-normal levels of G-6-PD, and the assay may be spuriously normal. In this situation, blood can be centrifuged, and the denser, older RBCs from the bottom of the tube used for quantitative assay. Comparison should be made to similarly isolated cells from a "control" with equivalent reticulocytosis. Alternatively, it may be helpful to study male siblings of the patient for G-6-PD deficiency or to wait until later for testing. Demonstration of Heinz bodies also may be useful in suspected G-6-PD-deficient patients during the early phase of an acute hemolytic episode.

Drug-induced hemolytic anemia with unstable Hgb variants is very similar in clinical and laboratory features to G-6-PD deficiency. Thus, if the G-6-PD activity is normal (in a specimen without reticulocytosis), tests for unstable Hgb (Hgb electrophoresis, isopropanol denaturation test, heat stability test) should be

Table 17-18. Clinical Features of Representative Glucose 6-Phosphate Dehydrogenase Variants

	Variant			
	A⁻ (Africans)	Mediterranean (Greeks, Sardinians, Israelis, Iraqis)	Canton (Chinese)	Chicago (Northern Europeans)
Prevalence	10–15%	Common, variable %	~5%	Rare
G-6-PD activity	10–20%	0.5%	4–24%	0.5%
Neonatal jaundice	± (premature)	++	+++	++
Hemolysis with oxidants/infection	+	+	+	+
Increased activity in reticulocytes	+	Minimal	+	+
Chronic hemolysis without stress	0	+	0	+
Drop in Hgb (g/dL) with hemolysis	2–5	4–10	4–10	Chronically < 10
Fava bean sensitivity	0	++	0	++

(From Miller et al.,[31] with permission.)

performed. Other rare enzyme defects of the hexose monophosphate shunt and reduced glutathione formation, such as deficiency of glutathione synthetase and γ-glutamyl cysteine synthetase, may also mimic G-6-PD deficiency.

Test: Heinz Bodies (Heinz Body Stain, Heinz Body Preparation)[2,7,30,32]

Background and Selection

Heinz bodies are focal precipitates of oxidatively denatured hemoglobin within the RBC. They appear as single or multiple irregular inclusion bodies, usually adjacent to the cell membrane. Heinz bodies are not visible with Wright-Giemsa stain and require supravital stains to demonstrate their presence.

The demonstration of Heinz bodies may be a useful screening test in acute hemolytic episodes when oxidative denaturation of Hgb is suspected. This can occur when large amounts of oxidant chemicals or drugs have been ingested (e.g., phenylhydrazine, chlorate, naphthalene, dapsone). In addition, smaller doses of mild to strong oxidant drugs (e.g., primaquine or some sulfa derivative drugs) may lead to Heinz body formation in patients with deficient Hgb reduction capability or in patients with unstable Hgb variant. Heinz body testing may be useful in patients with high prevalence of G-6-PD deficiency (e.g., black males) who develop a hemolytic anemia after oxidant drug ingestion. In these patients, falsely normal G-6-PD levels may found attributable to the high amounts present in newly generated reticulocytes. Thus the presence of Heinz bodies provides evidence for the etiology, despite seemingly normal levels of red blood cell G-6-PD enzyme.

The blood smear may show cookie-bite RBCs with Heinz body formation, caused by the removal of the Heinz body by the spleen, but this finding is not a particularly sensitive or specific indicator of the presence of Heinz bodies. Because Heinz bodies are stained by the stain used for reticulocyte count (new methylene blue), their presence may be noted in the reticulocyte smear.

Heinz bodies are cleared rapidly in the unsplenectomized patient, and thus are detected only during the acute hemolytic episode. In the absence of acute oxidative drug challenge and rapid hemolysis, staining for Heinz bodies is not particularly useful in screening for RBC enzyme defects or most unstable Hgb variants, as the small numbers of Heinz bodies produced in these disorders are promptly removed by the spleen. However, Heinz bodies are readily identified in patients with these disorders after splenectomy.

Logistics

EDTA- or heparin-anticoagulated blood may be used and should be less than 24 hours old. Preformed Heinz bodies may be seen by mixing blood with a supravital dye (e.g., methyl violet, crystal violet, brilliant cresyl blue, brilliant green) and either examining a wet mount of the RBCs or wedge smears. The sensitivity to Heinz body detection may vary with different dye preparations and whether isotonic or hypotonic suspension solution is used. Methyl violet, crystal violet, and brilliant green are specific for Heinz bodies, but brilliant cresyl blue and other supravital dyes also stain reticulin and Howell-Jolly bodies.

One to 10 round to irregularly shaped Heinz body inclusions may be seen per RBC. They vary in size from

0.3–2 μm in diameter. Typically, Heinz bodies are found close to the RBC membrane and may protrude from it or even be attached by a stalk.

Interpretation

Only a rare preformed Heinz body should be detected in the healthy patient. The most common cause of Heinz body hemolytic anemia is administration of an oxidant drug to a patient with G-6-PD deficiency. Individual differences in metabolism and excretion of drugs and the severity of enzyme deficiency may influence the reaction to different drugs. Common oxidant drugs that may precipitate hemolysis include nalidixic acid, niridazole, nitrofurantoin, primaquine, sulfacetamide, sulfanilamide, sulfapyridine, sulfamethoxazole, and thiazolsulfone. Oxidant drugs would also be expected to cause Heinz body formation in patients who have hemolytic disorders caused by rarely occurring deficiencies of other enzymes necessary for the formation of reduced glutathione (i.e., glutathione reductase, glutathione synthetase, γ-glutamyl cysteine synthetase).

In rare cases, large doses of oxidant drugs or chemicals (e.g., phenylhydrazine, chlorate, naphthalene, dapsone, pyridium, or sulfa-containing medications) may induce Heinz bodies in healthy patients. In addition, Heinz bodies may occasionally be seen with vitamin E deficiency in the newborn (exacerbated by iron therapy), with phenacetin in splenectomized patients, and with unstable Hgb in a splenectomized patient.

Heinz bodies may be induced in susceptible patients by incubating the blood with a strong oxidant agent (e.g., phenylhydrazine) or incubation of sterile blood for 24–48 hours at 37°C before staining. Abnormal RBCs with a defective enzymatic pathway for reducing oxidized Hgb or unstable Hgb may show more than 50% of RBCs with 5 or more Heinz bodies. However, smaller numbers of Heinz bodies may form in healthy patients, and it is important for the laboratory to establish a reference range for the particular incubation and staining technique that is employed. In addition, splenectomized patients and neonates with decreased amounts of RBC-reducing enzymes may show significant Heinz body formation with oxidant or incubation stress. Because more reliable tests for RBC enzymatic activity and unstable Hgb values are available, the incubated Heinz body preparation is of limited value.

When Heinz bodies are demonstrated, a patient history for drug ingestion should be obtained. In addition, a family history of enzyme deficiency or hemoglobinopathy is useful. Further testing, depending on clinical situation, would include measurement of G-6-PD after the acute hemolytic period, tests for unstable Hgb variant (isopropanol denaturation test, heat stability test, Hgb electrophoresis), and tests for other enzyme deficiencies in the hexose monophosphate shunt (Fig. 17-7).

Test: Osmotic Fragility (Red Blood Cell Fragility)[7,10,12,33,34]

Background and Selection

The osmotic fragility test measures the susceptibility or resistance of the RBC to osmotic stress. Red blood cells placed in a hypotonic media will swell and eventually rupture as water enters the cell. Spherocytic RBCs, with a decreased surface-to-volume ratio, have a limited capacity to expand in hypotonic solutions, and thus lyse at a lesser degree of osmotic stress than do normal biconcave RBCs (increased osmotic fragility). Conversely, target cells, with a high surface to volume ratio, have an increased capacity to expand in hypotonic solutions and have decreased susceptibility to osmotic lysis.

The osmotic fragility test is important in the evaluation of congenital hemolytic anemia, particularly when hereditary spherocytosis is suspected. A positive test merely confirms the presence of spherocytic RBCs. Spherocytic anemias often have a normal to low MCV and increased MCHC. If a Hgb concentration curve is available from the hematology analyzer, the presence of the dense spherocytic RBCs may be seen. On a blood smear, spherocytes have a smaller diameter and are more intensely stained, often lacking central pallor. If spherocytes can be clearly identified on a well made peripheral blood smear, the expensive and time consuming osmotic fragility test is unnecessary.

In the past, the osmotic fragility test was used as a screening test for thalassemia, in which RBCs show decreased osmotic fragility. However, the measurement of MCV with widely available automated hematology instruments is a much easier means of screening for thalassemia.

Logistics

Freshly drawn heparinized or defibrinated blood is used. Blood must be sterile, and no hemolysis or clotting should be present. Red blood cells are incubated in buffered sodium chloride solutions of 0.30–0.85%, and an additional tube of distilled water is used for total

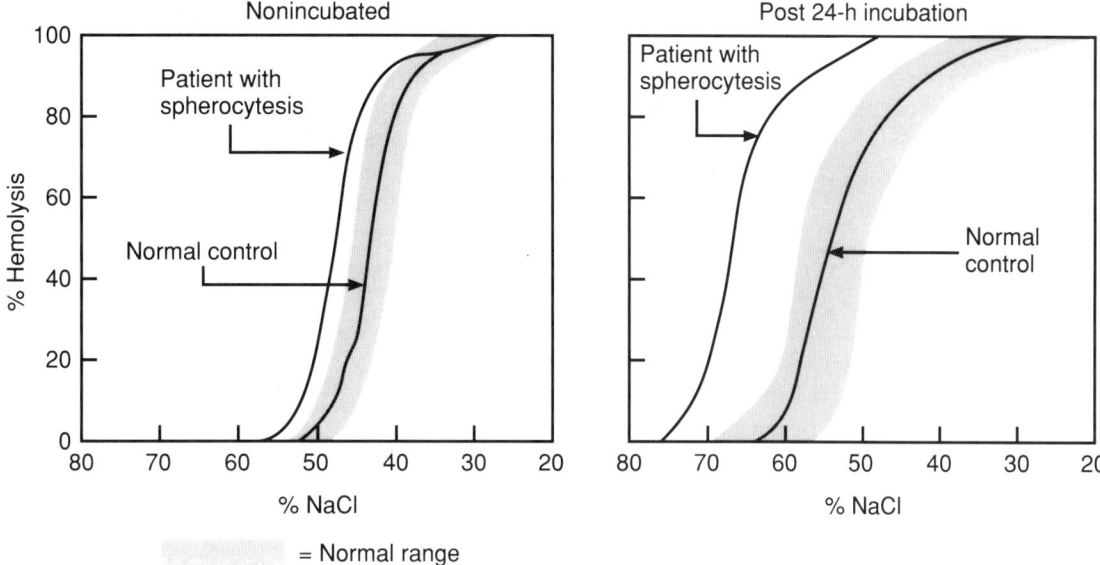

Fig. 17-8. Red blood cell osmotic fragility.

hemolysis. After centrifugation, the supernatent Hgb for each salt concentration can be measured and expressed as percentage hemolysis, related to the tube with complete hemolysis. The results are presented graphically (Fig. 17-8). The sensitivity of the test to smaller numbers of spherocytes may be greatly enhanced by incubating the blood at 37°C for 24 hours before testing. The incubated osmotic fragility test is usually performed if the osmotic fragility results for fresh blood are normal or borderline. A control blood specimen from a healthy donor should be assayed simultaneously with the patient specimen, and the control osmotic fragility curve should fall within the shaded reference range (Fig. 17-8).

A more recently described procedure uses EDTA-anticoagulated blood, which can be stored at 4°C for up to 4 days. Only four sodium chloride dilutions are used for both the unincubated and incubated osmotic fragility tests. The percentage hemolysis for each salt concentration is compared with the normal reference range; the test result is consistent with spherocytosis if the percentage hemolysis exceeds the reference limits in three of four of the salt concentrations.

Interpretation

In healthy persons, hemolysis of RBCs in unincubated blood begins at 0.45–0.50% sodium chloride and is complete by 0.35% sodium chloride. Spherocytes from any cause will show RBC lysis beginning at higher concentrations of salt (increased osmotic fragility), or a shift of the curve to the left (Fig. 17-8). When decreased osmotic fragility is present, lysis of RBCs requires a lower concentration of salt, and the curve is shifted to the right. After incubation, the width of the normal curve is expanded, and the entire curve is shifted toward increased osmotic fragility. However, spherocytic cells show an even greater increase in osmotic fragility with incubation (Fig. 17-8). At times, the abnormality in the osmotic fragility curve may be limited to a small population of cells that are unusually susceptible or resistant to lysis.

Although increased osmotic fragility is present in nearly all patients with hereditary spherocytosis, a positive test may be seen with any cause of spherocytic red cells. Immune hemolytic anemia is a common cause of spherocytic anemia, and a direct antiglobulin test is important to assess this possibility (Ch. 31). Decreased osmotic fragility is seen in disorders with large numbers of target cells, including iron deficiency, homozygous and heterozygous thalassemia, other hemoglobinopathies (especially Hgb C), and liver disease.

Test: Sucrose Hemolysis (Sugar Water Test, Test for PNH)[1,7,30,34]

Paroxysmal nocturnal hemoglobinuria is an acquired clonal stem cell disorder affecting the cell membrane structure of RBCs, WBCs, and platelets. It most commonly presents as a chronic hemolytic anemia, with increased sensitivity of the RBCs to lysis by complement. An isotonic sucrose solution of low ionic strength can enhance the binding of complement to RBCs, causing lysis of the PNH cells.

Background and Selection

The sucrose hemolysis test is very useful as a rapid screen for PNH. When both the sucrose hemolysis test and a stain for urine hemosiderin are negative, the diagnosis of PNH may be excluded. Paroxysmal nocturnal hemoglobinuria is suspected in the presence of chronic hemolysis, particularly intravascular type hemolysis with hemosiderinuria. Paroxysmal nocturnal hemoglobinuria patients may often be iron deficient because of the loss of large amounts of iron in the urine. Intermittent exacerbations of acute hemolysis caused by complement activation may be seen with infection, transfusion of unwashed RBCs, and surgery. The classic presentation of hemoglobinuria at night is caused by carbon dioxide retention during sleep and a fall in plasma pH that facilitates the activation of complement; however, this phenomenon is present in less than 25% of cases.

Paroxysmal nocturnal hemoglobinuria is often associated with marrow hypoplasia and pancytopenia, and the mutation associated with PNH may arise in idiopathic or drug-induced marrow aplasia. Thus, the sucrose hemolysis test may be a reasonable screen in the workup of any idiopathic hypoplastic anemia. Finally, venous thrombotic problems in unusual locations, such as the hepatic or mesenteric veins, or venous thrombosis in patients younger than age 40 may be associated with PNH.

Logistics

Citrate- or oxalate-anticoagulated blood, less than 4 hours old, is the preferred sample. Heparin or EDTA cannot be used, because complement is inactivated, resulting in false negative results. However, if the testing method uses washed patient RBCs and exogenous serum for a complement source, any anticoagulant may be used for collecting patient RBCs.

In the qualitative screen, patient blood is added to an isotonic sucrose solution, incubated, centrifuged, and observed for hemolysis. An equivalent amount of patient plasma should be added to another aliquot of sucrose to make sure that hemolysis is not present in the unincubated sample.

In the quantitative test, washed patient RBCs are mixed with ABO compatible or AB normal serum (fresh or properly stored to preserve complement activity). The tube is incubated and then centrifuged, and the percent hemolysis in the supernatant is determined. Any hemolysis or red color in the control tubes (omitting serum or the patient RBCs) is subtracted from the result in the calculation.

Interpretation

In the qualitative screen, no hemolysis should be noted in the supernatent beyond the amount present in the control tube. For the quantitative test, less than 5% hemolysis in the test specimen is negative, 5–10% is suspicious, and greater than 10% is very suggestive of PNH.

The sucrose hemolysis test is very sensitive for the detection of PNH. False negative results are rare and are usually due to the failure to use sufficient activated complement in the assay. In addition, a false negative result may occur if the clone of sensitive cells has been destroyed in a recent hemolytic episode or is diluted by transfusion. False positive results have occasionally been noted in many diverse conditions, including autoimmune hemolytic anemia, megaloblastic anemia, malignancy, infection, and renal failure. In the quantitative assay, these conditions usually cause less than 5% hemolysis. However, a positive sucrose hemolysis test should be followed by the more specific Ham's acid serum test for PNH. A direct antiglobulin test may be useful when a false positive sucrose hemolysis test occurs in the patient with hemolytic anemia. Patients with congenital dyserythropoietic anemia type II may have a positive Ham's acidified serum test similar to PNH, but the sucrose hemolysis test will be negative.

Test: Autohemolysis[7,12,30,34]

The autohemolysis test is performed by incubating sterile blood with and without the addition of glucose for 48 hours and then measuring the amount of Hgb released in the plasma. Normally less than 2.5% hemolysis occurs without glucose, and 0.6% with glucose. The primary use of autohemolysis testing is for hereditary spherocytosis, in which autohemolysis is greatly increased (7–15%) and is usually partially corrected by the addition of glucose. However, the autohemolysis test is variable in patients with acquired hemolytic anemias and an abnormal test does not distinguish hereditary spherocytosis from the spherocytosis of immune hemolytic anemia. Blood from patients with G-6-PD deficiency or other disorders of the pentose pathway may have slightly increased autohemolysis (corrected by glucose), whereas disorders of the glycolytic pathway (e.g., pyruvate kinase deficiency) have greatly increased autohemolysis on which glucose has no effect. The availability of specific RBC enzyme assays has made the autohemolysis test obsolete for the diagnosis of hereditary enzyme deficiencies.

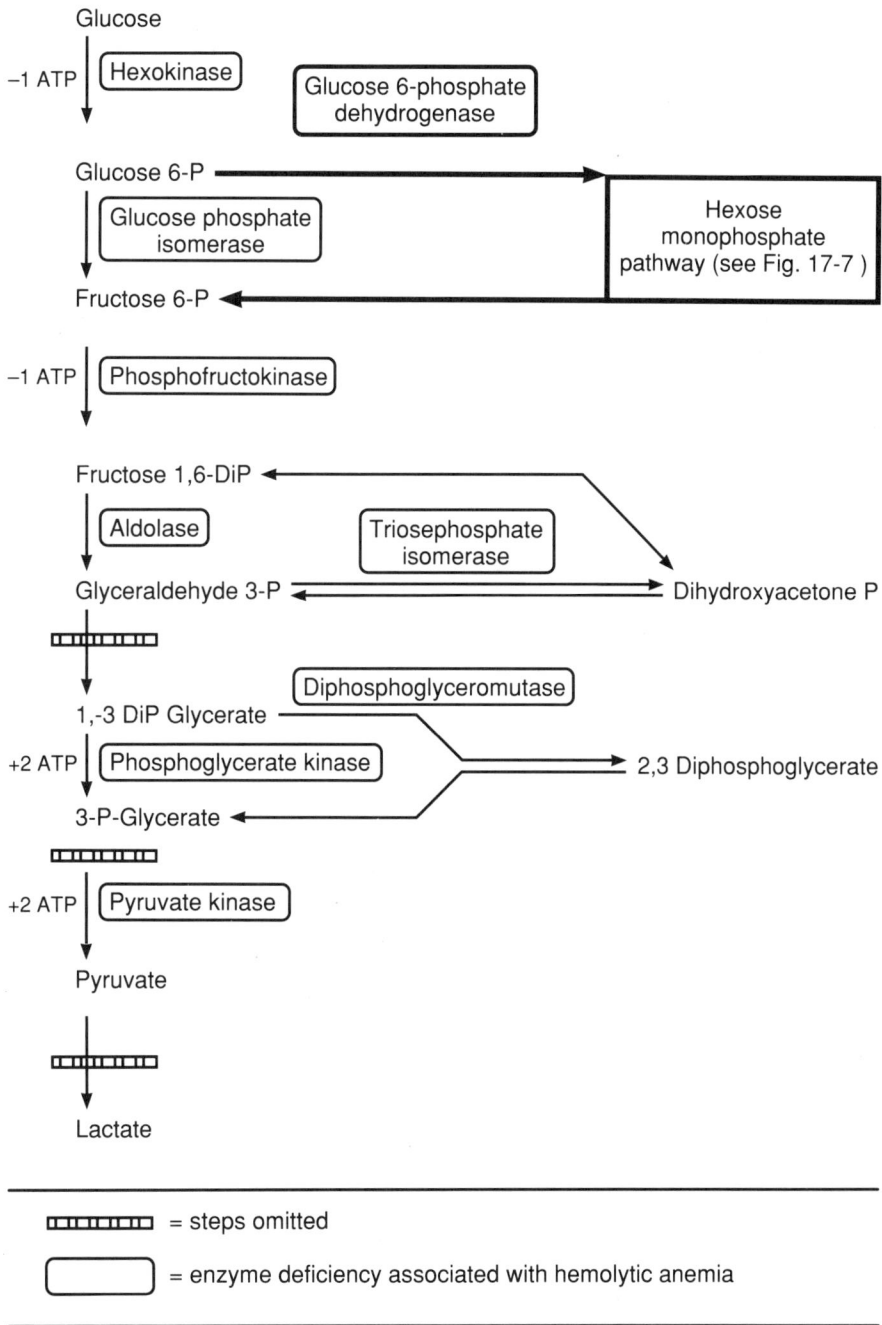

Fig. 17-9. Embden-Meyerhof glycolytic pathway. ATP, adenosine triphosphate; DiP, diphosphate; P, phosphate.

Test: Red Blood Cell Enzymes, Quantitative[3,30,31]

Hereditary hemolytic anemia can be caused by RBC enzyme disorders of the main glycolytic pathway, the hexose monophosphate shunt, or glutathione, metabolism (Figs. 17-7 and 17-9). Defects in the Embden-Meyerhof glycolytic pathway usually result in continuous, lifelong hemolysis; those in the hexose monophosphate shunt often show acute episodes of hemolysis with stress, during infection, with acidosis, or with oxidant drugs.

Most quantitative assays link RBC enzymatic activity to the formation or consumption of NADPH or NADH, which can be measured spectrophotometrically. Screening tests for pyruvate kinase and G-6-PD deficiency, the two most common abnormalities, are more widely available, whereas quantitative assays are usually performed in specialized research or reference laboratories. Falsely normal results for G-6-PD and hexokinase may occur in the presence of many reticulocytes, which exhibit increased activity of these enzymes.

Test: Red Blood Cell Half-life (RBC Life Span, RBC Survival Studies)[7,23]

Moderate to severe hemolysis leads to an increase in RBC catabolic products, as listed in Figure 17-1. In mild hemolytic states, however, these abnormalities may not occur. Chromium 51 (^{51}Cr) RBC survival studies may be useful in some cases to confirm decreased RBC half-life and determine the major site of RBC destruction. However, a decreased RBC half-life is observed with RBC loss because of bleeding as well as in a hemolytic process.

An aliquot of patient blood is collected into citrate anticoagulant and incubated in vitro with ^{51}Cr. A measured aliquot is infused into the patient. Serial blood samples are collected over 10–14 days and counted for ^{51}Cr activity. Counts per minute are plotted on semilogarithmic paper versus time to calculate the time for 50% of the RBCs to disappear. If gastrointestinal bleeding is suspected, the radioactivity of the stools can be counted. This provides a quantitative measure of gastrointestinal blood loss, as well as precludes an erroneous interpretation of the apparent decrease in RBC half-life. The normal half-life of ^{51}Cr labeled RBCs is 25–32 days. External scanning for radioactivity may detect the major sites of RBC destruction. The differential diagnosis of hemolytic anemia, along with useful laboratory tests, is presented in Table 17-5.

TESTS FOR ABNORMAL HEMOGLOBIN

Test: Heat Stability (Heat Denaturation, Thermolabile Hemoglobin, Unstable Hemoglobin Screen)[7,32,35,36]

Background and Selection

Unstable Hgb denatures more readily than normal Hgb when exposed to high temperature. Heat stability testing for unstable Hgb is usually performed when the isopropanol screen for unstable Hgb is positive. This somewhat more specific, but less sensitive, test for unstable Hgb provides confirmation of a presumptive positive by isopropanol denaturation. (See Test: Isopropanol Denaturation for discussion of clinical and laboratory findings suggesting the presence of an unstable Hgb.)

Logistics

EDTA-anticoagulated blood should be assayed on the day of phlebotomy. A hemolysate of the RBCs is incubated in buffer at 50°C for 1–2 hours and examined for turbidity. Quantitation of the percentage of unstable Hgb can be made if a precipitate forms. A normal blood should be assayed along with the patient specimen.

Interpretation

Normal blood should show little precipitation at 2 hours, and most unstable hemoglobins will show precipitation of more than 5%. In vitro methemoglobin formation may result in a small precipitate (less than 5%). More specific identification of the unstable Hgb variant requires very specialized research laboratory testing, such as globin chain electrophoresis or amino acid or peptide analysis. (See Test: Isopropanol Denaturation for further discussion of the unstable hemoglobins most frequently detected.)

Test: Hemoglobin Electrophoresis[1,2,6,30,32,36–39]

Background

Human Hgb is composed of four heme groups attached to four polypeptide chains (globin). The polypeptide chains consist of two identical α-chains and of two identical non-α-chains. Each globin chain has a separate autosomal genetic locus, with duplication of the α and γ genes. Normal Hgb molecules and the chromo-

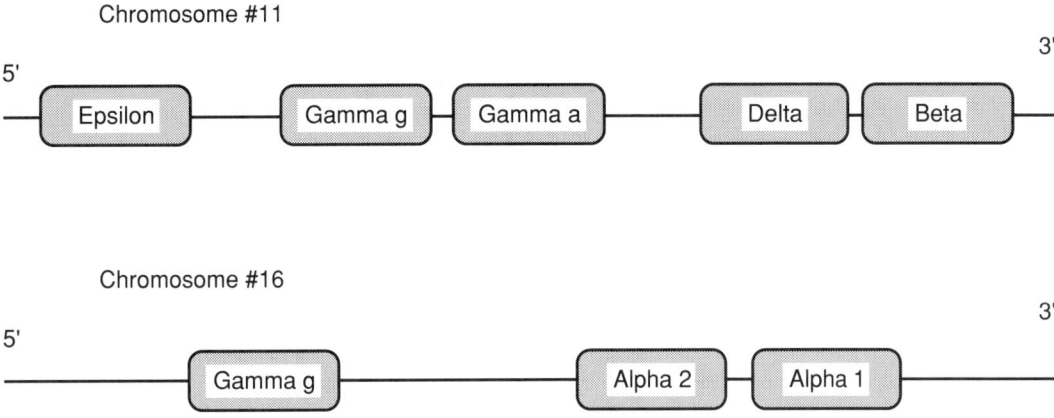

Fig. 17-10. Composition and genetics of globin chains.

somal origin of the globin chains are shown in Figure 17-10. A healthy adult has 95% or more Hgb A, with approximately 3% Hgb A_2 and 1% Hgb F.

> Normal Adult Hemoglobins (tetramers of 4 globin chains)
> A = $\alpha_2 \beta_2$
> F = $\alpha_2 \gamma_2$
> A_2 = $\alpha_2 \delta_2$

Disorders in Hgb synthesis may be divided into those caused by formation of abnormal globin polypeptides (hemoglobinopathies) and those associated with suppression of normal globin synthesis (thalassemias). Amino acid substitutions are responsible for most of the variant hemoglobins, whereas gene deletion or mutations that suppress the rate of transcription or translation lead to thalassemia syndromes. More than 400 variant Hgb molecules have been identified, but only a few cause disease in high incidence. Hemoglobin electrophoresis is the primary method for identifying structural abnormalities in the Hgb molecule.

The hemoglobinopathies may be classified functionally by the mechanism in which disease is produced (Table 17-19). A few abnormal hemoglobins, such as S and C, show decreased solubility and form rigid aggregates within the RBC. Some amino acid substitutions can result in an unstable Hgb molcule, which undergoes oxidative denaturation to Heinz bodies. A change in certain amino acids near the attachment point of heme allows reduction of heme iron and formation of methemoglobin. Other variants show increased or decreased affinity of the heme moiety for oxygen.

The various thalassemias are named for the globin chain affected (i.e., α-thalassemia, β-thalassemia, and $\beta\delta$-thalassemia). The clinical syndrome in α-thalassemia depends on the number of α genes deleted, as illustrated in Figure 17-11. β-Thalassemias comprise a more heterogeneous group of disorders. The β gene may be completely suppressed (β^0) or partially suppressed (β^+). The β gene alone may be affected, or the δ or δ and γ genes may also be suppressed. β-Thalassemias are sometimes referred to as thalassemia minor in the clinically asymptomatic heterozygous state and as thalassemia intermedia or major in the homozygous or double heterozygous condition, depending on clinical severity (Table 17-19). In hereditary persistence of fetal hemoglobin (HPFH), the β and δ genes are deleted, and normal suppression of γ-chain synthesis fails to occur, with resultant high levels of Hgb F. In a few cases, an abnormal Hgb molecule (e.g., Hgb E) is poorly synthesized and leads to a thalassemia-like syndrome. Double heterozygotes involving structural variants and the thalassemias also may be seen.

Selection

Clinical syndromes and RBC abnormalities associated with various categories of Hgb variants and thalassemic syndromes are given in Table 17-19. Hemoglobinopathy is part of the differential diagnosis in a patient with low MCV, unexplained hemolytic anemia, anemia precipitated by oxidant stress, or erythrocytosis. Thalassemia trait or abnormal Hgb with thalassemic production is suspected in patients with a mild decrease in Hgb, low MCV, and erythrocytosis. Homozygous thalassemia syndromes or a combination of thalassemia with a symptomatic structural variant are characterized by hemolytic anemia with a low MCV. Hemoglobin

Table 17-19. Functional Classification of Hemoglobinopathies and Thalassemic Syndromes: Clinical and Hematologic Features

Functional Defect/Syndrome	Autosomal Inheritance	Mechanism	Hematologic Symptoms	RBC Morphology	Examples
No defect	Heterozygous; occasionally homozygous	Mutation has no effect on function of Hgb	None	Normal, some may have target cells	Most low frequency heterozygotes; S, C, and D trait; homozygous D
Decreased solubility	Homozygous or double heterozygous	Polymerization of Hgb in RBC	Hemolytic anemia, splenic infarction in sickling disorders	Polychromasia, targets, sickle cells and/or Hgb C crystals, siderocytes, other changes if autosplenectomy	SS, CC, SC, SD, SO S-β thalassemia, C-β thalassemia
Unstable Hgb	Heterozygous	Oxidative denaturation of Hgb to Heinz bodies, with removal by spleen; some also have altered O_2 affinity	Mild to severe hemolytic anemia; may be exacerbated by oxidant stress	Polychromasia, hypochromia, nRBC if severe, Heinz bodies if splenectomized	Köln, Gun Hill, Hammersmith, Hasharon, E
High O_2 affinity	Heterozygous	Relative tissue hypoxia leads to increased erythropoietin	Erythrocytosis	Polychromasia	Chesapeake, Malmo
Low O_2 affinity	Heterozygous	Relative tissue O_2 excess leads to decreased erythropoietin	Anemia, cyanosis	Normocytic anemia	Kansas, Seattle

Silent thalassemia trait	Heterozygous	Deletion or mutation of 1 α gene	None	Silent α-thalassemia trait, Constant Spring
Thalassemia minor	Heterozygous occasionally homozygous	Deletion or mutation of 2 α genes; deletion, mutation, or suppression of 1 β gene	Mild decrease in Hgb and erythrocytosis without clinical symptoms	Microcytosis, hypochromia, targets, teardrops, coarse basophilic stippling	α-Thalassemia trait; silent α-thalassemia trait with Constant Spring; β^{+-}, β^{0-}, $\delta\beta^{0-}$, and $\gamma\delta\beta^{0}$-thalassemia trait; Lepore trait; homozygous HPFH or E; heterozygous E
Thalassemia intermedia	Homozygous or double heterozygous	Deletion or mutation of 3 α genes; near complete suppression of both β genes	Similar to thalassemia major, but milder	Similar to thalassemia minor, with more small, bizarre poikilocytes and polychromasia	Hgb H (β_4); homozygous β^+-thalassemia; double heterozygous for many types of β-thalassemia
Thalassemia major	Homozygous or double heterozygous	Deletion of 4 α genes (hydrops fetalis); complete suppression of both β genes	Unstable aggregates of 4 γ chains (Hgb Bart's) in α-thalassemia major and 4 α chains in β-thalassemia major leads to hemolytic anemia and ineffective erythropoiesis	Microcytosis, hypochromia, nRBC, targets, Howell-Jolly bodies, Cabot rings, nuclear fragments, siderocytes, small bizarre RBCs	Hgb Bart's (γ_4, hydrops fetalis); homozygous β^0- or $\delta\beta^0$-thalassemia; homozygous Lepore; E-β^0-thalassemia

Abbreviations: Hgb, hemoglobin; HPFH, hereditary persistence of fetal hemoglobin; RBC, red blood cell.

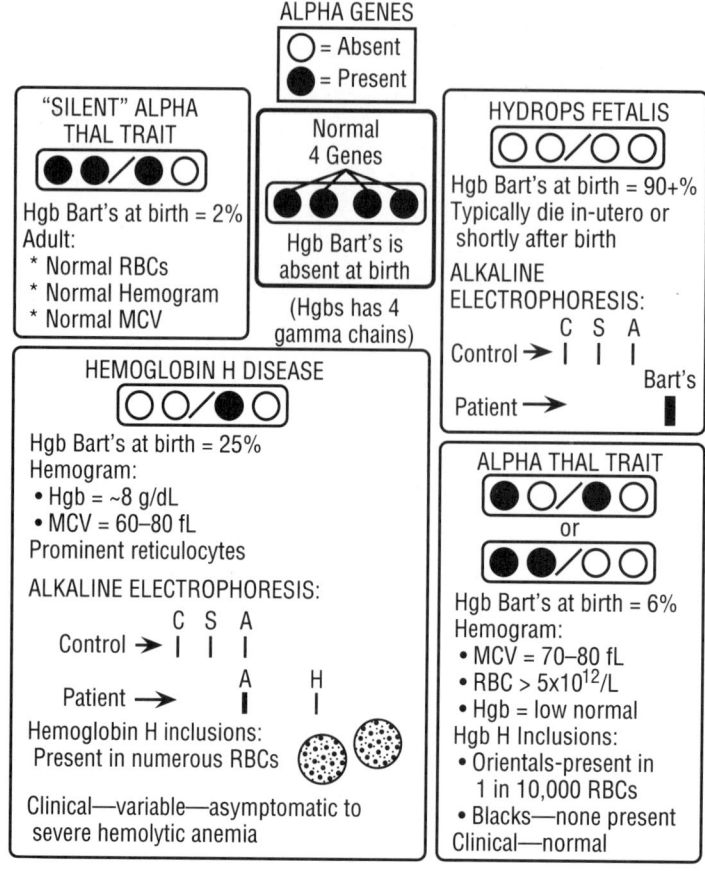

Fig. 17-11. Forms of α-thalassemia.

electrophoresis is sometimes ordered in relatives of patients with known abnormalities or to screen for carriers in populations with a high incidence of certain abnormalities. The most prevalent hemoglobins worldwide include S (8% incidence in American blacks), E (3–30% in various regions in southeast Asia), and C (2% in American blacks, more widely prevalent in the west African area of Nigeria). Hemoglobin G-Philadelphia, D-Los Angeles (also called D-Punjab), and O-Arab occur in low frequency in American blacks, but also may be seen in diverse ethnic groups. α- and β-Thalassemias are present in a broad geographic distribution, with high prevalence in the Mediterranean basin, the Middle East, Asia, northern and western Africa, and in American blacks. African-type HPFH is found in about 0.1% of American blacks. When a thalassemic syndrome is suspected, such as in a patient with a low MCV or microcytic RBC population, it is important to obtain an accurate quantitation of Hgb A_2 and Hgb F by nonelectrophoretic methods (see Test: Hemoglobin A_2 and Test: Hemoglobin F).

Terminology

Hemoglobin electrophoresis may include different combinations of tests in different laboratories. In some laboratories, quantitation of Hgb A_2 and Hgb F by nonelectrophoretic methods may be included as part of a quantitative Hgb electrophoresis panel, whereas in other laboratories they must be ordered separately. Alkaline electrophoresis on cellulose acetate media is usually the initial electrophoretic procedure; if an abnormal Hgb is detected, acid electrophoresis or neutral pH electrophoresis (for fast-migrating hemoglobins) should be performed to further identify the abnormal Hgb. Some laboratories automatically perform these specialized electrophoretic procedures when an abnormal Hgb is found on alkaline electrophoresis; in other cases, these more specialized electrophoreses must be ordered or sent to a reference laboratory.

Hemoglobin variants were initially given letter names, as they were identified by abnormal electrophoretic mobility. When more variants were discovered than letters of the alphabet, different variants with the same mobility were usually distinguished by adding the place of discovery to the letter name. The word *disease* is frequently used to designate the homozygous or double heterozygous condition, whereas, *trait* refers to the asymptomatic heterozygote.

Logistics

EDTA-anticoagulated blood is preferred and may be stored for several days at room temperature and even for 1 month in the refrigerator. Heparinized blood, including fingerstick capillary blood collected in heparinized tubes, also may be used and is stable for at least 1 week. Capillary blood absorbed onto filter paper is sometimes used for screening of newborns. If an unstable Hgb is suspected, the sample should be run within 24 hours.

Packed RBCs are washed and lysed with water. The hemolysate can be clarified by extracting the RBC membranes with organic solvent; this may give a cleaner electrophoretic pattern but should not be performed if an unstable Hgb is suspected. The Hgb is converted to the cyanmethemoglobin form. The hemolysate also may be stored for several weeks in the refrigerator.

A small amount of hemolysate is used for alkaline electrophoresis on a cellulose acetate membrane. Controls containing Hgb A, F, S, and C are also assayed. At alkaline pH, Hgb has a negative charge and migrates toward the anode (Fig 17-12). The distance the Hgb bands travel depends on the net negative charge, which can be affected by amino acid substitution. For example, Hgb S contains valine (no charge) rather than glutamic acid (negative charge) in the sixth position of the β chain and thus does not migrate as rapidly as Hgb A.

Hemoglobin C has lysine (positive charge) replacing the glutamic acid (negative charge) in the sixth position, decreasing its migration even more than S. After staining the electrophoretic membrane (usually with a protein-staining dye), the various Hgb bands can be quantitated with a densitometer. However, densitometry is not sufficiently sensitive to quantitate the small amounts of Hgb A_2 and Hgb F normally present (see discussion of Hgb A_2 and Hgb F as analytes).

When abnormal hemoglobins are seen with alkaline electrophoresis, electrophoresis at acid pH on agar (acid citrate agar electrophoresis) can aid in identification (Fig. 17-12). Adsorption of the Hgb to the agar, in addition to hemoglobin charge, plays a role in the migration of the Hgb. Better separation of Hgb F and A is obtained, and hence acid electrophoresis is useful in newborns. The agar media is usually stained with a dye detecting the peroxidative activity of Hgb. Electrophoresis at neutral pH on cellulose acetate membrane may be performed when a hemoglobin migrating faster than Hgb A is detected on alkaline electrophoresis, or when Hgb H or Hgb Bart's are suspected.

Newer methods for detection of abnormal hemoglobins include electrophoresis by isoelectric focusing and high pressure liquid chromatography (HPLC). These techniques may be particularly useful in detection of small amounts of abnormal hemoglobin in neonates.

Interpretation

In the healthy adult, alkaline Hgb electrophoresis shows a predominant band in the A position and a small band of Hgb A_2. A band of Hgb F is seen in the neonate or young child but is not usually detected in the adult unless Hgb F exceeds 1%. With the more sensitive acid citrate electrophoresis, a large band of Hgb

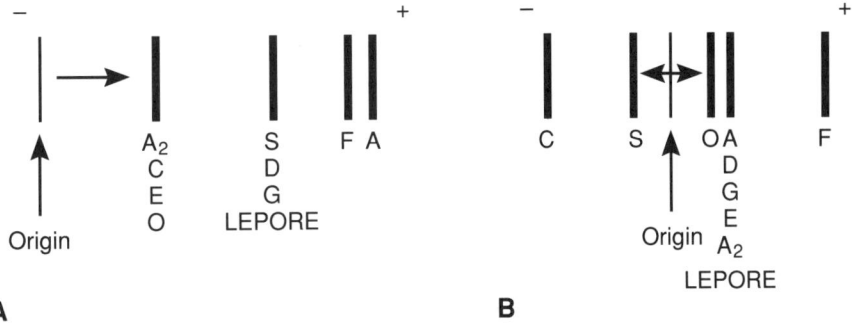

Fig. 17-12. Normal mobilities for hemoglobin electrophoresis. **(A)** Alkaline electrophoresis (cellulose acetate). **(B)** Acid electrophoresis (citrate agar).

A/A₂ and a small band of Hgb F is present in the healthy adult.

The electrophoretic patterns of the most frequently encountered abnormal hemoglobins are shown in Figure 17-5. With alkaline electrophoresis, Hgb D, G, and Lepore migrate in the same position as Hgb S, whereas Hgb C, E and O migrate the same as Hgb A₂. Hemoglobin mutants with a greater negative charge than Hgb A also occur and are called fast hemoglobins, examples of which are Hgb H, I, N, J, and Bart's.

Confirmatory tests are performed to differentiate among the various hemoglobins. When an abnormal Hgb is found in the S position, a positive sickle Hgb solubility test is sufficient for confirmation. With acid citrate electrophoresis (Fig. 17-12), Hgb S, C, and O are distinctly separate from other abnormal hemoglobins and from Hgb A. Neutral electrophoresis is useful when a fast-migrating Hgb is found. When a fast-migrating Hgb in the H region is noted, a test for Hgb H inclusions in the RBCs is confirmatory. Knowledge of the ethnic background, clinical and laboratory features, and quantitative measurement may aid in distinguishing other abnormal hemoglobins. In patients with a low MCV, quantitative measurement of the amount of variant Hgb and the amount of Hgb A is helpful in determining double heterozygousity for an abnormal Hgb and thalassemia trait. Characteristic proportions of various hemoglobins in representative disorders are shown in Table 17-20.

The main limitation of Hgb electrophoresis is the inability to detect many of the Hgb variants that do not affect the charge of the molecule. For example, approximately 50% of unstable Hgb variants may migrate with Hgb A on electrophoresis. Thus, isopropanol or heat denaturation tests are also indicated when an unstable Hgb is suspected. Similarly, measurement of the oxygen dissociation curve and P_{50} should be performed when a high or low O_2 affinity Hgb is suspected.

Specialized testing procedures may be performed when a conclusive diagnosis cannot be made. Further tests to identify an unknown variant include isoelectric focusing, immunologic assays, globin chain electrophoresis, fingerprinting peptide mapping, and even structural analysis of the globin chain. Globin chain synthesis studies and DNA hybridization are useful in distinguishing thalassemic conditions and elucidating genotypes of patients with combined hemoglobinopathy and thalassemia. For unusual cases, these studies are available from the National Reference Laboratory (NRL) for hemoglobinopathy detection at the Centers for Disease Control (CDC). In specialized research laboratories, DNA from fetal cells can be analyzed using restriction endonucleases, in order to establish the prenatal diagnosis of Hgb SS and β^0-thalassemia major.

Test: Hemoglobin A₂ (Quantitive Hgb A₂, Hgb A₂ by Column Chromatography)[1,2,6,30,32,36,37,40]

Background and Selection

Hemoglobin A_2 ($\alpha_2\delta_2$) is present in small amounts in healthy adults. In β-thalassemia trait, there is a decreased production of normal β-chains; thus, Hgb A ($\alpha_2\beta_2$), the major Hgb form in adults, is decreased. Relatively, and also apparently on an absolute basis, the amount of Hgb A_2 increases.

β-Thalassemias are a heterogeneous group of disorders, sometimes referred to as thalassemia minor in the clinically asymptomatic heterozygous state and as thalassemia intermedia or major in the homozygous or double heterozygous state. A variety of molecular mechanisms can be involved in suppressing β gene function, and the β gene may be partially (β^+) or completely (β^0) suppressed.

Quantitation of Hgb A_2 is performed in patients with persistent microcytosis to determine the presence of β-thalassemia (β^+ or β^0) trait (Table 17-20). β-Thalassemia trait (a form of thalassemia minor) is particularly suspected when the MCV is low with normal to elevated RBC count and Hgb above 10.0 g/dL (100 g/L) (Table 17-19). β-Thalassemia is present in a broad geographic distribution, from the Mediterranean basin to India, the Middle East, Asia, and northern and western Africa. A particularly high prevalence is seen in Italy and Greece. The frequency of β-thalassemia trait in the American black population is estimated to be 0.5–3.3%. Hgb A_2 is variable in homozygous β-thalassemia syndromes (Table 17-20), and measurement may not be useful in differentiating these disorders.

Logistics

In some laboratories, Hgb A_2 may be ordered as a separate test, while in others, it may be included as part of a quantitative Hbg electrophoresis panel. EDTA-anticoagulated blood is stable when refrigerated for up to 10 days. The preferred method of analysis is separation by affinity column chromatography. By regulating the pH value and ionic strength, most hemoglobins, including

Table 17-20. Quantitative Hemoglobin Proportions in Representative Hemoglobinopathies and Thalassemias

Condition	Genetic Defect	% Hgb A	% Variant	% Hgb A_2	% Hgb F
Normal adult		>95	0	<3.5	<2
Normal newborn		20–40	0	0–1.0	60–80
S trait (AS)	Mutation of 1 β gene	60	40	<4.5	<2
C trait (AC)	Mutation of 1 β gene	60	40	[a]	<2
D trait (AD)	Mutation of 1 β gene	60	40	<3.5	<2
E trait (AE)	Mutation of 1 β gene	70	30	[a]	<2
O-Arab trait (AO)	Mutation of 1 β gene	60–70	30–40	[a]	<2
G-Philadelphia trait (AG)					
with 1 α gene	Mutation of 1 α gene	75	25	<3.5	<2
with 2 α genes	Mutation of 2 α genes	70	30	<3.5	<2
with 3 α genes	Mutation of 3 α genes	65	45	<3.5	<2
Köln (A-Köln)	Mutation of 1 β gene	70–80	20–25	<3.5	<10
α-Thalassemia trait	Deletion of 2 α genes	>95	0	<3.5	<2
H disease ($β_4$)	Deletion of 3 α genes	60–90	5–20	1.5–2.5	5–15
Bart's ($γ_4$, hydrops fetalis)	Deletion of 4 α genes	0	100	0	0
Constant Spring trait (A-CS)	Terminator codon mutation of α gene, poorly expressed	>95	1–2	<3.5	<2
$β^+$- or $β^0$-Thalassemia trait	Reduced to absent expression of 1 β gene	85–95	0	3.5–7.0	<5
$δβ^0$-Thalassemia trait	Deletion of 1 δβ gene	80–95	0	1.0–2.5	5–20
Lepore trait (A-Lepore)	One composite δβ chain	75–85	5–15%	1.5–2.5	<5
$β^+$-Thalassemia	Reduced expression of 2 β genes	5–40	0	Variable	20–95
$β^0$-Thalassemia	Absent expression of 2 β genes	0	0	Variable	>90
$δβ^0$-Thalassemia	Deletion of 2 δβ genes	0	0	0	100
African HPFH trait	Deletion of 1 δβ gene with continued γ gene function	65–85	0	1–2.1	15–45
African HPFH homozygote	Deletion of 2 δβ genes with continued γ gene function	0	0	0	100
S disease (SS)	Mutation of 2 β genes	0	>85	<6.0	<10
S-$β^+$-Thalassemia	Combination of above	5–30	>50	Variable	1–20
S-$β^0$-Thalassemia	Combination of above	0	75–90	Variable	5–20
S-$δβ^0$-Thalassemia	Combination of above	0	75–90	Variable	10–25
S-α-Thalassemia	Mutation of 1 β gene and deletion of 1 to 2 α genes	65–75	25–35	<4.5	<2
S-HPFH	Combination of above	0	65–85	Variable	15–45
S-C disease (SC)	Combination of above	0	Approximately equal	[a]	<10
C disease (CC)	Mutation of 2 β genes	0	>85	[a]	<10
C-$β^+$-Thalassemia	Combination of above	5–30	>50	[a]	1–20
E disease (EE)	Mutation of 2 β genes	0	>85	[a]	<10
E-$β^0$-Thalassemia	Combination of above	0	60–85	[a]	15–40

[a] Hgb A_2 cannot be quantitated in the presence of these variant hemoglobins.
Abbreviations: Hgb, hemoglobin; HPFH, hereditary persistence of fetal hemoglobin.
(Data from Fairbanks,[32] Centers for Disease Control,[36] and Bunn et al.[37])

A, F, and S, remain attached to the column, while Hgb A_2 is eluted. Quantitation of Hgb A_2 also may be satisfactorily performed by elution from the electrophoretic membrane and spectrophotometric measurement. However, the Hgb band cannot be measured with sufficient precision by direct densitometry of the electrophoretic pattern.

Hemoglobins C, E, O, and S/G hybrids are eluted with A_2 in column chromatography and comigrate with A_2

on electrophoresis. Thus, Hgb A_2 cannot be quantitated in the presence of abnormal Hgb C, E, O, or S/G hybrids. If the reported Hgb A_2 value from the laboratory is greater than 8–10%, interference from these abnormal hemoglobins should be suspected. Patients with Hgb E trait plus iron deficiency occasionally have markedly reduced percentages of Hgb E to 10–15%, which may be mistaken for elevated Hgb A_2.

Interpretation

The reference range is 1.8–3.5% for adults. The percentage of Hgb A_2 is very low at birth, gradually rising to normal levels before 1 year of age. Hgb A_2 appears to be slightly elevated in the presence of Hgb S (1.7–4.5% with Hgb S trait, 1.7–5.9% with Hgb S disease), but it is unclear whether this phenomenon is physiologic or is related to methodologic interference.

An elevated value is diagnostic of β-thalassemia in a patient with a low MCV. The accompanying clinical presentation and hematologic data or knowledge of the complete hemoglobin phenotype are necessary to distinguish heterozygous β-thalassemia trait from homozygous or doubly heterozygous β-thalassemia major and intermedia syndromes (Tables 17-19 and 17-20). In addition, interaction of β-thalassemia with other hemoglobins with β mutations can lead to significant hematologic disease (Table 17-20). For these reasons, it is best to order Hgb A_2 in combination with a Hgb electrophoresis. An elevated Hgb A_2, accompanied by Hgb A and normal to slightly elevated levels of Hgb F, is consistent with the clinically benign β-thalassemia trait. Because of mild elevation of Hgb A_2 in the presence of Hgb S, the diagnosis of S/β-thalassemia is usually made from the finding of Hgb S greater than 50% (by densitometry of Hgb electrophoresis) in a patient with a low MCV (Table 17-20).

Decreased levels of Hgb A_2 occur with severe iron deficiency, sideroblastic anemia, $\delta\beta^0$-thalassemia, Hgb Lepore trait, Hgb H disease, and aplastic anemia. A falsely normal Hgb A_2 may be seen when β-thalassemia trait is accompanied by iron deficiency. If the patient remains microcytic after appropriate iron therapy, the Hgb A_2 should be repeated.

When the hemogram is suggestive of thalassemia trait, yet the Hgb A_2 is normal, other causes of unbalanced globin chain synthesis should be considered. Some abnormal hemoglobins (e.g., Hgb E, Hgb Lepore) are synthesized at a reduced rate and may thus give rise to a thalassemia-like syndrome. Deletion or reduced activity of the δ gene, as seen in $\delta\beta^0$-thalassemia or HPFH, will result in an increase in Hgb F, but not Hgb A_2 (Table 17-20). In α-thalassemia trait, the relative percentage of Hgb A_2 and Hgb F remains normal, as the α-globin chain is found in all the adult hemoglobins. α-Thalassemia trait, with a normal quantitative Hgb electrophoresis, is therefore frequently a diagnosis of exclusion for persistent microcytosis, when other causes of microcytic anemia (e.g., iron deficiency, anemia of chronic disease, microangiopathic hemolysis) have been excluded. The presence of rare Hgb H inclusions (present in approximately 1 in 10,000 RBCs) frequently occurs in α-thalassemia trait and is useful in confirming the diagnosis. Although deficient α chains may be demonstrated by globin synthesis studies or abnormal gene fragments by DNA analysis, these research laboratory studies are rarely necessary for diagnosis.

Test: Hemoglobin F (Fetal Hemoglobin)[1,2,6,30,32,36,37,41]

Background and Selection

Hemoglobin F ($\alpha_2\gamma_2$), the major Hgb in fetal life, is present in small amounts in healthy adults. The percentage of Hgb F may be elevated in various β- or $\delta\beta^0$-thalassemic syndromes, where the rate of production of other non-γ-globin chains is reduced. In addition, continued production of Hgb F occurs in the adult in HPFH.

Quantitation of Hgb F is performed in patients with persistent microcytosis to aid in the diagnosis of $\delta\beta^0$-thalassemia (high F thalassemia) or HPFH. African-type HPFH is present in approximately 0.1% of American blacks; other rare variants (e.g., Greek and Swiss-type, Hgb Kenya trait) of HPFH also are seen. Large amounts of Hgb F may be seen in juvenile chronic granulocytic leukemia, erythroleukemia, and PNH and quantitation may be a useful clue to these disorders.

Terminology

In some laboratories, Hgb F may be ordered as a separate test, whereas in others it may be included as part of a quantitative Hgb electrophoresis.

Logistics

EDTA-anticoagulated blood can be stored refrigerated for up to 1 week before analysis. Although Hgb F can be visualized as a separate band on electrophoresis, densitometry of the electrophoretic membrane overestimates small amounts of Hgb F because of the close migration of Hgb A and Hgb S. Hgb F may be accurately determined by immunologic methods, column chromatography, or resistence to alkaline denaturation. The widely used alkaline denaturation assay measures residual Hgb F after precipitation of other hemoglobins by strong alkali. Of other abnormal hemoglobins, only Hgb Ranier is resistant to alkaline denaturation. Because carboxyhemoglobin A (present in increased amounts in smokers) is also resistant to akaline precipitation, the method should initially convert carboxyhemoglobin to cyanmethemoglobin, to avoid spurious elevation of Hgb F. Many methods for Hgb F measurement may be nonlinear at high levels and may underestimate Hgb F levels greater than 30–60%. A semiquantitative estimate of Hgb F by densitometry of alkaline electrophoresis should be made if Hgb F levels exceed the limits of method linearity.

Interpretation

Most adults have less than 1% Hgb F, but a few healthy adults (particularly blacks) may have 1–2% Hgb F. Neonates have approximately 60–80% Hgb F and 20–40% Hgb A, with a steady decline of Hgb F to approximately 5% at 6 months, and normal adult levels in about 1 year. However, some children may have mildly elevated Hgb F levels for several years.

A thalassemic syndrome involving the β- or β- and δ-globin chains should be suspected when persistent microcytosis is present, accompanied by elevation of Hgb F. Clinical correlates of these syndromes and typical Hgb F levels can be seen in Table 17-20. Hemoglobin F levels of 90–100% are seen in homozygous HPFH and homozygous β^0- or $\delta\beta^0$-thalassemia. High levels of Hgb F (more than 10%) may be seen with heterozygous HPFH (15–40%), β^+-thalassemia major, or with an abnormal β chain Hgb variant combined with β^0-, β^+-, or $\delta\beta^0$-thalassemia trait. Heterozygous $\delta\beta^0$-thalassemia trait may show a Hgb F level of 5–20%. Occasionally, homozygous SS disease may show a Hgb F level of 10–20%, but most homozygous hemoglobinopathies have only mild elevation of Hgb F (less than 10%). Approximately one-half of patients with β-thalassemia trait (high A$_2$ thalassemia) or Hgb Lepore will show mild elevation of Hgb F (usually less than 5%).

There are also numerous acquired malignant and nonmalignant conditions associated with a elevated Hgb F, although the elevation is rarely a clue to unexpected disease. Mild elevations (less than 10%) are seen in many anemias, leukemias, myeloma, and malignancies metastatic to the bone marrow and with marrow fibrosis. Larger elevations may be present in erythroleukemia, juvenile chronic myelocytic leukemia (CML), and PNH.

A small rise in Hgb F levels occurs in some pregnant women, particularly during the second trimester. This increase is probably not a result of leakage of fetal cells into the maternal circulation but may represent activation of the maternal hematopoietic system by hormones.

With Hgb F levels of 10–20%, particularly in combination with Hgb S, a Kleihauer-Betke stain for RBC fetal HgB may be useful to distinguish HPFH from $\delta\beta^0$-thalassemia trait or homozygous SS disease. African-type HPFH causes pancellular staining, while the various β- or $\beta\delta$-thalassemia syndromes or elevated Hgb F in homozygous hemoglobinopathy give heterocellular staining. The combination of Hgb S with HPFH produces a clinically mild sickling disorder, mitigated by the protective effect of Hgb F in every RBC.

Test: Hemoglobin H Inclusions (Brilliant Cresyl Blue Test for Hemoglobin H)[7,6,30]

Background and Selection

Hemoglobin H is a tetramer of β-globin chains formed when α-globin production is severely reduced. Hemoglobin H disease is an α-thalassemia, resulting from the deletion of three of the four α genes (Fig. 17-11), or, less frequently, the deletion of two α chains with mutation of a third α chain. An unstable Hgb, Hgb H, forms numerous characteristic RBC inclusions when incubated with brilliant cresyl blue.

Moderately severe hemolytic anemia and persistent microcytosis occur in Hgb H disease. The presence of a fast moving Hgb on alkaline electrophoresis comprising approximately 10% of the total Hgb is also suggestive of Hgb H. Rare inclusions may be found in 1 in 10,000 RBCs in patients with α-thalassemia trait (two out of four α genes deleted), particularly in patients of Southeast Asian origin. α-Thalassemia trait is suspected in patients with persistent microcytosis and elevated RBC count, after β-thalassemia trait and iron deficiency have been excluded.

Deletion of the α gene is very prevalent in Southeast Asia and along the west coast of Africa. However, despite the high prevalence in black Americans (7% single gene deletion, 28% two gene deletion), Hgb H disease is rare. This is because the deletion of the two α genes nearly always occurs on opposite chromosomes in the *trans* position, rather than the *cis* position deletion frequently seen in patients of Southeast Asian origin (Fig. 17-11).

Logistics

EDTA-anticoagulated blood should be used less than 24 hours after phlebotomy. Equal amounts of blood are incubated with brilliant cresyl blue at 37°C for 1 hour and slides prepared. Hemoglobin H is precipitated as multiply speckled, evenly spaced, greenish blue inclusions, described as resembling a golf ball. The Hgb H inclusions should be distinguished from reticulocytes, Howell-Jolly bodies, and Heinz bodies, which also will stain with brilliant cresyl blue. Prolonged incubation may result in the production of Heinz bodies rather than Hgb H inclusions.

Interpretation

In Hgb H disease, 10–100% of the RBCs will contain characteristic inclusions. Patients who have been splenectomized may show numerous Heinz bodies as well as Hgb H inclusions. A rare inclusion may be seen in α-thalassemia trait in Southeast Asian persons. Alkaline and neutral pH Hgb electrophoresis should be ordered to confirm the presence of fast-migrating Hgb H.

Patients with Hgb H disease produce Hgb Bart's (γ_4) rather than Hgb H during the neonatal period. Hemoglobin Bart's also appears as a fast-moving Hgb on alkaline Hgb electrophoresis, but may not produce Hgb H inclusions with brilliant cresyl blue.

Test: Isopropanol Denaturation (Unstable Hemoglobin Screen)[7,30,32,35,36]

Background and Selection

Mutations in the globin-heme region of the Hgb molecule result in an unstable Hgb variant. These hemoglobinopathies are characterized by a chronic hemolytic anemia, with methemoglobin and Heinz body formation. The unstable hemoglobins are more easily denatured and precipitated by chemical agents that weaken the internal bonding of heme.

The isopropanol denaturation test should be ordered for patients with documented chronic nonspherocytic hemolytic anemia and suspected unstable Hgb variant.

Approximately 100 unstable hemoglobins have been identified; they are symptomatic in the heterozygous form, hence inherited in a dominant fashion. Clinical severity varies from severe hemolytic anemia in the first year of life to well compensated hemolysis with mild anemia. Hemolysis may be exacerbated with the use of oxidant drugs. The anemia may be macrocytic (from increased reticulocytes) and hypochromic (from removal of Hgb from the RBC in the form of Heinz bodies). Patients often have splenomegaly and occasionally may show dark urine, caused by an abnormal dipyrrole pigment, from catabolism of heme within precipitated Hgb aggregates. Because the spleen rapidly removes the Heinz bodies formed from the precipitated Hgb, they may be not detected until after splenectomy. One-fourth of all unstable Hgb variants may show a normal electrophoresis pattern, but the percentage of Hgb A_2 and Hgb F may be elevated because of the loss of the unstable Hgb.

Logistics

EDTA-anticoagulated blood should be assayed within 4 hours. A RBC hemolysate is incubated in buffered isopropanol. Unstable hemoglobins precipitate in 5–20 minutes, whereas normal hemoglobins will not precipitate until 30–40 minutes. Because pH value and alcohol concentration are critical in this screening test, a freshly drawn normal control blood should be assayed with the patient.

Interpretation

Isopropanol is a very sensitive, but somewhat nonspecific, test for unstable Hgb. False positive results occur with Hgb F greater than 4% and with increased methemoglobin (seen in older specimens or hemolytic anemias caused by oxidant chemicals or RBC enzyme deficiencies). A positive isopropanol screen should be followed by the more specific heat stability test. More specific identification of the unstable Hgb variant requires very specialized research laboratory testing such as globin chain electrophoresis or amino acid or peptide analysis.

Hemoglobins Köln, Zurich, and Hasharon are the most common unstable hemoglobins reported; they migrate as a smudged band in the Hgb S region on alkaline electrophoresis. In addition, Hgb H, a tetramer of β-globin (β_4) seen with deletion of three α genes, and Hgb E, a β-chain mutant with poor production, are unstable with laboratory testing. However, anemia is more likely the result of a thalassemic-like syndrome than clinical hemolysis in Hgb H disease or homozygous Hgb E.

Test: Kleihauer-Betke (Acid Elution for Fetal Hemoglobin)[7,30,32]

Background and Selection

The Kleihauer-Betke test is used for staining of postpartum Rh-negative maternal blood specimens when fetal maternal hemorrhage is suspected. Preliminary screening for fetal cells in maternal blood is performed with an immune rosetting procedure for D-positive cells. This test may be positive in 2% of cases, and the Kleihauer-Betke stain is then used for confirmation (approximately 20% of positive screens are confirmed). Additional doses of RhoGam can be administered, depending on the number of fetal cells present. In addition, the test is useful in distinguishing African HPFH with Hgb F in every RBC from $\beta\delta$-thalassemia trait and other hemoglobinopathies with increased Hgb F (Hgb F isolated to one population of RBCs).

Logistics

The patient should not have received a recent transfusion. EDTA- or heparin-anticoagulated blood should be less than 6 hours old. Smears should be fixed with alcohol within 1 hour after preparation to precipitate the RBC Hgb. Hemoglobin A is eluted with citric acid buffer, while Hgb F remains insoluble. After eosin counterstain is applied, cells with Hgb A appears as ghosts, whereas cells with Hgb F retain pink coloration. The percentage of cells with Hgb F can be determined. For assessment of fetal-maternal hemorrhage, 10,000 RBCs are counted and the percentage positive cells multiplied by 5000 mL (average maternal blood volume) to estimate the volume of fetal blood loss.

Interpretation

Healthy adults have no positive RBCs. One vial of Rh immunoglobulin neutralizes approximately 30 mL of fetal blood. If larger amounts of fetal blood are present, a larger dose of Rh immunoglobulin should be administered to prevent maternal sensitization. The African type of homozygous or heterozygous HPFH is the only hemoglobinopathy in which nearly all the RBCs have Hgb F. Since Hgb F ameliorates the sickling tendency of Hgb S, double heterozygotes for Hgb S and HPFH will not have hemolytic anemia. If test interpretation is difficult in a patient with suspected S-HPFH, Hgb F determination of the parent's blood would indicate whether HPFH trait could be inherited in the patient.

Test: Sickle Hemoglobin Solubility (Sickle Cell Preparation, Dithionite Test, Sickledex)[6,7,32,36,42]

Background and Selection

Hemoglobin S and a few other rarely encountered abnormal hemoglobins are insoluble in the presence of concentrated buffer and reducing agent. This test is used primarily as a screening test for the presence of Hgb S, whether in S trait (AS), S disease (SS), or in combination with another abnormal hemoglobin or with thalassemia trait. Infants younger than 6 months of age may not produce sufficient quantity of non-F Hgb to give a positive result. Many laboratories also use the solubility test to confirm the identity of a presumptive Hgb S found on alkaline Hgb electrophoresis, as an alternative to confirmation by acid electrophoresis analysis. Such confirmation of initial electrophoretic findings is important, because 1% of patients with typical S trait pattern on alkaline electrophoresis have non-S Hgb D or G.

Logistics

EDTA-anticoagulated blood is preferred, although any anticoagulant may be used. The EDTA-anticoagulated sample may be stored refrigerated for at least 3 weeks. Whole blood is added to a mixture of phosphate buffer, reducing agent (usually dithionate), and RBC lysing agent. Sickling Hgb forms insoluble tactoids in this mixture, resulting in a turbid solution. The test is sensitive to approximately 10–20% or 2 g/dL (20 g/L) of Hgb S.

With some solubility tests, a toluene organic phase is added to the buffer mixture to distinguish between homozygous and heterozygous sickling Hgb. Homozygous SS disease (without transfusion) causes a dark red layer at the organic-aqueous interface with absence of Hgb in the lower aqueous layer (which will be amber colored). Mixtures of sickling and nonsickling Hgb (e.g., AS, SD, SC, S-β-thalassemia trait, SS with transfusion) give rise to both a red interface Hgb-layer and varying shades of red Hgb in the lower aqueous layer.

False positive results may occur with turbid plasma due to lipemia or abnormally precipitable γ-globulins. In these cases, the blood may be tested after the plasma has been replaced with saline. Polycythemia and a large number of nucleated RBCs also may cause false positive results. False negative tests occur with Hgb below 7–8 g/dL, extensive transfusion to low levels of Hgb S, and in the presence of inhibitors of sickling, such as very high concentrations of Hgb F and phenothiazines.

In the past, the sickling phenomenon was also demonstrated by microscopically observing sickled RBCs after the addition of a reducing substance (usually metabisulfite). However, crenated cells or other poikilocytes may produce problems in test interpretation, and this method of screening for sickling hemoglobins is now rarely used.

Interpretation

A positive result is highly suggestive of the presence of Hgb S. Other rare hemoglobins that give a positive result include the unstable hemoglobins (particularly when Heinz bodies are present), and abnormal hemoglobins with one amino acid substitution identical to Hgb S (substitution of valine for glutamic acid in the sixth position of the β chain) plus one additional amino acid substitution. Examples are Hgb C-Harlem (also called C-Georgetown) and C-Ziguinchor, which migrate in the C position on alkaline electrophoresis and Hgb S-Travis.

A positive result does not differentiate between Hgb S trait (AS), Hgb S disease (SS), or double heterozygotes for S-β-thalassemia trait, S-HPFH, and S plus another abnormal Hgb. Even when a solubility test with toluene shows the presence of sickling and nonsickling hemoglobins, a doubly heterozygous hemoglobinopathy involving S cannot be excluded. A normal hemogram and blood smear morphology are seen in benign Hgb S trait, whereas anemia and RBC abnormalities are common in the clinically symptomatic disorders. A positive sickle Hgb solubility test should be followed by confirmatory identification with Hgb electrophoresis.

MISCELLANEOUS TESTS

Test: RBC Mass and Plasma Volume (^{51}Cr-Labeled Red Blood Cell Volume)[1,6,7,30]

Background and Selection

Measurement of RBC mass and plasma volume can distinguish between absolute and relative polycythemia. Red blood cell mass is increased in absolute polycythemia, whereas RBC mass is normal to borderline and plasma volume is decreased in relative polycythemia. Measurement of RBC mass and plasma volume may help in establishing the cause of polycythemia when the diagnosis is clinically obscure. When the Hgb is greater than 20 g/dL or the Hct is greater than 60%, an increase in RBC mass can be assumed. A decreased arterial pO_2 implicates hypoxia as the cause for absolute polycythemia. When neutrophilia, thrombocytosis, and splenomegaly accompany polycythemia, polycythemia vera is the likely diagnosis. In these situations, the measurement of RBC mass is not necessary. The measurement of RBC mass may be important to identify patients with stress erythrocytosis (Gaisböck syndrome) who have a relative polycythemia. However, a more useful manuever is for the patient to abstain from smoking, which often leads to disappearance of the polycythemia within a few weeks.

Logistics

Radiation from isotopic scanning procedures may interfere with the determination. Thus, at least 3 days should elapse after a liver, spleen, bone, or brain scan. The patient should not be receiving antibiotics or ascorbic acid, which can inhibit chromium binding to the RBCs. Blood for RIA tests should be drawn before the blood volume determination, because the ^{51}Cr may cause interference. The patient will not be able to drink or eat during the testing period, which may be several hours in duration.

Blood is collected into citrate anticoagulant, and the RBCs are separated and incubated with ^{51}Cr. Excess free isotope is removed by washing, and ascorbic acid is often added to inhibit any residual free ^{51}Cr from binding to RBCs in vivo. A measured aliquot of labeled RBCs in normal saline is reinfused into the patient, taking great care to make sure that it all enters the vein. After a period of mixing, usually 15 minutes, a venous sample is removed from the opposite arm. Splenomegaly or congestive heart failure may cause delayed equilibration, and another sample should be taken after 60 minutes. Red blood cell volume is calculated by dividing the total radioactivity of the injected cells, by the radioactivity/mL of RBCs in the venous circulation.

On occasion, the subsequent rate of disappearance of ^{51}Cr radioactivity can be measured to assess RBC life span, and external scanning for radioactivity can detect major sites of RBC destruction. Plasma volume is similarly determined by incubating plasma with iodine 125 (^{125}I) labeled albumin and intravenously injecting a measured aliquot into the patient. The measurement of plasma volume may not be as accurate as the RBC mass because of the leakage of albumin from the vascular compartment. An important cause of error is the failure to inject all the labeled RBCs or plasma back into the patient. Any leakage into tissues or residual in the syringe gives a falsely high value for RBC mass or plasma volume. Meticulous attention to detail is necessary to obtain accurate results.

Interpretation

Normal erythrocyte volume for men is 26–32 mL/kg, and for women and children, 23–29 mL/kg. A representative reference range for plasma volume is 36–44 mL/kg for both men and women. Spuriously low values may occur with obesity, because fat has less vascularity than lean body mass. The use of height/weight nomograms for RBC mass may give a more useful reference range.

Red blood cell mass is the only means of differentiating a relative versus an absolute polycythemia. Diagnostic considerations for these situations are given in Table 17-6 and discussed in the Introduction.

Red blood cell mass is usually elevated more than two times normal in polycythemia vera. In stress erythrocytosis (Gaisböck syndrome), the RBC mass is often high normal and the plasma volume is low or low-normal. Carbon monoxide from tobacco smoking may be an important factor in the etiology, leading to both tissue hypoxia and decreased plasma volume.

Test: Erythropoietin (EPO)[5,43]

Erythropoietin (EPO) is a glycoprotein produced in peritubular cells (perhaps endothelial) in the renal cortex. It is released in response to renal hypoxia, and accelerates erythropoiesis in the bone marrow. In the past, in vivo bioassays or in vitro cell culture assays for EPO were performed that were imprecise and lacking in sensitivity. With the availability of purified recombinant EPO, competitive RIAs have been developed. Theoretically, measurement of EPO might be useful in differentiating secondary polycythemia (EPO increased) from polycythemia vera (EPO normal or decreased). However, many patients with secondary polycythemia may have normal EPO values, and EPO may have limited value in this discrimination. Measurement of EPO may be of value in monitoring therapy of tumors with ectopic EPO production (Table 17-6). If recombinant EPO therapy proves useful in therapy for aplastic anemia or renal disease, EPO measurements may be of use in monitoring this treatment.

REFERENCES

1. Rapaport SI: Introduction to Hematology. 2nd Ed. Philadelphia, JB Lippincott, 1987.
2. Wintrobe MW, Lee GR, Boggs DR, et al: Clinical Hematology. 8th Ed. Philadelphia, Lea & Febiger, 1981.
3. Schumacher HR, Garvin DF, Triplett DA: Introduction to Laboratory Hematology. New York, Allen R Liss, 1984.
4. Abshire T, Reeves JD: Anemia of acute inflammation in children. J Pediatr 1983;103:869–871.
5. Zanjani ED, Ascensao JL: Erythropoietin. Transfusion 1989;29:46–57.
6. Henry JB: Clinical Diagnosis and Management by Laboratory Methods. 17th Ed. Philadelphia, WB Saunders, 1984.
7. Williams WJ, Beutler E, Erslev AJ, Lichtman MA: Hematology. 3rd Ed. New York, McGraw-Hill, 1983.
8. Cornbleet J: Spurious results from automated hematology cell counters. Lab Med 1983;14:509–514.
9. Bessman JD, Gilmer PR, Gardner FH: Improved classification of anemias by MCV and RDW. Am J Clin Pathol 1983;80:322–326.
10. Hillman RS, Finch CA: Red Cell Manual. 5th Ed. Philadelphia, FA Davis, 1985.
11. National Committee for Clinical Laboratory Standards: Method for Reticulocyte Counting. Proposed Standard. NCCLS document H16-P. Villanova, PA, NCCLS, 1985.
12. Dacie JV, Lewis SM: Practical Hematology. Edinburgh, Churchill Livingstone, 1975.
13. National Committee for Clinical Laboratory Standards: Reference Procedure for the Erythrocyte Sedimentation Rate (ESR) test. Approved Standard. HCCLS document H2-A2. Villanova, PA, NCCLS, 1988.
14. Sox HC, Liang MH: Erythrocytes and the sedimentation rate. Guidelines for rational use. Ann Intern Med 1986;104:515–523.
15. Cook JD: Clinical evaluation of iron deficiency. Semin Hematol 1982;20:61–80.
16. Crosby WH: Hemochromatosis: current concepts and management. Hosp Pract 1987;1:173–192.
17. Skikne BS, Cook JD: Serum ferritin in the evaluation of iron status. Lab Management 1981;5:31–35.
18. Witte DL, Anstadt DS, Davis SH, Schrantz RD: Predicting bone marrow iron stores in anemic patients in a community hospital using ferritin and erythrocyte sedimentation rate. Am J Clin Pathol 1988;90:85–87.
19. Witte DL, Kraemer DF, Johnson GF et al: Prediction of bone marrow iron findings from tests performed on peripheral blood. Am J Clin Pathol 1986;85:202–206.
20. Edwards CQ, Griffin LM, Goldgar DJ: Prevalence of hemochromatosis among 11,065 presumably healthy blood donors. N Engl J Med 1988;318:1355–1362.
21. Piomelli S: The diagnostic utility of measurements of erythrocyte porphyrins. Hematol Oncol Clin North Am 1987;1:419–443.
22. Carmel R: Pernicious anemia. The expected findings of very low serum cobalamin levels, anemia, and macrocytosis are often lacking. Arch Intern Med 1988;148:1712–1714.
23. Hoffbrand AV, Pettit JE: Essential Haematology. 2nd Ed. Oxford, Blackwell Scientific, 1984.
24. Lindenbaum J: Status of laboratory testing in the diagnosis of megaloblastic anemia. Blood 1983;61:624–627.

25. Lindenbaum J, Healton EB, Savage DG et al: Neuropsychiatric disorders caused by cobalamin deficiency in the absence of anemia or macrocytosis. N Engl J Med 1988;318:1720–1728.
26. Wallerstein RO: Laboratory evaluation of anemia. West J Med 1987;146:443–451.
27. Herbert V: Making sense of laboratory tests of folate status: folate requirements to sustain normality. Am J Hematol 1987;26:199–207.
28. Herbert V: Experimental nutritional folate deficiency in man. Trans Assoc Am Physicians 1962;75:307–320.
29. Carmel R, Sinow RM, Siegel MD, Samloff IM: Food cobalamin malabsorption occurs frequently in patients with unexplained low serum cobalamin levels. Arch Intern Med 1988;148:1715–1719.
30. Kjeldsberg CR (ed): Practical Diagnosis of Hematologic Disease. Chicago, American Society of Clinical Pathologists, 1989.
31. Miller DR, Baehner RL, McMillan CW: Blood Diseases of Infancy and Childhood. 5th Ed. St. Louis, CV Mosby, 1984.
32. Fairbanks VF: Hemoglobinopathies and Thalassemias. Laboratory Methods and Case Studies. New York, BC Decker, 1980.
33. Larson CJ, Scheidt RK, Fairbanks VF: The osmotic fragility test for hereditary spherocytosis: objective criteria for test interpretation. Am J Clin Pathol 1988;90:508 (abst).
34. Sun NCJ: Hematology—An Atlas and Diagnostic Guide. Philadelphia, WB Saunders, 1983.
35. Carell RW: Hemoglobin stability tests. CRC Crit Rev Lab Sci 1974;5:62–69.
36. Centers for Disease Control: Laboratory Methods for Detecting Hemoglobinopathies. Washington, DC, U.S. Department of Health and Human Services, 1984.
37. Bunn HF, Forget BG: Hemoglobin: Molecular, Genetic, and Clinical Aspects. Philadelphia, WB Saunders, 1986.
38. National Committee for Clinical Laboratory Standards: Detection of Abnormal Hemoglobin Using Cellulose Acetate Electrophoresis. Approved Standard. NCCLS document H8-A. Villanova, PA, NCCLS, 1986.
39. National Committee for Clinical Laboratory Standards: Citrate Agar Electrophoresis for Confirming Identifications of Mutant Hemoglobins. Proposed Guideline. NCCLS document H23-P. Villanova, PA, NCCLS, 1981.
40. National Committee for Clinical Laboratory Standards: Chromatographic (Microcolumn) Determination of Hemoglobin A_2. Tentative Standard. NCCLS document H9-T. Villanova, PA, NCCLS, 1980.
41. National Committee for Clinical Laboratory Standards: Quantitative Measurement of Fetal Hemoglobin by the Alkali Denaturation Method: Tentative Guideline. NCCLS document H13-T. Villanova, PA, NCCLS, 1986.
42. National Committee for Clinical Laboratory Standards: Solubility Test for Confirming the Presence of Sickling Hemoglobins: Approved Standard. NCCLS document H10-A. Villanova, PA, NCCLS, 1986.
43. Cotes PM, Dore CJ, Yin JA: Determination of serum immunoreactive erythropoietin in the investigation of erythrocytosis. N Engl J Med 1986;315:283–287.
44. Rudoph AM, Barnett HL, Einhorn AH (eds): Pediatrics. East Norwalk, CT, Appleton-Century-Crofts, 1977.

18 Hemostasis

John T. Brandt

INTRODUCTION

Hemostasis is a multicomponent system that serves two major functions; the first is to stem blood loss from sites of vascular disruption, whereas the second is to prevent pathologic thrombosis by limiting hemostatic plug formation to sites of vascular damage. Hemostasis thus can be thought of as a balanced system composed of opposing procoagulant and regulatory (anticoagulant) forces. The procoagulant side of the balance is responsible for formation of a stable hemostatic plug and involves the response of circulating platelets and plasma proteins. The regulatory system is responsible for limiting hemostatic plug formation to sites of vascular damage and depends on the interaction of endothelial cells and circulating plasma proteins. Many, if not most, clinical problems involving this system arise because of shifts in this balance (Fig. 18-1). This discussion briefly reviews the contribution of these various components to the hemostatic response and then outlines an approach to the evaluation of clinical hemostatic problems. Several excellent textbooks provide details on this system for the interested reader.[1-5]

Formation of the Hemostatic Plug

Disruption of the vessel wall initiates a sequence of events that culminates in the formation of a stable hemostatic plug.[6] The first detectable response is the arrival of platelets that stick to the site of damage and spread over the exposed subendothelial tissues in a process referred to as *adhesion*. These adhering platelets release chemical mediators that recruit additional platelets to the site; the responding platelets stick to the platelets that are already present, resulting in the formation of a platelet plug or aggregate. As the platelet plug is forming thrombin is generated and converts fibrinogen to fibrin; the fibrin monomers then polymerize around and through the aggregating platelets, adding strength to the growing hemostatic plug. Factor XIII is activated by thrombin and forms covalent crosslinks between the fibrin monomers, making the fibrin clot less susceptible to lysis by plasmin. The entire hemostatic plug ultimately retracts around the site of damage because of an active contractile mechanism in platelets.

Platelet Plug Formation

The platelet response can be divided into three major phases: adhesion (platelet-nonplatelet interaction), shape change and secretion, and finally aggregation (platelet-platelet interaction). Both adhesion and aggregation are mediated by molecular "glues" (referred to as adhesive proteins) that crosslink the platelet surface to other surfaces. The most important protein mediating platelet adhesion at sites of high shear rates, such as in the capillary bed, is von Willebrand factor (VWF). von Willebrand factor, present in plasma, platelets, and subendothelial tissue, binds to a specific receptor on the platelet surface, glycoprotein Ib (GP Ib), and to receptors in the connective tissue of the vessel wall. von Willebrand factor is produced as a polymer of varying molecular weight; it is the larger polymers (or high molecular weight multimers as they are often called) that are particularly effective at mediating platelet adhesion, perhaps because they most effec-

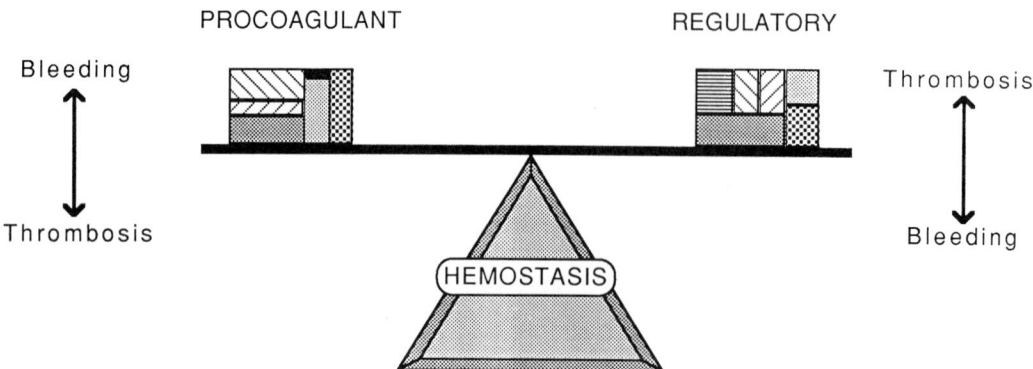

Fig. 18-1. Hemostasis is a balanced multicomponent system. The potent procoagulant side, which is responsible for formation of a stable hemostatic plug, is balanced by the regulatory system. Either a decrease in the procoagulant side (e.g., hemophilia A) or an increase in the regulatory side (e.g., heparin therapy) may cause clinical bleeding. Similarly, an increase in the activity of the procoagulant side (e.g., metastatic tumor) or a decrease in the regulatory side (e.g., antithrombin III deficiency) may predispose to thrombosis.

tively maximize the amount of platelet membrane–subendothelial surface contact (Fig. 18-2).

Adhesion of platelets to the vessel wall activates several metabolic pathways in the platelet, leading to a rapid increase in cytoplasmic calcium levels. Changes in calcium flux lead to shape change, which is dependent on a contractile mechanism, and to secretion, resulting in release of platelet granular contents to the external environment of the platelet. Two major biochemical pathways that promote calcium flux have been identified: the thromboxane A_2 (TxA_2) and phosphatidylinositol (PI) pathways. Thromboxane A_2 is a potent stimulator of platelet aggregation that is synthesized by platelets in response to a variety of stimuli. It is a product of the prostaglandin pathway initiated by release of arachidonic acid from platelet membranes (Fig. 18-3).

The PI pathway is initiated by activation of membrane associated phospholipase C, which splits phosphatidylinositol bisphosphate into two important intermediates: diacylglycerol (DAG) and inositol trisphosphate (IP_3). Diacylglycerol associates with an enzyme called protein kinase C, increasing its affinity for calcium and thus its enzymatic activity (Fig. 18-4). Protein kinase C then phosphorylates target proteins, including a 40,000-da protein involved in platelet secretion. Phosphorylation results in activation of the target proteins. IP_3 functions as a calcium ionophore, resulting in movement of calcium from its storage site in the dense tubular system into the cytoplasm. The increased calcium levels activate calmodulin-dependent phosphorylation of the actin-myosin system proteins, leading to the formation of active contractile units and shape change.

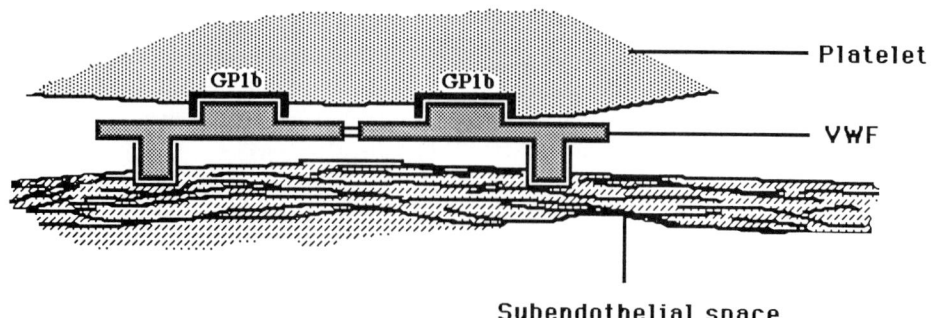

Fig. 18-2. Platelet adhesion to the damaged vascular wall is mediated by von Willebrand factor (VWF). VWF binds to glycoprotein Ib (GP Ib) on the platelet surface and to an unidentified receptor in the subendothelial matrix. Very large multimers of VWF are necessary for effective adhesion, presumably to increase the area of surface contact. Patients who are deficient in VWF (von Willebrand's disease) or in the platelet receptor for VWF (Bernard-Soulier syndrome) have abnormal platelet adhesion and usually present clinically with recurrent mucocutaneous bleeding caused by the abnormal platelet plug formation.

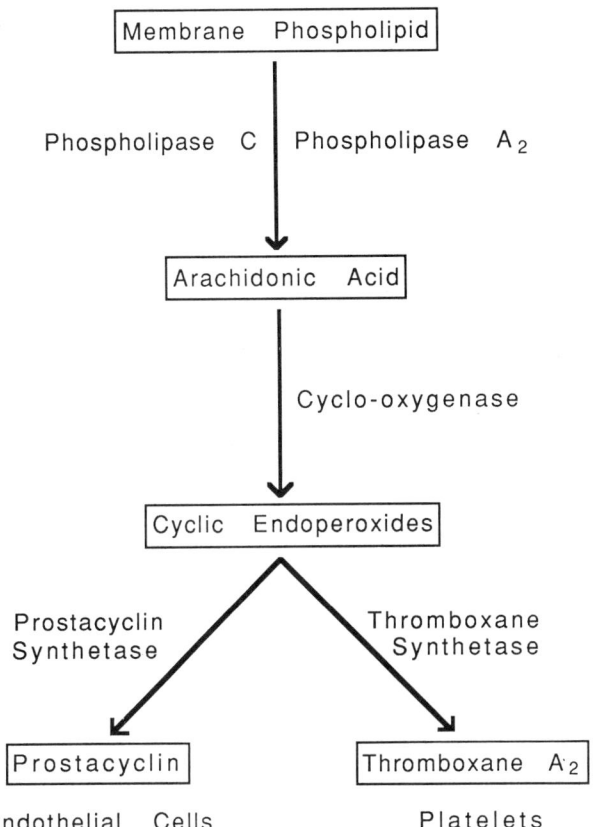

Fig. 18-3. The prostaglandin pathway is initiated by the release of arachidonic acid from membrane phospholipids by either phospholipase A_2 or phospholipase C. Arachidonic acid is then converted to unstable cyclic intermediates by the enzyme cyclo-oxygenase. Within platelets, these cyclic endoperoxides are converted to thromboxane A_2 (TxA_2), a potent platelet agonist. However, in endothelial and other vessel wall cells, the cyclic endoperoxides are converted to prostacyclin, a potent vasodilator and inhibitor of platelet aggregation. Aspirin irreversibly inhibits cyclo-oxygenase, thus blocking formation of TxA_2 and prostacyclin. Other nonsteroidal anti-inflammatory drugs reversibly block cyclo-oxygenase and are also capable of inhibiting platelet function.

A third metabolic pathway involving cyclic adenosine monophosphate (cAMP) is necessary for regulation of these calcium-dependent responses. cAMP inhibits the activity of phospholipase C and also increases storage of calcium; high cAMP levels thus inhibit platelet function (Fig. 18-4). The level of cAMP is modulated by both synthesis and degradation; synthesis is dependent on membrane-associated adenylate cyclase, and degradation is dependent on the enzyme, phosphodiesterase. Interaction of platelet agonists, such as thrombin, with their surface receptor, can lead to simultaneous activation of phospholipase C and to inhibition of adenylate cyclase, a combination that potentiates the platelet response. Natural and pharmacologic inhibitors of platelet function often work by stimulating adenylate cyclase activity or by inhibiting phosphodiesterase activity, leading to increased platelet cAMP levels.

There are two major types of storage granules in platelets: the α- and dense granules. α-Granules store a large number of proteins, some of which are homologues of plasma proteins, but others, such as β-thromboglobulin, are only found in platelets (Table 18-1). By contrast, dense granules are storage sites for adenosine diphosphate (ADP), adenosine triphosphate (ATP), serotonin, small amounts of calcium, and other small molecules; the most important constituent of the dense granules is ADP. When ADP is secreted it acts as a potent platelet agonist, inducing surrounding platelets to aggregate. The contents of both types of granules are released during the secretory process, as is TxA_2. The released products stimulate additional platelets to respond, resulting in the positive feedback loop of platelet stimulation and aggregation.

The final stage of platelet plug formation is platelet-platelet interaction known as *aggregation*. As with adhesion, this process is mediated by adhesive proteins. The major molecular "glue" mediating platelet aggregation is fibrinogen, a large dimeric protein. Fibrinogen binds to a specific membrane receptor, the glycoprotein IIb-IIIa complex that is exposed only after the platelet has been activated by agonists such as ADP. Once the receptor has been exposed, fibrinogen binds to receptors on adjacent platelets, crosslinking the platelet membranes (Fig. 18-5).

Fibrin Clot Formation

Fibrin clot formation is a complex process that can be divided into two major phases: formation of thrombin and formation of a stable fibrin clot.[6,7] Thrombin formation is a phospholipid dependent process that usually takes place on the surface of stimulated platelets but that may take place on a variety of other phospholipid membranes (e.g., stimulated monocytes and endothelial cells). It is dependent on the conversion of inactive proteins to active proteins at the site of vascular damage. This activation is accomplished by selective cleavage of critical amino acid bonds, which permits a change in the conformation of the target protein. By contrast, fibrin formation is a fluid phase process that, under appropriate conditions, leads to formation of a semisolid gel. Thrombin is formed by proteolytic cleavage of its circulating precursor, prothrombin; the enzyme responsible for this is factor Xa (the a after a Roman numeral designation indicates an activated

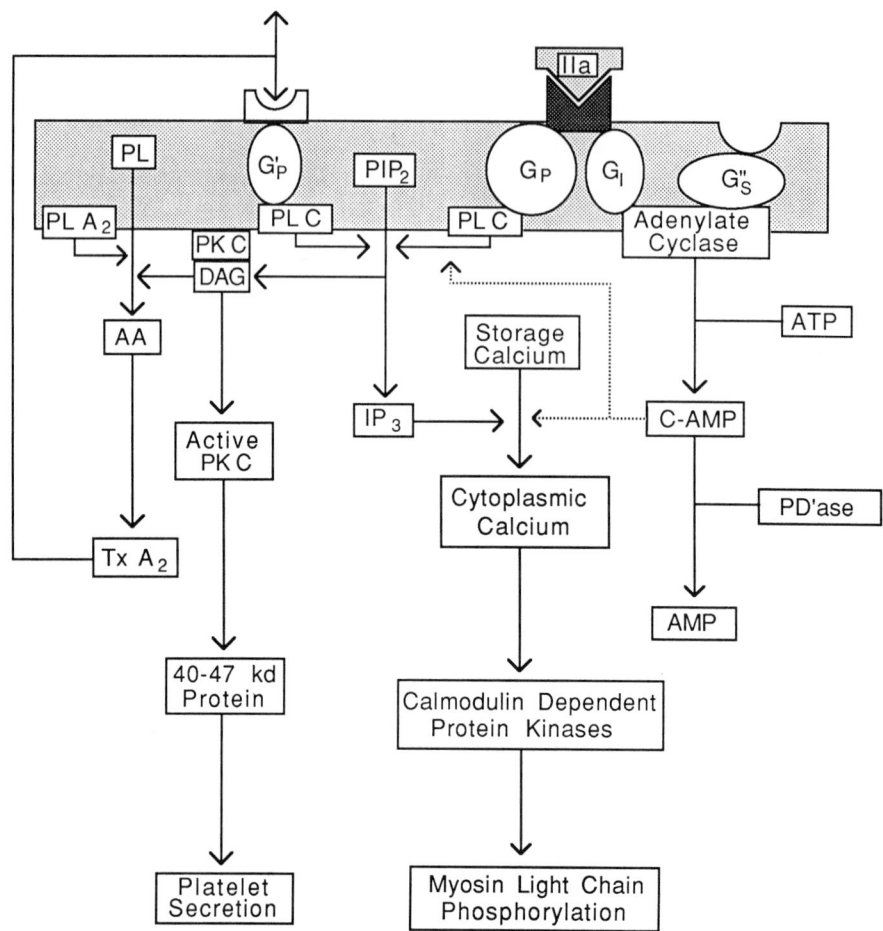

Fig. 18-4. Activation of the platelet leading to platelet secretion and shape change involves several metabolic pathways. A key component is activation of phospholipase C (PL C). This involves interaction between a platelet agonist such as thrombin (IIa) and its membrane receptor. This signal is transmitted to PL C by membrane G proteins (G_P) and results in cleavage of membrane phosphatidyl inositols including phosphatidyl inositol bisphosphate (PIP_2). Cleavage of PIP_2 releases diacylglycerol (DAG) and inositol trisphosphate (IP_3), two important intracellular mediators. DAG activates the protein kinase C system, resulting in phosphorylation of cytoplasmic proteins, including a 40,000–47,000-da protein involved in platelet secretion. DAG may also serve as a source of arachidonic acid (AA). IP_3 releases calcium from intracellular storage sites, resulting in a sudden increase in cytoplasmic calcium concentration which activates calmodulin dependent protein kinases. This pathway is essential for myosin light chain phosphorylation and assembly of the contractile mechanism necessary for shape change and contraction. The platelet response is regulated by cyclic adenosine monophosphate (C-AMP), which inhibits the activity of PL C and the release of calcium into the cytoplasm. The level of C-AMP is controlled by the relative rates of its synthesis (adenylate cyclase) and degradation (phosphodiesterase; PD'ase).

form of a coagulation protein). The story of thrombin formation is thus the story of factor Xa formation, which may be summarized as follows.

Two pathways lead to formation of factor Xa: the *intrinsic system* (because all necessary factors are present in circulating blood), and the *extrinsic system* (because one critical factor is not present in normal circulating blood). The major physiologic pathway is probably the extrinsic system, which is activated when plasma factor VIIa comes into contact with tissue factor (Fig. 18-6). Tissue factor is composed of a membrane protein (apoprotein III) and phospholipid and serves as a cofactor for the activation of factors IX and X by factor VIIa. This pathway is measured by the prothrombin time (PT).

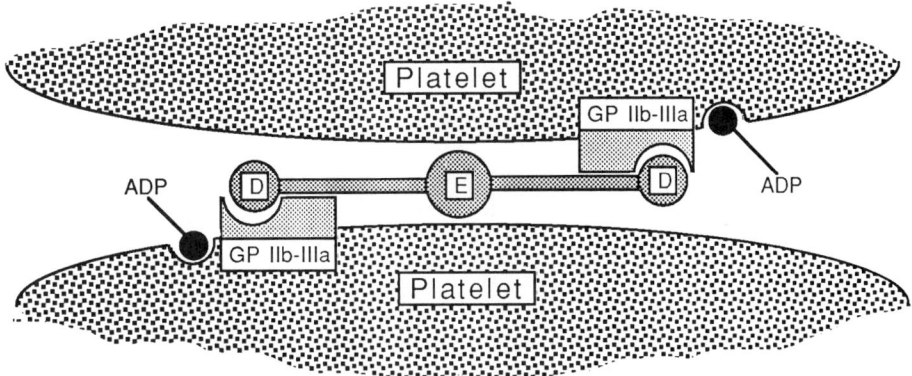

Fig. 18-5. Platelet aggregation is mediated by intact fibrinogen which binds to a specific membrane receptor, glycoprotein IIb-IIIa (GP IIb-IIIa). Under resting conditions GP IIb-IIIa can not bind fibrinogen. However, after the platelet membrane has been stimulated, for example, by adenosine diphosphate (ADP), the binding sites are opened and fibrinogen binds. Fibrinogen is a large homodimer with a central E domain and two identical terminal D domains. The D domain of fibrinogen binds to the GP IIb-IIIa receptor on adjacent platelets, crosslinking their surfaces. Platelets lacking the GP IIb-IIIa receptor (Glanzmann's thrombasthenia) are unable to aggregate resulting in a bleeding disorder. Monomeric fibrin degradation products, containing only a single D domain, can actually block platelet aggregation by competitively binding to a GP IIa-IIIb receptor but not crosslinking it to an adjacent platelet.

Once factor Xa is formed, it can activate prothrombin to thrombin. Its ability to activate prothrombin is greatly enhanced by a nonenzymatic cofactor, factor V, which appears to help concentrate the enzyme and its substrate on the phospholipid surface (Fig. 18-7). The ability of factor V to accelerate prothrombin activation is greatly enhanced by limited cleavage of the native protein by thrombin, resulting in an activated two-chain form designated Va. Thus, initial thrombin formation is slow until enough thrombin is formed to permit feedback activation of the nonenzymatic cofactors factors V and VIII; once this happens, there is an ex-

Table 18-1.	Platelet α-Granule Proteins
Homologues of Plasma Proteins	**Platelet-Associated Proteins**
Fibrinogen	Platelet factor 4
Fibronectin	β-Thromboglobulin
Albumin	Platelet-derived growth factor
Factor V	Thrombospondin
High molecular weight kininogen	
von Willebrand factor	
Plasminogen	
Factor D	
β₁-H-globulin	
Protein S	
Factor XIIIa	

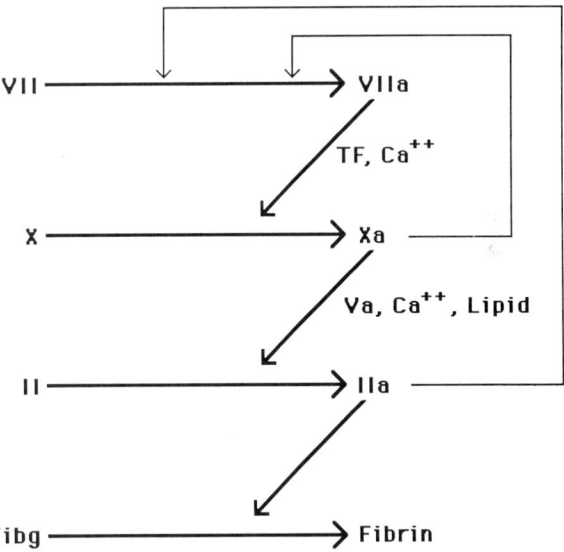

Fig. 18-6. The extrinsic pathway of coagulation is initiated by interaction of factor VIIa with tissue factor (TF) in the presence of calcium and a phospholipid surface. VIIa converts factor X to its active form, Xa, which in turn activates prothrombin (factor II) to thrombin (IIa). Factor Va, calcium (Ca^{++}), and a phospholipid surface are necessary for this second step. Thrombin then removes fibrinopeptides A and B from fibrinogen (fibg) to form fibrin; the fibrin monomers then polymerize to form the fibrin gel (clot). Both thrombin and Xa activate more factor VII to VIIa through a positive feedback loop, further accelerating the process. The extrinsic pathway is measured by the prothrombin time (PT). Although VIIa can also activate factor IX of the intrinsic pathway, this step is not measured by PT.

504 • Laboratory Medicine

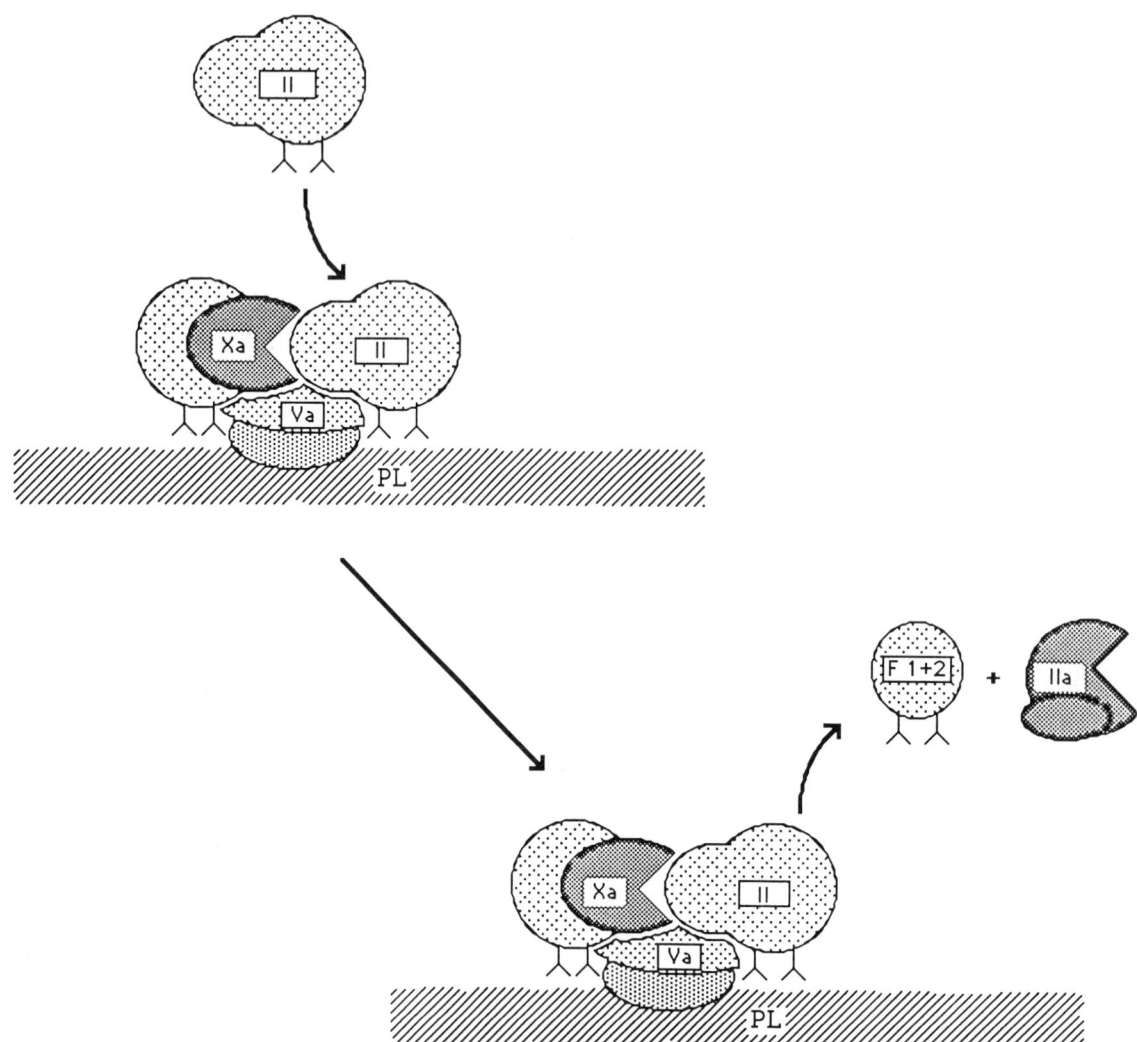

Fig. 18-7. Formation of the "prothrombinase" complex. Factor Xa activates prothrombin in the presence of factor Va, phospholipid and calcium. The phospholipid surface and Va serve to localize and accelerate the interaction between Xa, an active enzyme, and its substrate, prothrombin. The activation of prothrombin results in the release of a large peptide (activation peptide) designated F_{1+2} and thrombin. Many other reactions involved in the coagulation cascade involve analogous phospholipid-dependent activation complexes.

plosive formation of thrombin at the site of platelet plug formation.

The *intrinsic pathway* of coagulation is initiated by contact of factor XII with negatively charged surfaces, which results in expression of factor XIIa activity. Factor XIIa proteolytically activates both prekallikrein and factor XI, with high molecular weight kininogen serving as a cofactor for both steps (Fig. 18-8). In a positive feedback loop, kallikrein activates more factor XII, which further enhances activation of factor XI. In turn, factor XIa activates factor IX, which in the presence of factor VIIIa activates factor X. As with factor V, the procoagulant activity of factor VIII is enhanced by limited proteolytic cleavage resulting in a two chain protein. The remainder of the pathway is the same as for the extrinsic pathway and is often designated the *final common pathway*. The intrinsic pathway of coagulation is measured by the activated partial thromboplastin time.

Activation of thrombin can be viewed as the result of the formation of several enzyme-cofactor-substrate complexes on phospholipid surfaces. This approach permits division of the involved coagulation factors into two major groups on the basis of their function

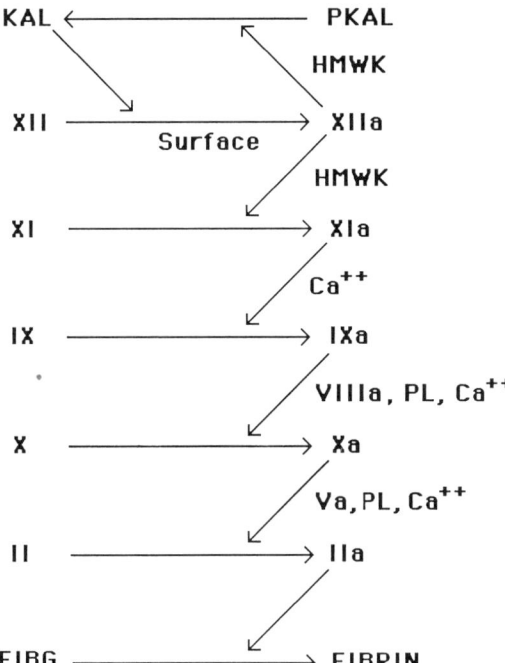

Fig. 18-8. The intrinsic system begins with the conversion of factor XII to an active enzyme, XIIa. This change occurs when factor XII binds to negatively charged surfaces. XIIa then activates prekallikrein (PKAL) and factor XI. Kallikrein (KAL) activates more factor XII to XIIa, forming a positive feedback loop. XIa activates factor IX to IXa, which then converts factor X to Xa in the presence of factor VIIIa (a nonenzymatic cofactor), phospholipid, and calcium (Ca^{++}). The remainder of the cascade is the same as for the extrinsic system and is known as the final common pathway. The intrinsic system is measured by the activated partial thromboplastin time (APTT). HMWK, high molecular weight kallikrein; PL, phospholipid; FIBG, fibrinogen.

Table 18-2. Classification of Coagulation Factors by Function

Proenzymes	Cofactors
Contact family	
Factor XI	High molecular weight
Factor XII	kininogen
Prekallikrein	
Vitamin K family	
Factor II	Protein S
Factor VII	
Factor IX	
Factor X	
Protein C (regulatory)	
Miscellaneous	
Factor XIII	Factor V
	Factor VIII
	Fibrin (for plasmin activation)

(Table 18-2). All the enzymes involved in thrombin generation are serine proteases that may be subdivided into two groups: the vitamin K dependent and independent groups. The vitamin K dependent proteases (factors II, VII, IX, and X) are all characterized by the presence of 8–12 γ-carboxyglutamic acid residues near the NH_2-terminal portion of the molecule. These unique amino acids are produced by post-translational modification of intrachain glutamic acid residues, for which vitamin K is an obligatory cofactor (Fig. 18-9). The γ-carboxyglutamic residues are necessary for the calcium binding and phospholipid surface interaction characteristics of these proteins. A unique aspect of prothrombin is that this region of the prothrombin molecule, designated F_{1+2}, is removed during activation, altering the surface binding properties of thrombin and allowing it to become a fluid phase enzyme (Fig. 18-7).

The second stage of fibrin clot formation begins with the conversion of fibrinogen to fibrin by thrombin. Fibrinogen is a homodimer composed of 6 peptide chains (2 Aα-, 2 Bβ-, and 2 γ-chains) linked by disulfide bonds (Fig. 8-10). Thrombin removes a short peptide from the central, NH_2-terminal portion of each Aα- and Bβ-chain, releasing fibrinopeptides A and B and exposing binding sites for the COOH-terminal D domain of other fibrin monomers (Fig. 8-10). If the concentration of fibrin monomers is high enough, they polymerize spontaneously into long protofibrils that associate to form the fibrin gel encompassing the platelet plug (Fig. 18-11). Factor XIIIa, which is formed from circulating factor XIII by thrombin, then covalently crosslinks D domains, giving strength to the latticework and making the clot more resistant to digestion by plasmin.

Regulation of Hemostasis

Formation of the hemostatic plug is normally limited to sites of vascular damage by a potent regulatory system that is dependent on intact endothelial cells (Table 18-3). Both the platelet response and fibrin formation are regulated by this system.[6,8] A major regulator of the platelet response is production of prostacyclin by endothelial and vascular wall cells. Prostacyclin is derived from arachidonic acid metabolism in the vessel wall, which contains prostacyclin synthetase rather than thromboxane synthetase (Fig. 18-3). Prostacyclin inhibits platelets through stimulation of adenylate synthetase and increased cAMP levels. Endothelial cells release ADPase, which breaks down ADP, a potent

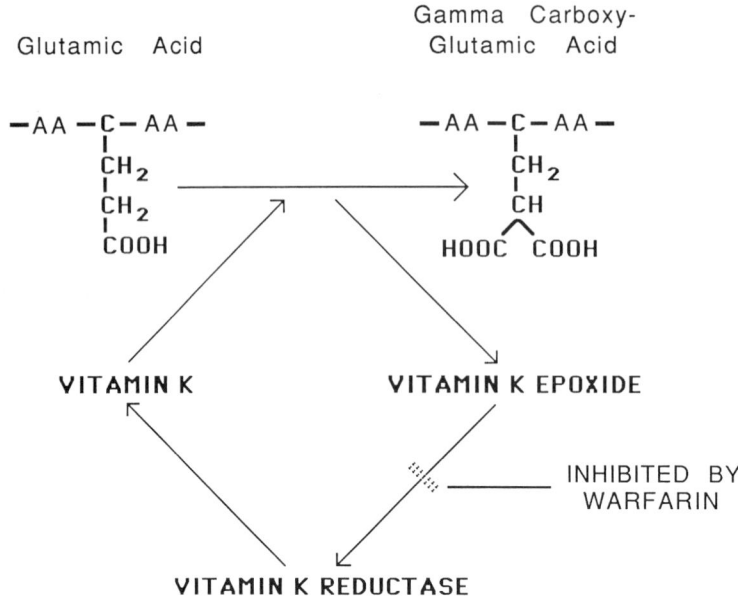

Fig. 18-9. Synthesis of the vitamin K dependent factors involves the formation of γ-carboxyglutamic acid residues after the basic protein is constructed. These dicarboxylic acid groups are necessary for calcium binding and interaction with phospholipid surfaces. The formation of these groups is dependent on vitamin K, which is oxidized in the process. Vitamin K is regenerated through a reductase system; it is this process that is inhibited by oral anticoagulants such as warfarin.

platelet agonist that is released from platelets and damaged red blood cells (RBCs). A third limiting factor in platelet plug formation is the normal endothelium surrounding a vascular defect that does not support platelet adhesion. In addition, endothelial cells produce endothelium cell-derived relaxing factor (EDRF), which inhibits both platelet adhesion and aggregation.[9]

Regulation of fibrin formation involves at least four systems (Table 18-3). The serine protease inhibitors (SERPINS) are responsible for inhibition of the major enzymes of the coagulation cascade: factor Xa and thrombin. Antithrombin III (AT III) is the most critical of these inhibitors, but heparin cofactor II may have an important role as well. Antithrombin III inhibits

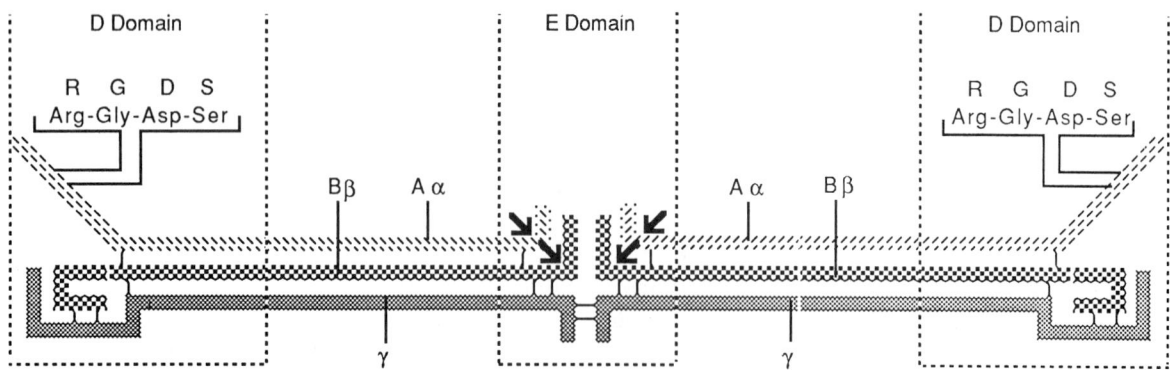

Fig. 18-10. Fibrinogen is a large protein composed of six peptide chains: two Aα, two Bβ, and two γ-chains. The intact fibrinogen molecule is a homodimer, with each half of the molecule composed of one Aα-, one Bβ-, and one γ-chain linked by disulfide bonds. The NH$_2$-terminal ends of each half are linked by disulfide bonds between the γ-chains to form a central region known as the E domain. The COOH-terminal portions on each side of the homodimer are thus mirror images of each other and are designated D domains. Each D domain is linked to the central E domain by a long helical portion composed of α-, β-, and γ-chains. The thrombin susceptible bonds are present in the central E domain (arrows). Thrombin cleaves a bond in each Aα- and Bβ-chain, releasing fibrinopeptides A and B. The COOH-terminus of the α-chain contains an arginine-glycine-asparagine-serine sequence (RGDS), a recognition site on fibrinogen for the interaction with the platelet receptor GP IIb-IIIa.

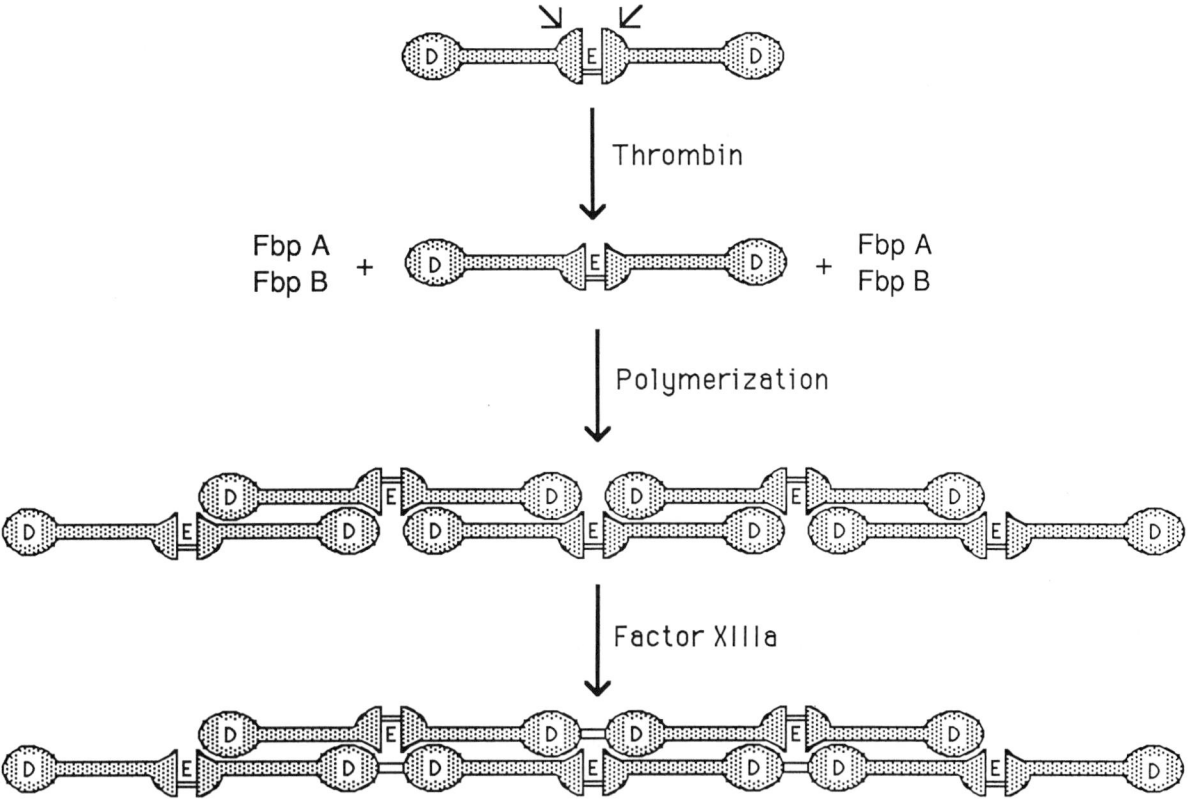

Fig. 18-11. Thrombin removes a portion of the Aα and Bβ (fibrinopeptides [Fbp] A and B) from each NH$_2$-terminus in the E domain. This opens binding sites for D domains in this region of the molecule. The fibrin monomers polymerize by interaction of D domains with the exposed binding sites, form long protofibrils that associate to form the complex fibrin gel. Factor XIIIa stabilizes the clot by forming covalent bonds between the adjacent D domains of individual fibrin monomers. The crosslinking of the fibrin matrix by factor XIIIa makes the clot relatively resistant to proteolysis by plasmin.

thrombin and factor Xa by forming a covalent bond with the active site serine of the enzyme. The interaction of AT III with these enzymes is greatly accelerated by heparin and heparan sulfate, which are present on normal endothelial cell surfaces; neutralization of thrombin and Xa thus probably takes place on endothelial cell surfaces (Fig. 18-12).

Protein C is a vitamin K dependent serine protease that is activated by thrombin in the presence of a cofactor called thrombomodulin. Thrombomodulin is a endothelial surface membrane protein that functions as a binding site for thrombin. Once thrombin binds to thrombomodulin it is no longer capable of converting fibrinogen to fibrin or activating factors V, VIII, and

Table 18-3. Regulation of Hemostasis

Regulatory System	Endothelial Contribution	Component Regulated
Prostacyclin	Synthesis	Platelet aggregation
ADPase	Synthesis	Platelet aggregation
Endothelium-derived relaxing factor	Synthesis	Platelet aggregation
SERPINS (antithrombin III and heparin cofactor II)	Heparin and heparan sulfate	Thrombin and factor Xa
Protein C system	Thrombomodulin	Factors Va and VIIIa
Fibrinolytic system	Tissue plasminogen activator	
	Plasminogen activator inhibitor	Fibrin clot deposition
Extrinsic pathway inhibitor	Synthesis	VIIa-tissue factor

Abbreviations: ADPase, adenosine diphosphatase; SERPINS, serine protease inhibitors.

508 • Laboratory Medicine

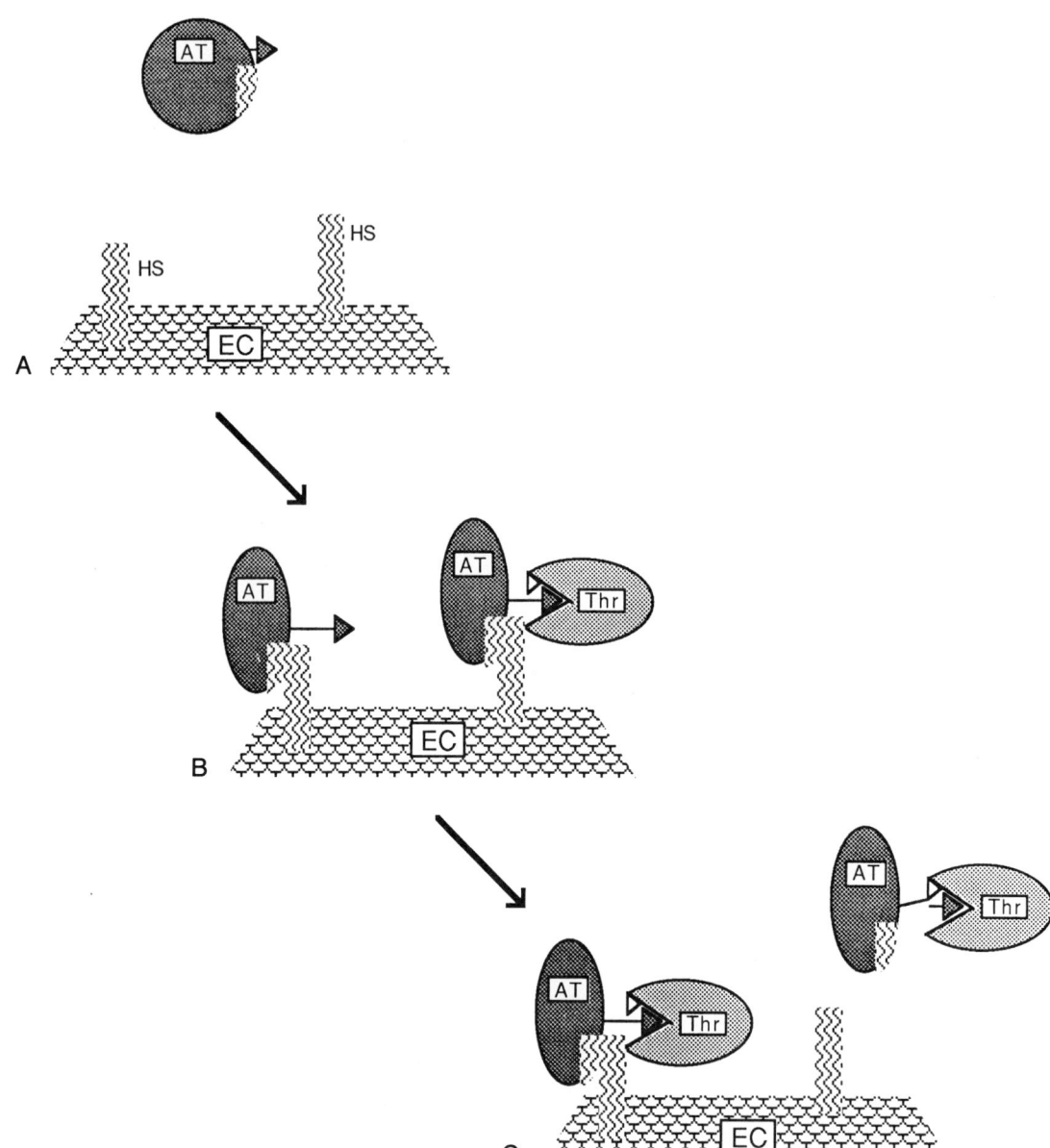

Fig. 18-12. Neutralization of thrombin (Thr) by antithrombin III (AT) is accelerated by heparin in vitro. (**A**) In vivo heparan sulfate (HS) on the surface of endothelial cells (EC) probably mediates and accelerates the interaction between AT and thrombin. (**B**) When AT binds to heparin or HS, it undergoes a conformational change, opening up the inhibitor site for interaction with thrombin. Interaction with thrombin leads to formation of a covalent bond between the active enzyme site and the inhibitor. (**C**) The thrombin-AT complex loses its affinity for HS and dissociates into circulating blood, from which it is removed by the liver. The EC site is then available to catalyze another thrombin-AT interaction.

XIII. However, thrombin bound to thrombomodulin is an efficient activator of protein C (Fig. 18-13). Activated protein C degrades factors Va and VIIIa, the major cofactors of the coagulation cascade. A protein cofactor and phospholipid surface are necessary for this activity; the cofactor is another vitamin K dependent protein, protein S (which is not an enzyme), and the phospholipid surface can be the platelet membrane or the surface of other cells, such as endothelium (Fig. 18-14).

The fibrinolytic system is dependent on the formation of plasmin from its circulating precursor plasminogen at the site of fibrin clot formation. The major physio-

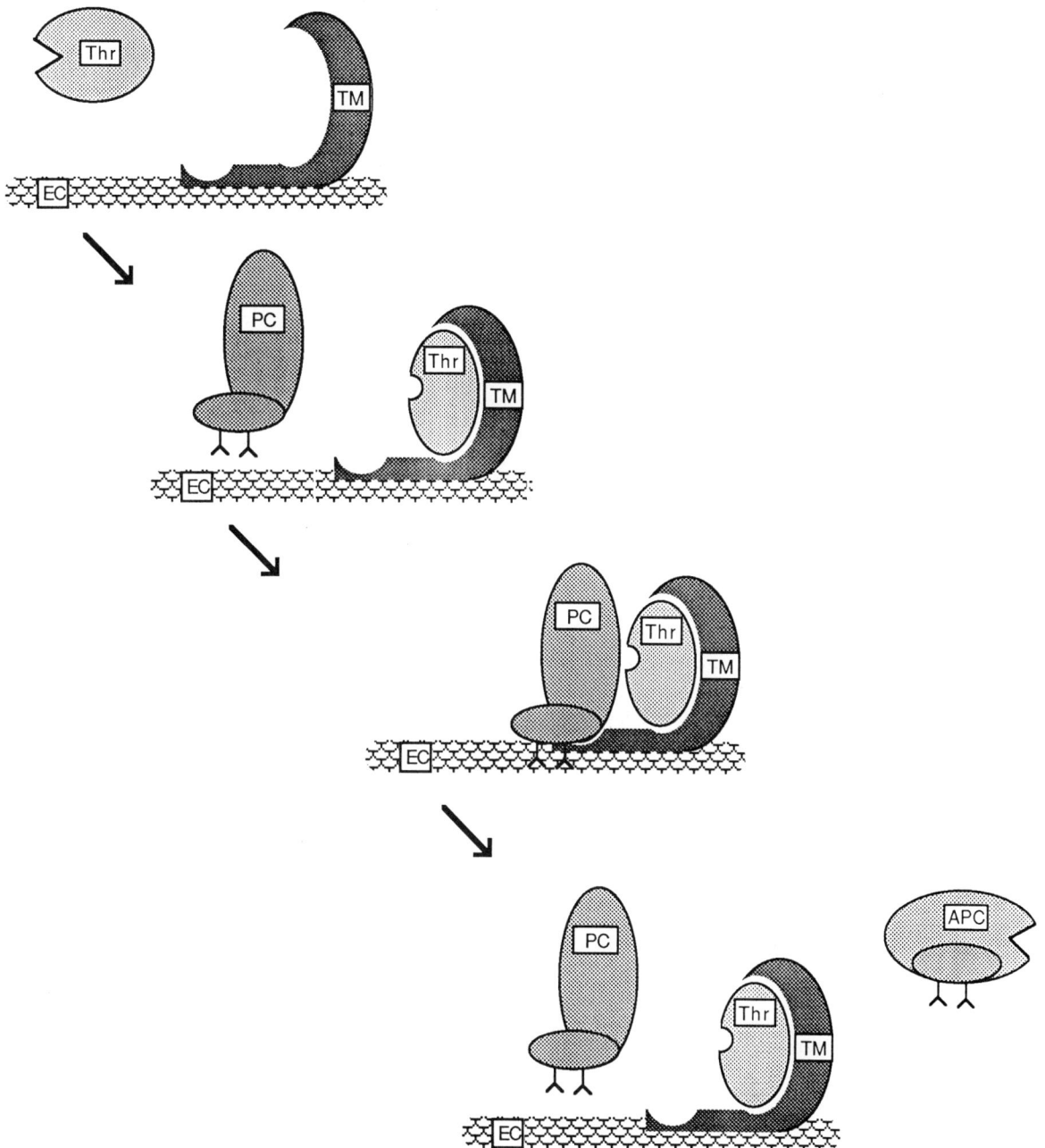

Fig. 18-13. Thrombin (Thr) activates protein C (PC) on endothelial cell (EC) surfaces in the presence of calcium and the cell surface cofactor thrombomodulin (TM). A conformational change occurs in thrombin when it binds to TM, altering its substrate specificity. The Thr-TM complex recognizes PC and rapidly converts it to activated protein C (APC). The amount of TM on the surfaces of ECs can be modulated by a variety of inflammatory stimuli.

logic activator of plasminogen is tissue plasminogen activator (tPA). Activation of plasminogen by tPA is greatly enhanced by fibrin, which serves as a surface or receptor for these proteins (Fig. 18-15). The plasmin generated within the clot matrix can then degrade the fibrin matrix. Plasmin activity is tightly regulated by its SERPIN, α_2-antiplasmin, which rapidly neutralizes any free plasmin (Fig. 18-16). Through selective activation of plasmin at sites of fibrin formation and rapid inhibition of any free plasmin, the activity of this potent enzyme is normally confined to sites of thrombus formation.

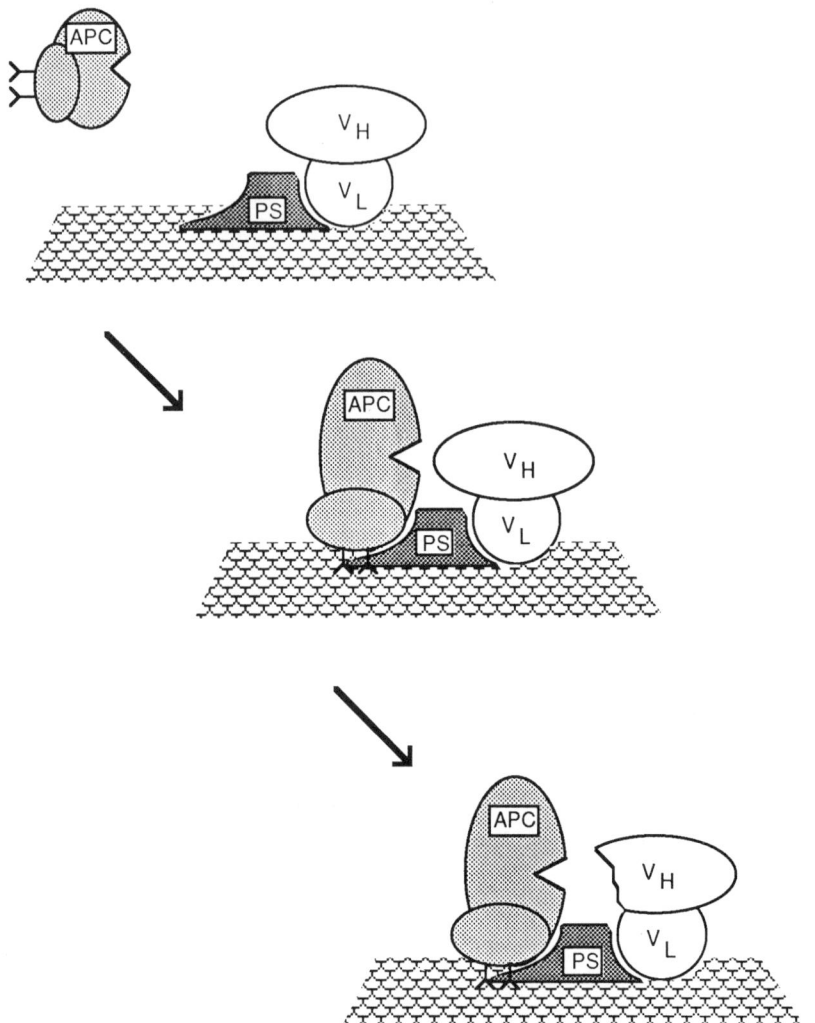

Fig. 18-14. The natural substrates for activated protein C (APC) are factors Va and VIIIa, which have a similar structure, with each composed of a light and heavy chain (here designated V_H and V_L for factor Va). APC proteolytically degrades the heavy chain of each protein. A cofactor, designated protein S (PS) is necessary for APC degradation of factors Va and VIIIa. PS is a vitamin K-dependent protein, which functions as a nonenzymatic cofactor, approximating APC with its substrates on a phospholipid surface.

More recently, a novel mechanism regulating initiation of the coagulation cascade has been described.[10] Factor Xa can combine with a protein that normally circulates with the lipoprotein fraction of plasma; this protein has been designated *extrinsic pathway inhibitor*. The factor Xa-inhibitor complex then binds to the factor VIIa-tissue factor complex, inhibiting its activity (Fig. 18-17). This reversible process is dependent on the presence of free factor Xa, but early clinical studies suggest that it may be a major regulatory pathway.

The activity of each of these regulatory components is complementary. A defect in any one component of the system is sufficient to alter the hemostatic balance in favor of a thrombotic process (Fig. 18-1). By contrast, increased activity of these components, as occurs with pharmacologic activation of plasmin or heparin therapy can tip the balance of hemostasis in favor of hemorrhage. Compared with the procoagulant side of hemostasis, there appears to be much less functional reserve on the regulatory side. Levels of procoagulant clotting factors down to approximately 10% of usual values are often well tolerated unless there is a major hemostatic challenge; by contrast, decreases in levels of regulatory proteins to the 50% range are commonly associated with a thrombotic tendency.

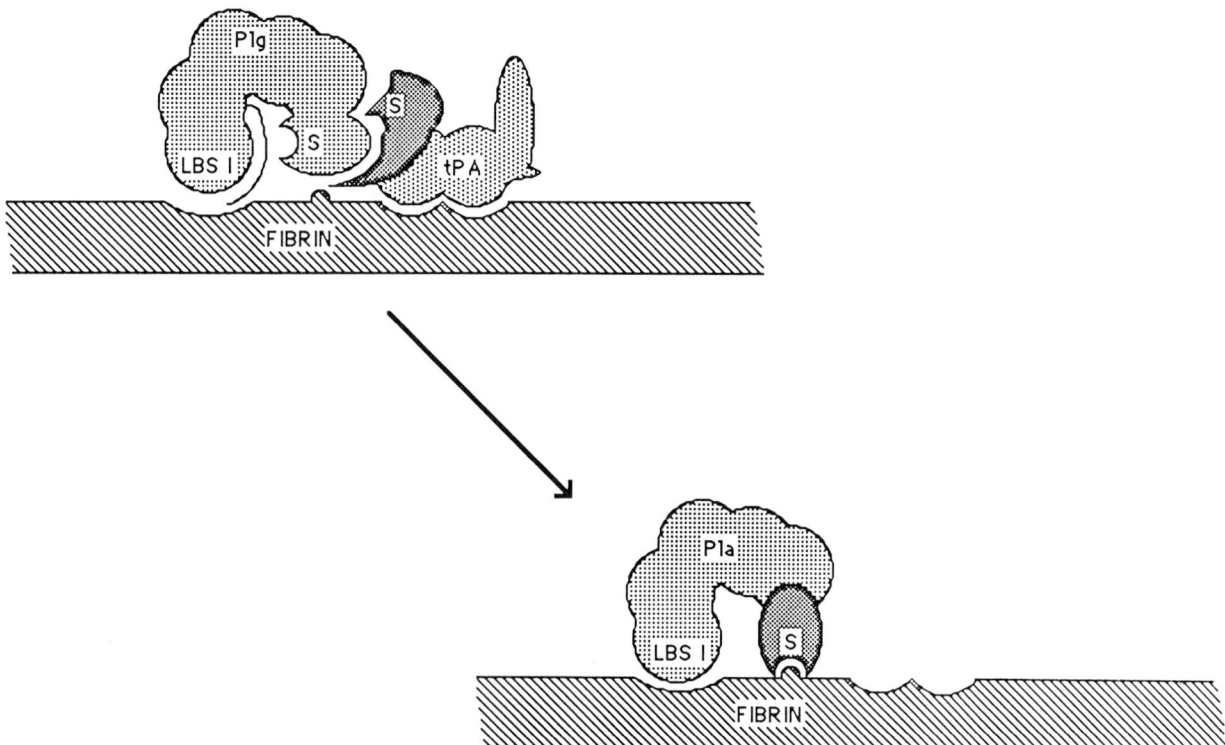

Fig. 18-15. Physiologic activation of plasminogen (Plg) by tissue plasminogen activator (tPA) occurs within the matrix of a fibrin clot. Tissue plasminogen activator is a serine protease which has relatively high affinity for fibrin. Plasminogen also binds to fibrin, which serves as a cofactor, localizing the activator with its substrate. Tissue plasminogen activator converts plasminogen to plasmin (Pla) by clipping a single amino acid bond. Plasmin continues to bind to the fibrin clot through its lysine binding sites (LBS) and is relatively protected from its inhibitor, α_2-antiplasmin, as long as it remains bound to fibrin.

CLINICAL ASSESSMENT OF HEMOSTATIC PARAMETERS

Assays of the hemostatic system are generally ordered for one of three reasons: to account for a patient's symptoms, to assess the risk of hemostatic complications during iatrogenic intervention (e.g., will my patient bleed during surgery?), or to assess the pharmacologic effect of a therapeutic agent on the hemostatic system (therapeutic monitoring). Abnormalities of hemostasis may present clinically as a bleeding disorder, as a thrombotic disorder, or as a complex disorder involving simultaneous bleeding and microvascular thrombosis. A thorough clinical history combined with a family history, physical examination, and a few screening tests of the hemostatic system is usually sufficient to arrive at either a presumptive diagnosis or a limited differential diagnosis. Appropriate specific assays to confirm the clinical impression can then be performed. The goal of this section is to provide the background necessary for arriving at a correct differential diagnosis for the more common hemostatic disorders and for monitoring therapeutic manipulation of the hemostatic system.

Approach to Bleeding Disorders

The assessment of a potential bleeding disorder begins with a good clinical history. The objective is to determine whether (1) the patient has a significant bleeding problem, (2) the problem is congenital or acquired, and (3) the problem is likely due to a platelet defect or to abnormal fibrin clot formation. At times it is difficult to ascertain whether there has actually been significant bleeding. Questions regarding amount of blood loss, length of bleeding (e.g., did epistaxis last 5 minutes or 5 days?), the need for transfusion to replace blood loss, development of iron deficiency anemia secondary to chronic blood loss, or blood loss during any previous invasive procedures or major trauma can be useful in establishing the significance of any symptoms. Questions regarding the age of onset, family history of simi-

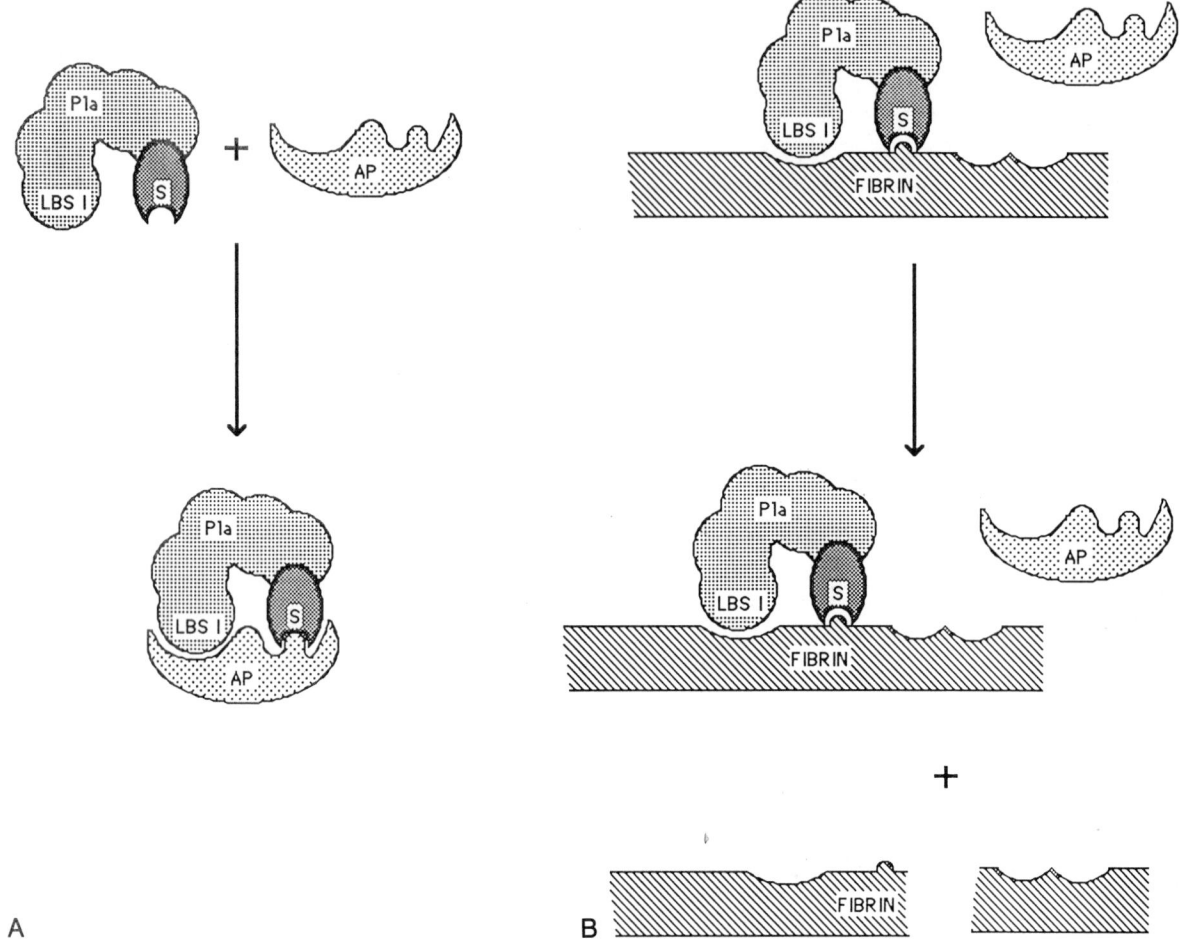

Fig. 18-16. The major regulator of plasmin (PLA) is the serine protease inhibitor α_2-antiplasmin (AP). (**A**) In the fluid phase, AP very rapidly neutralizes plasmin; no cofactor such as heparin is required for this process. (**B**) If plasmin remains bound to fibrin, AP cannot bind to and neutralize plasmin. Thus, fibrinolysis continues as long as plasmin is protected by the clot matrix. Once the clot matrix is degraded, the plasmin is rapidly neutralized, effectively limiting normal fibrinolysis to sites of fibrin clot formation.

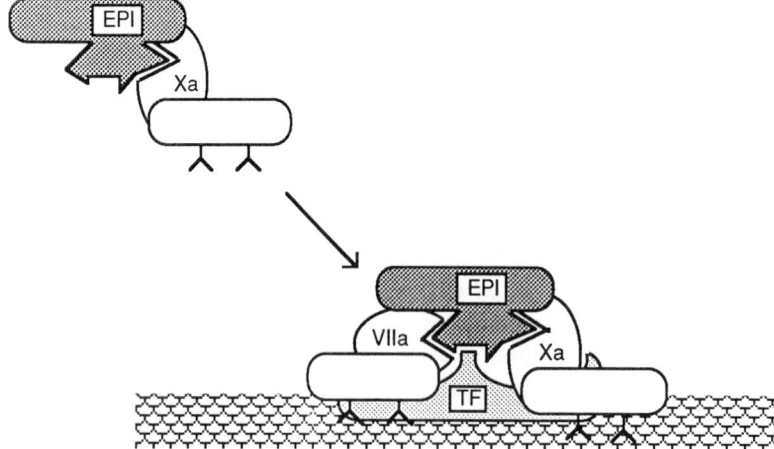

Fig. 18-17. Activation of the coagulation cascade through the extrinsic system is regulated by extrinsic pathway inhibitor (EPI). EPI forms a complex with factor Xa (Xa). The EPI-Xa complex then forms a reversible complex with the tissue factor (TF)-factor VIIa complex. Binding of EPI-Xa to TF-VIIa inhibits the ability of VIIa to activate factor X or IX.

lar problems, history of other medical problems, and drug history are useful in distinguishing a potential congenital problem from an acquired defect. The nature of bleeding is often helpful in separating platelet disorders from fibrin clot defects. Platelet disorders are most commonly characterized by mucocutaneous and post-traumatic bleeding, whereas fibrin clot defects are commonly associated with soft tissue bleeding, such as hemarthrosis and intramuscular hematoma formation (Table 18-4). It should be remembered, however, that there can be considerable overlap in the clinical manifestations of bleeding disorders.

The four screening assays that are widely used to assess the integrity of hemostatic plug formation are the prothrombin time (PT), activated partial thromboplastin time (APTT), platelet count, and bleeding time (BT). If there is no history of excessive bleeding and none of these tests is abnormal, a significant hemostatic defect is extremely unlikely. If the clinical history suggests a significant hemostatic defect, however, additional investigation is usually indicated. The PT and APTT measure fibrin clot formation; thus, prolongation of either or both of these tests suggests a fibrin clot defect. The platelet count and BT assess the platelet contribution to hemostatic plug formation and abnormalities of either or both of these tests indicate a platelet disorder. Below a platelet count of 50,000/μL (50 × 10^9/L), the BT is generally of little use in assessing hemostasis, because it will be greatly prolonged simply because of the thrombocytopenia. The combination of a long BT and a platelet count greater than 100,000/μL (100 × 10^9/L) is indicative of abnormal platelet function. The combination of a long BT and APTT with PT and platelet count within the reference range should raise the possibility of von Willebrand's disease (VWD).

Platelet Disorders

Quantitative Platelet Problems

Quantitative platelet problems may be separated into those with an increased count (thrombocytosis) and those with a decreased count (thrombocytopenia). Reactive (secondary) thrombocytosis is usually clinically silent. By contrast, primary thrombocytosis seen with myeloproliferative disorders, such as essential thrombocythemia, chronic myelocytic leukemia, and polycythemia vera, may be associated with either bleeding or thrombosis. Thrombocytopenia is usually clinically silent until the count is less than 50,000–70,000/μL (<50–70 × 10^9/L), unless there is an associated qualitative platelet defect. Below a platelet count of 50,000–70,000/μL (50–70 × 10^9/L) excessive bleeding may occur with invasive procedures, trauma, or sur-

Table 18-4. Patterns of Clinical Bleeding

Platelet-type Bleeding	Fibrin-Formation Bleeding
Petechiae	Hemarthrosis
Ecchymoses	Intramuscular hematomas
Epistaxis	Soft tissue hematomas
Mucosal bleeding	Intracranial hemorrhage
Bleeding with trauma	Bleeding with trauma

gery. Major spontaneous bleeding caused by thrombocytopenia alone usually does not occur until the platelet count is less than 10,000–20,000/μL (<10–20 × 10^9/L). Platelet counting and quantitative platelet disorders are more thoroughly discussed in Chapter 19.

Hereditary Qualitative Platelet Problems

Hereditary qualitative platelet problems may be separated into those affecting adhesion, secretion/release, or aggregation[11] (Table 18-5). von Willebrand's disease, the most common hereditary bleeding disorder, is due to abnormal platelet adhesion. A decrease in concentration or a qualitative abnormality in von Willebrand factor results in the clinical symptoms characteristic of this disorder (Fig. 18-2). von Willebrand factor also functions as a carrier for factor VIII in plasma; thus, when VWF is decreased, factor VIII is decreased, resulting in the long APTT characteristic of VWD. The tests used to assess possible VWD include the BT, APTT, platelet aggregation with ristocetin, VWF antigen, ristocetin cofactor assay (a functional measure of VWF), factor VIII assay, and VWF crossed immunoelectrophoresis (a measure of VWF multimeric structure). von Willebrand factor multimeric analysis and platelet VWF analysis can be used in special circumstances to further delineate the defect in this common disorder.

Bernard-Soulier syndrome is a rare autosomal recessive disorder characterized by mild thrombocytopenia, giant platelets, and a deficiency of membrane GP Ib, the binding site for VWF (Fig. 18-2). Bernard-Soulier syndrome can be separated from VWD by demonstrating factor VIII, VWF antigen, and ristocetin cofactor activity within the reference range in conjunction with decreased response of patient platelets to ristocetin. In Bernard-Soulier syndrome, the usual response occurs to other platelet agonists, such as ADP and thrombin.

Platelet aggregation studies are used to identify patients with disorders of platelet secretion and aggregation. Glanzmann's thrombasthenia is a rare autosomal

Table 18-5. Hereditary Platelet Disorders

Disorders	Laboratory Assessment
Abnormal adhesion	
von Willebrand syndrome	VWF, platelet aggregation (R)[a]
Bernard-Soulier syndrome	VWF, platelet aggregation (R)[a]
Collagen disorders	BT, normal platelet aggregation
Abnormal aggregation (primary wave)	
Glanzmann's thrombasthenia	BT, platelet aggregation, GP IIB-IIIA
Afibrinogenemia	BT, platelet aggregation, fibrinogen
Abnormal aggregation (secondary wave)	
Abnormal granules (storage pool defects)	
Idiopathic	
Hermansky-Pudlak syndrome	
Wiskott-Aldrich syndrome	BT, platelet aggregation, EM
Chediak-Higashi syndrome	
Thrombocytopenia-absent radii syndrome	
Gray platelet syndrome	
Abnormal secretion (release defects)	
Cyclo-oxygenase deficiency	
Thromboxane A_2 synthetase deficiency	
Abnormal release of arachidonic acid	
Deficiency of α_2-adrenergic receptors	BT, platelet aggregation, ATP release
Impaired responsiveness to thromboxane A_2	
Defective calcium mobilization (?)	
Defective myosin phosphorylation (?)	

[a] Platelet aggregation with ristocetin.
Abbreviations: VWF, von Willebrand factor; GPIIB-IIIA, glycoprotein IIB-IIIA; BT, bleeding time; EM, electron microscopy; ATP, adenosine triphosphate.

recessive disorder characterized by a normal aggregation response to ristocetin, but absolutely no response to agonists such as ADP, collagen, and epinephrine (Fig. 18-18). Platelets from patients with Glanzmann's thrombasthenia lack the GP IIb-IIIa complex and thus can not be crosslinked by fibrinogen (Fig. 18-5). In patients with defects involving platelet secretion there is usually an initial wave of platelet aggregation in response to ADP and epinephrine, but no complete, secondary wave response (Fig. 18-18). The defect in such patients may be due to lack of storage granules or inability to release the contents of otherwise normal granules (Table 18-5).

Acquired Qualitative Platelet Disorders

Acquired qualitative platelet disorders are the most common cause of abnormal platelet function. A variety of abnormalities may cause abnormal platelet function, but the most common is drug therapy (Table 18-6). The most common drug associated with abnormal platelet function is aspirin, but many others (particularly cardiac drugs) have been shown to affect platelet function either in vivo or in vitro, or both (Table 18-7). The initial clinical history may be negative for drug use until the patient is questioned in specific detail. Many patients do not regard aspirin as a drug; in addition, aspirin is in many over-the-counter medications that the patient may be taking without realizing they contain aspirin. Aspirin irreversibly blocks cyclo-oxygenase, the initial enzyme in the TxA_2 pathway (Fig. 18-3). Therefore, the effect of aspirin persists for several days after cessation of the drug, while new platelets are being made to restore platelet function. The effect on platelet function may vary considerably between patients for many of the drugs listed in Table 18-6. The inhibitory effect of drugs other than aspirin is usually reversible and persists only as long as the drug remains in the circulation. Of the drugs listed in Table 18-6, bleeding has been most frequently encountered with aspirin, other nonsteroidal anti-inflammatory drugs, and antibiotics.

The diagnosis of acquired qualitative disorders is generally made on the basis of clinical history and the demonstration of an abnormal BT. Platelet aggregation studies are usually not indicated, as all these disorders can result in abnormalities of the secondary wave response to ADP and epinephrine. Thus, the acquired disorders

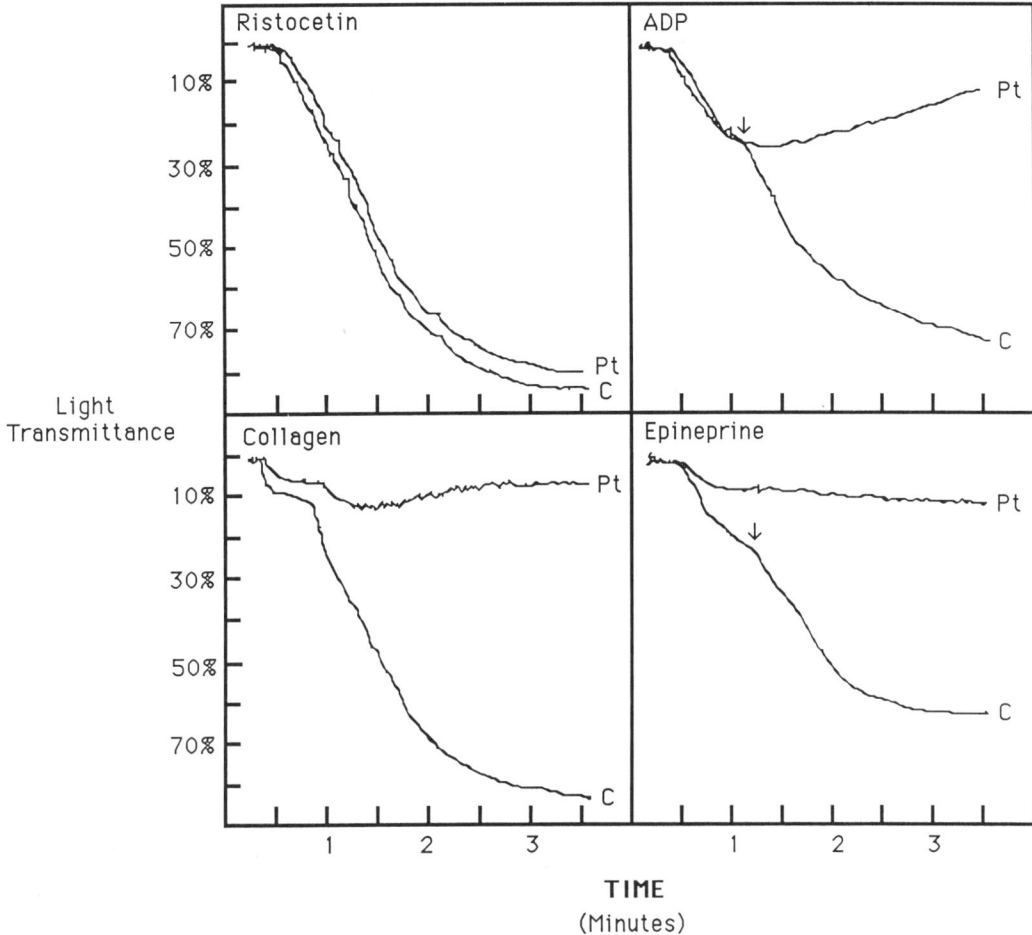

Fig. 18-18. Platelet aggregation is usually measured by monitoring the change in light absorbance or transmittance as the platelets form large aggregates. Formation of large aggregates is associated with a large increase in light transmittance. Adenosine diphosphate (ADP) and epinephrine usually induce a biphasic wave of aggregation as shown by the control curves (C). The second wave of aggregation with these agents (arrow) is dependent upon an intact platelet release mechanism. If release does not occur, the platelets show only a primary wave, followed by disaggregation (shown by Pt). Similarly the response to collagen may be blunted. Ristocetin induces binding of von Willebrand factor to platelets and is not dependent on an intact release mechanism. Patients with Bernard-Soulier syndrome or von Willebrand syndrome typically have abnormalities of ristocetin induced aggregation but a normal response to other agonists. If patients lack the receptor for fibrinogen (GP IIb-IIIa), there will be no response at all to epinephrine or ADP.

Table 18-6. Acquired Disorders Associated with Impaired Platelet Function

Drugs
Platelet antibodies
Renal disease
Myeloproliferative disorders
Myeloma
Fibrinolysis
Macromolecules
Fibrin split products
Monoclonal proteins
In vivo "release"
Hypothyroidism

cannot be distinguished from each other or from hereditary disorders on the basis of platelet aggregation studies alone.

Disorders of Fibrin Clot Formation

Hereditary Disorders of Fibrin Formation

Hereditary disorders of fibrin formation most commonly present as soft tissue bleeding early in childhood. The two most common disorders are hemophilia A (caused by a deficiency of factor VIII) and hemophilia B (caused by a deficiency of factor IX) (Table 18-8). Together with VWD, these two disorders proba-

Table 18-7. Drugs Associated with Abnormal Platelet Function In Vivo or In Vitro

Anti-inflammatory agents
    Aspirin
    Indomethacin
    Ibuprofen
    Phenylbutazone
    Sulfinpyrazone
    Naproxen
Antibiotics
    Penicillin
    Carbenicillin
    Ticarcillin
    Mezlocillin
    Piperacillin
    Cephalosporins
Tricyclic antidepressants
    Imipramine
    Desipramine
    Amitriptyline
    Nortriptyline
β-Blockers
    Propranolol
    Timolol
    Metoprolol
Calcium channel blockers
    Verapamil
    Nifedipine
    Diltiazem
Lipid-lowering drugs
    Clofibrate
    Halofenate
    Cyproheptadine
Antihistamines
    Theophylline
    Aminophylline
    Chlorpheniramine
    Diphenhydramine
Miscellaneous
    Ethanol
    Dipyridamole
    Ticlopidine
    Sodium valproate
    Hydralazine
    Dextran
    Papaverine
    Suloctidil
    Furosemide
    Ethacrynic acid
    Acetazolamide
    Hydroxychloroquine
    Hydrocortisone
    Methylprednisolone
    Daunorubicin
    Mithramycin
    Nitrofurantoin
    Chlorpromazine
    Triprolidine
    Reserpine
    Nitrates
    Dazoxidine
    Nafazatrom

Table 18-8. Frequency of Hereditary Coagulation Disorders

Disorder	Frequency
von Willebrand syndrome	1:200–1:5000
Hemophilia A (factor VIII deficiency)	1:5000–10,000
Hemophilia B (factor IX deficiency)	1:50,000–100,000
Factor XI deficiency	1:100,000–500,000
Factor II deficiency	$<1:10^6$
Factor V deficiency	$<1:10^6$
Factor VII deficiency	$<1:10^6$
Factor X deficiency	$<1:10^6$
Factor XII deficiency	$<1:10^6$
Prekallikrein deficiency	$<1:10^6$
High molecular weight kininogen deficiency	$<1:10^6$
Afibrinogenemia	$<1:10^6$

bly make up more than 95% of hereditary bleeding disorders. Severe hemophilia A and B are clinically indistinguishable; thus, the diagnosis depends on the demonstration of the specific defect by factor assays. Mild factor deficiency can pose serious problems, as the clinical history may be negative until the hemostatic system is severely challenged (e.g., surgery) and the screening tests may be within the reference range.

Acquired Disorders of Hemostasis

A number of acquired disorders of hemostasis can affect fibrin clot formation; they can be divided into acquired deficiency states and acquired inhibitors of hemostasis (Table 18-9). Mixing studies, which test a mixture of patient and normal plasma, are used to distinguish a simple factor deficiency from the presence of a circulating inhibitor. If the prolonged clotting time is due to factor deficiency, it will shorten when the patient's plasma is mixed with normal plasma. If the clotting time does not correct after mixing with normal plasma, an inhibitor is present in the patient's plasma. The most common inhibitor encountered is heparin, usually given therapeutically. However, a rare patient may release endogenous heparin into the circulation, leading to a bleeding diathesis. The classic inhibitors of blood coagulation are antibodies directed at some component of the hemostatic mechanism. Lupus anticoagulants, directed at phospholipid, are the most common of the immunoglobulin inhibitors encountered. Paradoxically, lupus anticoagulants do not cause a bleeding diathesis, perhaps because they do not intefere with thrombin formation on platelet surfaces; instead, lupus anticoagulants are associated with a thrombotic tendency.

Table 18-9. Acquired Disorders of Fibrin Clot Formation

Acquired Deficiency States	Inhibition of Clot Formation
Liver disease	Heparin
Vitamin K deficiency	Lupus anticoagulants[a]
Oral anticoagulants	Neutralizing factor inhibitors
Amyloidosis	Non-neutralizing factor inhibitors
Consumptive coagulopathies	Macromolecules (e.g., Dextran)
Hematin	Dysfibrinogenemia
Snake venoms	

[a] Generally not associated with bleeding.

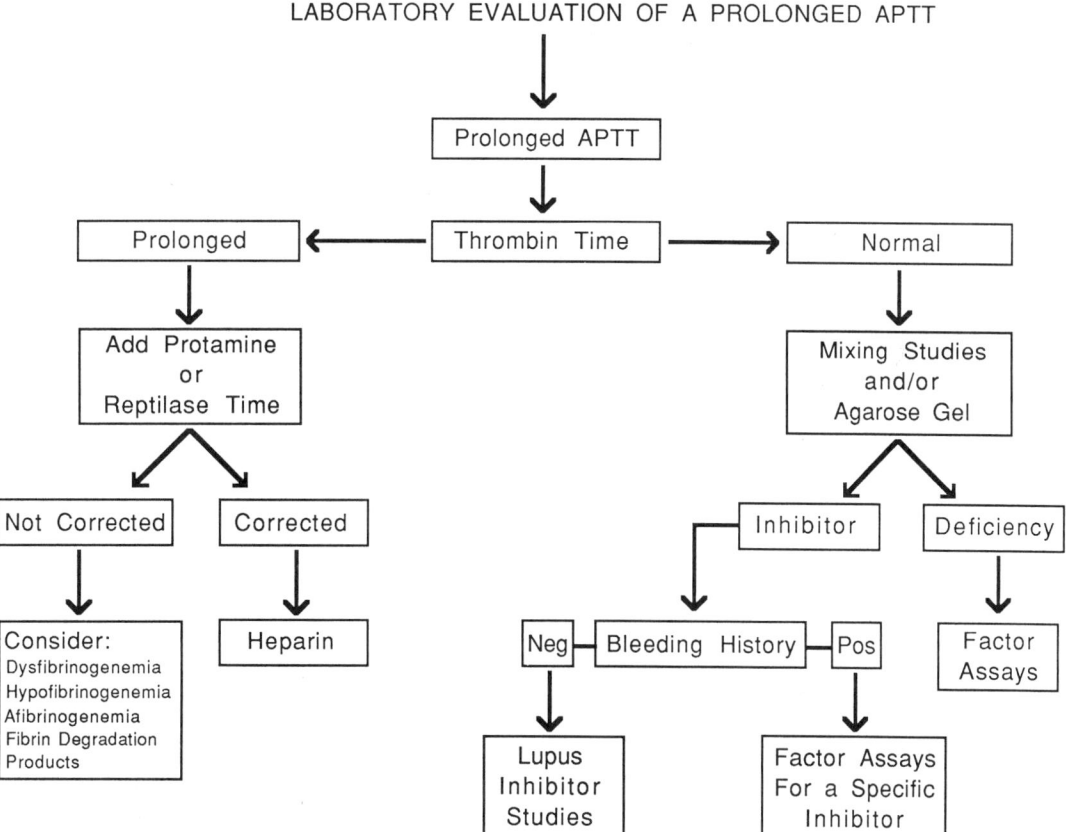

Fig. 18-19. Flow diagram for a laboratory approach to the evaluation of a prolonged activated partial thromboplastin time (APTT). One of the first steps is to repeat the APTT to rule out artifacts that may interfere with the assay. A thrombin time is a very helpful procedure as heparin is one of the most common causes of a long APTT. If the thrombin time is prolonged, mixing studies with normal plasma and protamine sulfate can be used to document the presence of heparin or suggest the possibility of a fibrinogen abnormality. The Reptilase time may be substituted for mixing studies with protamine. If the thrombin time is normal, mixing studies of the patient plasma with normal plasma are used to differentiate between a circulating anticoagulant and a factor deficiency. If mixing studies show correction of the APTT, factor assays are performed to determine the deficient factor. If the mixing studies document an inhibitor, then further workup is guided by the clinical history and presentation. If there is any evidence of bleeding, a specific factor inhibitor must be ruled in or out. If there is no evidence of bleeding, studies to document a lupus anticoagulant are often helpful.

Other inhibitors are directed at one of the specific coagulation proteins, most commonly factor VIII. These specific factor inhibitors are usually associated with a serious bleeding diathesis. Factor VIII inhibitors occur in about 10% of patients with severe hemophilia A. They also occur spontaneously in the elderly, in association with pregnancy (usually around the time of parturition), in patients with autoimmune or lymphoproliferative disorders, and in association with some drugs (e.g., penicillin). Specific factor antibodies can be either neutralizing (the most common) or non-neutralizing (relatively uncommon) inhibitors. With neutralizing inhibitors, the antibody blocks the procoagulant activity of the coagulation factor; with non-neutralizing inhibitors, the antibody binds to a nonfunctional part of the protein, maintaining its function (Fig. 18-19). Both inhibitors lead to a deficiency of the target coagulation factor in circulating blood, because the antibody-antigen complex is removed from the circulation. However, mixing studies with a non-neutralizing antibody often suggests a simple factor deficiency, because the antibody does not neutralize the target factor in the normal plasma in vitro.

Acquired factor deficiency, in contrast to the hereditary disorders, usually affects multiple factors and can be due to decreased synthesis or increased consumption. The three common causes of decreased synthesis are liver disease, vitamin K deficiency, and oral anticoagulant therapy. The defects in vitamin K deficiency and oral anticoagulant therapy result from diminished or absent post-translational carboxylation of γ-carboxyglutamic acid residues and thus result in a deficiency of factors II, VII, IX, and X as well as the regulatory proteins, protein C, and protein S (Fig. 18-9). By contrast, liver disease affects all the procoagulant proteins except VWF, which is synthesized by endothelial cells. The level of factor VIII is commonly within the reference range or increased until late in liver disease, but the ratio of factor VIII to VWF is decreased even in early liver disease, suggesting an abnormality of factor VIII synthesis. With unregulated activation of the hemostatic system, as in disseminated intravascular coagulation (DIC), multiple factors may be rapidly consumed (see under Approach to Complex Hemostatic Disorders). An unusual cause of increased destruction of a single coagulation factor is amyloidosis, which may result in isolated factor X deficiency. The factor X appears to be rapidly removed from the circulation by binding to extravascular amyloid; as a result, replacement therapy is often ineffective.

The pattern of screening test results is very helpful in developing a differential diagnosis to account for the abnormality detected by the clinical history and screening tests (Table 18-10). The most common cause of a long APTT in hospitalized patients is heparin; the second most common cause is the lupus anticoagulant. The laboratory workup of a long APTT should take these common problems into consideration (Fig. 18-19). The most common causes of a prolonged PT with an APTT within the reference range or mildly prolonged are oral anticoagulant therapy, vitamin K deficiency, and liver disease; coagulation inhibitors are an uncommon cause of this pattern. Because the clinical history can often provide the necessary clues for the diagnosis of these entities, further laboratory investigation is often not needed, except to guide potential replacement therapy in a bleeding patient with liver disease. The easiest way to confirm the diagnosis of

Table 18-10. Differential for Abnormal Screening Tests of Coagulation

Prolonged APTT	Prolonged PT	Prolonged PT and APTT
Common		
Heparin	Vitamin K deficiency	Vitamin K deficiency
Lupus Anticoagulants	Oral anticoagulants	Oral anticoagulants
Hemophilia A	Liver disease	Liver disease
Hemophilia B		Consumptive coagulopathies
VWD (+ long BT)		
Uncommon		
Specific factor inhibitors	Factor VII deficiency	Factor II, V, or X deficiency
Factor XI or XII deficiency		Hereditary dysfibrinogenemia
Prekallikrein deficiency		Afibrinogenemia
High molecular weight kininogen deficiency		Specific factor inhibitors
		Amyloidosis

APTT, activated partial thromboplastin time; PT, prothrombin time; VWD, von Willebrand factor; BT, bleeding time.

vitamin K deficiency is parenteral administration of vitamin K; in uncomplicated deficiency, the PT usually corrects in less than 24 hours.

Bleeding Disorders Without Abnormalities in Screening Tests

Patients may give a history that strongly suggests a significant bleeding disorder, and yet no screening assays are abnormal. A variety of disorders, affecting either platelet function or fibrin clot formation, can present in this manner (Table 18-11). Therefore, if the history is positive, additional laboratory investigation aimed at identifying a specific disorder is indicated. Laboratory parameters in mild VWD may fluctuate over time or may be within the reference range, particularly if the platelet VWF is normal. A syndrome of mild platelet dysfunction characterized by a BT within the reference range or nearly so and mild clinical symptoms has been described. Both disorders may be unmasked by the aspirin tolerance test.

The PT and APTT are not sensitive to defects in fibrin stabilization or fibrinolysis. Abnormalities of this part of the hemostatic response, such as factor XIII deficiency (either hereditary or acquired as a result of an inhibitor), α_2-antiplasmin deficiency, dysfibrinogenemia, and enhanced fibrinolytic activity may be associated with excessive clot lysis and a bleeding tendency. The bleeding in such patients is often delayed and responds well to fibrinolytic inhibitors such as ϵ-aminocaproic acid. Occasionally, a patient with a mild deficiency of either factor VIII or IX may present with a history of excessive bleeding; most of the patients are women who are heterozygous for the factor deficiency, and there may be a history of hemophilia affecting male members of the family.

Approach to Thrombotic Disorders

In recent years, it has become clear that there is a group of patients with a hereditary predisposition to thrombosis. The tendency in most families is transmitted as an autosomal dominant trait with a relatively high rate of expression. Recurrent thromboembolic events usually begin in adolescence or young adulthood (most affected patients are symptomatic by age 40–45), and any event may be life threatening. A thrombotic event in a young patient should prompt a thorough family history and clinical/laboratory investigation. Most of the hereditary defects associated with thrombosis affect the regulatory system of hemostasis; others include dysfibrinogenemia and a poorly defined and difficult to diagnose "hyperactive" platelet syndrome (Table 18-12). Because there are no screening tests that assess overall function of the regulatory system, the evaluation of this type of patient involves measurement of each of the possible causes of thrombosis. When selecting assays to assess the regulatory system, functional assays are generally superior to antigenic assays, because the latter

Table 18-11. Evaluation of the Patient with a History of Bleeding and Normal Screening Assay Results

Disorder	Laboratory Evaluation
Platelet Disorders	
Mild von Willebrand syndrome	Repeat BT, ASA tolerance test, VWF
Mild platelet dysfunction	Repeat BT, ASA tolerance test, platelet aggregation
	Serotonin release studies
Fibrin clot disorders	
Factor XIII Deficiency	Factor XIII assay
Hereditary	
Acquired	
α_2-Antiplasmin deficiency	α_2-Antiplasmin assay
Hereditary dysfibrinogenemia	Clottable and antigenic fibrinogen, TT, fibrin polymerization
Mild factor IX deficiency	Factor IX assay
Mild factor VIII assay	Factor VIII assay
Plasminogen activator inhibitor deficiency (?)	Plasminogen activator inhibitor assay

Abbreviations: ASA, aspirin; BT, bleeding time; TT, thrombin time; VWF, von Willebrand factor.

Table 18-12. Hereditary Disorders Associated with Thrombosis

System	Disorders
Serine protease inhibitors (SERPINS)	Antithrombin III deficiency Heparin cofactor II deficiency[a]
Protein C system	Heterozygous protein C deficiency Homozygous protein C deficiency Heterozygous protein S deficiency
Fibrinolytic system	Plasminogen deficiency Tissue plasminogen activator deficiency Dysfibrinogenemia
Platelets	Hyperactive platelet syndrome
Miscellaneous	Variant factor VII deficiency Factor XII deficiency[a] Prekallikrein deficiency[a] Homocystinuria

[a] Association has been suggested, but not documented, by a sufficient number of cases.

yield no apparent abnormalities in the presence of an abnormal, nonfunctional protein. The demonstration of familial transmission of the abnormality is very helpful in establishing the diagnosis of a hereditary thrombotic tendency.

A number of systemic disorders (Table 18-13) are associated with an increased risk of thrombosis, and a thorough clinical history is usually sufficient to identify such patients; most of these disorders affect patients older than 40–45 years of age, another helpful factor in distinguishing these patients from those with a hereditary thrombotic tendency. Recurrence of thrombosis in the face of therapeutic oral anticoagulation may be a clue to the presence of an occult tumor, whereas recurrence of thrombosis during therapeutic heparin therapy should raise the possibility of a heparin dependent antiplatelet antibody. An unexplained prolongation of the APTT in a patient with thrombosis should suggest the possibility of a lupus anticoagulant, although the mechanism of thrombosis in such patients is still poorly understood. The diagnosis of a lupus anticoagulant depends on demonstrating the phospholipid dependence of the inhibitory activity. The latter may be achieved with tests such as the tissue thromboplastin inhibition assay and platelet neutralization procedure.

Increased activation of the hemostatic system on a chronic basis may predispose the patient to thrombosis. A series of assays are emerging from research laboratories that can indicate whether such activation is occurring in vivo. These assays can detect components formed by thrombin activation, activity, and neutralization; evidence for increased levels of thrombin activation has been found in patients with hereditary deficiency of regulatory proteins predisposed to thrombosis[8,12] (Fig. 18-20). Using a panel of such assays, it may be possible to identify patients with increased ac-

Table 18-13. Acquired Disorders Associated with Thrombosis

Systemic conditions
    Atherosclerotic vascular disease
    Diabetes mellitus
    Malignant neoplasms
    Myeloproliferative disorders
    Paroxysmal nocturnal hemoglobinuria
    Estrogens and oral contraceptives
    Pregnancy
    Venous stasis
    Nephrotic syndrome
    Hyperlipidemia
    Artificial vascular prostheses
    Hyperviscosity
Hemostatic disorders
    Lupus anticoagulants
    Heparin dependent antiplatelet antibodies
    Disseminated intravascular coagulation
    Thrombotic thrombocytopenic purpura
    Hemolytic-uremic syndrome
    Snake venoms
    Coagulation factor concentrates

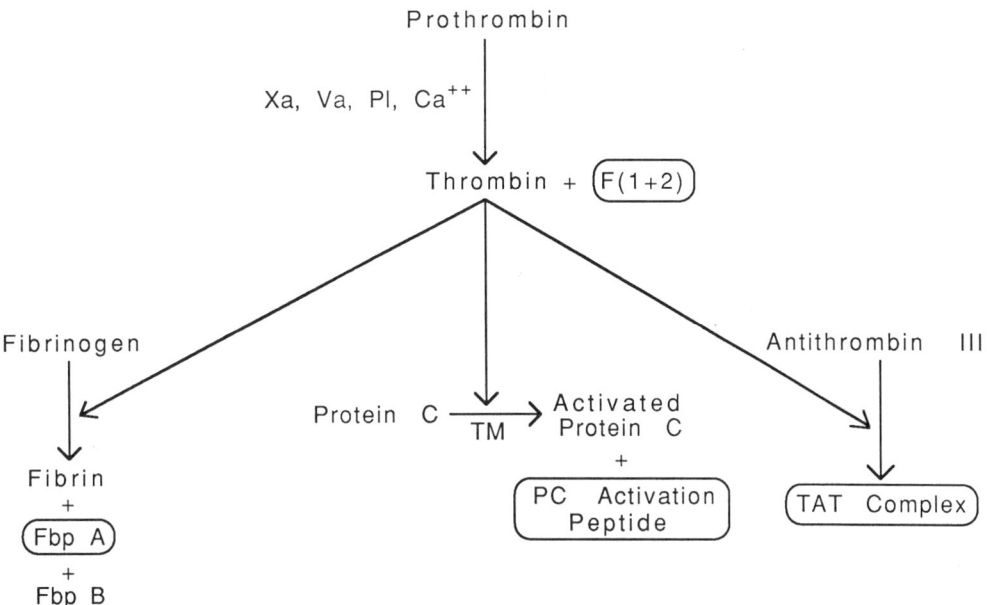

Fig. 18-20. The formation of thrombin and its associated activities are accompanied by generation of marker proteins, which can be used to assess the degree of activation of the coagulation cascade. Conversion of prothrombin to thrombin is associated with release of a large peptide designated F_{1+2} (see Fig. 18-7). Cleavage of fibrinogen by thrombin results in release of fibrinopeptides (Fbp) A and B; of these fibrinopeptide A is the more commonly measured peptide. Activation of protein C (PC) by thrombin and thrombomodulin (TM) results in release of a short peptide from the heavy chain of protein C. This activation peptide can be measured with a sensitive radioimmunoassay. Neutralization of thrombin by antithrombin III results in formation of thrombin-antithrombin III (TAT) complexes. Although assays for these markers are very sensitive, they do not differentiate between physiologic and pathologic activation of the coagulation cascade. Thus, these results need to be interpreted with caution and always in light of the clinical situation.

tivation attributable to acquired diseases such as malignancy and whether intervention (e.g., anticoagulant therapy) has been successful in decreasing the level of thrombin activation.

Approach to Complex Hemostatic Disorders

Several complex, acquired disorders of hemostasis may present clinically with simultaneous bleeding and microvascular thrombosis (Table 18-14). The classic example of this group is acute DIC. The basic pathogenesis of DIC is excessive activation of thrombin and plasmin that overwhelms usual regulatory mechanisms, leading to simultaneous microvascular thrombosis and bleeding (Fig. 18-21). The diagnosis of DIC depends on the clinical setting and manifestations and on laboratory documentation of excessive thrombin and plasmin activity. Excessive thrombin generation results in consumption of fibrinogen, presence of circulating fibrin monomers, consumption of AT III and protein C, and thrombocytopenia. By contrast, excessive plasmin generation results in formation of fibrin degradation products (FDPs) and consumption of fibrinogen, factor V, and factor VIII. Clinical manifestations vary from patient to patient, depending in part on the extent and relative degree of thrombin and plasmin activation.

In contrast to the predominant involvement of the coagulation system by DIC, thrombotic thrombocytopenic purpura (TTP) and the hemolytic uremic syndrome (HUS) primarily involve platelets. These disorders are characterized by extensive microvascular thrombosis and consumption of platelets but minimal activation of the coagulation cascade and fibrinolytic system. The presence of a microangiopathic peripheral blood picture (see Ch. 16), thrombocytopenia, and APTT, PT, and fibrinogen within the reference range should raise the possibility of TTP or HUS.

Liver disease is associated with many abnormalities of the hemostatic system (Table 18-15) caused by decreased production of essential hemostatic factors or production of abnormal proteins such as dysfibrinogenemia. Both procoagulant and regulatory components are affected in patients with liver disease, reduc-

Table 18-14. Complex Hemostatic Disorders	
Disorder	**Laboratory Manifestations**
Disseminated intravascular coagulation	Thrombocytopenia, low fibrinogen, long PT, long APTT, increased FDPs, low AT III
Thrombotic thrombocytopenic purpura Hemolytic uremic syndrome	Thrombocytopenia, microangiopathic peripheral blood film, normal fibrinogen, normal AT III
Liver disease	Long PT, normal to low fibrinogen, low AT III

Abbreviations: PT, prothrombin time; APTT, activated partial thromboplastin time; FDPs, fibrin degradation products; AT III, antithrombin III.

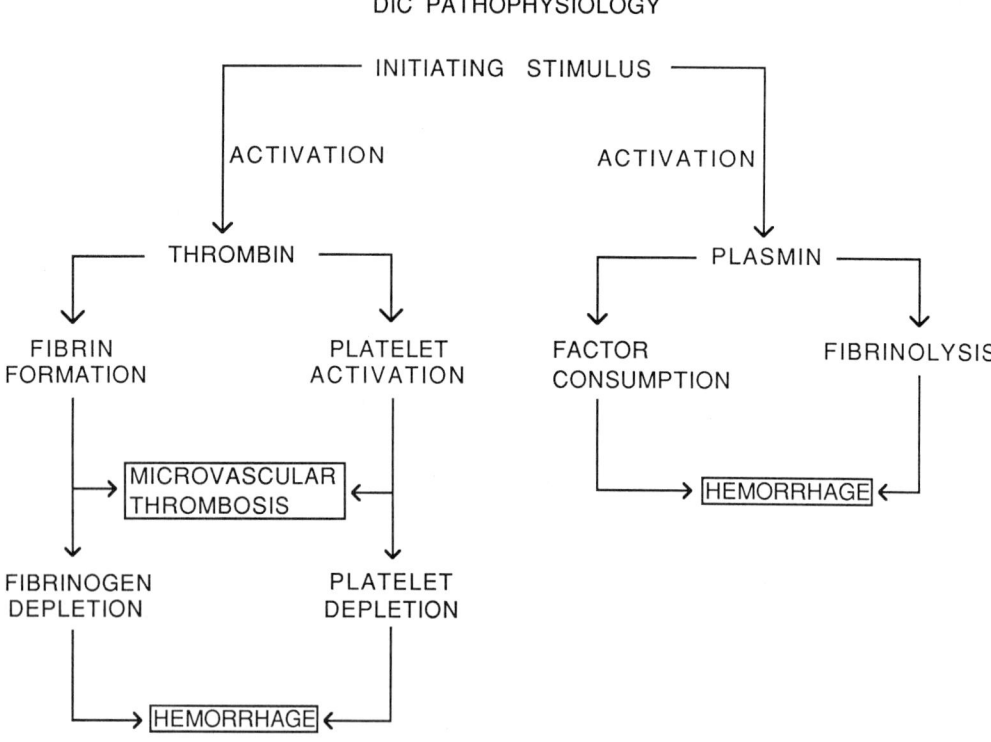

Fig. 18-21. Disseminated intravascular coagulation (DIC) is a complex process involving many systems. The basic pathology of DIC involves unregulated activation of plasmin and thrombin. Thrombin activity leads to activation of platelets and formation of fibrin thrombi. These hemostatic plugs tend to form in the microcirculation where the fibrin strands can shear passing RBCs, resulting in the fragmentation of RBCs commonly seen in DIC. Once platelet and fibrinogen are depleted, the patient may not be able to form physiologic thrombi at sites of vascular disruption, contributing to the bleeding tendency. Active plasmin can degrade hemostatic plugs giving rise to the diffuse bleeding commonly seen in association with DIC. In addition, plasmin can degrade factors V and VIII as well as fibrinogen and platelet membrane proteins. The degradation products derived from fibrin and fibrinogen can also inhibit platelet aggregation by competing for the glycoprotein IIb-IIIa binding sites. The result of excessive plasmin activation is thus a serious bleeding diathesis. In a patient with DIC, both microvascular thrombosis and fibrinolysis may occur simultaneously. The clinical manifestations in any given patient thus depend on the relative balance of thrombin and plasmin activation and the underlying condition of the patient.

Table 18-15. Hemostatic Abnormalities Associated with Liver Disease

Abnormality	Laboratory Manifestation	Clinical Manifestation
Thrombocytopenia	Thrombocytopenia	Bleeding
Decreased synthesis of coagulation factors	Prolonged PT, APTT	Bleeding
Decreased synthesis of regulatory proteins	Decreased AT III, protein C	Thrombosis, DIC
Dysfibrinogenemia	Prolonged TT, PT, APTT, false positive FDPs	None or mild bleeding
Abnormal vitamin K dependent proteins	Prolonged PT	Bleeding (?)

Abbreviations: PT, prothrombin time; APTT, activated partial thromboplastin time; AT III, antithrombin III; DIC, disseminated intravascular coagulation; TT, thrombin time; FDPs, fibrin degradation products.

ing the functional reserve of the hemostatic system. Such patients often respond poorly or abnormally to challenges to the hemostatic system that healthy individuals would handle without any problem. For example, excessive bleeding from a vascular defect may be encountered caused by diminished hemostatic response or DIC may be precipitated by minor stimuli secondary to an inability to regulate thrombin and plasmin generation adequately. The approach to patients with liver disease should include a careful evaluation of the clinical problems (e.g., are there anatomic lesions that should be repaired to control bleeding?) and measurement of the degree of hemostatic compromise. The PT, APTT, and fibrinogen are most useful for the latter, but other specific factor assays may be necessary to clarify the situation. In some cases, it may be very difficult to distinguish the coagulopathy of liver disease from DIC on the basis of laboratory results; in such cases, repeat determination of the platelet count and fibrinogen level over time is often useful for determining if any active consumption is taking place.

Approach to Therapeutic Monitoring of Hemostatic Agents

Oral Anticoagulant Therapy

Oral anticoagulants commonly are used for therapy of deep venous thrombosis and prophylaxis against thrombosis in high risk patients such as those with artificial heart valves or undergoing hip surgery.[13] These drugs inhibit carboxylation of glutamic acid residues in the vitamin K dependent proteins (Fig. 18-9); thus, their anticoagulant effect results principally from a decrease in the procoagulant side of hemostasis. The major complication of oral anticoagulant therapy is bleeding, the risk of which is proportional to the degree of anticoagulant effect or factor deficiency. Other complications of oral anticoagulant therapy include teratogenic effects, warfarin-induced skin necrosis, atheroembolization caused by bleeding into atherosclerotic plaques, and hypersensitivity reactions. The response to oral anticoagulants varies from patient to patient and is also affected by diet and concurrent medications. The list of drugs that can inhibit or potentiate the effect of oral anticoagulants is quite long; perhaps the best approach to a change in medication in a patient receiving oral anticoagulants is to monitor the PT carefully after the change has been made. Furthermore, substituting one brand for another brand of oral anticoagulant may affect the biologic response; such changes also need to be closely monitored.

The major goals of monitoring oral anticoagulant therapy are to ensure an adequate therapeutic response and to minimize the potential risk of bleeding caused by excessive anticoagulation. The most common test used to monitor oral anticoagulant therapy is the PT; others that are used occasionally include the PT and proconvertin time, amidolytic (chromogenic substrate) assays for vitamin K dependent proteins, and immunologic assays for these factors. Recent studies have focused on the optimal therapeutic range and the variability in PT response measured by different PT reagents. These studies have led to the development of the international normalized ratio (INR), a method for comparing the PT result obtained with one reagent to that obtained with other reagents. The INR is the ratio of patient PT to the mean PT of the reference range that would be obtained if an international reference thromboplastin were used to perform the PT measurement. By converting PT results obtained with working reagents to INRs (see under Test: Prothrombin Time), it is possible to compare the relative degree of anticoagulant effect measured by individual laboratories. Targets for therapeutic ranges in various clinical situations have been recommended by a recent consensus conference sponsored by the National Institutes of Health and the American College of Chest Physicians[14] (Table 18-16).

524 • Laboratory Medicine

Table 18-16. Recommendations for Oral Anticoagulant Therapy

Clinical Condition	Therapeutic Range		
	INR	PT Ratio[a]	Time[a] (sec)
Prophylaxis of venous thromboembolism	2.0–3.0	1.2–1.5	14–18
Treatment of venous thromboembolism	2.0–3.0	1.2–1.5	14–18
Prophylaxis of systemic embolization in patients with atrial fibrillation, valvular heart disease, acute myocardial infarction, or bioprosthetic heart valve	2.0–3.0	1.2–1.5	14–18
Recurrent systemic embolization	3.0–4.5	1.5–2.0	18–24
Prophylaxis of systemic embolization in mechanical prosthetic heart valve patients	3.0–4.5	1.5–2.0	18–24

Abbreviations: INR, international normalized ratio; PT, prothrombin time.
[a] Based on a PT performed with a typical North American rabbit brain thromboplastin; times are an approximation only. (Based on Dalen and Hirsh.[14])

Heparin Therapy

Heparin is frequently administered to hospitalized patients. Clinical uses include therapy for acute thromboembolic problems, prophylaxis against thrombosis in high risk patients, maintenance of extracorporeal circulation (e.g., renal dialysis and cardiopulmonary bypass), and maintenance of vascular access (e.g., arterial lines and intravenous catheters). Heparin potentiates the anticoagulant activity of AT III and thus the major effect of heparin is to enhance normal regulatory mechanisms (Fig. 18-12). Heparin is not a benign drug and is associated with a number of potential complications, including hemorrhage, thrombocytopenia with paradoxical thrombosis, skin necrosis, elevated liver enzymes, osteoporosis, alopecia, and hypersensitivity reactions.[13] The major complications of heparin therapy are bleeding and heparin-induced thrombocytopenia. Bleeding is directly related to dose, but a number of other factors can increase the risk of bleeding, including age (the elderly are more susceptible to bleeding), other defects in the hemostatic system (e.g., drug-induced platelet dysfunction), vascular defects resulting from recent surgery or trauma, and a history of alcoholism.

Heparin therapy is most often monitored when the drug is used to treat acute thrombosis or maintain extracorporeal circulation. The most common assay used to assess therapy for thrombosis is the APTT, but other tests such as the whole blood activated clotting time (ACT), modified thrombin time, and heparin concentration assays also can be used effectively. The therapeutic range in terms of the APTT response is usually given as 1.5–2.5 × the reference range, but there are a number of variables which impinge on the response of any given patient[13] (Table 18-17). In terms of heparin concentration, this therapeutic range corresponds to approximately 0.2 to 0.5 U/mL. Two of the most important variables affecting apparent heparin response are the shortened half-life of heparin during acute thrombotic events and the effect of increased factor VIII levels on the response to heparin measured by the APTT. Use of the patient's preheparin APTT as a guide to response can be useful to counteract the effect of increased factor VIII. The maintenance of extracorporeal circulation requires a higher concentration of heparin than therapy of acute thrombosis. The ACT is the most common test used to monitor heparin effect in these situations, as the APTT is usually unreadable at such high concentrations of heparin.

Heparin-induced thrombocytopenia is caused by an antibody that develops in some patients treated with heparin. The antibody binds to platelets in the pres-

Table 18-17. Variables Affecting the APTT Response to Heparin

Patient Variables	Analytic Variables
Route of administration	Specimen collection
Variation in infusion rate	Specimen storage
Diurnal variation in heparin	Specimen processing (centrifugation)
Body weight	Anticoagulant used for collection
Platelet count and PF4	
Antithrombin III	Factor VIII level
Recent thromboembolic events	APTT reagent
Natural variation in heparin half-life	Instrument used for the APTT

Abbreviations: APTT, activated partial thromboplastin time; PF4, platelet factor 4.

ence of heparin and induces in vivo platelet aggregation, which can result in thrombosis of the major arteries.[13] The development of thrombocytopenia, arterial thrombosis, or recurrent venous thrombosis while at a therapeutic level of heparin anticoagulation should raise the possibility of this disorder. The antibody usually does not appear until after several days of therapy, unless there has been a previous exposure to heparin. Once present, only small amounts of heparin (e.g., from periodic flushes of indwelling lines) are necessary to cause significant clinical problems. The platelet count should be monitored periodically in patients receiving heparin therapy.

Fibrinolytic Therapy

There has been a marked increase in the use of fibrinolytic therapy during recent years, particularly for treatment of acute myocardial infarction.[15] Three agents are available for use, and each has a different mechanism of action. Streptokinase is a bacterial product that combines with plasminogen to form a plasminogen activator complex; the streptokinase-plasminogen complex then activates other plasminogen molecules both in plasma and in association with blood clots. Urokinase is an enzyme that directly activates plasminogen, both in plasma and in association with blood clots. Therefore, both agents are systemic plasminogen activators and are consequently associated with depletion of circulating fibrinogen. Tissue plasminogen activator, which is produced by recombinant DNA technology, is a direct activator of plasminogen that requires fibrin as a cofactor. Fibrinolysis induced by tPA thus tends to be more clot specific than with the other two agents; despite this clot specificity, depletion of systemic fibrinogen and bleeding may occur during tPA therapy.

The major complication of fibrinolytic therapy is bleeding; fibrinogen depletion and lysis of physiologic thrombi at sites of vascular access appear to be major contributing factors to this complication. The presence of recent damage to vessels (e.g., surgery, arterial catheterization, recent stroke) augments the bleeding tendency associated with fibrinolytic therapy. The major goals of laboratory monitoring of fibrinolytic therapy are to determine whether excessive fibrinolysis and fibrinogen depletion have occurred and whether there has been an adequate fibrinolytic response. The only way to document lysis of the pathologic thrombus is with angiographic procedures; there are no laboratory assays that tell whether this thrombus has been lysed. Determination of fibrinogen levels is perhaps the most useful procedure for monitoring patients undergoing fibrinolytic therapy. The level of fibrinogen should be maintained above 50 mg/dl (0.5 g/L); if it falls below this level, fibrinolytic therapy should probably be decreased or stopped.

The thrombin time is sensitive to both fibrinogen depletion and generation of FDPs and may be useful in monitoring therapy with either streptokinase or urokinase. The level of FDPs increases markedly during fibrinolytic therapy but does not correlate very well with therapeutic effectiveness. A D-dimer assay may provide information regarding in vivo lysis of cross-linked fibrin clots, but the assay does not distinguish the lysis of pathologic thrombi from physiologic thrombi (e.g., at the site of a previous venipuncture). Measurement of α_2-antiplasmin and plasminogen may be of use in selected patients treated with urokinase or streptokinase who have an atypical response; excessive activation and consumption of plasminogen may lead to a suboptimal therapeutic outcome.

ASSAYS OF HEMOSTASIS

FIBRIN CLOT FORMATION

Test: Prothrombin Time[1-5,16]

Background and Selection

The PT measures the extrinsic portion of the coagulation cascade initiated by the interaction between factor VII and tissue factor (Fig. 18-6). The PT is used to screen for hemostatic disorders involving fibrin formation (Table 18-10) and to monitor the effectiveness of oral anticoagulant therapy.

Logistics

The PT is performed on citrated, platelet-poor plasma usually obtained by venipuncture; without special equipment, it cannot be performed on capillary blood samples. The National Committee on Clinical Laboratory Standards (NCCLS) has recommended that specimens for PT determination be placed on ice immediately after venipuncture and stored at 4°C until the PT is performed.[16] Whole blood is mixed with either 109 mM (3.2%) or 129 mM (3.8%) trisodium citrate in a blood to citrate ratio of 9:1; to preserve the pH value, buffered citrate is generally preferred. If multiple tubes are being collected at the time of blood sampling, the first tube *should not* be used for coagulation testing. The specimen should be processed promptly and the platelet-poor plasma placed in plastic. The PT may show artifactual shortening if the plasma is left in contact with glass at 4°C for long periods. The PT should be performed within 2 hours from the time the specimen is drawn; the specimen may be stored at −30°C or less for testing at another time.

The test is performed at 37°C by mixing platelet-poor plasma with a thromboplastin reagent (a mixture of tissue factor and calcium chloride) and measuring the time to clot formation. The source and concentration of tissue factor vary between commercially available thromboplastins. Formation of the clot may be detected by manual observation (tilt tube method), electromechanical sensors or photo-optical instruments. The PT result should be reported in seconds along with a reference range for the laboratory performing the assay. An older method of reporting results compared the patient's clotting time with that of a series of plasma samples diluted with various amounts of buffer. The PT result with this system was reported as the percentage activity; this method is no longer recommended.[16]

The PT time of specimens obtained from patients on stable, oral anticoagulant therapy can be converted to INR values in order to assess the effectiveness of oral anticoagulant therapy against accepted standards. The INR represents the ratio of patient PT to the mean PT of the normal population that would be obtained if an international standard thromboplastin (PT reagent) were used to perform the PT. An international sensitivity index (ISI) value for the working thromboplastin reagent is necessary to calculate the INR. The ISI represents the slope of the line relating the log PT obtained with the working reagent to the log PT of the standard reagent; the ISI is generally provided by the reagent manufacturer. The INR is calculated from the following equation:

$$INR = \left(\frac{PT_{patient}}{PT_{normal}}\right)^{ISI}$$

where $PT_{patient}$ is the PT of the patient plasma using the working thromboplastin, PT_{normal} is the mean PT of a healthy population using the working thromboplastin and ISI is the sensitivity index determined for the working thromboplastin. The effectiveness of oral anticoagulant therapy can then be judged by the INR value (Table 18-16). Because most thromboplastins used in the United States have similar ISIs, the therapeutic range is still occasionally expressed in terms of the ratio of the PTs for the patient and mean of healthy subjects (Table 18-16). The use of the INR reporting system should be limited to patients on stable oral anticoagulant therapy; it is not designed for monitoring the initiation of therapy or evaluation of other hemostatic disorders that may affect the PT.

Interpretation

The reference range and response to specific coagulation abnormalities vary depending on the reagent and technique employed by the laboratory. Generally, the PT is prolonged, when one or more of the extrinsic system factors is less than 50% of normal or clottable fibrinogen is less than 80–100 mg/dL (0.8–1.0 g/L). The most common causes of a prolonged PT include liver disease, oral anticoagulant therapy, vitamin K deficiency, and acute DIC (Table 18-10). Vitamin K deficiency occurs most commonly in hospitalized patients who are receiving systemic antibiotics and have poor oral intake; it may be associated with serious bleeding from multiple sites. Vitamin K deficiency may be rapidly reversed by parenteral administration of vitamin K. The response to oral anticoagulants may be judged in terms of the ratio of the patient PT to the mean of normals or the INR (Table 18-16). Abnormal proteins, such as descarboxy vitamin K dependent factors (those that have not been carboxylated) (Fig. 18-9), and dysfibrinogenemia may also cause a mild prolongation of the PT. Congenital deficiency of coagulation factors affecting the PT is uncommon and is usually detected early in childhood (Table 18-8). Lipemia and hyperbilirubinemia may affect the results with some photo-optical instruments. Heparin in high concentration may affect the PT. A shortened PT may be seen in patients transfused with activated coagulation products or in samples that have been activated in vitro. Occasionally, short PTs are seen in patients with in vivo activation of the coagulation system; a common clinical setting for this is metastatic tumor.

Test: Activated Partial Thromboplastin Time[1-5,16]

Background and Selection

The APTT measures the intrinsic portion of the coagulation cascade that is initiated by the interaction of factor XII with negatively charged surfaces (Fig. 18-8). It is frequently used to screen for disorders of fibrin formation and to monitor heparin therapy. It is also used to monitor replacement therapy in hemophilia A and B.

Logistics

The APTT is performed on citrated, platelet-poor plasma usually obtained by venipuncture. If a specimen is obtained from an indwelling catheter, an aliquot of blood (5–20 mL) should be discarded or used for other purposes; a plasma specimen obtained after such a discard may still show evidence of heparin contamination if heparin has been administered through the line or used to keep the line open. The blood sample is anticoagulated by mixing blood with either 109 mM (3.2%) or 129 mM (3.8%) trisodium citrate in a ratio of 9:1. An inappropriate relationship between plasma volume and citrate may result in a spurious APTT. This may occur as a result of under- or overfilling of the tube or to extreme alteration of the hematocrit (e.g., more than 55%). The APTT should be performed within 2 hours of sampling with platelet-poor plasma; the plasma specimen may be stored frozen in a plastic tube at $-30°C$ or less for testing at another time.

The APTT is a two-stage assay performed at $37°C$; during the first stage, plasma is incubated with a reagent containing phospholipid and a surface activator of factor XII. After this incubation, which varies in length for different reagents, $CaCl_2$ is added and the time to clot formation is measured. Clot formation may be detected by manual observation (tilt tube method), an electromechanical instrument, or a photo-optical instrument. Lipemia and hyperbilirubinemia may interfere with the APTT determination on some photo-optical instruments. The APTT is reported as the time (seconds) for clot formation after addition of $CaCl_2$.

Interpretation

The reference range varies considerably between reagents and clot detection systems; it should be reported with the APTT result. A number of coagulation abnormalities may result in a long APTT (Table 18-10). Among hospitalized patients, heparin and lupus anticoagulants are the most common causes of a long APTT with PT within or nearly within the reference range. Liver disease, vitamin K deficiency, and oral anticoagulants, which may result in prolongation of both the APTT and PT are also common. Intrinsic pathway factor levels below 40–50% of the reference range usually result in prolongation of the APTT (Fig. 18-8); the most common hereditary deficiencies in this pathway affect factors VIII and IX (Table 18-8). Factor deficiency may be distinguished from a factor inhibitor on the basis of mixing studies and inhibitor assays. The APTT may be prolonged when the fibrinogen concentration is less than 80–100 mg/dL (0.8–1.0 g/L) and in the presence of dysfibrinogenemia or descarboxy vitamin K dependent factors. A shortened APTT may be seen during an acute phase reaction or other conditions associated with an increased level of factor VIII and with activation in vitro because of poor specimen handling.

Perhaps the most common reason for performance of an APTT is to monitor heparin therapy given for an acute thromboembolic event. A number of variables affect the APTT response to heparin (Table 18-17). Among the more important are the reagent used for the APTT, the level of factor VIII, the size of the patient, and preparation of the sample. The therapeutic range is often given as prolongation of the APTT to 1.5–2.5 times the mean of the reference range.[13] However, this range should be adjusted for the reagent in use and perhaps for the patient's own baseline APTT. Failure to achieve a "therapeutic" response to a standard dose of heparin can be caused by one or more of several factors (see under Heparin Therapy). Comparison with the baseline APTT, measurement of factor VIII, and measurement of plasma heparin level may be of use in evaluating the adequacy of therapy.

Test: Thrombin Time (TT)[1–5]

Background and Selection

The TT is used to screen for abnormalities of fibrinogen and to determine whether heparin is the cause of a long APTT (Fig. 18-19).

Logistics

The TT is performed on citrated, platelet-poor plasma; specimen collection and handling is as described for the APTT assay. The TT measures thrombin conversion of fibrinogen to fibrin and polymerization of fibrin polymers to a fibrin gel; it does not measure fibrin stabilization or fibrinolysis. It is performed at $37°C$ by the addition of thrombin (often of bovine origin) to citrated plasma and determining the time to clot formation. Determination of the endpoint is usually by manual observation, thus, lipemia and hyperbilirubinemia do not interfere. Results of the TT are reported in seconds. If the TT is prolonged, mixing studies with normal plasma and protamine sulfate can be useful to differentiate heparin effect from other causes of a long TT.

Interpretation

The reference range is dependent on the source and concentration of thrombin and is determined by each laboratory. The most common cause of a prolonged TT is heparin; other causes include dysfibrinogenemia (common in liver disease), hypofibrinogenemia, increased levels of FDPs, and uremia (for unclear reasons). The presence of heparin is easily confirmed by correction of the TT with protamine sulfate, which neutralizes the anticoagulant effect of heparin. A Reptilase time may also be used to distinguish heparin effect from other causes of a long TT. The TT usually will be corrected to normal by mixing patient and normal plasma in a 1:1 ratio if the cause is hypofibrinogenemia, whereas the TT may remain prolonged after mixing with either protamine or normal plasma in the case of dysfibrinogenemia or elevated FDPs.

Test: Reptilase Time[1-5]

Background and Selection

A Reptilase time is most commonly used to evaluate the cause of a long TT. It is also used to assess the possibility of dysfibrinogenemia.

Logistics

A Reptilase time is performed on citrated, platelet-poor plasma, prepared as described for an APTT, by addition of the reagent to the plasma at 37°C and determining time to clot formation. Reptilase (Batroxobin) is an enzyme derived from the venom of *Bothrops atrox*, which clots human fibrinogen by cleavage of fibrinopeptide A from fibrinogen (Fig. 18-10). The advantage of Reptilase is that it is not inhibited by heparin or AT III.

Interpretation

The Reptilase time is reported in seconds with the reference range determined by the laboratory performing the test. A long TT and Reptilase time within the reference range is evidence of heparin in the sample. The Reptilase time is sensitive to dysfibrinogenemia; thus if both the TT and Reptilase time are prolonged, hypo- or dysfibrinogenemia should be suspected.

Test: PTT, APTT, and TT Correction Tests (Mixing Studies)[1-5]

Background and Selection

Patient plasma that gives an abnormal result with the PT, APTT, or TT may be mixed with normal plasma to separate a simple factor deficiency from a circulating inhibitor.

Logistics

The patient specimen is obtained as described for performance of an APTT. It is then mixed with normal plasma and the clotting assay repeated on the mixture. The usual mixture tested consists of 1 part patient plasma to 1 part normal plasma; a mixture of 4 parts patient plasma to 1 part normal plasma may be a more sensitive indicator of the presence of an inhibitor if the original clotting time is only mildly prolonged.

The mixture of patient and normal plasma may also be incubated together for 1–2 hours at 37°C to detect time dependent inhibitors. These antibodies require a longer period of time to interact with their target component of the hemostatic system; the most common example is a factor VIII inhibitor. The clotting time is repeated after the incubation. To control for the potential loss of labile factors during the incubation (which may cause a prolongation suggesting a time dependent inhibitor), patient specimens and normal plasma are also incubated at 37°C for the same period. A new mixture is made after incubation and its clotting time is compared with the clotting time of the incubated mixture. Progressive or time dependent inhibitors result in a significant prolongation of the clotting time of the incubated mixture compared to the new mixture of the plasmas incubated separately.

Interpretation

A factor deficiency is the likely cause of the prolonged PT or APTT if the clotting time of the mixture returns to the reference range. Confirmation of the factor deficiency is accomplished by measurement of the involved factor(s). Failure of the clotting time to return to the reference range is indicative of an inhibitory substance. Possibilities include heparin, circulating inhibitors (antibodies), dysfibrinogenemia, descarboxy vitamin K dependent proteins, and FDPs. The presence of heparin can be confirmed with a TT or Reptilase time. Specific factor inhibitors need to be distinguished from lupus inhibitors, because they are usually associated with a serious bleeding diathesis, but lupus inhibitors are not. With a specific factor inhibitor, one factor is affected and its level is very low (less than 10%); with lupus inhibitors, specific factor levels may be within the reference range or several factors may appear to be mildly reduced (to about 20–50%). Additional tests that may be of help in distinguishing specific factor inhibitors from lupus anticoagulants include the tissue thromboplastin inhibition, the platelet neutralization procedure, and the dilute Russell viper venom time (see Test: Dilute Russell Viper Venom Time). The presence of dysfibrinogenemia is usually documented by a discrepancy between clottable (functional) fibrinogen and antigenic fibrinogen (see below). Immunologic assays can be used to demonstrate the presence of fibrin(ogen) degradation products (see below).

Test: Prothrombin and Proconvertin Test (P and P)[4]

Background and Selection

The prothrombin (factor II) and proconvertin (factor VII) assay is a modified PT in which the test plasma is diluted and mixed with an exogenous source of factor V and fibrinogen. The assay is thus sensitive only to defects in II, VII, and X and can be used to monitor oral anticoagulant therapy. The results are usually reported in terms of percentage activity in reference to series of normal plasmas diluted with saline. It is not widely used and offers no significant advantage over the PT. Results from the P and P cannot be converted to INR values.

Test: Thromboelastography (TEG)[1-5]

Thromboelastography provides a picture of clot formation, stabilization, and fibrinolysis. The assay requires whole blood obtained with meticulous technique to avoid in vitro artifacts and a specialized instrument. An abnormal TEG can suggest defective procoagulant function or increased fibrinolysis but it is difficult to gain insight into the more specific nature of the defect from the assay results. The TEG is more sensitive to factor XIII function than is the more commonly employed urea clot solubility test (see below). Today TEG is most commonly used as an aid in monitoring the status of the hemostatic system during cardiopulmonary bypass and liver transplantation.

PLATELET FUNCTION

Test: Bleeding Time (BT)[1-5,17]

Background and Selection

The BT measures the interaction between platelets and the vessel wall; a defect in either component may result in a prolonged bleeding time. It is the most commonly used test to measure in vivo platelet function and is often included as part of a battery of tests used to screen for hemostatic disorders. The BT is sensitive to the platelet count as well as abnormalities of platelet function; if the platelet count is less than $50,000/\mu L$ ($<50 \times 10^9/L$), there are few reasons to perform a BT because it is usually greatly prolonged in such cases.

Logistics

The BT is an in vivo test performed directly on the patient by an experienced technologist or physician. A standardized incision is made on the volar surface of the forearm with a blood pressure cuff on the upper arm inflated to 40 mmHg to provide uniform capillary pressure. Disposable equipment permitting reproducible incisions is now commerically available from several sources. The incision may be made parallel or perpendicular to the long axis of the arm, but the results will be affected by the direction of the incision. Thus the same direction should always be used by the laboratory to ensure reproducible results. The length of time for the incision to stop bleeding is determined and reported as the BT. A BT may be performed on the legs if a suitable blood pressure cuff is available and the laboratory has developed a reference range for this site. A true end point for the BT may be difficult to determine in the elderly because they may bleed into or under the skin because of aging-related changes in skin tone. The BT may leave a small scar; a more significant scar may form in those prone to keloid formation.

Interpretation

The reference range, determined by each laboratory performing the procedure, should be provided with the test result. The most common cause of a long BT with a platelet count within the reference range is drug therapy affecting platelet function (Table 18-7) and thus proper interpretation depends on a thorough clinical history. The most common drug causing abnormal platelet function is aspirin, which irreversibly inhibits circulating platelets; the BT may thus be prolonged for several days after cessation of aspirin. However, the ability of aspirin to affect platelets is short-lived because of the rapid in vivo deacetylation of aspirin. Thus platelet transfusion may be effective in patients with platelet-type bleeding caused by aspirin. Other drugs usually cause reversible platelet inhibition, and the duration of their effect is dependent on the drug half-life. Other acquired disorders (Table 18-6) are more common than hereditary disorders of platelet function; the clinical history and other laboratory tests usually provide the information necessary for diagnosis of these disorders. Platelet aggregation studies are usually not indicated in the evaluation of acquired platelet disorders, because they add little diagnostic information regarding the etiology of the defect. If the clinical history suggests a hereditary disorder, evaluation with aggregation studies (see below) and measurement of VWF (see below) are in order. The development of petechiae on the arm distal to the blood pressure cuff during performance of the bleeding time is further evidence of abnormal platelet function.

Test: Aspirin Tolerance[17]

The aspirin tolerance test is a modification of the bleeding time that is useful in patients with a clinical history of platelet-type bleeding and a BT within the reference interval.[17] After the routine bleeding time is performed, the patient takes 650 mg of aspirin and a repeat BT is performed 2 hours later. Most healthy subjects show a prolongation of 1–4 minutes; a more marked prolongation is suggestive of a mild platelet abnormality. Platelet function studies, including VWF and platelet aggregation assays, on a specimen obtained before aspirin ingestion can confirm the presence of such a defect.

The aspirin tolerance test is not performed if the initial BT is abnormal.

Test: Capillary Fragility (Tourniquet Test)[1-5]

The capillary fragility test is a crude measure of platelet-vessel wall interaction. A blood pressure cuff is inflated to the midpoint between the diastolic and systolic pressures (but not greater than 100 mmHg) and the development of petechiae over a 5-minute period is monitored. The development of petechiae under these conditions suggests an abnormality of vessel wall-platelet interaction. If petechiae develop during performance of the BT, there is no indication to do a capillary fragility test.

Test: Platelet Count

See Chapter 19.

ASSAYS OF PLATELET FUNCTION

PLATELET ADHESION

Test: von Willebrand Factor Antigen (VWF: Ag)[1-5,18,19]

Background and Selection

von Willebrand factor is necessary for platelet adhesion to damaged vessel walls (Fig. 18-2). A deficiency or abnormality in the function of VWF is the etiology of VWD, the most common hereditary bleeding disorder (Table 18-6). This assay measures the concentration of VWF in plasma independent of its functional activity and is most commonly performed in conjunction with other assays to assess the possibility of VWD in a patient with a history of platelet defect-type bleeding. Patients with VWD most often have a prolonged BT and APTT with a PT and platelet count within the reference range. Other assays that are commonly performed with VWF: Ag include ristocetin-induced platelet aggregation, ristocetin cofactor activity, and factor VIII coagulant activity.

Terminology

The terminology for factor VIII and VWF has changed during recent years. These are two distinct proteins under different genetic control. Factor VIII was formerly designated factor VIIIC to denote its procoagulant function, whereas VWF was formerly designated with the abbreviation VIIIR, indicating VIII-related protein. Currently, the abbreviation VWF is used to designate the von Willebrand protein; it may be modified to indicate which property of the VWF is being measured (e.g., VWF: Ag).

Logistics

von Willebrand factor is usually measured in citrated platelet-poor plasma prepared as described for an APTT. The sample may be frozen at $-30°C$ or less prior to assay. The antigen concentration is most commonly determined by the Laurell rocket immunoelectrophoresis technique and results are reported in terms of percentage VWF relative to pooled normal plasma, which is assumed to have 100% VWF. Antigen concentration may also be determined by other immunologic assays, including enzyme-linked immunosorbent assays (ELISA).

Interpretation

The reference range for many procoagulant proteins is often given as 50–150% of "normal" where "normal" is defined as the amount of the factor present in plasma pooled from healthy donors. The reference range for VWF increases with increasing age and is also dependent on blood type. For example, the lower limit in persons who are blood group O is considerably lower than for other blood groups and may be as low as 35% of pooled normal plasma. To avoid overdiagnosis of VWF in blood group O patients and underdiagnosis in other blood groups,[18] the patient's blood group must be considered in the interpretation of VWF: Ag results in the range of 35–60%. The results of the VWF: Ag assay must be interpreted with results obtained from other measurements of VWF in order to establish a diagnosis of VWD (Table 18-18).

von Willebrand's disease is divided into three major types based on the results of multiple assays.[19] Type I VWD is inherited as an autosomal dominant trait and is characterized by a quantitative decrease of an otherwise normal VWF. Laboratory results typically show a parallel reduction in VWF: Ag, ristocetin cofactor activity (VWF: Rcof), and factor VIII with a normal distribution of high molecular weight multimers. Type II VWD is characterized by a deficiency of high molecular weight multimers; the BT is prolonged, but results of other VWF assays are variable, and concentrations of VWF: Ag within the reference range are often present. Type II VWD thus represents production of an abnormal VWF, which is not capable of mediating platelet adhesion (Fig. 18-2); it is usually inherited as an autosomal dominant trait. Multiple subtypes of type II VWD have been identified on the basis of the multimeric pattern and involvement of platelet VWF. The IIb subtype is of interest, because it is often associated with thrombocytopenia. Distinction between the type I and II subtypes is significant in that type I VWD can often be treated with the vasopressin analogue 1-deamino-8-arginine vasopressin (DDAVP), which causes a transient increase in VWF levels. DDAVP is generally not effective in type II VWD, because the abnormal VWF released does not correct the hemostatic defect. In type IIb VWD, the administration of DDAVP is associated with further thrombocytopenia.

A related disorder is pseudo-VWD, also known as platelet-type VWD. This disorder is characterized by an abnormality of the platelet membrane GP Ib, which functions as the binding site for VWF (Fig. 18-2). The abnormal GP Ib on unstimulated circulating platelets is capable of binding high molecular weight VWF multimers. The platelets and VWF multimers are then rapidly cleared from the circulation resulting in thrombocytopenia and a decrease in plasma high molecular weight VWF multimers. As a result, laboratory evaluation usually shows a long BT, mild thrombocytopenia, and an abnormal VWF multimeric distribution; the pattern looks very much like the type IIb defect. These two disorders can be distinguished by evaluation of the patient's platelets; with pseudo-VWD, the platelets bind an increased amount of normal VWF at low concentrations of ristocetin.

Type III VWD is characterized by very low to unmeasurable amounts of VWF and factor VIII; it is usually transmitted as an autosomal recessive trait. Patients with type III VWD tend to bleed like hemophiliacs because of the very low levels of factor VIII. This disorder may be misdiagnosed in infancy as severe hemophilia A if VWF is not measured. In contrast to the symptoms that accompany heterozygous type I VWD, the heterozygous parents of type III VWD patients are often asymptomatic.

Acquired VWD caused by an autoantibody to VWF has been reported, most commonly in association with lymphoproliferative disorders. von Willebrand factor antigen is usually reduced in acquired VWD, but type II defects with normal VWF: Ag have been reported. Increased levels of VWF: Ag are commonly seen in preg-

Table 18-18. Comparison of Laboratory Results in Hemophilia A and von Willebrand Syndrome

Assay	Hemophilia A	Type I VWD	Type II VWD	Type III VWD
APTT	Increased	Increased	Often normal	Increased
PT	Normal	Normal	Normal	Normal
Bleeding time	Normal	Increased	Increased	Increased
Factor VIII	Decreased	Decreased	Normal	Decreased
VWF: Ag	Normal	Decreased	Normal or decreased	Absent
VWF: Rcof	Normal	Decreased	Normal or decreased	Absent
VWF: CIE	Normal	Normal	Abnormal	Not performed
VWF: multimers	Normal	Normal	Decreased high molecular weight multimers	Not performed
RIPA	Normal	Variable	Variable	Decreased

Abbreviations: APTT, activated partial thromboplastin time; PT, prothrombin time; VWF: Ag, von Willebrand factor antigen; VWF: Rcof, von Willebrand factor ristocetin cofactor activity; VWF: CIE, crossed immunoelectrophoresis of von Willebrand factor; RIPA, ristocetin induced platelet aggregation.

nancy and liver disease. The rise in VWF: Ag during pregnancy may obscure the diagnosis of VWD during this period. Alterations in the multimeric distribution and antigen concentration of VWF have been reported in uremia, thrombotic thrombocytopenic purpura, and adult respiratory distress syndrome (ARDS).

Test: Ristocetin Cofactor Activity (VWF: Rcof)[1-5,18,19]

Background and Selection

Ristocetin is an antibiotic that facilitates the interaction of human VWF and platelets; the addition of ristocetin to a suspension of normal platelet-rich plasma will induce agglutination or aggregation of the platelets. The test is used to assess the functional activity of VWF during the evaluation of possible VWD.

Terminology

The property of VWF that permits its interaction with platelets was formerly designated VIIIR: ristocetin cofactor.

Logistics

The VWF: Rcof assay is performed on citrated platelet-poor plasma prepared as described for the APTT; stored plasma may be used if it is kept at $-30°C$ or less. The assay is performed using formalin-fixed platelets and a standard concentration of ristocetin. A standard curve is determined from the degree or rate of agglutination of these platelets in the presence of varying concentrations of VWF supplied by the standard or patient plasma. Results are expressed in terms of percentage activity, with 100% defined as the activity of pooled normal plasma.

Interpretation

As with VWF: Ag, the level of VWF: Rcof is dependent on blood type and the reference range increases with age. People with blood group O have lower levels of VWF than do those with other blood types; a level of 35-40% of pooled normal plasma may occur normally in patients with blood group O (see Test: VWF: Ag). von Willebrand's disease is characterized by a deficiency or abnormal function of VWF and may be subtyped based on the defect in VWF (see Test: VWF: Ag). Reduced levels of VWF: Rcof that parallel the changes in VWF: Ag and factor VIII are characteristic of type I VWD with very low to absent VWF: Rcof seen in type III VWD (Table 18-18). The results of the VWF: Rcof assay are quite variable in type II VWD and may be low, increased, or within the reference range. This occurs because intermediate to lower molecular weight multimers may be active in the ristocetin cofactor assay but unable to mediate platelet adhesion in vivo. Thus, patients with type II VWD who are missing the high molecular weight multimers may have a discrepancy between in vivo function and in vitro VWF: Rcof activity. Increased levels of VWF: Rcof may be seen in liver disease and pregnancy; the rise in VWF during pregnancy may obscure the diagnosis of VWD.

Test: Ristocetin-Induced Aggregation[1-5,19]

Background and Selection

Ristocetin will induce binding of VWF to platelets, initiating an aggregation response. This antibiotic is used to assess the interaction between VWF and platelets in patients suspected of having a platelet disorder, on the basis of clinical history or an abnormal BT. This assay is used for the diagnosis of VWD and Bernard-Soulier syndrome; it can be used to distinguish between these two syndromes.

Logistics

The Ristocetin-induced aggregation is usually performed in conjunction with platelet aggregation response to other agonists such as ADP, collagen, and epinephrine. The assay is performed on a blood specimen drawn into a plastic tube containing either 109 mM (3.2%) or 129 mM (3.8%) trisodium citrate in a blood to citrate ratio of 9:1. The amount of citrate should be adjusted if the hematocrit (Hct) is very abnormal (less than 30% or more than 50%). Because of the sensitivity of platelet function studies to artifacts introduced by sampling technique, the specimen is generally obtained by an experienced coagulation technologist at the time the assay is to be performed. Testing must be completed in 2-4 hours, and the specimen cannot be stored for delayed testing. A platelet count within the reference range is generally required for performance of this assay but, with special techniques, the assay may be performed with platelet counts within the $50,000-100,000/\mu L$ ($50-100 \times 10^9/L$) range. The aggregation response is determined by the change in light transmittance through a continuously stirred plasma suspension of platelets in an instrument called a platelet aggregometer (Fig. 18-18). A normal control platelet-rich plasma is generally run in parallel to ensure that all reagents are working satisfactorily. The response to low (less than 1.0 mg/mL), intermediate (1.0–1.2 mg/mL), and high (1.5 mg/mL) concentrations of ristocetin is generally measured. Results are usually reported as an increased, normal, or absent response.

Interpretation

An absent response to intermediate or high concentrations of ristocetin (1.0–1.5 mg/mL) combined with a normal response to other platelet agonists is classically seen in VWD and Bernard-Soulier syndrome. However, up to 30–40% of patients with VWD may have a normal or only mildly decreased aggregation response to ristocetin; thus, this assay is not very sensitive for the diagnosis of VWD. Bernard-Soulier syndrome and VWD are differentiated by demonstrating a plasma defect in VWD and a platelet defect in Bernard-Soulier syndrome. For example, addition of normal platelet-poor plasma to the specimen from a patient with Bernard-Soulier syndrome would not correct the defective response to ristocetin, because the abnormality in this syndrome involves GP Ib on the platelet surface (Fig. 18-2). By contrast, the addition of normal plasma to the platelet-rich specimen from a patient with VWD should restore the response to ristocetin. In Bernard-Soulier syndrome, other measures of VWF such as VWF: Ag and VWF: Rcof are within the reference range.

Decreased or absent aggregation to ristocetin is occasionally seen in patients with secretory platelet defects; these patients are identified by the presence of additional abnormalities in the aggregation response to other platelet agonists and VWF: Ag and VWF: Rcof within the reference range. A lack of response to ristocetin may be seen in black patients with no history of bleeding, an otherwise normal VWF, and no other evidence of VWD.

Aggregation in response to low concentrations (less than 1.0 mg/dL) of ristocetin is typically seen only in type IIb VWD and pseudo-VWD. Type II VWD is due to a deficiency of high molecular weight VWF multimers (see Test: VWF: Ag). Type IIb is a specific subtype caused by binding of an abnormal VWF to normal circulating platelets with clearance of the bound VWF multimers and platelets. Laboratory assays usually reveal intermittent thrombocytopenia, normal VWF: Ag concentration, variable VWF: Rcof activity, and an abnormal VWF: CIE (see below), indicating loss of the larger multimers. The defect in pseudo-VWD is an abnormality in platelet GP Ib resulting in increased affinity for normal plasma VWF. As with type IIb VWD, the platelet-VWF complexes are cleared from the circulation resulting in a decrease in the platelet count and high molecular weight VWF multimers. Analogous to the situation with Bernard-Soulier syndrome and type I VWD, type IIb VWD can be distinguished from pseudo-VWD by mixing the patient's platelet-poor plasma with normal platelets. Induction of platelet aggregation in this mixture by low concentrations of ristocetin would indicate a defect in plasma VWF and support a diagnosis of type IIb VWD.

Test: Crossed Immunoelectrophoresis of VWF (VWF: CIE)[1-5]

Background and Selection

Because of the variation in molecular weight of the VWF multimers in plasma, VWF gives an assymetric pattern on crossed immunoelectrophoresis with higher molecular weight multimers moving more cathodally. This assay is used to assess the multimeric composition of VWF in plasma, with an abnormal VWF: CIE indicating an absence of high molecular weight multimers. Absence of the high molecular weight multimers is characteristic of type II VWD (see Test: VWF: Ag). This assay is performed as part of the evaluation of possible VWD in patients who present with a long BT and/or a history of platelet-defect type bleeding.

Logistics

Crossed immunoelectrophoresis is performed on citrated, platelet-poor plasma collected as described for APTT determination. It may be performed on stored plasma kept below −30°C. Plasma is first electrophoresed in agarose to separate proteins on the basis of charge and, in the case of VWF, multimeric size. The agarose adjacent to this strip is then replaced with agarose containing antibody to VWF and electrophoresis is repeated with the field perpendicular to the original migration. The protein binds the antibody and precipitates, analogous to the Laurell technique. Because of the large variation in the size and relative concentration of VWF polymers in plasma, VWF forms an asymmetric precipitin arc (Fig. 18-22).

Interpretation

The VWF: CIE assay is a qualitative measurement of the multimeric distribution of VWF in plasma and is usually reported as normal or abnormal. Interpretation

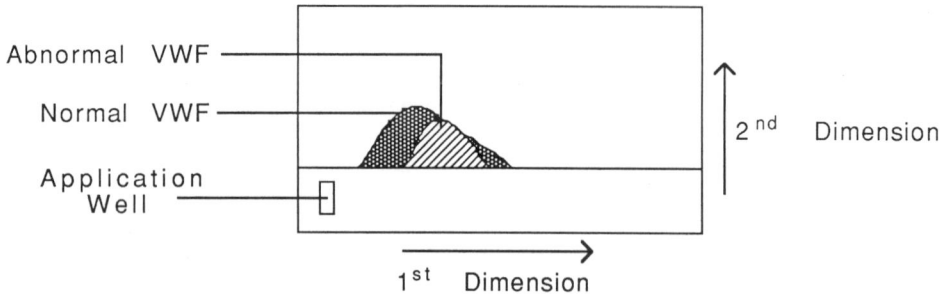

Fig. 18-22. Crossed immunoelectrophoresis is commonly performed to assess the multimeric structure of von Willebrand factor (VWF). Sample is first placed in a well cut in agarose and electrophoresed. VWF migrates based in part on size, with the larger multimers migrating more slowly. The agarose next to the strip used for migration in the first dimension is then replaced with agarose containing antibody to VWF. The plate is then electrophoresed perpendicular to the first dimension. As the VWF migrates into the antibody containing agarose, a precipitin arc forms. Normal VWF displays an asymmetrical arc due to the large distribution of monomers. The more slowly moving (anodal) portion of the arc is missing in patients deficient in high molecular weight multimers (abnormal pattern). This pattern is characteristic of type II von Willebrand's disease.

is difficult at low levels of VWF: Ag (e.g., less than about 25% of normal). An abnormal VWF: CIE usually indicates a decrease in high molecular weight VWF multimers and is typically seen in type II VWD and pseudo-VWD (see VWF: Ag). Subclassification of type II VWD requires performance of a multimeric analysis by SDS-agarose electrophoresis. An abnormal VWF: CIE may also be seen in some cases of acquired VWD and in other hemostatic disorders, including TTP, ARDS, and uremia.

Test: Multimeric Analysis of VWF[1-5]

The reference procedure for analysis of the multimeric composition of plasma VWF is SDS-agarose gel electrophoresis. This procedure permits resolution of VWF into distinct bands corresponding to polymers of increasing molecular weight. With high resolution electrophoresis, each of the major bands can be separated into several minor bands. Type II VWD is characterized by a decrease in the bands corresponding to high molecular weight multimers. Type II VWD may be subclassified, in part, on the basis of changes in the minor bands comprising each of the major bands.[19] The assay is generally available only from major coagulation reference laboratories. It is usually not needed to establish a clinical diagnosis of VWD, but it may be used to confirm a diagnosis of type II VWD. The distinction of type I from type II VWD is important because it affects therapy. In general, the drug DDAVP, which causes a transient rise in plasma VWF, cannot be used in type II VWD.

Test: Platelet VWF[19]

Platelets contain a significant amount of VWF. Some patients with VWD have a discordance between plasma and platelet VWF; in patients with type I VWD and normal platelet VWF, the BT is shorter and clinical symptoms are milder than in patients with a concordant decrease in platelet and plasma VWF. Platelet VWF may be measured by any of the previously described assays for VWF. A sample of platelets must be obtained and separated from plasma, either by washing or by gel filtration. The platelets are then lysed and the released VWF analyzed. At this time analysis of platelet VWF is usually only done for research purposes.

Test: Platelet Binding of VWF[19]

This assay is used to help distinguish type IIb VWD from pseudo- (platelet-type) VWD (see Test: VWF: Ag). The assay is performed using the patient's platelets, normal VWF, and ristocetin. Binding of normal VWF to the patient's platelets with increasing concentrations of ristocetin is determined by measuring the residual, nonbound VWF in the supernate after centrifugation. In pseudo-VWD, there is increased binding of normal VWF at low concentrations of ristocetin because of an abnormality of platelet GP Ib, the platelet receptor for VWF (Fig. 18-2). This assay is usually performed by reference coagulation laboratories in an attempt to distinguish between type IIb VWD and pseudo-VWD; it has little role in the usual clinical evaluation of VWD. Patients with pseudo-VWD may be more effectively treated with platelet concentrates than with cryoprecipitate.

Test: Glass Bead Retention Time (Solzman Test, Platelet Adhesion Test)[1-5]

The glass bead retention time was one of the first tests of platelet adhesion to be introduced; it has been largely replaced by direct assays of VWF. Whole blood is passed through a column of glass beads at a standardized flow rate and pressure. The platelet count is determined before and after passage through the column. In healthy persons, generally about 75% of the platelets are retained in the column. Patients with abnormal platelet adhesion do not retain as many platelets. The assay is difficult to standardize, and there is often considerable variation in results between laboratories and between persons performing the test in the same laboratory. It is infrequently used now.

PLATELET SECRETION AND AGGREGATION

Test: Platelet Aggregation[1-5]

Background and Selection

The platelet aggregation response to various agonists is used to assess the possibility of intrinsic platelet dysfunction. The test is used primarily for evaluation of patients with a possible hereditary defect based on a clinical history of platelet-type bleeding and/or an abnormal bleeding time (Table 18-4). Because the results obtained with acquired defects of platelet function are nonspecific, platelet aggregation studies are of little help in these disorders. Platelet aggregation is occasionally used in the evaluation of patients with a possible myeloproliferative disorder because in vitro responses are often abnormal in such patients. By contrast, platelet aggregation studies are usually within the reference range in patients with reactive thrombocytosis in the absence of drug effect or other problems affecting platelet function.

Logistics

Platelet aggregation studies are usually performed on platelet-rich plasma, although more recent technology permits performance on diluted whole blood. The specimen must be carefully obtained and placed in plastic throughout the evaluation period, to avoid in vitro activation of platelets. Whole blood is anticoagulated with either 109 mM (3.2%) or 129 mM (3.8%) trisodium citrate in a blood to citrate ratio of 9:1. The amount of anticoagulant should be adjusted if the Hct is abnormal (less than 30% or more than 50%). The studies should be completed within 2–4 hours of the time the specimen is drawn. The specimen is usually obtained by specially trained personnel at the time the procedure is to be performed; a control specimen from a healthy volunteer is normally processed in parallel. The patient and control subject should be free of any medication that might affect the platelet aggregation response (Table 18-7).

A variety of platelet agonists may be used; common agonists include ADP, collagen, epinephrine, arachidonic acid, and thrombin. Arachidonic acid is effective for detecting an aspirin-like defect, whereas ADP and epinephrine are useful for assessing platelet secretion. The aggregation response is usually determined by monitoring the change in light transmittance through a constantly stirred suspension of platelets. As large platelet aggregates form, the light transmittance increases (Fig. 18-18). Results are generally reported as a narrative interpretation of function that takes into consideration other clinical and laboratory data. Occasionally, the rate of aggregation is interpolated from the maximal slope of change in light transmittance. The aggregation of platelets can also be monitored in diluted whole blood by an electrical impedance technique or by monitoring the change in apparent platelet count in the platelet-rich plasma (which decreases as platelets aggregate).

Interpretation

Two major abnormal patterns may be observed with platelet aggregation studies. Primary wave defects are characterized by a total lack of response to all agonists except ristocetin; this pattern is seen with afibrinogenemia and with Glanzmann's thrombasthenia (Table 18-5). Secondary wave defects are characterized by an initial primary wave response to epinephrine and/or ADP but by a lack of a secondary wave (Fig. 18-18). A similar pattern may be seen with arachidonic acid, and the response to collagen may be delayed and/or decreased in amplitude in such samples. A secondary wave defect is typical of hereditary platelet secretory problems and of most acquired qualitative platelet defects (Tables 18-5 and 18-6). Occasionally, the response to an agonist is increased, in terms of either a decreased concentration of agonist necessary for maximal response or an increased rate of aggregation. The clinical significance of this finding is still uncertain, but it has been suggested that it might correlate with in vivo platelet hyperactivity and a thrombotic tendency.

Test: Serotonin Release Assay[1-5]

In the serotonin release assay, platelets take up radiolabeled serotonin from the surrounding medium into the dense granules. After a period of equilibration, the platelets are washed to remove external serotonin and the release of radiolabeled serotonin in response to agonists is measured. Decreased release of radiolabeled serotonin is seen in disorders characterized by abnormal secretion of platelet granules. Such a defect may be due to an abnormality of the granules themselves or to an abnormality of the secretory process (Table 18-5). A modification of this assay for detection of heparin dependent antiplatelet antibodies was recently described.[20]

Test: ATP Release Assay[1-5]

In the ATP release assay, the contents of the platelet dense granule, including ATP, are discharged into the surrounding medium during the normal release reaction. The released ATP can be quantitated by the generation of chemiluminescence with the luciferase assay. With a specialized instrument, ATP release and platelet aggregation can be monitored simultaneously. The assay is used to demonstrate an abnormality of platelet secretion (Table 18-5).

Test: Clot Retraction[1-5]

After formation, a normal hemostatic plug contracts in size in response to a metabolically active platelet contractile mechanism. Clot retraction is diminished in Glanzmann's thrombasthenia, perhaps related to the deficiency of GP IIb-IIIa, which appears to serve as a membrane anchor site for the contractile proteins. The assay is performed by clotting platelet-rich plasma in a test tube and incubating the clot at 37°C. The clot is observed manually for clot retraction, which usually occurs within minutes of clot formation.

Test: Platelet Factor III Assay (Platelet Phospholipid Assay)[1-5]

Platelet factor III refers to the ability of the stimulated platelet phospholipid membrane to support thrombin formation. Various assays to measure this property have been described, but they have little clinical value. Only one patient with an apparent intrinsic defect in platelet mediated thrombin activation has been described.

IN VIVO PLATELET ACTIVATION

Test: Circulating Platelet Aggregates Assay (Hyperaggregate Assay)[1-5]

Background and Selection

Under conditions associated with increased activation of the coagulation system in vivo, it appears that small aggregates of platelets may circulate in peripheral blood. Such aggregates spontaneously dissociate when EDTA, the usual anticoagulant for performance of platelet counts, is added. This method is designed to preserve such aggregates. The assay is generally used to assess the possibility of increased in vivo platelet activation and a thrombotic tendency, particularly in patients with atypical arterial thrombosis.

Logistics

The specimens must be obtained by the laboratory; one sample is anticoagulated with EDTA, whereas another is anticoagulated with a mixture of formalin and EDTA; platelet counts are performed on each sample. The platelet aggregates are fixed by the formalin-EDTA tube, whereas they dissociate in the regular EDTA tube. The presence of in vivo platelet aggregates is thus reflected by a difference in platelet counts between the two samples. The results are usually expressed as a ratio of the two counts.

Interpretation

In healthy persons, the ratio of platelets in formalin-EDTA to platelets in EDTA only is usually greater than 0.8; a lower ratio is indicative of circulating platelet aggregates. There are few data concerning the clinical specificity and sensitivity of this test for a thrombotic tendency.

Test: Platelet Factor 4 (PF4)[1-5]

Background and Selection

Platelet factor 4 is normally present only in platelet α-granules. Once released during the secretory phase of the platelet response, it is rapidly but reversibly cleared from the circulation; endothelial cell binding appears to play a major role in PF4 clearance. Increased levels of PF4 are indicative of increased platelet release; thus, this assay is used to assess in vivo platelet activation. The clinical value of this assay is limited by its extreme sensitivity to artifacts related to in vitro release and the nonspecific implications of increased PF4 levels. For these reasons, performance of the assay is usually limited to research studies.

Logistics

Levels of PF4 are usually very low to absent. However, there can be significant release of PF4 during venipuncture and/or specimen processing. Therefore, specimens for PF4 assay must be drawn carefully by experienced phlebotomists and placed immediately into specialized tubes containing anticoagulants and antiplatelet agents to prevent in vitro release. Once the plasma has been separated from platelets, the PF4 is stable at −30°C, and specimens can be batched. While PF4 is measured most frequently by a very sensitive radioimmunoassay (RIA), ELISA can also be used.

Interpretation

Increased levels of PF4 are associated with active in vivo thrombosis from whatever cause. The assay is so sensitive to platelet activation that it may be difficult to distinguish physiologic from pathologic responses. Heparin therapy may falsely increase plasma PF4 levels by displacement of endothelial bound PF4. The major problem with this assay is reliable specimen acquisition and processing.

Test: β-Thromboglobulin (BTG)[1-5]

Background and Selection

β-thromboglobulin is another platelet-specific α-granule protein that can be used to monitor platelet release. The clearance of BTG is slower than for PF4 and is primarily dependent on renal clearance. Increased levels of BTG are indicative of increased platelet release; thus, this assay is used to assess in vivo platelet activation. The clinical value of this assay is limited by its extreme sensitivity to artifacts related to in vitro release and by the nonspecific implications of increased BTG levels. For these reasons, performance of the assay is usually limited to research studies.

Logistics

The assay for BTG is also a sensitive RIA and subject to the same collection and processing problems as the PF4 assay. Because these assays are most commonly performed together, the specimen is processed identically to that for PF4.

Interpretation

Increased levels of BTG are seen with any disorder characterized by in vivo platelet activation. Increased levels may also be seen in renal disease caused by decreased clearance. As with PF4, the major problem is distinguishing in vivo from in vitro release.

Test: Membrane Glycoprotein Expression[1-5]

New glycoproteins appear on the surface of stimulated platelets. Sensitive methods for detecting platelets expressing such glycoproteins using flow cytometers and monoclonal antibodies have recently been described. It is still unclear whether such assays will be of clinical importance.

Test: Glycocalicin[21]

Glycocalicin is a proteolytic degradation product derived from GP Ib. Increased plasma levels of glycocalicin have been found to correlate with in vivo turnover rate.[21] Thrombocytopenic disorders characterized by increased destruction are associated with high levels of glycocalicin. At this time the assay is not widely available.

FIBRIN CLOT FORMATION

COAGULATION FACTORS

Test: Factor VIII Procoagulant Assay[1-5,22]

Background and Selection

Quantitation of factor VIII functional activity is usually performed as part of an evaluation of a long APTT (Fig. 18-19) or evaluation of possible VWD (Table 18-18). The possibility of factor VIII deficiency (hemophilia A) is raised by a history of soft tissue bleeding with a long APTT and PT within the reference range (Table 18-4). Factor VIII assays may be performed as a part of a battery of assays used to determine the cause of a long APTT; such a battery often includes factor IX, XI, and XII assays. Factor VIII assays are also performed to monitor replacement therapy in patients deficient in this factor and to quality control blood products such as cryoprecipitate which are used to treat patients with factor deficiencies. There is little role for factor VIII assays in the evaluation of possible acute DIC.

Terminology

In the past, factor VIII has been designated factor VIIIC; with the clarification of the relationship between factor VIII and VWF, it is now referred to as factor VIII. Other names that have been used for this protein include antihemophilic factor, factor VIII procoagulant protein, and factor VIII coagulant antigen (VIIIC: Ag).

Logistics

Factor VIII assays are performed on citrated platelet-poor plasma.[22] The specimen should be obtained as described for the APTT and the plasma placed into a plastic container as soon as possible. If the assay can not be performed within 2–4 hours, the specimen may be stored frozen at −30°C or less for up to 1–2 months. Factor VIII (and factor V) are relatively unstable in plasma and care must be exercised in the handling of the specimen. The procoagulant cofactor activity of factor VIII is increased by limited proteolytic cleavage by thrombin. The one-stage factor VIII assay, based on a modified APTT system, is sensitive to such pre-assay activation and gives a higher activity value when such activation is present. This type of activation may occur in pathologic conditions in vivo or in vitro as a result of suboptimal specimen handling. The two-stage and amidolytic (chromogenic substrate) assays for factor VIII activity, which are not widely used in the United States, are not as sensitive to pre-assay or in vivo factor VIII activation.

The one-stage factor VIII assay is performed by determining the APTT of a 1:1 mixture of diluted patient plasma and substrate plasma with no factor VIII. Under these conditions, the APTT is dependent on the amount of factor VIII present in the diluted patient specimen. This APTT is compared with the APTT values of 1:1 mixtures of serially diluted reference plasma with a known factor VIII concentration and substrate plasma. The activity of the patient plasma is deter-

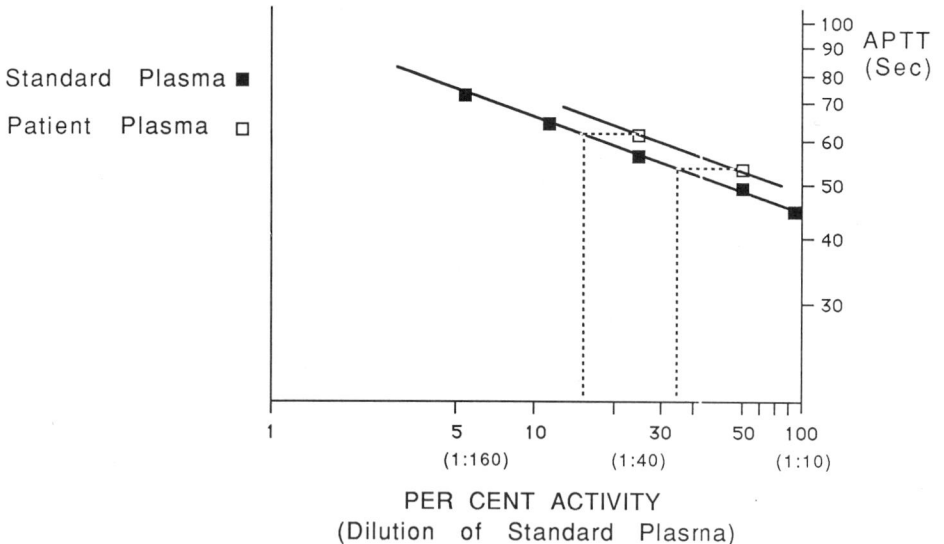

Fig. 18-23. One-stage factor assays are performed using a modification of either prothrombin time (PT) or activated partial thromboplastin time (APTT) as shown in this example of a factor VIII assay. Dilutions of plasma containing a known amount of factor VIII are mixed with plasma deficient in factor VIII. An APTT is determined on this mixture and is proportional to the amount of factor VIII in the diluted sample. A standard curve is then plotted relating the clotting time to the assigned factor activity. In this example, a 1:10 dilution of the curve corresponds to 100% factor VIII activity. The patient sample is then diluted, mixed with deficient plasma, and an APTT determined. The corresponding activity is read from the standard curve by visual interpolation or, more commonly, linear regression analysis of the standard curve. In this example, visual interpolation is indicated by the dashed lines. The APTT for the patient dilution is linked to the standard curve and the corresponding activity read from the graph (dashed lines); this value must then be corrected for the relative dilution. The activity in this example would thus be ~68% (34% × 2 and 17% × 4). Two or more patient dilutions are routinely tested to document that the line through the patient dilutions parallels the standard curve. If the lines are not parallel, the assay is not valid.

mined from regression analysis of the standard curve relating the concentration of VIII in the mixture to the APTT (Fig. 18-23). The accuracy of the method is largely dependent on the validity of the assigned activity in the reference plasma.

Interpretation

The reference range for factor VIII activity is about 50–150%. Low levels of factor VIII are characteristic of hemophilia A, VWD, and the rare hereditary disorder, combined deficiency of factors V and VIII. Very low levels of factor VIII are seen in acquired deficiency states caused by autoantibodies; these antibodies are usually of the neutralizing type. Antibodies to factor VIII occur in about 10% of severe hemophiliacs and sporadically in elderly patients, in pregnant women near parturition, in association with other autoimmune diseases, and in association with some drugs such as penicillins. Decreased levels of factor VIII may be seen in acute DIC, but this finding occurs in fewer than 25% of patients with this disorder. Although recent evidence indicates that factor VIII is synthesized in the liver, normal to increased levels of factor VIII are commonly seen in liver disease until the terminal stages of the disease. However, in patients with liver disease the ratio of factor VIII to VWF is often decreased, suggesting that production is suboptimal. The ratio of factor VIII to VWF has also been used to evaluate the possibility of carrier status for hemophilia A. Women who are heterozygous carriers for hemophilia tend to have a lower factor VIII:VWF ratio than is found in healthy women. Today this approach has been supplanted by direct analysis of the factor VIII gene and in utero diagnosis of hemophilia.

Factor VIII assays are used to guide replacement therapy in patients with hemophilia A. A level of more than 50% is necessary to maintain hemostasis for invasive procedures and other major challenges to the hemostatic system. A lack of response to an adequate dose of factor VIII suggests the presence of a factor VIII inhibitor.

Factor VIII is an acute-phase reactant and increased levels are commonly seen in acute inflammatory disorders. Increased factor VIII activity, which is common in patients with acute deep venous thrombosis, decreases the prolongation of the APTT in response to heparin and may contribute to heparin resistance early in the course of anticoagulant therapy. Increased factor VIII activity is also seen in pregnancy and in patients with atherosclerotic vascular disease. Lupus anticoagulants may interfere with performance of the one-stage factor VIII assay, leading to spuriously low results.

Test: Factor IX Procoagulant Activity[1-5,22]

Background and Selection

Factor IX activity is most commonly measured with a one-stage factor assay as part of the evaluation of a long APTT. Hereditary deficiency of factor IX occurs in hemophilia B, which is clinically indistinguishable from hemophilia A. The possibility of hemophilia is suggested by a history of soft tissue bleeding and a long APTT with a PT within the reference range (Table 18-4). Factor IX assays may be performed as part of a battery of assays used to determine the cause of an unexplained prolongation of the APTT; factor VIII, XI, and XII assays are frequently part of such a battery. Acquired inhibitors of factor IX are encountered much less frequently than factor VIII inhibitors and occur principally in patients with severe (less than 1% activity) hemophilia B. Reduced factor IX levels are also seen in liver disease, vitamin K deficiency, and oral anticoagulant therapy, although measurement of factor IX activity usually adds little to the management of such patients.

Terminology

Other names for factor IX include Christmas factor and plasma thromboplastin component.

Logistics

Factor IX assays are performed on citrated plasma prepared as described for an APTT. The activity is determined by a modified APTT assay analogous to that used for factor VIII assays (Fig. 18-23). The only difference is that the substrate plasma is deficient in factor IX rather than factor VIII.

Interpretation

The reference range for factor IX is 50–150% of the activity in pooled normal plasma. Reduced levels are seen in hemophilia B, liver disease, vitamin K deficiency, and oral anticoagulant therapy. Inhibitors to factor IX are uncommon and usually occur in patients with a history of severe factor IX deficiency. Lupus anticoagulants may interfere with the assay and give spuriously low results.

Factors XI and XII, Prekallikrein, and High Molecular Weight Kininogen[1-5]

Factors XI and XII, prekallikreins and high-molecular-weight kininogen are most commonly measured as part of an evaluation of an unexplained prolongation of the APTT with a PT within the reference interval. The APTT is very sensitive to deficiency of these four factors and mildly prolonged APTT values may be seen in heterozygotes with 35–60% of normal activity. These factors may also be measured by a one-stage APTT assay method (see discussion of factor VIII). Hereditary deficiency of these factors is uncommon to rare (Table 18-8); deficiency of factor XII, prekallikrein, or high-molecular weight kininogen is not associated with a bleeding tendency. Rather, such patients may have an increased risk of thrombosis. Factor XI deficiency, sometimes designated hemophilia C, is associated with a mild to moderate bleeding tendency and occurs principally among people of Ashkenazi Jewish ancestry. Lupus anticoagulants may interfere with the assays of these factors, resulting in spuriously low values.

Test: Prekallikrein Activity Screen (Fletcher Factor Assay)[1-5]

The prekallikrein activity assay is used to screen for prekallikrein deficiency, because the deficient plasma necessary for performance of a one-stage assay may be difficult to obtain or too expensive to keep in stock for a rarely performed assay. The initial stages of the intrinsic system of coagulation involve a positive feedback loop in which factor XIIa generates kallikrein, which in turn generates more XIIa (Fig. 18-9). A deficiency of prekallikrein may be detected as a prolonged APTT; the degree of prolongation may be significantly decreased if the initial period of activation before addition of $CaCl_2$ is increased. This enables the slowly forming factor XIIa to generate more factor XIa, compensating for a lack of prekallikrein. A prolonged APTT caused by a deficiency of the other contact system factors (factors XI and XII and high molecular weight kininogen) will not shorten, because each is necessary for factor XI activation, and prolonged incubation does not counteract the deficiency. The assay is performed by determining an APTT after two periods of activation; a significant shortening of the APTT with the prolonged incubation is indicative of prekallikrein deficiency.

Test: Factor Assay for II, V, VII, and X[1-5]

Measurement of factors II, V, VII, and X is usually performed as part of an evaluation of a long PT or combined prolongation of the APTT and PT. A combination of factor V and VII determination can differentiate liver disease from vitamin K deficiency.

These assays are performed on citrated platelet-poor plasma prepared as described for a PT. Care should be taken to avoid in vitro activation of factor VII, which may cause a spurious increase in its apparent activity; such activation usually occurs when plasma is stored in glass tubes at 4°C. Assays for II, V, and X can be performed by a modification of either the PT or APTT; the modified PT is used most commonly. A modified PT system is used for a factor VII assay. The assays are similar to the one-stage factor VIII assay. A dilution of patient plasma is mixed 1:1 with a substrate plasma deficient only in the factor being assayed. The PT (or APTT) is compared with the clotting times of serially diluted reference plasma with known factor activity mixed 1:1 with the substrate plasma (Fig. 18-23). These coagulation factors may also be measured by amidolytic (chromogenic) substrate assays which tend to be insensitive to pre-assay activation of the proteins.

The reference range for each of these factors is 50–150% of pooled normal plasma. Hereditary deficiency of each of these factors is uncommon (Table 18-8) thus acquired deficiency is most commonly encountered. Acquired deficiency, as with liver disease and vitamin K deficiency, most often affects multiple factors, but may affect only one factor in the case of a specific factor inhibitor (Table 18-15). Assay of both factor VII and factor V may be of use in differentiating liver disease from vitamin K deficiency; both factors are reduced in liver disease, but only factor VII is reduced in vitamin K deficiency. Although any of the vitamin K factors (II, VII, IX, X, protein C, protein S) can be used for this purpose, factor VII is useful because it has the shortest half-life, accurately reflecting the patient's current status. A more cost-effective technique of differentiating vitamin K deficiency from liver disease is a trial course of parenteral vitamin K. If the PT has not corrected within 24 hours, vitamin K deficiency is essentially ruled out.

Increased in vivo or in vitro activation of factor VII results in increased apparent activity by a one-stage factor assay. Increased cold activation of factor VII occurs commonly in plasma obtained during pregnancy or from women taking estrogen-containing oral contraceptives. Increased levels of factor VII have been seen in patients with atherosclerosis and are related to prognosis. The higher the level of factor VII activity, the higher the risk of cardiac mortality.[23]

Test: Factor Antigen Concentration[1-5]

The protein concentration of most coagulation factors can be determined by a variety of immunologic techniques, including Laurell rocket immunoelectrophoresis, ELISA, and RIA. These assays usually do not add to the clinical management of patients with factor deficiency. However, they have been useful in assessment of protein C and protein S levels in patients on oral anticoagulant therapy (see under Assessment of the Protein C System). Determination of antigenic levels of coagulation factor is helpful in identifying patients who have a functionally/structurally abnormal factor; such patients usually have a low ratio of activity to antigen concentration. Such variants are not uncommon among patients with a hereditary deficiency of a vitamin K dependent protein.

Test: Clottable Fibrinogen (Fibrinogen Activity)[1-5]

Background and Selection

Fibrinogen is necessary to support hemostatic plug formation. Hereditary disorders of fibrinogen production are relatively uncommon, but acquired disorders affecting fibrinogen are very common. Fibrinogen determination is very useful in evaluating patients with possible consumptive coagulopathies, major hemorrhage, major surgery (e.g., cardiopulmonary bypass), and liver disease and perhaps in patients with atherosclerotic vascular disease. Fibrinogen determination also is useful in monitoring patients receiving fibrinolytic therapy.

Logistics

Fibrinogen assays are performed on citrated platelet-poor plasma prepared as described for an APTT. The most common procedure uses a modification of the thrombin time. When present in very high concentrations, heparin and FDPs may interfere with the assay, particularly if the concentration of fibrinogen is low. Specimens may be stored below $-30\,°C$ for testing at an alternate time. If the patient is receiving fibrinolytic therapy, the specimen may have to be collected in a specialized tube containing fibrinolytic inhibitors, such as aprotinin, soybean trypsin inhibitor, or D-Phe-Pro-Arg-chloromethylketone (PPACK) to prevent in vitro digestion of fibrinogen by an activated fibrinolytic system.

A variety of other methods are also used clinically. These include measurement of the change in absorbance after addition of thrombin to plasma, precipitation and weighing of fibrinogen and formation of a fibrin clot, followed by determination of the protein content of the clot. The various assays give different results in both normal and abnormal samples.

Interpretation

Low fibrinogen values are seen in association with consumptive coagulopathies, major hemorrhage, dysfibrinogenemia, fibrinolytic therapy, and the uncommon hereditary disorders hypofibrinogenemia and afibrinogenemia. A level of 50–100 mg/dL (0.5–1.0 g/L), where the reference range is approximately 170–400 mg/dL (1.7–4.0 g/L) is usually sufficient to maintain hemostasis in the absence of additional hemostatic defects. A level below 50 mg/dL (0.5 g/L) in a patient receiving fibrinolytic therapy should probably cause a change in therapy, because such patients appear to be at increased risk of bleeding. Fibrinogen synthesis is well maintained in liver disease until the terminal stages are reached. A gradually declining fibrinogen in a patient with liver disease may indicate progression of the disease. Dysfibrinogenemia, with a discrepancy between clottable and antigenic fibrinogen concentration, is very common in liver disease and may cause a mild prolongation of the PT, APTT, and TT (Table 18-15). Cryoprecipitate is an excellent source of fibrinogen for replacement therapy.

Fibrinogen is an acute-phase reactant and increased levels are commonly seen during inflammatory reactions. Increased levels are also seen during pregnancy and in patients with atherosclerosis. The fibrinogen concentration correlates with risk of cardiac mortality, with higher levels associated with a higher risk.[23] Increased levels of fibrinogen may also be seen in patients with chronic or low-grade consumptive disorders; a common example is in association with metastatic tumor.

Test: Fibrinogen Antigen[1-5]

Several immunologic techniques are available for determination of the amount of fibrinogen antigen present. The assay is usually performed to confirm the presence of dysfibrinogenemia suggested by an unexplained abnormal thrombin time that does not correct with the addition of protamine (Fig. 18-19). The Reptilase time will also be prolonged in the presence of dysfibrinogenemia. A low (less than 0.75–0.80) ratio of clottable to antigenic fibrinogen is consistent with dysfibrinogenemia. The clinical significance of acquired dysfibrinogenemia is unsettled, but it does not appear to be associated with a significant bleeding tendency. By contrast, hereditary dysfibrinogenemia, may be associated with a significant bleeding diathesis, thrombosis, or no clinical symptoms at all.

Test: Factor XIII Screen[1-5]

Factor XIII is necessary for stabilization of fibrin thrombi (Fig. 18-11) but it is not measured with routine screening tests of hemostasis, such as the PT and APTT (Table 18-11). Only a small amount (2–5% of normal) of factor XIII is necessary to maintain adequate hemostasis. The presence of factor XIII is usually assessed by the stability of a clot in 5 M urea. Plasma is allowed to clot in vitro and is incubated for a period of time to permit factor XIIIa to stabilize the clot, which is then placed in the urea. If factor XIII is present in adequate amounts, the clot will not dissolve in the urea, but if factor XIII is absent, the clot will dissolve. Results are thus usually reported as factor XIII present or absent. Hereditary factor XIII deficiency is a rare, autosomal recessive disorder associated with a moderate to severe bleeding tendency. Acquired factor XIII deficiency caused by autoantibodies also occurs and is associated with significant bleeding. These patients are usually adults who present with the sudden onset of a bleeding diathesis without any abnormalities in the screening tests of hemostasis.

ACQUIRED INHIBITORS

Test: Agarose Gel Inhibitor Screening[1-5]

The assay is useful for confirming the presence of an inhibitor as a cause of a long PT or APTT (Fig. 18-19). To perform the assay, normal plasma is mixed with agarose as it is cooling and the mixture is poured on a glass plate. After the gel has solidified, a citrated platelet poor plasma specimen is placed in a well cut in the gel and allowed to diffuse into the agarose. The plate is then immersed in $CaCl_2$ and clot formation followed visually as opacification of the gel. In the presence of an inhibitor, there will be a clear zone around the application well (Fig. 18-24). The assay is usually reported as positive or negative for the presence of an inhibitor. Any inhibitor of coagulation, including lupus inhibitors, specific factor inhibitors, and heparin, may give a positive result. Non-neutralizing antibodies will not be detected by this method. This method may be useful in detecting weak inhibitors, which are not apparent with mixing studies.

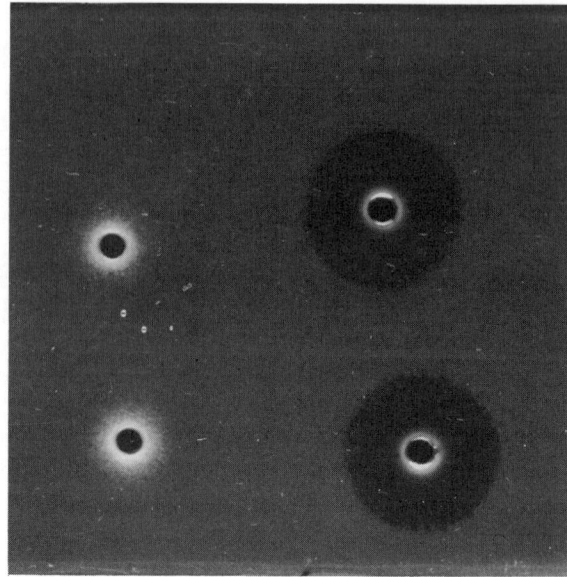

Fig. 18-24. The agarose inhibitor plate is a useful technique for documenting the presence of a circulating inhibitor. Normal plasma is added to agarose as it is cooling; the mixture is then poured onto a glass plate. After the agarose cools, wells are cut in the agarose and the sample added to the wells. The sample is allowed to diffuse into the surrounding agarose and the plate is then immersed in $CaCl_2$ to initiate coagulation. As clot forms, the agarose becomes opaque (left wells). If an inhibitor is present, there will be a clear zone around the sample wells (right wells).

Test: Bethesda Assay for Factor VIII Inhibitors (Quantitative Factor VIII Inhibitor Assay)[1-5,24]

Background and Selection

The Bethesda assay is used to titer the strength of anti-factor VIII antibodies. Although the assay was introduced in an attempt to standardize the titers of such antibodies, there is still significant interlaboratory variation in results from this assay.

Logistics

The Bethesda assay is performed on a platelet-poor plasma specimen obtained as for an APTT determination. The principle of the assay is to determine the amount of factor VIII in a normal plasma that is neutralized by a dilution of the patient's plasma. Because most factor VIII inhibitors require time to neutralize factor VIII, a 2-hour incubation is included. The factor VIII activity in a mixture of normal plasma and diluted patient plasma is compared with the activity in a mixture of normal plasma and buffer; the ratio of these two activities is designated the residual factor VIII activity. Results are then interpolated from a standard graph relating inhibitor activity to residual factor VIII activity and expressed in terms of Bethesda units. One Bethesda unit is the inhibitor activity capable of neutralizing 50% of the factor VIII activity in a normal plasma. The assay may be modified to quantitate the inhibitor activity of antibodies directed at other coagulation factors.

Interpretation

Two major types of factor VIII inhibitors have been recognized.[24] The first type is characteristically found in patients with hemophilia A, complicated by a factor VIII inhibitor; these inhibitors tend to show an anamnestic response to subsequent exposure to factor VIII, and high titers of antibody may be found. By contrast, the acquired factor VIII inhibitors found in other conditions often do not show an anamnestic response and tend to have a low titer of activity. Factor VIII inhibitor assays are used to diagnose the presence and follow the clinical course of these inhibitors. For example, a patient may be treated with intensive plasma exchange to decrease the titer of the antibody before a surgical procedure is performed. Determination of antibody titer can also be helpful in guiding selection of therapy; patients with high titer antibodies generally do not respond to infusions of factor VIII concentrate, even at very large doses.

Test: Tissue Thromboplastin Inhibition Assay (TTI)[1-5]

Background and Selection

The TTI is a modification of the PT and is commonly used in the evaluation of possible lupus anticoagulants suspected on the basis of a prolonged APTT that does not correct on mixing studies (Fig. 18-19).

Logistics

The TTI is performed using platelet-poor plasma obtained as described for APTT. Thromboplastin (PT reagent) is diluted and a modified PT performed; dilution of the thromboplastin makes the assay more dependent on the availability of phospholipid, which is in excess in the usual PT assay. Lupus anticoagulants are directed at phospholipid and can cause a relative prolongation of the clotting time when lower concentrations of phospholipid are used. Results are usually expressed as the ratio of the clotting time of the patient plasma to the clotting time of normal plasma for each dilution tested.

Interpretation

A ratio of 1.3 or more is generally regarded as a positive result. The TTI is positive with about 90% of lupus anticoagulant samples and can therefore be a useful assay for confirmation of the presence of this inhibitor. A number of other hemostatic defects can also give a positive TTI, including heparin, factor VIII inhibitors, factor V inhibitors, factor deficiencies, and oral anticoagulant therapy. Indeed, a significant percentage of healthy persons may also give a positive result. Thus, a positive TTI is not a very specific finding and must be interpreted in light of the results of other coagulation assays. A diagnosis of a lupus anticoagulant should never be made on the basis of an isolated positive TTI.

Test: Platelet Neutralization Procedure (PNP)[1-5]

Background and Selection

The PNP is used as a confirmatory test in the diagnosis of lupus anticoagulants suspected on the basis of a long APTT (Fig. 18-19).

Logistics

Lupus inhibitors interfere with phospholipid-dependent coagulation reactions by binding to the phospholipid in the test reagent. Somewhat paradoxically, they do not interfere with the ability of platelet phospholipid membranes to promote coagulation reactions either in vivo or in vitro. Thus, the addition of platelets to a coagulation system in the presence of a lupus anticoagulant can lead to shortening of the clotting time. The PNP is designed to work with the APTT, but it can also be modified to work with the dilute Russell viper venom time. The procedure is performed by mixing equal portions of freeze-thawed platelets and patient-platelet poor plasma (the platelet count should be less than $10,000/\mu L$ [$< 10 \times 10^9/L$]) or saline and patient plasma and repeating the APTT on the mixture. The assay is designed for performance on specimens with a long APTT that either do not correct with mixing studies or have positive agarose gels. The procedure should not be performed on specimens with APTT values within the reference range or when there is no evidence of an inhibitor present. The assay is reported as positive or negative.

Interpretation

Generally, a greater than 5-second shortening of the APTT with addition of platelets is regarded as a positive result. A positive PNP is seen in about 90% of lupus anticoagulant specimens. The assay is more specific than the TTI, but false positive results may be seen with heparin, factor V inhibitors, and perhaps oral anticoagulant therapy. In contrast with the TTI, the PNP is negative with factor VIII inhibitors.

Test: Dilute Russell Viper Venom Time (RVVT)[1-5]

Background and Selection

The RVVT is used to screen for and confirm the presence of lupus anticoagulants. The test may be ordered in patients suspected to have a lupus anticoagulant on the basis of clinical history (recurrent thrombosis or failed pregnancies) or other laboratory findings (prolonged APTT).

Logistics

The assay is performed on platelet poor plasma (the platelet count should be less than $10,000/\mu l$ [$<10 \times 10^9/L$]), prepared as for an APTT. Russell viper venom contains an enzyme that proteolytically activates factor X, bypassing the intrinsic and extrinsic pathways. The venom activated factor X then activates prothrombin in the presence of factor V and phospholipid. In the dilute RVVT, the amount of phospholipid is diluted to the point where the clotting time is very sensitive to changes in availability of phospholipid. Lupus anticoagulants bind to the phospholipid, blocking its participation in activation of prothrombin and causing a prolongation of the clotting time. The assay may be modified by using platelets instead of phospholipid to provide the surface for prothrombin activation. As lupus anticoagulants do not interfere with the procoagulant activity of platelet membranes, the dilute RVVT is significantly shorter with platelets if the initial cause of a prolonged time was a lupus anticoagulant.

Interpretation

The dilute RVVT is reported in seconds with the patient result compared with a reference range determined by the individual laboratory. Prolonged RVVTs may be further evaluated with mixing and platelet substitution studies; failure to correct the long RVVT after mixing normal and patient plasma and correction after substitution of platelets for phospholipid is evidence for a lupus anticoagulant. A false positive result may be seen with heparin; deficiency or inhibition of factor II, V, or X should give a long RVVT but no correction with platelets. Factor VIII inhibitor specimens have a dilute RVVT within the reference range.

MEASUREMENT OF HEPARIN

Test: Factor Xa Inhibition Assay[1-5,13]

Background and Selection

An occasional patient receiving therapeutic heparin may have a suboptimal response in terms of prolongation of the APTT. Determination of heparin concentration can be used to document that a therapeutic level of heparin has been achieved.

Logistics

Heparin accelerates the neutralization of factor Xa and thrombin by AT III. In the Xa inhibition assay, residual factor Xa activity is determined after incubation with AT III and patient plasma (as a source of heparin); the more heparin present, the less residual factor Xa activity. The Xa activity may be determined with either a clot endpoint technique or by use of an amidolytic (chromogenic) substrate specific for Xa. A platelet-poor plasma sample (less than $10,000/\mu L$ [$<10 \times 10^9/L$]) should be used, because platelets contain PF4, which is capable of neutralizing heparin in vitro. The ability of heparin to accelerate neutralization of Xa by AT III is dependent only on its ability to induce the appropriate conformational change in AT III. By contrast, the ability of heparin to accelerate the neutralization of thrombin by AT III is dependent on its ability to induce a conformational change in AT III as well as its ability to approximate the AT III to thrombin. This latter function requires a larger (higher molecular weight) heparin molecule. Thus, in contrast to thrombin-based heparin assays, the Xa assay is sensitive to both high and low molecular weight fractions of heparin.

Interpretation

The therapeutic range is considered to be 0.2 to 0.5 U/mL.[13] It is still unclear whether heparin concentration or APTT prolongation more accurately reflects effectiveness of therapy. However, risk of bleeding increases with total dose of heparin, and higher doses tend to be given to patients with a poor APTT response. Monitoring heparin concentrations may be more effective in preventing bleeding complications in such patients. The clearance of heparin is complex, and there are differences based on molecular weight. High molecular weight heparin fractions are cleared more rapidly than are low molecular weight fractions. This may lead to differences in the apparent heparin concentration determined by Xa and thrombin methods.

Test: Thrombin Inhibition[1-5,13]

The thrombin inhibition assay is analogous to the Xa inhibition assay, except that it depends on the ability of heparin to accelerate AT III neutralization of thrombin. Because this takes a larger heparin molecule than is required for Xa neutralization, this assay is relatively insensitive to low molecular weight fractions of heparin (see above). As with Xa assays, the residual thrombin activity can be determined with specific amidolytic (chromogenic) substrates or by a clot endpoint. The therapeutic range for heparin therapy is 0.2 to 0.5 U/mL. Discrepancies may be noted between results obtained with thrombin-based and Xa-based assays because of their different sensitivities to low molecular weight heparin.

INTRAVASCULAR COAGULATION

Test: Fibrin Degradation Products (FDP)[1-5,15]

Background and Selection

Activation of plasmin in vivo results in the breakdown of fibrinogen and fibrin clots. These proteolytic fragments are designated FDPs (Fig. 18-25). Assays for FDPs are used to assess the possibility of in vivo plasmin activation in a patient suspected of having disseminated intravascular coagulation (DIC). This assay also is used to judge whether a fibrinolytic response to streptokinase or urokinase has been achieved.

Logistics

Specialized tubes have been designed for collection of specimens for FDP determination and careful attention must be paid to the volume of blood placed in the tube or else spurious results may be obtained. The most commonly performed FDP assays use a latex agglutination technique, in which an antibody that recognizes FDPs is coated on the surface of the latex particles. The particles agglutinate in the presence of FDPs; the concentration of FDPs is determined by the dilution of serum that sustains agglutination. Because the antibodies used in this assay cross-react with fibrinogen, fibrinogen must be completely removed from the patient specimen. This is accomplished by clotting the blood specimen with thrombin or a snake venom in the presence of a plasmin inhibitor (to prevent in vitro generation of split products). These reagents are present in the special collection tubes.

Interpretation

A positive result is generally regarded as agglutination of the latex particles by at least a 1:5 dilution of patient serum. The presence of FDPs indicates in vivo fibrinolytic activity; positive results are typically seen in acute DIC and during fibrinolytic therapy, but they may also be seen in other conditions, particularly liver disease, after recent surgery, or after recent thrombosis (Table 18-14). Chronic DIC is often characterized by mild to moderately elevated FDPs, increased fibrinogen levels, and a thrombotic tendency. An increase in FDPs may also be seen in patients with TTP or HUS. False positive results may be seen any time that fibrinogen is not completely removed from the sample; common causes of this are heparin, dysfibrinogenemia, and specimen collection problems (too little or too much blood in the collection tube). A titer greater than 1:160 is uncommon unless the patient is receiving fibrinolytic therapy or there is a spurious result. The FDP assay does not distinguish between fibrinogenolysis and fibrinolysis (Fig. 18-25).

Test: D-Dimer[1-5,15]

The D-dimer assay is similar to the FDP assay, except that the antibody used to detect the breakdown products is specific for covalently crosslinked fragments derived from fibrin (Fig. 18-25); there is no cross-reactivity with fibrinogen. Thus, this assay can be performed on a plasma specimen obtained for other coagulation tests without removal of fibrinogen; no specialized collection tubes are required, and dysfibrinogenemia does not interfere. A positive D-dimer result is indicative of in vivo fibrinolytic activity. Positive results are seen in DIC and other conditions associated with activation of the fibrinolytic system (e.g., fibrinolytic therapy, postoperative, acute thrombosis, pre-eclampsia). A positive D-dimer assay does not distinguish between lysis of pathologic and physiologic thrombi, but it does distinguish between fibrinogenolysis and fibrinolysis (Fig. 18-25).

Test: Euglobulin Lysis Time[1-5,15]

The euglobulin lysis assay is a screening assay for increased fibrinolytic activity. Plasminogen and its activators are separated from their natural inhibitors by acid precipitation. The ability of this precipitate to lyse a clot in vitro is then recorded. Increased in vivo fibrinolytic activity results in a shortened euglobulin lysis time. This is a relatively crude technique that is difficult to standardize and quite time consuming for the laboratory. Consequently, it is used infrequently.

Test: Protamine Sulfate and Ethanol Gelation[1-5]

The protamine sulfate and ethanol gelation assays are used to demonstrate in vivo generation of thrombin particularly in cases of possible acute DIC. Thrombin removes fibrinopeptides A and B from fibrinogen to form fibrin monomers (Fig. 18-11). If the concentration of fibrin monomers is too low for spontaneous gelation, they may associate with fibrinogen or large FDPs and circulate in blood. These monomers can be precipitated out by either ethanol or protamine sulfate. The assay is reported as either positive or negative. A positive result indicates in vivo fibrin monomer formation. The assay is neither 100% specific or sensitive for DIC; results of this assay must be interpreted with other findings, such as PT, APTT, fibrinogen, platelets, and FDPs.

ASSESSMENT OF THE SERPIN FAMILY

Test: Antithrombin III Activity[1-5,12]

Background and Selection

Antithrombin III is the major regulator of thrombin and factor Xa in vivo (Fig. 18-12). Hereditary deficiency of AT III is associated with a thrombotic tendency; thus, AT III frequently is measured to evaluate a patient for a possible hereditary thrombotic tendency (Table 18-12). Functional assays are always preferred when screening for thrombophilia, because variant AT III molecules have been described. Variant AT III molecules are characterized by production of normal or near-normal quantities of protein, but the protein does not function normally. An assay that measures protein

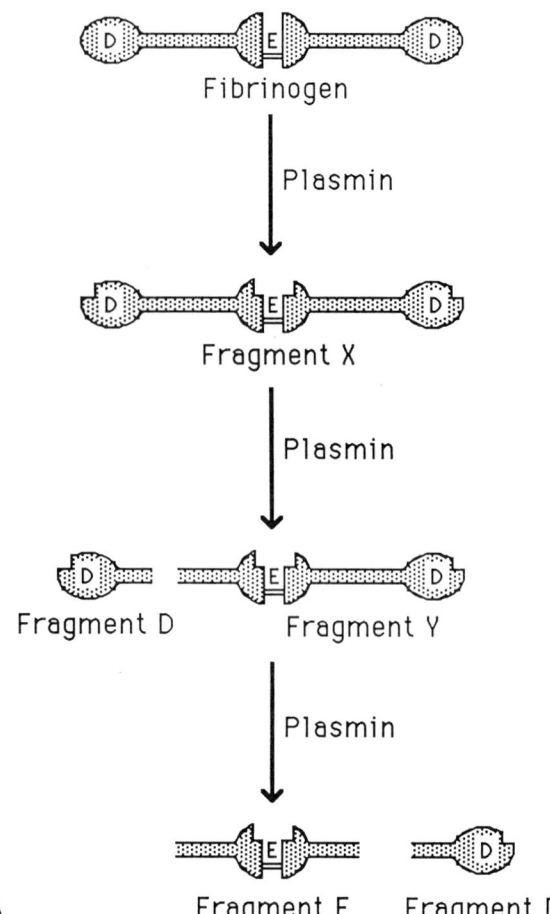

Fig. 18-25. (A) Plasmin degrades fibrinogen and fibrin in a predictable pattern. Plasmin cleavage of fibrinogen (fibrinogenolysis) is shown. Initially a large COOH-terminal portion of the Aα-chain and an NH$_2$-terminal peptide of the Bβ-chain (Bβ 1-42) are removed. This derivative is called fragment X and is still slowly clottable. This is followed by cleavage of the long helical connecting segment between the terminal D domain and the central E domain, giving rise to a large fragment designated fragment Y, and a D fragment. A reciprocal cleavage then frees another D domain and the central E domain. (*Figure continues*).

concentration rather than protein function could miss such a variant. Additionally, AT III is depleted in consumptive coagulopathies and is sometimes measured to evaluate the possibility of DIC or pre-eclampsia.

Logistics

Although AT III activity can be measured in citrated plasma or serum, plasma assays are always preferred, because there is a variable and uncontrolled loss of AT III in the conversion of blood to serum. Most assays measure neutralization of thrombin or factor Xa in the presence of added heparin. Activity is expressed in

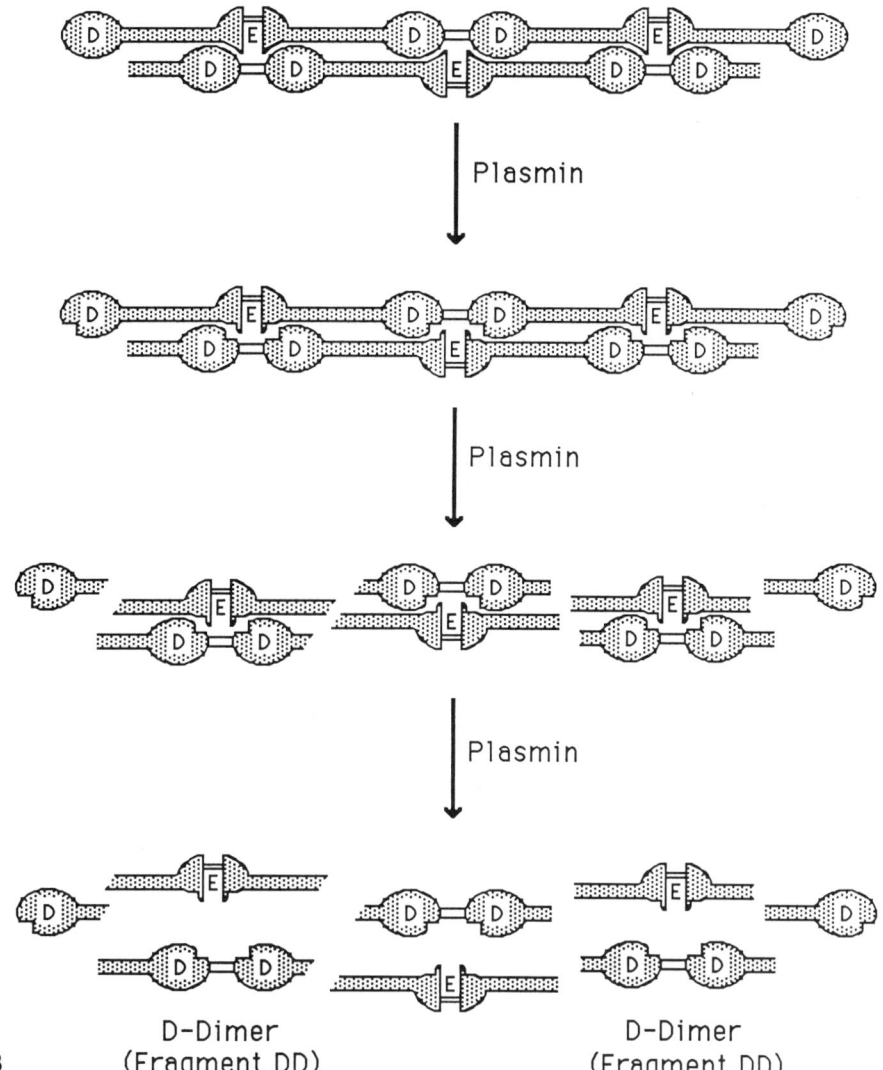

Fig. 18-25 *(Continued).* **(B)** The cleavage of crosslinked fibrin (fibrinolysis) proceeds along similar lines except that the terminal products are E domains and the crosslinked adjacent D domains known as D-D-dimers. Antibodies are available that specifically recognize the D-D-dimer; such antibodies are useful for recognizing true fibrinolysis. Note that if thrombin has converted fibrinogen to fibrin, the initial step will release a different peptide designated Bβ 15-42. This latter peptide may be measured by radioimmunoassay.

terms of percentage activity, with pooled normal plasma assigned an activity of 100%. Heparin and oral anticoagulants do not interfere with the measurement of plasma AT III.

Interpretation

Because the reference range varies from technique to technique, data must be interpreted in terms of the reference range established by the laboratory performing the assay. Hereditary AT III deficiency is an autosomal dominant disorder with symptomatic expression in heterozygotes; the AT III activity in affected persons is usually 40–70% of normal.[12] Involvement of other family members should be documented and other potential acquired causes of AT III deficiency eliminated before a diagnosis of hereditary deficiency is established. Acquired deficiency of AT III occurs in liver disease, during heparin therapy, in consumptive coagulopathies (e.g., DIC, pre-eclampsia), in the nephrotic syndrome (where it may contribute to thrombosis), during major thrombotic episodes, and in association with drugs (e.g., asparaginase). Although AT III is frequently decreased during heparin therapy, it is rarely decreased to the level that would interfere with an effective anticoagulant response; this does not usually occur until AT III is around 25 to 30% of normal. Patients with hereditary deficiency of AT III and acute thrombosis usually have sufficient AT III to respond adequately to heparin therapy. In contrast to fibrinogen and factor VIII, the level of AT III decreases relatively early during the course of parenchymal liver disease. In contrast to acute DIC, levels of AT III are usually within the reference range in TTP and HUS.

Test: Antithrombin III Antigen[1-5,12]

Antithrombin III protein concentration can be measured by a variety of immunologic techniques. Variant AT III deficiency, characterized by an abnormal relationship between activity and antigen concentration has been described. An immunologic assay can be used to evaluate the possibility of such a variant. This assay should not be used as a screening assay for hereditary AT III deficiency, because such variants are not detected.

Test: Heparin Cofactor II (HC II)[1-5]

Heparin cofactor II is a serine protease inhibitor (SERPIN) that is capable of neutralizing thrombin but not factor Xa. The activity of HC II is accelerated by heparin and dermatan sulfate. Decreased levels of HC II are seen in consumptive coagulopathies and liver disease. Hereditary deficiency of HC II may be associated with a thrombotic tendency (Table 18-12). Measurement of HC II does not currently add to the evaluation of other clinical disorders.

ASSESSMENT OF THE PROTEIN C SYSTEM

Test: Protein C Activity[1-5,12]

Background and Selection

Protein C is the major regulator of the key cofactors of the coagulation cascade, factors Va and VIIIa (Figs. 18-13 and 18-14). Hereditary deficiency of protein C is associated with a thrombotic tendency. Protein C is usually measured as a part of an evaluation of a possible thrombotic tendency (Table 18-12).

Logistics

Assays for protein C activity are performed on platelet-poor plasma that may be stored below −30°C. There are no functional assays available to clinical laboratories that totally reflect the function of protein C. A snake venom that activates protein C in vitro can be used to estimate protein C activity. The endpoint of the assay can be measured in terms of either clotting time (effect on factors V and VIII) or protein C cleavage of an amidolytic (chromogenic) substrate. The former type of assay more closely corresponds to in vivo function and variants (abnormal forms of protein C) with normal amidolytic activity, but deficient neutralization of factors V and VIII has been described. Oral anticoagulants result in a marked decrease in protein C activity and limit the ability to establish the diagnosis of hereditary deficiency by functional assays while patients are on anticoagulant therapy. Heparin and lupus anticoagulants interfere with the clot endpoint venom assay; they do not affect most other functional assays.

Interpretation

The reference range depends on the method used by the laboratory performing the assay. Two major hereditary forms of protein C deficiency have been described.[12] The autosomal recessive disorder is rare and usually presents as neonatal purpura fulminans with undetectable protein C. The parents are heterozygotes and, in contrast to the autosomal dominant form of the disease, tend to be asymptomatic. Autosomal dominant protein C deficiency presents as recurrent thrombosis in adolescence or young adulthood; affected persons are heterozygotes with 40–60% of normal protein C activity. Decreased levels of protein C are also seen in liver disease, oral anticoagulant therapy, vitamin K deficiency, and consumptive coagulopathies. In contrast to AT III, protein C is usually elevated or within the reference range in the nephrotic syndrome. As with AT III deficiency, acquired causes of deficiency should be ruled out and familial transmission documented before a diagnosis of hereditary protein C deficiency is established. Increased levels of protein C have been found in patients with the nephrotic syndrome.

Test: Protein C Antigen[1-5,12]

Because of the technical problems with functional protein C assays, antigenic protein C assays are still commonly used to screen for protein C deficiency. Protein C concentration may be determined by a number of immunologic techniques. The most commonly used methods are Laurell rocket immunoelectrophoresis assay and ELISA. The results are expressed as either a percentage of pooled normal plasma or concentration (e.g., μg/mL or mg/L) of protein. The reference range varies between laboratories and should be reported with the results obtained by the individual laboratory. Interpretation of results is analogous to protein C functional assays (see above); however, abnormal or dysfunctional protein C molecules will not be detected by antigenic assays. Protein C antigen determinations can also be used to assess possible protein C deficiency in patients on stable oral anticoagulant therapy. This is accomplished by simultaneous measurement of several vitamin K dependent proteins. In patients on oral anticoagulants, there is a concordant decrease in the level of the various vitamin K dependent factors and thus the ratio of protein C to factor II or X would be normal (~1.0). If the patient is congenitally deficient in protein C, the ratio of protein C to other vitamin K dependent proteins is abnormally low (~0.5), even on anticoagulant therapy. It should be remembered, however, that this technique does not detect patients with dysfunctional protein C molecules.

Test: Protein S Antigen[1-5, 12]

Background and Selection

Protein S is an essential cofactor for protein C (Fig. 18-14). Hereditary deficiency of protein S is associated with a thrombotic tendency; therefore, it is most frequently measured as part of an evaluation for a possible hereditary predisposition to thrombosis (Table 18-12).

Logistics

Because good functional assays for protein S are currently not available, measurement is usually done by an immunologic technique on citrated platelet-poor plasma, prepared as for a PT. The most common methods are Laurell rocket immunoelectrophoresis assay and ELISA. Interpretation of reduced levels of protein S is complicated because there appear to be at least two "pools" of protein S in plasma.[12] Some protein S circulates in a complex with C4b binding protein (C4b-BP); this fraction appears to be inactive. Other protein S circulates free and is fully active. The level of total protein S may vary as a result of changes in either the level of C4b-BP or free protein S. As C4b-BP decreases, total protein S may decrease with no change in free protein S; conversely, if C4b-BP increases, total protein S may increase without a change in free (functional) protein S. Such changes in C4b-BP can mask a significant change in free protein S, making a diagnosis of hereditary deficiency of protein S difficult on the basis of total protein S concentration.

Interpretation

The results are reported as a percentage of pooled normal plasma or protein concentration (e.g., $\mu g/mL$ or $mmol/L$). A laboratory is likely to report both free and total protein S; a decrease in both would be consistent with hereditary deficiency. Reduced levels of protein S can be seen in liver disease, consumptive coagulopathies, oral anticoagulant therapy, vitamin K deficiency, and a variety of other conditions that affect C4b-BP. Increased levels of total protein S may be seen when C4b-BP is increased. When a patient is on stable oral anticoagulant therapy, a presumptive diagnosis of protein S deficiency may be made by comparing the level of protein S with that of other vitamin K dependent proteins. In patients on oral anticoagulants, there is a concordant decrease in the level of the various vitamin K dependent factors, and thus the ratio of protein S to factor II or X would be normal (~1.0). If the patient is congenitally deficient in protein S, the ratio of protein S to other vitamin K dependent proteins is abnormally low (~0.5), even on anticoagulant therapy. Protein S antigen assays do not detect patients with abnormal, dysfunctional forms of protein S.

ASSESSMENT OF THE FIBRINOLYTIC SYSTEM

Test: Plasminogen Activity[1-5,15]

Background and Selection

Plasmin is the effector enzyme of the fibrinolytic system (Figs. 18-15, 18-16, and 18-25). Hereditary deficiency of plasminogen, the precursor of plasmin, is associated with a thrombotic tendency, but the incidence appears to be much lower than either AT III, protein C, or protein S deficiency. Plasminogen activity is often determined as part of an evaluation of a possible thrombotic tendency (Table 18-12) or to assess the effects of fibrinolytic therapy on the fibrinolytic system.

Logistics

Platelet-poor plasma, prepared as for an APTT, is used for the plasminogen assay; it may be stored frozen below $-30°C$ before assay. If the patient has received fibrinolytic therapy (streptokinase, urokinase or tPA), a fibrinolytic inhibitor should be added to the anticoagulant to prevent further in vitro activation and neutralization of plasmin (see Test: Clottable Fibrinogen). The most common clinical assay is based on the ability of plasmin to cleave an amidolytic (chromogenic) substrate after the specimen plasminogen has been completely activated to plasmin by streptokinase or tPA. Heparin and oral anticoagulant therapy do not interfere with measurement of plasminogen.

Interpretation

Results are expressed in terms of percentage activity, with 100% being the activity of pooled normal plasma. The reference range depends on the assay methodology and should be reported with the result. Hereditary disorders of plasminogen are characterized by a reduction of plasminogen activity to the 40–60% range of normal. Fibrinolytic therapy with systemic activators of plasminogen such as urokinase and streptokinase typically results in a marked decrease in plasminogen levels. However, there is little relationship between effectiveness of fibrinolytic therapy and degree of plasminogen consumption. Reduced levels of plasminogen are also seen in liver disease (Table 18-15) and consumptive coagulopathies (e.g., DIC) (Fig. 18-21).

Test: α_2-Antiplasmin (α_2AP)[1-5,15]

α_2-Antiplasmin is the key regulator of plasmin in vivo (Fig. 18-16). Hereditary deficiency of α_2AP is associated with a mild to moderate bleeding tendency and is an example of a hereditary bleeding disorder that presents with normal screening assays (Table 18-11). The test is usually performed in a reference laboratory. Both functional and immunologic assays for α_2AP are available, and the results are usually reported in terms of percentage of normal. Decreased levels of α_2AP also are seen during fibrinolytic therapy, liver disease, and consumptive coagulopathies, which must be distinguished from a hereditary problem.

Test: Tissue Plasminogen Activator[1-5,15]

Tissue plasminogen activator is the major physiologic activator of plasminogen in vivo (Fig. 18-15). It differs from most of the other coagulation proteins in that it is not an endogenous plasma protein; rather, it is secreted by endothelial cells in response to stimuli such as vasoocclusion and thrombin. Decreased tPA release, apparently on a hereditary basis, has been associated with a thrombotic tendency but measurement of tPA by clinical laboratories is difficult. Both immunologic and functional assays for tPA have been described. Immunologic assays for tPA measure both free (active) and complexed (inactive) tPA; free tPA appears to be the most critical. Normal, unstimulated tPA levels are at the level of detection of most assay systems making it difficult to measure a decrease in basal tPA. Stimulation of tPA release is difficult to standardize and is also affected by previous vascular disease, including previous venous thrombosis. For these reasons, measurement of tPA is not commonly performed in the clinical setting, although useful information is being gained in the research setting.

Test: Plasminogen Activator Inhibitor-1 (PAI-1)[1-5,15]

Plasminogen activator inhibitor-1 is a SERPIN released from endothelial cells that neutralizes tPA and urokinase. Resting levels are quite low, but increased levels have been reported in a variety of conditions including post myocardial infarction. It has been suggested that increased PAI-1 levels may decrease the effectiveness of tPA as a fibrinolytic agent. The role of PAI-1 measurement in clinical medicine is still not established. It is usually measured by an immunologic method.

Test: Plasmin-α_2-Antiplasmin Complex (P-AP)[1-5,15]

After plasmin has been neutralized by its inhibitor, the inactive plasmin-α_2-antiplasmin complex (P-AP) circulates in peripheral blood until it is cleared by the liver (Fig. 18-16). Increased levels of P-AP thus indicate increased in vivo fibrinolytic activity. The assay is used primarily for research purposes; it currently adds little clinical information of value.

Test: Bβ 1-42 and Bβ 15-42[1-5,15]

Plasmin digests the β-chain of fibrinogen and fibrin, releasing a portion of the NH$_2$-terminal portion of this chain. The Bβ 1-42 peptide is derived from fibrinogen, whereas the Bβ 15-42 peptide is derived from fibrin (fibrinopeptide B, released by thrombin, consists of Bβ 1-14). Radioimmunoassays (RIAs) for these two peptides have been developed and can be used to differentiate between fibrinolysis and fibrinogenolysis. The assays are generally used for research purposes, as they add little relevant clinical information.

IN VIVO THROMBIN ACTIVATION

Test: Thrombin-Antithrombin III Complex (T-AT)[1-5,8]

The inactive complex formed by AT III neutralization of thrombin (Fig. 18-12) circulates in the blood for a short time before it is removed by the liver. It may be measured by sensitive immunologic assays; an increased level of T-AT is indicative of increased thrombin activation in vivo (Fig. 18-20). This can be seen in patients with hereditary disorders of the regulatory system, consumptive coagulopathies, and active thrombosis (Tables 18-12 and 18-13). This assay is currently used primarily for research purposes.

Test: Prothrombin Fragment 1 + 2 (F_{1+2}; Fragment 1 + 2 Assay)[1-5,8]

Activation of prothrombin by factor Xa is associated with release of a large peptide from the NH_2-terminal end of prothrombin; this peptide is designated F_{1+2} (Fig. 18-20). The plasma level of this peptide can be measured by immunologic techniques. Careful specimen handling and processing are required to prevent artifacts because of in vitro activation of thrombin. Increased levels of F_{1+2} are seen in patients with hereditary disorders of the regulatory system (Table 18-12) even during periods not associated with active thrombosis and in other disorders characterized by increased activity of the coagulation system (Table 18-13). Of clinical interest, the level of F_{1+2} decreases during effective anticoagulant therapy.[8] Although still a research assay, in the future this method may prove useful for documenting the effectiveness of anticoagulant therapy.

Test: Fibrinopeptide A[1-5,8]

Thrombin conversion of fibrinogen to fibrin is associated with the release of two peptides from the NH_2-terminal portion of each side of the dimer; these peptides are designated fibrinopeptides A and B (Fig. 18-10). Fibrinopeptide A may be measured by a sensitive RIA; increased levels are associated with any active thrombosis. This assay can document an increased activity of thrombin on one of its principal substrates. Careful specimen handling and processing are required to prevent artifacts due to in vitro activation of thrombin. Currently it is used primarily for research purposes.

Test: Activation Peptide of Protein C[1-5,8]

Thrombin activation of protein C is associated with release of a peptide from the NH_2-terminal portion of the heavy chain of protein C (Fig. 18-13). This peptide can be measured by sensitive immunologic assays. The plasma level reflects ongoing thrombin interaction with protein C, one of its critical substrates. Increased levels are found in patients with active thrombosis and in those with a thrombotic tendency (Tables 18-12 and 18-13). It is used primarily for research purposes.

REFERENCES

1. Bloom AL, Thomas DP (eds): Haemostasis and Thrombosis. 2nd Ed. London, Churchill Livingstone, 1987.
2. Bowie EJW, Sharp AA (eds): Hemostasis and Thrombosis. London, Butterworths, 1985.
3. Colman RW, Hirsh J, Marder VJ, Salzman EW (eds): Hemostasis and Thrombosis: Basic Principles and Clinical Practice. 2nd Ed. Philadelphia, JB Lippincott, 1987.
4. Sirridge MS, Shannon R: Laboratory Evaluation of Hemostasis and Thrombosis. 3rd Ed. Philadelphia, Lea & Febiger, 1983.
5. Triplett DA (ed): Laboratory Evaluation of Coagulation. Chicago, American Society of Clinical Pathologists, 1982.
6. Hawiger J: Formation and regulation of platelet and fibrin hemostatic plug. Hum Pathol 1987;18:111.
7. Furie B, Furie BC: The molecular basis of blood coagulation. Cell 1988;53:505.
8. Bauer KA, Rosenberg RD: The pathophysiology of the prethrombotic state in humans: insights gained from studies using markers of hemostatic system activation. Blood 1987;70:343.
9. Moncada S, Radomski MW, Palmer RMJ: Endothelium-derived relaxing factor. Biochem Pharmacol 1988;37:2495.
10. Rapaport SI: Inhibition of factor VIIa/tissue factor-induced blood coagulation: with particular emphasis upon a factor Xa-dependent inhibitory mechanism. Blood 1989;73:359.
11. White JG: Inherited abnormalities of the platelet membrane and secretory granules. Hum Pathol 1987;18:123.
12. Rosenberg RD, Bauer KA: Thrombosis in inherited deficiencies of antithrombin, protein C and protein S. Hum Pathol 1987;18:253.
13. Raskob GE, Carter CJ, Hull RD: Anticoagulant therapy for venous thromboembolism. p. 1. In Coller BS (ed): Progress in Hemostasis and Thrombosis. Vol. 9. Philadelphia, WB Saunders, 1989.
14. Dalen JE, Hirsh J: American College of Chest Physicians and the National Heart, Lung, and Blood Institute National Conference on Antithrombotic Therapy. Arch Intern Med 1986;146:462.
15. Verstraete M, Collen D: Thrombolytic therapy in the eighties. Blood 1986;67:1529.
16. National Committee for Clinical Laboratory Standards: Collection, Transport and Preparation of Blood Specimens for Coagulation Testing and Performance of Coagulation Assays. Approved Guideline. NCCLS document H21-A. Villanova, PA, NCCLS, 1986.
17. Stuart MJ, Miller ML, Davey FR, Wolk JA: The post-aspirin bleeding time: a screening test for evaluating haemostatic disorders. Br J Haematol 1979;43:649.
18. Gill JC, Endres-Brooks J, Bauer PJ et al: The effect of ABO blood group on the diagnosis of von Willebrand disease. Blood 1987;69:1691.
19. Ruggeri ZM, Zimmerman TS: von Willebrand factor and von Willebrand disease. Blood 1987;70:895.

20. Kelton JG, Sheridan D, Santos A et al: Heparin-induced thrombocytopenia: laboratory studies. Blood 1988; 72:925.
21. Steinberg MH, Kelton JG, Coller BS: Plasma glycocalicin: an aid in the classification of thrombocytopenic disorders. N Engl J Med 1987;317:1037.
22. National Committee for Clinical Laboratory Standards: Determination of Factor VIII Coagulant Activity (VIII:C). NCCLS document H-34. Villanova, PA, NCCLS, 1986.
23. Meade TW: Thrombosis and ischemic heart disease. Br Heart J 1985;53:473.
24. Hoyer LW: Molecular pathology and immunology of factor VIII (hemophilia A and factor VIII inhibitors). Hum Pathol 1987;18:153.

19 White Blood Cell and Platelet Disorders

P. Joanne Cornbleet
Robert Astarita
Paul L. Wolf

INTRODUCTION

White blood cell (WBC) and platelet disorders include nonmalignant and malignant abnormalities of granulocytes (neutrophils, eosinophils, basophils), monocytes, lymphocytes, and megakaryocytes/platelets. Nonmalignant abnormalities consist of reactive quantitative changes, benign morphologic alterations, and functional disorders. The origin, production, distribution, and function of WBCs and platelets is thoroughly discussed in Chapter 16. The diagnosis of these disorders is often made on the basis of morphology, which is also presented in Chapter 16.

White blood cells are produced in the bone marrow and migrate through the blood to the tissues, where they perform their functions. Although granulocytes survive only a short time in the blood and tissues, monocytes and lymphocytes may persist for days to years. The monocytes differentiate in tissues to macrophages, which may be "wandering," scattered throughout the tissues and body cavities, or "fixed," lining the sinuses of the liver, spleen, lymph nodes, and bone marrow, and the alveoli of the lung. Lymphocytes are present in large numbers in peripheral lymphoid tissue, including lymph nodes, spleen, tonsillar tissue, and submucosal accumulations in the gastrointestinal, respiratory, and urinary tracts. Thus, reactive or malignant disorders of monocytes and lymphocytes may involve not only the blood and bone marrow, but any tissue in which these cells reside, particularly lymph nodes and spleen.

Platelets are formed in the bone marrow from the cytoplasm of megakaryocytes. They circulate for 8–10 days and are removed by splenic macrophages. About one-third of the circulating platelets are normally present in the red pulp of the spleen; with marked hypersplenism, up to 85% of platelets may be sequestered.[1]

White blood cells have an important role in host defense against infection. Neutrophils are required for phagocytic killing of microorganisms and participate in the tissue inflammatory response. Eosinophils and basophils may interact to combat tissue invasion by parasites too large to be ingested by phagocytic cells.[1] Monocytes appear to have a role both in phagocytic killing of some types of microorganisms and in the immune response.[1] Lymphocytes are required for humoral (B lymphocytes) and cellular (T lymphocytes) immune response to foreign antigens. Platelets play a vital role in hemostasis by forming a mechanical plug at the site of vascular injury.

A significant decrease in either the number or functional ability of neutrophils or lymphocytes is associated with severe recurrent infections. Bacterial infections are primarily seen in neutrophil or B-lymphocyte deficiency, whereas a deficiency in T lymphocytes results in viral, fungal, mycobacterial, and protozoal infections. In addition, patients who are deficient in T lymphocytes may have a high incidence of secondary malignancies and autoimmune disorders. Decreased or dysfunctional platelets results in a bleeding tendency. Only a brief overview of the many disorders of WBCs and platelets is given in this chapter. The reader is referred to current hematology textbooks for a more thorough discussion of these disease entities.[1-4]

Quantitative and Morphologic Abnormalities of White Blood Cells and Platelets

Changes in the number of WBCs and platelets in the peripheral blood accompany a wide variety of infectious, inflammatory, neoplastic, and metabolic diseases. Although these quantitative changes do not provide a definitive diagnosis, they may serve as a guide to a list of associated disorders, as enumerated in Tables 19-1 to 19-11. Likewise, alteration in WBC morphology can occur as a reaction to many systemic disorders. For example, toxic granulation and Döhle bodies can be found in neutrophils with infections, burns, trauma, pregnancy, and cancer and after administration of

Table 19-1. Causes of Neutrophilia

Physiologic neutrophilia
    Neonates (1–2 days), pregnancy (third trimester), labor, emotional stress, moderate to severe exercise, excessive cold or heat, epinephrine release or injection, convulsions, nausea and vomiting
Infection
    Bacterial, fungal, viral (first few days), spirochetal, rickettsial, endotoxin
Inflammation or tissue necrosis
    Myocardial infarction, neoplastic necrosis, trauma, surgery, anoxia, thrombosis or infarction, chemical or electrical injury, burns, collagen vascular disorders, drug hypersensitivity reaction, gout, dermatitis, thyroiditis
Metabolic disturbances
    Diabetic acidosis, uremia, eclampsia
Drugs
    Chlorpropamide, clioquinol, corticosteroids, digitalis, epinephrine, etiocholanolone, heparin, histamine, lithium, may toxins, vaccines
Hematologic disorders
    Acute hemorrhage, hemolysis, myeloproliferative disorders
Hereditary
    Chronic idiopathic neutrophilia, cyclic neutrophilia, familial neutrophilia

(Data from Kjeldsberg[4] and Wintrobe.[65])

Table 19-2. Causes of Lymphocytosis

Physiologic
    From first week of life to fourth or fifth year of childhood
Infections
    Infectious lymphocytosis, Epstein-Barr virus, cytomegalovirus, viral exanthems, hepatitis, many other viral infections, pertussis, brucellosis, typhoid-paratyphoid, *Mycoplasma*, toxoplasmosis, rickettsial, syphilis
Drug sensitivity
    Diphenylhydantoin, p-aminosalicylic acid, sulfonamides, phenothaizines
Toxins
    Lead, arsenicals, TNT, tetrachlorethane
Autoimmune disorders
Endocrine disorders
    Thyrotoxicosis, adrenal insufficiency
Dermatitis
Graft rejection
Hematopoietic malignancies
    Acute lymphocytic leukemia, chronic lymphocytic leukemia, prolymphocytic leukemia, large granular lymphocytic leukemia, adult T-cell leukemia/lymphoma, leukemia phase of lymphoma, hairy cell leukemia (rarely), Sézary cell syndrome (rarely), Hodgkin's disease, immunoblastic lymphadenopathy

(Data from Kjeldsberg,[4] Koepke,[18] and Wood and Frankel.[26])

Table 19-3. Causes of Monocytosis

Normal newborn (first 2 weeks)
Infections
    Subacute bacterial endocarditis, tuberculosis, brucellosis, *Salmonella*, leprosy syphilis, rickettsial, many protozoan
Recovery from acute infection
Recovery from neutrophil suppression
Many nonhematopoietic malignancies
Hematologic malignancies
    Chronic myeloproliferative disorders, myelodysplastic syndromes, monocytoid forms of AML, Hodgkin's disease, lymphoma, malignant histiocytosis
Collagen vascular disorders
    Especially SLE and rheumatoid arthritis
Granulomatous disease
    Especially sarcoidosis
Gastrointestinal disease
    Especially ulcerative colitis, regional enteritis
Radiation therapy
Chronic high dose corticosteroids
Lipid storage disorders
    Gaucher's, Niemann-Pick

Abbreviations: AML, acute myelocytic leukemia; SLE, systemic lupus erythematosus.
(Data from references 4, 18, 24, and 65.)

Table 19-4. Causes of Eosinophilia
Neonates
Allergic reactions
Asthma, atopic dermatitis, allergic rhinitis, sensitization to foreign proteins, drug hypersensitivity reaction, graft rejection, graft-versus-host disease
Skin diseases
Especially pemphigus, pemphigoid, dermatitis herpetiformis
Infections
Metazoan (particularly with tissue invasion), *Pneumocystis carinii*, fungal (bronchopulmonary aspergillosis, coccidioidomycosis, mucocutaneous candidiasis), scabies, occasionally in bacterial and viral infections (although eosinopenia is produced acutely)
Collagen vascular diseases
Especially rheumatoid arthritis, periarteritis nodosa
Neoplasms
Particularly with metastasis, in mucin-secreting epithelial malignancies, with involvement of serous surfaces or bone, with necrosis, or postirradiation therapy
Hematologic malignancies
Myeloproliferative disorders, eosinophilic leukemia, lymphoma, Hodgkin's disease, systemic mastocytosis
Other hematologic disorders
Pernicious anemia, acute hemolysis or hemorrhage, postsplenectomy (first few months), acquired or cyclic neutropenia, returning bone marrow function
Idiopathic pulmonary eosinophilic syndromes
Tropical eosinophilia (hypersensitivity to filaria degenerating in lungs), Löffler syndrome (migratory pulmonary infiltrates), pulmonary infiltration with eosinophila (pulmonary infiltrates with high fever), hypereosinophilic syndrome (with widespread tissue infiltration)

(Data from Koepke[18] and Wintrobe.[65])

Table 19-5. Causes of Basophilia
Hematologic malignancies
Chronic myeloproliferative disorders, myelodysplastic syndromes, mastocytosis, basophilic leukemia, Hodgkin's disease
Allergic or hypersensitivity reactions
Hypothyroidism, antithyroid drugs
Radiation therapy
Postsplenectomy
Chickenpox, smallpox
Ulcerative colitis

(Data from Kjeldsberg[4] and Koepke.[18])

Table 19-6. Causes of Neutropenia
Agents that suppress the bone marrow in all patients
Radiation, chemotherapeutic agents, azidothymidine (AZT), benzene, arsenicals, alcohol
Agents that suppress marrow or induce neutrophil antibodies in sensitive patients
Many antibiotics (particularly semisynthetic penicillins), sulfonamide-type drugs (bactericidals, diuretics, diabetic agents), analgesics, antithyroid drugs, anticonvulsants, antihistamines, tranquilizers
Infections
Typhoid, paratyphoid, many viral (including AIDS), rickettsial, many protozoal, transiently in many acute infections
Overwhelming infection
Especially in elderly or patients with limited marrow reserve
Bone marrow replacement
Hematologic malignancies, nonhematologic malignancies, fibrosis, necrosis, storage diseases
Hematologic disorders with suppressed or ineffective marrow production
Aplastic anemia, pernicious anemia, folate deficiency, paroxysmal nocturnal hemoglobinuria, myelodysplastic syndromes, Chédiak-Higashi syndrome
Inherited disorders
Infantile genetic agranulocytosis, Fanconi's anemia, familial cyclic neutropenia
Hypersplenism
Systemic lupus erythymatosus, rheumatoid arthritis (Felty syndrome), cirrhosis, Gaucher's disease
Immune-mediated
Antineutrophil antibody
Cachexia
Dialysis
Pump-oxygenator in open heart surgery

(Data from Koepke[18] and Wintrobe.[65])

many cytotoxic agents and granulocyte colony stimulating factors.[3] Large, stimulated reactive lymphocytes are prominent in viral infection or drug hypersensitivity reaction.

Inherited morphologic abnormalities (Table 19-12) of WBCs can result in abnormal cytoplasmic inclusions (May-Hegglin or Adler-Reilly anomalies) or in abnormal nuclear segmentation (Pelger-Huët anomaly or hereditary hypersegmentation). White blood cell function is usually normal in these disorders, and the clinical course is often benign. However, the Chédiak-Higashi syndrome, which shows giant fusion granules in the WBCs, is associated with severe neutrophil dysfunction.

> **Table 19-7.** Causes of Lymphopenia
>
> Inherited immunodeficiencies
>   Bruton-type agammaglobulinemia, Di George syndrome, severe combined (Swiss-type) immunodeficiency, common variable hypogammaglobulinemia, Wiscott-Aldrich syndrome, ataxia telangiectasia
> Acquired immunodeficiency syndrome (AIDS)
> Increased destruction
>   Increased corticosteroids (stress, Cushing syndrome, administration), radiation therapy, alkylating agents, antilymphocyte antibody therapy, cyclosporine
> Severe cachexia (usually with advanced malignancy)
> Gastrointestinal loss (malabsorption states)
> Collagen vascular disorders
> Bone marrow aplasia
> Renal failure
> Sarcoidosis

(Data from Kjeldsberg.[4])

Functional Disorders of White Blood Cells and Platelets

Functional platelet and lymphocyte disorders are discussed in Chapters 18 and 30, respectively. Only functional disorders of neutrophils are considered here. Neutrophil dysfunction should be suspected in patients with chronic or recurrent pyogenic or fungal infections with a normal absolute neutrophil number. This is especially true if the infections are caused by unusual pathogens (e.g., *Serratia marcescens, Staphylococcus epidermidis, Pseudomonas* spp.) or if multiple sites are involved.[5] Because neutrophil functional defects are uncommon, attention first should be directed to excluding deficiencies in the immune system, including complement, humoral, and cell mediated immunity; useful screening tests for these components of the immune system include total hemolytic complement, quantitative immunoglobulins, and skin testing (see Ch. 30).

> **Table 19-8.** Causes of Monocytopenia, Eosinopenia, and Basopenia
>
> Monocytopenia
>   Corticosteroids, hairy cell leukemia
> Eosinopenia and basopenia
>   Acute stress, inflammation, or infection, drugs (epinephrine, ACTH, corticosteroids), Cushing syndrome

(Data from Henry.[33])

Effective neutrophil function in the killing of microorganisms requires a number of steps, including (1) adherence to the endothelial surface; (2) emigration from the blood vessel; (3) chemotaxis, or directed movement to the site of infection; (4) opsonization of microorganism by specific antibody and complement; (5) phagocytosis; (6) degranulation of lysosomes into phagocytic vacuoles; and (7) metabolic production of bactericidal oxidants.[6] Serum factors play an important role; for example, complement components are important for neutrophil adherence and chemotaxis, and coating of bacteria with immunoglobulin and complement facilitates neutrophil recognition and phagocytosis.

Oxidative metabolic pathways in neutrophils involve a membrane-associated oxidase system. The neutrophil oxidase complex contains a unique electron-transfer enzyme, cytochrome b_{558}.[7] During phagocytosis, oxygen uptake occurs in a respiratory burst. This oxygen is partially used by the hexose monophosphate shunt to generate NADPH. Using NADPH as the electron donor, a series of electron transfer steps occur, resulting in the reduction of additional oxygen to superoxide anion (O_2^-). The superoxide is rapidly converted (spontaneously or by the enzyme superoxide dismutase) to hydrogen peroxide and hydroxyl radicals, which provide most of the microbicidal activity within the phagosome.[7] Neutrophil myeloperoxidase (MPO) can use the hydrogen peroxide to form additional potent bactericidal compounds (e.g., hypochlorous acid or free chlorine), but these substances seem to be of lesser importance for effective killing.[7]

Inherited or acquired defects can occur at each step of neutrophil function, as listed in Table 19-13. Specialized functional assays can assess the various steps of the microbicidal process (see Tests of Neutrophil Function), but these tests are difficult to perform and interpret. Thus, it is important to exclude the many common acquired diseases (Table 19-13) that secondarily produce neutrophil dysfunction before pursuing the diagnosis of a rare inherited disorder. Examples of some of the inherited conditions are given in Table 19-14, along with more specific laboratory tests that may be useful in their diagnosis.

Malignant Disorders of WBCs and Platelets

Hematologic malignancies include (1) leukemias (originating in the hematopoietic cells of the bone marrow, with abnormal cells usually present in the periph-

Table 19-9. Causes of Thrombocytopenia

Failure of bone marrow production
    Congenital
        Fanconi syndrome, amegakaryocytic thrombocytopenia with congenital malformations, neonatal rubella, maternal ingestion of thiazide diuretics
    Acquired
        Aplastic anemia, megakaryocytic aplasia, marrow infiltration, radiation, myelosuppressive drugs, drugs acting specifically on platelet production (thiazide diuretics, interferon), viral and bacterial infections, paroxysmal nocturnal hemoglobinuria, cyclic thrombocytopenia, renal failure, hyperbaric exposure

Ineffective thrombopoiesis (normal to decreased megakaryocytes)
    Megaloblastic anemias, chronic alcoholism, myelodysplastic syndromes, hereditary thrombocytopenias (Wiskott-Aldrich syndrome, May-Hegglin anomaly)

Hypersplenism
    Cirrhosis (with portal hypertension and congestive splenomegaly), infiltrative disorders (e.g., Gaucher's disease, leukemia, lymphoma), myelofibrosis with myeloid metaplasia, Felty syndrome

Increased platelet destruction
    Congenital
        Nonimmune
            Erythroblastosis fetalis, prematurity, maternal pre-eclampsia, renal vein thrombosis, indwelling unbilical catheter, thrombocytopenia-hemangioma syndrome (Kasabach-Merritt)
        Immune or immune complex
            Maternal drug sensitivity, isoimmune neonatal thrombocytopenia, maternal idiopathic thrombocytopenic purpura, infection
    Acquired
        Nonimmune (or complex mechanisms)
            Disseminated intravascular coagulation, thrombotic thrombocytopenic purpura, hemolytic-uremic syndrome, hemangioma, heart valve, tumor emboli in microcirculation, adult respiratory distress syndrome
        Immune or immune-complex
            Infection (bacterial, viral, rickettsial, protozoan), idiopathic thombocytopenic purpura (acute and chronic), drug-related immune thrombocytopenia (quinidine, quinine, heparin, gold salts are common causes, vast numbers of other drugs can infrequently cause), secondary immune thrombocytopenia (lupus, lymphoma, chronic lymphocytic leukemia), post-transfusion purpura (P1^A1-negative recipient of P1^A1 platelets), anaphylaxis

Loss of platelets
    Massive transfusion, extracorporeal perfusion

(Data from Rapaport[1] and Williams et al.[3])

Table 19-10. Causes of Increased Platelets

Reactive thrombocytosis
    Trauma
    Postoperative
    Postpartum
    Splenectomy (transiently)
    Infection
    Chronic inflammation (including collagen vascular disease)
    Hemorrhage
    Hemolytic anemia, particularly with splenectomy
    Iron deficiency
    Malignancy
Primary thrombocythemia
    Essential thrombocythemia (as a predominant feature)
    Polycythemia vera
    Chronic myelocytic leukemia
    Myelofibrosis with myeloid metaplasia

(Data from Rifkind et al.[15] and Schumacher et al.[66])

Table 19-11. Causes of Leukemoid States

Neutrophilic leukocytosis, usually with WBC $> 50 \times 10^3/\mu L$ ($> 50 \times 10^9/L$)
    Severe infections
    Miliary tuberculosis
    Severe anoxia
    Acute hemorrhage or severe hemolysis
    Malignancy, with bone metastasis or superimposed infection
    Electric shock
    Severe burns
    Neonates with Down syndrome
Lymphocytic leukocytosis, often with reactive or variant lymphocytes
    Infectious lymphocytosis
    Infectious mononucleosis
    Tuberculosis
    Pertussis infection

(Data from Williams[3] and Henry.[33])

Table 19-12. Benign Abnormalities of Leukocyte Morphology

Disorder	Leukocyte Morphology	Other Associated Abnormalities	Pattern of Inheritance	Clinical Manifestations
May-Hegglin anomaly	Prominent Döhle-like bodies (representing alterations in RNA) in neutrophils and sometimes in eosinophils, basophils, and monocytes	Giant platelets; may have neutropenia and thrombocytopenia	Aut. dom.	Bleeding problems in some patients
Alder-Reilly anomaly	Large azurophilic granules in neutrophils, eosinophils, basophils, and some lymphocytes and monocytes; may be more prominent in bone marrow		Aut. rec.	May be a benign disorder, or may be associated with mucopolysaccharidoses
Pelger-Huët anomaly (see Plate 11A)	Hyposegmented neutrophils with pince-nez or dumbbell nuclei; hyperclumping of nuclear chromatin; homozygotes may show round to oval, single-lobed nuclei	Pseudo-Pelger-Huët neutrophils may be seen in myelodysplastic and myeloproliferative disorders, myeloid leukemias, and with some drugs	Aut. dom.	Neutrophils functionally normal
Hereditary hypersegmentation of neutrophils	Many large neutrophils, with ≥ 5 nuclear lobes		Aut. dom.	Neutrophils functionally normal

Abbreviations: Aut. dom., autosomal dominant; Aut. rec., autosomal recessive.
(Data from Miller et al.[6] and Brunning.[67])

Table 19-13. Causes of Neutrophil Dysfunction

Defective adherence and chemotaxis (cellular factors)
    Dermatitis with increased IgE (including Job syndrome)
    Dermatitis and respiratory with increased IgA
    Lazy leukocyte syndrome
    Neutrophil CR3 deficiency
    Newborns
    Chronic renal failure with dialysis
    Diabetes mellitus
    Rheumatoid arthritis
    Bone marrow transplant and graft-versus-host reaction
    Allergic rhinitis with staphylococcal furunculosis
    Malnutrition
    Corticosteroids
Defective adherence and chemotaxis (serum factors)
    C3 deficiency
    Chemotactic factor inactivators (seen in Hodgkin's disease, sarcoidosis, leprosy, lupus erythematosus)
    Antineutrophil inhibitors
Defective opsonization and ingestion
    Immunoglobulin deficiencies
    C3 or C5 deficiency
    Newborns
    Sickle cell disease
Defective bacterial killing by primary and specific granules
    Chédiak-Higashi syndrome
    Specific granule (lactoferrin) deficiency
    Thermal injury
Defective oxidative bactericidal mechanisms
    Chronic granulomatous disease
    Glucose 6-phosphate dehydrogenase deficiency (severe, < 1% activity)
    Myeloperoxidase deficiency

(Data from Williams et al.[3] and Miller et al.[6])

eral blood); (2) lymphomas (originating in peripheral lymphoid organs); (3) immunoproliferative malignancies (producing large amounts of monoclonal immunoglobulin); and (4) histiocytic malignancies (originating in tissue macrophages). Symptoms of these malignancies result from enlargement or compromise of the affected organs. With infiltration of the bone marrow, decreased production of normal hematopoietic cells results in anemia, infection, and impaired hemostasis. The diagnosis is made by detecting the characteristic malignant cells in the peripheral blood or in a biopsy of the involved tissue. Special techniques, such as cytochemistry, immunophenotyping, cytogenetics, and gene rearrangement studies, are useful in diagnosing and subclassifying these malignancies.

Acute Leukemia

Leukemias are traditionally classified by degree of differentiation and cell type. In acute leukemia, the marrow is infiltrated with blasts or cells of early differentiation. In chronic leukemias, the malignant proliferation consists of more differentiated cells. The two major cytologic categories of leukemia are lymphoid and nonlymphoid (or myeloid). Because granulocytes, monocytes, erythrocytes, and megakaryocytes originate in a common myeloid stem cell, it is not surprising that the acute myelocytic leukemias and chronic myeloproliferative disorders can show differentiation along these various cell lines. Even when one nonlymphoid cell line predominates, dysplastic features in the other myeloid lines may be noted. At times, mixed phenotype acute leukemia occurs, in which cells show differentiation along both myeloid and lymphoid lineages. This finding is consistent with the idea that a pluripotential stem cell is a common precursor for lymphoid as well as myeloid cells.

Although acute leukemia was once a rapidly fatal disease, combination chemotherapy can now produce partial or complete remissions in a high percentage of patients. With appropriate therapy, more than 50% of children with acute lymphocytic leukemia can be cured. Bone marrow transplantation shows promise in extending disease-free survival in the acute leukemia subgroups with a less hopeful prognosis. Therefore, it is important that acute leukemia accurately be classified, so that acute lymphocytic leukemia (ALL) can be distinguished from acute myelocytic leukemia (AML) and a correct subclassification of ALL can be made.

Acute myelocytic leukemia can often be distinguished from ALL on morphologic grounds (see Ch. 16). However, morphologic differences may often be subtle, and verification of lineage by cytochemistry and immunophenotyping is recommended. The characteristics of AML and ALL are compared in Table 19-15. Myeloperoxidase (positive in most AML), nonspecific esterase (positive in many monocytic AML), and terminal deoxynucleotidyltransferase (TdT) (positive in nearly all ALL, except B-ALL) are useful tests for determining cell lineage. Surface antigen patterns are useful both for differentiating and subclassifying AML and ALL. With high resolution banding and cell synchronization techniques, cytogenetic abnormalities can be found in many cases of acute leukemia (Table 19-16). Karyotypic abnormalities can define subgroups of AML or ALL with specific features or prognoses; they also can be used as markers after treatment or bone marrow transplant to detect residual leukemic cells.

Table 19-14. Examples of Inherited Neutrophil Dysfunction

Disorder	Dysfunction	Pattern of Inheritance	Clinical Manifestations	Laboratory Tests
CR3 deficiency	Lack of complement receptor on neutrophils, monocytes, lymphocytes; decreased adherence and phagocytosis	Autosomal recessive	Delayed umbilical cord separation; poor wound healing, early onset of recurrent bacterial infections; frequent neutrophilia (occ. > 100,000/μL [>100/L])	Flow cytometry for CR3 (CD11b) antigen on neutrophil surface[a]
Specific granule deficiency	Failure to synthesize specific neutrophil granules that have lactoferrin and that may regulate chemotaxis and oxidative burst	Autosomal recessive	Recurrent severe bacterial infections; decreased inflammatory response	WBC morphology[a] (lack of specific granules; may have bilobed nuclei with blebs and clefts) Immunoassay for lactorferrin
Chédiak-Higashi syndrome (see Plate 12)	Defective chemotaxis and lysosomal granules; fusion of cytoplasmic granules in WBCs and other cells	Autosomal recessive	Recurrent bacterial infections; accelerated phase with lymphoproliferative disorder; albinism, photophobia, and neurologic abnormalities	WBC morphology[a] (giant granules in neutrophils, monocytes and, lymphocytes)
Chronic granulomatous disease	Defective oxidative bactericidal killing in neutrophils and monocytes; cytochrome b_{558} deficient in X-linked form	X-linked: 66% autosomal recessive; 34% rare autosomal dominant	Recurrent infections with catalase-positive bacteria and with fungi	Nitroblue tetrazolium dye reduction test[a] Oxidative burst analysis by flow cytometry.[a]
Myeloperoxidase deficiency	Defective oxidative bacterial killing in vitro	Autosomal recessive	Usually asymptomatic; other oxidative mechanisms may compensate; may have increased susceptibility to systemic *Candida* infection	Leukocyte myeloperoxidase stain[a]
Glucose 6-phosphate dehydrogenase deficiency (G-6-PD)	Defective oxidative burst due to lack of NADH and NADPH	X-linked	Recurrent infections; occurs only with severe deficiency (<1% activity)	RBC G-6-PD

[a] See text for discussion of analytes.
(Data from Axtell[5] and Malech and Gallin.[7])

Table 19-15. Characteristics of Acute Leukemia

Factor	AML	ALL
Age	More common in adults	More common in children
Extramedullary disease	Common in liver and spleen; rare in nodes and CNS; may have granulocytic sarcoma (chloroma)	Common in liver, spleen, and nodes; may have CNS or gonadal involvement or relapse
Morphology	Smooth, fine nuclear chromatin, prominent often multiple nucleoli, moderate N/C ratio; may have cytoplasmic granules or Auer rods	Knobby, fine nuclear chromatin, 0–1 nucleoli high N/C ratio, no cytoplasmic granules
Cytochemistry[a]	Positive peroxidase or Sudan black; positive nonspecific esterase if monocytoid; negative TdT; megakaryocytic variant may be negative for all stains	Negative peroxidase or Sudan black; positive TdT (except for B-ALL)
Immunophenotype[a]	Positive for myeloid or monocytoid or megakaryocytic surface antigens	Positive for early B- or T-surface antigens or surface immunoglobulin

[a] See text for discussion of analytes.
Abbreviations: AML, acute myelocytic leukemia; ALL, acute lymphocytic leukemia; CNS, central nervous system; N/C ratio, nuclear to cytoplasmic ratio; TdT, terminal deoxynucleotidyl transferase; B-ALL, B-cell ALL.
(Data from Rapaport[1] and Kjeldsberg.[4])

The most commonly used classification system for AML is that proposed by the French-American-British (FAB) group[8,9] (Table 19-17). The FAB group distinguishes AML from myelodysplastic syndromes by requiring 30% of the myeloid lineage cells in the bone marrow to be blasts for a diagnosis of AML. Photomicrographs of the seven categories of AML are shown in Plates 13 to 19. FAB M1 is myeloblastic, with little evidence of maturation. M2 shows differentiation along the granulocytic line, which is often dysplastic. M3 is hypergranular promyelocytic leukemia (AProL), an entity also defined by a specific translocation, t(15;17). A hypo- or microgranular variant of M3 may also occur, which may morphologically resemble monocytoid forms of AML; however, the cells will still have strongly positive MPO and show the typical t(15;17) translocation. In FAB M4, or acute myelomonocytic leukemia (AMML), both granulocytic and monocytic differentiation occurs. Often the monocytic differentiation is more prominent in the peripheral blood, whereas the granulocytic differentiation predominates in the bone marrow. M5, or acute monocytic leukemia (AMoL), is divided into M5a (primarily immature monoblasts) and M5b (significant numbers of promonocytes and monocytes). FAB M6 (erythroleukemia) is characterized by more than 50% erythroid precursors in the bone marrow, with blasts comprising more than 30% of the nonerythroid myeloid lineage cells. Although dysplastic changes in the erythroid, granulocytic, or megakaryocytic series can be seen in any category of AML, they are most frequently found in M6. Erythroleukemia arises from a multipotential stem cell with broad myeloid potential and may transform, as the disease progresses, to M1, M2, or M4.[2] M7, or megakaryocytic leukemia, is characterized by highly pleomorphic blasts, varying from small lymphoblast-like to larger blasts with cytoplasmic blebs or vacuoles.[9] Patients may present with few circulating blasts and normal to elevated platelet count, sometimes with giant platelets and megakaryocytic fragments. The bone marrow often is inaspirable; the biopsy shows a mixture of fibrosis, abnormal megakaryocytes, and blasts. Classification of AML as M7 requires the demonstration of platelet-specific surface glycoproteins by immunophenotyping or platelet peroxidase by electron microscopy. Basophilic and eosinophilic leukemia are not recognized by the FAB classification. It is a matter of conjecture as to whether these occur as distinct entities, or as part of the acceleration phase of chronic myelocytic leukemia (CML).

The incidence of the various FAB subgroups of AML is roughly M1, 18%; M2, 28%; M3, 8%; M4, 27%; M5, 10%; M6, 4%; and M7, 5%.[2] The FAB classification does not affect therapy or prognosis, with a few exceptions. M3 is associated with disseminated intravascular coagulation (DIC) and bleeding, possibly caused by thromboplastic material in the promyelocytic granules. Heparin is frequently administered during the induction therapy of M3, and the chemotherapeutic regimen

Table 19-16. Common Chromosomal Abnormalities in Leukemia and Lymphoma

Disorder[a]	Chromosomal Abberations
AML-M1	t(9;22)(q34;q11)
AML-M2	t(8;21)(q22;q22)
AML-M3	t(15;17)(q22;q11)[b]
AML-M4, M5	Abnormalities involving chromosome 11
AML-M5	t(9;11)(p21-22;q23)
AML-M4 with eosinophila	inv(16)(p13;q22); del(16)(q22)
AML-M2, M4 with basophilia	t(6;9)(p23;q34)
AML, M1, M2, M4, M7 with normal to elevated platelets	inv(3)(q21;q26)
AML, any subclass	+8; −7; 7q 5q−;−5; −Y; +21; i(17q)(q11)
ALL, early B lineage	t(9;22)(q34;q11); 6q−; t/del 12p
ALL, early B lineage, hyperdiploid	+21; +6; +12; +14; +10; +4, +8; +18
ALL, pre-B lineage	t(1;19)(q23;p13); t(1;11)(p32;q23)
ALL, biphenotypic (early B lineage, monocytic)	t(4;11)(q21;q23)
ALL, L1 or L2	t(10;14)(q24;q11); t(11;14)(p13;q11); t(9;22)(q34;q11)
ALL, L3 (B-ALL)	t(8;14) or t(8;22) or t(2;8)[b]
ALL, T lineage	Abnormalities involving chromosome 11(q23) or 14; 6q−, 9q−
Myelodysplastic syndromes	−5; 5q−; −7; 7q−; inv(3)(q21;q26) with progression, often complex abnormalities
CML	t(9;22)(q34;q11)[b]
PV	1q+; 20q−; +8; +9; −5
ET	Variable
MMM	13q−; t(1;13)
B-CLL	+12; 14q+; t(11;14)(q13;q32)
B-PLL	14q+; t(11;14)(q13;q32); 6q−; t(6;12); frequent karyotypic evolution
T-PLL	Marked chromosomal instability with multiple deletions and hypoploidy
HCL	6q−
ML, small lymphocytic	+12; t(11;14)(q13;q32)
ML, follicular	t(14;18)(q32;q21)
ML, immunoblastic (B), or small noncleaved (Burkitt's or non-Burkitt's lymphoma)	t(8;14) or t(8;22) or t(2;8)[b]
Myeloma	t(11;14)(q13;q32)

[a] See text for discussion of subclassifications (M1, M2, etc.)
[b] Occurs in >90% of cases.

Abbreviations: AML, acute myelocytic leukemia; ALL, acute lymphocytic leukemia; CML, chronic myelocytic leukemia; PV, polycythemia vera; ET, essential thrombocythemia; MMM, myelofibrosis with myeloid metaplasia; B-CLL, B-cell chronic lymphocytic leukemia; B-PLL, B-cell prolymphocytic leukemia; T-PLL, T-cell PLL; HCL, hairy cell leukemia; ML, malignant lymphoma.

(Data from references 10, 13, 68, and 69.)

is sometimes modified for slower destruction of the leukemic cells. In addition, some of the promyelocytes may exist in a postmitotic state; complete eradication of leukemic cells from the marrow during induction therapy is unnecessary. Acute monocytic leukemia, M5, is associated with skin and gum infiltration and a higher incidence of central nervous system (CNS) involvement. M7 may have a poorer response to conventional induction therapy.

Although immunophenotyping is becoming widely used in acute leukemia, the FAB classification has not yet been modified to include surface antigen markers. Correlation of the FAB classification of AML with immunophenotypic features is presented in Table 19-18. Aneuploidy is found in most cases of AML, and specific chromosomal abnormalities can define recognizable syndromes of AML. Table 19-16 lists some common associations. Somewhat poorer responses to therapy may be seen with partial or complete deletions of chromosomes 5 or 7, trisomy 8, t(6;9), inv(3), and complex karyotypic changes.[10]

Acute lymphocytic leukemia is divided into three subsets (L1, L2, L3) on the basis of the FAB classification (Table 19-19). L1 is characterized by small blasts with a high nuclear to cytoplasmic ratio, whereas larger blasts are seen in L2. Cells of L3 ALL are large with

Table 19-17. French-American-British (FAB) Classification of Acute Myelocytic Leukemias[a]

Category	Morphologic Criteria (Bone Marrow)	Cytochemical Criteria
M1 Myeloblastic without maturation	≥90% of myeloid-line cells are blasts	≥3% of blasts positive for MPO or Sudan black
M2 Myeloblastic with maturation	30–89% of myeloid-line cells are blasts, >10% are promyelocytes to PMN (often dysplastic), <20% are monocytes	
M3 Promyelocytic	Hypergranular promyelocytes with heavy to dust-like granules, often Auer rods; nucleus often bilobed; microgranular variant may occur	Strongly MPO positive
M4 Myelomonocytic	30–80% of myeloid-line cells are myeloblasts plus maturing neutrophils; >20% of myeloid-line cells are monocytic lineage. In addition, >5000/µL monocytic cells in peripheral blood	If <5000/µL blood monocytes, can classify as M4 if >20% of myeloid-line cells in marrow are demonstrated to be monocytic lineage by nonspecific esterase stain
M4 With eosinophilia	As above, with ≥5% abnormal eosinophils that may have unsegmented nucleus and both eosinophilic and large basophilic granules	Eosinophils stain with both PAS and chloroacetate esterase
M5 Monoblastic, monocytic	>80% of myeloid-line cells are monoblasts, promonocytes, or monocytes; in M5a, 80% of myeloid-line cells are monoblasts; in M5b, <80% are monoblasts, and remainder are promonocytes and monocytes	Most cells are positive for nonspecific esterase
M6 Erythroleukemia	≥50% of bone marrow cells are erythroid precursors; ≥30% of nonerythroid myeloid-line cells are blasts	
M7 Megakaryocytic	Blasts in marrow or blood are identified as megakaryocytic lineage; if marrow inaspirable, biopsy shows large numbers of blasts, frequently with increased numbers of megakaryocytes and reticulin	Megakaryocytic lineage (>30% of blasts) is established by detection of factor VIII antigen, glycoproteins Ib, IIb/IIIa, or IIIa, or platelet peroxidase by EM; MPO negative, but nonspecific esterase may be focally positive with acetate substrate

[a] Definition of acute myelocytic leukemia: blasts ≥30% of total myeloid-line cells when <50% erythroid cells in bone marrow. Blasts ≥30% of nonerythroid myeloid-line cells when ≥50% erythroid cells in bone marrow (M6 leukemia). (Blast percentage does not include proerythroblasts; they are included with total erythroid cells. Myeloid-line cells includes blasts, maturing neutrophils, eosinophils, basophils, monocytic cells, megakaryocytes, and all erythroid precursors.)

Abbreviations: MPO, myeloperoxidase; PMN, polymorphonuclear leukocytes; PAS, periodic acid-Schiff; EM, electron microscopy. (Data from Rapaport[1] and Bennett et al.[8,9])

Table 19-18. Correlation of FAB Classification of Acute Myelocytic Leukemia with Immunophenotypic Features

FAB Subtype	M1	M2	M3	M4	M5	M6	M7
HLA-DR	+	+	−	+	+	+/−	+/−
CD33 (MY9)	+	+	+	+	+	+/−	+/−
CD13 (MY7)	+/−	+	+	+	+	−	NR
CD15 (MY1, M1)	+/−	+	+/−	+	+	+/−	NR
CD14 (MY4, M3)	−	+/−	−	+	+	−	NR
Glycophorin A	−	−	−	−	−	+	−
Platelet GP IB/IIB/IIIA	−	−	−	−	−	−	+

[a] The reaction in most of cases is noted, but exceptions may occur; for a review of the percentages of cases that have been reported as positive, see Keren.[41]

Abbreviations: FAB, French-American-British; NR, not reported; +, positive reaction in ≥ 20% of gated blasts; +/−, positive or negative; GP, glycoprotein.

(Data from the Second MIC Cooperative Study Group[10] and Keren.[41])

very basophilic cytoplasm, often with punctate vacuolization. The L3 morphology resembles Burkitt's lymphoma and correlates with the mature B-ALL phenotype. Photomicrographs of L1 and L3 types of ALL are shown in Plates 20 and 21.

Even with specific grading schemes, it is difficult to separate reproducibly the L1 and L2 subtypes. With the advent of monoclonal antibodies against a variety of lineage-specific cell antigens, ALL can be classified by immunologic criteria (Table 19-20) into "groups" corresponding to developmental stages of B- or T-cell differentiation (see also Fig. 16-2, Ch. 16). Early B-surface antigens and immunoglobulin gene rearrangements have been found in most cases of ALL that would have been classified as null cell in the past. Thus, these early B-lineage lymphocytes, with or without the common acute lymphocytic leukemia antigen (CALLA, known as CD10), constitute most cases of ALL (Table 19-20A, groups I–IV, sometimes termed *pre-pre-B ALL*). When μ heavy chain is detected in the cytoplasm, the leukemia is termed *pre-B ALL* (Table 19-20A, group 5); B-ALL (Table 19-20A, group VI) refers to Burkitt-type leukemia/lymphoma with identifiable surface immunoglobulin. Similarly, T-cell ALL (Table 19-20B) is divided into three groups on the basis of resemblance to stages of thymocyte development. T-cell ALL more commonly occurs in older children and adults, and is associated with a mediastinal mass, hepatosplenomegaly, early CNS involvement, and a high WBC count.[4]

To define the patients in need of more cytotoxic induction and postremission therapy, much attention is given to identifying high risk factors in children with ALL. In addition, very high risk children or adults may have an increased chance for long-term survival with bone marrow transplant in first remission. The best

Table 19-19. FAB Classification of Acute Lymphocytic Leukemia

Cytology	L1	L2	L3
Cell size	Small	Large	Large, homogeneous
Nuclear chromatin	Homogeneous	Variable	Finely stippled
Nuclear shape	Regular	Irregular	Oval to round
Nucleoli	Rare	Present	1–3
Cytoplasm	Scanty	Moderate	Moderate, vacuolated
Cytoplasmic basophilia	Moderate	Variable	Intense
Incidence in children	85%	13%	2%
Incidence in adults	35%	63%	2%
Immunologic markers	Early B or thymic T	Early B or thymic T	Differentiated B (SIg positive), Burkitt-type leukemia/lymphoma

Abbreviations: SIg, surface immunoglobulin.
(Data from Kjeldsberg.[4])

Table 19-20. Classification of Acute Lymphocytic Leukemia by Immunophenotypic Features

A. B-Lineage Acute Lymphocytic Leukemia Groups

Groups	Early B Lineage 1	Early B Lineage 2	Early B Lineage with CD10 3	Early B Lineage with CD10 4	Pre-B 5	B 6
DR	+	+	+	+	+	+
CD19 (pan-B)	−	+	+	+	+	+
CD10 (CALLA)	−	−	+	+	+	+ or −
CD20 (pan-B)	−	−	−	+	+	+
Cytoplasmic μ	−	−	−	−	+	+
Surface Ig	−	−	−	−	−	+

B. T-Lineage Acute Lymphocytic Leukemia Groups

Groups	Early Thymocyte 1	Common Thymocyte 2	Late Thymocyte 3
CD7 (early T)	+	+	+
Cytoplasmic CD3 (pan-T)	+ or −	+	+
CD5 (pan-T)	+ (75%)	+	+
CD2 (pan-T)	+ (90%)	+	+
CD1 (thymic T)	−	+	−
Surface CD3 (pan-T)	−	+ (25%)	+
CD4 (T helper)	−	+ (90%)	+ or −
CD8 (T suppressor)	−	+ (90%)	+ or −

[a] In addition, many cases of T-ALL (or lymphoblastic lymphoma) may express DR or CD10 (CALLA).
(Data from Deegan[42] and Foon and Tood.[43])

prognosis is seen in patients aged 2–9 years, WBC count less than $10 \times 10^3/\mu L$ ($<10 \times 10^9/L$), L1 morphology, early B lineage with CD10 and hyperdiploidy (more than 50 chromosomes).[11–13] Factors that indicate a particularly poor prognosis in ALL include WBC count more than $50 \times 10^3/\mu L$ ($>50 \times 10^9/L$), presentation with CNS involvement, mature B lineage (with surface immunoglobulin), and chromosomal translocations.[11–13] Specific chromosomal translocations associated with ALL are listed in Table 19-16.

Myelodysplastic Syndromes

The myelodysplastic syndromes (MDS) are a heterogeneous group of hematopoietic stem cell disorders, often resembling AML, but characterized by maturation abnormalities in one or more of the myeloid cell lines rather than by a preponderance of blasts. Other names previously used to describe subsets of these disorders include dysmyelopoietic syndrome, hematopoietic dysplasmia, preleukemia, smoldering leukemia, subacute myeloid leukemia, subacute myelomonocytic leukemia, chronic monocytic leukemia, acute myeloproliferative syndrome, primary acquired panmyelopathy with myeloblastosis, refractory megaloblastic anemia, chronic erythemic myelosis, Di Guglielmo syndrome, chronic erythremic myelosis, and acquired idiopathic sideroblastic anemia.

Typically, the bone marrow is normocellular to hypercellular, but ineffective hematopoiesis occurs, resulting in peripheral cytopenias. Dysplastic morphology is recognized in the erythroid, granulocytic, and megakaryocytic lines, as outlined in Table 19-21 (Plates 11B, 22A and B). Monocytosis may also occur. Most patients with MDS are over the age of 50 and have symptoms related to anemia, neutropenia, or thrombocytopenia. In many patients, MDS progresses to overt AML, whereas in others, the disorder may have a prolonged course or may result in death caused by infection or bleeding.

Secondary or therapy related MDS can occur in patients treated with alkylating agents and/or radiation therapy. Such cases differ from idiopathic MDS in that the marrow may be hypocellular with variable degrees of fibrosis. In addition, abnormal megakaryocytes and ringed sideroblasts are more frequently seen in secondary MDS.[4,14] Myelodysplastic features also may be found in bone marrows from patients with acquired immunodeficiency syndrome (AIDS), often with cytopenias.[4]

Table 19-21. Morphologic Evidence of Myelodysplasia

Peripheral Blood Smear	Bone Marrow

Dyserythropoiesis
    MCV often increased
    Prominent anisocytosis (large oval macrocytes plus small hypochromic cells)
    Small, bizarre poikilocytes with central pallor
    Coarse basophilic stippling, Pappenheimer bodies
    Nucleated RBCs
    Increased Hgb F
    Rarely, acquired HgB H or PNH
	Increased, left-shifted erythropoiesis
	Megaloblastic or megaloblastoid changes
	Nuclear abnormalities: lobation, budding, karyorrhexis, multinucleate
	Cytoplasmic vacuoles
	Uneven hemoglobinization
	Ringed sideroblasts
	Abnormal mitotic figures
	PAS-positive erythroids

Neutropenia
    Pseudo-Pelger-Huët changes (nuclear hyposegmentation, hyperclumping of chromatin)
    Hypogranular cytoplasm
    Döhle bodies close to nucleus
    Occasional blast or promyelocyte
    Monocytosis
	Left-shifted granulopoiesis, sometimes with partial arrest
	Binucleate or donut-shaped nucleus
	Rarely, myeloperoxidase deficient
	Abnormal cytoplasmic granulation (fusion of azurophilic granules)
	Nests of blasts, centrally located rather than next to bony spicule
	Paramyeloblasts (cells with characteristics of both promyelocytes and promonocytes)
	Eosinophilic and basophilic granules in same cell

Dysmegakaryocytopoiesis
    Thrombocytopenia
    Giant platelets
    Hypogranular platelets
    Vacuolization of platelets
    Micromegakaryocytes
    Megakaryocytic fragments
	Micro- or macromegakaryocytes
	Mononuclear or binuclear megakaryocytes
	Megakaryocytes with small, separated nuclei
	Vacuolization of megakaryocyte cytoplasm

Abbreviations: RBCs, red blood cells; Hgb, hemoglobin; PAS, periodic acid-Schiff; PNH, paroxysmal nocturnal hemoglobinuria. (Data from Kjeldsberg[4] and Bennett et al.[14])

The FAB group has classified MDS into five subgroups, based on morphologic criteria[4,14] (Table 19-22). The scheme stresses the importance of the percentage of blasts, calculated in the bone marrow from the nonerythroid myeloid-lineage cells. Refractory anemia (RA) is characterized by anemia, reticulocytopenia, and variable degrees of dyserythropoiesis; blasts are minimal in number, and dysplasias in other cell lines are usually absent. Refractory anemia with ringed sideroblasts (RARS) is synonymous with acquired idiopathic sideroblastic anemia; more than 15% of the erythroid cells are ringed sideroblasts, and dysplasias in the other cell lines are usually absent. When the peripheral blood shows greater than 5% blasts, or the bone marrow has 5–20% blasts, the syndrome is classified as refractory anemia with excess of blasts (RAEB), regardless of the number of ringed sideroblasts or the lineages involved. Chronic myelomonocytic leukemia (CMML) is a variant of refractory anemia with an excess of blasts, in which there is a prominent component of monocytes in the blood (more than $1.0 \times 10^3/\mu L$ [$>1.0 \times 10^9/L$]). Refractory anemia with excess of blasts in transformation (RAEB-IT) describes a group with more than 5% blasts in the peripheral blood and 20–30% blasts in the bone marrow, in which acute leukemia may be imminent. Repeated blood and/or marrow examinations can resolve whether MDS is to run a chronic course or is rapidly progressing to AML.

Transformation to AML occurs in approximately 15% of patients with RA or RARS, in 30% of patients with RAEB, in 40% of patients with CMML, and in nearly 100% of patients with RAEB-IT.[2] Severe granulocytic or megakaryocytic dysplasia with neutropenia and thrombocytopenia is also a poor risk factor for survival.

With high resolution banding analysis, approximately 80% of patients with de novo MDS have recurrent chromosomal defects.[2] Most have a loss of chromosomal material, rather than translocation or inversion. The most common abnormalities are shown in Table 19-16. The risk of transformation to AML is lowest with normal karyotype or a single chromosomal abnormality but very high when complex chromosomal abnormali-

Table 19-22. French-American-British (FAB) Classification of Myelodysplastic Syndromes

Refractory anemia
    Anemia with normo- to hypercellular bone marrow
    Variable dyserythropoietic change
    Usually reticulocytopenia, or ineffective erythropoiesis
    Less frequently, neutropenia or thrombocytopenia occurs, with or without dysplastic change; when this occurs, this category is sometimes termed *refractory cytopenia*
    Blasts should not exceed 1% in peripheral blood, or 5% in the bone marrow[a]

Refractory anemia with ringed sideroblasts
    As above, with >15% ringed sideroblasts in bone marrow

Refractory anemia with excess of blasts (RAEB)
    Variable degree of anemia, neutropenia, and thrombocytopenia with normo- to hypercellular bone marrow
    Variable degree of dyserythropoiesis, dysgranulopoiesis, and dysmegakaryocytopoiesis
    Blasts are <5% in peripheral blood, and 5–20% in bone marrow

Chronic myelomonocytic leukemia (CMML)
    As for RAEB, except peripheral blood monocytes >1000/μL
    Often associated with increase in mature granulocytes, rather than neutropenia

Refractory anemia with excess of blasts in transformation (RAEB-IT)
    As for RAEB, except >5% blasts in peripheral blood and/or 20–30% blasts in bone marrow and/or the presence of Auer rods

Therapy-related myelodysplastic syndrome (MDS)
    Additional features of MDS induced by chemotherapy and/or radiation therapy can include
    Hypocellular marrow
    Marrow fibrosis
    More frequent finding of numerous ringed sideroblasts and abnormal megakaryocytic precursors
    Higher proportion of blasts in peripheral blood than is expected from percentage in bone marrow

[a] Blasts as a percentage of total nonerythroid myeloid-line cells, including nonerythroid blasts, maturing neutrophils, eosinophils, basophils, monocytic cells, and megakaryocytes.
(Data from Kjeldsberg[4] and Bennett et al.[14])

ties arise during the course of the disease.[2] Impaired granulocyte-monocyte colony formation in culture systems has also been observed in the bone marrow of most patients with MDS, with deterioration of cloning efficiency accompanying progression to AML.[2]

Myelodysplastic syndrome must be distinguished from other, often treatable, disorders that may produce similar bone marrow and peripheral blood findings. In particular, vitamin B_{12} or folate deficiency resemble the refractory anemia category (with little granulocytic or megakaryocytic dysplasia). It is important to eliminate these entities as a cause of ineffective erythropoiesis with cytopenias before a diagnosis of MDS is made. Sideroblastic anemia can occur as an inherited X-linked disorder, or it can be secondary to drugs (including isoniazid, cycloserine, chloramphenicol), toxins, lead, and severe alcoholism.[1] Rarely, congenital dyserythropoietic anemias can resemble MDS, but these rare inherited disorders are usually recognized in childhood.

Myeloproliferative Disorders

Differentiated leukemias of the myeloid lineage are termed myeloproliferative disorders (MPD). These chronic disorders are characterized by an uncontrolled clonal proliferation of erythroid, myeloid, and megakaryocytic lines arising from malignant transformation of a pluripotent stem cell. They occur mainly in middle-aged to elderly adults. The four myeloproliferative disorders, named by the predominent cell proliferation, are CML, polycythemia vera (PV), essential thrombocythemia (ET), and myelofibrosis with myeloid metaplasia (MMM). Common features of these disorders include anemia, leukocytosis with immature neutrophils, eosinophilia, basophilia, thrombocytosis (in early stages), and qualitative platelet abnormalities. Hyperuricemia may result from increased cellular turnover, and patients with MPD have a high incidence of gout. Hepatosplenomegaly occurs because of infiltration and extramedullary hematopoiesis in these sites. The bone marrow shows trilineage hyperplasia with variable degrees of fibrosis. It is thought that normal fibroblasts in the marrow react to increased growth factor production by abnormally proliferating megakaryocytes. Differential characteristics between various myeloproliferative disorders are shown in Table 19-23. Characteristic blood and bone marrow findings are illustrated in Plates 23 to 25. However, hematologic findings may vary with the stage of the disease, and there may be considerable overlap between the different types of MPD. In addition, some patients may be classified as having atypical myeloproliferative disorder, because their clinical and laboratory findings do not clearly fit into a specific disease entity.[4] All the MPD, especially CML, can terminate in acute leukemia.

It is important to differentiate MPD, especially CML, from benign causes of marked neutrophilia or myeloid

Table 19-23. Chronic Myeloproliferative Disorders

	Polycythemia Vera	Chronic Myelocytic Leukemia	Essential Thrombocythemia	Myelofibrosis with Myeloid Metaplasia
Peripheral blood				
WBC × 10⁹/L[a]	Usually <20.0	Often >50.0	Usually <25.0	Usually <30.0
Immature neutrophils	Few	Myelocytes with occasional promyelocyte and blast	Few	Occasional immature neutrophils of all stages
RBCs	Often microcytic, hypochromic	Nonspecific findings	May be microcytic/hypochromic	Prominent anisocytosis and teardrop cells
nRBC	Occasional	Occasional	Occasional	Common
Platelet count[a]	Normal to increased	Variable	Marked increased	Variable
Leukocyte alkaline phosphatase[a]	Usually increased	Markedly decreased	Usually normal	Usually increased
Bone marrow[a]				
Cell types	Trilineage hyperplasia	Primarily granulocytic hyperplasia	Trilineage hyperplasia with markedly increased megakaryocytes	Trilineage hyperplasia with increasing fibrosis
Iron	Absent	Usually present	Present or absent	Usually present
Philadelphia chromosome	Absent	Present	Absent	Absent
Spleen				
Size	Mildly increased	Moderately increased (usually when WBC count >100.0)	Mildly increased	Markedly increased

[a] See text for discussion of analytes.
(Data from Jandl[2] and Kjeldsberg.[4])

leukemoid reaction (Tables 19-11 and 19-24). Although dysplastic morphology of granulocytes and platelets may occasionally be seen in MPD, the MPD are generally distinguished from myelodysplastic syndromes by effective release of WBCs and platelets to the peripheral blood rather than cytopenias. MPD usually shows all stages of neutrophil maturation in the peripheral blood with less than 5% blasts, in contrast to AML, in which there is a hiatus in cell types between blasts and mature neutrophils in the peripheral blood.[2]

Chronic Myelocytic Leukemia

Chronic myelocytic leukemia is characterized by a massive overproduction of granulocytes. More than 90% of patients with CML have the Philadelphia (Ph) chromosome, the presence of which may proceed CML by several years.[2] The Ph chromosome is present in the metastases of cells committed to the production of neutrophils, eosinophils, basophils, monocytes, platelets, erythroblasts, B lymphocytes, and some T lymphocytes.[2] The Ph chromosome is a small chromosome 22 (22q-) resulting from an unequal translocation between chromosomes 9 and 22. The *abl* oncogene on chromosome 9 is relocated to chromosome 22, adjacent to the residual part of the breakpoint cluster *(bcr)* gene; this results in a 210-kd chimeric *bcr-abl* protein product, a tyrosine kinase with increased enzymatic activity.[11] The mechanism by which this growth factor induces uncontrolled myelogenesis is unknown. Some patients with apparent Ph-negative CML have been shown to have the *abl-bcr* translocation on a molecular level, even through karyotypic analysis is normal.[11] Other Ph-negative patients, when critically assessed, are thought to have myelodysplastic syndrome (particularly chronic myelomonocytic leukemia) rather than CML. The presence of the Ph chromosome, as well as a very low level of leukocyte alkaline phosphatase, distinguishes CML from other MDSs and from leukemoid neutrophilic reactions. Although bone marrow examination is of little help in diagnosing CML, it is indicated to obtain cells for cytogenetic studies.

Survival with CML is variable, with a median of 3.5-4 years. Chronic myelocytic leukemia terminates in an accelerated phase, usually with transformation to acute leukemia. Signs of acceleration in CML include additional chromosomal abnormalities, an increasing or decreasing WBC count, thrombocytopenia, marked basophilia or eosinophilia, an increase in spleen size, or increased marrow fibrosis. The presence of more than 10% of blast forms in the peripheral blood generally signifies blast crisis.[2] Myeloid blast crisis, with a mixture of undifferentiated blasts, myeloblasts, megakaryoblasts, and erythroblasts is most common.[2] Approximately 20-30% of blast crises are early B lineage, with TdT and CD10-positive blasts.[2] These lymphoid blasts crises may respond to therapy with vincristine and prednisone, as opposed to the myeloid blast crises, which are refractory to chemotherapy.

Polycythemia Vera

Polycythemia vera predominantly affects the erythroid line, with an erythropoietin-independent increase in red blood cell (RBC) mass. The increase in blood volume and viscosity results in symptoms of headache, tinnitus, pruritis (particularly with bathing), and ruddy cyanosis, and complications of serious vascular hemorrhage and thrombosis.[15] Gastrointestinal dyspepsia

Table 19-24. Differentiation of Myeloid Leukemoid Reaction from Chronic Myelocytic Leukemia

	Leukemoid Reaction	CML
WBC count	$<100 \times 10^3/\mu L$ ($<100 \times 10^9/L$)	May be as high as $500 \times 10^3/\mu L$ ($500 \times 10^9/L$)
WBC differential[a]		
Eosinophils, basophils	Normal to decreased	Usually increased
Immature granulocytes	Few, usually to myelocyte	May have many myelocytes, occasional promyelocyte, blast
Nucleated RBCs	Rare	May be common
Toxic granulation, Döhle bodies	Frequent	Usually not present
Leukocyte alkaline phosphatase[a]	High	Usually very low
Ph chromosome[a]	Absent	Present >95%
Bone marrow M/E ratio[a]	6-8:1	15:1
Spleen	Rarely palpable	Usually enlarged

[a] See text for discussion of analytes.
Abbreviations: CML, chronic myelocytic leukemia; WBC, white blood cell; RBCs, red blood cells; Ph, Philadelphia; M/E ratio, myeloid to erythroid ratio.
(Data from Rapaport[1] and Kjeldsberg.[4])

with bleeding and hyperuricemia with secondary gout are more common in PV than in other MPD.[15] Most patients are iron deficient, because of increased iron use for RBC production and iron loss from gastrointestinal bleeding or phlebotomy therapy.

Polycythemia vera must be differentiated from other causes of relative and secondary erythrocytosis, as discussed in Chapter 17. The Polycythemia Vera Study Group has developed criteria for an unambiguous definition of PV (Table 19-25). However, determination of RBC mass, an expensive test fraught with interpretation problems, is often unnecessary, particularly if the hematocrit (Hct) exceeds 60%. The diagnosis of PV can usually be established clinically by observing splenomegaly, normal arterial oxygen saturation (or no clinical evidence for hypoxemia), neutrophilia, basophilia, thrombocytosis, and hyperuricemia in a patient with an elevated Hct. Bone marrow examination is not essential but will show trilineage hyperplasia with reduced to absent iron stores.[2]

Polycythemia vera is slowly progressive, with median survival in excess of 10 years.[2] Myelofibrosis with marrow failure develops late in the course of approximately 10% of PV patients and is termed the *spent phase* of PV.[2] Acute myelocytic leukemia also develops in a small percentage of patients, particularly with alkylator or radiation therapy.

Essential Thrombocythemia

Essential thrombocythemia is a myeloproliferative disorder with a persistent elevation in platelet count and a striking increase in bone marrow megakaryocytes. Platelet count is often in excess of $1000 \times 10^3/\mu L$ ($1000 \times 10^9/L$), accompanied by mild neutrophilia. Platelets are frequently dysfunctional, and both bleeding and thrombotic complications occur. As in PV, gastrointestinal bleeding and iron deficiency are common. However, approximately 20% of patients, particularly younger patients, remain free of symptoms for long periods of time.[2]

The Polycythemia Vera Study Group also has proposed criteria for the diagnosis of ET (Table 19-26). Most criteria are directed at differentiation of ET from other MPD and from reactive thrombocytosis. The causes of benign, reactive thrombocytosis are listed in Table 19-10. In particular, it is important to exclude iron deficiency, infection, and occult malignancy as a cause of thrombocytosis with anemia before reaching a diagnosis of ET. Although platelet counts also may be very high in reactive thrombocytosis, bleeding and thrombosis do not occur. Bone marrow aspirate and biopsy may be useful to exclude myelofibrosis and to perform chromosomal analysis to exclude CML. The bone marrow in ET shows panmyelosis with abundant megakaryocytes, which may occur in clusters and may be abnormally large and bizarre in appearance.[2,4]

Myelofibrosis with Myeloid Metaplasia

Myelofibrosis with myeloid metaplasia is characterized by increasing bone marrow fibrosis with extramedullary hematopoiesis. Symptoms relate to development of refractory anemia and bleeding tendency, along with massive hepatosplenomegaly. The peripheral blood shows polychromasia and marked anisopoikilocytosis with numerous teardrop forms. Giant and bizarre dysfunctional platelets and megakaryocytic fragments are common. A leukoerythroblastic reaction, that is, the presence of nucleated and immature neutrophils in the peripheral blood, is characteristically found. Neutrophilia and thrombocytosis may be seen in the early

---

Table 19-25. Polycythemia Vera Study Group Criteria for the Diagnosis of Polycythemia Vera

Increased total RBC mass
AND
Normal arterial oxygen saturation
AND
Splenomegaly or, if absent, two of the following
  Platelet count $>400 \times 10^3/\mu L$ ($>400 \times 10^9/L$)[a]
  WBC $> 12.0 \times 10^3/\mu L$ ($12.0 \times 10^9/L$)[a]
  Leukocyte alkaline phosphatase increased[a]
  $B_{12} > 900$ µg/L (>660 pmol/L)
  Unsaturated B_{12} binding capacity > 2200 µg/L (>1620 pmol/L)

[a] See text for discussion of analytes.
(Data from Berlin.[70])

Table 19-26. Polycythemia Vera Study Group Criteria for the Diagnosis of Essential Thrombocythemia

Platelet count $>600 \times 10^3/\mu L$ ($>600 \times 10^9/L$)[a]
Hemoglobin ≤ 13 g/dL (≤ 130 g/L) or normal RBC mass
Stainable bone marrow iron or failure of iron therapy[a] (<1 g/dL [<10 g/L] rise in hemoglobin after 1 month of iron therapy)
Philadelphia chromosome absent
Absent bone marrow collagen fibrosis, or fibrosis of less than one-third the marrow biopsy without both splenomegaly and leukoerythroblastic reaction
No known cause for reactive thrombocytosis

[a] See text for discussion of analytes.
(Data from Murphy et al.[71])

Table 19-27. Leukemias of Differentiated B Lymphocytes

Disorder	WBC ($\times 10^9/\mu L$)		Morphology	Clinical Manifestations	Surface Markers
Chronic lymphocytic leukemia	15.0–200.0	PB	Small to medium mature lymphocytes; often ruptured or smudged cells; variable number of prolymphocytes with prominent nucleolus	Onset late adulthood Variable lymphadenopathy, hepatosplenomegaly May be associated with hypogammaglobulinemia; autoimmune hemolytic anemia, low level monoclonal paraprotein Variable course, from months to >10 years May transform to more aggressive form Prolymphocytic (>20% prolymphocytes in PB) Richter syndrome (development of large cell lymphoma)	Pan-B, CD21 (C3dR), weak monoclonal SIg (usually IgM +/− IgD, but occasionally cytoplasmic Ig only), anomalous T (CD5) Similar phenotype occurs in prolymphocytic transformation In Richter syndrome, may see similar phenotype or loss of T (CD5) or change in type of SIg
		BM	Diffusely infiltrated, usually >40% lymphocytes (may be patchy in early stages)		
		LT	May be diffusely infiltrated; in prolymphocytic transformation, foci of large, immature cells; in Richter's transformation, diffuse proliferation of large cell type of lymphoma begins in lymph nodes and spleen		

(Continued)

Table 19-27. Leukemias of Differentiated B Lymphocytes *(Continued)*

Disorder	WBC (×10⁹/μL)		Morphology	Clinical Manifestations	Surface Markers
Prolymphocytic leukemia (Plate 26B)	Often >100.0	PB	Medium to large lymphocytes with eccentric nucleus, clumped nuclear chromatin, prominent single nucleolus	Onset late adulthood Minimal lymphadenopathy, marked hepatosplenomegaly May be associated with monoclonal paraprotein Aggressive course with short survival	Pan-B, CD21 (C3dR) +/−, strong monoclonal SIg (IgM, IgG, or IgA), anomalous T (CD5) +/−, FMC7 (experimental antibody) Occasional cases are T lineage of helper or suppressor phenotype
		BM	Diffuse, moderate to heavy infiltration		
		LT	Diffuse, heavy infiltration of spleen		
Hairy cell leukemia (Plate 26A)	Decreased to 30.0 Often pancytopenic, monocytopenic	PB	Small to medium lymphocytes with abundant cytoplasm containing hair-like projections; number of abnormal cells may be small	Onset middle-aged adulthood, male predominance Minimal lymphadenopathy, moderate to marked splenomegaly May be associated with monoclonal paraproteins May have chronic course (2–10 yr)	Pan-B, strong monoclonal SIg (may show multiple heavy chains), FcR for IgG, plasma cell associated antigens, IL-2R, strong anomalous monocytoid (CD11c). Contains tartrate resistant acid phosphatase; occasional cases T-lineage associated with HTLV-II infection
		BM	Focal or diffuse heavy infiltration; mononuclear cells with abundant clear cytoplasm; predominance of ovoid shaped has better survival in earlier years than convoluted or indented nuclei; reticulin fibrosis (often dry tap)		

Leukemic phase of B-lymphoma (lymphosarcoma cell leukemia) (Plates 27B and 28A & B)	Normal to 30.0	LT	Initially present in splenic red pulp; lymph nodes spared until late in course	Pan-B, CD21 (C3dR) +/−, strong monoclonal SIg; small cleaved follicular may be CD10 (CALLA) positive
		PB	Medium-size lymphocytes, often with high N/C ratio and clefted nucleus in small cleaved lymphoma; large cell types of lymphoma may appear as large monocytoid or immunoblastic cells	Typically occurs with small cleaved follicular center cell lymphomas but may occur with widespread lymphoma of many histologic types. Prominent lymphadenopathy, minimal to moderate slenomegaly. Leukemic conversion of small cleaved cell lymphomas has no effect on survival, but conversion of large cell lymphomas associated with a very poor prognosis
		BM	Usually nodular infiltrate, but may be heavy and diffuse with widespread disease; occasionally may not be involved	
		LT	Shows histologic pattern of underlying lymphoma	

Abbreviations: WBC, white blood cell; PB, peripheral blood; BM, bone marrow; LT, lymphoid tissue; C3dR, receptor for third component of complement; SIg, surface immunoglobulin; FcR, receptor for Fc portion of immunoglobulin; IL-2R: receptor for interleukin-2, HTLV-II, human T cell leukemia/lymphoma virus type II. (Data from Rapaport,[1] Jandl,[2] and Kjeldsberg.[4])

Table 19-28. Leukemias of Differentiated T Lymphocytes (Peripheral or Post-thymic T-Cell Malignancies)

Disorder	WBC (×10⁹/L)	Morphology	Clinical Manifestations	Surface Markers

Large granular lymphocyte leukemia	Decreased to 30.0	PM
		  Medium to large lymphs with mature nuclear chromatin and azurophilic cytoplasmic granules
		BM
		  Usually diffuse infiltrate, but occasionally forcal
		LT
		  Infiltration of splenic red pulp cords, often with prominent germinal centers; infiltration of hepatic sinusoids may occur
			Onset variable, usually late
			Minimal lymphadenopathy, hepatomegaly, and skin involvement; approximately 50% have splenomegaly
			Associated with neutropenia, recurrent pyogenic infections, and autoimmune disorders, particularly rheumatoid arthritis; may find polyclonal gammopathy, immunocomplexes, antibodies to platelets and neutrophils
			Slowly progressive, chronic course
				Heterogeneous phenotypes with variable expression of pan-T, suppressor, and NK-associated antigens (CD16, CD56, CD57)
				Most common phenotype is CD3+, CD2+, CD57+, CD16+, or CD16- with rearrangement of T-cell receptor

Cutaneous T-cell lymphoma (mycosis fungoides, Sézary syndrome) (Plate 27A)	Normal to 20.0	PB
		  Small to large lymphs with cerebriform nuclei
		BM
		  Usually not involved until terminal phase
		LT
		  Early: scattered clusters of convoluted lymphs in paracortical areas of nodes
		Late: diffuse infiltrates in nodes, liver, spleen
			Onset late adulthood, male predominance
			Initially, plaques or nodules in skin (*Mycosis fungoides*), progressing to erythroderma with malignant cells in peripheral blood (Sézary syndrome)
			Lymphadenopathy, hepatosplenomegaly as disease progresses
			Random chromosomal abnormalities, often aneuploid
			Often chronic course
				Pan-T, helper subset (CD4)

T-helper CLL	30.0–700.0	PB Small, mature lymphs with irregular nuclear shape; no nucleoli; most, but not all, have agranular cytoplasm	Onset usually in young adults (<40 yr), nonendemic Marked lymphadenopathy, hepatosplenomegaly; extensive skin invasion; frequently CNS involvement; no mediastinal mass	Pan-T, usually helper subset (CD4); rarely, hybrid helper/suppressor (CD4/CD8) Rarely, punctate acid phosphatase or nonspecific acetate esterase in cytoplasm

(Continued)

Table 19-28. Leukemias of Differentiated T Lymphocytes (Peripheral or Post-thymic T-Cell Malignancies) *(Continued)*

Disorder	WBC (×10⁹/L)	Morphology	Clinical Manifestations	Surface Markers

		BM
		  Diffusely infiltrated
		LT
		  Diffusely infiltrated
			Often have 14q abnormalities
			Aggressive course (median survival 15 months)	

Adult T-cell leukemia/lymphoma	Normal to 30.0	PB
		  Medium-size lymphs with lobated or knobby nuclei; may have cytoplasmic granules
		BM
		  May be normal or have scattered infiltrates, even with large number of malignant cells in peripheral blood
		LT
		  Diffuse infiltration of large, or small and large cells
			Onset middle to late adulthood; endemic in SW Japan, Carribean, and somewhat in blacks in SE United States
			Lymphadenopathy, no mediastinal mass, skin lesions, lytic bone lesions, approximately 50% hepatosplenomegaly, frequent CNS involvement; presents as lymphoma in leukemic phase
			Associated with HTLV-I seropositivity, hypercalcemia, opportunistic infections; often have trisomy 7 or 7q-
			Aggressive course with short survival
				Pan-T, usually helper subset (CD4), CD25 (IL-2R), associated with anomalous suppressor activity

Leukemic phase of T-cell lymphoma (lymphosarcoma cell leukemia)	Variable	PB
		  Large cell type of lymphoma, appearing as large monocytoid or immunoblastic cells
		BM
		  Usually diffusely infiltrated
		LT
		  Shows histologic pattern of underlying lymphoma
			Rarely seen, usually as a terminal event with widespread disease	Variable pan-T and helper and/or suppressor; anomalous phenotypes, with absence of 1 or more pan-T markers

Abbreviations: WBC, white blood cell; PB, peripheral blood; BM, bone marrow; LT, lymphoid tissue; NK, natural killer; IL-2R, receptor for interleukin-2; CNS, central nervous system; SW, southwest; SE, southeast; HTLV-I, human T cell leukemia/lymphoma virus type I.
(Data from references 1, 2, 4, and 44.)

cellular phase of this disorder, but pancytopenia develops as marrow fibrosis progresses.

Bone marrow aspiration is often unsuccessful (dry tap) because of marrow fibrosis. However, the bone marrow biopsy is important in distinguishing MMM from other causes of leukoerythroblastic reaction, including acute leukemia, other MPD, replacement of bone marrow by metastatic tumor, or disseminated tuberculosis.[2] In the early stages of MMM, a reticulin stain may be necessary to detect early collagen increase. In addition to myelofibrosis, osteosclerosis (bony thickening) may occur. Myelofibrosis with myeloid metaplasia follows a progressive downhill course, with an average survival of 3–4 years.[15] In approximately 20% of patients, this transforms to an acute blastic phase.[15]

Leukemias of Differentiated Lymphocytes

Leukemias of differentiated lymphocytes include those of both B and T subtypes. The B-cell leukemias usually have monoclonal surface immunoglobulin, whereas differentiated T-cell leukemias are TdT negative, possess a variable phenotype of pan-T and/or natural killer (NK)-related antigens, and often are either of the helper or suppressor subtype. Gene rearrangement studies can demonstrate monoclonality for the T-cell receptor gene when pan-T antigens are present. The morphology, clinical manifestations, and associated surface marker antigens for these leukemias are presented in Tables 19-27 and 19-28. These lymphocytic leukemias must be distinguished from marked reactive lymphocytosis or lymphoid leukemoid reaction (Table 19-29). Although blood cell morphology and clinical presentation may be sufficient in making this distinction, bone marrow examination and/or lymphoid tissue biopsy are useful when malignancy is strongly suspected. Immunophenotyping and gene rearrangement studies may be helpful in selected cases.

Lymphoma

Lymphomas are malignancies of immune-related cells originating in the lymphoid tissues. They are divided into Hodgkin's and non-Hodgkin's lymphomas. Lymphadenopathy often is the presenting feature, but involvement frequently extends to the liver, spleen, and bone marrow. Non-Hodgkin's lymphomas may involve, and even originate in, extranodal sites, particularly lymphoid collections in the gastrointestinal tract. When lymphadenopathy occurs, the clinician must distinguish between reactive and neoplastic causes (Table 19-30). Clinical history and selective noninvasive tests usually can document the underlying cause. However, when lymphadenopathy persists without adequate explanation, or if malignancy is suspected, a lymph node biopsy must be performed.

Table 19-29. Differentiation of Lymphoid Leukemoid Reaction From Hematopoietic Malignancy)

	Lymphoid Leukemoid Reaction	Lymphoproliferative Malignancy
WBC differential[a]	Lymphocytes have heterogeneous appearance	Lymphocytes have monotonous appearance
Bone marrow[a]	Variable number of lymphoid cells—often no increase	Usually shows lymphoid infiltrate
Lymph node biopsy[a]	Morphologic evidence for reactive process; pathogens may be cultured	Morphologic evidence for malignant disorder

Immunophenotyping[a]	Polyclonal surface Ig light chain on B lymphocytes
	Heterogeneous T lymphocytes, frequently with activation antigens
		Early B- or T-lineage antigens in ALL
		Monoclonal surface Ig light chains in B-LP malignancy
		Often inconclusive results in
		    Post-thymic or peripheral T-LP malignancy
		    NK or large granular LP malignancy

Gene rearrangement[a]	No clonal change	Clonal rearrangement of Ig or T-receptor genes
Chromosomal analysis[a]	Normal diploid	May show abnormality

[a] See text for discussion of analytes.
Abbreviations: LP, lymphoproliferative; WBC, white blood cell; NK, natural killer (cells); Ig, immunoglobulin.

Table 19-30. Causes of Lymphadenopathy

Localized
  Local infection
    Pyogenic (e.g., pharyngitis, dental abscess, otitis media)
    Viral (e.g., cat scratch fever, lymphogranuloma venereum)
    Fungal (e.g., actinomycosis)
    Tuberculous
  Dermatopathic lymphadenopathy
  Postvaccinial lymphadenitis
  Histiocytic necrotizing lymphadenitis (Kikuchi's disease)
  Lymphoma
    Hodgkin's disease
    Non-Hodgkin's lymphoma
  Malignant disorders of macrophages
  Metastatic carcinoma and melanoma

Generalized
  Disseminated infection
    Bacterial (e.g., brucellosis, syphilis, Salmonella, endocarditis)
    Viral (e.g., infectious mononucleosis, measles, rubella, hepatitis)
    Fungal (e.g., histoplasmosis)
    Protozoal (e.g., toxoplasmosis)
    Tuberculous
  Inflammatory diseases
    Collagen vascular disorders (e.g., rheumatoid arthritis, lupus)
    Hyperthyroidism
    Sarcoidosis
    Serum sickness
  Drug reaction (e.g., hydantoins, beryllium)
  AIDS-related lymphadenopathy
  Kaposi sarcoma
  Leukemias, especially ALL, CLL
  Lymphoma
    Hodgkin's disease
    Non-Hodgkin's lymphoma
  Malignant disorders of macrophages
  Metastatic carcinoma and melanoma (rare)
  Benign immune proliferations
    Angioimmunoblastic lymphadenopathy
    Sinus histiocytosis with massive lymphadenopathy
    Castleman's disease
    Mucocutaneous lymph node syndrome (Kawasaki disease)

Abbreviations: AIDS, acquired immunodeficiency syndrome; ALL, acute lymphocytic leukemia; CLL, chronic lymphocytic leukemia.
(Data from Dorfman and Warnke[60] and Hoffbrand and Pettit.[72])

Hodgkin's Disease. Hodgkin's disease (HD) is a hematopoietic malignancy characterized by the presence of giant cells, called Reed-Sternberg cells, admixed with variable numbers of reactive elements (small lymphocytes, plasma cells, eosinophils, histiocytes, and fibrous tissue). The lineage of the malignant Reed-Sternberg cell is still a matter of controversy. The Reed-Sternberg cell is frequently aneuploid and may have multiple chromosomal abnormalities. It classically appears as a large binucleate cell, with a halo around a prominent nucleolus, giving the cell an owl eye appearance. Morphologic variants may occur, including multinucleate forms and mononuclear forms with similar nuclear features. Histologically, HD is classified into four types, as shown in Table 19-31, reflecting a variable proportion of malignant Reed-Sternberg cells and reactive cells. Lymphocyte predominance and nodular sclerosing HD carry the best prognosis, but this may be attributable to frequent presentation at an early disease stage (see below).[15] Lymph node biopsy is essential to distinguish Hodgkin's disease from non-Hodgkin's lymphoma and other reactive lymphadenopathies.

Hodgkin's disease has a bimodal age distribution, with a peak incidence between ages 25–30 and after 50 years.[15] Painless and progressive cervical node enlargement is the first manifestation of HD in 60–80% of patients.[15] Mediastinal and para-aortic nodes also are frequently involved. Reactive peripheral blood findings in HD can include neutrophilia, thrombocytosis, monocytosis, and eosinopenia.[4] With extensive bone marrow involvement, pancytopenia can occur. Defective T-cell function and cellular immunity can result in increased susceptibility to infection.

Hodgkin's disease starts in a single group of lymph nodes and spreads in a predictable manner from one lymph node area to the next or to adjacent organs.[15] With improved therapy for HD, prognosis is more dependent on the stage or extent of disease rather than on histologic classification. Accurate staging (Table 19-32) is necessary for planning of therapy and can include liver and spleen scans, abdominal imaging techniques, bone marrow biopsy, exploratory laparotomy with removal of suspicious abdominal nodes, liver biopsy, and splenectomy. Patients with stages IA, IIA, and III$_1$A can be successfully treated with radiation therapy (~80% 10-year survival rate).[1] Patients with stage III$_2$ or IV, or with B symptoms, are more often treated with combination chemotherapy, with or without irradiation (~50% 10-year survival rate).[1] Patients treated with alkylating agents, particularly in combination with radiation, are at increased risk of the development of AML and aggressive non-Hodgkin's lymphoma; therefore, chemotherapy should be used only as necessary for more extensive disease stages.

Non-Hodgkin's Lymphomas. The non-Hodgkin's lymphomas (NHLs) arise from a clonal proliferation of

Table 19-31. Rye Histologic Classification of Hodgkin's Disease

Finding	Description
Lymphocyte predominance	Mature lymphocytes plus varying number of histiocytes Few R-S cells, although may have many R-S variants Associated with especially good prognosis
Nodular sclerosis	Nodules of lymphoid tissue, separated by thick bands of collagen Many R-S variants present in lacunar spaces (lacunar cells) Necrosis may be common
Mixed cellularity	Variable numbers of lymphocytes, reactive histiocytes, neutrophils, eosinophils, and plasma cells R-S cells and variants readily apparent
Lymphocyte depletion	Few lymphocytes, with numerous R-S cells and variants Often prominent necrosis and fibrosis Rare occurrence, associated with least favorable prognosis
R-S cell	A large bi- or multinucleated cell with abundant cytoplasm and prominent nucleoli, surrounded by a characteristic clear halo
R-S variants	Variant mononuclear forms of R-S cells with similar nuclear features Occasionally, the variants may be smaller, with more lobulated nuclei, particularly in the lymphocyte predominant form

Abbreviation: R-S, Reed-Sternberg.
(Data from Rapaport[1] and Kjeldsberg.[4])

a malignant cell of lymphoid origin. Unlike HD, NHL does not show contiguous lymph node spread and may be found in widely separated nodes and in extranodal sites. Extranodal involvement occurs most frequently in liver, spleen, bone marrow, kidneys, and, for T-cell lymphomas, in the skin.[15] Although the clinical stage of NHL is defined by the same criteria as for HD, most patients with NHL have widespread disease at the time of diagnosis. In contrast to HD, where clinical staging is important, the histology of the involved lymph nodes is the major predictor of prognosis and therapy in NHL. Important considerations include the patterns of malignant proliferation (follicular or nodular versus diffuse) and the cytology of the malignant cells (small or large size; normal or cleaved or blastic nucleus). The heterogeneous NHLs may to some extent reflect stages of T- and B-lymphocyte transformation in response to antigen stimulation.

Table 19-32. Ann Arbor Staging System for Hodgkin's Disease[a]

Stage	Description
I	Involvement of a single lymph node region (I) or localized involvement of a single extralymphatic organ or site (Ie)
II	Involvement of two or more lymph node regions on the same side of the diaphragm (II) or localized involvement of one extralymphatic site and one or more lymph node regions on the same side of the diaphragm (IIe)
III	Involvement of lymph node regions on both sides of the diaphragm (III), which may be accompanied by involvement of spleen (IIIs), or localized involvement of one extralymphatic site (IIIe), or both (IIIse)
III$_1$	Upper abdominal nodes (splenic hilum, celiac, portal) and/or spleen involvement
III$_2$	Lower abdominal node involvement (para-aortic, iliac, mesenteric)
IV	Diffuse or disseminated involvement of one or more extralymphatic organs with or without associated lymph node enlargement

[a] In addition, absence or presence of symptoms (fever, night sweats, severe pruritis, loss of >10% of body weight) is designated by A (absent) or B (present).
(Data from Kjeldsberg[4] and Rifkind et al.[15])

Many classification systems for NHL have been proposed over the years. Most recently, an international panel has developed a Working Formulation of Non-Hodgkin's Lymphomas for Clinical Usage[16] (Table 19-33). The Working Formulation divides the NHLs into three groups, low grade, intermediate grade, and high grade based on clinical prognosis and rate of progression. Even though the classification system recognizes better prognosis for follicular pattern and small nonblastic cells, lymphocyte phenotype is not considered.

Table 19-33. Working Formulation of Non-Hodgkin's Lymphomas for Clinical Usage

Low grade
  ML: Small lymphocytic
    Consistent with CLL
    Plasmacytoid
    Mantle zone
    Intermediate differentiated
  ML: Follicular
    Predominantly small cleaved cell (diffuse areas, sclerosis)
  ML: Follicular
    Mixed, small cleaved and large cell (diffuse areas, sclerosis)

Intermediate Grade
  ML: Follicular
    Predominantly large cell (diffuse areas, sclerosis)
  ML: Diffuse
    Small cleaved cell (sclerosis)
  ML: Diffuse
    Mixed, small and large cell (sclerosis, epithelioid cell component)
  ML: Diffuse
    Large cell (cleaved cell, noncleaved cell, sclerosis

High grade
  ML: Large cell, immunoblastic (plasmacytoid, clear cell, polymorphous, epithelioid cell component)
  ML: Lymphoblastic (convoluted cell, nonconvoluted cell)
  ML: Small noncleaved cell (Burkitt's, follicular areas)

Miscellaneous
  Composite
  Mycosis fungoides
  Histiocytic
  Extramedullary plasmacytoma
  Unclassifiable
  Other

Abbreviations: ML, malignant lymphoma; CLL, chronic myelocytic leukemia.
(Data from the Non-Hodgkin's Lymphoma Pathologic Classification Project.[16])

Low grade lymphomas, all follicular lymphomas, and the Burkitt variant of high grade lymphomas are always B lineage; high grade lymphoblastic lymphomas are T lineage. Other intermediate or high grade lymphoma subtypes may be either B or T lineage. The T-lineage lymphomas may have a worse prognosis and may be more refractory to chemotherapy than B-lineage lymphomas of the same morphologic subtype.[2] Both B and T-cell lymphomas frequently have abnormalities involving chromosome 14, the site of the heavy chain immunoglobulin gene and the T-receptor α chain gene.

The median age for occurrence of lymphoma is 50–60 years. The most prevalent histologic subtypes in adults are small lymphocytic and follicular small cleaved cell (low grade lymphomas) and diffuse small cleaved and diffuse large cell (intermediate grade lymphomas).[2] By contrast, when lymphomas do occur in children or adolescents, they are most frequently high grade.[4] An increased incidence is seen in patients with immunodeficiency syndromes or in patients who have received immunosuppressive drug regimens.

Low grade lymphomas progress slowly over many years and may even show spontaneous regression in more than 20% of patients.[15] However, they are widely disseminated at presentation and are not curable with chemotherapy. At least 50% of low grade lymphomas eventually evolve to an intermediate or high grade lymphoma. Once conversion has occurred, the patients may respond poorly to further chemotherapy, in contrast to de novo intermediate and high grade NHL. Paradoxically, intermediate and high grade lymphomas can be successfully treated with aggressive combination chemotherapy, with approximately 30% of patients achieving an apparent cure.[2]

At times, the distinction between NHL and lymphocytic leukemia may be blurred. Leukemia initially involves the blood and bone marrow, whereas lymphoma arises in the lymphoid tissues. However, as NHL spreads, malignant lymphoma cells enter the blood from the infiltration of the bone marrow or even directly from lymphoid tissues. When this occurs, the terms *lymphosarcoma cell leukemia* or *leukemic phase of lymphoma* are used. In addition, some lymphomas and leukemias represent proliferation of the same cell type.[1] These include (1) malignant lymphoma, small lymphocytic, and CLL; (2) malignant lymphoma, lymphoblastic, and T-ALL; and (3) malignant lymphoma, small noncleaved (Burkitt's variant), and B-ALL (L3).

Immunoproliferative Malignancies

Immunoproliferative malignancies are clonal proliferations of immunoglobulin producing plasma cells or B lymphocytes. The resulting monoclonal gammopathy is helpful in classifying the disease. Multiple myeloma usually is associated with abnormal IgG, IgA, or free light chains; Waldenström's macroglobulinemia with IgM; and heavy chain disease with μ, α, or γ heavy chain. The primary laboratory tests used in the diagnosis of these disorders are serum and urine electrophoresis and immunoelectrophoresis (see Ch. 8).

Multiple Myeloma. Multiple myeloma typically involves proliferation of plasma cells in the bone marrow. Rarely, large numbers of plasma cells can escape into the blood; when they exceed 2000/μL, the patient is said to have plasma cell leukemia.[15] Pancytopenia occurs because of extensive marrow infiltration. The myeloma cells can secrete an osteoclast-activating factor, which leads to increased osteolytic activity, producing bony lesions and hypercalcemia. The synthesis of large amounts of abnormal immunoglobulin, often with excess of light chains (Bence Jones protein), causes additional clinical findings, which can include renal failure, neuropathy (caused by amyloid formation), circulatory abnormalities (from hyperviscosity), bleeding tendency (from coating of the platelets with abnormal protein), and Raynaud's phenomenon (from cryoglobulin formation). The presence in the plasma of large amounts of asymmetrically charged protein results in rouleaux formation of the RBCs on peripheral blood smear and an increase in erythrocyte sedimentation rate.

Most patients with myeloma are 50–70 years of age, with a common initial complaint of skeletal pain produced by a pathologic bone fracture.[1] The diagnosis is usually based on the presence of monoclonal serum immunoglobulin or urine Bence Jones protein in combination with plasma cell infiltration of bone marrow or lytic bone lesions. In most cases, bone marrow aspirate will show large numbers of mature and/or immature plasma cells. However, patchy infiltration of the bone marrow may occur, and the plasma cells may be increased in some parts of the marrow, yet absent from others. Increases in plasma cells of up to 20–30% can be seen in reactive conditions producing polyclonal gammopathy. Abnormal plasma cell morphology, such as binucleate cells and inclusions, may be seen in both reactive and malignant conditions. However, the presence of large numbers of immature proplasmacytes (larger plasma cells with prominent nucleoli) occurs primarily in myeloma. Immunophenotyping of the marrow cells may be helpful in some cases to demonstrate that the plasma cells contain monoclonal cytoplasmic immunoglobulin. This is particularly true for the small (less than 1) percentage of nonsecretory myelomas with no detectable monoclonal serum or urine protein.[15] Like B-cell lymphoma, myeloma frequently shows abnormalities in chromosome 14, the location of the immunoglobulin heavy chain gene.

The prognosis in myeloma is related to the extent of disease. A staging system has been proposed based on tumor cell load, using the level of monoclonal protein, the presence of lytic lesions, elevation of serum calcium, and degree of anemia. In addition, serum β_2-microglobulin elevation correlates with disease extent and may be an additional useful predictor of survival.[1] Other factors connoting a poorer prognosis include renal disease and the presence of Bence Jones proteinuria, particularly λ light chain subtype.[15]

Chemotherapy with an alkylating agent and prednisone results in clinical improvement but does not seem to lengthen the median survival of 2–2½ years.[15] Chemotherapy for myeloma is associated with a high risk of therapy-related AML, which approaches 20% at 4–5 years.[15] Occasionally, myeloma presents as a solitary plasmacytoma, found in bone marrow or extramedullary sites. Many of these tumors, particularly those arising in the nasopharynx, may be successfully treated with radiation. Approximately 50% of these patients, however, will subsequently develop widespread myeloma.[15]

Waldenström's Macroglobulinemia. Waldenström's macroglobulinemia is a variant of a low grade malignant lymphoma (small lymphocytic, plasmacytoid) in which the neoplastic cells synthesize large amounts of monoclonal IgM. Predominant symptoms are related to hyperviscosity caused by this abnormal macroglobulin, including retinal hemorrhages, CNS symptoms, congestive heart failure, and abnormal bleeding (caused by coating of platelets). At times, this IgM may exhibit antibody activity, as a cold agglutinin or as an anti-IgG antibody with rheumatoid factor activity.[1]

Waldenström's macroglobulinemia occurs primarily in older patients. As in other low grade lymphomas, lymphadenopathy and hepatosplenomegaly are common; the lytic lesions and bone pain characteristic of myeloma are not observed. The bone marrow is infiltrated with a mixture of small lymphocytes, plasma cells, and plasmacytoid lymphocytes, which may also appear in the peripheral blood in late disease. Treatment with alkylating agent and plasmapheresis can control disease activity for many years.[1]

Heavy Chain Diseases. Heavy chain diseases are rare lymphoma-like immunoproliferative disorders in which the monoclonal protein consists of only heavy chains or heavy chain fragments. γ-Heavy chain disease involves a plasmacytoid lymphocytic proliferation in lymph nodes, liver, and spleen, with a predilection for the tonsillar tissue. α-Heavy chain disease patients appear to be a subset of patients with the Mediterranean form of intestinal lymphoma. Patients with μ-heavy chain secretion have an atypical form of CLL.[1]

Monoclonal Gammopathy of Unknown Significance. Monoclonal gammopathy associated with chronic infection or inflammatory disorders (particularly rheumatoid arthritis) or with non-B-lymphoid malignancies is termed secondary monoclonal gammopathy. Monoclonal gammopathy occurring without evidence of myeloma, other B-cell malignancy, or associated underlying conditions is called benign monoclonal gammopathy (BMG) or monoclonal gammopathy of unknown significance (MGUS). MGUS is seen increasingly with age, occurring in more than 3% of people over 70 years of age.[2] The monoclonal paraprotein usually is IgG and has a concentration of less than 3.0 g/dL (30 g/L), without associated urinary Bence Jones protein.[4] The bone marrow shows a mild increase in plasma cells, with a predominant number producing the monoclonal protein. Because approximately 10% of these patients develop myeloma within 5 years, it is important to follow these patients for signs of increased paraprotein production or clinical symptoms.[2] With sensitive high resolution agarose electrophoresis, however, as many as 5% of adults of all ages may have very small amounts of monoclonal proteins, without an increased incidence of myeloma.[2]

Malignancies of Macrophages

True malignancies of macrophages are a heterogeneous group of disorders. The histiocytosis X or Langerhans cell histiocytosis group of disorders include the benign localized eosinophilic granuloma and more severe, systemic Hand-Schuller-Christian and Letterer-Siwe diseases. It is thought that these tissue proliferations of macrophages may be a reaction to immunodeficiency, rather than to neoplasia.[2] Malignant histiocytosis is a rare disease characterized by rapid onset, pancytopenia, lymphadenopathy, and hepatosplenomegaly. Atypical macrophages may be found in the sinusoids of lymph nodes, liver, spleen, and in small numbers, in the bone marrow and peripheral blood smear. These atypical-appearing macrophages often demonstrate erythrophagocytosis, but this finding must be distinguished from reactive hemophagocytosis involving morphologically benign macrophages. The reactive hemophagocytic syndrome is seen with a variety of infections, usually in the setting of immunodeficiency.

Mast Cell Proliferation

Mast cell proliferations may be localized to the skin (urticaria pigmentosa) or may be systemic with involvement of liver, spleen, lymph nodes, gastrointestinal tract, and bone marrow. Approximately 15% of patients with systemic mastocytosis may transform to mast cell leukemia.[2] Mast cells resemble basophils in containing metachromatic granules with heparin and histamine but have an ovoid rather than segmented nucleus.

CELL COUNTS

Test: White Blood Cell (WBC) Count, White Cell Count, Leukocyte Count)[3,17-20]

Background and Selection

The WBC count is a basic hematologic test usually included with the hemoglobin (Hgb), hematocrit (Hct), RBC count, and RBC indices. The WBC count is often ordered along with other blood cell measurements as a screening test on routine physical, in prenatal evaluation, with admission to the hospital, or before a surgical procedure. However, its usefulness has been questioned in these situations, particularly in the asymptomatic patient. The WBC count is most useful in the patient with suspected primary hematologic disorder or infection. It is also appropriate during treatment with chemotherapeutic drugs or radiotherapy, which are toxic to the bone marrow, and to check for possible idiosyncratic myelosuppressive reactions to other medications. The WBC count is determined to monitor return of bone marrow function after suppressive therapy or bone marrow transplant. In conjunction with the percentage of neutrophils from the WBC differential, the absolute number of neutrophils can be calculated, and the severely neutropenic patient placed in protective isolation.

Although the WBC count is frequently ordered in patients with suspected infection, the sensitivity and specificity of elevated WBC count for infection are low. Thus, elevation of WBC count cannot be used to confirm infection when clinical suspicion is low, and normal WBC count does not exclude infection when clinical suspicion is high. In particular, the WBC count (and neutrophilia or increased bands) should not be used as an indicator of infection when other causes for leukocytosis (and neutrophilia or increased bands) are present. Common causes in hospitalized patients include trauma, surgery (within 36 hours), hemorrhage, hemolysis, postpartum state, diabetic ketoacidosis, tissue necrosis (including myocardial infarction), sickle cell crisis, and many medications (see Table 19-1). Corticosteroids cause leukocytosis and neutrophilia, but the number of band forms remains normal.

Terminology

The WBC count is usually included with other routine blood cell measurements parameters in a panel that may be called a hemogram or complete blood count (CBC). In very small laboratories, manual methods may be used for the blood cell count; in this case, the WBC count may be ordered separately from the RBC parameters.

Logistics

EDTA-anticoagulated blood is the preferred specimen. Heparinized blood is not acceptable because of platelet agglutination in many specimens, which can cause an apparent increase in WBC count. In addition, heparin may polymerize with the lysing reagents in certain instruments to cause spurious leukocytosis. Citrate-anticoagulated blood is occasionally used when an EDTA dependent platelet agglutinin is present, to avoid spurious leukocytosis; WBC values are then multiplied by 1.1 to correct for anticoagulant dilution (see Platelet Count). Newer instruments use only a 0.10-0.25-mL sample. Thus, capillary blood from neonates or children can be collected directly into EDTA-coated microcollection vials. Alternatively, capillary blood may be diluted directly into a measured amount of normal saline. Blood should be promptly mixed in anticoagulant to prevent clotting. The sample should not be diluted by intravenous fluid or, in the case of capillary blood, obtained by squeezing the finger or heel, which may dilute the specimen with tissue fluid. The WBC count is stable for at least 24 hours at room temperature and for 24-48 hours when refrigerated.

White blood cells are enumerated after RBCs are removed by a lysing reagent. In very small laboratories, they may be counted microscopically on a hemocytometer chamber. However, this manual method is time consuming and has a large coefficient of variation (~15-20% within the normal range). More commonly, the WBC count is performed on an instrument that counts particles by electrical impedance or laser light scatter. After dilution and RBC lysis, the WBCs are drawn through a narrow aperture at a fixed rate. The cells impede the passage of electrical current or scatter light, producing electronic signals or pulses proportional to the cell count. Because the pulse height or intensity of light scattered at particular angles is related to cell size, platelets and RBC stroma can be ignored by excluding the smaller particles.

Older hematology cell counters use lysing agents that completely strip the cytoplasm from the WBC, leaving bare nuclei for counting. However, newer hematology analyzers use weaker lysing reagents, shrinking the WBC cytoplasm about the nucleus. This technique enables the generation of a WBC histogram (see Fig. 19-1), based on cell volume. The volume histogram can be divided into different cell fractions, giving a partial WBC differential (see White Blood Cell Screening Differential). Detection of a large number of small particles at the lower end of this volume histogram can provide a warning of spurious elevation of the WBC count. Interference can be caused by nucleated RBCs, platelet clumps, large platelets, cryoglobulin, unlysed RBCs (particularly found when a large number of acanthocytes are present), megakaryocytic fragments, malaria inclusions, and circulating microorganisms. Laboratories usually correct the WBC count for the presence of nucleated RBCs by counting the number of nRBCs per 100 WBCs on the peripheral blood smear, then using the formula

$$\text{True WBC count} = (\text{instrument WBC count} \times 100)/(100 + [\# \text{nRBCs}/100 \text{WBCs}]).$$

However, this formula presumes that the cell counter includes all the nRBCs as part of the total WBC count, a situation that may not occur with all the newer automated cell counters.

Interpretation

Reference values for the WBC count vary among different studies, possibly caused by differences among ethnic groups. Representative values for different ages are shown in Table 19-34. In infants, the WBC count is high at birth but decreases to near adult levels during the first few days of life. The upper level for the WBC range remains slightly higher in children than in adults. Black patients have a lower limit for the WBC range ($\sim 3.6-3.8 \times 10^3/\mu L$ [$\sim 3.6-3.8 \times 10^9/L$]) because of a decreased lower limit for neutrophils (~1.1–1.2 × 10³/μL [~1.1–1.2 × 10⁹/L]). In elderly adults (above 65 years of age), the total WBC count tends to be lower (reference range, ~3.1–8.5 × 10³/μL [~3.1–8.5 × 10⁹/L]) because of a decrease in lymphocytes. In addition, the leukocyte count may not rise as high in response to infection in the elderly caused by a diminished marrow reserve of neutrophils.

Except in hematologic malignancy, the total WBC count is usually an index of the neutrophil count, the most prevalent WBC. Thus, causes of leukocytosis and leukopenia are most likely to be causes of neutrophilia and neutropenia (Tables 19-1 and 19-6). Lymphocytosis occurs with viral infection, which is occasionally of sufficient magnitude to elevate the WBC count, particularly in children. When unexpected abnormalities in the WBC count occur, a WBC differential is performed to characterize the cells further. If a malignant WBC disorder is suspected after examination of the peripheral blood smear or if unexplained leukopenia (and neutropenia) persists, a bone marrow examination should be performed.

Test: White Blood Cell Slide Differential (Differential WBC Count, Leukocyte Differential, Manual Differential)[3,4,19–26]

Background and Selection

The WBC slide differential is a microscopic classification of the various WBC subtypes. Absolute numbers of the cell types are obtained by multiplying the percentage of each type by the WBC count. The WBC differential is an appropriate diagnostic test in the patient with a suspected primary hematologic disorder or with unexplained leukocytosis, leukopenia, anemia, polycythemia, thrombocytopenia, or thrombocytosis. Quantitative abnormalities also are used as evidence in support of suspected infection. The WBC differential is monitored at frequent intervals in patients treated with chemotherapeutic drugs or radiotherapy, which are toxic to the marrow, and after myelosuppressive therapy or bone marrow transplant, to assess return of marrow function. In patients with bone marrow suppression, the absolute number of neutrophils is important in determining the need for protective isolation.

Although the WBC differential is sometimes performed as a routine component of the CBC, its value as a screening test has been questioned. The 100-cell count manual differential is a labor-intensive (and expensive) test, is very imprecise, and has poor sensitivity and specificity. It appears to have little value as a screening procedure in the ambulatory care setting, in routine admission to the hospital, or in ambulatory surgery patients. Often, the WBC differential is ordered in suspected bacterial infection. However, the occurrence of neutrophilia is nonspecific and cannot be used as an indicator of bacterial infection when other causes of neutrophilia (and leukocytosis) are present (Table 19-1).

More recently, most larger automated hematology instruments are used to perform a screening WBC differential with the other hemogram parameters. The percentage and absolute values of total neutrophils (bands and segmented) and lymphocytes are reported; with some instruments, monocytes, eosinophils, and basophils can be reported as well. Cell fractions are more precisely enumerated, because a larger number of cells (usually 10,000 cells) are classified. The screening differential can replace the manual slide differential when enumeration of neutrophils is of interest, for example, in suspected infection or monitoring of therapy-related neutropenia. The presence of significant numbers of abnormal cells or immature granulocytes (usually more than 5%) or severe leukopenia (e.g., WBC count less than 1.0 × 10³/μL [<1.0 × 10⁹/L] on some instruments) may interfere with the automated differential and result in flagging of the specimen results. A manual differential will be necessary for these specimens to generate correct quantitative results and to assess the presence of abnormal cells.

Although the automated differential does not enumerate band neutrophils, the situations are limited in which the band count alone is significant. The reliability of the band percentage in the manual differential is extremely poor, because of both random variation in the 100-cell count and lack of consistency among technologists in identifying bands. This problem is illustrated by the wide variation in the reference range quoted for bands, the mean counts ranging from 3–9.5%. Elevation in bands generally parallels the elevation in neutrophils. Few cases of infectious or inflammatory disorders are seen in which elevation in bands is not accompanied by either neutrophilia, leukocytosis, or fever, parameters that are more precisely measured. However, enumeration of bands may be more useful than total neutrophils or WBC count in detecting infection or inflammation in a few specific groups of patients: (1) neonates, in whom the WBCs and neutrophils may be transiently elevated with crying; (2) elderly patients and patients treated with chemotherapy, who have limited bone marrow reserve and cannot respond to stimuli with an elevated WBC count or neutrophilia; and (3) patients receiving corticosteroid therapy, who consistently have elevation of segmented neutrophils with normal band neutrophils.

Terminology

In some laboratories, the WBC differential from the blood smear is included with the cell analyzer results when a hemogram or CBC is ordered, whereas in others a separate request is required, or the slide differential is performed only when certain parameters from the automated counts are abnormal. In laboratories with newer instruments that include the automated screening differential as part of the CBC, the slide differential may be performed only when certain abnormalities occur in the screening differential or hemogram or when the physician specifically requests a manual slide differential.

Logistics

Blood smears are prepared from either finger or heel puncture capillary blood or from EDTA-anticoagulated venous blood. Heparinized blood should not be used, because the basophilic anticoagulant will give a blue hue to the stained slide. If EDTA anticoagulant is used, smears should be prepared within 2 hours for best morphology; however, smears prepared even 6-12 hours after blood collection may be adequate for identification of normal cells. A small drop of blood is placed on one end of a slide and spread by means of another slide at a 30-45-degree angle. The well made smear has a wedge shape and covers approximately one-half of the slide. In a few laboratories, slides are produced with centrifugal devices. These blood smears may have a more random distribution of WBCs, as opposed to the wedge smears which tend to concentrate lymphocytes in the center and neutrophils toward the edges. In the leukopenic patient, buffy coat slides may be prepared to concentrate the WBCs. Blood is centrifuged in a long, narrow tube, and the WBC layer is aspirated, along with a small amount of plasma and RBCs. Wedge smears are prepared from this mixture. However, sedimentation of WBCs is not uniform, and these smears contain a much lower proportion of neutrophils than does the original blood.

Blood smears are stained with a Romanowsky stain, such as Wright or Wright-Giemsa. These stains contain various combinations of methylene blue, oxidation products of methylene blue, and eosin. Adjustment of time in the stain, in a stain-buffer mixture, and in the buffer alone as well as the buffer pH produces the optimal color characteristics. The nuclei of the leukocytes should be purplish blue (not violet), whereas the neutrophil cytoplasm should have tan nonspecific neutrophils granules and violet primary azurophilic granules.

The optimal area of the smear for the leukocyte differential is the area in which approximately 50% of the RBCs overlap to the region in which the RBCs show a tendency toward linear orientation. Examination of the thicker areas of the smear can result in misidentification of the WBC types.

The smear is examined in a "battlement" pattern, moving cross-wise from one lateral edge to another. Usually, 100-200 consecutive WBCs are identified and classified by the examiner. The results are expressed as a percentage of all WBCs counted. Nucleated RBCs or megakaryocytic fragments are reported as the number seen per 100 leukocytes. Other morphologic abnormalities are noted, including toxic granulation and Döhle bodies in neutrophils, bilobed nuclei or nuclear hypersegmentation of neutrophils, or dysplastic changes. Photomicrographs and descriptions of WBC types and morphologic variations are discussed in Chapter 16.

During the 1970s, pattern recognition or image analysis technology was introduced to automate the slide differential. These instruments classify cells by computer analysis of video images, storing abnormal or atypical cells for operator identification. Although accurate in cell classification, these instruments only count 100-200 cells and suffer from the same degree of imprecision as the manual differential. Since the introduction of screening differentials on automated cell counters, these image analysis instruments are no longer manufactured.

Interpretation

Reference values for the WBC slide differential vary greatly among different studies, because of the large imprecision of the 100-cell count differential. In addition, differences between ethnic groups and diurnal variation of neutrophils also may occur. Representative reference ranges for the various types of cells are given in Table 19-34. Black persons have a decreased lower limit for neutrophils ($\sim 1.1-1.2 \times 10^3/\mu L$ [$\sim 1.1-1.2 \times 10^9/L$]).

Quantitative changes in cell types have numerous etiologies, as presented in Tables 19-1 to 19-8. The most frequently encountered quantitative abnormality is neutrophilia (Table 19-1). Common causes of neutrophilia include infection (usually bacterial), inflammation, tissue necrosis (including myocardial infarction), trauma, surgery (within 36 hours), hemorrhage, hemolysis, postpartum state, diabetic ketoacidosis, sickle cell crisis, early viral infection, and many medications. The presence of an increased number of band or less mature neutrophils (with or without an increase in total neutrophils) is referred to as a left shift.

Neutrophilia can occur within minutes of stimulation caused by the redistribution of peripheral blood neutrophils from the marginated to circulating pool. The maximal response with demargination is a doubling of the number of neutrophils; this increase occurs without left shift or increase in band neutrophils. Acute demargination of neutrophils is seen with severe pain, exercise, or other transient stress and appears to be mediated by epinephrine and/or corticosteroid release (physiologic neutrophilia). With more prolonged stimuli or tissue damage, marrow storage pool neutrophils are released within 4–24 hours, capable of increasing the blood neutrophils up to 10-fold. A left shift may result from the release of immature neutrophils from the bone marrow storage pool. Chronic stimulus results in increased marrow granulopoiesis and hypercellular marrow within 1–2 weeks. With normal marrow function, neutrophilia can be sustained, despite increased flow of neutrophils to the inflammatory site. Finally, decreased egress of neutrophils from the circulation may produce neutrophilia and is thought to be a mechanism contributing to the neutrophilia caused by corticosteroids.

Neutrophilia may not occur in the presence of appropriate stimuli if tissue demand for neutrophils is extremely great or if the bone marrow has limited reserve (e.g., in patients receiving marrow-suppressive therapy or in elderly patients). In these cases, normal to decreased numbers of neutrophils with left shift will be present in the peripheral blood; with extreme marrow stress, an occasional blast and promyelocyte may be found as well.

Occasionally, a marked neutrophilic leukocytosis may occur with the WBC count exceeding $50.0 \times 10^3/\mu L$ ($>50.0 \times 10^9/L$), often accompanied by left shift. This is termed a *leukemoid reaction,* and it is important to distinguish this reactive response from malignant myeloproliferative disorders, particularly CML. Disorders associated with myeloid leukemoid reactions are listed in Table 19-11. Table 19-24 presents useful features to help differentiate leukemoid reaction from CML.

Causes of lymphocytosis are listed in Table 19-2. Children younger than 5 years of age have a predominance of lymphocytes in the peripheral blood; appropriate age-related normal values must be used in assessing lymphocytosis in this group. Lymphocytosis is often caused by viral infections; lasts 3–6 weeks; and is accompanied by fever, pharyngitis, exanthems, or malaise. Many causes of lymphocytosis are accompanied by various forms of atypical or reactive lymphocytes (Plate 10A & B). These represent stimulated lymphocytes that are responding to the presence of antigen. Reactive lymphocytes may be particularly prominent (more than 20% of WBC differential) in infectious mononucleosis, hepatitis, cytomegalovirus, (CMV) infections, and drug hypersensitivity reaction. Reactive lymphocytes in these viral infections are predominantly activated T lymphocytes, frequently containing cytoplasmic granules (lysosomes). In infectious mononucleosis, the Epstein-Barr virus (EBV) infects and transforms the B lymphocytes; the reactive lymphocytes in the peripheral blood represent activated suppressor T lymphocytes, which kill the EBV-transformed B cells. Serologic tests for viral agents, including the EBV, may be useful when viral infection is suspected as a cause of lymphocytosis (see Ch. 29).

High counts of normal lymphocytes or the presence many immature-appearing forms of reactive lymphocytes may simulate lymphocytic leukemias (lymphoid leukemoid reaction). Causes are listed in Table 19-11. Benign lymphocytosis can often be differentiated from malignant processes by the heterogeneous appearance of the reactive lymphocytes on the peripheral blood smear. However, persistent unexplained lymphocytosis may require further investigation, including immunophenotyping, bone marrow examination, and biopsy of enlarged lymph nodes.

Causes of monocytosis are shown in Table 19-3. Indolent infectious disease with tissue destruction (e.g., tuberculosis, subacute bacterial endocarditis) was a common cause of monocytosis in the past. Currently, monocytosis is most often associated with malignancies (hematologic and nonhematologic) and collagen vascular disorders. When infection is present, monocytes and tissue macrophages are activated and may phagocytose RBCs, WBCs, and platelets.

As shown in Table 19-4, eosinophilia has a multitude of causes. Most common causes are allergic reactions, skin diseases, and parasitic infection (particularly with tissue infestation). Persistent absolute eosinophilia, with eosinophils greater than 10%, can be evaluated by (1) serologic tests for parasites or stool examination;

Table 19-34. Reference Values for White Blood Cell Count and Slide Differential

Age	Leukocytes (total) (×10⁹/L)	Neutrophils (×10⁹/L) Total	Band	Segmented	Eosinophils	Basophils	Lymphocytes	Monocytes
At birth	18.1 (9.0–30.0)[a]	11.0 (6.0–26.0) 61%[b]	1.61 9.1%	9.4 52%	0.40 (0.02–0.85) 2.2%	0.10 (0–0.64) 0.6%	5.5 (2.0–11.0) 31%	1.05 (0.40–3.1) 5.8%
12 hours	22.8 (13.0–38.0)	15.5 (6.0–28.0) 68%	2.33 10.2	13.2 58%	0.45 (0.02–0.95) 2.0%	0.10 (0–0.50) 0.4%	5.5 (2.0–11.0) 24%	1.20 (0.40–3.6) 5.3%
24 hours	18.9 (9.4–34.0)	11.5 (5.0–21.0) 61%	1.75 9.2%	9.8 52%	0.45 (0.05–1.00) 2.4%	0.10 (0–0.30) 0.5%	5.8 (2.0–11.5) 31%	1.10 (0.20–3.1) 5.8%
1 week	12.2 (5.0–21.0)	5.5 (1.5–10.0) 45%	0.83 6.8%	4.7 39%	0.50 (0.07–1.10) 4.1%	0.05 (0–0.25) 0.4%	5.0 (2.0–17.0) 41%	1.10 (0.30–2.7) 9.1%
2 weeks	11.4 (5.0–20.0)	4.5 (1.0–9.5) 40%	0.63 5.5%	3.9 34%	0.35 (0.07–1.00) 3.1%	0.05 (0–0.23) 0.4%	5.5 (2.0–17.0) 48%	1.00 (0.20–2.4) 8.8%
4 weeks	10.8 (5.0–19.5)	3.8 (1.0–9.0) 35%	0.49 4.5%	3.3 30%	0.30 (0.07–0.90) 2.8%	0.05 (0–0.20) 0.5%	6.0 (2.5–16.5) 56%	0.70 (0.15–2.0) 6.5%
2 months	11.0 (5.5–18.0)	3.8 (1.0–9.0) 34%	0.49 4.4%	3.3 30%	0.30 (0.07–0.85) 2.7%	0.05 (0–0.20) 0.5%	6.3 (3.0–16.0) 57%	0.65 (0.13–1.8) 5.9%
4 months	11.5 (6.0–17.5)	3.8 (1.0–9.0) 33%	0.45 3.9%	3.3 29%	0.30 (0.07–0.80) 2.6%	0.05 (0–0.20) 0.4%	6.8 (3.5–14.5) 59%	0.60 (0.10–1.5) 5.2%
6 months	11.9 (6.0–17.5)	3.8 (1.0–8.5) 32%	0.45 3.8%	3.3 28%	0.30 (0.07–0.75) 2.5%	0.05 (0–0.20) 0.4%	7.3 (4.0–13.5) 61%	0.58 (0.10–1.3) 4.8%
8 months	12.2 (6.0–17.5)	3.7 (1.0–8.5) 30%	0.41 3.3%	3.3 27%	0.30 (0.07–0.70) 2.5%	0.05 (0–0.20) 0.4%	7.6 (4.5–12.5) 62%	0.58 (0.08–1.2) 4.7%
10 months	12.0 (6.0–17.5)	3.6 (1.0–8.5) 30%	0.40 3.3%	3.2 27%	0.30 (0.06–0.70) 2.5%	0.05 (0.–0.20) 0.4%	7.5 (4.5–11.5) 63%	0.55 (0.05–1.2) 4.6%

Age							
12 months	11.4 (6.0–17.5)	3.5 (1.5–8.5) 31%	0.35 3.1%	3.2 28%	0.30 (0.05–0.70) 2.6%	0.05 (0–0.20) 0.4%	7.0 (4.0–10.5) 61%	0.55 (0.05–1.1) 4.8%
2 years	10.6 (6.0–17.0)	3.5 (1.5–8.5) 33%	0.32 3.0%	3.2 30%	0.28 (0.04–0.65) 2.6%	0.05 (0–0.20) 0.5%	6.3 (3.0–9.5) 59%	0.53 (0.05–1.0) 5.0%
4 years	9.1 (5.5–15.5)	3.8 (1.5–8.5) 42%	0.27 (0–1.0) 3.0%	3.5 (1.5–7.5) 39%	0.25 (0.02–0.65) 2.8%	0.05 (0–0.20) 0.6%	4.5 (2.0–8.0) 50%	0.45 (0–0.8) 5.0%
6 years	8.5 (5.0–14.5)	4.3 (1.5–8.0) 51%	0.25 (0–1.0) 3.0%	4.0 (1.5–7.0) 48%	0.23 (0–0.65) 2.7%	0.05 (0–0.20) 0.6%	3.5 (1.5–7.0) 42%	0.40 (0–0.8) 4.7%
8 years	8.3 (4.5–13.5)	4.4 (1.5–8.0) 53%	0.25 (0–1.0) 3.0%	4.1 (1.5–7.0) 50%	0.20 (0–0.50) 2.4%	0.05 (0–0.20) 0.6%	3.3 (1.5–6.8) 39%	0.35 (0–0.8) 4.2%
10 years	8.1 (4.5–13.5)	4.4 (1.8–8.0) 54%	0.24 (0–1.0) 3.0%	4.2 (1.8–7.0) 51%	0.20 (0–0.60) 2.4%	0.04 (0–0.20) 0.5%	3.1 (1.5–6.5) 38%	0.35 (0–0.8) 4.3%
12 years	8.0 (4.5–13.5)	4.4 (1.8–8.0) 55%	0.25 (0–1.0) 3.0%	4.2 (1.8–7.0) 52%	0.20 (0–0.55) 2.5%	0.04 (0–0.20) 0.5%	3.0 (1.2–6.0) 38%	0.35 (0–0.8) 4.4%
14 years	7.9 (4.5–13.0)	4.4 (1.8–8.0) 56%	0.24 (0–1.0) 3.0%	4.2 (1.8–7.0) 53%	0.20 (0–0.50) 2.5%	0.04 (0–0.20) 0.5%	2.9 (1.2–5.8) 37%	0.38 (0–0.8) 4.7%
16 years	7.8 (4.5–13.0)	4.4 (1.8–8.0) 57%	0.23 3.0%	4.2 54%	0.20 (0–0.50) 2.6%	0.04 (0–0.20) 0.5%	2.8 (1.2–5.2) 35%	0.40 (0–0.8) 5.1%
18 years	7.7 (4.5–12.5)	4.4 (1.8–7.7) 57%	0.23 3.0%	4.2 54%	0.20 (0–0.45) 2.6%	0.04 (0–0.20) 0.5%	2.7 (1.0–5.0) 35%	0.40 (0–0.8) 5.2%
20 years	7.5 (4.5–11.5)	4.4 (1.8–7.7) 59%	0.23 (0–0.07) 3.0%	4.29 (1.8–7.0) 56%	0.20 (0–0.45) 2.7%	0.04 (0–0.20) 0.5%	2.5 (1.0–4.8) 33%	0.38 (0–0.8) 5.2%
21 years	7.4 (4.5–11.0)	4.4 (1.8–7.7) 59%	0.22 (0–0.7) 3.0%	4.2 (1.8–7.0) 56%	0.20 (0–0.45) 2.7%	0.04 (0–0.20) 0.5%	2.5 (1.0–4.8) 34%	0.30 (0–0.8) 4.0%

[a] Mean (95% confidence) for most absolute values.
[b] Mean only for percentage values.
(Data from Altman and Dittmer.[30])

(2) determination of IgE, which is usually elevated in allergic eosinophilia; (3) chest x-ray to look for sarcoidosis or pulmonary eosinophilic syndromes; and (4) biopsy of lymph nodes, if enlarged, to exclude Hodgkin's disease. Bone marrow examination is rarely helpful except to obtain material for chromosomal analysis, if CML is suspected.

Disorders associated with basophilia are shown in Table 19-5. The presence of increased basophils in association with neutrophilic proliferation suggests a myeloproliferative disorder, such as CML or polycythemia vera. In the terminal or acceleration phase of CML, very large numbers of basophils (more than 30%) sometimes may be found.

Mechanisms producing neutropenia include bone marrow suppression, ineffective granulopoiesis (often caused by intramedullary destruction of the more mature granulocytes), reduced survival in peripheral blood (caused by increased demand in tissues or destruction by antineutrophil antibody), and pseudoneutropenia (with shift from the circulating to the marginal neutrophil pool). Increased risk of infection is present when neutrophils are less than $1.0 \times 10^3/\mu L$ ($<1.0 \times 10^9/L$) and the risk of severe infection is pronounced when neutrophils are less than $0.5 \times 10^3/\mu L$ ($<0.5 \times 10^9/L$). Causes for neutropenia are shown in Table 19-6. Drugs are an important cause of neutropenia and may act by multiple mechanisms. Thus, the neutropenia of drug toxicity is associated with a hypocellular bone marrow or a hypercellular marrow, particularly with a partial arrest in granulocytic maturation. Bone marrow examination may be indicated in persistent neutropenia when accompanied by anemia and thrombocytopenia or when immature WBCs, dysplastic WBCs or nucleated RBCs are seen in the peripheral blood smear.

Lymphocytopenia may be seen in hereditary syndromes or AIDS, but most frequent causes are stress, collagen vascular disease, and severe cachexia (Table 19-7). Treatment with corticosteroids, alkylating agents, and radiation also decreases the number of lymphocytes. Even localized irradiation can lead to destruction of circulating lymphocytes as they pass through the affected area. Immunodeficiency syndromes are discussed further in Chapter 29.

Monocytopenia, eosinopenia, and basopenia are difficult to assess by the routine blood smear differential, because these cells normally occur in low numbers. When direct chamber counting or special cytochemical techniques have been used, low numbers of these cells have been associated with the conditions listed in Table 19-8.

The significance of day-to-day quantitative changes in the WBC differential must be interpreted in light of the large sampling variation. Confidence limits of 95% for the percentage of cells obtained in the 100-cell count differential are illustrated in Table 19-35. For example, if 5% of a cell type is reported, the true value could be 1–12% and, if 50% is reported, the true value would be 39–61%. These confidence ranges are based solely on chance variation in the cells selected for counting on the slide. For cell classifications with large intraobserver variability (e.g., identification of band neutrophils), even larger confidence intervals are seen.

Leukoerythroblastic reaction refers to the presence of both nucleated RBCs and immature granulocytes (blasts, promyelocytes, or myelocytes) in the peripheral blood smear (Table 19-36). Proposed mechanisms for this finding include (1) infiltration of the marrow by malignant cells, "forcing out" immature cells of the myeloid and erythroid line; (2) damage of the sinusoidal blood-marrow barrier, by infiltration or fibrosis of the marrow; (3) extramedullary hematopoiesis (e.g., in spleen or liver), occurring with either marrow infiltration or severe marrow stress. In one prospective study, 63% of leukoerythroblastic reactions were associated

Table 19-35. Confidence Limits (95%) for Percentages of Cells Reported in the 100-Cell Count Manual Differential

% Reported	Range	% Reported	Range
0	0–4	100	96–100
1	0–6	99	94–100
2	0–8	98	92–100
3	0–9	97	91–100
4	1–10	96	90–99
5	1–12	95	88–99
6	2–13	94	87–100
7	2–14	93	86–98
8	3–16	92	84–97
9	4–17	91	83–96
10	4–18	90	82–96
15	8–24	85	76–92
20	12–30	80	70–88
25	16–35	75	65–84
30	21–40	70	60–79
35	25–46	65	54–75
40	30–51	60	49–70
45	35–56	55	44–65
50	39–61	—	—

(Data from Rumke.[73])

Table 19-36. Causes of Leukoerythroblastic Reaction
Infancy
Hematologic malignancies: AML, ALL, chronic myeloproliferative disorders, myelodysplastic syndromes, lymphoma (with marrow involvement)
Solid tumors, with bone marrow metastases
Gaucher's disease
Hemorrhage
Hemolytic anemia
Severe anoxia
Severe infection
Recovery from bone marrow suppression or transplant
Postsplenectomy (rare)

Abbreviations: AML, acute myelocytic leukemia; ALL, acute lymphocytic leukemia.
(Data from Koepke[18] and Weick et al.[25])

with malignancy, including acute leukemia, myeloproliferative disorders, and other malignancies involving the bone marrow. In patients with known metastatic malignancy, the development of a leukoerythroblastic reaction invariably signifies bone marrow metastases. Common nonmalignant causes include hemolysis and blood loss. Leukoerythroblastic reaction also may occur acutely with severe anoxic stress or severe infection, presumably caused by marrow storage pool release.

Toxic granulation and Döhle bodies (Plate 9A & B) are found in neutrophils in a variety of infections, or with burns, trauma, pregnancy, cancer, and many cytotoxic agents. Toxic granulation (an increase in azurophilic lysosomal granules) may be caused by stimulation of bone marrow production with decreased marrow transit time or increased granule permeability to stain. Döhle bodies (pale blue inclusions near the neutrophil periphery) represent liquified endoplasmic reticulum. Toxic granulation and Döhle bodies are particularly numerous in severe, systemic infection, and may be accompanied by phagocytic vacuoles in the cytoplasm.

Inherited morphologic abnormalities (Table 19-12) of WBCs include May-Hegglin anomaly (Döhle-like bodies in neutrophils with giant platelets), Alder-Reilly anomaly (prominent azurophilic granules in WBCs), Pelger-Huët anomaly (hyposegmented neutrophils with hyperclumping of chromatin), and hereditary hypersegmentation (hypersegmented neutrophils). Neutrophil function is usually normal in these disorders, and the clinical course is often benign. White blood cells with prominent azurophilic granules similar to those found in the Alder-Reilly anomaly can be associated with the mucopolysaccharidoses. Inherited disorders of neutrophil function (Table 19-14) usually have normal-appearing neutrophils. The exception is the Chédiak-Higashi syndrome, which shows giant fusion granules in neutrophils, monocytes, and lymphocytes. Large numbers of blasts or other abnormal cells may appear in the blood in malignant diseases of WBCs. Descriptions of peripheral blood findings in various acute and chronic leukemias can be found in Tables 19-22, 19-24, 19-26, and 19-27 to 19-30.

When abnormal cells are found on a slide differential, their identification should be confirmed by an experienced technologist or physician. A bone marrow examination is usually performed when a hematologic malignancy is suspected or when neutropenia persists without explanation. Immunophenotyping and leukocyte cytochemistry are helpful in identifying the blast lineage in acute leukemia or in evaluation of persistent lymphocytosis in the adult. Leukocyte alkaline phosphatase and cytogenetics for the identification of the Philadelphia chromosome are helpful in distinguishing a myeloid leukemoid reaction from CML.

Test: White Blood Cell Screening Differential (Screening Differential, Automated Differential)[18-21,28-31]

Background and Selection

The WBC screening differential classifies the major cell types by physicochemical properties in solution rather than by morphologic appearance. These characteristics may include electronic pulse height (related to volume), light scatter at various angles (related to volume and cytoplasmic content), radiofrequency pulse height (related to nuclear complexity), cytochemistry (related to lysosomal peroxidase content), and resistance to various lysing solutions. The instruments report the percentage and absolute values of total neutrophils (bands and segmented) and lymphocytes; some instruments can also enumerate monocytes, eosinophils, and basophils. Precision for quantitative results is much better than the manual differential, because a large number of cells (usually 10,000) are classified.

A screening differential should be ordered, rather than the slide differential, when a primary hematologic disorder is not suspected and quantitative differential results are of interest. This includes assessment of neutrophilia for evidence of infection and monitoring neutropenia when myelosuppressive therapy is given or when the WBC count is falling. Although the automated differential does not measure band neutrophils, the situations are limited in which the band count is elevated without neutrophilia. However, enumeration of bands on the slide differential may be useful in (1) neonates, where the WBC count and neutrophils may be transiently elevated with crying; (2) elderly patients and patients treated with chemotherapy, who have limited bone marrow reserve and cannot respond to stimuli with an elevated WBC count or neutrophilia; and (3) patients receiving corticosteroid therapy, who consistently have elevation of segmented neutrophils with normal band neutrophils.

Terminology

Some laboratories include the WBC screening differential with the cell analyzer results when a hemogram or CBC is ordered, whereas others require a separate request. Laboratories that include the automated screening differential as part of the CBC may perform the slide differential only when certain abnormalities occur in the screening differential or hemogram or when the physician specifically requests a manual slide differential.

Logistics

EDTA-anticoagulated blood is used. Other anticoagulants are not acceptable because they alter the expected WBC volume and light scattering properties. Blood should be mixed promptly to prevent clotting, which also alters the physicochemical characteristics of the WBCs. Screening differentials based on electronic pulse volume measurements may require an equilibrium period of 15–30 minutes in anticoagulant before valid results can be obtained, and blood usually cannot be analyzed after 5–6 hours of storage. However, the cytochemical screening differential parameters are stable for a minimum of 24 hours at room temperature and 54 hours when refrigerated.

The electrical impedance methods use a weak lysing reagent, which shrinks the lymphocytes to one-half the original volume and granulocytes to two-thirds the original volume (due to the cytoplasmic granules). With normal blood, three separate volume fractions are obtained (lymphocyte, mononuclear, and granulocyte), as illustrated for the Coulter S-Plus IV instrument in Figure 19-1. When valleys are not found at the appropriate R regions, incomplete separation between the fractions occurs. The affected cell fractions are R flagged and will not have valid screening differential results. Abnormalities causing interference at each R region are also shown in Figure 19-1. In particular, R1 flags at the lower WBC counting threshold should initiate a search for platelet clumps and nRBC on the blood smear.

In the cytochemical screening differential (Technicon H-1), WBCs are stained for myeloperoxidase activity after lysis of RBCs. A plot of light absorbance (from the intensity of precipated stain) and forward angle light scatter (a measure of cell size) is constructed (Fig. 19-2). Distinct cell clusters of neutrophils, monocytes, eosinophils, and lymphocytes can be identified. Abnor-

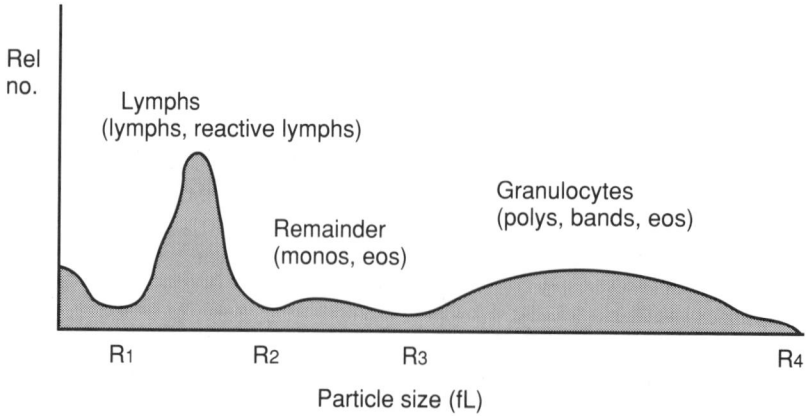

Fig. 19-1. White blood cell screening differential (volumetric method). With various abnormalities, the R1-R4 valleys are obliterated and the sample flagged. Causes of interference at the various R-regions are as follows. R1: nRBC, platelet clumps, large platelets, fibrin, cryoglobulin, small lymphocytes (as in CLL), unlysed red blood cells, malaria, microorganisms. R2: Reactive lymphocytes, malignant lymphoid cells, blasts, basophilia, stored sample, clotted sample. R3: Eosinophilia, monocytosis, immature granulocytes, ingested microorganisms, blasts, stored sample, clotted sample. R4: High granulocyte count.

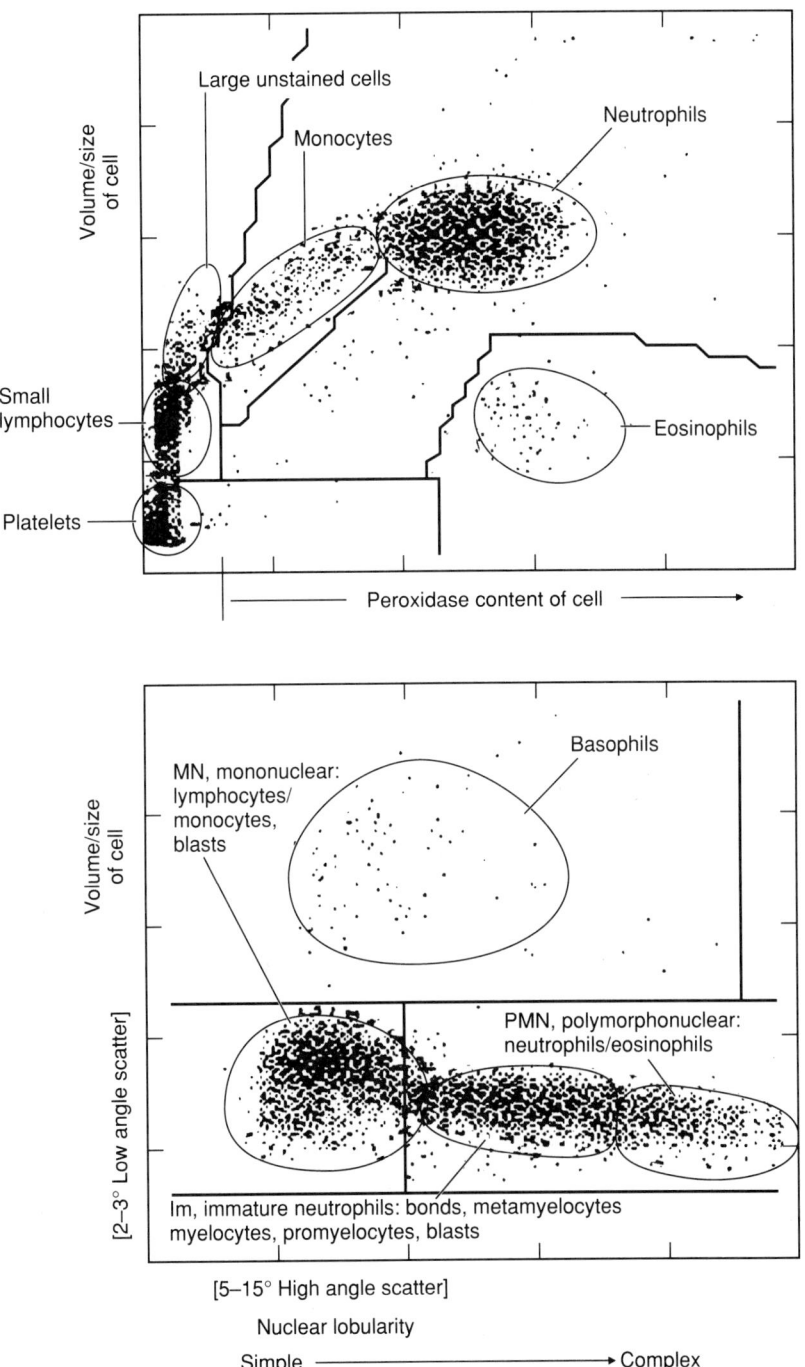

Fig. 19-2. White blood cell screening differential (cytochemical method).

mal peroxidase-containing cells, such as immature granulocytes or myeloblasts, obliterate the expected cluster separation, whereas abnormal peroxidase-negative cells appear as large unstained cells (LUC). Basophils are identified by their unique resistance to a separate lysing reagent.

The recently released generation of electronic impedance instruments have enhancements such as laser light scatter, radiofrequency current, or special lysing reagents that enable counting of neutrophils, lymphocytes, monocytes, eosinophils, and basophils. Significant numbers of immature granulocytes and other abnormal cells are flagged, because they alter the expected appearance of cell clusters on the scattergram plots of multiple parameters. Although some of these automated instruments have algorithms to flag for increased band neutrophils, sufficient sensitivity and specificity of these flags for clinical use have not as yet been demonstrated.

Interpretation

Reference values for the total neutrophil, lymphocyte, monocyte, eosinophil, and basophil cell types recognized by the automated screening differentials vary between instruments, but are similar to those shown for the manual differential in Table 19-34. Causes of quantitative abnormalities in the various cell types are presented in Tables 19-2 to 19-12 and are discussed in the interpretation of the White Blood Cell Slide Differential.

The presence of significant numbers of abnormal cells or immature granulocytes (usually more than 5%) or severe leukopenia (e.g., less than $1.0 \times 10^3/\mu L$ [$<1.0 \times 10^9/L$] on some instruments) may result in flagging of the specimen results. The automated differential results also may be invalid, depending on the particular instrument and the extent of the specimen abnormality. At times, a normal specimen may be flagged for unknown reasons. A manual differential will be necessary for these specimens to assess the presence of abnormal cells and, in some cases, to generate correct quantitative results. If hematologic malignancy is suspected, a slide differential should always be performed, even when the screening differential is normal. However, in the absence of abnormalities in the WBC count, screening differential, Hct, or platelet count, hematologic malignancy is very unlikely.

Test: Eosinophil Count (Absolute Eosinophil Count, Total Eosinophil Count)[4,32,33]

Background and Selection

Accurate documentation of eosinophilia may be desirable before subsequent evaluation is undertaken. The absolute eosinophil count can be calculated from the percentage of eosinophils and the WBC count. However, the percentage of eosinophils from the manual differential is very imprecise. A more precise absolute eosinophil count can be obtained by a direct hemocytometer count of stained eosinophils. The hemocytometer eosinophil count is not necessary if the percentage of eosinophils is obtained from an automated screening differential that classifies a large number of WBCs.

Logistics

EDTA-anticoagulated blood is used. The count is performed on a hemocytometer after lysing the RBCs and staining the eosinophils with phloxine.

Interpretation

Eosinophilia is present when the absolute eosinophil count is greater than $0.35-0.40 \times 10^3/\mu L$ ($>0.35-0.4 \times 10^9/L$) by direct hemocytometer count or automated differential, as compared with approximately $0.5-0.7 \times 10^3/\mu L$ ($\sim 0.5-0.7 \times 10^9/L$) when calculated from the manual differential count. Diurnal variation occurs, with highest results in the morning and lowest at night. In the chronic hypereosinophilic syndromes, eosinophil levels are persistently greater than $1.5 \times 10^3/\mu L$ ($>1.5 \times 10^9/L$). Causes of eosinophilia are numerous and are listed in Table 19-4. Persistent absolute eosinophilia can be evaluated by (1) serologic tests or stool examination for parasites; (2) determination of IgE, which is elevated in allergic eosinophilia; (3) chest x-ray for sarcoidosis or pulmonary eosinophilic syndromes; and (4) biopsy of lymph nodes, if enlarged, to exclude Hodgkin's disease. Bone marrow examination is rarely helpful, except for determination of Philadelphia chromosome, if CML is suspected.

Test: Platelet Count[1,3,17-19,33,34]

Background and Selection

The platelet count frequently is ordered in patients with a suspected bleeding disorder or as part of a screen for bleeding abnormalities before major surgery. It is indicated in malignancies and other disorders that infiltrate the bone marrow and suppress platelet production or with splenomegaly, in which platelets are sequestered in the spleen. The platelet count often is repeated daily in patients receiving marrow suppressive therapy. It also is measured to assess the effectiveness of platelet transfusion or of drug therapy (e.g., steroid treatment) for immune thrombocytopenia. Because the platelet count can be determined simultaneously by newer cell analyzers, some laboratories may include it with the other hemogram parameters. However, other laboratories require a separate order for platelet count, because low platelet counts or specimens with potential interferences are verified by examination of the blood smear or by manual methods.

Logistics

EDTA-anticoagulated blood is preferred and is stable at room temperature for at least 5 hours and for 24 hours if refrigerated. Blood should be placed in anticoagulant promptly and mixed thoroughly to prevent partial clotting with platelet clumping, which will spuriously lower the platelet count. Free-flowing capillary blood should be collected quickly to avoid an apparent decrease in platelet count caused by adhesion of platelets to the margins of injured vessels. Heparinized blood is unacceptable, because of platelet clumping in some samples. Citrate anticoagulated blood is used when the patient has an EDTA dependent platelet agglutinin. These cold-reacting immunoglobulins irreversibly agglutinate platelets in vitro at room temperature and are not associated with any particular clinical disorders. When collecting citrate anticoagulated blood for platelet count, it is important to fill the tube with the appropriate amount of blood and multiply by a dilution factor to correct for the anticoagulant volume. If platelet clumping still occurs with citrate anticoagulant, blood can be directly diluted into ammonium oxalate lysing reagent for counting by phase microscopy.

Methods for counting platelets have improved over the years, progressing from manual hemocytometer methods with phase microscopy, to semiautomated electronic impedance counters for platelet-rich plasma, to the present whole blood platelet counting instruments. Increased precision has been achieved, with a coefficient of variation for whole blood platelet counts of usually less than 5% in the reference range, and 5–10% for platelet counts of less than $50 \times 10^3/\mu L$ ($<50 \times 10^9/L$). However, manual hemocytometer counts with phase microscopy after lysis of RBCs by ammonium oxalate is still the reference method. It is used in small laboratories and for specimens showing interference and thus inaccurate counts with automated methods. The coefficient of variation for hemocytometer counts is approximately 10–20% within the reference range and often greater than 20% for platelet counts of less than $50 \times 10^3/\mu L$ ($<50 \times 10^9/L$).

Platelet counting and sizing in whole blood pose a number of technical problems, because platelets can overlap in size with debris and small RBCs and are outnumbered 20:1 by the RBC component. Initially instruments used RBC lysing reagents, but accurate low platelet counts could not be determined because of interference by cellular debris. New refinements that enable platelet counting in the presence of RBCs include hydrodynamic focusing (centering the cells as they pass through the counting aperture for more accurate sizing), sweep-flow fluid (preventing the RBCs from partially reentering the aperture and being counted as platelets), and pulse editing (eliminating the aberrant electronic pulses from the count, which represent off-axis RBCs rather than platelets). One instrument (Coulter S-Plus series) counts platelets within the 2–20-fL size range to eliminate interference by RBCs, stores and fits the channelized data to a log-normal curve, then extrapolates the curve to cover the normal platelet range of 0–70 fL.

Despite improvements in precision and speed, some specimens give erroneous results with automated whole blood platelet counters. Most instruments have warning flags or alarms to detect these samples (Fig. 19-3). When a large percentage of the platelet-size particles are at the small end of the counting size range or the mode of the lognormal platelet histogram is low, interference from debris (RBC or WBC fragments) or electronic noise is suspected. When a large percentage of the platelet-size particles are at the large end of the counting size range or the mode or standard deviation

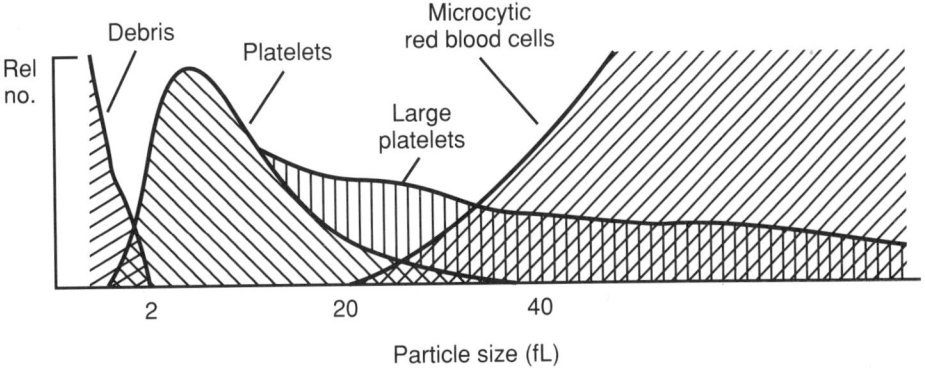

Fig. 19-3. Log-normal platelet distribution and interferences.

of the log-normal platelet histogram is high, interfering microcytic RBCs or giant platelets beyond the upper counting size threshold are suspected. These samples should be counted visually with phase microscopy to obtain accurate counts.

Platelet clumping is an important cause of spurious thrombocytopenia on automated instruments. The clumps of platelets usually exceed the upper size threshold for platelets and are thus excluded from the platelet count. The clumps may be so large that they are not recognized in the error detection systems of the instruments. Frequently, they are the size of small WBCs and thus also may cause spurious leukocytosis. Instruments with WBC sizing histograms can detect most cases of platelet clumps by noting interference in the lower threshold area of the WBC count. If phase microscopy counts are performed, the clumped platelets are seen on the hemocytometer chamber. Platelet clumping most often is caused by poor collection technique with partial clotting. Thus blood should be recollected for the platelet count when platelet clumping occurs. Occasionally, the cause is an EDTA dependent platelet agglutinin, and blood can be collected in citrate for the platelet count. Platelet satellitosis is a rare cause of spurious thrombocytopenia, in which platelets both clump and adhere to neutrophils in vitro. Most instances of platelet satellitosis also are EDTA dependent.

Estimates of platelet count can be made from the peripheral blood wedge smear in an area in which the RBCs barely overlap. The average number of platelets per 100× oil power field times $20 \times 10^9/L$ is an estimate of the platelet count, with approximately 7–21 platelets per field corresponding to the quantitative reference range.

Interpretation

The reference range is $150-400 \times 10^3/\mu L$ ($150-400 \times 10^9/L$) for adults and children. Neonates may have slightly lower platelet counts (i.e., a lower range to $100 \times 10^3/\mu L$ [$100 \times 10^9/L$]) during the first 2 days of life. When the platelet count falls to $60 \times 10^3/\mu L$ ($60 \times 10^9/L$), the patient has enough thrombocytes to prevent spontaneous bleeding but could bleed excessively after surgery or traumatic injury. A serious bleeding tendency develops when the platelet count is up to $20 \times 10^3/\mu L$ ($\leq 20 \times 10^9/L$), characterized by petechiae, small ecchymoses, bleeding from mucosal surfaces, increased blood loss following any surgical procedure, and a threat of CNS bleeding. With a platelet count below $5 \times 10^3/\mu L$ ($<5 \times 10^9/L$), the patient is in imminent peril of fatal CNS or gastrointestinal bleeding. Patients with platelet counts of $20-60 \times 10^3/\mu L$ ($20-60 \times 10^9/L$) vary in their risk of serious bleeding. If the patient is thrombocytopenic because of increased platelet destruction, with stimulated marrow megakaryocytes, the newly produced platelets are large with increased hemostatic effectiveness. The risk of bleeding is substantially increased if drugs (particularly aspirin) that impair the function of the remaining platelets are administered.

Causes of thrombocytopenia are presented in Table 19-9. They can be divided into thrombocytopenias with failure of bone marrow production, ineffective marrow production, increased peripheral platelet destruction, hypersplenism, or loss of platelets. Mechanisms of increased peripheral platelet destruction include (1) IgG coating of platelets (by direct binding of Fab segment to the platelet antigen determinant or to platelet-bound drug or chemical, or nonspecific binding of Fc fragment of immune complexes to platelets), (2) intravascular clotting with thrombin damage to platelets, and (3) blood flow through small vessels with fibrin or denuded endothelium. Important information in delineating the etiology of thrombocytopenia would include the time of onset or history of previous episodes; exposure to drugs and toxins, particularly those with a high incidence of immune induced platelet destruction (e.g., quinidine, sulfa-derived antibiotics or diuretics, rifampicin, gold salts, valproic acid, and heparin) or those that can cause marrow aplasia; heavy alcoholism; recent infection or blood transfusions; evidence for collagen vascular disease; evidence for AIDS; and splenomegaly. The peripheral blood smear always should be examined in newly diagnosed thrombocytopenia to confirm the automated result by platelet slide estimate. In addition, the blood smear may reveal clues to etiology, such as macrocytic RBCs with hypersegmented neutrophils in megaloblastic anemia, abnormal leukocytes in leukemia, schistocytes in consumptive coagulopathies, and large agranular platelets in myelodysplastic syndrome. The finding of an increased mean platelet volume or large (granular) platelets on the peripheral smear is evidence for stimulated platelet production by marrow megakaryocytes. A bone marrow examination is frequently performed in cases of thrombocytopenia to evaluate the number of megakaryocytes and assess the presence or absence of marrow infiltration. Platelet-associated IgG may be determined to identify immune thrombocytopenia with immunoglobulin binding to the platelet surface. However, platelet-associated IgG often occurs in other thrombocytopenias caused by increased platelet destruction. If the platelet count is normal with history or physical evidence of bleeding, a bleeding time (BT) test, activated partial thromboplastin time (APTT), and partial thromboplastin time (PTT) should be performed to assess other aspects of hemostasis.

Causes of increased platelets are shown in Table 19-10. Reactive thrombocytosis is common and occurs secondary to numerous disorders. Primary thrombocythemia results from malignant myeloproliferative disorders with unregulated control of platelet production. Clinical and laboratory findings useful in the diagnosis of myeloproliferative disorders are listed in Tables 19-23 to 19-26. Evidence for myeloproliferative disorders includes a platelet count in excess of 1000×10^9/L, splenomegaly, eosinophilia or basophilia, circulating nucleated RBCs or immature neutrophils, and an increased Hct (in polycythemia vera). The platelets in myeloproliferative syndromes may appear large, bizarre shaped, and agranular on the blood smear and are frequently dysfunctional.

Test: Mean Platelet Volume (MPV)[35–40]

Background and Selection

Megakaryocytes occur in 8N to 64N polyploid classes. With intense thrombopoietin stimulation, the proportion of higher ploidy megakaryocytes increases. These megakaryocytes produce larger platelets, and thus elevate the mean platelet volume (MPV). The MPV may be useful in thrombocytopenia, to aid in distinguishing marrow suppression from peripheral destruction. It also may be measured in suspected hereditary platelet disorders, especially Wiscott-Aldrich syndrome, a sex-linked disorder associated with thrombocytopenia, very small platelets, eczema, and recurrent infections. The MPV can be monitored after bone marrow transplant or cessation of chemotherapy, to predict the return of megakaryocyte function.

Logistics

EDTA-anticoagulated blood usually is used when the MPV is analyzed along with the platelet count by automated hematology analyzers. The mean platelet volume is derived from the histogram of platelet volume measurements (Fig. 19-4), after log-normal conversion of the data. Mathematically, this represents the geometric MPV. However, many technical problems can occur in routine measurement of MPV with clinical hematology analyzers. Platelets exist in vivo as disc-shaped particles. Activation transforms them to a spheroid shape, which has a higher electronic volume than a disc of the same size. This shape change and apparent increase in electronic impedance MPV also occurs with EDTA anticoagulant. Approximately 1–3 hours are required for complete equilibration of platelet volume in EDTA, during which time the MPV may increase from 5–50%, depending on the particular sample. For instruments that measure platelet volume with light scatter, MPV can either increase or decrease with EDTA anticoagulation. Thus, in order to obtain a constant MPV measurement, blood must be allowed to remain at room temperature for 1–3 hours before analysis. After that, the MPV appears to be stable for at least 6 hours at room temperature. The MPV value is very dependent on the type of anticoagulant. Different values are obtained with liquid tripotassium EDTA (used in the United States) than with disodium EDTA (used in Europe).

The MPV is accurate only if the histogram from the cell analyzer has the characteristic log-normal distribution, with a return to baseline at both the lower and upper ends. The MPV, as well as platelet count, is not reliable if (1) cytoplasmic fragments or electronic noise exceeds the platelet signal in a thrombocytopenic sample, (2) giant platelets are present, or (3) microcytic RBCs interfere (Fig. 19-3). The MPV is most useful in thrombocytopenia, but unfortunately, thrombocytopenic specimens have a high incidence of flagged results because of these problems. In some cases of thrombocytopenia with an unreliable value for MPV, inspection of the platelet histogram may indicate whether small or large platelets are predominating.

An additional problem with MPV is the lack of standard calibration, even among instruments from the same manufacturer. There is no guarantee that an instrument from a given laboratory is calibrated in the same manner as the instrument that generated the reference range nomogram, or that the same instrument does not vary in calibration over time.

In research laboratories, MPV can be measured with special electronic impedance instruments with channelizers that are calibrated to standardized spherical latex particles. Citrate-anticoagulant mixtures are used that stabilize the in vivo volume and platelet-rich plasma is isolated so that severely thrombocytopenic samples can be analyzed.

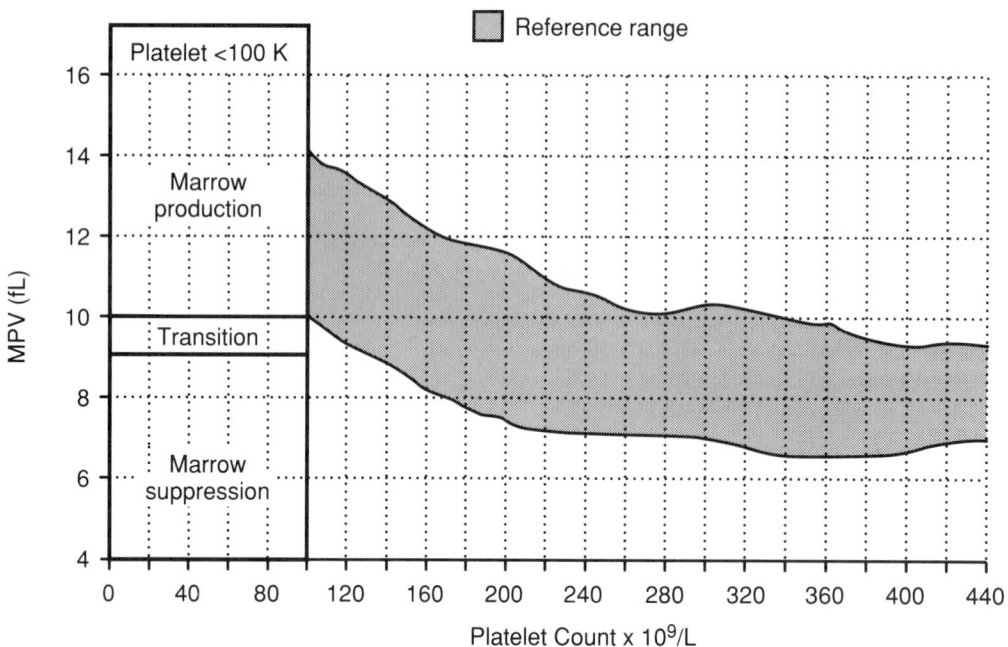

Fig. 19-4. Mean platelet volume (MPV). Mean platelet volume varies inversely (and nonlinearly) with platelet count. This nomogram was constructed from 530 normal employees at Stanford University Hospital. The hematology instrument (coulter s-plus IV) was calibrated to the mode of polyvinyl toluene spheres (Seragen Diagnostics #47807), with a measured diameter of 2.124 ± 0.0163 μm, mean/mode of 5.233 fL. Regions representing marrow production and suppression for low platelet counts were compiled from a study of patients undergoing bone marrow aspiration/biopsy who had not received chemotherapy in the past 60 days. (Stanford University Hospital, unpublished data.)

Interpretation

The reference range for MPV is inversely and nonlinearly related to platelet count, as shown in the nomogram in Figure 19-4. Clinical correlation with MPV is shown in Table 19-37. The MPV is high in patients with thrombocytopenia caused by ITP and other platelet-destructive processes, with a continued inverse relationship between MPV and platelet count. By contrast, patients with thrombocytopenia caused by marrow suppression have a decreased MPV. With recovery from bone marrow suppression, a rise in MPV may precede the rise in platelet count by a few days. Hypersplenism occasionally results in a lower MPV because the spleen selectively sequesters larger platelets. The MPV is elevated in some cases of myeloproliferative disorders, but considerable overlap in MPV values between reactive and malignant causes of thrombocytosis occurs. Although the MPV may be somewhat useful in predicting megakaryocytic function, a bone marrow examination frequently is performed in unexplained cases of thrombocytopenia to evaluate the number of megakaryocytes and assess the presence or absence of marrow infiltration.

Newer automated cell analyzers also calculate other indexes of platelet size, including (1) platelet distribution width (PDW), a measure proportional to the standard deviation of the log-normal platelet curve (analogous to RDW); (2) platelet-crit (PCT), the MCV times the platelet count, or total platelet mass (analogous to Hct; and (3) P-LCR, the percentage of platelets larger than a set size threshold. The clinical value of these platelet parameters has not been established.

TESTS OF NEUTROPHIL FUNCTION

Neutrophil dysfunction is an uncommon cause of recurrent infection. Laboratory testing initially should be directed toward excluding more common etiologies, such as neutropenia (including cyclic neutropenia) and deficiencies in complement, immunoglobulin, and cell mediated immunity (see Ch. 30). The causes of neutrophil dysfunction are listed in Table 19-13. Acquired neutrophil dysfunction, secondary to other clinical disorders, should be eliminated before pursuing the diagnosis of an inherited defect. Functional assays are ex-

Table 19-37. Clinical Correlations with Mean Platelet Volume

Low MPV for platelet count
    Marrow suppression
        Chemotherapy
        Megaloblastic anemia
        Aplastic anemia
        Marrow infiltration
        Sepsis
    Hypersplenism (variable)
    Hereditary disorders
        Wiscott-Aldrich

Normal to high MPV for platelet count
    Hyperdestruction with marrow compensation
        Immune-related (ITP, drug-induced)
        Mechanical (consumptive coagulopathies, vasculitis)
        Hemorrhage (major)
        Sepsis (without marrow suppression)

High MPV for platelet count
    Hereditary disorders
        Bernard-Soulier
        May-Hegglin
        Mediterranean macrothrombocytopenia
    Miscellaeous
        α- and β-Thalassemia trait (unknown cause)
        Myelodysplastic syndrome
        Myeloproliferative disorders (in some cases)

Abbreviations: MPV, mean platelet volume; ITP, idiopathic thrombocytopenic purpura.
(Data from references 19, 35, 37, and 38.)

pensive, labor intensive, and difficult to perform and interpret. Thus, patient history and test availability may play a role in test selection. Tests listed in Table 19-14, focusing on specific congenital defects, give more consistent results.

Test: Functional Assay of Adherence and Chemotaxis (Rebuck Skin Window)[5]

The Rebuck skin window is a qualitative in vivo functional test that assesses neutrophil adherence and chemotaxis. A small patch of skin is denuded down to the papillary layer of the epidermis, and a glass slide is taped over the lesion. Normally, at least 300 cells should migrate to the slide within 3 hours, 90% of which should be neutrophils. If the Rebuck skin window test is normal, a significant defect in adherence or chemotaxis is unlikely. If the skin window test is abnormal, the next test to be performed is a determination of neutrophil surface CR3.

Test: Neutrophil CR3 (Cr3bi Receptor Complement Receptor, CD11b/CD18 Glycoprotein)[5,7,41]

Neutrophil adherence is dependent on a surface receptor for complement, CR3. CR3 is a glycoprotein heterodimer with subunits recognized by monoclonal antibodies CD11b and CD18. Neutrophils can be analyzed for the surface expression of CR3 using a monoclonal antibody to CD11b with flow cytometry. Test sensitivity is enhanced by stimulation of the neutrophils with a calcium ionophore (A23187), which increases surface expression of CD11b/CD18. Both complete and partial deficiencies of CR3 can be identified.

Test: Functional Assays of Chemotaxis[5]

Neutrophil chemotaxis can be assessed by observing migration through a micropore filter (Boyden chamber technique) or through agarose in response to chemotactic agents. Both assays suffer from inherent variability and require careful control to ensure valid results.

Test: Functional Assays of Phagocytosis and Intracellular Killing[5]

These assays are performed sequentially, using patient neutrophils and target bacteria. The cells are incubated with bacteria and serum and, at various time intervals, aliquots of sedimented cells and supernatant are cultured. The disappearance of viable bacteria from the supernatant is evidence for phagocytosis, while the disappearance from the cell sediment is evidence for intracellular killing. Newer techniques employ radioactive particles, ^{3}H-thymidine bacteria, or latex beads to simplify assessment of phagocytosis. However, determination of intracellular killing still requires bacterial culture.

Test: Functional Assays of Degranulation[5]

The two major disorders of neutrophil degranulation—Chédiak-Higashi syndrome and specific granule deficiency—are readily diagnosed by light or electron microscopy. To assess other defects in neutrophil degranulation, release of granule contents (e.g., β-glucuronidase for primary granules, lactoferrin for specific neutrophilic granules) can be measured after stimulation of the neutrophils. More recently, degranulation has been measured using right angle light scatter on the flow cytometer, which varies directly with the cytoplasmic granularity of the cell.

Test: Oxidative Burst Analysis (Nitroblue Tetrazolium Test, NBT Test)[4,5,41]

Neutrophils generate bactericidal products through the uptake of oxygen (oxidative burst) and reduction of molecular oxygen to free radicals and cellular oxidants. Defective oxidative metabolism is associated with the chronic granulomatous diseases but also occurs in specific granule deficiency and in severe glucose 6-phosphate dehydrogenase (G-6-PD) deficiency.

The nitroblue tetrazolium (NBT) method is the standard method of assessing oxidative burst activity. Neutrophils are incubated with glucose and NBT and stimulated with endotoxin or phorbol myristate acetate. Smears are prepared and counterstained. With oxidative burst activity, the colorless NBT dye is reduced to a blue-black formazen precipitate in the cytoplasm of neutrophils and monocytes. Normal subjects will have more than 90% positive neutrophils, whereas patients with chronic granulomatous disease and other severe defects in oxidative burst activity will show few, if any, positively staining neutrophils. Present, but reduced, percentages of positive cells may be seen in carriers of X-linked chronic granulomatous disease and in patients receiving antibiotics, steroids, phenylbutazone, or aspirin.

Recently, flow cytometric procedures have been used to determine the intracellular oxidative burst capacity of neutrophils. A nonfluorescent compound, DCFH-DA (2'-7'-dichlorofluorescein diacetate), enters the neutrophil and is oxidized to a fluorescent compound by the hydrogen peroxide generated in the oxidative burst.

CYTOCHEMICAL AND IMMUNOLOGIC TESTS

Test: Immunophenotyping (Cell Surface Antigens, Cell Surface Markers, Immunologic Cell Marker Studies, Immunohistochemistry, Immunoperoxidase, Flow Cytometry, Leukemia Typing, Lymphoma Typing)[10,41-44] (See Also Ch. 30)

Background and Selection

Characterization of surface antigens and surface and cytoplasmic immunoglobulin is an important tool in the diagnosis and classification of WBC malignancies. With the advent of commercial monoclonal antibodies and user-friendly flow cytometers, immunophenotyping is available in many clinical laboratories. Whenever malignancy is suspected, it is important to store bone marrow or lymph node samples for immunophenotyping at the time of biopsy. A decision regarding appropriate testing can be made after inspection of tissue morphology.

Immunophenotyping is useful in distinguishing reactive lymphoid proliferations in blood, bone marrow, or lymph node from leukemia or lymphoma. It is performed in acute leukemia, to distinguish myeloid from lymphoid lineage. In addition, immunologic subclassification of ALL has therapeutic and prognostic significance in children. Immunophenotyping can aid in the differential diagnosis of the differentiated lymphoid leukemias (Tables 19-27 and 19-28). It is frequently performed on lymph node biopsies with anaplastic malignant cells, to distinguish lymphoma from carcinoma, sarcoma, or melanoma. Lymphomas may be subclassified into B- or T-cell types, but the prognostic significance is controversial.

Terminology

Because monoclonal antibody clones have been produced by many research and commercial laboratories, multiple names have been given to antibodies with similar specificity. International workshops were held during the 1980s to formulate cluster designations (CD) for antibodies recognizing similar leukocyte differentiation antigens. A list of many of the monoclonal antibodies used in leukocyte immunophenotyping, along with their expected reaction pattern, is given in Table 19-38.

Logistics

Immunophenotyping by flow cytometry can be performed on cell suspensions from peripheral blood, bone marrow aspirate, body fluids, tissue aspirates, or disaggregated tissue. Immunoenzymatic methods (most frequently immunoperoxidase) are used for tissue sections, blood smears, touch preparations, or cytocentrifuge slide preparations. It is imperative that the clinician consult the laboratory before obtaining the specimen to determine the preferred sample and how it is to be handled.

Tissue never should be placed in routine fixatives if immunophenotyping is a consideration, because fixatives destroy many of the surface antigens of interest. Most frequently, tissue is transported to the laboratory

Table 19-38. Selected WBC Antigen Markers

Cluster Designation	Common Names	Cells Identified
T, NK lymphocytes		
CD1	T6, Leu 6	Common thymocytes
CD2	T11, Leu 5	Pan-T, some NK
CD3	T3, Leu 4	Pan-T, TcR complex
CD4	T4, Leu 3	Helper-inducer subset
CD5	T1, Leu 1	Pan-T, anomalous on CLL
CD6	T12	Pan-T
CD7	Leu 9	Early T, many NK, some AML
CD8	T8, Leu 2	Cytotoxic/suppressor subset; some NK
CD25	Tac	IL-2R, activated T cells
CDw29	4B4	Inducer of B-cell function; B cells, monocytes
CDw38	T10, Leu 17	Activated T, B; plasma cells
CDw45R	2H4, Leu 18	Inducer of cytotoxic/suppressor cells; B cells, monocytes
HNK-1	Leu 7	NK cells, some T-suppressor cells; neuroectodermal tissue and tumors
CD56	Leu 19, NKH-1	NK cells; may be expressed in both AML and ALL
B lymphocytes		
HLA-DR	Ia, DR	Pan-B, activated T/NK, monocytes, granulocytes
CD10	J5, CALLA	Early B, some T-ALL
CD19	B4, Leu 12	Pan-B
CD20	B1, Leu 16	Pan-B
CD21	B2, Leu	B-subset, C3dR
CD22	Leu 14	Pan-B
CD24	BA-1	Pan-B, granulocytes
Surface Ig		Mature B, plasma Ig bound to Fc receptor on some lymphocytes (especially NK), granulocytes, monocytes
PCA-1, PC-1		Some plasma cells; weakly on monocytes, granulocytes, hairy cell leukemia, Waldenström's and other plasmacytoid lymphomas
Granulocytes, monocytes		
CD11b	Mo1, OK M1, Leu 15	C3biR on granulocytes, monocytes, some Ts/c
CD11c	Ki-M1, Leu M5	Monocytes, granulocytes, NK, hairy cell leukemia, weakly on CLL/lymphoma
CD13	MY7	Granulocytes, monocytes
CD14	Mo 2, MY4, Leu M3	Monocytes
CD15	MY1, Leu M1	Granulocytes, monocytes, some T lymphomas, R-S cells, some carcinomas
CD16	VEP-13, Leu 11, a, b, or c	Fc receptor for IgG; granulocytes, NK Granulocytes, monocytes
CD33	MY9, Leu My 9	
Other		
CD30	Ki-1	Activated T, B; R-S cells
CD34	MY10, HPFC	Immature precursors, many leukemias
CD41a	Glycoprotein IIb/IIIa	Megakaryocytes, platelets
CD42b	Glycoprotein Ib	Megakaryocytes, platelets
Factor VIII-related Ag		Megakaryocytes platelets
CD45	T200, LCA, HLE-1	Pan-leukocyte
Glycophorin		RBCs and precursors; some erythroblasts
TdT		Early B, thymic T

Abbreviations: NK, natural killer (cell); CLL, chronic lymphocytic leukemia; AML, acute myelocytic leukemia; IL-2R, receptor for interleukin 2; ALL, acute lymphocytic leukemia; CD3R, receptor for CD3; Ig, immunoglobulin; C3biR, receptor for C3bi; Ts/c, T cytotoxic/suppressor; R-S, Reed-Sternberg; RBCs, red blood cells; TdT, terminal deoxynucleotidyl transferase.

(Data from Keren[41] and Deegan.[42])

in saline, where it is snap-frozen, preferably within 1 hour of removal. Storage in cold phosphate-buffered saline for up to 7 days often is acceptable if tissue must be transported.

Blood, bone marrow, and body fluids are most often collected in heparin anticoagulant. EDTA anticoagulant may be used if the sample is to be processed the same day. Storage at room temperature for 24 hours is usually acceptable for a heparinized specimen. If longer storage is anticipated, specimens are placed in various media containing azide, antibiotics, and serum. Similar media may be used for tissue aspirates. Delay in analysis may result in partial antigen loss and cell death, but the predominant immunophenotype often may be identified after 48–72 hours of storage. The best preservation of viability is obtained with a homogeneous malignant population, whereas poor viability results when a substantial number of granulocytes are admixed with the malignant cells.

For flow cytometry, viable cells are concentrated by Ficoll-Hypaque density gradient isolation, which removes dead cells, debris, RBCs, and mature granulocytes. Alternatively, with peripheral blood, lysing agents can be used to remove interfering RBCs. Cell surface antigens are stained by antibodies conjugated to fluorescent compounds, usually fluorescein isothionate (FITC) or phycoerythrin (PE), which emit green or red fluorescence, respectively. In the flow cytometer, the cells pass single file in a fluid stream through a beam of light generated by a laser. Light scattered by each cell in discrete directions, as well as fluorescent light emitted by each cell at particular wavelengths, is measured and the information is stored in a computer. Correlated plots can be made of the parameters from the stored information. Light scattered at low forward angle is proportional to cell size, whereas light scattered at 90 degrees is a reflection of cell granularity. As shown in Figure 19-5, a plot of forward versus 90-degree light scatter can separate the

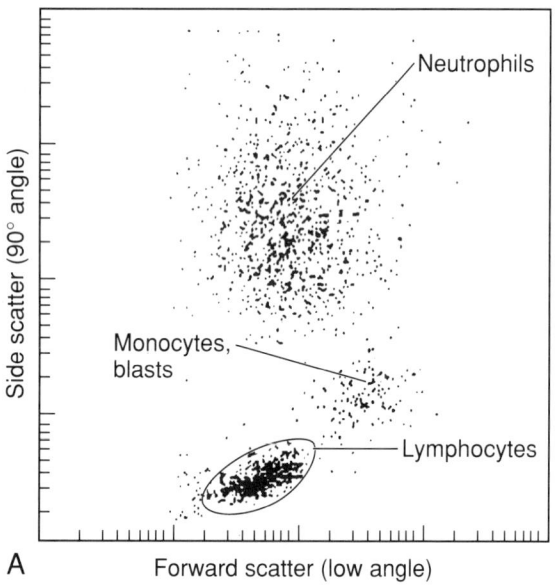
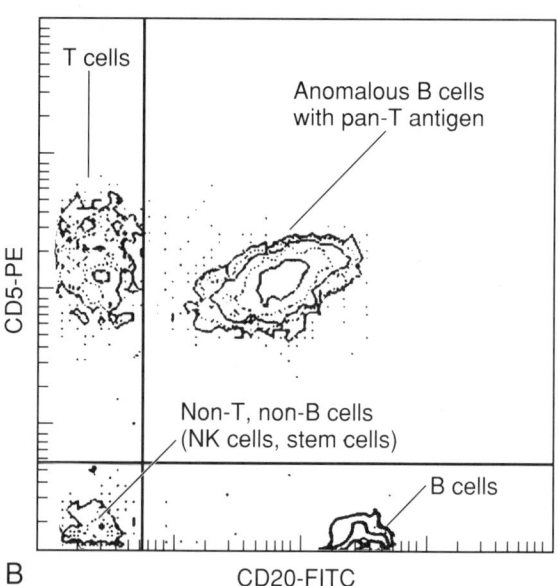

Fig. 19-5. Immunophenotyping by flow cytometry. The white blood cells (WBCs) are incubated with monoclonal antibody conjugated to fluorescein isothiocyanide (FITC, green fluorescence) directed against a pan-T (CD5) surface antigen and with a monoclonal antibody conjugated to phycoerythrin (PE, red fluorescence) directed against a pan-B (CD20) surface antigen. Red blood cells (RBCs) are removed by a lysing reagent. **(A)** The plot of low foward angle scatter (related to cell size) and 90-degree angle side scatter (related to cell granularity) shows clusters of various WBC populations. The lymphoid cluster region is gated for further analysis. **(B)** Analysis of fluorescence on these lymphoid cells shows a population of T lymphocytes with strong red fluorescence (quadrant 1), a population of B lymphocytes with strong green fluorescence (quadrant 4), a population of presumed natural killer (NK) or stem cells with only autofluorescence (quadrant 3), and a population of abnormal cells with strong dual red and green fluorescence (quadrant 3). These abnormal B lymphocytes, bearing the anomalous T-cell antigen CD5, are characteristically seen in chronic lymphocytic leukemia.

lymphoid, monocytoid, and granulocytic cell fractions. When malignant cells or atypical lymphoid cells are present, a discrete cluster will be identified by light scatter properties. This cluster is then gated and subsequent analysis performed on the cells of interest. In dual color analysis, pairs of antibodies are combined, one with FITC and one with PE. A plot of the intensity light emitted in the green (FITC) and red (PE) regions, also shown in Figure 19-5, can identify the percentage of cells positive for one or both antibodies. Nonreactive antibody conjugates also are analyzed to control for nonspecific binding to the cells. The gated malignant cells are considered to be positive for a given antibody when up to 20% of the population is reactive. Although flow cytometry primarily detects surface antigens, cytoplasmic or nuclear antigens can be detected after special treatment of the cells. Advantages of flow cytometry include high sensitivity, the ability to test for two antigens on the same cell, and expression of objective, quantitative results on a large number of cells.

Tissue procedures use indirect methods of analysis, in which the primary antibody (usually a mouse monoclonal antibody) is unlabeled. In the immunoperoxidase method (Fig. 19-6), a biotinylated secondary antibody is used with specificity for the primary antibody (e.g., horse antimouse). An avidin-biotin-peroxidase enzyme complex is added, which binds tightly to the biotinylated antibody. Color is localized to the reacting cells by reaction with hydrogen peroxide and a dye. Alkaline phosphatase-based immunohistochemical procedures are sometimes used for blood and bone marrow, with the addition of an inhibitor for endogenous enzyme. Immunophenotyping of tissues or blood smears detect both surface and cytoplasmic antigens. Advantages of tissue immunohistochemistry are the preservation of architectural features of the tissue, permitting anatomic localization of the positive staining cells, and detection of cytoplasmic antigens without sample treatment.

Interpretation

Although immunophenotyping is an important tool in solving diagnostic problems, it is only an adjuvant to classic morphologic criteria. Expected patterns of antigen expression do not occur in 100% of cases. It is important to examine the histologic morphology of the original specimen in conjunction with the immunophenotyping results to arrive at a final diagnosis. In addition, it is important to examine slides of cell suspension preparations to be sure that a sufficient number of malignant cells are present.

Malignant lymphoproliferations are distinguished by the presence of monoclonality. Monoclonality of B lymphocytes is defined by restriction of neoplastic cells to the production of either κ or λ light chain. In blood or bone marrow, a κ/λ ratio of greater than 3 or less than

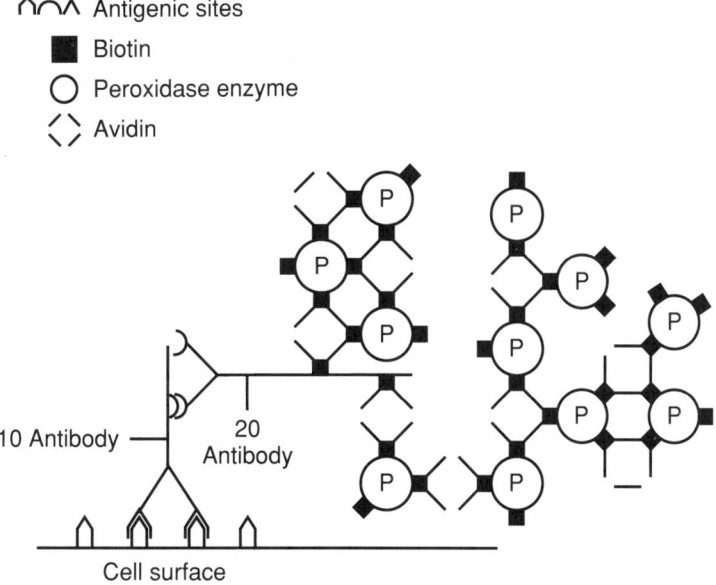

Fig. 19-6. Immunophenotyping by immunoenzymatic methods (the avidin-biotin-peroxidase complex (ABC) interacts with exposed biotin on the secondary antibody. Development of the peroxidase enzyme with colored chromogen marks the positively reacting cells.

0.5 is evidence for a monoclonal population. In frozen sections, greater than 90% of the putative cells should belong to a single light chain class. No immunologic marker is available to assess T-cell clonality, although various pan-T or T-subset reagents can be used to determine whether an obvious malignant infiltration is of T-cell origin. Clonal rearrangement of the T-cell genes is tested by Southern blot analysis of DNA and is considered the molecular equivalent of B-cell monoclonality. Atypical B or T phenotypes can occur and are an indirect sign of malignant lymphoproliferation. These anomalous phenotypes include the loss of one or more pan-B or T antigens, loss of the leukocyte common antigen, coexpression of pan-T antigen CD5 on B cells, coexpression of NK antigen CD16 on large numbers of T cells, dual expression of helper/suppressor antigens, or appearance of immature antigens on peripheral blood cells (e.g., CD10 or CD1-common thymocyte antigen). A small battery of antibodies can help distinguish large cell lymphoma from nonlymphoid malignancies and can be used with fixed paraffin-embedded tissue. These include leukocyte common antigen (positive in most hematolymphoid malignancies), epithelial membrane antigen or cytokeratins (positive in carcinoma), vimentin (positive with sarcoma), and S100 protein (reactive with melanoma).

Assessment of myeloid and lymphoid antigens can distinguish AML from ALL and indicates when an acute leukemia is bilineage or biclonal. Immunophenotyping is also helpful in blast crisis of chronic myelogeneous leukemia; approximately 20–30% of cases are early B-lymphoid lineage and may respond to therapy with vincristine and prednisone. Although the FAB classification of AML does not consider surface antigen expression, some degree of correlation with immunophenotyping results occurs, as shown in Table 19-18. For ALL, it is postulated that leukemic cells express antigens corresponding to various developmental stages of T- or B-cell differentiation (Fig. 16-2, Ch. 16). With the development of monoclonal antibodies to early B-surface antigens, many cases of ALL that would have been classified as null cell ALL in the past have been found to be early B lineage. As shown in Table 19-20A, B-lineage ALL can be divided into six groups, each representing the acquisition of B-differentiation antigens. The presence of early B-lineage markers, with or without CD10, constitute the majority of cases of ALL (groups 1–6). When cytoplasmic μ heavy chain is detected, the leukemia is termed pre-B ALL (group 5). B-ALL, or Burkitt-type leukemia-lymphoma, has clonal surface immunoglobulin, usually IgM (group 6). T-lineage ALL resembles stages of thymocyte development (Table 19-20B). Groups 2 and 3 often show dual expression of helper and suppressor antigens. CD10 may be weakly expressed in T-ALL. In children, the best prognosis is associated with early B-lineage ALL with CD10 (groups 3 and 4). A significant number of cases of ALL in both children and adults show weak expression of myeloid antigens CD13, CD14, and/or CD33, which appears to be associated with a poorer prognosis.

Immunophenotyping is helpful in distinguishing among the leukemias of differentiated lymphocytes. The chronic leukemias of differentiated B lymphocytes (Table 19-27) usually have monoclonal surface immunoglobulin, although it is expressed very weakly in CLL. The typical case of CLL has weak surface IgM or IgM and IgD, reacts with most pan-B antibodies, and expresses the anomalous pan-T cell antigen, CD5. Prolymphocytic leukemia (PLL) has stronger monoclonal surface immunoglobulin of any type, reacts with most pan-B antibodies, may or may not express CD5, and reacts with FMC7, an experimental antibody that reacts with approximately one-half the lymphocytes in the normal peripheral blood, but only rarely with CLL. Hairy cell leukemia (HCL) has strong monoclonal surface immunoglobulin, which can show multiple heavy chains. The cells react with plasma cell-associated antigens and FMC7 as well as the pan-B antibodies and strongly express CD11c (M5), a monocyte and NK-associated antigen. Other differentiated B leukemias and lymphomas also may anomalously express CD11c, but only weakly. Occasional cases of CLL, PLL, and HCL may be of T-helper or suppressor phenotype. The leukemic phase of a B lymphoma most often is seen in small cleaved follicular lymphoma, which expresses strong monoclonal surface immunoglobulin, various pan-B antigens, and weak CD10.

The leukemias of differentiated T lymphocytes include three entities (i.e., T-helper CLL, Sézary syndrome, and adult T-cell leukemia/lymphoma) of T-helper phenotype (Table 19-28). Thus, clinical and morphologic features are more important in distinguishing among these disorders. Large granular lymphocyte leukemia (LGL) or T-γ lymphoproliferative disease is characterized by proliferation of medium to large lymphocytes with prominent azurophilic granules in the blood and bone marrow. It has an indolent clinical course with neutropenia, recurrent infection, and autoimmune disorders. The phenotype is heterogeneous, most often T suppressor with variable expression of NK-associated antigens such as CD16, CD11b, CD11c, CD56 and CD57. Because an increase in T-suppressor cells and granulated lymphocytes may occur in reactive processes (e.g., viral infections, other malignancies), clonality may be established by gene rearrangement studies in unclear cases. Approximately 15% of LGL may be of NK phenotype, lacking pan-T or suppressor antigens and the T-cell receptor gene rearrangement. Chromosomal abnormalities can be demonstrated in some of these cases as evidence of a malignant rather than reactive process.

In non-Hodgkin's lymphomas, it is difficult to correlate immunologic findings with morphologic classification, but several patterns have emerged. Low grade small lymphocytic lymphomas are immunologically similar to CLL, with weak surface immunoglobulin, various pan-B antigens, and anomalous expression of pan-T antibody CD5. Follicular lymphomas of both small and large cells are uniformly of B phenotype. Monotypic immunoglobulin is strongly expressed in most cases of small cell follicular lymphoma, but surface immunoglobulin is occasionally absent from the follicular mixed and large types. More than one-half of the low grade small cleaved follicular lymphomas express CD10. Diffuse intermediate grade lymphomas and immunoblastic high grade lymphomas are immunologically heterogeneous, and the prognostic significance of B versus T subtypes is controversial. The diffuse B lymphomas may show loss of surface immunoglobulin or one or more pan-B antigens, and usually do not express CD10. Diffuse T lymphomas have a post-thymic phenotype (TdT, CD1 negative) and frequently show loss of one or more pan-T antigens. Among the high grade lymphomas, lymphoblastic lymphoma is thymic derived and shares many features with T-lineage ALL; like T-ALL, its membrane phenotype recapitulates the three stages of thymocyte maturation (Table 19-20B). Similarly, high grade small noncleaved lymphoma (both Burkitt's and non-Burkitt's morphologic subtypes) are B-cell malignancies with surface IgM analogous to that of B-ALL.

The malignant Reed-Sternberg cells in Hodgkin's disease react with CD30 (Ki-1) and CD15. However, many post-thymic T-cell lymphomas and some carcinomas are also reactive with these antibodies. Failure to demonstrate CD30 and CD15 reactivity is evidence against Hodgkin's disease, because both antibodies are reactive with Reed-Sternberg and mononuclear Hodgkin's cells in most cases.

Both malignant and benign plasma cells have a characteristic phenotype. These cells show loss of surface pan-B antigens, HLA-DR, surface immunoglobulin, and the common leukocyte antigen. Only CD38 and plasma cell associated antigens (e.g., PCA-1, PC-1) are expressed. Monoclonal cytoplasmic immunoglobulin is present in multiple myeloma, as opposed to polyclonal cytoplasmic immunoglobulin in reactive plasmacytosis. The presence of CD10 antigen on myeloma cells has been associated with a more aggressive tumor. The plasma cells in Waldenström's macroglobulinemia contain monoclonal cytoplasmic IgM, whereas the malignant lymphocytes show pan-B antigens, plasma cell-associated antigens, and monoclonal surface IgM.

If the diagnosis of malignancy is still in question after correlation of morphologic and immunophenotyping results, gene rearrangement studies may be useful in establishing clonality of a B- or T-lymphoid malignancy. In addition, the demonstration of abnormal cytogenetic karyotype or DNA aneuploidy suggests a malignant process.

Test: Myeloperoxidase Stain (MPO, Leukocyte Peroxidase)[3,6,45–47]

Background and Selection

Myeloperoxidase is present in the azurophilic or primary lysosomal granules of granulocytes and monocytes. Using hydrogen peroxide as a substrate, MPO can catalyze the oxidation of microorganisms in the phagolysosome. Although the enzyme is thought to contribute to microbial killing, it is not essential for the microbicidal activity of these cells. Myeloperoxidase staining is performed to determine the lineage of blasts in acute leukemia. The test may also be useful in the diagnosis of hereditary myeloperoxidase deficiency, in which increased susceptibility to *Candida albicans* infections may occur.

Logistics

Slides for MPO cytochemistry may be prepared from blood, bone marrow, body fluids, or the buffy coat or Ficoll density cell isolates of these specimens. A sufficient number of blasts (e.g., more than 20%) should be present. Both EDTA- or heparin-anticoagulated specimens are acceptable for slide preparation. Slides from body fluids or density gradient isolates of WBCs are best prepared using a cytocentrifuge. Tissue imprints can be stained, but MPO activity will not be present in paraffin-embedded tissue. Slides should be prepared the same day of collection and protected from light. When slides are stored in the dark, the enzymatic activity is stable for several days at room temperature and several weeks at 4°C. Enzymatic activity can be preserved for a very long time if slides are wrapped in foil and frozen.

Slides are fixed, usually with buffered formalin or glutaraldehyde, and incubated with hydrogen peroxide and dye. The dye is initially in a reduced colorless form but, when oxidized, forms an insoluble colored product at the site of the MPO enzymatic activity. Benzidine was widely used as the substrate dye for MPO in the past but has been found to be carcinogenic. 3-Amino-9-ethylcarbazole, which gives a red color on oxidation, is the most widely used dye. Other alternate chromogens for MPO include diaminobenzidine, 4-chloronaphthol, tetramethylbenzidine dihydrochloride, and p-phenylenediamine with pyrocatechol (Hanker-Yates reagent). The incubation mixture for MPO cytochemistry must be freshly prepared, with the hydrogen peroxide added immediately before staining. Slides are often counterstained, typically with hematoxylin, to visualize the cell nucleus. After staining, slides should be protected from light to prevent color fading.

Interpretation

Peroxidase activity is present in all stages of neutrophil development (Table 19-39). It is moderately positive in monocytes and weak to absent in basophils. Intensely positive cyanide-resistant MPO activity is seen in eosinophils. A positive MPO reaction is useful to differentiate these cells from lymphocytic or erythroid cells, which are MPO negative.

In acute leukemia, only the blasts are assessed for MPO reactivity. When more than 3% of the blasts are positive, a diagnosis of myeloid lineage leukemia is made by the FAB classification (Table 19-17). Even when blast cells or microgranular promyelocytes fail to show azurophilic granules on the Wright-Giemsa stain, the MPO may be positive, presumably staining peroxidase activity that is not yet packaged into lysosomal granules. Auer rods, thought to be fused lysosomal granules, are MPO positive. If MPO activity is absent in the blasts, other tests must be performed to determine the type of leukemic cells. These include leukocyte esterase (for the monocytoid forms of AML), TdT (for lymphoid lineage), platelet peroxidase by electron microscopy (for megakaryocytic lineage), and immunophenotyping (all types of leukemia). At times, the blasts of myeloid leukemia may be negative for MPO but show surface antigens characteristic of the myeloid lineage by immunophenotyping.

Table 19-39. Reactions of Commonly Used Leukocyte Stains in Acute Leukemia

Cell	MPO	Esterase Naphthol AS-D Chloroacetate	α-Naphthyl Butyrate	α-Naphthyl Acetate	TdT
Granulocyte (promyelocyte) to poly	Pos	Pos	Neg	Neg	Neg
Eosinophil	Pos (CN resistant)	Neg	Neg	Neg	Neg
Basophil	Neg to weakly pos	Neg to weakly pos	Neg	Neg	Neg
Mast cell	Neg	Pos	Neg	Neg	Neg
Monocyte	Weakly to moderately pos	Neg	Pos	Pos	Neg
Histiocyte	Neg	Neg	Pos	Pos	Neg
Lymphocyte	Neg	Neg	Neg[a]	Neg[a]	Neg
Plasma cell	Neg	Neg	Neg	Pos	Neg
Megakaryocyte	Neg	Neg	Neg to weakly pos	Pos	Neg
Erythroblast	Neg	Neg	Neg	Neg[b]	Neg
Myeloblast	Pos	Pos	Neg	Neg	Neg[c]
"Monoblast"	Neg to pos	Neg	Pos	Pos	Neg[c]
Lymphoblast	Neg	Neg	Neg[a]	Neg[a]	Pos[d]
Lymphoma cell	Neg	Neg	Neg[a]	Neg[a]	Neg
Hairy cell	Neg	Neg	Pos (crescent-like)	Pos (crescent-like)	Neg

[a] Occasionally may have focal polar large granule, particularly in T-lineage lymphoid cells.
[b] May be positive in megaloblastic erythroids.
[c] A variable number of blasts in AML may be positive, depending on the sensitivity of the assay for TdT.
[d] B-cell acute lymphocytic leukemia (with surface immunoglobulin) is TdT negative.
Abbreviations: MPO, myeloperoxidase; TdT, terminal deoxynucleotidyl transferase; Pos, positive; Neg, negative; AML, acute myelocytic leukemia.
(Data from Williams et al.,[3] ICSH,[45] and Bell et al.[48])

Hereditary myeloperoxidase deficiency is an autosomal recessive disorder with absent neutrophil and monocyte MPO in the homozygote, and diminished enzyme in the heterozygote. Eosinophil MPO activity is unaffected. Most patients are asymptomatic, but an occasional patient with increased susceptibility to infection with *C. albicans* has been described. Occasionally, MPO activity may be diminished or absent in some of the mature neutrophils of patients with myelodysplastic syndrome or AML.

Test: Sudan Black B Stain (SBB)[3,48]

Sudan black B is a lipid stain that appears to stain a lipid component present only in neutrophils, monocytes, and eosinophils. Sudanophilia roughly parallels the MPO reaction. The Sudan black B stain is as sensitive and specific as MPO in distinguishing myeloid from lymphoid leukemias. It may be especially useful when fresh blood smears are not available, because the stain can be used on slides several years old.

Test: Esterase Stain (Chloroacetate Esterase, Naphthol AS-D Chloroacetate Esterase, Specific Esterase, α-Naphthyl Acetate Esterase, α-Naphthyl Butyrate Esterase, Nonspecific Esterase, NSE, Naphthol AS-D Acetate Esterase, Fluoride Sensitive Esterase)[3,47,48]

Background and Selection

The leukocyte esterase enzymes are present in the azurophilic or primary lysosomal granules of neutrophils, monocytes, and some lymphocytes. They hydrolyze ester bonds of a variety of aliphatic and aromatic esters. Nine isoenzyme forms exist, many of which are cell type specific. Reaction with a given substrate depends on the isoenzyme forms present in the cell and on the reaction conditions (e.g., fixative, pH, and temperature). Esterase stains are performed to determine the lineage of the blasts in acute leukemia. The nonspecific esterase stains (monocytic esterase) are particularly useful to demonstrate the monocytoid variants of myelocytic leukemia (AML-M4, myelomonocytic leukemia; AML-M5, monocytic leukemia). The chloroacetate (neutrophilic) esterase reaction is not as sensitive as MPO and Sudan black B for the myeloblasts of AML, and thus is not frequently used. However, the chloroacetate esterase is the only leukocyte enzyme that can be tested on paraffin-embedded tissue and may be useful when this is the only specimen available for study.

Terminology

Leukocyte esterase reactions with different substrates have been termed specific or nonspecific, depending on lineage restriction. Naphthol AS-D chloroacetate esterase is present only in neutrophils and is thus sometimes referred to as specific esterase or neutrophilic esterase. Esterase reactivity with other substrates is found in both neutrophils and monocytes and is called nonspecific. However, the nonspecific esterase activity with these substrates can be made specific for monocytes by appropriate adjustment of pH value or by the use of fluoride inhibitor. For example, the activity of α-naphthyl acetate esterase and α-naphthyl butyrate at pH 6.0–6.3 is strong in monocytes but weak to negative in neutrophils. Naphthol AS-D acetate esterase activity is seen in both neutrophils and monocytes, but only the monocyte enzyme is inhibited by fluoride. Thus, under appropriate reaction conditions, the nonspecific esterase is often referred to as monocytic esterase.

Logistics

Slides for esterase cytochemistry may be prepared from blood, bone marrow, body fluids, or the buffy coat or Ficoll density cell isolates of these specimens. A sufficient number of blasts (e.g., greater than 20%) should be present. Both EDTA- and heparin-anticoagulated specimens are acceptable for slide preparation. Slides from body fluids or density gradient isolates of WBCs are best prepared using a cytocentrifuge. Tissue imprints can be stained, but only activity with chloroacetate substrate (in neutrophils) will be present in paraffin tissue. Slides should be prepared the same day of collection and protected from light. When slides are stored in the dark, the enzymatic activity is stable for 2 weeks at room temperature. Enzymatic activity can be preserved for a very long time if slides are wrapped in foil and frozen.

Slides are fixed, usually with buffered formalin, and incubated with an ester derivative of naphthalene. The naphthol compound is liberated and rapidly couples with a diazonium salt in the mixture, giving a colored precipitate at the site of enzyme activity. Chloroacetate (neutrophil) esterase is incubated at pH 7.4, whereas the nonspecific (monocyte) esterase reaction is optimally performed at pH 6.1. In the past, monocyte esterase was often demonstrated by inhibition with fluoride. However, fluoride is unnecessary with α-naphthyl acetate or butyrate substrates at with acid pH, because the neutrophils are negative or very weakly positive. To visualize the cell nucleus, slides are often counterstained, typically with hematoxylin. After staining, slides should be protected from light to prevent color fading. Some techniques use sequential reactions for neutrophilic and monocytic esterases with different color dye detectors. In this manner, the blasts can be assessed for differentiation along both the neutrophil and monocyte pathways.

Interpretation

Chloroacetate (neutrophilic) esterase activity with naphthol AS-D chloroacetate substrate is present in neutrophils, beginning with the promyelocytic stage. It is not as sensitive as MPO and Sudan black B in detecting myeloblasts in AML. Eosinophils, lymphocytes, plasma cells, megakaryocytes, and monocytes are negative, but mast cells and histiocytes are positive (Table 19-39). A positive reaction for chloroacetate esterase in the blasts of acute leukemia is thus seen in AML-M1, M2, M3, and M4, but AML-M5 (monocytic leukemia) is negative.

Nonspecific (monocytic) esterase activity with α-naphthyl acetate substrate is seen in monocytes, macrophages, megakaryocytes, platelets, plasma cells, basophils, hairy cell leukemia, and megaloblastic or leukemic erythroblasts. α-Naphthyl butyrate substrate is somewhat less sensitive than α-Naphthyl acetate, but is more specific for monocytes and macrophages (Table 19-39). Both substrates show focal dot positivity in a small number of cases of ALL or lymphoma, particularly those of T-cell origin.

A positive reaction for α-naphthyl acetate or butyrate esterase in the blasts of acute leukemia is seen in AML-M4 (myelomonocytic) and AML-M5 (monocytic) and occasionally, with acetate substrate, in AML-M7 (megakaryocytic). Demonstration of a monocytic component of the bone marrow with esterase stain is required in the FAB criteria for AML-M4 (Table 19-17), unless easily recognizable mature monocytic forms are present in the peripheral blood. In the bone marrow, promyelocytes and promonocytes have a similar appearance, and the monocyte esterase stain is very useful to establish monocytic lineage.

Dual staining techniques for neutrophilic and monocytic esterases optimally demonstrate granulocyte esterase only in AML-M1, M2, and M3; monocyte esterase only in AML-M5; and blasts with dual staining for both esterase types in AML-M4. However, this technique suffers from lack of sensitivity of the neutrophilic chloroacetate esterase.

If esterase activity is absent in the blasts, other tests must be performed to determine the type of leukemic cells. These include myeloperoxidase (MPO), TdT, platelet peroxidase by electron microscopy, and immunophenotyping. At times, the blasts of monocytic variants of AML may be negative for monocytic esterase but show surface antigens characteristic of the monocytic lineage by immunophenotyping.

Test: Lysozyme (Muramidase)[46]

Lysozyme or muramidase is present in many mammalian tissues, including lung, kidney, and blood cells. In human leukocytes, monocytes contain large amounts, whereas granulocytes have a moderate quantity of lysozyme. Marked elevation of lysozyme in serum or urine has been used in the past to verify an increase in monocytoid cells in suspected myelomonocytic (AML-M4) or monocytic (AML-M5) acute leukemia; currently, esterase stains or immunophenotyping for specific monocytic surface antigens are more useful tests. However, immunologic detection of lysozyme antigen in paraffin tissue sections is occasionally used to demonstrate granulocytes and monocytes when appropriate material is not available for other tests.

Test: Terminal Deoxynucleotidyl Transferase (TdT)[2,49-53]

Background and Selection

Terminal deoxynucleotidyl transferase is a DNA polymerase that is normally expressed in early T (pre-T) and early B (pre-B) lymphoid cells of the bone marrow and thymus. Differentiated T and B lymphocytes lack TdT. TdT can catalyze terminal incorporation of up to 600 nucleotides onto the free 3' hydroxyl end of single-stranded DNA without template instruction. The enzyme is postulated to function as a somatic mutagen, vital to the generation of immunoglobulin or T-cell receptor gene diversity in immature lymphoid cells. The TdT test is performed to aid in determination of the lineage of blasts in acute leukemia and in blast crisis of CML. TdT should not be used to assess persistence of small numbers of residual lymphocytic leukemic cells in the bone marrow; regenerating bone marrow cells after chemotherapy or bone marrow transplant can also be TdT positive. However, TdT may be very useful in blood or CSF to detect minimal leukemic involvement, because nonleukemic TdT-positive cells are not found in these fluids.

Logistics

When immunofluorescent or immunocytochemical methods are used for TdT, slides may be made directly from bone marrow aspirates or body fluids. They may be prepared from the buffy coat or Ficoll density cell isolates of bone marrow or peripheral blood specimens. A sufficient number of blasts (e.g., greater than 20%) should be present. Both EDTA- or heparin-anticoagulated specimens are acceptable for slide preparation. Slides from body fluids or density gradient isolates of WBCs are best prepared using a cytocentrifuge. Direct smears of peripheral blood are not used because the excessive number of RBCs interfere with assessment of positive reaction. Tissue imprints or frozen sections can be assayed, but TdT activity will not be present in paraffin-embedded tissue. Slides should be prepared the same day of collection and protected from moisture. TdT is stable in unfixed slides for 1 week at room temperature or for at least 6 months if slides are wrapped in foil and stored refrigerated or frozen.

Polyclonal antibodies have generally been more sensitive than single monoclonal antibodies for TdT. In the indirect immunofluorescent assay, fixed slides are incubated with rabbit anticalf TdT, then with fluorescein-tagged goat antirabbit antibody. Cells positive for TdT show bright nuclear fluorescence, whereas cytoplasmic fluorescence is nonspecific. Immunocytochemical methods have employed cocktails of multiple mouse monoclonal antibodies to TdT, resulting in increased sensitivity but decreased specificity.

A sensitive solid-phase enzyme immunoassay for TdT in extracts of mononuclear cells is available but is rarely used. This assay uses cell isolates of bone marrow or whole blood (EDTA anticoagulated), separated by Ficoll density gradient centrifugation. The samples should be frozen until assayed. A disadvantage of this assay is the inability to quantitate the percentage of cells containing TdT and to assess the morphology of the TdT-positive cells. More recently, TdT has also been assessed by flow cytometry, with pretreatment of the cells to allow entry of the anti-TdT antibody into the nucleus. However, the performance of this assay method has not been adequately evaluated.

Interpretation

Normal or reactive cells in blood and body fluids do not have TdT (Table 19-39). Bone marrows in nonleukemic disorders may show up to 20% of cells positive for TdT. In many instances, the positively staining marrow cells are lymphoid-like, with very high nuclear to cytoplasmic ratio, hyperchromatic nuclear chromatin, and nuclear clefts. These cells are sometimes referred to as hematogones and are postulated to be a pluripotential or early lymphoid stem cell of the bone marrow. Abundant numbers of these hematogones can be seen in regenerating bone marrows and in young children, particularly during the newborn period. Increased numbers of hematogones (and potentially TdT-positive cells) also have been seen in a variety of hematologic disorders, including idiopathic thrombocytopenic purpura, iron deficiency, erythrogenesis imperfecta, and amegakaryocytosis.

Results for the enzyme immunoassay for TdT in extracts of mononuclear cells are expressed in $ng/mL/10^8$ mononuclear cells. In patients with nonhematologic disorders, the range is 0–160 for bone marrow mononuclear cells, and 0–50 for blood mononuclear cells or whole blood extracts.

TdT is positive in more than 90% of cases of acute lymphocytic leukemia, (of T and early B (pre-B) lineage. Typically, more than 40% of the blasts are positive. A negative TdT (less than 10% of blasts positive) is evidence against ALL (except for B-ALL). TdT is also positive in lymphoblastic lymphoma and in 30% of patients with blast crisis of CML. In contrast to the myeloid blast crisis, the lymphoid TdT-positive blast crisis in CML may respond to treatment with vincristine and prednisone. TdT is usually negative in B-ALL (Burkitt's or L3 leukemia) and in differentiated T and B lymphomas or leukemias. Initially, TdT positivity was thought to be rare in AML. Subsequently, many investigators have found a variable frequency of TdT-positive AML, from 5% to more than 40%. The frequency of TdT-positive AML cases appears to be dependent on the percentage of positive blast cells taken by the investigator as a cutoff value for positivity and on the sensitivity of the assay. The immunocytochemical and enzyme immunoassay procedures show a higher incidence of positivity in AML than does the less sensitive immunofluorescent assay. It is likely that there is a continuous spectrum of TdT activity in AML, ranging from undetectable levels to values comparable to those of ALL.

Patients with AML and large numbers of TdT-positive blasts (more than 30%) by the immunofluorescent assay seem to represent a subgroup of AML (often monocytoid variants) that respond poorly to the usual chemotherapeutic regimens. Most of these cases of TdT-positive AML are biphenotypic, with the blasts simultaneously displaying myeloid lineage antigens and TdT. Although detection TdT was once considered essential in characterizing acute leukemia, it is now clear that a positive TdT does not adequately separate lymphoid from myeloid leukemias. With increasing use of immunophenotyping for antigen characterization of the leukemic cells, TdT testing has diminished in importance.

Test: Periodic Acid-Schiff Stain (PAS)[3,4,48]

In the past, PAS was useful in identifying some cases of acute lymphocytic leukemia. However, TdT and immunophenotyping are now more useful tests. Abnormal staining is seen in erythroleukemia (AML-M6) and myelodysplastic syndromes, and this stain is still occasionally used in suspected cases. Both air-dried formalin-fixed slides and tissue sections can be stained with PAS. This stain reacts with intracellular carbohydrates, such as the glycogen in the blood and bone marrow cells. Periodic acid oxidizes carbohydrates to aldehydes, which then react with the Schiff reagent (leukofuchsin) to release fuchsin and stain the cellular component a magenta color.

The cytoplasm of neutrophils, monocytes, and platelets/megakaryocytes stains diffusely with PAS, occasionally with superimposed fine or coarse granules. Mature lymphocytes may contain a few small granules. Normal erythroid precursors do not stain. In erythroleukemia (AML-M6), a variable number of erythroid precursors show intense, granular to diffuse cytoplasmic PAS staining. Other disorders with erythroid PAS positivity include myelodysplastic syndromes, acquired sideroblastic anemia, iron deficiency, and thalassemia. Lymphoblasts of ALL show variability in PAS staining. Many have coarse granules or large blocks of PAS-staining material in the cytoplasm. Myeloid blasts show diffuse cytoplasmic positivity; however, granular to block positivity against a background of diffuse staining can be seen in many cases, particularly in the monocytic forms of AML. The PAS stain also shows granular positivity in Sézary cell leukemia.

Alkaline Phosphatase Stain (Leukocyte Alkaline Phosphatase, LAP)[3,4,54]

Background and Selection

Leukocyte alkaline phosphatase is present in the specific secondary granules of neutrophils, from the myelocyte stage to the polymorphonuclear cell. Stimulated neutrophils contain increased amounts of LAP. LAP is diminished in CML and is useful in distinguishing this disorder from reactive neutrophilia and from other myeloproliferative syndromes (Tables 19-23 and 19-24). An elevated LAP is found in polycythemia vera and is one of the criteria used in distinguishing this syndrome from secondary polycythemia (Table 19-25).

Logistics

Blood smears can be prepared from unanticoagulated blood or from heparinized blood. A sufficient number of neutrophils (e.g., greater than 20%) should be present. EDTA anticoagulant inhibits the enzyme reaction and cannot be used. Slides should be fixed (usually with alkaline citrate acetone) within 4 hours for optimal activity. Fixed slides may be stored frozen for at least 6 months without loss of enzymatic activity. Slides are incubated with naphthol AS-BI phosphate at alkaline pH. The hydrolyzed naphthol derivative is coupled to a soluble diazonium dye, which forms an insoluble colored precipitate at the site of enzymatic activity in the cells. Slides are counterstained with methylene blue or hematoxylin to visualize the cell nucleus.

To obtain the LAP score, 100 segmented and band neutrophils are counted and graded from 0 to 4+, depending on the amount and intensity of the granular staining. The LAP score is the sum of the grades of the 100 cells (and thus can range from a minimum of 0 to a maximum of 400). A spuriously low LAP may occur in eosinophilia, if the negative-staining eosinophils are mistakenly counted as segmented neutrophils.

The normal LAP score may vary, depending on the diazonium dye, within a typical range of 10–100. Low LAP scores are seen in CML, some cases of myelodysplastic syndrome and AML, paroxysmal nocturnal hemoglobinuria, idiopathic thrombocytopenic purpura, pernicious anemia, and infectious mononucleosis. Elevated LAP scores occur with any neutrophilic response to infection, inflammation, tumor, or necrosis; with administration of granulocyte colony stimulating factor, steroids, or contraceptives; or in polycythemia, agnogenic myeloid metaplasia, or essential thrombocythemia. A low LAP score with neutrophilia and left shift is very suggestive of CML. Demonstration of the Philadelphia chromosome in aspirated bone marrow cells provides the definitive diagnosis.

Test: Acid Phosphatase Stain, Tartrate Resistant (Tartrate Resistant Acid Phosphatase, [TRAP], Leukocyte Acid Phosphatase)[3,4,46,55]

Background and Selection

The acid phosphatases are a group of enzymes that hydrolyze phosphate esters at an acid pH. They are located in lysosomes and within the Golgi endoplasmic reticulum. The acid phosphatase of most normal and malignant cells is inhibited by tartrate, but the acid phosphatase form (isoenzyme 5) of hairy cell leukemia is resistant to tartrate inhibition. When hairy cell leukemia is suspected on the basis of morphologic criteria, tartrate resistant acid phosphatase cytochemistry is performed for confirmation.

Logistics

Blood smears can be prepared from unanticoagulated blood or from heparin or EDTA-anticoagulated blood. A buffy coat preparation of blood or marrow should be used if the specimen is leukopenic or contains a small number of suspected hairy cells. Good quality smears with intact cells are essential for proper interpretation of inhibition of staining. A sufficient number of suspect cells (e.g., greater than 20%) should be present. Unfixed slides can be stored at room temperature for 2–4 weeks, whereas fixed slides can be stored at 4°C or −20°C for longer periods of time.

Slides are fixed (usually with acid citrate acetone) and incubated with naphthol AS-BI phosphate at acid pH, with and without tartrate. The hydrolyzed naphthol derivative is coupled to a soluble diazonium dye, which forms an insoluble colored precipitate at the site of enzymatic activity in the cells. Slides are counterstained with hematoxylin, to visualize the cell nucleus. Careful timing and regulation of tartrate concentration are necessary to obtain inhibition of most acid phosphatase activity, except for isoenzyme 5 of hairy cells. Control slides must show acid phosphatase staining of neutrophils when tartrate is not present in the incubation mixture, and near absence of acid phosphatase in neutrophils with tartrate.

Interpretation

Strong enzyme activity is seen in macrophages, monocytes, Gaucher cells, megakaryocytes, plasma cells, osteoclasts, and hairy cells. Weak activity occurs in neutrophils, lymphocytes, basophils, erythroblasts, and platelets. Transformed T lymphocytes and T-cell-derived malignancies may have strong focal acid phosphatase activity confined to the Golgi area. However, focal acid phosphatase staining is not a reliable test in distinguishing T-ALL from B-ALL.

With tartrate, only macrophages, Gaucher cells, osteoclasts, and hairy cells exhibit acid phosphatase activity. However, weakly positive tartrate resistant acid phosphatase activity may be seen occasionally in CLL, prolymphocytic leukemia, Sézary syndrome, B-lymphoma cells, and reactive lymphocytes. Immunophenotyping of hairy cells shows a characteristic surface antigen pattern. The hairy cells are B lymphocytes with monoclonal surface light chain, yet have large amounts of the monocytoid antigen, CD11c. In addition, bone marrow biopsy shows the characteristic infiltration pattern of lymphoid cells with copious clear cytoplasm.

Test: Toluidine Blue Stain[46]

Toluidine blue binds with acid mucopolysaccharides to give metachromatic staining. It is occasionally useful in identifying basophils and their precursors and mast cells.

Test: Platelet Peroxidase (PPO)[9]

The platelet peroxidase reaction is used to demonstrate the megakaryocytic lineage of blasts in acute leukemia. Leukocytes are isolated, fixed, then incubated with hydrogen peroxide and diaminobenzidine to form an electron-dense product. Transmission electron microscopy is required to demonstrate the site of peroxidase reactivity. Megakaryocytes and their precursors show PPO activity in the nuclear envelope and/or endoplasmic reticulum. Myeloperoxidase activity mainly occurs in the lysosomal granules, but sometimes in the Golgi area and endoplasmic reticulum of granulocytes, monocytes, and their precursors. The myeloperoxidase activity is largely inhibited by the glutaraldehyde-formaldehyde fixative mixture. The PPO test is difficult to perform. More recently, platelet-specific monoclonal antibodies have been used to establish the diagnosis of megakaryocytic leukemia. When megakaryocytic lineage is seen in up to 30% of blasts, megakaryocytic leukemia (AML, M7) is the diagnosis.

TISSUE BIOPSIES

Test: Bone Marrow Aspirate and Biopsy (Bone Marrow Examination)[18,33,56-58]

Background and Selection

The bone marrow is examined when hematologic malignancy is suspected; for example, when abnormal cells are present in the peripheral blood smear, in cases of unexplained leukopenia or thrombocytopenia, or in patients with unexplained lymphadenopathy or hepatosplenomegaly. The bone marrow also may be involved with metastasis in nonhematopoietic malignancies, which can be manifested in the peripheral blood by pancytopenia, teardrop RBCs, and/or a leukoerythroblastic reaction. Staging of Hodgkin's disease or lymphoma often requires a bone marrow biopsy. Repeated bone marrow examinations are performed to monitor therapy for hematologic malignancies, particularly acute leukemia, and after bone marrow transplantation.

Bone marrow examination is helpful in unexplained thrombocytopenia, distinguishing between suppression of platelet production with low numbers of megakaryocytes and peripheral platelet destruction or splenic sequestration with adequate bone marrow megakaryocytes. Occasionally, the examination of trabecular bone in the biopsy specimen is useful in metabolic bone disease. Bone marrow culture is a low-yield procedure, but it may be useful in fever of unknown origin when initial tests have proven negative, particularly when infection with *Histoplasma*, *Cryptococcus*, or *Mycoplasma* is suspected.

Bone marrow examination is not helpful in the workup of most patients with anemia. Iron deficiency usually can be assessed by ferritin levels rather than bone marrow iron stores, and folate and vitamin B_{12} levels or a Schilling test can be performed when megaloblastic anemia is suspected. Biochemical testing should be used to elucidate the etiology of hemolytic anemias. Most cases of unexplained anemia with no abnormality in WBCs or platelets are secondary to systemic disease (anemia of chronic disease) rather than a hematologic disorder. A bone marrow examination may be indicated in unexplained macrocytic anemia to look for evidence of myelodysplastic syndrome (e.g., ineffective erythropoiesis or dysplasia of RBC precursors).

Terminology

Several preparations of bone marrow may be studied as part of a complete examination.

Trephine Biopsy

The tissue biopsy, which includes both marrow and bone, is usually fixed in Bouin's or Zenker's fixative, decalcified, and embedded in paraffin. Sections are stained with hematoxylin and eosin (H&E). In some histology laboratories, the biopsy is embedded in plastic and stained with tissue Giemsa. The biopsy is a good preparation for assessing cellularity and quantitative cellular relationships and for detecting fibrosis, granulomas, or focal infiltration with lymphoma, Hodgkin's disease, or metastatic carcinoma. It is a poor preparation for appreciating the morphology of individual cells or for evaluating iron stores, which are diminished by the decalcification treatment. In addition, it is difficult to perform special enzyme cytochemistries and immunophenotyping.

Touch Preparation of Biopsy

The touch preparation is an imprint of the trephine biopsy on a glass slide, usually stained with Wright-Giemsa. When an aspiration cannot be obtained, the touch preparation provides a specimen for assessment of individual cell morphology and special enzyme stains. In general, the bone marrow must be heavily infiltrated with abnormal cells to obtain an adequate touch preparation.

Aspirate Particle Smears

One to two spicule particles are selected from the EDTA-anticoagulated bone marrow aspirate and placed on a coverslip or slide. A second coverslip or slide is placed on top, and the smear is made by gently pulling the coverslips/slides apart. These particle slides are routinely stained with Wright-Giemsa and Prussian blue (for iron content). These slides also can be used for enzyme cytochemistry and TdT. The aspirate smear is a good preparation for assessing the morphology of individual cells. However, focal malignant infiltration and granulomas may not be detected.

Direct Aspirate Smears

A push smear of the aspirated bone marrow can be rapidly prepared at the bed side, but will include a variable mixture of aspirated particles and blood. These are sometimes good preparations for cytologic detail but do not permit quantitative cellular assessment or detection of focal infiltration.

Clotted or Concentrated Particle Sections

After slides of marrow aspirate particles have been prepared, the remaining spicules from the aspirate are concentrated, fixed, and embedded in paraffin. Sections are stained with H&E. Like the biopsy, the particle sections can demonstrate quantitative cellular relationships, and focal collections of abnormal cells (if they are aspirated), but are less useful in assessing the cytology of individual cells. Bone marrow iron content can also be evaluated on particle sections.

Leukocyte Isolates

The WBCs from the bone marrow aspirate can be concentrated by simple centrifugation or centrifugation over a density gradient (e.g., Ficoll-Hypaque). These preparations are useful for enzyme cytochemistries, immunophenotyping, and other special studies. Wright-Giemsa morphology of these preparations can be examined on slides prepared with the cytocentrifuge.

Logistics

The bone marrow is always interpreted in conjunction with the peripheral blood findings. Accordingly, the blood cell counts and peripheral blood smear should be examined on the same day of the marrow study. The laboratory should be notified of the impending marrow, so that a technologist can assist in handling the bone marrow specimen and preparing the slides. In addition, careful thought should be given to the special studies that may be required, including culture, enzyme cytochemistries, immunophenotyping, cytogenetics, gene rearrangement studies, or electron microscopy. The laboratory personnel should be consulted concerning the proper sample to obtain for these tests.

For most patients, concurrent bone marrow aspirate and trephine biopsy is the best approach for a thorough morphologic study. Bone marrow aspiration without biopsy often is performed in pediatric patients, whereas biopsy without aspiration is performed to assess bone marrow involvement in the patient with solid malignancy, lymphoma, or Hodgkin's disease. Bilateral biopsies often are performed in the staging of lymphoma or Hodgkin's disease. The location of choice for marrow aspiration and biopsy is the posterior iliac crest. The anterior iliac crest sometimes is aspirated if the patient is obese or if the posterior crest has been exposed to irradiation. Occasionally, a focal bony lesion, localized by radiography, is sampled. In the past, the sternum was used for aspiration, but a biopsy cannot be performed at this site. In infants, the proximal anterior aspect of the tibia can be used for bone marrow aspiration.

The Jamshidi needle frequently is used for bone marrow biopsy. The bone marrow aspiration also can be obtained through this needle before the biopsy if the needle is advanced 2–3 cm between the aspiration and biopsy. Alternatively, some physicians obtain the trephine biopsy first and perform aspirate with a smaller University of Illinois sternal needle at least 1 cm away from the biopsy site.

Marrow must be aspirated into syringes containing anticoagulant to prevent clotting. The first 0.5 mL of marrow is aspirated into EDTA anticoagulant for slide preparation. This initial sample is the most concentrated in spicules and least diluted with blood. Additional marrow should be aspirated in a separate anticoagulated syringe at this point for special studies (e.g., chromosomal analysis, immunophenotyping, gene rearrangement studies) and placed in the appropriate anticoagulant or media. Slides are prepared from the aspirate as described under Terminology. An adequate bone marrow biopsy should be at least 1–1.5 cm in length.

Interpretation

The bone marrow report includes the following findings.

Overall Cellularity

Cellularity is best estimated on the biopsy or particle section slides. The cellularity is an estimate of the area occupied by the cells as a percentage of the total area occupied by cells, background substance, and fat. Normal cellularity is age dependent. The marrow is approximately 60–100% cellular in the newborn, 40–90% cellular in the child, 30–80% cellular in the adult, and 15–60% cellular in the older adult (over age 65). Increased cellularity is caused by granulocytic or erythroid hyperplasia or by bone marrow infiltration. Decreased cellularity is invariably accompanied by a decrease in the number of granulocytes, the most numerous cell line in the marrow.

Adequacy of Megakaryocytes

The number of megakaryocytes is best estimated on the biopsy or particle section slides, although an adequate impression often can be gained from the aspirate particle smear. An overall average of one megakaryocyte per 40–50× objective field is usually seen in the biopsy or particle section slides. Thrombocytopenia with decreased megakaryocytes occurs with bone marrow suppression or infiltration, whereas thrombocytopenia with normal to increased megakaryocytes is seen with peripheral platelet destruction, splenic platelet sequestration, or ineffective megakaryopoiesis (e.g., in myelodysplastic syndrome).

Relative Number of Myeloid and Erythroid Precursors

The quantitative relationship of myeloid and erythroid cells can be ascertained in many ways. Differential cell counts frequently are performed on bone marrow aspirate slides; however, most experienced pathologists or hematologists can make a reasonable estimate of the quantitative cell relationships. Occasionally, a 500-cell differential may be useful in the subclassification of myeloid leukemia (Table 19-17) or myelodysplastic syndrome (Table 19-22). Reference values for the adult bone marrow differential are given in Table 19-40, although published values for these numbers vary widely. As a rule of thumb, approximately 25% of marrow cells should be segmented or band neutrophils, and 10–15% should be erythroid precursors. The myeloid to erythroid (M/E) ratio also is computed. In the adult, the normal range is approximately 2:1–4:1.

As for megakaryocytes, quantitative changes in bone marrow myeloid and erythroid precursors is interpreted in conjunction with peripheral blood findings. Anemia and neutropenia can be due to diminished bone marrow production or infiltration, peripheral consumption with normal to increased bone marrow production, or ineffective bone marrow poiesis (often accompanied by morphologic dysplasia).

Individual Cell Morphology

Cell morphology is best seen with Wright-Giemsa preparations of the aspirate. Maturation sequence (normal or dysplastic) of neutrophils, erythroids, and megakaryocytes is assessed, and any abnormal cells are identified. Increases in other cells, such as small lymphocytes, plasma cells, eosinophils, mast cells, or histiocytes, are noted.

Status of Iron Stores

Prussian blue staining for iron content can be performed on the aspirate particle smears or particle sections. Iron stores in the bone marrow biopsy may be spuriously low because of the use of decalcification agents. Iron is graded as absent, decreased, normal, increased, or markedly increased. In addition, the location of iron is assessed. Ringed sideroblasts (abnormal location of iron in mitochondria surrounding the nucleus) can sometimes be found in erythroid dysplasia.

Focal Lesions

Focal lesions are best appreciated in the bone marrow biopsy or particle section. Examples of focal lesions that can be found in the marrow include metastatic tumor, lymphoma, Hodgkin's disease, granulomas, benign lymphoid follicles, myeloma, hairy cell leukemia, systemic mastocytosis, fibrosis, necrosis, serous fat atrophy, vasculitis or thromboses, and storage disease (e.g., Gaucher's disease).

Bone Lesions

Examination of bony trabeculae in the biopsy may be important in evaluation of hyperthyroidism, osteoporosis, osteomalacia, or Paget's disease.

All these findings are interpreted in light of the peripheral blood findings and clinical history. When possible, a diagnosis is made. On the basis of the morphologic findings, further testing may be indicated. A silver stain can demonstrate an increase in reticulin fibers when marrow fibrosis is suspected. Cytochemistry, immunotyping, and cytogenetics are useful in classifying acute leukemia. Immunotyping and sometimes gene rearrangement studies may be indicated to distinguish reactive from malignant lymphoproliferation or hematopoietic from nonhematopoietic malignancy. When granulomata or necrotic areas are found, special stain-

Table 19-40. Reference Values for Bone Marrow Differential

Cell Type	Adult Reference Range (%)
Myeloblasts	0–3.5
Promyelocytes	1–6
Myelocytes	8–15
Metamyelocytes	9–25
Bands and segmented cells	15–27
Neutrophils	7–25
Eosinophils	0–4
Basophilic	0–1
Erythroblasts	0–3
Basophilic normoblasts	1–5
Polychromatophilic normoblasts	5–20
Orthochromic normoblasts	1–15
Lymphocytes	3–20
Plasma cells	0–3.5
Monocytes and precursors	0–2
Myeloid to erythroid ratio	1.5–3.5

(Data from Koepke.[18])

ing for microorganisms, such as Gram stain, acid fast for mycobacteria, or methanamine silver for fungi, should be performed.

Test: Lymph Node Biopsy[1,4,15,45,59-64]

Background and Selection

Clinical indications for lymph node biopsy include the following: (1) diagnosis of metastatic carcinoma, Hodgkin's disease, non-Hodgkin's lymphoma, infection, granulomatous lymphadenitis, abnormal immune reactions, and other conditions in patients presenting with persistent lymph node enlargement without an obvious clinical explanation; (2) confirmation of suspected metastatic tumor in patients with known malignancies; (3) staging of patients with known malignant neoplasm, including Hodgkin's and non-Hodgkin's lymphoma; (4) assessment of tumor remission or recurrence after treatment; (5) assessment of the evolution of non-Hodgkin's lymphoma from low grade to high grade neoplasms; (6) complementing the hematologic workup of a patient presenting with unexplained lymphadenopathy and abnormal peripheral blood WBCs; and (7) determination of the need for further procedures, including exploratory laparotomy, thoracotomy, mediastinoscopy, and surgical staging.

Lymph node biopsy is ordered by the patient's physician, usually after consultation with a hematologist-oncologist and a surgeon. Lymph node biopsy is considered only after other relevant noninvasive studies have been explored. Useful serologic tests for diagnosis of infectious disorders that may cause lymphadenopathy (e.g., infectious mononucleosis, toxoplasmosis) are discussed in Chapter 29.

Today, fine needle aspiration (FNA) of lymph nodes is gaining favor as a useful diagnostic procedure that may be performed rapidly, economically, and with minimal discomfort in an outpatient setting. Lymph node FNA is employed in staging of patients with previously diagnosed Hodgkin's disease and non-Hodgkin's lymphoma and in evaluating these patients for suspected new sites of involvement or for recurrence. Although a primary diagnosis of non-Hodgkin's lymphoma or of Hodgkin's disease may be made by lymph node FNA alone, confirmatory surgical biopsy is performed at most medical centers. In questionable cases, the application of lymphocyte marker techniques to cytologic specimens has enhanced our ability to make a definitive diagnosis of malignant lymphoma from cytologic smears or cytospin preparations.

Logistics

Surgical lymph node biopsy requires close communication between the surgeon and the pathologist to ensure that an optimal specimen is obtained. To increase the likelihood of a diagnostic biopsy, the surgeon should biopsy the largest lymph node possible. Lymph nodes should be handled carefully, avoiding crushing, drying, and heat artifacts caused by cautery. Ideally, a small portion of the specimen should be submitted for bacterial, fungal and mycobacterial culture at the time of surgery (while sterile technique is being observed). The fresh lymph node biopsy specimen should then be submitted to the pathologist in a sterile Petri dish on saline dampened gauze for immediate processing (Fig. 19-7). Priority should be given to immediate fixation of representative sections in 10% neutral buffered formalin and B-5 or Zenker's fixative for routine light microscopic examination. Frozen sections may be prepared to exclude obvious metastatic carcinomas and granulomatous lymphadenitis. Most hematopathologists will defer the diagnosis of malignant lymphoma until permanent sections are available for examination. Frozen tissue must be saved, however, for subsequent cell marker and/or gene rearrangement studies, if indicated. Cytologic imprints may be air dried and/or fixed appropriately (e.g., 95% ethanol for cytoplasmic antigens, cold buffered acetone for surface antigens) to allow for subsequent immunocytochemistry studies. A small piece of tissue (1–2 mm^3) may be fixed in cold phosphate-buffered glutaraldehyde for electron microscopic study as well. Lymphocyte suspensions, collected in culture media such as RPMI with fetal calf serum, may be employed for evaluation of surface membrane immunoglobulin and other monoclonal antibody studies by flow cytometry. Improper handling of the specimen usually precludes definitive diagnosis, requiring re-biopsy.

Interpretation

The clinician ordering a lymph node biopsy is looking for an explanation for the patient's lymph node enlargement. Is the condition benign or malignant? Specifically, how will the diagnosis affect the patient's management, therapy, and survival? A variety of conditions may cause lymphadenopathy (Table 19-30) and it is the pathologist's responsibility to make an accurate diagnosis. Most diagnoses are straightforward, but some remain elusive and require a battery of ancillary studies and careful clinical correlation to classify precisely.

The pattern of lymph node involvement and cytology of infiltrating cells offer important clues to the patholo-

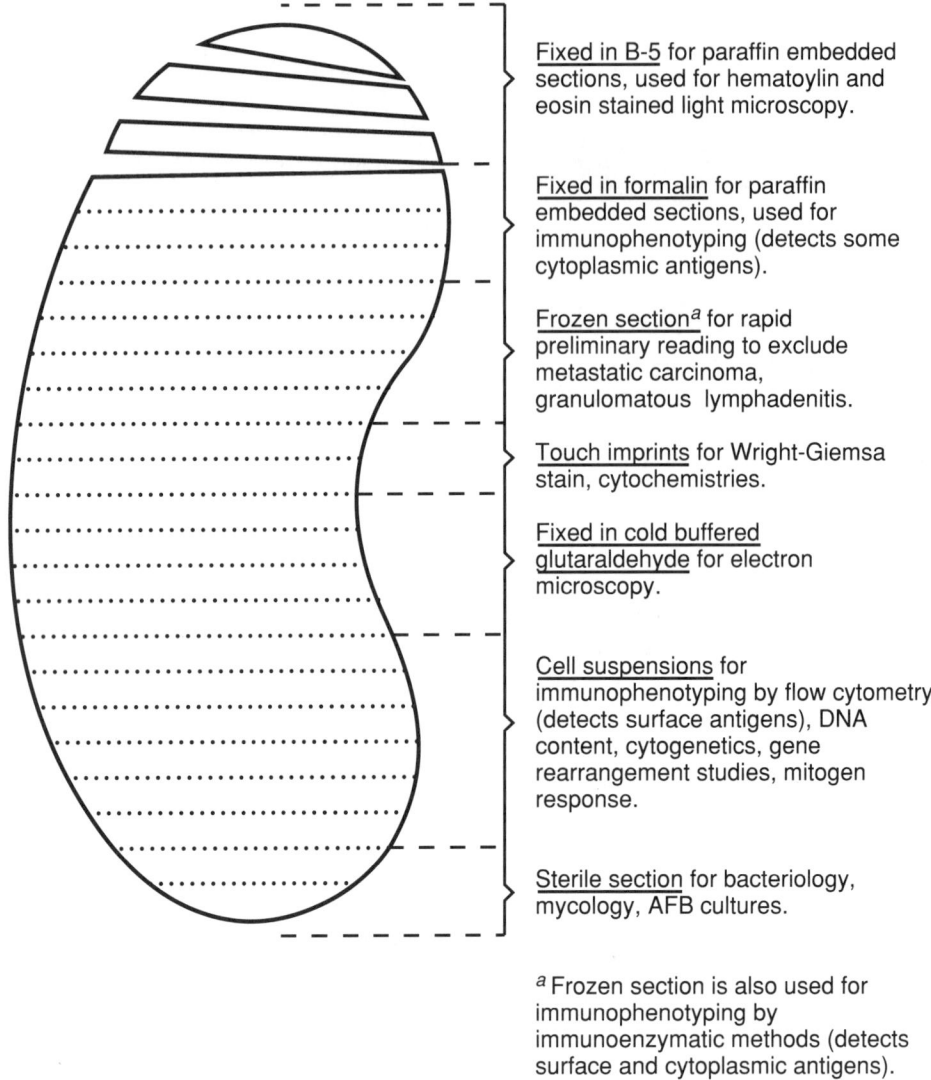

Fig. 19-7. Processing of the lymph node biopsy. AFB, acid-fast bacteria.

gist in examination of the lymph node. Most lymphadenopathies show follicular (nodular) proliferation of cells, diffuse proliferation of cells, mixed interfollicular/follicular proliferation of cells, or proliferation of cells beginning in the lymph node sinuses (Fig. 19-8). The cell populations may be monomorphous (relatively uniform population of one cell type) or heterogeneous (proliferation of a mixture of cell types). Cells may be of hematologic origin (e.g., lymphocytes, plasma cells, immunoblasts, myeloid cells) or of nonhematologic origin (e.g., carcinoma, sarcoma). In most malignant cases, neoplastic cells mimic their normal counterparts, allowing for easy recognition. When neoplasms are poorly differentiated, their cell of origin may not be recognizable by light microscopy alone, requiring additional study (special histochemical stains, immunophenotyping, electron microscopy).

A variety of benign and malignant conditions that demonstrate follicular, diffuse, mixed interfollicular/follicular, or sinus patterns of nodal involvement are enumerated in Table 19-41. In general, benign or reactive conditions show preservation of normal cortical, medullary, and sinusoidal architecture, with a heteromorphous mixture of cells. Reactive lymph nodes usually demonstrate follicular hyperplasia (expansion of the B-cell areas) characterized by prominent germinal centers and tingible body macrophages (histiocytes phagocytosing nuclear debris), a spectrum of small and larger lymphocytes, and a mixture of other cell types, including plasma cells, histiocytes, eosinophils, and neutrophils. Reactive lymph nodes may show interfollicular or paracortical hyperplasia (expansion of T-cell areas) as well. By contrast, malignant lymphomas usually demonstrate effacement of nodal architecture and

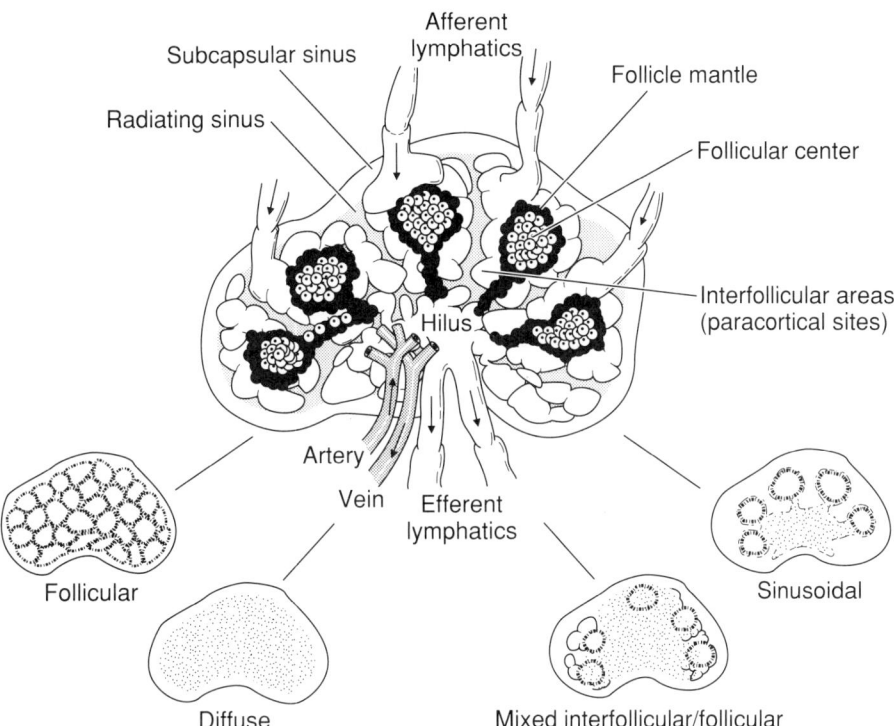

Fig. 19-8. Basic architecture of lymph node and patterns of infiltration. (See Table 19-41 for reactive and malignant causes of these infiltrative patterns.) (Adapted from Tindle,[64] with permission.)

contain a relatively monomorphous population of lymphocytes. Lymphomas may demonstrate a follicular or diffuse pattern of involvement.

Classification systems for non-Hodgkin's lymphoma have proved confusing for clinicians and pathologists alike. Dr. Henry Rappaport first offered a simplified reasonable classification in 1956 based on size and pattern of infiltrate. However, the diffuse histiocytic lymphoma in his classification was found most often to represent a lymphoma of large, transformed lymphocytes rather than to be of histiocytic origin. Along with rapid advances in immunology came combined morphologic and immunologic classifications of lymphomas introduced by Lennert, Lukes and Collins, and others. These investigators proposed that different types of lymphoma could arise from T- and B-lymphoid cells of the node at various steps in the sequence of immune stimulation or transformation (see Fig. 16-2, Ch. 16). In 1982 the National Cancer Institute (NCI) Working Formulation was published, culminating in an exhaustive study of non-Hodgkin's lymphomas by a worldwide panel of experts. Non-Hodgkin's lymphomas were divided into clinically prognostic groups on the basis of morphologic criteria and survival data (Table 19-33).

The panel did not assess the clinical significance of the B- and T-cell immunologic subsets of malignant lymphomas. The Working Formulation correlates more favorable survival with a follicular pattern as an independent variable from cell type as compared with a diffuse pattern of infiltration. Cell type also correlates with the biologic behavior of the lymphoma. Generally, lymphomas of small, cells have a slow course, whereas those of larger cells are more aggressive. Blast-like lymphomas (e.g., large immunoblastic, T-lymphoblastic lymphoma, small noncleaved or Burkitt-like) with a high proliferative rate have the most rapidly progressive course. The Working Formulation provides a useful mechanism for translating terms from different classification systems into prognostic groups, allowing for comparative assessment of clinical therapeutic trials throughout the world.

Lymph node biopsy diagnosis of Hodgkin's disease is based on the recognition of classic Reed-Sternberg cells (the origin of which is still unknown) or their variants and an appropriate cellular background, usually composed of irregular small lymphocytes and a varying number of plasma cells, eosinophils, and neutrophils. Because Hodgkin's disease may be focal, with reactive

Table 19-41. Architectural Patterns of Reactive and Malignant Lymphadenopathies

Pattern	Reactive	Malignant

Follicular/nodular pattern	Reactive follicular hyperplasia
	   Nonspecific
	   Florid
	AIDS-related lymphadenopathy
	Syphilis
	Rheumatoid arthritis
	Castleman's disease
	   Hyaline-vascular type
	   Plasma cell type
		ML, follicular types
		ML, some variants of small lymphocytic (e.g., intermediate, mantle zone)
		
		HD, some cases of lymphocyte predominant and nodular sclerosing

Diffuse pattern	Viral lymphadenitis
	   Infectious mononucleosis
	   Herpes zoster
	Postvaccinial lymphadenitis
	Dilatin and other drug-induced hypersensitivities
	Atypical lymphoplasmacytic and immunoblastic proliferation
	Angioimmunoblastic lymphadenopathy
		ML, diffuse types
		Hodgkin's disease, all types
		Metastatic tumors
		Leukemias

Mixed interfollicular/follicular pattern	Dermatopathic lymphadenopathy
	Toxoplasmosis
	Necrotizing granulomatous inflammation
	   Cat scratch disease
	   Lymphogranuloma venereum
	   Yersinia
	Histiocytic necrotizing lymphadenitis (Kikuchi's disease)
	Systemic lupus erythematosus
	Mucocutaneous lymph node syndrome (Kawasaki disease)
		ML, diffuse, T-cell subtypes
		Mycosis fungoides
		HD, some cases of mixed cellularity and nodular sclerosing
		Leukemias
		Hairy cell leukemia
		Malignant histiocytosis
		Histiocytosis X
		Mast cell disease
		Metastatic carcinomas

Sinus pattern	Sinus histiocytosis
	Sinus histiocytosis with massive lymphadenopathy
	Hemophagocytic syndromes
	   Viral associated
	   Bacterial associated
	Langerhans cell histiocytosis
	Whipple's disease
	Lymphangiogram effect
		Vascular transformation of sinuses
		ML, diffuse large cell type (rare)
		Leukemias
		Hairy cell leukemia
		Malignant histiocytosis
		Histiocytosis X
		Mast cell disease
		Metastatic carcinomas
		Kaposi's sarcoma

Abbreviations: ML, malignant lymphoma; HD, Hodgkin's disease; AIDS, acquired immunodeficiency syndrome. (Data from Burke.[59])

hyperplasia elsewhere in the node, it is imperative that all areas of the lymph node be carefully examined so that the diagnosis is not missed. Focal disease also presents a problem for fine needle aspiration diagnosis because of the limited sample obtained. The types of Hodgkin's disease and morphologic criteria for diagnosis are summarized in Table 19-31. Before advances in radiation therapy and chemotherapy, the morphologic type was considered predictive of biologic behavior. Lymphocyte predominant Hodgkin's and nodular sclerosing Hodgkin's disease correlated with a favorable prognosis, mixed cellularity was less favorable, and lymphocyte-depleted Hodgkin's disease had the least favorable prognosis. Today, both the clinical (Table 19-32) and pathologic stage of the disease determine therapy and prognosis, with many centers reporting overall cure rates exceeding 80%.

A definitive lymph node biopsy diagnosis may be made in most cases on the basis of morphology alone; however, when the diagnosis is in doubt, additional studies may be performed. Sometimes profound reactive lymphoid hyperplasia mimics follicular (nodular) lymphoma. In such cases, the lymphoid proliferations can be phenotyped with panels of antibodies. Generally, a monoclonal B-cell population (e.g., all cells with one type immunoglobulin light chain) is equated with a diagnosis of malignant lymphoma, whereas a polyclonal lymphocyte population (e.g., cells with both κ- and λ-light chains) indicates a benign reactive process. Phenotyping also can be useful in some cases of florid diffuse lymphoid proliferations, in which benign polyclonal proliferations caused by drug reactions, infectious mononucleosis, influenza, and other immune reactions may mimic histiocytic or immunoblastic lymphoma. Recognition of T-cell lymphomas on the basis of morphology alone is difficult and often requires confirmation by lymphocyte marker studies. In addition, gene rearrangement studies of DNA can indicate monoclonality for T cells by demonstrating clonal rearrangement of the T-cell receptor.

In other cases of large cell proliferations within lymph nodes, it may be difficult to differentiate histiocytic lymphoma or immunoblastic sarcoma from undifferentiated or poorly differentiated carcinomas. In such cases, special histochemical stains and monoclonal antibody panels, including cytokeratin, carcinoembryonic antigen (CEA), common leukocyte antigen, α-fetoprotein, β-human chorionic gonadotropin (hCG), S100, and vimentin should unmask the cell of origin. In rare cases, electron microscopy may be necessary to resolve the question of malignant cell origin.

REFERENCES

1. Rapaport SI: Introduction to Hematology. Philadelphia, JB Lippincott, 1987.
2. Jandl J: Blood. Textbook of Hematology. Boston, Little Brown, 1987.
3. Williams WJ, Beutler E, Erslev AJ, Lichtman MA: Hematology. New York, McGraw-Hill, 1984.
4. Kjeldsberg C (ed): Practical Diagnosis of Hematologic Disorders. Chicago, ASCP Press, 1989.
5. Axtell RA: Evaluation of the patient with a possible phagocytic disorder. Hematol Oncol Clin North Am 1988;2:1–12.
6. Miller DR, Baehner RL, McMillan CW: Blood Diseases of Infancy and Childhood. St. Louis, CV Mosby, 1984.
7. Malech HL, Gallin JJ: Current concepts: immunology. Neutrophils in human diseases. N Engl J Med 1987;317:687–694.
8. Bennett JM, Catovsky D, Daniel MT et al: Proposed revised criteria for the classification of acute myeloid leukemia. Ann Intern Med 1985;103:626–629.
9. Bennett JM, Catovsky D, Daniel MT et al: Criteria for the diagnosis of acute leukemia of the megakaryocyte lineage (M7). A report of the French-American-British cooperative group. Ann Intern Med 1985;103:460–462.
10. Second MIC Cooperative Study Group: Morphologic, immunologic and cytogenetic (MIC) working classification of the acute myeloid leukaemias. Br J Haematol 1988;68:487–494.
11. Champlin R, Gale RP: Acute lymphoblastic leukemia: recent advances in biology and therapy. Blood 1989;73:2051–2066.
12. Smithson WA: Childhood acute leukemia. Curr Hematol Oncol 1987;5:45–76.
13. Sobol RE, Bloomfield CD, Royston I: Immunophenotyping in the diagnosis and classification of acute lymphoblastic leukemia. Clin Lab Med 1988;8:151–162.
14. Bennett JM, Catovsky D, Daniel G: Proposals for the classification of the myelodysplastic syndromes. Br J Haematol 1982;51:189–199.
15. Rifkind RA, Band A, Marks PA et al: Fundamentals of Hematology. Chicago, Year Book Medical Publishers, 1986.
16. The Non-Hodgkin's Lymphoma Pathologic Classification Project: National Cancer Institute sponsored study of non-Hodgkin's lymphomas. Summary and description of a working formulation for clinical usuage. Cancer 1982;49:212–235.
17. Van Assendelft OW, England JM: Advances in Hematologic Methods: The Blood Count. Boca Raton, FL, CRC Press, 1982.
18. Koepke JA (ed): Laboratory Hematology. New York, Churchill Livingstone, 1984.
19. Schoentag RA: Hematology analyzers. Clin Lab Med 1988;8:653–673.
20. Shapiro MF, Greenfield S: The complete blood count and leukocyte differential count. An approach to their rational application. Ann Intern Med 1987;106:65–74.
21. Bentley SA: Alternatives to the neutrophil band count. Arch Pathol Lab Med 1988;112:883–884.
22. Koepke JA (ed): Differential Leukocyte Counting. Aspen, College of American Pathologists, 1977.
23. Koepke JA: Standardization of the manual differential leukocyte count. Lab Med 1980;11:371–375.
24. Maladonado JE, Hanlon DG: Monocytosis: A current appraisal. Mayo Clin Proc 1965;40:246–251.
25. Weick JK, Hagedorn AB, Linman JW: Leukoerythroblastosis: Diagnosis and prognostic significance. Mayo Clin Proc 1974;49:110–113.
26. Wood TA, Frankel EP: The atypical lymphocyte. Am J Med 1967;42:923–936.
27. DeCresce R: The Technicon H-1: A discrete, fully automated complete blood count and differential analyzer. Lab Med 1986;17:17–21.
28. Griswald DJ, Champagne EV: Evaluation of the Coulter S-Plus IV three-part differential in an acute care hospital. Am J Clin Pathol 1985;84:49–57.
29. Pierre RV, Payne BA, Lee WK, et al: Comparison of four leukocyte differential methods with the National Committee for Clinical Laboratory Standards (NCCLS) reference method. Am J Clin Pathol 1987;87:201–209.
30. Altman PL, Dittmer DS (eds): Blood and Other Body Fluids. Bethesda, Federation of American Societies for Experimental Biology, 1961.
31. Cornbleet J, Kessinger S: Evaluation of Coulter S-Plus three-part differential in a population with a high prevalence of abnormalities. Am J Clin Pathol 1985;84:620–626.
32. Dacie JV, Lewis SL: Practical Haematology. 5th Ed. Edinburgh, Churchill-Livingstone, 1975.

33. Henry JB: Clinical Diagnosis and Management by Laboratory Methods. Philadelphia, WB Saunders, 1984.
34. Cornbleet J: Spurious results from automated hematology cell counters. Lab Med 1983;14:509–514.
35. Bessman JD: New parameters on automated hematology instruments. Lab Med 1983;14:488–491.
36. Corash L: Measurement of platelet volume in the clinical hematology laboratory. ASCP Check Sample H 88-7. Chicago, American Society of Clinical Pathologists, 1988.
37. Corash L: Platelet sizing: Techniques, biologic significance, and clinical applications. Curr Top Hematol 1983;4:99–122.
38. Levin J, Bessman JD: The inverse relation between platelet volume and platelet number. J Lab Clin Med 1983;101:295–307.
39. Nelson RB, Kehl D: Electronically determined platelet indices in thrombocytopenic patients. Cancer 1981;48:954–956.
40. Threatte GA, Adbrados C, Ebbee S, Brecher G: Mean platelet volume: The need for a reference method. Am J Clin Pathol 1984;81:769–772.
41. Keren DF: Flow Cytometry in Clinical Diagnosis. Chicago, American Society of Clinical Pathologists, Press, 1989.
42. Deegan MJ: Membrane antigen analysis in the diagnosis of lymphoid leukemias and lymphomas: Differential diagnosis, prognosis as related to immunophenotype, and recommendations for testing. Arch Pathol Lab Med 1989;113:606–618.
43. Foon KA, Todd RF: Immunologic classification of leukemia and lymphoma. Blood 1986;68:1–31.
44. Loughran TP, Starkebaum G: Large granular lymphocytic leukemia. Medicine (Baltimore) 1987;66:397–405.
45. International Committee for Standardization in Haematology (ICSH): Recommended methods for cytological procedures in haematology. Clin Lab Haematol 1985;7:55–74.
46. Li C-Y: Morphologic, cytochemical, and immunologic diagnosis of hematologic malignancies. Curr Hematol 1981;1:308–342.
47. Yam LT, Li C-Y, Crosby WH: Cytochemical identification of monocytes and granulocytes. Am J Clin Pathol 1971;55:283–290.
48. Bell MS, Hippel T, Goodman H: Use of cytochemistry and FAB classification in leukemia and other pathologic states. Am J Med Technol 1981;6:437–471.
49. Barr RD, Koekebakker M: Storage and transportation of samples for analysis of terminal transferase by indirect immunofluorescence. Am J Clin Pathol 1984;81:660–661.
50. Erber WN, Mason DY: Immunoalkaline phosphatase labeling of terminal transferase in hematologic samples. Am J Clin Pathol 1987;88:43–50.
51. Fairbands TR, King WJ, Coleman MS et al: Solid-phase enzyme immunoassay for terminal deoxynucleotidyl transferase (Abbott TdT-EIA) in extracts of whole blood and mononuclear cells isolated from bone marrow and blood. J Clin Lab Anal 1987;1:175–183.
52. Lanham GR, Melvin SL, Stass SA: Immunoperoxidase determination of terminal deoxynucleotidyl transferase in acute leukemia using PAP and ABC methods: Experience in 102 cases. Am J Clin Pathol 1985;83:366–370.
53. Muehleck SD, McKenna RW, Gale PF, Brunning RD: Terminal deoxynucleotidyl transferase (TdT)-positive cells in bone marrow in the absence of hematologic malignancy. Am J Clin Pathol 1983;79:277–284.
54. Kaplow LS: Leukocyte alkaline phosphatase cytochemistry: Applications and methods. Ann NY Acad Sci 1968;155:911–947.
55. Janckila AJ, Li C-Y, Lam K-W, Yam LT: The cytochemistry of tartrate resistant acid phosphatase. Technical considerations. Am J Clin Pathol 1978;70:45–55.
56. Batjer JD: Preparation of optimal bone marrow samples. Lab Med 1979;10:101–106.
57. Brynes RK, McKenna RW, Sundberg RD: Bone marrow aspiration and trephine biopsy. An approach to a thorough study. Am J Clin Pathol 1978;70:753–759.
58. Hyun BK, Gulati GL, Ashton JK: Bone marrow examination: Techniques and interpretation. Hematol Oncol Clin North Amer 1988;2:513–523.
59. Burke JS: Reactive lymphadenopathies. Semin Diagn Pathol 1988;5:312–316.
60. Dorfman RF, Warnke R: Lymphadenopathy simulating the malignant lymphomas. Hum Pathol 1974;5:519–550.
61. Lieberman PH, Filippa DA, Straus DJ et al: Evaluation of malignant lymphomas using three classifications and the Working Formulation—482 cases with median follow-up of 11.9 years. Am J Med 1986;81:365–380.
62. Lukes RJ, Parker JW, Taylor CR et al: Immunologic approach to non-Hodgkin's lymphoma and related leukemias. An analysis of the results of multiparameter studies of 425 cases. Semin Hematol 1978;15:322–351.
63. Rappaport H: Tumors of the hematopoietic system. pp. F8-97–F8-98. In Atlas of Tumor Pathology. Section 3, Fascicle 8. Washington, DC, US Armed Forces Institute of Pathology, 1986.
64. Tindle BH: Teaching monograph. Malignant lymphomas. Am J Pathol 1984;116:119–170.
65. Wintrobe MM: Clinical Hematology. 8th Ed. Philadelphia, Lea & Febiger, 1981.
66. Schumacher HR, Barvin DF, Triplett DA: Introduction to Laboratory Hematology and Hematopathology. New York, Allen R Liss, 1984.
67. Brunning RD: Morphologic alterations in nucleated blood and marrow cells in genetic disorders. Hum Pathol 1970;1:99–124.
68. First MIC Cooperative Study Group: Morphologic, immunologic, and cytogenetic (MIC) working classification of acute lymphoblastic leukemias. Cancer Genet Cytogenet 1986;23:189–197.
69. Trent JM, Kaneko Y, Mitelman F: Report of the committee on structural chromosome changes in neoplasm. Cytogenet Cell Genet 1989;51:553–562.
70. Berlin NI: Diagnosis and classification of the polycythemias. Semin Hematol 1975;12:339–351.
71. Murphy S, Iland H, Rosenthal D, Laszlo J: Essential thrombocythemia: An interim report for the Polycythemia Vera Study Group. Semin Hematol 1986;23:177–182.
72. Hoffbrand AV, Pettit JE: Essential Haematology. London, Blackwell Scientific, 1984.
73. Rumke CL: The statistically expected variability in differential leukocyte counting. In Koepke JA (ed): Differential Leukocyte Counting. Aspen, College of American Pathologists, 1977.

20 Blood and Bone Marrow

Thomas R. Fritsche
Gerald Lancz
Ron B. Schifman
Steven Specter

INTRODUCTION

The detection of microorganisms in blood is always an important finding requiring prompt assessment. Its clinical significance comprises a wide spectrum, ranging from a benign transient condition to life-threatening septicemia.

Bacteremia and fungemia are generally detected by culturing an aseptically collected peripheral blood specimen. Although most pathogens are detected by standard methods, some organisms require special conditions for isolation or are recognized as the cause of infection by serologic testing. Viral cultures usually are limited to a few circumstances, for example, suspected herpesvirus infection in the newborn or cytomegalovirus (CMV) infection in the immunosuppressed patient. Despite the rapid development of serologic and DNA probe techniques for the diagnosis of blood parasite infections, detection of parasitemia is made by direct examination of the patient's blood smear.

BASIC TESTS

Test: Blood Culture

Background[1]

Serious bloodstream infections generally are caused by normal inhabitants of the patient's body. Microorganisms gain access to the blood when there is deterioration in host defenses related to immunosuppression, a break in skin or mucosal barriers, intravascular lesions, presence of a foreign body, or alteration of commensal flora by antibiotic therapy. Certain conditions such as cirrhosis, sickle cell anemia, and diabetes mellitus are associated with increased risk of infection. Some bloodstream infections are preventable by conscientious attention to the proper use of invasive devices that serve as a source of infection. Organisms also may gain access to the blood as a consequence of infection at another site (e.g., urinary tract) or by direct inoculation from an insect vector or blood transfusion. Microbial virulence factors (i.e., endotoxin and adherence properties) also may play a role in precipitating infection and causing the clinical manifestations and complications associated with bloodstream infections.

Nearly any organism can infect the blood. Members of the Enterobacteriaceae family and *Pseudomonas aeruginosa* generally invade the blood from infected foci associated with hospital-acquired pulmonary, wound, or urinary tract infections.[2] Coagulase negative staphylococci originating from contaminated intravascular catheters are the most frequently isolated gram-positive bacteria.[3] Bloodstream infections are a major cause of morbidity and mortality among hospitalized patients, with survival directly related to the severity of the underlying disease. Although the mechanisms are not well understood, these infections tend to produce serious complications including coagulopathy, respiratory distress syndrome, hypotension, shock, and metastatic abscesses.

Selection

Blood cultures should be performed on any patient having signs and symptoms suggestive of a bloodstream infection, either as a primary condition (i.e., endocarditis) or as a secondary condition when organisms enter the blood from another site of infection (i.e., acute bacterial pneumonia). Fever and chills are the fundamental manifestations of bacteremia. Occasionally, bacteremia without fever occurs in the elderly, newborn, or immunosuppressed patient, and in patients with acute alcoholism, renal failure, or hypothyroidism. Other signs of bacteremia are tachycardia, hypotension, leukocytosis, thrombocytopenia, and changes in mental status. Bacteremia also can cause ophthalmic and peripheral vascular lesions, particularly in association with endocarditis. When secondary bacteremia or fungemia develops as a consequence of infection at another site, blood cultures are useful for establishing the causative organism, especially when direct examination is difficult or undependable (Table 20-1). Follow-up blood cultures can be useful for monitoring the success of therapy in bacteremic patients.

Special blood culture procedures are required when disseminated *Mycobacterium avium* complex is suspected in the acquired immunodeficiency syndrome (AIDS) patient or when the history and findings suggest infection with *Brucella* spp., or *Streptobacillus moniliformis*. Serologic testing rather than blood culture is indicated when tularemia, leptospirosis, or rocky mountain fever are suspected (see Special Procedures).

Terminology

Bacteremia, fungemia, or *viremia* are terms used to indicate the presence of microorganisms in the bloodstream. *Sepsis* or *septicemia* refers to the constitutional symptoms and physical signs and other damaging consequences of bloodstream infection.

Logistics

Specimen Requirements

Proper collection of venous blood samples is crucial for obtaining valid results. The phlebotomy procedure, collection volume, and frequency of testing are important variables that affect test results. Aseptic blood collection is necessary to avoid contamination by commensal skin flora. This is done by disinfecting the skin with alcohol, followed by iodophor or chlorhexidine. Because skin decontamination is not instantaneous, phlebotomy should be delayed for 1 or 2 minutes after preparing the venipuncture site. Blood may be collected into special transport tubes containing the anticoagulant sodium polyanetholsulfonate (SPS) and immediately delivered to the laboratory for processing. Alternatively, specimens can be inoculated directly into broth culture bottles at the bedside. Specimens collected through intravascular lines are inferior to venipuncture collections because of a higher frequency of contamination. Collection of blood from the peripheral vein of neonates can be problematic. In this situation, blood collected from the umbilical artery catheter

Table 20-1. Infections Associated With Bacteremia

Abscess, perirectal (with granulocytopenia)
Abscess, pyogenic liver
Abscess, spleen
Cellulitis
Cholangitis
Endocarditis
Endomyometritis
Enteric fever
Fever of unknown origin
Pneumonia
Pyelonephritis
Meningitis
Necrotizing fascitis
Osteomyelitis
Peritonitis, spontaneous bacterial
Peritonitis, traumatic
Salpingo-oophoritis
Septic arthritis
Suppurative phlebitis

Table 20-2. Comparative Sensitivity of Blood Culture Methods

Method	Enterobacteriaceae	Staphylococcus	Streptococcus	Haemophilus	Neisseria	Anaerobe	Fungi	Contaminant
Broth/radiometric (aerobic)	++	++	+++	+++	++	++	++	++
Broth/radiometric (anaerobic)	++	++	+++	++	++	+++	+	++
Lysis centrifugation[a]	+++	+++	++	++	+	+	+++	+++
Biphasic	+++	++	+++	+++	+++	+	+++	++

[a] Only method that provides quantitative results.
Abbreviations: +, Low; ++, average; +++, high sensitivity.

at the time of placement or from a heel stick is an acceptable alternative for culture. Even though animal experiments suggest that fungal cultures may be more sensitive when arterial blood is examined, the significance of this finding for fungemia detection in clinical practice is unclear.

Timing

Because bacteremia is not always continuous, more than one blood culture specimen must be obtained to optimize sensitivity. Additionally, the pattern revealed from performing two or three separate blood culture tests has interpretive value. About 80–90% of bacteremias will be detected with one culture and the addition of one or two more will detect nearly all bacteremic episodes. It is rarely necessary to obtain more than three specimens. Specimen collections should be spaced apart by 30–60 minutes, but it may be necessary at times to shorten this interval to have at least two cultures performed before antibiotic therapy is initiated. Bacteremia typically occurs before an episode of fever and chills. Because this stage is impossible to determine before it occurs, the best alternative is to collect a specimen at the onset of fever.

Volume

During episodes of bacteremia, the number of microorganisms in the bloodstream is often low. Consequently, the sensitivity of bacteremia detection depends on the quantity of blood cultured. As a general rule, sensitivity will increase by about 3% for each milliliter of blood collected between 5 and 20 mL. Blood culture sensitivity also is related to the patient's underlying disorder. For example, blood cultures are almost always positive in patients with endocarditis, but infrequently positive in disseminated candidiasis. In most cases, 10–20 mL of blood per culture is sufficient. In pediatric patients, this collection volume is obviously not attainable and in premature neonates it may only be suitable to collect a few milliliters of blood.

Analysis

There are three primary methods of culturing blood for bacteria: broth, biphasic, and lysis centrifugation. There are substantial differences between method sensitivity, specificity, time to detection, time to identification, and ability to provide quantitative results (Table 20-2). Methods should provide both aerobic and anaerobic conditions and have the capacity to eliminate antibiotic effects. Cultures showing growth are usually evident within 48 hours. In rare instances 1 week or longer may be required to demonstrate the presence of certain fastidious organisms, many of which are contaminants. Although most fungi can be detected with routine culture conditions, incubation at lower temperatures (30°C) is recommended and some (e.g., *Histoplasma capsulatum*) require longer incubation times (up to 8 weeks). Unfortunately, blood cultures are frequently negative in patients with fungemia.

Special procedures are required to detect *Leptospira*, *Francisella tularensis*, *Brucella*, rickettsiae, *M. avium* complex, *S. moniliformis*, and *Spirillum minor*. The laboratory should be notified if infection caused by any of these organisms is suspected (see Special Procedures).

Interpretation[4,5]

The pattern of bacteremia, type of microorganism(s), and clinical circumstance all have a bearing on the significance of blood culture results. Bacteremia may show a continuous, intermittent, or transient pattern. Continuous bacteremia is typically seen with intravascular infections (i.e., endocarditis, intravascular catheter infection, thrombophlebitis) and in the early stages of infection caused by *Brucella* spp. and *Salmonella typhi*. Intermittent bacteremia may accompany pneumonia, abscess, or any localized or early systemic infection. Transient bacteremia occurs with momentary breaks in the skin, mucosal surfaces, or colonized tissue associated with regular activities (teeth brushing, bowel movement) or trauma (dental extraction, childbirth), and is generally inconsequential except in patients with heart valve lesions or an intravascular prosthetic device. Bacteremia may continue while the patient is receiving therapy. This can be caused by antimicrobial resistance, sequestered infection (abscess), or impaired host defenses. Recurrent bacteremia is another pattern in which bacteremia is separated by extended periods of sterile blood cultures and is often associated with malignancy.

A common problem with blood culture interpretation is distinguishing between truly significant and false positive results. False positive results range from about 2–10% of all tests performed, and about 25% of all positive results are false positive. Differentiation is made by evaluating key test results and clinical features (Table 20-3). Although false positive results are generally attributed to contamination caused by skin flora, recent evidence indicates it also may be caused by benign, transient bacteremia. Therefore, isolation of the same organism from two simultaneously collected samples does not necessarily imply a clinically significant result. This is one reason for spacing apart specimen collections.

Table 20-3. Factors Associated With the Interpretation of False Positive Blood Culture Results

Contamination
    Skin flora or transient bacteremia (*Staphylococcus epidermidis*, diphtheroids)
    Environmental (*Bacillus* spp.)
Pattern of bacteremia and growth characteristics
    Single positive from multiple specimens
    Single positive result from two or more different cultures on same specimen
    Positive growth of nonfastidious organism after 48 hours
    Low level bacteremia (<1 organism/mL) by pour plate or lysis centrifugation
Incompatible clinical findings
    Isolate not appropriate for clinical syndrome (*Enterococcus* spp. and pneumonia)
    Isolate not identical with organism recovered from primary infection site

The lysis centrifugation method provides quantitative results and this may aid the analysis. The magnitude of bacteremia tends to correlate with severity of disease, high counts associated with a worse outcome. Likewise, serial quantitative cultures showing a decline in bacterial counts generally indicate an improving clinical course.

Polymicrobial results are obtained in 5–20% of all positive blood cultures. This type of septicemia is associated with a higher mortality risk. Predisposing conditions include neutropenia, invasive procedures, obstruction of the gastrointestinal or urinary tract, and gynecologic infections. Anaerobic gram-negative bacilli are often part of the polymicrobial bacteremia in the latter two conditions.

Identity of the blood culture isolate can help ascertain the source of infection, and certain organisms have special significance when detected in the blood (Table 20-4).

Endocarditis

Blood culture is the most important laboratory test for the etiologic diagnosis of infective endocarditis. More than 95% of untreated patients with this disease have continuous bacteremia. An intrinsic heart valve lesion, intracardiac prosthesis, infected intravascular catheter or shunt, and intravenous drug addiction are predisposing conditions. Members of the *Streptococcus viridans* group are the most common organisms infecting damaged heart or prosthetic valves that have been in place for more than 1 year. *Staphylococcus epidermidis* is the most frequent agent in early prosthetic valve infections and catheter-induced, nosocomial endocarditis. A variety of microorganisms such as *Staphylococcus aureus*, *P. aeruginosa*, Enterobacteriaceae, and *Candida* infect heart valves (usually tricuspid) in the intravenous drug abuser. Associated laboratory findings in patients with endocarditis are elevated erythrocyte sedimentation rate (95%), anemia (80%), rheumatoid factor (50%), polyclonal hypergammaglobulinemia (25%), proteinuria, and hematuria.

About 3% of patients with infective endocarditis have negative bacterial cultures.[6] This may be caused by right-sided infection, antibiotic therapy before culture, fastidious bacteria, and other agents that cannot be isolated with routine blood culture procedures (Table 20-5). Noninfectious causes for endocarditis also must be considered when blood cultures are negative (e.g., myxoma, rheumatic fever, and carcinoid). Negative culture in a patient suspected of having endocarditis often presents a difficult management problem, because therapy must be given without an etiologic diagnosis. It is essential that the laboratory be aware of such cases so that special procedures can be initiated. In this situation, blood cultures should be incubated for at least 3 weeks and an antimicrobial removal procedure should be used if the patient is receiving antibiotics. Subcultures with coculture of *S. aureus* may show satellite colony formation indicative of nutritionally deficient streptococci. Likewise, incubation in special media such as hypertonic sucrose, or with vitamin B_6 and cysteine supplements, should be considered. Subcultures and special stains for acid fast bacilli, fungi, and *Legionella* should be performed. Serologic tests are helpful for the diagnosis of endocarditis caused by *Coxiella burnetii*, *Brucella* spp., and *Chlamydia* infections. Bone marrow culture also may help identify the etiologic agent in other cases (e.g., *Histoplasma capsulatum*). Embolic specimens also should be cultured when present and obtainable.

Fungemia

Candida albicans and other *Candida* species are the most common etiologic agents of fungemia. The gastrointestinal tract is the main source of infection. Candidemia, an increasing frequent nosocomial infection, is often a manifestation of local or disseminated infection in patients who are immunosuppressed or receiving prolonged antibiotic therapy. Characteristic nodular skin lesions and endophthalmitis generally signify disseminated infection, although this is infrequently seen with *Candida (Torulopsis) glabrata* infection. Candidemia also may occur as a transient condition, associated with intravenous catheter contamination or break in

Table 20-4. Secondary Infections and Findings Associated With Bacterial and Fungal Blood Culture Results

Result	Interpretation, Associated Findings
Acinetobacter spp.	Pneumonia, catheter infection, malignancy, contamination, bacteremia from contaminated equipment or solutions
Actinobacillus actinomycetemcomitans	Endocarditis
Aeromonas hydrophilia	Opportunistic infection (malignancy, cirrhosis), wound infection, endocarditis, exposure to fresh water
Aspergillus	Opportunistic infection, contaminant
Bacillus	Contamination, nosocomial bacteremia from contaminated equipment, catheters, or fluid, opportunistic infection
Bacteroides fragilis and other *Bacteroides* spp.	Abdominal trauma, neoplasm, transient bacteremia, gynecologic infection, decubitus ulcer, suppurative thrombophlebitis, septic abortion, puerperal bacteremia, pleuropulmonary infection, dental abscess
Brucella	Brucellosis, fever of unknown origin, atypical lymphocytosis
Candida	Prostatic valve endocarditis, intravenous catheter infection, opportunistic infection
Campylobacter fetus	Opportunistic infection, cellulitis, thrombophlebitis
Clostridium perfringens and other *Clostridium*	Abdominal trauma, neoplasm, septic abortion, gynecologic infection, disseminated intravascular coagulation, hemolysis with acute tubular necrosis, contaminant
Clostridium septicum	Hematologic or colonic malignancy, neutropenia, ischemic bowel
Cardiobacterium hominis	Endocarditis
Corynebacterium diphtheriae	Endocarditis
Corynebacterium jeikeium, (formerly group JK)	Opportunistic infection (granulocytopenia), sepsis, intravenous catheter infection, contamination
Corynebacterium spp.	Contamination, endocarditis, misidentified *Listeria monocytogenes*
Cryptococcus neoformans	Meningitis, immunosuppression, AIDS
DF-2	Septicemia or endocarditis associated with dog bite in asplenic patient
Enterobacteriaceae	Urosepsis, abdominal trauma, nosocomial bacteremia, nosocomial pneumonia, prostatic valve endocarditis, cholangitis, solid tumor neoplasia, gynecologic and postpartum infection
Enterococcus	Urosepsis, abdominal trauma, endocarditis, endometritis, nosocomial bacteremia
Erysipelothrix rhusiopathiae	Endocarditis (aortic valve), history of animal exposure
Fusobacterium	Suppurative thrombophlebitis *(F. necrophorum)*, upper respiratory and oral cavity infection, see *Bacteroides*
Haemophilus influenzae	Pneumonia, meningitis, epiglottitis, primary bacteremia, cellulitis, septic arthritis
Haemophilus parainfluenza, Haemophilus aphrophilus, Haemophilus paraphrophilus	Endocarditis
Listeria monocytogenes	Meningitis, neonatal sepsis, granulomatosis infantiseptica, puerperal infection, septic abortion, opportunistic infection (lymphoma, leukemia, renal transplant), ingestion of contaminated dairy products
Malassezia furfur	Therapy with lipid-containing hyperalimentation fluid, especially in neonates
Mycobacterium avium-complex	Opportunistic infection especially with AIDS
Neisseria gonorrhoeae	Disseminated gonorrhea, salpingitis, septic arthritis, neonatal sepsis, dermatitis, pharyngitis
Neisseria meningitidis	Meningitis, complement deficiency, chronic meningococcemia, primary bacteremia, transient bacteremia

(Continued)

Table 20-4. Secondary Infections and Findings Associated With Bacterial and Fungal Blood Culture Results (Continued)

Result	Interpretation, Associated Findings
Neisseria spp.	Endocarditis
Pasteurella multocida	Cat bite, wound infection, malignancy
Peptococcus magnus and *Peptococcus* spp.	Polymicrobial infection, soft tissue, head and neck, female genital tract infections, surgical wound infection, endocarditis
Pseudomonas aeruginosa	Opportunistic infection (hematologic malignancy), urosepsis, catheter infection, burn infection, pneumonia, tracheostomy, nosocomial bacteremia from contaminated equipment or fluids, wound infection, abdominal trauma, ecthyma gangrenosum, cellulitis
Pseudomonas cepacia	Nosocomial bacteremia outbreak from contaminated equipment or solutions, pseudobacteremia from contaminated iodine solution
Pseudomonas pseudomallei	Severe melioidosis
Propionibacterium acnes	Contamination
Salmonella	Gastroenteritis, typhoid fever *(S. typhi)*
Staphylococcus aureus	Skin and soft tissue infection, intravenous catheter infection, phlebitis, wound infection, endocarditis, pneumonia, pyelonephritis, abscess, osteomyelitis, septic arthritis, prostatic valve endocarditis, abscess, contamination
Staphylococcus epidermidis	Intravenous catheter infection, granulocytopenia, shunt infection, prostatic valve endocarditis, contamination
Streptobacillus moniliformis	Rat bite fever, endocarditis
Streptococcus anginosus (milleri)	Endocarditis, oral cavity infection, abdominal trauma, occult abscess
Streptococcus agalactiae (group B)	Neonatal sepsis, pneumonia, meningitis, gynecologic infection, cellulitis
Streptococcus bovis	Gastrointestinal neoplasm, endocarditis
Streptococcus pneumoniae	Pneumonia, meningitis, osteomyelitis, sinusitis, peritonitis
Streptococcus pyrogenes (group A)	Skin and soft tissue infection, thrombophlebitis, puerperal sepsis
Streptococcus (β hemolytic, not group A or B)	Endocarditis, wound infection, gynecologic infection, meningitis, transient bacteremia, malignancy (group G)
Streptococcus viridans	Endocarditis, transient bacteremia, contaminant
Vibrio vulnificus	Wound contamination with salt water, raw oyster ingestion, cellulitis, liver disease
Yersinia enterocolitica	Iron overload, cirrhosis
Yersinia pestis	Septicemic or bubonic plague

skin or mucosal barriers. Less often, other fungi, including *Aspergillus, Geotrichum,* Zygomycetes, and *Rhodotorula,* disseminate and infect the blood of patients with defective cell-mediated immunity. Unfortunately, blood cultures are usually negative during these infections and may be difficult to interpret when positive, because these fungi also may be laboratory contaminants. Fungemia also may occur as a consequence of infection at another site, such as with cryptococcal meningitis or acute pulmonary *Histoplasma* infection.

Special Procedures

Leptospirosis

This zoonotic infection is caused by spirochetes transmitted to humans by contact with infected urine of domestic and wild animals. Infection is often subclinical, but severe disease with hepatocellular injury (Weil's syndrome) occurs in about 5% of cases. Leptospira are present for up to 1 week in the patient's blood

Table 20-5. Organisms Associated With Culture Negative Endocarditis
Actinobacillus actinomycetemcomitans
Aspergillus spp.
Brucella spp.
Candida spp.
Cardiobacterium hominis
Corynebacterium spp.
Coxiella burnetii (Q fever)
Chlamydia psittaci
Chlamydia trachomatis
Eikenella corrodens
Haemophilus aphrophilus
Haemophilus parainfluenzae
Histoplasma capsulatum
Legionella spp.
Mycobacterium spp.
Neisseria spp.
Nocardia spp.
Spirillum minor
Streptobacillus moniliformis
Streptococcus spp. (nutritionally deficient, B$_6$ or cysteine)
Zygomycetes spp.

and spinal fluid during the first stage of disease, but during the second stage, which may last for several months, organisms are present only in urine. Leptospiras occasionally can be detected in the blood, urine, or cerebrospinal fluid (CSF) by dark-field examination or by culture on special media (Fletcher's, Tween 80-albumin). However, by the time a diagnosis of icteric leptospirosis is considered (fever, jaundice, renal failure, hemorrhage, myocarditis, meningitis), the spirochete is ordinarily not present in blood. Serologic testing or urine culture is usually the most suitable method for laboratory diagnosis of this disease.

Tularemia

Francisella tularensis infection is acquired by contact with wild animals, particularly rabbits or ticks, or by contaminated water. The most common presentation is ulcerglandular infection with painful ulcers at the site of inoculation and tender, enlarged regional lymph nodes. Bacteremia is transient, the organism is difficult to grow, and is highly infectious to laboratory workers. The laboratory diagnosis of tularemia should be made by serologic testing.

Brucella

Brucellosis is a febrile and frequently occult illness, acquired by contact with infected domestic animals (i.e., *Brucella abortus*, cattle; *Brucella melitensis*, sheep; *Brucella suis*, swine) and unpasteurized milk or milk products. The infection presents with acute fever, chills, headache, atypical peripheral lymphocytes, generalized lymphadenopathy, and hepatosplenomegaly. Osteomyelitis is one of the most serious complications, but occurs infrequently. *Brucella* is present in blood only during the acute phase of disease. Blood culture should be considered before therapy for patients with appropriate occupational or exposure history who present with acute febrile illness of undetermined etiology. *Brucella* is slow-growing and may require up to 4 weeks of incubation before it is detected. A biphasic culture system with 10% CO_2 enrichment improves sensitivity. Because the organism does not readily produce turbidity in broth, frequent subcultures are necessary to identify positive results. Only about 25% of patients with serologically confirmed brucellosis have positive blood cultures. Therefore, although blood cultures should be performed in all suspected cases, serologic testing is the most reliable procedure for laboratory diagnosis.

Rickettsiae

Rickettsial infections are transmitted by insects and produce fever, headache, and rash. There is a significant mortality if untreated. *Rickettsia rickettsii*, transmitted by tick bites, is the cause of rocky mountain spotted fever, an endemic infection in the United States, whereas other species account for infections in other parts of the world. Although bacteremia is a consistent feature of infection, isolation of the organism requires special techniques (yolk sac culture) and is extremely hazardous to laboratory workers. Laboratory diagnosis is therefore made by serologic testing. Unfortunately, serologic responses may not become evident until late in the course of disease. The diagnosis of rocky mountain spotted fever also may be made by demonstrating rickettsia in skin biopsy tissue by immunologic staining.

Mycobacterium Avium Complex

Mycobacterium avium complex is a common, opportunistic, systemic infection in patients with advanced AIDS. Even though the organism can be recovered from stool and most body fluids, blood culture using special media and growth conditions is one of the best methods for establishing the diagnosis. Direct examination of a buffy coat smear has poor sensitivity.

Rat Bite Fever

This manifests as an acute febrile illness accompanied by rash and arthritis; is caused by *S. moniliformis* or the spirochete *S. minor*; and is transmitted by contact with rodents. *S. moniliformis* infection is associated with a false positive VDRL (Venereal Disease Research Laboratory) result. Because the anticoagulant, SPS, used for routine blood culture collections is inhibitory to *S. moniliformis*, sterile blood collected in citrate should be cultured. Recovery is enhanced by adding ascitic fluid or horse serum to broth medium. Growth in broth is characteristically seen as "fluff balls." *Spirillum minor* also can be recovered from blood but requires animal inoculation. It is critical that this test be performed under properly controlled conditions, because *S. minor* infections are endemic in laboratory animals. Direct detection of the spirochete in blood smears by dark-field examination is possible, but is insensitive and artifacts, mistaken as spiral organisms, may produce false positive results.

Test: Direct Examination of Blood

Background and Selection

Although potentially advantageous for rapid confirmation of bacteremia or fungemia, direct examination of whole blood or buffy coat smears is inefficient and lacks diagnostic sensitivity.[7] Positive smears occur with fulminant bacterial pulmonary or wound infections (e.g., *Clostridium perfringens*) and are associated with a poor prognosis. Asplenic and severely immunosuppressed patients also tend to have large numbers of circulating organisms. There are, however, a few special circumstances where direct microscopic examination is worthwhile: detection of the bacillemia of lepromatous leprosy, Bartonellosis, and *Borrelia* spp. spirochetemia in relapsing fever. Direct examination for the identification of parasitemia in malaria, *Babesia*, trypanosome, and filarial infections is discussed on page 629.

Interpretation

Bartonellosis (Oroya Fever, Carrion's Disease)

Bartonellosis is caused by infection with *Bartonella bacilliformis*, transmitted to humans by sandflies, and is endemic to South America. The organism infects endothelial and red blood cells. Patients present with intermittent fever, anemia, hepatosplenomegaly, and lymphadenopathy. Characteristic hemangiomatous nodular skin lesions (verruga peruana) appear several weeks later. Infection is frequently complicated by *Salmonella* bacteremia. This infection should be considered with presence of fever and anemia associated with appropriate travel or exposure history. During the febrile stage, organisms can generally be identified within red blood cells. Blood culture for *Bartonella* and *Salmonella* also should be performed.

Borrelia

Relapsing fever is an acute febrile systemic disease caused by various species of *Borrelia*. The spirochete is transmitted either by the human body louse with rodents serving as the natural reservoir or by *Ornithodoros* ticks. The infection presents as an acute febrile illness with headache and tender splenomegaly several days to 2 weeks after a bite. Febrile episodes of declining intensity may recur weekly. *Borrelia* infection is rare in the United States although outbreaks have been associated with habitation of rustic cabins. Examination of blood for *Borrelia* spirochetemia should be performed when relapsing fever symptoms occur and there is an appropriate exposure history. Detection of *Borrelia* spirochetemia in a Wright or Giemsa stained peripheral blood smear or dark-field examination during the febrile phase of relapsing fever provides a definitive diagnosis. In suspected cases where the smear examination is negative, demonstration of spirochetemia after intraperitoneal inoculation of the patient's blood into mice can be performed to improve diagnostic sensitivity. Serologic testing is not reliable.

Test: Viral Blood Culture

Background

The relationship between viremia and clinical disease varies widely from asymptomatic or mild transient infection to severe life-threatening disease. Some viruses such as herpesvirus, human immunodeficiency virus (HIV), and rubeola persist in leukocytes, in contrast to others such as enteroviruses, which exhibit a biphasic viremia that occurs before and during clinical symptoms. In most other infections where viremia tends to be transient, virus is cleared from the blood before the onset of clinical disease. The value of examining blood for virus detection is therefore limited to only a few special circumstances.

Selection

Viremia, unlike bacteremia, is not generally associated with constitutional symptoms like fever and chills. In addition, for most commonly encountered viral infections, the agent is generally present in higher quantities in alternative, readily accessible sites. For example, acute enterovirus infection may produce a prolonged viremia, but there will be a much greater amount of virus present in the throat and feces. Consequently, blood is not a preferred specimen for virus isolation in this circumstance. In a few instances, however, culture

Table 20-6. Interpretation of Viral Blood Culture Results

Result	Interpretation, Associated Disease
Cytomegalovirus	Opportunistic infection in immunocompromised patient, congenital infection, pneumonitis, retinitis, mononucleosis
Viral infections causing viremia, not routinely tested for in blood samples	
Adenovirus	Pneumonia (children)
Bunyaviruses	Encephalitis, hemorrhagic fever
Enterovirus	Gastrointestinal infection, meningitis, respiratory infection (children)
Hepatitis B virus	Acute or chronic hepatitis
Epstein-Barr virus	Infectious mononucleosis, chronic infection, immunosuppression, X-linked proliferative disease
Human herpesvirus 6	Chronic fatigue syndrome?, neoplasia
Herpes simplex virus	Exanthem, encephalitis, meningitis, keratitis, genital lesions, hepatitis
Varicella-zoster virus	Chickenpox, shingles
Mumps virus	Parotitis, orchitis, oophoritis, encephalitis, pancreatitis
Rubella	Congenital rubella syndrome, arthritis, encephalitis
Rubeola	Measles
Human immunodeficiency virus	Asymptomatic, AIDS-related complex (ARC), AIDS
Human T lymphotrophic viruses I and II	Neoplasia, tropical spastic paraparesis?

may be worthwhile for assessing systemic viral infections (such as CMV and varicella-zoster virus) in immunocompromised individuals or newborns, as well as the workup of aseptic meningitis, encephalitis, and hemorrhagic fevers. Blood culture should always be supplemented with culture of specimens from other appropriate sites.

Unfortunately, chemotherapy is not currently available for most viral infections. The importance of pursuing virus isolation and identification other than CMV assumes importance primarily in the practice of community health medicine. This may be critical for effective control of virus spread by the institution of public health measures, for example patient isolation, mosquito control, and water treatment. Viruses that may be detected in blood are listed in Table 20-6.

Logistics[8]

Specimen

Blood specimens for viral culture are collected aseptically by venipuncture. Ten milliliters of blood is collected into sterile heparin or citrate tubes. Detection of congenital infection with CMV and other viruses is readily accomplished by sampling cord blood. Transport fluid is not required, but specimens should be delivered to the laboratory and processed as quickly as possible. Specimens whose delivery is temporarily delayed should be stored cold (refrigerated or on ice), but not frozen.

Selecting the appropriate blood component (leukocytes or serum) is critical for viral cultures. Ficoll/Hypaque prepared leukocyte fractions are more sensitive as compared with buffy coat cultures when attempting to recover viruses that have a tendency to remain cell associated (e.g., CMV and varicella-zoster virus).[9] Enteroviruses tend not to be cell associated and are more readily isolated from whole blood or serum.

Methods

The presence of virus in the blood is detected by development of cytopathogenic effects, hemadsorption, or immunologic procedures performed on tissue culture cells that have been inoculated with the blood specimen. Positive results may be seen as soon as 1 day after culture, but specimens should be incubated for 3 weeks before they are declared negative. Negative results, however, do not necessarily indicate that there was no viral infection. The quality of the specimen, type of infection, time in the disease course, and conditions of transport influence culture results.

In the special case of human retrovirus detection, the patient's leukocytes are cocultured with susceptible cells. The conditions of this assay require lymphocyte stimulation and proliferation. Virus is detected by observing cytopathic effects, increased levels of viral reverse transcriptase, or by immunoassay for specific viral antigens. Because HIV is hazardous to laboratory workers, cultures are performed only in specialized facilities. HIV in blood can now be detected by polymerase chain reaction techniques (see Ch. 29).

Interpretation[10]

The presence of virus in the blood is a significant finding for individuals displaying clinical disease (Table 20-6). In the neonate or immunocompromised host, the presence of virus in the blood is often associated with central nervous system (CNS) infection or systemic disease, which may be life-threatening. If available, chemotherapeutic intervention is dictated. When herpes simplex or varicella-zoster virus is isolated from the blood of individuals with clinical disease, acyclovir treatment should be instituted. For the actively immunosuppressed patient (such as transplant recipients), it may be necessary to modify immunosuppressive therapy to permit the patient to develop an effective natural immune response to the virus (usually CMV) causing the infection.

Test: Examination of Blood for Parasites[11,12]

Background and Selection

Malaria, *Babesia*, trypanosomes, and various species of microfilariae are important causes of parasitemia. Infection and its complications are distinct for each, as described below. In general, disease is transmitted to humans by the bite of an infected insect vector. Appropriate travel history is an important component of the diagnostic evaluation, because parasitemic infections are generally confined to specific geographic locations and are not endemic to the United States (except for *Babesia*).

Logistics

When requests for blood examination for malaria, *Babesia*, trypanosomes, and microfilariae are submitted, the initial evaluation usually includes both the thick and thin blood smears that ideally should be stained with Giemsa. In addition, examination of fresh blood or buffy coat preparation may be useful, especially for trypanosome or microfilariae. A variety of concentration procedures also has been described and are used primarily for recovering trypanosomes, leishmaniae, and microfilariae when their presence is suspected, but not confirmed, by the examination of blood smears (Table 20-7).[11]

Thick and Thin Smears

The thin smear is prepared in routine fashion such that a single layer of intact red blood cells predominates on the smear. The thick smear, in which blood is dehemoglobinized before staining, serves to concentrate the blood 20–40 times, thus increasing the sensitivity of the examination and decreasing the time necessary to detect the presence of parasites. Although a species diagnosis of malaria may often be made from the thick smear, the thin smear offers a cleaner field in which to make this determination. Repeated examinations should be performed when parasitemia is suspected, but not detected. The use of concentration procedures may be indicated when smear evaluations are negative, but the index of suspicion for filarial infection remains high.

Wet Preparation

Fresh blood may be examined for the presence of trypanosomes or microfilariae because of the motility, relative large size, and typical morphology. Specific identification, however, must be made from a stained blood smear.

Buffy Coat

Anticoagulated blood may be centrifuged and the resulting buffy coat examined in a wet preparation for motile trypanosomes. Alternatively, thin smears may

Table 20-7. Common Procedures Used to Examine Blood for Parasites

	Malaria	*Babesia*	Trypanosomes	*Leishmania donovani*	Microfilariae
Thick/thin smear	X	X	X	X	X
Blood wet preparation			X		X
Buffy coat			X	X	
Other concentration					X

be prepared from the buffy coat and stained with Giemsa to examine for either *Leishmania donovani* or trypanosomes.

Concentration Techniques for Microfilariae

A variety of concentration procedures including concentration cell lysis, Knott concentration technique, membrane filtration, gradient centrifugation, and others are used to recognize the presence of microfilariae in blood samples.[11] Usually the concentrated material is examined as a wet preparation (except for the membrane filtration techniques) although permanent stained slides must be examined for species identification.

Interpretation

Malaria

Malaria is a disease endemic to many of the developing countries in the world and occurs in immigrants or travelers returning from known malarious areas. The number of malaria cases reported to the Centers for Disease Control have increased dramatically in recent years. Individuals who have an appropriate travel history should be evaluated for possible malaria if they present with fever, chills, myalgias, anemia, splenomegaly, or some combination of symptoms. Because life-threatening complications may develop in nonimmune individuals exposed to *Plasmodium falciparum,* a rapid and correct laboratory diagnosis is essential to initiate appropriate chemotherapy.

The diagnosis of malaria is usually made on the basis of the characteristic paroxysm (periodic rigors, fever, and sweats), signs (anemia and splenomegaly), and examination of thick and thin blood smears. Malarial organisms are most numerous in the peripheral blood just prior to the onset of a febrile paroxysm. Blood specimens obtained by venipuncture, finger stick, or ear lobe puncture should ideally be collected at that time. When collecting blood using the finger stick method, care should be taken to avoid milking the finger as serous fluids will dilute the capillary blood. Multiple blood smears may need to be examined if blood is drawn between paroxysms. Smears prepared directly from fresh blood are best. When this is not practical, EDTA-anticoagulated blood may be examined. Problems arise with other anticoagulants because of distortion occurring to the parasites and interferences with their staining characteristics. Care must be taken to avoid exposing blood cells to the alcohol used to disinfect the finger stick or venipuncture site. Unintentional fixation of blood cells will prevent their lysis in the preparation of thick blood smears.

The single most important task faced by laboratory technicians in examining malaria smears is differentiating between *P. falciparum* and the other plasmodia, *P. vivax, P. ovale,* and *P. malariae.* Usually significant morphologic differences are apparent; early infections containing few parasites often occur, however, and may make identification more difficult. In these cases, multiple smears taken at different time intervals may be necessary to identify additional diagnostic stages. The differentiation of platelets lying on top of erythrocytes also may cause problems for the inexperienced observer and are controlled for by examination of platelets in the field separate from erythrocytes.

The clinical pattern of fever relates to the maturation of erythrocytic schizonts, and release of merozoites helps to identify the species responsible for the infection (Table 20-8). Fever spikes tend to be irregular early in the infection, but become more synchronized as the disease progresses. High parasitemias may occur with *P. falciparum* infection because of the parasites' ability to infect erythrocytes of any age. *P. vivax* and *P. malariae* infect predominantly young and senescent red blood cells, respectively, and the levels of parasitemia rarely approach those seen with *P. falciparum.*

Babesia

Babesiosis is a malarial-like disease caused by *Babesia microti* and is transmitted by the same species of hard ticks that transmit Lyme borreliosis. Transfusion associated cases also are described. Human infections occur worldwide, and in the United States are found

Table 20-8. *Plasmodium* Species Infecting Humans

Species	Malarial Disease	Length of Asexual Cycle	Relapse Potential
P. vivax and *P. ovale*	Benign tertian	48	Yes
P. falciparum	Malignant tertian	48	No
P. malariae	Quartan	72	No

primarily in the northeast, although a few cases have been reported on the west coast. Infections are characterized by myalgias, fatigue, hemolytic anemia, and hemoglobinuria and may be particularly severe in splenectomized patients. The laboratory diagnosis of *Babesia* is identical to that for malaria given the appropriate clinical and geographic histories, especially a recent history of tick bite. The organisms tend to be distributed sparsely in peripheral blood where they resemble early ring trophozoites of *P. falciparum* and care must be exercised in making this distinction. The presence of pairs and tetrad forms, lack of pigment, and absence of schizonts and gametocytes helps make the differentiation. Serologic testing can be performed for the diagnosis, but crossreaction with *Plasmodium* render these tests useless in endemic malarious areas.

Trypanosomiasis

Trypanosoma brucei rhodesiense and *Trypanosoma brucei gambiense,* the causes of acute and chronic African trypanosomiasis, respectively, are transmitted via the saliva or bite of the tsetse fly. Once inoculated, the dividing trypomastigote form multiplies in the bloodstream and subsequently invades lymph nodes, liver, and spleen. During this time, irregular fever, sweats, and headaches may appear and trypomastigotes may be plentiful in the peripheral blood, especially during febrile episodes. Invasion of the CNS results in characteristic "sleeping sickness," a combination of behavioral and psychological changes associated with the infection that ultimately may lead to death. Infection with *T. b. rhodesiense* is a more fulminant process, with death often occurring before extensive CNS invasion. The two diseases are transmitted by different species of tsetse flies occurring in different habitats. The Gambian form of sleeping sickness occurs primarily in west and west-central portions of Africa where humans are the predominant reservoir. By contrast, Rhodesian trypanosomiasis occurs in East Africa primarily as a zoonosis. The ability of both species to express variable antigen types enables them to evade the host's immune response. This leads to marked antigenic stimulation with characteristically high IgM levels in blood and CSF that may be useful in diagnosis.

African trypanosomiasis (Chagas' disease) is a zoonosis caused by *Trypanosoma cruzi* and is transmitted via the feces of blood sucking insects in the family Reduviidae, known as "kissing" bugs. When the infectious organisms are inoculated into the bite wound or exposed to mucosal surfaces, they invade a variety of tissues and multiply intracellularly as the rounded, nonmotile amastigote form. Following rupture of cells, the amastigotes elongate and circulate as motile trypomastigotes that characteristically assume a C or U shape in stained blood smears. Acute disease may be symptomless, and the diagnosis delayed until the infection becomes chronic. Symptoms when present may include fevers, myalgias, hepatosplenomegaly, lymphadenopathy, and myocarditis. Chronic infection may result in additional myocardial injury, and disturbances in esophageal and colonic function caused by inflammatory destruction of nerve ganglia.

Direct examination of blood, as well as lymph node aspirate, bone marrow, or CSF is used to detect the presence of African trypanosomes in individuals suspected of having this infection based upon appropriate clinical findings and geographic history. Motile trypomastigotes seen in wet blood smears, Wright or Giemsa stained thick and thin smears, or buffy coat smears confirm the diagnosis. Lymph node aspirates and spinal fluid examinations are important not only for diagnosing the disease but also in following its progression. Similarly, examination of blood smears for trypomastigotes or lymph node aspirates for amastigotes are indicated for the diagnosis of *T. cruzi*. Animal inoculations, serology, and xenodiagnosis also are used to confirm the diagnosis of this disease in chronic cases. Serologic testing for all trypanosomes is hampered by crossreactions with related protozoa and some viruses.

Leishmaniasis

The *Leishmania* comprise a group of species related to trypanosomes and are transmitted by the bite of infected sandflies. Unlike the trypanosomes, leishmaniae are obligate intracellular parasites in their mammalian host and only assume a flagellated stage in the insect vector. Following inoculation, the organisms proliferate in reticuloendothelial cells causing inflammation and necrosis. Classically, three forms of the disease have been described; they include cutaneous, mucocutaneous, and visceral involvement. Only those organisms comprising the *L. donovani* complex and causing visceral leishmaniasis (known as kala-azar) may be recovered from peripheral blood. Onset of infection with this species may be subclinical or acute. Severe disease is often characterized by twice a day fever, hepatosplenomegaly, lymphadenopathy, pancytopenia, hypoalbuminemia, and hypogammaglobulinemia. Death usually results from secondary infections. The disease is primarily a zoonosis and is endemic to portions of Europe, Africa, Asia, and Central and South America.

Tissue specimens submitted for diagnosis may include liver, spleen, or bone marrow biopsies. Stained buffy coat preparations of peripheral blood may reveal the amastigotes of *L. donovani* in monocytic cells. Cultivation of specimens on special media in addition to smear evaluation provides highest sensitivity.[11] The other species of *Leishmania* infect primarily histiocytes and are not recovered from the peripheral blood.

Microfilarial Parasitemias

When filariasis is suspected given appropriate clinical findings and geographic history, the diagnosis is confirmed by demonstrating microfilariae in the peripheral blood (Table 20-9). Eosinophilia is a prominent, but nonspecific finding in most filarial diseases and may be the only sign suggestive of a helminthic infection. At least seven filarial species are known to infect humans with *Wuchereria bancrofti* and *Brugia malayi*, causative agents of Bancroftian and Malayan filariasis, respectively, causing the most serious disease. Following transmission of the infectious *Wuchereria* or *Brugia* microfilariae via mosquitoes, the filariae grow and mature in inguinal and other lymphatics causing chronic inflammation and lymphatic obstruction with subsequent lymphedema in severe cases. Lymphatic rupture may result in chyluria or chylous ascites. Elephantiasis or hydrocele are possible complications that tend to occur after many years of infection and re-infection.

Among the pathogenic filariae, *Onchocerca volvulus* is especially prominent, causing a disease known as "river blindness" in portions of Africa, and Central and South America. These worms are transmitted by species of black flies and mature in subcutaneous tissues where they form characteristic nodules. Most of the pathologic effects result from the constant migration of microfilariae through the skin rather than through the blood, with the development of hypersensitivity to microfilarial antigens. Dermatitis, lymphadenitis, and eventually, ocular lesions leading to blindness are the principal serious sequelae. The African eye worm *Loa Loa* is another pathogenic filarial worm, which, unlike the other filariae, migrates as the adult through subcutaneous and deeper connective tissues. The microfilariae circulate in the peripheral blood and are transmitted by biting tabanid flies of the genus *Chrysops*. Clinically, disease symptoms relate to the migrations of the worms, which result in localized subcutaneous edema referred to as "Calabar" or "fugitive" swellings. Often the migrations may go unnoticed until a worm appears beneath the conjunctiva of the eye.

The remaining species of Filaria known to infect humans include *Mansonella perstans*, *Mansonella ozzardi*, and *Mansonella streptocerca*, which are generally thought to result in asymptomatic infections. Pruritic dermatitis has been described, however, as a prominent feature in some cases of human streptocerciasis.

Microfilariae of all these species except *Onchocerca* are generally present in the blood during intermediate stages of disease, but tend to be absent in both early and advance stages of infection. Proper timing of blood sampling is often important for the diagnosis of filarial infections, because of the predictable periodicity seen with microfilariae in the peripheral blood for some species (Table 20-9). Generally, *Wuchereria* and *Brugia* display nocturnal periodicity with microfilariae most plentiful in peripheral blood between the hours of 2200 hours and 0200 hours. *L. loa* has a diurnal periodicity and sampling for larvae is best performed around noon. The *Mansonella* are nonperiodic and may be seen in the blood at any time. Microfilariae of *Onchocerca* also are nonperiodic, but are usually detected in skin snips and early in the course of disease.[12]

Test: Antigenemia, Endotoxemia

Procedures to detect microbial antigens in blood are less sensitive than culture, limited to a narrow spectrum of pathogens, and are not widely employed for

Table 20-9. Filarial Species Infecting Humans

Species	Distribution	Periodicity of Microfilariae
Wuchereria bancrofti	Widely spread in tropics and subtropics	Nocturnal
Brugia malayi	India, Asia, southwest Pacific	Nocturnal
Onchocerca volvulus	Africa, Central and South America	Nonperiodic (in tissue)
Loa loa	Tropical Africa	Diuranal
Mansonella perstans	Tropical Africa and America	Nonperiodic
Mansonella streptocerca	Tropical Africa	Nonperiodic
Mansonella ozzardi	Tropical Africa	Nonperiodic

diagnosis. These include tests for pneumococcal capsular polysaccharide, group B streptococcus, *N. meningitidis,* polyribophosphate polysaccharide *(Haemophilus influenzae),* K2 capsule *(Klebsiella* spp.), mannan, *(Candida* spp.), and *Aspergillus* antigenemia. Test sensitivity is related to the quantity of organisms present. Nonspecific, false positive results may occur when blood or blood culture broth is tested. The primary use of these tests is for rapid, preliminary identification. Detection of gram-negative bacteremia by testing for endotoxin with the limulus lysate test lacks adequate specificity.

Test: Intravascular Catheter Culture

Background

Nosocomial bacteremia secondary to insertion wound infection or suppurative phlebitis is a significant complication associated with the use of peripheral and central intravascular catheters, especially those with plastic cannulas. The duration of catheterization and amount of inflammation at the insertion site correlate with bacteremia risk. This has become one of the most important predisposing factors responsible for nosocomial bacteremias owing to the large proportion of hospitalized patients who have indwelling vascular lines. The remedy as well as the laboratory diagnosis of these infections is accomplished by removing the intravascular device(s). Semiquantitative culture of a removed catheter helps distinguish insertion wound infection from benign contamination and thus helps differentiate catheter related from other sources of bacteremia.

Selection

Semiquantitative catheter culture should be considered for all patients with indwelling catheters who develop septicemia without an identified source of infection. This is particularly important for *S. epidermidis* bacteremia, which is most often caused by intravascular catheter infections. Rapid, direct methods for diagnosis of catheter-related bacteremia by direct examination of the tip, either with impression smears or by direct staining and microscopic examination are described but not widely used. The methods are impractical, and the clinical value of a rapid preliminary diagnosis in this setting is questionable.

It would be desirable to identify the source of infection without having to remove an intravascular catheter when bacteremia is present or suspected. Theoretically, if two simultaneous blood cultures are obtained, one from a vein and the other from the catheter, interpretation of quantitative cultures from both might help differentiate catheter-related infection (high counts from catheter and low counts from the vein) from another source (low colony counts from catheter). However, the reliability of this method has not been verified.[13] This approach should only be considered in the evaluation of sepsis when quantitative blood cultures are available and when venous access is poor and replacement of the catheter is a significant problem.

Logistics

A variety of methods are described for culturing intravascular devices. The first one reported and perhaps the most widely used is the roll plate method described by Maki in 1977. The catheter is removed with sterile forceps, placed in a dry container, and immediately transported to the laboratory. Long central catheters must be aseptically cut to culture the distal 5–10 cm tip. The catheter is rolled back and forth onto nonselective plated media, which is then incubated at 35°C.

The roll plate method lacks the ability to detect organisms within the catheter's lumen. Newer methods have subsequently been described for measuring bacterial and fungal growth from the entire catheter tip with precise quantitative measurements. This is done by using centrifugation, vortexing, or sonication to dislodge bacteria from the catheter into a specified amount of broth or other solution, and then culturing a precise aliquot of this liquid on plated media. Studies using these methods confirm the association between quantitative culture results and risk of infectious complications. Although these newer methods help confirm the pathogenesis of catheter-related bacteremias, it is still unclear whether these techniques provide any more useful clinical information that the roll plate method.

Interpretation

A semiquantitative culture with ≥15 colonies is associated with colonization and inflammation at the insertion site, while greater than 1000 is associated with catheter-related septicemia.[14] Interpretation of quantitative catheter cultures also depends on the type of organism recovered and antecedent therapy. For example, isolation of *C. albicans* and *S. aureus* from intravascular devices is more likely to be associated with bacteremias regardless of the colony count, while antibiotic therapy is more likely to prevent bacteremia even in the presence of high quantitative culture results. If culture results show that the catheter is not implicated as the source of infection, a search for other causes of bacteremia must be initiated. Catheter tip cultures may also be used to monitor the quality of catheter care, especially central lines. That is, a high or increasing prevalence of bacterial and fungal contamination of intravascular catheters (corrected for time the device is in place) might indicate a breakdown in technique for their proper care with concomitant increased risk of nosocomial bloodstream infection.

Simultaneous blood culture from an intravascular catheter and peripheral vein is an alternative but much less reliable method for assessing catheter colonization. Blood from infected catheters will have significantly higher numbers of organisms (10 times or more) than blood collected at the same time from a venous sample.

Test: Bone Marrow Culture

Background and Selection

Systemic infection with certain fungi (i.e., *Coccidioides immitis*, *H. capsulatum*, *Candida* spp., *Cryptococcus neoformans*), *Mycobacterium* sp., *Brucella* spp. and *S. typhi* may be identified by culturing bone marrow. This test should be considered in the evaluation of granulomatous disease involving the bone marrow or when blood cultures are negative in suspected cases of *S. typhi*. Histologic examination with special stains (periodic acid-Schiff [PAS], Gomori methenamine-silver [GMS], acid fast) may reveal organisms. Microscopic examination of bone marrow also may be useful when peripheral blood evaluations are negative in suspected infections with malaria, trypanosomes, and *L. donovani*.

Logistics

A few milliliters of bone marrow is aspirated and placed in a sterile heparinized tube. For fungal culture, brain heart infusion broth and blood containing plated media are incubated at 30°C for up to 8 weeks. Culture on appropriate media of buffy coat preparations may be more sensitive for isolating mycobacteria. *Brucella* and *S. typhi* can be recovered with routine blood culture methods, although *Brucella* generally requires prolonged incubation.

Interpretation

Bone marrow cultures are often negative in systemic infections, and when positive, the diagnosis is commonly already established by microbiologic evaluation of another site. Bone marrow culture is of greatest diagnostic value for the initial detection of occult, disseminated histoplasmosis and coccidiomycosis.

REFERENCES

1. Harris RL, Musher DM, Blood K et al: Manifestations of sepsis. Arch Intern Med 1987;147:1895–1906.
2. Weinstein MP, Reller LB, Murphy JR, Lichtenstein KA: The clinical significance of positive blood cultures: a comprehensive analysis of 500 episodes of bacteremia and fungemia in adults. I. Laboratory and epidemiology observations. Rev Infect Dis 1983;5:35–70.
3. Kirchhoff LV, Sheagren JN: Epidemiology and clinical significance of blood cultures positive for coagulase-negative *Staphylococcus*. Infect Control Hosp Epidemiol 1985;6:479–486.
4. Bryan CS: Clinical implications of positive blood cultures. Clin Microbiol Rev 1989;2:329–353.
5. Strand CL, Shulman JA: Bloodstream infections: laboratory detection and clinical considerations. Chicago, American Society of Clinical Pathologists Press, 1988.
6. Van Scoy RE: Culture negative Endocarditis. Mayo Clin Proc 1982;57:149–154.
7. Reik H, Rubin SJ: Evaluation of the buffy-coat smear for rapid detection of bacteremia. JAMA 1981;245:357–359.
8. Specter S, Lancz GJ: Clinical Virology Manual. New York, Elsevier Science Publishing, 1986.
9. Howell CL, Miller MJ, Martin WJ: Comparison of rates of virus isolation from leukocyte population separated from blood by conventional and Ficoll-Paque/Macrodex methods. J Clin Microbiol 1979;10:533–537.
10. Friedman HM: Cytomegalovirus: subclinical infection or disease? Am J Med 1981;70:215–217.
11. Ash LR, Orihel TC: Parasites: A Guide to Laboratory Procedures and Identification. Chicago, American Society of Clinical Pathologists, 1987.
12. Beaver PC, Jung RC, Cupp EW: Clinical Parasitology. 9th Ed. Philadelphia, Lea & Febiger, 1984.
13. Paya CV, Guerra L, Marsh HM et al: Limited usefulness of quantitative culture of blood drawn through the device for diagnosis of intravascular-device-related bacteremia. J Clin Microbiol 1989;27:1431–1433.
14. Brun-Buisson C, Abrouk F, Legrand P et al: Diagnosis of central venous catheter-related sepsis. Critical level of quantitative tip cultures. Arch Intern Med 1987;147:873–877.

21 Eye, Ear, Nose, and Throat

Joseph M. Campos   Ron B. Schifman
Thomas R. Fritsche Steven Specter
Gerald Lancz

INTRODUCTION[1]

The upper respiratory tract is the most common site of infection in humans. The syndromes include rhinitis, pharyngitis, gingivostomatitis, laryngitis, tracheitis, bronchitis, and laryngotracheobronchitis (croup), and most are caused by viruses (Tables 21-1 and 21-2). Etiologic diagnosis is usually unnecessary because these infections are typically mild and self limiting. However, laboratory evaluation may be required if infection progresses into the sinuses or lower respiratory tract, causing severe or even life-threatening disease.

Bacterial infections of the upper respiratory tract include pharyngitis, tonsillar abscess, retropharyngeal abscess, diphtheria, and epiglottitis. In the majority of cases, specific microscopic and culture examinations are indicated for identifying the pathogen and guiding therapy. Infections that occur in the lower respiratory tract but are best diagnosed by examination of specimens from the nasopharynx, include pertussis (whooping cough) as well as viral and neonatal chlamydia pneumonias.

Bacterial and fungal infections of the ear most often develop in the outer and middle regions. Outer ear infections (otitis externa) occur in all age groups, whereas middle ear infections (otitis media) are primarily limited to children younger than 10 years of age. Most ear infections are diagnosed clinically and treated empirically. The need to obtain an etiologic diagnosis is generally limited to special cases involving chronic infections or acute infections of the newborn or immunosuppressed patient. Despite the ears being involved during some viral infections, obtaining specimens from the middle ear for viral culture is rarely indicated.

The eye is a remarkably complex organ with many potential sites for infection. Bacterial and fungal infections that affect tissues immediately adjacent to the eyes (conjunctivitis, blepharitis), the eye surface (keratitis), the intraocular space (endophthalmitis), and periorbital soft tissue (cellulitis) are more common than viral etiologies. Serious eye disease and possible loss of vision may also result from infection with certain protozoa or helminths.

Despite almost constant contact with a microbe laden environment, ocular infections are much less common than respiratory infections. Laboratory examination of eye specimens is often required, not only for identifying the specific etiologic agent, but for distinguishing between noninfectious causes of eyelid inflammation, corneal infiltrates, and intraocular diseases.

Table 21-1. Viruses Causing Upper Respiratory Tract Infection

Adenovirus	Rhinitis, pharyngitis, pharyngoconjunctival fever (3,4,7), acute respiratory disease (military recruits)
Coronavirus	Rhinitis
Coxsackieviruses	Rhinitis (A21,24), pharyngitis, herpangina (group A serotypes)
Cytomegalovirus	Pharyngitis
ECHOvirus	Rhinitis (types 11,20)
Epstein-Barr Virus	Pharyngitis, infectious mononucleosis
Herpes Simplex Virus	Pharyngitis, gingivostomatitis
Influenza	Rhinitis, pharyngitis, croup
Parainfluenza (<2 years old)	Rhinitis, pharyngitis, croup
Respiratory syncytial virus (<2 years old)	Rhinitis, pharyngitis, croup
Rhinovirus	Rhinitis, pharyngitis
Rubeola	Koplik spots, measles

BASIC TESTS

Test: External Ear Examination

Background

The external ear canal is normally colonized with *Staphylococcus epidermidis* and diphtheroids. Infections are caused by the same spectrum of organisms associated with skin and wound infections at other body sites. The most common bacterial pathogens are *Staphylococcus aureus* and *Pseudomonas aeruginosa*. Fungi, particularly *Aspergillus* spp. and less often, *Candida* spp., account for about 10% of external ear infections (otomycosis). The presence of large amounts of cerumen (earwax) or trapped moisture in the outer ear as well as swimming and diving activities predispose to infection. Trauma or sloughing of epithelial cells lining the ear canal leads to secondary infection. Diabetes mellitus and other disorders associated with poor blood circulation in tissues surrounding the ears may lead to malignant otitis externa.[2] This is a life-threatening, necrotizing infection caused by incursion of *P. aeruginosa* or less often, other opportunistic organisms that is sometimes heralded by cranial nerve palsies and that may progress to parotitis, meningitis, or osteomyelitis.[3]

Selection

The diagnosis of outer ear infection is largely made on clinical grounds. Because management usually involves cleansing and administration of empirically chosen topical or systemic antimicrobial therapy, laboratory identification of the etiologic agent is unnecessary. Cultures should be reserved for patients who fail antimicrobial therapy or who have complications such as cellulitis or malignant otitis externa. Isolates should be tested for antimicrobial susceptibility to guide therapy.

Logistics

Outer ear specimens for culture must be carefully collected to minimize contamination with the cutaneous flora normally inhabiting the ear canal. Dried flakes and chunks of cerumen present in the outer ear should be removed and discarded. A thin-tipped sterile swab should be introduced into the ear without touching the walls of uninfected sections and used to absorb exudative material. The swab should be removed from the ear with equal care and sent in transport media for culture. A separate swab specimen should be obtained for microscopic examination. Specimens are inoculated to 5% sheep blood, chocolate, and MacConkey (or EMB) agar media for bacterial culture, and to Sabouraud dextrose agar for fungal culture.

Interpretation

Presumptive laboratory diagnosis of otitis externa is obtained by examination of Gram stained smears of scrapings from the cellular surface of the ear canal that is visibly inflamed. Microscopic appearance of large numbers of homogeneously appearing bacteria or fungi with inflammatory cells indicate otitis externa. *Pseudomonas aeruginosa*, *S. aureus*, and *Streptococcus pyogenes* are the most likely bacterial pathogens, whereas *Aspergillus* spp., *Penicillium* spp., and *Candida albicans*

Table 21-2. Relative Frequency of Respiratory Viruses in Human Infections

Infection	Percent of All Infections
Rhinoviruses	25
Parainfluenza and respiratory syncytial virus	20
Influenza	10
Enterovirus, adenovirus, coronavirus	10
Other viruses	25–30
All bacterial causes	5–10

are the most likely causes of fungal infection. Specimens from children with ruptured tympanic membranes may reveal growth of pathogens associated with otitis media (see below). Growth of mixed cutaneous flora such as coagulase negative *Staphylococcus* spp. or diphtheroids in any amounts indicates a poorly collected specimen and is nondiagnostic.

Test: Inner Ear Cultures

Background[4]

The middle ear is susceptible to infection by organisms that gain entry from the nasopharynx via the eustachian tube or rarely by hematogenous spread. Anatomic deviations of the nasopharynx may be a predisposing condition for recurrent infections. Ordinarily, the middle ear is protected by the ciliated epithelial cells lining the eustachian tube that sweep organism laden secretions back into the nasopharynx. Obstruction of the eustachian tube by secretions or inflammation produces increased pressure and trapping of organisms within the middle ear, suppuration, and more pressure. This produces severe ear pain often accompanied by fever, although infants with acute otitis media may be asymptomatic. In some cases, infection leads to spontaneous tympanic membrane rupture and otorrhea (spillage of organisms and pus into the outer ear). Mastoiditis is a rare complication associated with progression of untreated otitis media into the air spaces of the adjoining mastoid bone, eventually forming an abscess. This is a serious infection that may progress to meningitis. The major causes of acute otitis media and mastoiditis are *Streptococcus pneumoniae, Haemophilus influenzae, Moraxella* (formerly *Branhamella*) *catarrhalis, S. pyogenes,* certain viruses (such as respiratory syncytial virus, influenza virus, enterovirus, adenovirus, and rhinovirus), and mixed anaerobic bacteria. Fungi and other bacteria or viruses are unusual causes of infection. In addition to the organisms listed above, neonatal otitis media may be caused by enteric gram-negative bacilli or *Chlamydia trachomatis*. The role of *Mycoplasma pneumoniae* in otitis media is unclear.

Viral pathogens cause mild otitis media often in association with upper respiratory infections.[5] Viral infection of the upper respiratory tract also may be complicated by bacterial otitis media, either as a single infection of the middle ear, combined with, or secondary to viral otitis media. These infections may cause bullous myringitis, a condition identified by painful vesicular blebs on the tympanic membrane. *Chlamydia trachomatis* pneumonia in children younger than 6 months of age may be complicated by otitis media. Congenital infection of the inner ear with rubella or cytomegalovirus (CMV) may rarely cause deafness. Mumps may cause unilateral nerve deafness, or deafness may ensue in the aftermath of viral encephalitis. Reactivation of varicella-zoster infection may involve the external ear canal, auditory nerves, or tympanic membrane.

Middle ear effusion causing limited mobility of the tympanic membrane is a common feature of otitis media and frequently remains several weeks or more after therapy. Subacute infection, referred to as otitis media with effusion (OME), develops when fluid persists within the middle ear for 3 weeks or more and is a frequent and often asymptomatic aftermath of infection. The effusion generally lacks purulence, is more often culture negative than in acute infections, and in many cases it resolves spontaneously. Protracted effusions, lasting more than 3 months, may cause fibroblast proliferation within the middle ear (cholesteatoma) and increasingly viscus effusion that may permanently damage the ossicles. Besides the typical pathogens that cause acute infection, Enterobacteriaceae, *P. aeruginosa,* and anaerobic bacilli tend to be more commonly associated with chronic otitis media.

Selection

Because the spectrum of organisms causing acute otitis media in children is limited and of predictable antimicrobial susceptibility and because invasive methods are generally required for specimen collection, laboratory diagnosis is not routinely performed. However, the pathogens that cause otitis media in neonates and chronic otitis media in all age groups are unpredictable, and in these cases, middle ear aspirates should be obtained for bacterial culture and Gram stained smear. Other indications for culture include failure to eradicate the infection with antimicrobial therapy or the occurrence of complications such as mastoiditis. Nasopharyngeal cultures are not indicated because they correlate poorly with the etiologic agents recovered by tympanocentesis. Fungal culture is indicated when the patient fails therapy, bacterial cultures are negative, or the patient is immunosuppressed. Anaerobic cultures should be considered in cases of chronic otitis media or with treatment failures. Acid-fast smears and culture for *Mycobacterium tuberculosis* should be attempted when a patient fails empirical antimicrobial therapy and has other evidence of tuberculosis or has a history of close contact with a tuberculous individual.

Immunologic methods, such as counter immunoelectrophoresis or latex agglutination, for detecting polysaccharide antigens of *S. pneumoniae* and *H. influenzae* in middle ear effusions can provide an etiologic diagnosis, and may be particularly helpful for evaluating partially treated infections that are culture negative. However, the value and indications for performing this test are limited because the diagnostic spectrum of the method is narrow, it requires invasive specimen collections, most strains of *H. influenza* that cause otitis media are untypable (they do not possess the capsular polysaccharide), and infection generally responds well to empiric therapy.

Generally, viral infections involving the ear are accompanied by other disease symptoms and if cultures are indicated, they should be obtained from another source, most commonly the throat or nasopharynx.

Logistics

Collection of middle ear effusion by tympanocentesis should be accomplished using aseptic techniques to prevent contamination of specimens with organisms colonizing the external ear canal. The walls of the ear canal and the tympanic membrane itself should be disinfected with alcohol before the procedure. When rupture of the tympanic membrane has already occurred, fluid residing in the ear canal may be absorbed on a swab and submitted to the laboratory for testing. Aspirates of mastoid abscess fluids should be collected aseptically and transported to the laboratory for aerobic and anaerobic culture.

Middle ear and mastoid abscess effusions submitted to the laboratory should be analyzed microscopically and by culture. A Gram stained smear that reveals abundant neutrophils suggests bacterial infection and the etiologic diagnosis can generally be made without difficulty by culture.

Middle ear and mastoid abscess fluids should be inoculated to 5% sheep blood, chocolate, MacConkey (or EMB) agar, and a nonselective enrichment broth such as tryptic soy broth supplemented with 5% Fildes reagent. Cultures for anaerobic bacteria should be reserved only for specimens obtained aseptically by tympanocentesis and transported to the laboratory under conditions assuring the survival of anaerobes. Specimens that may harbor *M. tuberculosis* should be inoculated to Lowenstein-Jensen medium, Middlebrook 7H10 or 7H11 agar, and Middlebrook 7H9 or Dubos Tween 80 broth. Detection of *C. trachomatis* in neonatal otitis media is achieved by shell vial culture in cycloheximide treated McCoy cells.

Interpretation[6]

In order of frequency, acute otitis media in children is caused by *S. pneumoniae*, *H. influenzae*, *M. catarrhalis*, respiratory viruses, *S. pyogenes*, and *S. aureus*. Isolation of any of these organisms is diagnostic. Results from culturing material discharged from a ruptured tympanic membrane should be interpreted with the assumption that the fluid was contaminated with normal ear canal (mixed cutaneous) flora. Sterile cultures or organisms of uncertain diagnostic relevance, such as *S. epidermidis* and diphtheroids, may be seen in 20–40% of middle ear aspirates obtained from children with otitis media. The significance of this finding is often unclear, but may implicate viral or partially treated bacterial infections. Besides culture, there are no useful clinical or laboratory findings that will differentiate viral from bacterial infection. Expected pathogens to be recovered in chronic otitis media include anaerobes, Enterobacteriaceae, and *P. aeruginosa*, as well as typical pathogens found with acute infections.

Some physicians culture the external ear canal at the time of tympanocentesis to help differentiate between external ear canal contamination and genuine middle ear pathogens. This practice has limited value because the pathogens that typically cause otitis media usually differ from those inhabiting the external ear canal.

Test: Nasal Cultures

Background[7]

Bacterial and fungal infections of the nose occur rarely in the immunocompetent patient. Scleroma (Slavic leprosy) is a chronic granulomatous infection of the cells lining the respiratory tract caused by *Klebsiella rhinoscleromatis* that usually also involves nasal mucosal surfaces. The infection is endemic to Eastern Europe, Africa, Asia, and Central and South America. In severe cases, expansion of infection into bony tissue or obstruction of nasal passages ensues. Ozena is an uncommon infection of the nasal mucosa characterized by chronic atrophic rhinitis. Patients produce a foul-smelling nasal discharge from which *Klebsiella ozaenae* is frequently isolated. However, *K. ozaenae* probably only colonizes the affected nasal mucosa and is considered a doubtful cause of the infection.

Clinically significant nasal infection or colonization, especially by fungi, occurs almost exclusively in immunocompromised patients. Growth of *Aspergillus fumigatus* or *Aspergillus flavus* in a nasal culture from a febrile, neutropenic patient is often the first evidence of disseminated aspergillosis. The nose is a frequent site for colonization by *S. aureus*. Individuals suffering from recurrent *S. aureus* infections or health care workers serving as vectors for nosocomial infections may have nasal reservoirs of the organism. Infection of sites contiguous to the nose (see paranasal sinuses and nasopharynx below) is much more common than infection of the nose itself.

Selection

Examination of purulent nasal discharges from patients who may have scleroma or ozena should include Gram stain and culture. Individuals who may serve as nasal reservoirs of *S. aureus* should be cultured specifically for the organism. The role of performing surveillance cultures of the nose in immunocompromised patients is controversial but if done, the specimen should be cultured for fungi. A biopsy of nasal mucosa is the preferred specimen when infection is suspected in the immunocompromised host. Besides routine bacterial and fungal culture, special stains for fungi (e.g., calcofluor white or methenamine silver nitrate) should be performed. Culture of nasal discharge to establish the etiology of sinusitis or otitis media is unreliable and therefore inappropriate.

Logistics

Specimen Collection

Nasal discharge or surveillance specimens of nasal mucosa should be collected with sterile swabs and delivered promptly to the laboratory for bacterial and fungal cultures. Anaerobic culture is not appropriate.

Analysis

Gram Stain. Thin smears should be prepared from nasal discharge specimens, fixed with heat or methanol, stained, and examined for microorganisms and inflammatory cells.

Fungal Stain. Touch preparations from nasal biopsy specimens from immunocompromised patients should be stained with calcofluor white or methenamine silver nitrate and examined for fungal elements.

Bacterial Culture. Nasal discharge specimens should be inoculated to 5% sheep blood agar, chocolate agar, and when scleroma or ozena are suspected, MacConkey (or EMB) agar. Blood and chocolate agar cultures should be incubated at 35°C in an atmosphere enriched with 5–10% CO_2 for 48–72 hours. MacConkey (or EMB) cultures should be incubated aerobically at 35°C for 24 hours. Nasal surveillance cultures for *S. aureus* colonization should be inoculated to a selective medium such as mannitol salt agar and incubated aerobically at 35°C for 24 hours.

Fungal Culture. Nasal biopsies and surveillance swabs should be inoculated to Sabouraud dextrose agar and a fungal medium containing antibacterial agents such as brain heart infusion agar with chloramphenicol and gentamicin. Cultures should be incubated at 25–30°C in an aerobic atmosphere for 21–28 days. Selective fungal media containing cycloheximide should not be used exclusively because growth of *Aspergillus* spp. and other opportunistic fungi may be inhibited. When *Zygomycetes* spp. is suspected in biopsy material, a portion should be cultured without grinding.

Interpretation

Mucoid, lactose fermenting colonies on MacConkey or EMB media, recovered from patients with possible scleroma or ozena, should be identified on the basis of biochemical reactions. Both *K. rhinoscleromatis* and *K. ozaenae* are readily identified by conventional test systems. Unlike other *Klebsiella* spp., most isolates of *K. rhinoscleromatis* and *K. ozaenae* are susceptible to ampicillin and carbenicillin.

Growth of large numbers of *S. aureus* from nasal surveillance cultures is evidence of nasal colonization. The organism should be saved on an agar slant for possible bacteriophage typing, plasmid analysis, or other methods appropriate for epidemiologic investigations.

Detection of *A. fumigatus* or *A. flavus* in a nasal surveillance culture from an immunocompromised patient should be reported to the patient's physician without delay. The result may prompt immediate institution of antifungal therapy if the patient is febrile and neutropenic.

Test: Sinus Aspirate Cultures

Background[8]

Acute and chronic sinusitis usually occur as the result of an upper respiratory tract viral infection but may also complicate dental infections, allergic rhinitis, anatomic defects, or indwelling nasal cannula. The infection is responsible for millions of physician visits each year. Although usually self limited, sinus infection can advance into the central nervous system (brain abscess) or frontal bone and may go unrecognized if symptoms are obscured by the primary disease. Orbital cellulitis, often caused by *S. aureus*, *S. pneumoniae*, or *H. influenzae*, is another complication.

The bacterial agents responsible for acute sinusitis are predictable and consist of various members of the upper respiratory flora (e.g., *S. pneumoniae;* nontypable *H. influenzae;* and less often, *M. catarrhalis, S. aureus,* group A *Streptococcus;* and mixed anaerobes, which are associated with dental disease and upper respiratory viruses. Fungal sinusitis is uncommon in the normal host, whereas infection can also be a major problem in patients who are diabetic, immunocompromised, or who have had recent orofacial surgery.[9] Infection is potentially life-threatening because of the predilection of fungi to invade the central nervous system from the facial sinuses. Etiologic agents include *Aspergillus* spp., *Pseudoallescharia boydii,* and *Zygomycetes* spp. In immunosuppressed patients, *Zygomycetes* spp. may cause a rapidly invasive and difficult to cure infection, termed *rhinocerebral mucomycosis,* involving the nose, sinuses, and frontal lobes.

Selection

The evaluation of patients with sinusitis first involves nonlaboratory test modalities. Transillumination (in acute infections) and more often, radiographic examination of the sinuses provide sufficient information to establish the diagnosis. Antimicrobial treatment of acute sinusitis is fairly standardized without requiring laboratory diagnosis of the etiologic agent for patient management.

Sinus puncture with aspiration for identification of bacterial and fungal infectious agents is indicated for patients with acute or chronic sinusitis who are immunosuppressed, do not respond to standard antimicrobial agents, have suspected intracranial invasion, or have nosocomial infections from indwelling nasal tubes. Although various viral etiologies account for about 25% of acute paranasal sinus infections in adults, culture for these agents is usually not helpful for patient therapy or management.

Logistics

Specimen Requirements

When laboratory examination is indicated, a sinus aspirate is the specimen of choice. The aspirate should be collected with needle and syringe by piercing the cartilage surrounding the sinus cavity after aseptically preparing the puncture site. If necessary, the sinus cavity may be rinsed with sterile nonbacteriostatic saline to facilitate aspiration. The specimen should be conveyed promptly to the laboratory with request for Gram stain, routine bacterial culture, and anaerobic culture. The aspirate can be sent in a syringe with a leak-proof cap, or placed in an anaerobic transport device to ensure the survival of anaerobes.

Analysis

Microscopy. Smears from needle aspirates of patients with sinusitis should be Gram stained and examined for microorganisms and inflammatory cells. Specimens from patients with possible fungal sinusitis should be stained with calcofluor white or methenamine silver nitrate and examined for fungal elements.

Culture. Sinus aspirates for bacterial culture should be inoculated to 5% sheep blood, chocolate, and MacConkey (or EMB) agar media and incubated aerobically at 35°C for 24 hours. Quantitative cultures using either a calibrated loop or pipet may be helpful in differentiating contamination (<50,000 colonies/mL) from genuine infection.

Cultures for anaerobic bacteria should be performed only on specimens transported to the laboratory under conditions assuring the survival of anaerobes. Anaerobic specimens should be inoculated to selective and nonselective prereduced blood containing media supplemented with vitamin K and hemin. Selective media for enhancing recovery of *Bacteroides* spp. (laked blood agar with kanamycin and vancomycin), and gram-positive anaerobes colistin-naladixic acid (CNA) agar should be included. Cultures should be incubated at 35°C in anaerobic atmosphere for 5–7 days.

Sinus aspirates for fungal culture should be inoculated to Sabouraud dextrose agar and a medium containing antibacterial agents (such as brain heart infusion agar with chloramphenicol and gentamicin). Selective media containing cycloheximide should not be used exclusively because growth of *Mucor, Rhizopus, Absidia* and other opportunistic fungi are usually inhibited. Cultures should be incubated at 25–30°C in an aerobic atmosphere for 21–28 days.

Interpretation

Sinus infections, especially if chronic, are often polymicrobial in nature. It then becomes difficult to determine whether the results indicate an infectious process or merely a poorly collected specimen contaminated with nasal flora. Interpretation of culture and smear results from patients with anatomic lesions is particularly difficult since they typically are colonized with bacteria. Infection is almost invariably associated with large numbers of inflammatory cells on gram smear and greater than 50,000 colony forming units (CFU)/mL on culture. This and correlation between the smear and culture findings help to substantiate a diagnosis of infection. When obligate anaerobes are recovered, the patient should be carefully examined for abscesses of the upper teeth, because dental infections are the usual source for anaerobic bacteria in sinusitis. Chronic sinusitis may be caused by enteric gram-negative bacilli and nonfermentative gram-negative bacilli as well as by upper respiratory flora. Growth of fungal colonies from a sinus aspirate should be considered significant when obtained from an individual with chronic infection or who is immunosuppressed and at risk of invasive disease.

Test: Throat (Oropharynx) Culture

Background

Pharyngitis is caused by a large number of different viral and bacterial etiologies. Most throat infections are self limited and have no post infectious sequelae.

Viral Infections

Rhinitis caused by viral infection is the most common of all human viral diseases. This infection, better known as the common cold, usually causes mild symptoms but may be accompanied by pharyngitis and a slight fever. The most commonly involved agents are rhinovirus (of which there are more than 110 serotypes), coronavirus, and adenovirus. In addition, colds with or without pharyngitis may be caused by coxsackieviruses (the cause of herpangina), Echoviruses, influenza viruses, parainfluenza viruses, adenoviruses, and respiratory syncytial virus (RSV). If there are no complications and no progression of infection down the respiratory tract, culture for virus is unnecessary and the patient recovers without assistance. Laryngitis, tonsillitis, or tracheitis are less frequent complications of the viruses responsible for pharyngitis. The etiology is seldom determined because cultures are not routinely performed. Conjunctivitis may complicate adenovirus pharyngitis. In military recruits, this virus is also known to cause acute respiratory disease, which has a prominent pharyngitis. Herpes simplex virus (HSV), CMV, and Epstein-Barr virus (EBV) also may cause pharyngitis, often associated with fever, anorexia, and malaise, and in the case of the latter two viruses, infectious mononucleosis.

Bacterial Infections

Bacteria for which cultures are performed and antimicrobial therapy is administered are *S. pyogenes, Neisseria gonorrhoeae,* and *Corynebacterium diphtheriae.* Possible pathogens for which laboratory testing is not yet commonly practiced include *Corynebacterium haemolyticum* and *Chlamydia psittaci* TWAR. The majority of bacterial infections of the pharynx occur in children.[10] However, *N. gonorrhoeae, C. haemolyticum,* and *C. psittaci* TWAR primarily affect adolescents and young adults. Gonococcal pharyngitis does not display a seasonal peak, whereas *S. pyogenes* and other pathogens cause infection predominately during the fall and winter months. Not all strains of *S. pyogenes* and *C. diphtheriae* recovered from the oropharynx are pathogens. These bacteria and possibly *C. haemolyticum* produce extracellular bacteriophage mediated toxins that are essential for pathogenicity. Visible signs of infection include frank inflammatory exudate that covers the throat and/or tonsils during streptococcal pharyngitis and a pseudomembranous coat of bacteria, and inflammatory and epithelial cells that appear in the throat during diphtheria. *Francisella tularensis* and *Legionella pneumophila* are rare causes of pharyngitis for which a strong index of suspicion is needed before a search for the pathogen is attempted.

Ulcerative gingivitis (trench mouth) and infections involving the peritonsillar (Quinsy throat), submandibular (Ludwig's angina), and retropharyngeal (Vincent's angina) spaces are usually polymicrobial and include various anaerobes from the upper respiratory flora and less often, *S. pyogenes* and *S. aureus.* Infection results from direct invasion of organisms from the upper respiratory tract and, in rare instances (especially with *Fusobacterium necrophorum* involvement), progresses to septic thrombophlebitis of the jugular vein, sepsis, and metastatic infection.

Bacterial epiglottitis is a childhood disease and is almost exclusively caused by *H. influenzae* type b.[11] The organism invades the epiglottal mucosa and is frequently associated with bacteremia. Observation of the tip of the inflamed epiglottis (maraschino cherry sign) behind the tongue is the most direct evidence of infection. Epiglottal swelling can be severe enough to cause asphyxiation and require emergency airway management. Occasional, less serious cases are caused by *S. pyogenes.* Infection in adults is unusual and is usually attributable to bacteria other than *H. influenzae.*[12]

Fungal Infections

Candida albicans and less often other *Candida* spp. cause mucous membrane infections of the mouth and throat of neonates (thrush) and patients with deficient cell mediated immunity. These yeasts, which are common members of the respiratory flora, first colonize, then infect the mucous membranes of immunodeficient individuals. Oral candidiasis is often one of the first manifestations of acquired immunodeficiency syndrome (AIDS).

Other Infections

Two additional types of lesions are seen in the mouth that are not respiratory infections. Primary HSV infection, most commonly type 1, causes gingivostomatitis. Vesicular lesions may be extensive in the oral cavity, involving the gingiva, labia, and buccal mucosa, last for about 2 weeks, and can be extremely painful. Lesions are readily cultured for confirmation of HSV infection. Rubeola (measles) also produces lesions in the buccal mucosa called Koplik spots, characterized by bluish white lesions with a red halo. They appear during the prodrome phase of the disease, preceding the rash by about 3 days and are pathognomonic for rubeola. Viral culture is rarely required to diagnose measles.

Selection[13]

The primary purpose of using the microbiology laboratory in routine cases of acute pharyngitis is to differentiate *S. pyogenes* (group A) infection from other etiologies. Although cervical adenitis, sore throat, and palatal petechiae are frequent findings in streptococcal pharyngitis, the diagnosis cannot be reliably determined solely on clinical grounds. The potential postinfectious complications of *S. pyogenes* pharyngitis, such as rheumatic fever and glomerulonephritis, can be prevented by treating the patient with antibiotics (usually penicillin). After therapy, repeat testing of an asymptomatic patient to confirm eradication of *S. pyogenes* is not indicated, because the organism will still be present in 10–25% of treated and even retreated patients. In almost all such cases, acute infection is not present and the patient is in no danger of developing postinfectious complications.

Commercially available antigen detection tests presently are not sufficiently sensitive to replace culture. Diagnosis of *S. pyogenes* infection should either rely exclusively on culture or on antigen detection plus culture of antigen negative specimens. The latter approach requires collection of duplicate specimens from each patient and testing of both specimens in the majority of instances. Dual testing is both time consuming and expensive.

Communication with the laboratory is an absolute requirement for detecting other pathogens in pharyngeal specimens. In the absence of special instructions, a throat swab submitted for culture will be tested for *S. pyogenes* only. There is no hope of detecting *N. gonorrhoeae*, *C. diphtheriae*, or *C. haemolyticum* in a culture routinely processed only for detection of *S. pyogenes*.

Culture for virus is warranted when pharyngitis is severe and complicated by high fever or occurs in infants, the elderly, or immunocompromised patients. If infection is caused by RSV, parainfluenza, or influenza viruses in a hospital nursery, the child should be isolated to limit the spread of infection to others. It is more common to culture individuals at the beginning of an epidemic season to establish the presence of a particular virus in the community. If a patient expresses classic symptoms during an established epidemic, it is seldom necessary to culture for virus.[14] Additional studies may be considered in special circumstances, depending on history, symptoms, and seasonal considerations. The presence of constitutional symptoms such as fever, myalgia, malaise, headache, and lethargy suggest the possibility of influenza A, adenovirus, infectious mononucleosis (EBV or CMV) or acute human immunodeficiency virus (HIV) infection. Influenza A infections are seasonal (winter) and associated with community outbreaks. The diagnoses of infectious mononucleosis and HIV are made by serologic testing. Culture examination of the eye for bacteria and adenovirus may be useful when conjunctivitis accompanies pharyngitis. The presence of vesicles and ulcers of the palate or buccal mucosa suggest HSV infection, which is easily identified by culture. When *N. gonorrhoeae* is suspected from the patient's history, specimens from pharyngeal, urethral, and rectal sites should be cultured with appropriate selective medium.[15] Special examination for *C. diphtheria* detection should be performed when a pharyngeal or tonsillar membrane is seen and the patient has no history of vaccination.

The major difficulty faced in identifying the etiologic agents of tonsillar and retropharyngeal abscesses is collection of specimens that are not contaminated with upper respiratory flora. Once obtained, specimens should be referred to the laboratory for aerobic and anaerobic cultures.

Examination and specimen collection from the inflamed epiglottis is contraindicated because of the risk of inducing airway obstruction and the predictability of the offending pathogen *(H. influenza)*. Only under circumstances in which patients can be rapidly intubated should microbiologic examination of the epiglottis be considered. Because children with epiglottitis often are bacteremic, blood cultures should be obtained as an aid for confirming the etiologic diagnosis.

Logistics

Specimen Collection and Analysis

A pharyngeal specimen is collected from a widely opened mouth, the tongue is depressed to improve visibility, and the swab inserted so that the tip makes contact with exudative, inflamed regions of the posterior pharynx and tonsils. The value of a carefully collected specimen, especially in children, cannot be overemphasized. Poorly collected specimens in which material from the tongue or buccal mucosa are on the swab compromises test sensitivity. Such specimens, even when collected from genuinely infected patients, are usually antigen negative, or at best, weakly culture positive. Cotton, rayon, or dacron swabs are suitable for culture; swabs for *S. pyogenes* antigen detection should be rayon or dacron. Cotton swabs may interfere with antigen testing. Moistening or inserting pharyngeal swabs into transport medium, such as modified Stuarts's or Amie's medium, is recommended for survival of pathogens other than *S. pyogenes*, which can endure for long periods on dry swabs. Table 21-3 lists the proper specimens that should be collected for isolating viral agents, although this is seldom indicated.

Aspirates of tonsillar and retropharyngeal abscesses must be collected in an aseptic fashion. The surface of the abscess should be disinfected to reduce the quantity of commensal upper respiratory flora. The aspirate is then collected, taking care that the syringe needle does not contact any nondisinfected oral surfaces. Aspirates should be submitted for Gram stain and both aerobic and anaerobic culture. The specimen for anaerobic culture must be transported to the laboratory under conditions that ensure survival of anaerobic bacteria.

Table 21-3. Appropriate Specimens to Collect for Isolating Virus in Upper Respiratory Infections

Rhinitis	Nasopharyngeal swab, wash, or aspirate (especially in young children)
Pharyngitis	Nasopharyngeal swab, throat swab, oropharyngeal wash
Croup	Nasopharyngeal swab, throat swab, nasopharyngeal aspirate
Gingivostomatitis	Swab of buccal mucosa
Rubeola (Koplik spots)	Swab of lesion, nasopharyngeal swab, throat swab

Epiglottal swabs from patients with epiglottitis should be collected only when absolutely required. Equipment necessary for providing an emergency airway for the patient should be immediately at hand during the procedure. An epiglottal swab, if deemed necessary, should be accurately identified so that the laboratory will include chocolate agar among the media inoculated so that recovery of *H. influenzae* is possible.

Oropharyngeal mucocutaneous candidiasis (thrush) in the neonate or immunodeficient patient is readily recognized by visual examination. When laboratory documentation is deemed important, scalpel scrapings from the plaque should be examined microscopically to establish the presence of yeast, and cultured to identify the specific agent. Surveillance of immunodeficient patients for fungal colonization of the upper respiratory tract is best achieved by fungal culture.

Antigen Detection

Dozens of rapid assays for detection of *S. pyogenes* antigen are commercially available. Almost all use either latex particle agglutination or rapid enzyme immunoassays. Prior to testing, the assays require chemical or enzymatic extraction of the *S. pyogenes* antigen from bacteria enmeshed in the throat swab. Latex particle agglutination assays are performed by mixing extracted antigen with antibody coated, microscopic latex particles. A positive result is signaled by macroscopic clumping of the latex particle suspension. The rapid enzyme immunoassay relies on the reaction of extracted antigen with antibody that is attached to a solid phase (such as a nitrocellulose membrane or a plastic paddle). The solid phase is bathed with an antibody enzyme conjugate, washed thoroughly to remove unbound conjugate, and then exposed to enzyme substrate. A positive result is depicted by conversion of the substrate to a colored end product.

Microscopic Examination

Because of the plethora of upper respiratory flora present in the pharynx, Gram stains are not recommended for screening specimens except to use the examination for diagnosis and early management of tonsillar and retropharyngeal abscesses. Direct examination for *S. pyogenes* with fluorescent labeled antibody has been largely replaced by more convenient antigen detection methods. Microscopic examination of KOH preparations, Gram or calcofluor white stained smears prepared from plaque-like lesions of the roof of the mouth can confirm the clinical diagnosis of oropharyngeal yeast infection. Scalpel scrapings of material from the plaque should be placed on a microscope slide and brought to the laboratory for examination.

Culture

Cultures for *S. pyogenes* should be inoculated to 5% sheep blood agar. Agar containing selective antimicrobial and/or chemical agents is recommended. Culture plates may be incubated aerobically or anaerobically. Anaerobic or "stab" cultures are more likely to show characteristic β-hemolysis. To maximize the test's sensitivity, the length of incubation should be at least 24 and preferably 48 hours. Identification of β-hemolytic colonies as *S. pyogenes* should be verified by detection of group A-specific antigen in colonies or by demonstration of L-pyrrolidonyl-B-naphthylamide (PYR) hydrolytic activity in the colonies. Reliance upon bacitracin susceptibility to distinguish group A from other streptococcal groups is much less reliable than use of the aforementioned methods.

Specimens for *C. diphtheriae* culture should be inoculated to an enrichment medium (e.g., Löffler or Pai agar slant) as well as to a selective plate (e.g., cystine-tellurite agar). After inoculation of the selective and enrichment media, the swab should be left on the surface of the enrichment agar. Cultures should be incubated aerobically overnight at 35°C. Growth on the enrichment agar should be smeared, stained with methylene blue, and examined for metachromatic granules. Observation of metachromatic granules is presumptive evidence of *C. diphtheriae*. Colonies from positive slants should be subcultured to selective agar. Selective agar should be incubated for 48 hours and examined each day for gray to black colonies. Suspicious colonies are subcultured to 5% sheep blood agar in preparation for biochemical test identification and toxicology testing.

Pharyngeal swabs for culture of *N. gonorrhoeae* should be inoculated to selective medium (modified Thayer-Martin). Culture plates must be incubated in an aerobic atmosphere enriched with 5–10% CO_2 for 48–72 hours. Growth of oxidase positive gram-negative diplococci should be biochemically or immunologically confirmed as *N. gonorrhoeae*.

Cultural detection of *C. haemolyticum* is best achieved by inoculation of pharyngeal specimens onto 5% rabbit or human blood agar. Cultures should be incubated aerobically or anaerobically at 35°C for at least 48 hours. *Corynebacterium haemolyticum* colonies are strongly β-hemolytic on rabbit or human blood agar, but grow poorly on standard sheep blood agar.

Epiglottal swabs should be inoculated onto 5% sheep blood and chocolate agar. Cultures should be incubated at 35°C in a 5–10% CO_2 enriched aerobic atmosphere for 48 hours. Tonsillar and retropharyngeal abscess aspirates should be inoculated to aerobic and anaerobic culture media. Aerobic media should include 5% sheep blood and chocolate agars; anaerobic media should be prereduced and include anaerobic blood agar enriched with vitamin K and hemin, a selective blood agar for members of the *Bacteroides melaninogenicus* group (laked blood agar with kanamycin and vancomycin), and a selective blood agar for gram-positive anaerobes (CNA agar). Aerobic cultures should be incubated at 35°C in an atmosphere supplemented with 5–10% CO_2 for 48 hours. Anaerobic cultures should be incubated at 35°C for 5–7 days.

Fungus

Specimens for fungal culture should be inoculated to media that discourage the growth of bacteria (e.g., Sabouraud dextrose agar). All specimens collected from the upper respiratory tract contain large amounts of commensal bacteria, many of which grow at a faster rate than fungi. Even though most yeasts and opportunistic fungi are able to grow on nonselective bacterial media, heavy growth of bacteria very easily could mask the presence of young fungal colonies. Cycloheximide-containing media should be used with caution, because they may inhibit the growth of some fungi.

Virus

Laboratory methods for direct and culture detection of viruses are described in Chapter 22.

Interpretation *(Table 21-4)*

A positive rapid antigen detection test for *S. pyogenes* in a throat swab is convincing evidence for the presence of the organism in the specimen. Because detection by these assays require at least 1000 CFU in the specimen, a positive result indicates the presence of relatively large numbers of *S. pyogenes*. Although crossreactions with other respiratory bacteria are very rare, a negative test result does not rule out infection by *S. pyogenes* because the method is capable of detecting only 80% or less of culture positive specimens. Not all laboratories, however, utilize sensitive culture methods. In physician office laboratories, antigen detection tests actually provide more sensitive results than culture. Nevertheless, negative antigen detection tests should be confirmed by culture.

Although the diagnosis appears obvious when *S. pyogenes* is recovered from patients with acute pharyngitis,

Table 21-4. Important Bacterial and Fungal Pathogens Causing Upper Respiratory Tract Infection

Pathogen	Infection, Associated Disease
Aspergillus spp.	Contaminant, pharyngeal colonization, sinusitis in the immunocompromised host
Bordetella pertussis	Pertussis (whooping cough)
Moraxella (Branhamella) catarrhalis	Pharyngeal colonization, sinusitis
Candida spp.	Pharyngeal colonization, thrush
Chlamydia trachomatis	Neonatal pneumonia, pharyngeal colonization associated with sexual transmission
Corynebacteria diphtheriae	Diphtheria (toxin-producing strains)
Corynebacteria hemolyticum	Pharyngitis with rash
Enterobacteriaceae	Pharyngeal colonization in hospitalized patients, sinusitis
Fusobacterium necrophorum	Tonsillitis, peritonsillar abscess, complicated by jugular vein thrombophlebitis
Haemophilus influenzae	Sinusitis, epiglottitis, orbital cellulitis, pharyngeal colonization
Mycoplasma spp.	Pharyngeal colonization, sinusitis?
Neisseria gonorrhoeae	Pharyngeal colonization associated with sexual transmission, mild pharyngitis
Neisseria spp. other than *N. gonorrhoeae*	Pharyngeal colonization, sinusitis *(N. meningitidis)*
Pseudoallescharia boydii	Sinusitis in the normal or immunocompromised host
Pseudomonas aeruginosa	Pharyngeal colonization in hospitalized patients
Staphylococcus aureus	Pharyngeal colonization, sinusitis, orbital cellulitis
Streptococcus pyogenes	Pharyngitis, tonsillitis, with risk of postinfectious rheumatic fever or glomerulonephritis, pharyngeal colonization, sinusitis, orbital cellulitis
Streptococcus spp., β-hemolytic, not group A	Pharyngitis, tonsillitis, pharyngeal colonization
Streptococcus pneumoniae	Pharyngeal colonization, sinusitis, periorbital cellulitis
Yersinia enterocolitica	Pharyngitis, abdominal pain
Zygomycetes spp.	Sinusitis in immunocompromised host

only about one-half have a serologic response to extracellular *S. pyogenes* antigens that is indicative of invasive disease. Unfortunately, there is no accurate way to distinguish infection from colonization simply by examining culture plates. The popular notion that cultures displaying 10 or fewer colonies always represent colonization is fallacious. The number of colonies that appear in positive cultures is greatly affected by the cooperation of the patient and the care with which the specimen was collected. Children can be especially uncooperative patients, and fewer than 10 colonies could very well be the result of sampling the tongue or the roof of the mouth of a genuinely infected child. Although many specimens yielding fewer than 10 colonies indeed reflect colonization rather than infection, the most cautious approach, especially in the childhood age group most susceptible to acute rheumatic fever, is to regard all positive cultures in the symptomatic patient as clinically significant and administer antimicrobial agents accordingly. The significance of finding the organism in the throat after appropriate antibiotic therapy is less clear and occurs in 10–25% of patients, even when therapy is repeated.[16] If the patient is asymptomatic, this finding nearly always denotes a carrier state rather than genuine infection. Infection may be demonstrated by a rising anti-streptolysin-O titer on acute and convalescent serum specimens or a single abnormal result with the streptozyme test.[17] However, it should be recognized that therapy can blunt the immunologic response.

Microscopic examination of appropriately selected and collected pharyngeal and oral specimens yields clinically valuable information. Observation of bacteria, spirochetes, and inflammatory cells in swabs from ulcerative gingivitis or aspirates of retropharyngeal or peritonsillar abscesses helps confirm bacterial infection, and empirical antimicrobial therapy should be started pending definitive culture results.[18] The presence of budding or mycelial yeast forms in scrapings from oral plaques collected from neonates or immunodeficient patients is diagnostic of mucocutaneous candidiasis (thrush). Diagnosis of syphilis by microscopic examination of ulcerative mouth lesions is notoriously difficult because of confusion of the spirochete with normal mouth flora. Direct smear of throat lesions is insensitive for identifying *S. pyogenes* or *C. diphtheriae* infections.

Isolation of toxigenic *C. diphtheriae* from the throat of a symptomatic patient is definitive evidence of infection. The clinical significance of recovery of *C. haemolyticum* from the throat is still being elucidated. Growth of colonies resembling *N. gonorrhoeae* from throat specimens inoculated to selective media must be carefully identified, because related members of the resident throat flora (such as *Neisseria meningitidis*, *Neisseria lactamica*, *Neisseria cinerea*, and *Kingella* spp.) may be confused with *N. gonorrhoeae*. Detection of confirmed *N. gonorrhoeae* in the throat signifies infection and in the nonsexually active child, is evidence of sexual abuse until proven otherwise. Identification of *H. influenzae*, *S. aureus*, or other pyogenic bacteria in large numbers from epiglottal cultures is indicative of infection in symptomatic patients. Growth of aerobic and/or anaerobic bacteria from properly collected retropharyngeal or peritonsillar aspirates denotes infection. Polymicrobial infections are the rule rather than the exception. Yeasts, especially *C. albicans*, are part of the normal flora and are frequently identified in routine upper respiratory tract cultures. Recovery of large numbers of yeasts from patients with evidence of mucous membrane infection, however, is highly suggestive of infection.

Test: Nasopharynx Culture

Background

Although the pathogenic process is centered in the lower respiratory tract, examination of nasopharyngeal specimens is key to the definitive diagnosis of pertussis and viral or neonatal chlamydia pneumonia. Rapid antigen detection and culture are widely available for both pathogens in hospital or reference laboratories. The nasopharynx is also a site frequently colonized by bacteria of epidemiologic importance. Cultures specifically for *S. aureus*, *N. meningitidis*, and *H. influenzae* can be inoculated to identify asymptomatic carriers of these potential pathogens.

Pertussis (whooping cough) is an infection of the ciliated epithelial cells of the lower respiratory tract. The etiologic agent is *Bordetella pertussis*. Infection is most common in infants and young children; when disease occurs in adults, it follows a much milder course. *Bordetella parapertussis* and *Bordetella bronchiseptica* cause a pertussis-like syndrome that is much milder than pertussis. *Bordetella pertussis* is spread by respiratory droplets to susceptible individuals. There is no distinct seasonality to the infection; however, slightly higher numbers of cases have been observed during the late summer and early fall months. The organism possesses or elaborates several factors that aid in adherence to epithelial cells and evasion of host defense mechanisms. The paroxysmal cough is caused by the host's attempt to expel mucous and secretions from the site of infection. Encephalopathy is the most serious complication of infection and is thought to result from anoxia occurring during paroxysmal coughing.

Chlamydia trachomatis is an important cause of interstitial neonatal pneumonia. Disease follows contact with infected secretions during or soon after birth. Most cases are preceded by inclusion body conjunctivitis, which, if untreated, spreads to the respiratory tract. The most obvious sign of infection is development of a staccato-like cough in an afebrile child.

Laryngotracheobronchitis (croup) characterized by fever, cough, and respiratory distress with respiratory stridor is a serious manifestation of viral infection in young children. The infection is caused by parainfluenza virus types 1 and 2 in about 50% of all cases and less often, influenza viruses, and RSV. Fall epidemics are most frequently caused by parainfluenza, whereas influenza and RSV infections tend to occur more commonly during the winter months.[19]

Selection

Evaluation of nasopharyngeal specimens is appropriate when pertussis or pneumonia caused by respiratory viruses, mycoplasma, or chlamydia is suspected. In young children, this is the preferred specimen for viral culture and for direct examination for virus by immunofluorescence, whereas the throat swab is just as satisfactory for isolating viruses from adult patients with viral rhinitis, pharyngitis, or lower respiratory tract infections. In late stages of viral pneumonia, antigens often can be demonstrated in nasopharyngeal cells by direct immunoflourescence antibody (DFA) testing when the culture is negative.[20] Bacterial cultures are unrewarding in children with croup or laryngotracheobronchitis since nearly all cases are caused by viruses. Although virus can be isolated or detected by DFA in nasopharyngeal specimens from the majority of cases, there is often little value in pursuing an etiologic diagnosis.

Differentiation of pertussis from respiratory syncytial viral bronchiolitis can be difficult when the decision is based solely on clinical findings. Results of microbiologic, hematologic, and radiographic examinations are all important for the diagnosis. Nasopharyngeal swabs should be sent to the microbiology laboratory for DFA detection and culture. Culture is decidedly more sensitive than antigen detection and should always be performed. Neonatal chlamydia interstitial pneumonia is best diagnosed by documenting carriage of *C. trachomatis* in the nasopharynx by DFA and culture. Parallel testing of DFA and culture are equal in sensitivity and specificity for detecting of *C. trachomatis* in nasopharyngeal specimens.

Logistics

Specimen Collection

Nasopharyngeal specimens should be collected using a flexible, wire-shafted swab composed of calcium alginate fibers. The swab is introduced into one of the nares and inserted until the tip reaches the posterior wall of the nasopharynx. After insertion into the nasopharynx, the swab should be left in place for 45–60 seconds. The swab is then gently rotated to mechanically remove ciliated epithelial cells and withdrawn from the nose. Specimen collection using two swabs is encouraged when both direct smear examination and culture are performed.

Culture

B. pertussis is exquisitely sensitive to toxic material found in routine bacteriologic media. Therefore, specimens should be inoculated to selective charcoal blood agar (Regan-Lowe formulation) or freshly prepared (same day) Bordet-Gengou agar, with and without added antimicrobial agents. The charcoal and potato starch in these media, respectively, neutralize the toxic substances found in the base media. Cultures should be incubated at 35°C for 7 days in a humid environment. Colonies comprised of plump gram-negative rods should be confirmed as *B. pertussis* by direct immunofluorescence. *B. parapertussis* and *B. bronchiseptica* also grow well on the above mentioned media.

C. trachomatis is an obligate intracellular parasite dependent upon its host cell for energy in the form of adenosine triphosphate (ATP). Chlamydiae do not grow at all on artificial media and, therefore, cycloheximide treated McCoy cells are used instead. Specimens are inoculated to two sets of McCoy cells growing either on a coverslip inside a vial or on the base of a flat bottomed microtiter tray well by centrifuging the specimen onto the cells. Cultures are incubated aerobically in an atmosphere enriched with 5–10% CO_2 for 48–72 hours, and the first set of cultures examined microscopically for evidence of growth. *C. trachomatis* inclusion bodies are visualized by staining the McCoy cells with iodine, Giemsa, or immunofluorescence reagents. The latter stain is the most sensitive. If the examination is negative, the second set of cultures may be blindly passed to fresh McCoy cells and incubated an additional 48–72 hours.

The only commercially available immunoassay for *B. pertussis* or *C. trachomatis* in the respiratory tract is DFA. Nasopharyngeal smears are prepared on microscope slides, methanol or acetone fixed, and stained with appropriate fluorescent antibody conjugates. To heighten contrast, Evans blue can be used as a counterstain. After thorough rinsing, smears are coverslipped using glycerol based mounting medium, and examined microscopically using ultraviolet light illumination.

Interpretation

A positive DFA result for *B. pertussis*, if reported by experienced laboratory personnel, is reliable evidence of infection. A negative result does not rule out infection, because DFA detects only 60–70% of culture positive specimens. Likewise, negative cultures may be obtained in patients with positive DFA results as the only indication of infection.

A positive DFA for *C. trachomatis* is indicative of infection. The examiner must be careful not to confuse nonspecifically fluorescing bacteria such as protein A containing staphylococci with chlamydial elementary bodies. Elementary bodies are smaller than bacteria, and will display homogenous fluorescence, instead of the peripheral fluorescence characteristic of bacteria. A negative DFA result is as reliable as a negative culture result when testing nasopharyngeal specimens from neonates.

Positive surveillance cultures for *S. aureus*, *N. meningitidis*, and *H. influenzae* establish that the patient is nasopharyngeally colonized with the organism in question.

Test: Eye Cultures

Background[21]

Low numbers of bacteria that may be present in normal conjunctiva without any consequence include organisms normally found on the skin, such as *S. epidermidis* and diphtheroids, and less often bacteria that colonize the upper respiratory tract, such as *M. catarrhalis* or *H. influenzae*. Infection is prevented by the continuous rinsing action of tears as well as their aseptic properties mediated by lysozyme, immunoglobulin, and lymphocytes. These barriers may be penetrated with subsequent infection if defenses break down, are penetrated, or if organisms that come in contact with the eye possess certain pathogenic mechanisms, such as the ability to attach to epithelium via pili, to produce toxins, or to directly invade. Damage also may be done to the eye by the host's own inflammatory reaction to infection.

Conjunctivitis is an inflammation of the membranes between the eyelids and the eye. Pathogens reach the conjunctival membranes directly from the environment, usually via hand-to-eye contact or airborne fomites. Although a large proportion of cases are caused by allergic reactions, infections can be produced by bacteria (nontypable *H. influenzae, S. pneumoniae, S. aureus, M. catarrhalis,* and *N. gonorrhoeae*), as well as viruses, particularly HSV and adenovirus. Less common agents causing conjunctivitis include β-hemolytic streptococci, *C. diphtheria, Moraxella lacunata, Moraxella tuberculosis, Treponema pallidum,* and *Francisella tularensis*.

Adenovirus types 8, 11, 19, and 37 typically cause epidemic keratoconjunctivitis, whereas types 3, 4, and 7 produce a bilateral follicular conjunctivitis in children or may be seen in association with pharyngitis (pharyngoconjunctival fever). Keratoconjunctivitis caused by HSV is sporadic and may be either a primary or recurrent infection. Infections that are allowed to progress untreated can involve the stroma beneath the cornea leading to disciform keratitis, scarring, and ultimately to blindness. Less commonly, varicella-zoster virus in the form of shingles may affect the fifth cranial (ophthalmic) nerve leading to ophthalmic zoster, which can cause permanent damage to the cornea or other parts of the eye. Conjunctivitis is a common complication of exanthematous rashes such as rubella and rubeola. Congenital rubella infection may have severe ocular consequences resulting in cataracts, glaucoma, microphthalmia, and retinopathy, all of which can cause blindness. Coxsackievirus A24 and enterovirus 70 are two notable causes of acute hemorrhagic conjunctivitis that usually occur in epidemics. Symptoms include subconjunctival hemorrhage, keratitis, uveitis, and on rare occasions, neurologic complications. Healing is spontaneous, and there are seldom any long-term effects. Other causes of conjunctivitis that are found almost exclusively in the Third World include dengue, ebola, and marburg viruses.

Neonatal conjunctivitis is a serious infection typically spread by contact with infected cervical secretions during birth and caused by *N. gonorrhoeae* (occurring 3–5 days after birth), *C. trachomatis* (occurring 5–7 days after birth), and less often other bacteria *(S. aureus, S. pyogenes, H. influenzae, P. aeruginosa)*. Adult inclusion conjunctivitis is a sexually transmitted infection caused by secondary spread of *C. trachomatis* serotypes D through K from the urethra. Trachoma is a blinding eye infection occurring primarily in developing countries and is caused by *C. trachomatis* serotypes A through C. Blepharitis is an infection of the margin of the eyelid acquired primarily by hand-to-eye contact and is almost always caused by either *S. aureus* or *S. epidermidis*.

Infections of the cornea (keratitis) may arise from preexisting blepharitis or conjunctivitis, develop after trauma to the eye, or occur at the site of a preexisting defect in the corneal epithelium. Improper disinfection of soft contact lenses also leads to infection. *P. aeruginosa* is the most likely agent followed by *S. aureus, S. pneumoniae, S. epidermidis,* diphtheroids, *N. gonorrhoeae,* and members of the Enterobacteriaceae family. A large variety of other pathogens have been associated with keratitis including *Mycobacterium* spp., and anaerobes. The cornea is the most common site of fungal eye infections. Pathogens tend to be rapidly growing opportunists and include *C. albicans, Aspergillus, Fusarium, Curvularia,* and *Cephalosporium* spp.

Most bacterial or fungal infections of the intraocular chamber (endophthalmitis) are caused by traumatic inoculation of the eye (such as during an accident or ocular surgery), whereas about 25% occur from hematogenous spread during sepsis. Exogenously acquired bacterial and fungal endophthalmitis is most often caused by the same agents involved in keratitis. The more common agents of endogenous bacterial infections are *S. aureus, S. epidermidis, S. pneumoniae, H. influenzae* type b, *N. meningitidis;* less frequent ones are *Bacillus cereus,* anaerobes, *T. pallidum, M. tuberculosis,* and *Nocardia* spp. Endogenous fungal infection may be caused by *C. albicans, A. fumigatus, Cryptococcus neoformans, Blastomyces dermatitidis, Coccidioides immitis*, and *Sporothrix schenckii*. Fungi tend to cause less acute symptoms than bacterial infections but are just as serious. Endophthalmitis is often the first sign of disseminated *C. albicans* or other fungal infections in debilitated patients with long hospital stays and exposure to surgery, broad spectrum antibiotics, or immunosuppressive therapy. Chorioretinitis caused by CMV in immunocompromised individuals or as a congenital disease is a serious and potentially blinding infection. This condition is usually seen following or during the course of a systemic infection. In Africa, chorioretinitis caused by Rift Valley fever virus infection also has been reported. A wide variety of other viral infections may involve the eye (Table 21-5).

The eye also may be infected with certain parasites. External ocular disease is most commonly caused by the free-living amoeba Acanthamoeba or by microfilariae of the nematode *Onchocerca volvulus*. Serious retinal disease may be caused by the coccidian parasite *Toxoplasma gondii*, or by larval dog and cat nematodes of the genus *Toxocara*. *Taenia solium* cysticerci also occasionally localize in the eye and may be found either within or adjacent to ocular structures. The presence of a nematode migrating just underneath the conjunctiva usually suggests the presence of the African eye worm, *Loa loa*.

Ulcerative keratitis caused by various species of Acanthamoeba are becoming more commonplace as popularity of soft and extended wear contact lenses increases. The diagnosis is made by detecting the amoebae in corneal specimens. The disease may actually be under-reported due to the similarity of this infection to keratitis caused by herpesvirus and other pathogens. Acanthamoebae are ubiquitous in the environment and may be present in tap water or contaminate the fingers, and be transferred to the lenses and lens case. Presumably, transmission occurs following minor corneal trauma with inoculation of amoebic cysts or trophozoites into the abrasion. The keratitis tends to be recalcitrant and, despite reports of medical

Table 21-5. Viral Infections of the Eye

Culture Result	Interpretation, Associated Disease
Adenovirus 3, 4, 7 (others less common)	Pharyngoconjunctival fever
Adenovirus 8, 19, 37 (others less common)	Epidemic keratoconjunctivitis
Coxsackievirus A24	Acute hemorrhagic conjunctivitis
Cytomegalovirus	Chorioretinitis in immunosuppressed patient and congenital infection
Enterovirus 70	Acute hemorrhagic conjunctivitis
Herpes simplex virus	Primary or recurrent keratoconjunctivitis
Influenza virus	Conjunctivitis
Molluscum contagiosum	Molluscum (nodules) on eyelids
Parainfluenza type 1	Conjunctivitis
Rubella (German measles)	Conjunctivitis (with exanthem)
Rubella (in congenital rubella syndrome)	Microphthalmia, retinopathy
Rubeola (measles)	Keratitis, conjunctivitis (with exanthem), photophobia
Varicella zoster virus	Ophthalmic zoster (exanthem)
Seldom encountered viral infections of the eye	
Dengue (Tropics)	Conjunctivitis
Ebola (Africa)	Conjunctivitis, hemorrhagic fever
Epstein-Barr virus	Conjunctivitis, keratitis
Marbug (Africa)	Conjunctivitis, hemorrhagic fever
Mumps virus	Dacryoadenitis, optic neuritis, oculomotor palsy, keratitis, uveitis, scleritis, conjunctivitis, retinitis
Newcastle disease virus	Conjunctivitis (associated with working with chickens or their eggs)
Papillomaviruses	Papillomas on eyelid or conjunctiva
Rift valley fever virus (Africa)	Chorioretinitis

cures, often requires corneal transplantation to prevent perforation and subsequent loss of vision. Careful handling of lens cleaning and soaking solutions is necessary to prevent contamination. Thermal disinfection systems have been shown to be more effective in killing the organisms than chemical systems.[22]

Onchocerca volvulus is a filarial nematode transmitted by the bite of black flies of the genus *Simulium*. Adult worms usually remain localized within fibrous tissue capsules in either the dermis or subcutaneous tissues and are called onchocercomas. Unsheathed microfilariae migrate principally through the skin, rather than in the blood, and are responsible for most of the associated pathology including dermatitis and ocular lesions. Immune responses including hypersensitivity reactions to microfilarial antigens appear to be responsible for much of the tissue damage. Clinical disease is best treated by reducing the numbers of microfilariae either with surgical removal of detectable nodules or through drug therapy. Individuals living in areas endemic for *O. volvulus* (principally central and west Africa, and portions of Mexico and Central America) may develop ocular manifestations of onchocerciasis depending on the duration and severity of the infections. Initial symptoms often include photophobia and gradual blurring of vision that may progress to blindness. The presence of microfilariae in the corneal stroma causes sclerosing keratitis, anterior uveitis, and variable iridocyclitis. Retinal involvement and optic atrophy may also occur with heavy infections. Ocular lesions usually occur in conjunction with other manifestations of the disease including onchocercal dermatitis and lymphadenitis.

Ocular infections with *T. gondii* usually occur as part of a primary systemic infection in the neonatal period, often with involvement of the heart, lungs, and central nervous system. Reactivation of eye disease alone may occur years later. While less common, chorioretinitis may occur during acute acquired infection in the immunocompetent host. Such eye infections usually appear unilaterally, whereas in congenital infections the lesions are often bilateral.

Visceral larval migrans caused by the migration of the dog and cat round worms, *Toxocara canis* and *Toxocara cati*, respectively, may involve the eye and appear as a granulomatous reaction within the retina or a diffuse chronic endophthalmitis. This infection is usually seen in small children with a history of pica, and results from the ingestion of Toxocara eggs. The second stage larvae hatch in the upper small bowel and initiate a somatic migration to the liver, heart, lungs, and central nervous system, among others, which may be either symptomatic or asymptomatic. High peripheral eosinophilia is a typical reaction accompanying the infection. When ocular involvement is noted, visceral symptoms are often absent. Such patients tend to be older children (7–8 years of age) in which pica is less common. Fortunately, toxocariasis is usually a self-limited disease, since the available antilarval therapy is not very effective.

Ocular infection with the cysticerci of *T. solium* occurs in 10–15% of patients with cysticercosis. These cestode larvae may occur most anywhere within the eye or in the subchoroidal space, be visibly apparent, or they may present as a tumor.

The subcutaneous migrations of the filarial nematode *L. loa* may be noticed when the worm passes through the conjunctiva. Such migrations may occur anywhere in the body and are usually painless, although angioedema often is noticed and referred to as *Calabar* or *fugitive* swellings.

Selection[23-25]

Conjunctivitis and Blepharitis

Infection of the eyelid is typically accompanied by itching, burning, tearing, and irritation with foreign body sensation. Other symptoms include eyelid edema, hyperemic and red conjunctiva, and purulent exudate. Infection is usually unilateral although autoinoculation frequently leads to bilateral involvement. The usual infections, caused by *S. aureus*, *H. influenzae*, *S. pneumoniae*, and viruses, are mild, self limited, and can be treated empirically without laboratory diagnosis. However, viral keratoconjunctivitis may persist for up to 1 year. Purulent material from the eye should be cultured in sexually active individuals and in neonates suspected of having *N. gonorrhoeae* or *C. trachomatis* conjunctivitis. Gram stain and culture are the most appropriate tests for determining specific causes of bacterial conjunctival and eyelid infections. Diagnosis of *C. trachomatis* infection is made by antigen detection and culture. The use of Giemsa stain to demonstrate basophilic inclusion bodies has poor sensitivity. When vesicular eruptions on the eyelid with follicular conjunctivitis are present together with a pattern of dendritic or "geographic" ulcers on the cornea, the diagnosis of HSV infection can often be made on clinical grounds without laboratory confirmation. Because HSV infection is readily treated with antivirals, it is sensible to confirm the diagnosis by laboratory examination. Viral culture and isolation also are recommended for the immunocompromised patient who may benefit from experimental therapy with antiviral therapy.

Keratitis and Endophthalmitis

Keratitis is associated with pain, and unlike conjunctivitis, there is a decrease in vision, and discharge is typically absent. Because bacterial or fungal keratitis can be a sight imperiling infection causing corneal scarring or perforation, the diagnosis and selection of appropriate therapeutic intervention should be attempted in every case without delay. Clinical suspicion of infective keratitis can be confirmed by laboratory analysis of corneal scrapings. Microscopic examination of Gram stained smears provides a rapid, presumptive diagnosis, and culture offers definitive evidence in bacterial keratitis. Laboratory personnel should be forewarned when corneal scrapings are to be submitted, so that specimens can be processed and examined immediately.

Endophthalmitis is suggested by appropriate history (e.g., trauma), ocular pain, decreased vision, and eye examination. A tentative diagnosis of bacterial or fungal endophthalmitis may be substantiated by laboratory examination of intraocular fluid. Specimens should be conveyed to the laboratory for Gram stain, acid-fast stain (if mycobacterial infection is a possibility), fungal stain, and the corresponding cultures.

Orbital Cellulitis

Isolation of the pathogen in orbital cellulitis is difficult because there is usually no drainage and aspiration is contraindicated. Collection of a specimen from another involved site, such as the sinus, should be considered but is usually not necessary for management. Blood culture is also indicated.

Parasitic Infection[26]

Corneal scraping or biopsy should be performed when Acanthamoeba infection is considered in the differential diagnosis of progressive ulcerative keratitis, especially in users of soft and extended wear contact lenses. The presence of eye pain, a corneal ring infiltrate, and recurrent epithelial breakdown are suggestive of amebic keratitis, and specific tests should be performed to assist in its diagnosis.

Diagnosis of onchocerciasis is usually made by detecting the presence of microfilariae in skin, not in the blood as with other filarial worms.

Serologic testing for toxoplasmosis is indicated in cases of chorioretinitis, the majority of which are the result of congenital infection. Such symptoms are often seen at birth or later and often include involvement of the central nervous system. Reactivation of ocular infections in the second and third decades of life are not uncommon. The lesion often appears as a focal necrotizing retinitis with extension to the choroid. More severe ocular involvement, including panuveitis, may eventually require enucleation.

Peripheral eosinophilia is a typical reaction accompanying visceral larval migrans infection. Because of the similarity of a toxocara retinal granuloma to retinoblastoma, careful differentiation of the two is extremely important. The nematodes responsible for visceral larval migrans rarely mature in humans, obviating the need for stool examinations. Direct visualization of larvae on biopsies also is of little value. Diagnosis rests of the basis of appropriate clinical findings and use of serologic procedures. The latter usually involve the use of excretory-secretory products of larval worms as the antigen in enzyme immunoassays. Such tests are only performed at a few reference laboratories, including the Centers for Disease Control, but are known to be both sensitive and specific.

Diagnosis of cysticercosis may be made from radiographs or computed tomography (CT) scans, which will reveal multiple space occupying lesions or calcifications within the skull or extremities. An individual cysticercus may be present within the eye on occasion and may be visible on routine examination. Serologic tests are available from reference laboratories but may give false negative results or false positive cross-reactions with other cesodes.[27]

Loiasis is often diagnosed on the basis of clinical history including appropriate geographic residence, angioedema, detection of worm migrations, and eosinophilia. Additionally, blood may be examined for the parasite. Sheathed microfilariae may be found in the peripheral blood during the daytime.

Logistics

Specimen Collection

Bacteria and Fungi. Conjunctival specimens should be collected before ocular instillation of preservative containing medications. Specimens are best collected by scraping conjunctival membranes with a flexible-tipped, Kimura platinum spatula, although a swab or purulent discharge is also acceptable. Exudative material should be first removed with a swab, enabling good visualization of the conjunctiva. Scrapings should be smeared upon a glass slide for microscopy or antigen detection and inoculated directly to growth media for culture. Alternatively, ocular discharge may be collected with a cotton, rayon, dacron, or calcium alginate swab and submitted to the laboratory for Gram stain, antigen detection, and culture. Although rarely indicated, a nasopharyngeal or throat swab is the specimen of choice for isolating the etiologic agents of pharyngoconjunctival fever and epidemic keratoconjunctivitis.

Corneal scrapings are the specimens of choice for diagnosis of keratitis. Specimens should be collected by a trained individual (such as an ophthalmologist) with a platinum spatula. Swabs of infected corneal sites usually contain a much lower number of organisms than scrapings.

Intraocular fluid should be obtained by an ophthalmologist via needle aspiration. Fluid from both the anterior chamber and the vitreous cavity should be collected. Specimens should be transferred aseptically to a sterile tube or delivered to the laboratory immediately in a capped syringe. If anaerobic cultures are indicated, a portion of the fluid should be placed in an anaerobic transport vial to guarantee survival of organisms.

Virus. Subsequent to the development of keratitis, diagnosis of infection by viral isolation or direct examination using immunofluorescence can be accomplished using a conjunctival swab or corneal scrapings. Ocular discharge may also be submitted for viral culture.

Analysis

Direct Examination. Conjunctival, eyelid, and corneal specimens should be prepared at the bedside or in the outpatient setting by the individual collecting the specimen. Smears should be Gram stained prior to examination. Methanol fixed smears for fungal pathogens may be stained with a fluorescent stain (such as calcofluor white) or methylene blue. The former stain requires the use of a microscope equipped for ultraviolet light illumination. Giemsa stain is useful for identifying multinucleated giant cells and intranuclear or intracytoplasmic inclusions that may signify CMV or adenovirus.

Both DFA and enzyme immunoassays (EIA) exist for diagnosis of *C. trachomatis* inclusion body conjunctivitis and trachoma. The DFA assay is more rapid than EIA, enables the microscopist to assess the quality of the specimen simultaneously while examining for *C. trachomatis,* but accurate readings depend on experience. The EIA is more sensitive than DFA and is less labor intensive when large batches of specimens are tested.

Bacterial and some fungal pathogens are readily detected by Gram stain of intraocular fluid smears. The sensitivity of the Gram stain can be enhanced by centrifugation of the fluid and examining the sediment. This technique presupposes that there is sufficient fluid to make centrifugation worthwhile and that the fluid is not overly viscous. The Ziehl-Neelsen, Kinyoun carbolfuchsin, and rhodamine-auramine stains are all appropriate for detecting mycobacteria in intraocular fluid. Calcofluor white or methylene blue stain can be used to detect fungi that are not stained well with Gram reagents.

Culture. Conjunctival and eyelid specimens should be inoculated to 5% sheep blood and chocolate agars. A selective medium for *N. gonorrhoeae* is required when gonococcal conjunctivitis is suspected. Culture plates should be incubated at 35°C for 48–72 hours in an aerobic atmosphere enriched with 5–10% CO_2.

Cultures for *C. trachomatis* should be inoculated to cycloheximide treated McCoy cell cultures and incubated in a CO_2 enriched atmosphere for 48–72 hours. McCoy cells are examined for *C. trachomatis* inclusion bodies after staining with iodine, Giemsa, or fluorescent-labeled antibody stains. Negative cultures may be passed to fresh McCoy cells and reincubated for an additional 48–72 hours to increase sensitivity.

Corneal scrapings should be inoculated to culture media by the person collecting the specimen. Media on hand should include 5% sheep blood and chocolate agars and a tube of nonselective, nutrient enriched broth. Agar media should be inoculated directly with the platinum spatula, taking care to touch both sides of the spatula to the agar surface. In the laboratory, bacterial cultures should be incubated at 35°C in an aerobic atmosphere containing 5–10% CO_2 for 48–72 hours. If the enrichment broth becomes turbid, it should be Gram stained and subcultured to agar media. If fungal pathogens are a consideration, Sabouraud dextrose agar should be inoculated and incubated at 25–30°C in an aerobic atmosphere for at least 21 days.

Intraocular fluid for bacterial culture should be incubated to 5% sheep blood and chocolate agar plates.

Additionally, a tube of nonselective nutrient rich broth also should be inoculated. Cultures should be incubated at 35°C in an atmosphere enriched with 5–10% CO_2 for 48–72 hours. Anaerobic culture should also be performed by inoculating the specimen onto nonselective, prereduced blood agar enriched with vitamin K and hemin and prereduced chopped meat glucose broth. The use of media selective for gram-positive anaerobes (such as prereduced CNA agar) or gram-negative anaerobes (such as prereduced laked blood agar with kanamycin and vancomycin) is necessary when there is concern of polymicrobial infection or specimen contamination. Cultures should be incubated at 35°C in an anaerobic atmosphere for 5–7 days. Turbid broth cultures should be Gram stained and subcultured aerobically and anaerobically. When mycobacteria are suspected, intraocular fluid should be inoculated to Lowenstein-Jensen medium, Middlebrook 7H10 or 7H11 agar, and 7H9 or Dubos Tween 80 broth. Cultures should be incubated at 35°C in an aerobic atmosphere containing 5–10% CO_2 for 8–12 weeks. Cloudy broth cultures should be acid-fast stained and subcultured to mycobacterial solid media. Fluid for fungal culture should be inoculated to Sabouraud dextrose and brain heart infusion agars. When dimorphic fungi are suspected, a blood-containing media should be included. Media containing cycloheximide should not be used without including a nonselective fungal media. The growth of many opportunistic fungi capable of causing endophthalmitis are inhibited by cycloheximide. Cultures should be incubated at 25–30°C in an aerobic atmosphere for 21–28 days.

Examination for Parasites.[27] When indicated, corneal scrapings or biopsies should be examined directly for the typical trophozoites or double walled cysts of Acanthamoeba and cultured. Direct examinations may be made with saline wet mounts or with the use of permanent stains including Giemsa or trichrome. Acanthamoeba grow easily on non-nutrient agar plates containing an overlay of *Escherichia coli* and may be more reliably detected with this method than by direct examination. Following inoculation of the center of the plate with tissue, plates are examined daily for up to 1 week under the low power objective (10×) with diminished light. The amoebae rapidly multiply and leave "trails" as they meander through the bacterial lawn.

When onchocerciasis is suspected, small skin "snips" should be taken without blood contamination and incubated in saline on a slide with a coverslip. If present, the microfilariae will escape from the skin after 30 minutes to 1 hour and be visible under a low power objective. When larvae are present, the slide should be allowed to dry and then stained with Giemsa for definitive identification.

Interpretation

Gram stained smears of conjunctival and eyelid specimens that reveal large numbers of inflammatory cells are concrete evidence of infection. A predominance of neutrophils suggest acute bacterial infection, whereas lymphocytes and monocytes are the major cell types in viral and chronic bacterial infections. Intracellular gram-positive diplococci suggest *N. gonorrhoeae* infection. A mixed cellular pattern is typical of *C. trachomatis* conjunctivitis. Observation of small numbers of organisms displaying a variety of Gram stain morphologies likely represent mixed cutaneous flora. Lack of bacteria or presence of small numbers of organism of mixed morphologies suggests viral or chlamydial infection.

Bacterial culture results must be interpreted with care. Many of the organisms that cause conjunctivitis and blepharitis are cutaneous or respiratory tract organisms that may be present in low numbers in specimens from uninfected individuals. Recovery of nontypable *H. influenzae*, *S. pneumoniae*, *S. aureus*, or *M. catarrhalis*, in pure culture or obvious predominance, generally reflects infection. Detection of any amount of *N. gonorrhoeae* or *C. trachomatis* is regarded as documentation of infection.

The presence of any organism in a corneal ulcer is a potential pathogen. Detection of inflammatory cells along with microorganisms by microscopy or isolation of microorganisms in pure culture is evidence of infection. Caution is advised when interpreting the results of cultures yielding growth of multiple organisms. Such results can be caused by either contamination of the specimen/culture or bona fide polymicrobial infection. Because intraocular fluid is a sterile body fluid, observation or growth of any microorganisms is clinically significant until proven otherwise.

The presence of Acanthamoeba in a corneal specimen is diagnostic.

The diagnosis of Toxoplasma chorioretinitis in the newborn is complicated by the similarity of this infection to that of HSV, CMV, and rubella. Toxoplasma chorioretinitis may be suspected on clinical grounds including fundoscopic findings. If serologic titers are positive and retinal lesions are characteristic, the diagnosis may be made with confidence. IgG titers are often low with this syndrome, however, and IgM titers are usually negative. When the test is performed on undiluted serum, the infection may be excluded if serologic tests for IgG antibodies are negative. Further details may be found in Chapters 27 and 29.

A positive serologic test for visceral larva migrans with the appropriate clinical setting is diagnostic.

REFERENCES

1. Chow AW: Infectious syndromes of the head and neck. Infect Dis Clin North Am, 1988; 2:1–277.
2. Rubin J, Yu VL: Malignant external otitis: insights into pathogenesis, clinical manifestations, diagnosis, and therapy. Am J Med 1988; 85:391–398.
3. Doroghazi RM, Nadol JB, Hyslop NE et al: Invasive external otitis: report of 21 cases and review of the literature. Am J Med 1981;71:603–613.
4. Henderson FW, Collier AM, Sanyal MA et al: A longitudinal study of respiratory viruses and bacteria in the etiology of acute otitis media with effusion. N Engl J Med 1982;306:1377–1383.
5. Chonmaitree T, Howie VM, Truant AL: Presence of respiratory viruses in middle ear fluids and nasal wash specimens from children with acute otitis media. Pediatrics 1986;77:698–702.
6. Bluestone CD, Klein JO: Otitis Media in Infants and Children. Philadelphia, WB Saunders, 1988.
7. Altman G, Ostfeld E, Zohar S et al: Rhinoscleroma. Isr J Med Sci 1977;13:62–64.
8. Gwaltney JM Jr, Sydnor A Jr, Sande MA: Etiology and antimicrobial treatment of acute sinusitis. Ann Otol Rhinol Laryngol 1981;90(suppl):68–71.
9. Washburn RG, Kennedy AW, Begley MG et al: Chronic fungal sinusitis in apparently normal hosts. Medicine 1988;67:231–247.
10. McMillan JA, Sandstrom C, Weiner LB et al: Viral and bacterial organisms associated with acute pharyngitis in a school-aged population. J Pediatr 1986;109:747–752.
11. Sendi K, Crysdale WS: Acute epiglottis: Decade of change–a 10 year experience with 242 children. J Otolaryngol 1987;16:196–202.
12. Mustoe The, Strome M: Adult epiglottis. Am J Otolaryngol 1983;4:393–399.
13. Komaroff AL: A management strategy for sore throat. JAMA 1978;239:1429–1432.
14. Ray CG, Minnich LL: Efficiency of immunofluorescence for rapid detection of common respiratory viruses. J Clin Microbiol 1987;25:355–357.
15. Hutt DM, Judson FN: Epidemiology and treatment of oropharyngeal gonorrhea. Ann Intern Med 1986;104:655–698.
16. Kaplan EL, Gastanaduy AS, Huwe BB: The role of the carrier in treatment failures after antibiotic therapy for group A streptococci in the upper respiratory tract. J Lab Clin Med 1981;98:326–355.
17. Peter G, Smith AL: Group A Streptococcal infections of the skin and pharynx. N Engl J Med 1977;297:365–370.
18. Baker AS, Montgomery WW: Oropharyngeal space infections. p. 227–265. In Remington JS, Swarts MN (eds): Current Clinical Topics in Infectious Disease. New York, McGraw-Hill, 1987.
19. Denny FW, Murphy TF, Clyde WA Jr et al: Croup: an 11 year study in a pediatric practice. Pediatrics 1983;71:871–876.
20. Arens MQ, Swierkisz EM, Schmidt RR et al: Strategy for efficient detection of respiratory viruses in pediatric clinical specimens. Diagn Microbiol Infect Dis 1986;5:307–312.
21. Tabbara KF, Hyndiuk RA (eds): Infections of the Eye. Boston, Little Brown, 1986.
22. Ludwig IH, Meisler DM, Rutherford I et al: Susceptibility of Acanthamoeba to soft contact lens disinfection systems. Invest Ophthalmol Vis Sci 1986;27:626–628.
23. Karcioglu ZA (ed): Laboratory Diagnosis in Ophthalmology. New York, Macmillan, 1987.
24. Darell RW: Viral Diseases of the Eye. Philadelphia, Lea & Febiger, 1985.
25. Baker AS, Paton B, Haaf J: Ocular Infection: clinical and laboratory considerations. Clin Microbiol Newsletter 1989;11:97–101.
26. Beaver PC, Jung RC, Cupp EW: Clinical Parasitology. 9th Ed. Philadelphia, Lea & Febiger, 1984.
27. Garcia LS, Bruckner DA: Diagnostic Medical Parasitology. New York, Elsevier, 1988.

22 Lower Respiratory Tract Specimens

Henry D. Isenberg
Thomas R. Fritsche
Gerald Lancz
Steven Specter
Ron B. Schifman
Leonard Rossoff

INTRODUCTION

Pneumonia is the most common cause of infectious mortality in the United States, affecting over 2.5 million individuals per year. Community-acquired pneumonia is frequently treated empirically, often without attempting to make a specific etiologic diagnosis. When the laboratory diagnosis is sought, the principal means is still direct examination and culture of an expectorated sputum. However, for various reasons, fewer than one-half of patients with pneumonia have an accurate microbiologic diagnosis made by sputum examination alone. Sputum may not be obtainable, and organisms retrieved may not be the true pathogens. Antibiotic use is changing the typical microbiota to more unusual or inherently resistant strains. New microbiologic techniques are uncovering new pathogens as well as previously overlooked etiologies of pneumonia. There is also a larger population of immunocompromised patients susceptible to organisms previously not recognized as pathogens. On the other hand, newer albeit more invasive procedures are available to obtain a satisfactory specimen for routine and special diagnostic studies. These factors together with the development of new technologies for laboratory diagnosis highlight the importance of maintaining close communication and cooperation between physicians and the clinical microbiology laboratory.

BASIC TESTS

Test: Culture of Sputum and Other Lower Respiratory Tract Specimens

Background[1,2]

Predisposing Factors for Infection

The lower respiratory tract is protected from the abundant microbial flora of the oropharynx by several mechanisms including mucosal secretions, mucociliary clearance, cough reflex, secretory antibodies, and alveolar macrophages. Any breakdown in these defenses has the potential to cause infection by organisms colonizing the upper respiratory tract (Table 22-1). For example, defective mucociliary function in patients with cystic fibrosis causes susceptibility to pulmonary infections by *Pseudomonas aeruginosa* and *Staphylococcus aureus*. Drugs, alcohol, or neurologic dysfunction may make patients unable to protect airways, especially during bouts of vomiting or instrumentation. The epithelial cell surface is frequently altered in severely ill patients, leading to colonization and subsequent infection by gram-negative bacilli. These selective defects are broadened by the immunosuppressive and chemotherapeutic agents used to treat disease, thereby mark-

Table 22-1. Pathogens Associated With Conditions Altering Host Defenses and Predisposing to Pneumonia

Disorder	Pathogen
Qualitative and quantitative leukocyte disorders Drug induced, hypersplenism, radiation, chronic granulomatous disease, myelocytic leukemia, corticosteroids, acidosis, burns, uremia, viral infection	*Aspergillus* spp., *Candida* spp., Enterobacteriaceae, *Nocardia* spp., *Pseudomonas aeruginosa*, *Staphylococcus aureus*, *Zygomyces* spp.
Altered humoral response Lymphoproliferative disorders, radiation, multiple myeloma, congenital hypogammaglobulinemia, chemotherapy, splenectomy, malnutrition, large tumor burden	*Haemophilus influenzae*, *Pneumocystis carinii*, *Pseudomonas aeruginosa*, *Streptococcus pneumoniae*
Altered cellular immunity Hodgkin's disease, chemotherapy, corticosteroids, large tumor burden, uremia, AIDS, viral infection	Fungi, herpesviruses, *Listeria monocytogenes*, measles, *Mycobacterium* spp., *Nocardia* spp., *Pneumocystis carinii*, *Salmonella* spp., *Strongyloides stercoralis*, *Toxoplasma gondii*
Altered barrier function Decreased ability to protect airway (seizure, coma, alcohol, drugs, oropharyngeal topical anesthetics), regurgitation (esophageal disease, bowel obstruction, nasogastric tube), respiratory instrumentation (endotracheal and tracheostomy tubes, ventilatory humidifiers, bronchoscopy/suctioning)	Anaerobes, *Candida* spp., *Escherichia coli*, *Klebsiella* spp., *Pseudomonas aeruginosa*, *Staphylococcus* spp.

Table 22-2. Diseases Associated With Recurrent Pneumonia

Respiratory	Diffuse airways disease
	    Chronic bronchitis, bronchiectasis, cystic fibrosis, asthma, ciliary dysmotility syndromes
	Focal airways disease
	    Bronchogenic carcinoma, carcinoid, endobronchial metastasis, broncholithiasis, foreign body, extrabronchial compression, tracheobronchial fracture, endotracheal/tracheostomy tube
	Air pump dysfunction
	    Kyphoscoliosis, rib fracture/splinting, neuromuscular disorders, quadriplegia
	Miscellaneous
	    Sequestration, bronchogenic cyst, fibrocystic disease, right middle lobe syndrome

Pulmonary edema	Congestive heart failure
Gastrointestinal	Bulbar dysfunction, motility disorders, reflux/emesis, tracheoesophageal fistula, diverticulum, achalasia
Neurologic	Seizures
Drug	Alcohol, narcotic analgesics, sedatives, tranquilizers

Immunodeficiency	Primary
	    B cell, T cell, complement, phagocytosis
	Secondary
	    AIDS, immunosuppressive drugs and sera, steroids

Miscellaneous	Diabetes mellitus, renal failure, sickle cell disease, multiple antibiotics, multiple organ failure, stress, burns, trauma, ventilator dependence, endotracheal/tracheostomy tubes

edly expanding the spectrum of potential pathogens and severity of infection. Acquired immunodeficiency syndrome (AIDS) clearly is the major representative of this problem today. Pulmonary infections also may be caused by inhalation of small airborne infectious particles that bypass the normal protective mechanisms. This may cause virulent pathogens to be spread person to person (e.g., tuberculosis and influenza), or from the environment (e.g., coccidiomycosis and histoplasmosis). Certain chronic diseases also predispose to frequently recurrent infections (Table 22-2). Finally, pulmonary infection may occur via hematogenous spread from septic emboli as occurs with left sided *S. aureus* endocarditis.

Types of Infection

A large variety of pathogens may infect the lower respiratory tract (Table 22-3), although most infections are caused by only a few. *Streptococcus pneumoniae* and *Mycoplasma pneumoniae* account for the majority of community-acquired pneumonias. By contrast, less frequently encountered pathogens include *Legionella pneumophila, Haemophilus influenzae, Klebsiella pneumoniae*, and even less often encountered are *Moraxella* (formerly, *Branhamella*) *catarrhalis, S. aureus*, and *Neisseria meningitidis*. Community-acquired pneumonia caused by Enterobacteriaceae usually occurs in the elderly and in disease compromised individuals, whereas mixed anaerobic infections develop as a consequence of aspiration. With the exception of influenza, viral pneumonia in immunocompetent adults is infrequent. Viral pneumonia in the immunosuppressed host is often a manifestation of systemic infection with involvement at other sites such as skin, liver, and bone marrow. Preexisting pulmonary disorders, alcoholism, diabetes mellitus, and ethnic background predispose to chronic pneumonias (Table 22-4).

Hospital-acquired bacterial pneumonias account for about 10–20% of all nosocomial infections and are primarily caused by Enterobacteriaceae, *P. aeruginosa, S. aureus*, and *Acinetobacter* spp., and in pediatric patients, respiratory syncytial, influenza, and parainfluenza viruses. Infection in adults is usually the result of occult or obvious aspiration of gastric and oropharyngeal contents into the lung. Predisposing factors include immunosuppression, advanced age, sedation, airway instrumentation, H_2-receptor antagonists, surgery, diabetes mellitus, and underlying illness (Table 22-1). The frequency of pneumonia by inhalation of small droplet aerosols with respirators has declined with the improved sanitation of equipment.

Table 22-3. Bacteria and Fungi Isolated From Lower Respiratory Tract Specimens

Routine Sputum Culture	Special Procedure Required
Isolated With Some Frequency	
Acinetobacter spp.	*Actinomyces* spp.
Moraxella catarrhalis	*Bacteroides* spp.
Candida albicans	*Chlamydia psittaci* (TWAR agent)
Enterobacteriaceae, especially *Klebsiella pneumoniae*	*Fusobacterium* spp.
Haemophilus influenzae	*Legionella pneumophila*
Neisseria meningitidis	*Mycobacterium avium* complex
Pseudomonas aeruginosa	*Mycobacterium tuberculosis*[c]
Staphylococcus epidermidis[b]	*Mycoplasma pneumoniae*
Staphylococcus aureus	
Streptococcus pneumoniae	
Torulopsis glabrata	
Viridans streptococci[b]	
Infrequently Isolated	
Aspergillus spp.	*Arachnia propionica*
Candida spp., not *albicans*	*Bifidobacterium ericksonii*
Corynebacterium spp.[b]	*Blastomyces dermatitidis*[c]
Geotricum candidium	*Coccidioides immitis*[c]
Neisseria spp., not *meningitidis*[b]	*Cryptococcus* spp.
Pseudomonas, not *aeruginosa*	*Francisella tularensis*
Saccharomyces spp.	*Histoplasma capsulatum*[c]
Streptococcus, serogroups A, B, C, and F	*Legionella* spp., not *pneumophila*
	Mycobacterium spp., not *tuberculosis*
	Nocardia spp.
	Penicillium spp.
	Peptococcus spp.
	Trichosporon spp.
	Yersinia pestis
	Zygomyces

[a] Isolation does not reflect clinical significance of most microorganisms. Repeated isolation and/or clinical evidence of specific disease are required to establish the etiologic significance of the isolate.
[b] Rarely a significant pathogen.
[c] Always a significant pathogen.

Compared with other hospital-acquired infections, pneumonias tend to be the least avoidable and most life-threatening. Permanent lung dysfunction is common. Infections occurring in the intensive care unit have a mortality rate of about 30%, which rises to 70% in patients infected with *P. aeruginosa*. Regardless of the setting, the broadest range of infectious etiologies involving the lung is encountered in the immunosuppressed patient, with *Pneumocystis carinii* and cyto-

Table 22-4. Bacteria and Fungi Causing Chronic Pneumonia
Bacteria
Mycobacterium tuberculosis, M. kansasii, M. avium complex
Actinomyces israelii
Nocardia asteroides
Pseudomonas pseudomallei
Anaerobic/polymicrobial aspiration pneumonia
Fungi
Blastomyces dermatitidis
Coccidioides immitis
Cryptococcus neoformans
Histoplasma capsulatum
Paracoccidioides brasiliensis
Sporothrix schenckii

megalovirus (CMV) being two of the most serious and prevalent agents.

Streptococcus agalactiae (group B) is an important cause of pneumonia in newborns, whereas Enterobacteriaceae can infect the lung of neonates with compromised defenses. Pneumonia may present as part of certain congenital infections, including syphilis, CMV, herpes simplex virus (HSV), toxoplasmosis, or rubella. In the first year of life, *Chlamydia trachomatis* is a major cause of pneumonia in vaginally born infants, whereas respiratory syncytial virus (RSV), parainfluenza viruses, influenza viruses, and adenoviruses predominate as lower respiratory tract pathogens, causing bronchiolitis and pneumonia from infancy through 5 years of age.

Chronic pneumonias develop gradually over a period of weeks to months with symptoms of low grade fever, anorexia, weight loss, cough, hemoptysis, dyspnea, and chest pain. These infections may be associated with a wide variety of causes including anaerobic abscess, *Mycobacterium* spp., *Pseudomonas pseudomallei*, *Nocardia*, actinomycosis, coccidiomycosis, and histoplasmosis. The routine sputum culture is rarely beneficial in determining the etiology. Skin testing, serology, and specific microbiologic examination studies should be considered based on the pathogen suspected from the patient's history and clinical findings.

Selection[3]

Frequently, the clinical presentation of the patient and the radiographic findings substantially narrow the field of suspected etiologic pathogens and suggest both how best to acquire and to process a specimen. Routine microscopic and culture examination of sputum as well as blood cultures are generally indicated as the initial diagnostic approach for patients presenting with signs and symptoms of lower respiratory tract infection. Examination for fungi in sputum by direct examination of a KOH preparation and special culture is not indicated as part of the initial examination, unless the patient is immunosuppressed or presents with chronic pneumonia. The decision to use invasive specimen collection techniques and special diagnostic procedures depends on the patient's presentation, suspected pathogens, degree of illness, and sometimes, response or lack of response to empiric therapy. Special procedures that are available include cytology for virus and protozoa, special cultures (e.g., *Legionella*, chlamydia, mycobacteria, virus, and fungi), and direct immunofluorescence studies (e.g., CMV and *Legionella*). Serologic confirmation may be required for the diagnosis of certain pathogens that are not readily isolated by clinical laboratories, such as infections caused by *Mycoplasma* and *Coxiella burnetii* (Q-fever).

Clinical Presentation

Typical Pneumonia. Usually a patient with pneumonia presents with a characteristic group of symptoms that may be classified as either typical or atypical. A typical presentation is acute onset of fever and chills, with temperatures frequently peaking in the evening; a cough of recent onset, producing mucopurulent sputum, is present, and the peripheral blood leukocyte count is increased. There may be hemoptysis, although a massive amount suggests lung abscess, necrotizing pneumonia, bronchiectasis, or neoplasm. Tachypnea, pleuritic pain, or signs of sepsis related to secondary bloodstream infection may be present. There may be evidence of pulmonary consolidation with dullness to percussion, increased tactile and auditory fremitus, egophony, bronchial breath sounds, and crackles.

Table 22-5. Etiologic Agents of Typical and Atypical Pneumonia	
Typical	**Atypical**
Anaerobes	*Chlamydia* spp.
Moraxella catarrhalis	*Legionella* spp.
Haemophilus influenzae	*Mycoplasma pneumoniae*
Klebsiella pneumoniae	*Pneumocystis carinii*
Staphylococcus aureus	*Rickettsia* spp.
Streptococcus pneumoniae	Viruses
Streptococcus pyogenes	

Table 22-6. Incidence of Empyema Associated With Bacterial Pneumonias

Organism	%
Anaerobes	80
Streptococcus pyogenes (group A)	60
Klebsiella pneumoniae	30
Streptococcus agalactiae (group B)	30
Haemophilus influenzae	20
Staphylococcus aureus	15
Streptococcus pneumoniae	1
Neisseria meningiditis	<1

Typical pneumonias (Table 22-5) are frequently bacterial and require sputum culture. Pleuritic pain and/or clinical evidence of pleural effusion usually denotes extension of inflammation to the pleural space. This occurs in about 50% of bacterial (Table 22-6) and 20% of viral pneumonias. Most are sterile and resolve with the underlying pneumonia (parapneumonic effusion) whereas some are actively infected by the pathogen (empyema). The latter may require prompt chest tube drainage before loculation and formation of a thick chronic restrictive pleural peel. Thus prompt thoracentesis is indicated both to secure a reliable etiologic diagnosis and to indicate the need for drainage. It may also allow for the identification of uncommon pathogens such as actinomycetes or *Nocardia* spp. prior to their extension through the chest wall.

Once clinical findings suggest the possibility of pneumonia, the patient's age and where the disease was contracted become relevant. The history should include the patient's residence, travel, occupation, hobbies, animals, and other exposures (Table 22-7). It is also significant to know if the pneumonia was acquired in the community or in the hospital and the immune status of the host. The question of when the pneumonia has occurred is also helpful. An individual with influenza or other viral respiratory infection may begin to improve only to suffer a secondary bacterial superinfection. Pneumococcal infections are frequent in the winter, *Legionella* has peak incidence in the late summer and fall, and *Mycoplasma* in the early summer. Table 22-8 shows the seasonal occurrence of viral infections in temperate climates. Consideration of these factors helps to narrow the diagnostic possibilities and focuses the laboratory examination on specific etiologic agents.

Atypical Pneumonia. A nonproductive cough with minimal findings on examination of the chest is characteristic of an atypical pneumonia. Disease onset is more gradual and there may be a relative bradycardia in febrile patients. Chills and rigors are uncommon. The peripheral blood leukocyte count is normal or, with viral infection, may be depressed. The response to antibiotics may be absent or slow. Atypical pneumonias (Table 22-5) may be associated with mycoplasma, viruses, and other organisms that generally require spe-

Table 22-7. Bacterial and Fungal Pneumonia Associated With Environmental and Geographical Exposure

Pathogen	Exposure
Bacillus anthracis (Anthrax)	Cattle, horses, swine, goats, sheep (wool and hides)
Brucella spp. (Brucellosis)	Cattle, swine, goats, sheep
Coccidioides immitis (Coccidiomycosis)	Travel to southwest United States and northern Mexico
Francisella tularensis (Tularemia)	Rabbits, game animals, ticks, deer flies, mosquitoes; travel to southern states
Histoplasma capsulatum (Histoplasmosis)	Bats, bird droppings, travel to Mississippi and Ohio river valleys
Legionella pneumophila	Contaminated air coolers, water systems, whirlpools
Leptospira interrogans (Leptospirosis)	Rodents, opossums, skunks, raccoons, foxes, dogs, cats, pigs, cattle, horses, contaminated water
Pseudomonas pseudomallei (Melioidosis)	Travel to West Indies, Southeast Asia, Australia, New Guinea, Borneo, South and Central America, Africa, Iran, Turkey
Yersinia pestis (Plague)	Travel to western United States, squirrels, mice, wood rats, prairie dogs, chipmunks, rabbits

Table 22-8. Seasonal Prevalence of Disease Due to Viruses Causing Lower Respiratory Tract Infections (Temperate Climate)

Virus	Season
Adenovirus	None
Influenza virus	Late fall and winter
Parainfluenza 3	Fall to spring
Parainfluenza 1 and 2	Fall
Respiratory syncytial virus	Winter and early spring

cial examination (i.e., viral cultures, specific direct immunofluorescent examination, *Legionella* culture, and cytology). Occasionally extrapulmonary findings aid in the diagnosis of atypical pneumonias (Table 22-9).

Community-acquired atypical pneumonia in the normal host is seldom life-threatening. Therefore, special procedures may not be indicated because a precise diagnosis may be difficult, costly, and delayed. Patients may be treated empirically (with erythromycin) and followed closely. *Mycoplasma pneumoniae*, for example, accounting for 20% or more of community-acquired pneumonias, is usually a self-limiting illness, and results of serology or special culture may be delayed 2–3 weeks — well into the patient's convalescence.

Table 22-9. Extrapulmonary Findings in Pneumonia

Finding	Pathogen
Pharyngitis	Adenovirus, RSV, *Chlamydia psittaci*
Gingivitis	Anaerobes, parainfluenza, *Actinomyces* spp.
Herpes labialis	*Streptococcus pneumoniae*
Furuncles	*Staphylococcus aureus*
Buboes	*Francisella tularensis, Yersinia pestis*
Diarrhea	*Legionella* spp., *Mycoplasma pneumoniae, Mycobacterium avium* Complex
Jaundice	*Coxiella burnetii, Streptococcus pneumoniae*
Mental confusion	*Legionella pneumophila, Mycoplasma pneumoniae*, influenza A and B
Phlebitis	*Blastomycosis dermatitidis, Chlamydia psittaci*
Adenopathy	*Francisella tularensis, Chlamydia psittaci, Mycobacterium* spp.

Viral Disorders. Viral bronchitis is characterized by cough, fever, and rhonchi, often with pain under the sternum. It may be accompanied by pharyngitis or rhinitis, and usually both the trachea and bronchi are affected. Bronchiolitis, generally seen in children under 2 years of age, is characterized by wheezing, grunting, irritability, nasal flaring, retractions, tachypnea, and sometimes dehydration caused by voluntary denial of liquids. The majority of cases are caused by RSV, with parainfluenza type 3 the second leading cause. Other but infrequent causes include adenoviruses, rhinoviruses, influenza, and enteroviruses. A pertussis-like syndrome is associated with infection by adenovirus types 1–3, 5, 12, and 19. In such cases, care must be taken to exclude *Bordetella pertussis* as the cause of infection. The decision to perform diagnostic virology testing in these cases depends on how the information will be used to manage the patient. Results may guide specific therapy either by helping to exclude a bacterial etiology or by demonstrating a treatable viral infection. For example, in a hospital setting, confirmation of RSV infection by viral culture or direct examination of infected tissue is extremely important, since this virus is known to cause epidemic outbreaks in the nursery and the infection is treatable with ribavirin. Likewise, viral cultures for influenza A are indicated for recognizing infectious outbreaks in the community, since this disease can be controlled with amantadine chemotherapy. Awareness of a local epidemic caused by a particular agent, such as *Mycoplasma* or RSV, may allow the diagnosis of similar cases on clinical evidence only.

Radiology

The chest x-ray plays a critical role in test selection and management. Its initial purpose is to confirm or deny the clinical diagnosis. However, the radiograph is nonspecific; a variety of noninfectious disorders may mimic pneumonia including pulmonary vasculitis, neoplasia, thromboembolic disease, and pulmonary edema. These diseases may also manifest with dyspnea, fever, cough, sputum production, hemoptysis, and consolidation. In the intensive care unit, more than one-half of patients mechanically ventilated and meeting criteria for bacterial pneumonia subsequently may prove to have no significant bacterial infection.

Although a specific diagnosis cannot be made from a radiograph, pathogens can be suspected by the pattern of involvement. Two basic patterns are recognized. The first is caused by alveolar or air space infiltration that appears as localized, heterogeneous, fluffy densities with "air bronchograms." This pattern of typical pneumonia is frequently caused by bacteria, and in this setting routine smear and culture examination of a properly collected sputum sample will often provide an etiologic diagnosis. The second basic pattern is that of a diffuse reticular or reticulonodular distribution often referred to as interstitial pneumonia. In this case, the inflammation appears largely confined to the interalveolar septa, and both lungs may be involved. This pattern is commonly seen with the atypical pneumonia of *Pneumocystis, Mycoplasma,* and viruses. In this setting, examination of expectorated sputum is infrequently productive. When an etiologic diagnosis is urgently sought, more invasive specimen collection procedures are usually required. Other radiologic patterns may be seen with lower respiratory infections. Multiple nodular lesions are associated with granulomatous infections (e.g., histoplasmosis and mycobacteria) or septic emboli with multiple abscesses, whereas cavitary lesions suggest either tuberculosis or necrotizing pneumonia caused by *S. aureus,* anaerobes, or *P. aeruginosa.*

In as many as one-fourth of radiographically confirmed pneumonias, there may be little or nothing found on clinical chest examination. In the past, a normal radiograph virtually precluded the pathologic diagnosis of pneumonia, because significantly neutropenic or volume depleted patients only infrequently had initially normal chest x-rays. The incidence of negative chest x-rays with pathologically proven pneumonias has increased substantially in the AIDS population.

Serial radiographs also play an important role in judging the efficacy of therapy and complications of infection and diagnostic interventions (Table 22-10). The computed tomography (CT) scan may allow earlier detection of pneumonic infiltrates particularly of the interstitial atypical type as well as revealing underlying associated predisposing diseases such as bronchiectasis or endobronchial tumors. A number of radiographic techniques (e.g., fluoroscopy, CT scan, and sonography) aid both in the choice of diagnostic intervention and guidance for invasive specimen collections.

Blood Culture

Blood cultures are indicated in all cases of suspected bacterial pneumonia and are virtually without serious contraindications or complications. The isolation of any organism from blood, with the exception of contaminants, such as *Staphylococcus epidermidis* or *Bacillus* spp., implicates it as the pathogen.

Logistics[4,5]

Specimen Requirements

The technique of specimen collection is first determined by the presence or absence of a productive cough. If an adequate sputum specimen is obtained in the presence of a typical pneumonia, it usually is sufficient if a likely organism is retrieved and the patient responds to therapy. If the cough is nonproductive as in a community-acquired atypical pneumonia, the patient may be treated empirically. In the more toxic or immunocompromised host who is rapidly deteriorating, an initial more aggressive approach may be indicated. Table 22-11 lists techniques of specimen collection roughly in order of increasing invasiveness.

Sputum. The least invasive technique is collection of a sputum specimen. Three major approaches for col-

---

Table 22-10. Radiographic Detection of Complications of Pneumonia

Pleural effusion/empyema
Cavitation
Abscess
Pyopneumothorax
Gangrene of lung
Pneumatocele

Table 22-11. Techniques of Specimen Collection for Etiologic Diagnosis of Bacterial Pneumonia

Sputum expectoration
   Spontaneous
   Induced
Nasopharyngeal and throat swab
Blood culture
Thorancentesis
Transtarcheal aspiration
Fiberoptic bronchoscopy
   Bronchoalveolar lavage
   Protected brush
   Transbronchial biopsy
Transthoracic needle aspiration
Open lung biopsy

Table 22-12. Criteria for Grading the Quality of Sputum Specimens by Microscopic Findings

Squamous Epithelial Cells/ 100× Field	Leukocytes/ 1000× Field	Interpretation
>25	—	Improper specimen collection, culture not indicated
>10	<10	Poor specimen, culture results unlikely to be of diagnostic value; consider repeat specimen
<10	<25	Acceptable specimen
<10	>25	High quality specimen; culture results are most likely to have diagnostic significance.

lection exist: spontaneous cough, induced cough, and nasopharyngeal suctioning. Technical problems that can lead to misinterpretation of test results include improper collection, inadequate sputum, and delays in transport to the laboratory. Expectorated sputum is always contaminated with oropharyngeal flora that may overgrow more fastidious pathogens if the specimen is held at the bedside for even a brief period. Sputum induction should be considered for patients unable to produce an adequate specimen and is especially helpful for the identification of *P. carinii* and other infections in the AIDS patient. A history and clinical impression should accompany each specimen to alert laboratory personnel of suspected organisms requiring special procedures that are not included in the routine search (Table 22-3).

A series of three or more first morning specimens are appropriate for fungal and mycobacterial cultures. Occasionally it may be necessary to collect specimens via gastric lavage in infants, children, or adults who are unable to produce adequate expectorated sputum. Because prolonged exposure to the acidity of stomach contents is harmful to mycobacteria, gastric specimens must be buffered if processing is delayed.

Microscopic examination of a gram stained sputum for epithelial cells and leukocytes provides preliminary information about the specimen's quality and etiologic diagnosis (Table 22-12). Specimens containing more than 10 epithelial cells per low power field indicate significant oropharyngeal contamination. These specimens should ordinarily not be subjected to routine bacterial culture, although this degree of oropharyngeal contamination does not affect the sensitivity of recovering *Mycobacterium* spp. Less than 10 epithelial cells per low power field suggest that the majority of the specimen is from the lower respiratory tract, whereas specimens with greater than 25 leukocytes per ×1000 field have the greatest probability of producing diagnostically meaningful culture results. Unfortunately, less than one-fourth of sputum specimens submitted meet these criteria. It must be remembered that on Gram stain eosinophils are indistinguishable from neutrophils and may be misinterpreted as indicators of bacterial infections in asthmatic patients. They can be easily distinguished on a wet mount preparation or Wright stained smear.

Nasopharyngeal and Throat Swab. Lower respiratory tract infections caused by viruses, chlamydia, or mycoplasma may be detected in most instances by using specimens obtained from the upper regions of the respiratory tract (Table 22-13). In cases where this approach is nonproductive and making the diagnosis is important (i.e., in the rapidly deteriorating, immunocompromised patient), collection of lower respiratory tract specimens by more invasive procedures becomes necessary. The specimen type depends on the suspected agent (Table 22-7). *Mycoplasma* may be recov-

Table 22-13. Specimens Appropriate for Isolation of Special Lower Respiratory Tract Pathogens

Organism	Specimen(s)	Examination
Virus	Nasopharyngeal swab or washing, nasal aspirate, throat swab, BAL fluid, lung biopsy	Cell culture or direct immunofluorescence
Chlamydia	Tracheobronchial or lung aspirate, nasopharyngeal swab, lung biopsy	Cell culture or direct immunofluorescence
Mycoplasma	Expectorated sputum, nasopharyngeal swab, tracheal aspirate, lung biopsy	Bacteriologic culture (special medium) or direct immunofluorescence

Abbreviation: BAL, bronchoalveolar lavage.

Table 22-14.	Thoracentesis and Pleural Biopsy	
Indications	Contraindications	Complications
Pleural effusion Malignancy suspected as alternative diagnosis	Uncooperative patient Paroxysmal cough Bleeding disorder Mechanical ventilatory support	Pneumothorax Hemoptysis Empyema Implantation metastasis Air embolism

ered from expectorated sputum samples, but laboratory personnel must be notified because identification requires the use of specialized growth medium or specific immunologic or gene probe techniques.

Most viruses and chlamydia that cause lower respiratory infections can be recovered by nasopharyngeal swab. This is the best method for obtaining ciliated respiratory epithelial cells, the specimen of choice to detect virus both by direct examination with immunofluorescence reagents or by cell culture. Swabs should be cotton or dacron tips on a flexible aluminum shaft. The swab must be inserted deeply into the nasopharynx for approximately 60 seconds, then placed in a sterile container and sent as soon as possible to the laboratory or stored at 4°C for no more than 24 hours. If longer storage is necessary, the specimen should be frozen at −70°C. When both direct examination and culture for virus and chlamydia are desired, two swabs should be collected. A nasal aspirate or wash is an alternative specimen collection method that can be used in place of a swab, especially with young children from whom a nasopharyngeal swab may be difficult to obtain.

A throat swab has less sensitivity for viral studies than a nasopharyngeal swab, particularly if direct examination is to be performed. However, for detecting viruses such as influenza, enteroviruses, HSV, and CMV a throat swab is usually sufficient. A higher rate of isolation can be expected if throat and nasopharyngeal swabs are combined for study. For viral cultures, a throat swab or wash is often as good as a nasopharyngeal swab or wash.

Thoracentesis. Parapneumonic effusion or empyema is common in pneumonias (Table 22-6) and, if present, thoracentesis can provide a useful diagnostic specimen. The efficacy of this technique has been improved by the use of fluoroscopy and more recently ultrasonography. The latter allows the safe acquisition of even very small loculated effusions. The fluid can be examined grossly, stained, and cultured. A simultaneously closed pleural biopsy using one of several techniques may increase the positive yield of a suspected mycobacterial infection to as high as 80%. Rarely, one might proceed to direct inspection of pleural surface with a rigid or flexible thoracoscope allowing pleural and even lung biopsy under direct vision. Some indications, contraindications, and complications of thoracentesis are listed in Table 22-14.

Transtracheal Aspiration[6] Transtracheal aspiration was introduced to bypass the problem of nasopharyngeal contamination of sputum. The technique most widely used today is to insert a plastic catheter-sheathed needle percutaneously through the cricothyroid membrane; the needle is flushed with 2–3 mL of sterile saline that is then retrieved either by syringe or other suction device. Compared with expectorated sputum, the method yields fewer different organisms, and

Table 22-15. Transtracheal Aspiration

Indications
    Nonproductive cough
    Obtunded patient
    Indeterminant expectorated sputum Gram stain
    Anaerobic infection suspected
Contraindications
    Uncooperative patient
    Ineffective cough
    Uncontrolled coughing
    Bleeding disorder
    Hypoxemia
    Arrythmia/myocardiopathy
    Hypotension
    Recent antibiotics
Complications
    Hemoptysis (possibly fatal)
    Hematoma
        Skin, neck, tracheal wall
    Cutaneous or paratracheal infection
    Barotrauma
        Subcutaneous emphysema
        Pneumomediastinum
        Pneumothorax
        Pneumopericardium
    Respiratory distress
    Vasovagal reaction

when properly done, 80% of specimens are sterile or contain a single organism. The technique is also superior if anaerobes are suspected, for example, in patients with aspiration pneumonia. Patient discomfort, reported complications, and availability of bronchoscopy have now made transtracheal aspiration an infrequently used technique (Table 22-15).

Transthoracic Needle Biopsy. This technique, although initially introduced for the diagnosis of neoplastic disease, has been applied to specimen collection in pneumonia because it bypasses the problem of nasopharyngeal contamination. Several technical variations have been described ranging from a trephine to "skinny" needle technique. The needle is inserted percutaneously through the most appropriate intercostal space, guided by fluoroscopy, CT scan, or, when the infiltration is adjacent to the chest wall, ultrasonography. Listed in Table 22-16 are suggested indications, contraindications, and complications of this technique. Although few serious complications are reported and it shows diagnostic efficacy in animal models of focal pneumonia, the method does not yet show wide clinical application. It is less useful when infection is associated with diffuse infiltrations (e.g. *Pneumocystis*).

Bronchoscopy and Bronchial Alveolar Lavage.[7] Specimen collection via the flexible fiberoptic bronchoscope is ordinarily well tolerated and permits selective sampling from involved sites identified radiographically and by direct visualization. Topical anesthesia and some sedation are all that is usually required. This technique may be used to collect a variety of specimens by aspiration, washings, brushings, bronchoalveolar lavage (BAL), and transbronchial forceps biopsy. The biopsy is sensitive for the diagnosis of *Pneumocystis, Mycobacterium, Nocardia,* and fungi, although about one-half show only nonspecific inflammation. Collection of specimens through the bronchoscope by aspiration or BAL has fewer complications than does transtracheal aspiration. Contamination of the specimen by commensal flora as the bronchoscope is passed through the upper airway is a limiting factor, although this may be reduced by using a distal occluding polyethylene glycol plug at the end of the double sheathed, telescoping catheter. Experience with variation of this protected brush have been quite disparate, and it seems most efficacious when there is evidence of diffuse infiltration on the radiograph. Bronchoalveolar lavage performed by wedging the bronchoscope in as distal a segment as possible and washing the subtended lung has proven superior to transtracheal aspiration for the recovery of *Pneumocystis, Legionella,* CMV, HSV, influenza virus, and *Histoplasma*. Bronchoscopy may provide an etiologic diagnosis in more than 50% of cases.

Open Lung Biopsy. The gold standard for the diagnosis of pneumonia remains the open lung biopsy, usually performed under general anesthesia. It is reserved for the very rapidly deteriorating, usually immunocompromised patient or as an alternative to other invasive methods when more effective hemostasis is required. Still, in approximately one-third of patients, no specific etiologic diagnosis is made, and its usefulness in meaningfully extending quality or length of life, particularly in the immunocompromised patient, has been questioned.

Analysis[3]

Microscopic Examination for Bacteria and Fungi. The most diagnostically promising portions of sputum containing blood or pus should be selected for microscopic evaluation. Preprocessing the specimen by washing or with mucolytic agents is not necessary. To assure the adequacy of the specimen, there should be fewer than 10 epithelial cells per low power field and more than 25 leukocytes per low power field (100×). The morphologic appearance and Gram stain reaction of microorganisms are reported. Although yeast can generally be identified with the Gram smear, examination of the sediment of a digested sputum specimen by 10% KOH preparation or calciflor is helpful for recognizing hyphae and other fungal elements in sputum.

Table 22-16. Transthoracic Needle Aspiration

Indications
    Nonproductive cough
    Indeterminate expectorated sputum Gram stain
    Bronchoscopy contraindicated
    Peripheral lung infiltration (bronchoscopy unreliable)
    Malignancy suspected as alternative diagnosis
Contraindications
    Uncooperative patient
    Paroxysmal cough
    Bleeding disorder
    Pulmonary hypertension
    Bullous ling disease
    Severe chronic airflow limitation
    Mechanical ventilatory support
    Vascular lesion suspected
    Echinococcal cyst suspected
Complications
    Pneumothorax
    Hemoptysis
    Empyema
    Implantation metastasis
    Air embolism

Mycobacterium spp. can be demonstrated by various acid-fast staining methods including Ziehl-Nelson, Kinyoun, and fluorochrome. Sputum specimens should first be digested with a mucolytic agent and concentrated by centrifugation (3800g) before staining and reading. Direct acid-fast smear (without concentration) of sputum for identifying *Mycobacterium* spp. is insensitive. When the gram stained smear suggests *Nocardia* spp. (thin, filamentous, branching, beaded gram-positive organisms), a modified acid-fast stain, using 1% sulfuric acid as the decolonizing solution, is appropriate to confirm the diagnosis.

Routine Culture. The routine bacterial culture is generally performed by plating the specimen on sheep blood agar, a medium selective for gram-negative bacilli (eosin, methylene blue, or MacConkey), and supplemented chocolate agar for the isolation of fastidious organisms, such as *H. influenzae*. Cultures are grown in 5–10% CO_2. All gross culture findings should be documented and predominate growth identified. Anaerobic culture is not appropriate for expectorated sputum specimens. When anaerobic infection is suspected (e.g., in lung abscess), specimens must be obtained by one of the more invasive techniques previously described. Routine bacterial cultures generally demonstrate a wide mixture of organisms from the oropharynx, typically including α-hemolytic streptococci and nonpathogenic neisseriae. It is inappropriate to isolate and identify all organisms present on culture. Those that predominate are more likely to be diagnostically significant. If the sputum culture is deemed unreliable, a higher quality specimen collection may be indicated. Transtracheal aspirate, BAL, needle biopsies, and thoracentesis contain a lower diversity of microorganisms. In these cases predominating microorganisms are more likely to indicate the genuine etiologic agent.

Special Procedures. *Nocardia.* The organism grows on routine blood agar media, but may be difficult to detect because colonies are quickly overgrown by contaminating flora that may be suppressed by the use of fungal media. Cultures should be inspected after 3–7 days for small, heaped-up, pearly white, dry colonies. *Nocardia* is more likely to be identified in higher quality respiratory specimens obtained by bronchoscopy. The organism also survives the digestion decontamination procedure used for processing mycobacterial cultures and grows well on mycobacterial media. This procedure should be considered when trying to isolate *Nocardia* spp. from sputum specimens.

Actinomyces. Actinomyces pulmonary infections are notable for producing sulfur granules that may appear in sputum or, with advanced disease, in drainage from chest wall sinuses. On smear, these appear as large clumps of gram-positive, branched filamentous rods with peripheral clubs. This finding, however, is not specific; *Nocardia* and other organisms may produce sulfur granules. *Actinomyces* spp. is difficult to isolate; strict anaerobic conditions during transport, processing, and culture are required to recover the organism.

Mycobacteria.[8] Sputum specimens for *Mycobacterium* spp. culture must first be digested and decontaminated, because the organisms are readily overgrown by commensal flora. The most common method employs *N*-acetyl-L-cysteine and sodium hydroxide. After decontamination, the specimen is buffered and concentrated by centrifugation (3800g). The sediment is inoculated onto egg-based (Lowenstein-Jensen) and agar-based (Middlebrook) media at 35°C in 5–10% CO_2 and inspected at least weekly for a minimum of 8 weeks. This culture procedure also may be supplemented, but not replaced, with a radiometric method (BACTEC) that can detect growth within 1 or 2 weeks. The identification and speciation of *Mycobacterium* spp. is performed by biochemical testing, growth characteristics, and pigment production. Recently introduced molecular probes permit the rapid identification of *Mycobacterium tuberculosis* group and *M. avium* complex in sputum specimens and as culture isolates. Because working with *M. tuberculosis* presents an infectious hazard to laboratory personnel, all processing and culture inspections must be performed with proper precautions, in an approved, negative pressure, biologic safety cabinet.

Legionella.[9] The laboratory identification of legionella infection can be made by culture, direct immunofluorescence staining, or indirect immunofluorescence serology. Isolation requires special media, such as charcoal yeast extract agar, with or without antimicrobial additives. Sputum is generally an inadequate specimen for culture since organisms tend to be scant and are inclined to be overgrown or inhibited by contaminating flora. Direct examination of sputum or other respiratory specimens by immunofluorescence staining may be used for making a rapid diagnosis. Specimens obtained by BAL provide the greatest sensitivity. Although specific antisera reagent reacts with only the common serogroups, false negative results may occur with atypical strains, and infrequently, false positive results occur from cross-reactions with other organisms. Identification of the species from isolated colonies is made by immunologic and biochemical characteristics. Recently introduced molecular probes also may be used for *Legionella* spp. identification, but this method is not applicable for direct specimen examination. A single titer of 256 or more or a fourfold or greater rise in specific serum antibodies 3 weeks after onset of infection provides a presumptive diagnosis.

Fungal Culture. Specimens for fungal culture are inoculated onto a primary fungal medium (e.g., Sabouraud dextrose agar); an enriched medium (e.g., brain heart infusion agar), with and without blood; and medium that contains bacteria-inhibiting antibiotics (e.g., chloramphenicol, gentamicin, or cycloheximide). Media are incubated at 30°C for 4 weeks. Cultures should be held for 12 weeks if *Histoplasma capsulatum* or *Blastomyces dermatitidis* is suspected. Ordinarily, tissue specimens should be ground before being cultured, although zygomycetes are more readily isolated from specimens that are not ground. Because working with fungi has the potential to create infectious hazards to laboratory personnel, all processing and culture inspections should be performed with proper precautions in a biologic safety cabinet.

Pneumocystis carinii. See parasite examination below.

Virus, Chlamydia and Mycoplasma.[10] Detection of viruses and *C. trachomatis* is most reliably done with cell culture (by standard methods or shell vials), with enhanced detection by immunofluorescence or immunoperoxidase (for chlamydia, CMV, HSV, adenovirus, and influenza). Mycoplasma culture requires specialized medium and the organism is difficult to detect. *Chlamydia psittaci* is not routinely cultured, as it has low sensitivity and handling this organism creates a significant infectious hazard. Thus, specimens suspected of containing *C. psittaci* should be processed only by laboratories with appropriate containment facilities. It is possible to detect viruses, chlamydia, or mycoplasma by direct examination, but this approach usually has much less sensitivity than cell culture. Direct examination may be achieved using immunofluorescence or, in the case of mycoplasma, probes specific for its ribonucleic acid for which commercially prepared kits are available. Alternatively, cytologic examination of stained cells from bronchoscopy specimens for viral inclusion bodies (adenovirus and CMV) may provide a presumptive diagnosis.

Serologic analysis of paired acute and convalescent sera may be applied for diagnosis of any of these organism. Evidence of acute infection is suggested when a fourfold or higher rise in antibody titer is detected.

Serologic testing is the method of choice for the diagnosis of *C. psittaci* infection (see Ch. 29).

Interpretation[3]

As discussed earlier, the initial examination of the sputum may provide clues towards interpretation. Color and odor of purulent sputum may even suggest a specific pathogen ("rusty" sputum is associated with *S. pneumoniae,* "currant jelly" sputum with *K. pneumoniae,* "apple green" sputum with *H. influenzae,* and foul-smelling sputum with anaerobic bacterial infections). The Gram stain may presumptively identify gram-positive, lancet-shaped *S. pneumoniae,* or branched, filamentous *Nocardia* (Fig. 22-1), but its usefulness in identifying bacteria in other pneumonias is less reliable. Interpretation of the KOH preparation may also provide a rapid and accurate diagnosis for certain fungal infections involving the lung (Table 22-17).

The organisms listed in Tables 22-3 and 22-18 may all be involved in causing or complicating lower respiratory tract disease. The mere isolation of most of the organisms listed, however, does not confirm their etiologic role. The clinical circumstance, radiographic findings, type of specimen, smear results, and predominance of growth on culture are factors used in analyzing the significance of culture results. Repeat specimens may be warranted to confirm the original findings unless the patient has been placed on antibiotic therapy. A positive blood culture (excluding contaminants such as *S. epidermidis* and diphtheroids) in a patient with acute pneumonia nearly always provides the etiologic diagnosis.

Special Pathogens

Tularemia. Pneumonia is a potential complication of *Francisella tularensis* infection, occurring in about 10% of ulceroglandular and 70% of septicemic tularemia cases. Infection, which is usually sporadic, is acquired following contact with tissues of infected game animals (notably rabbits), the bite of an infected arthropod (ticks, deerflies, and mosquitoes), or ingestion of contaminated food or water. Primary pleuropulmonary infections may occur in laboratory workers exposed to infectious aerosols. Infection is characterized by abrupt onset of fever, nonproductive cough, and pleural effusion. A characteristic ulcerated skin lesion, painful lymphadenopathy, and exposure history are key clinical findings. It is uncommon to see the organism on sputum Gram stained smear. Isolation requires special media and is hazardous to laboratory

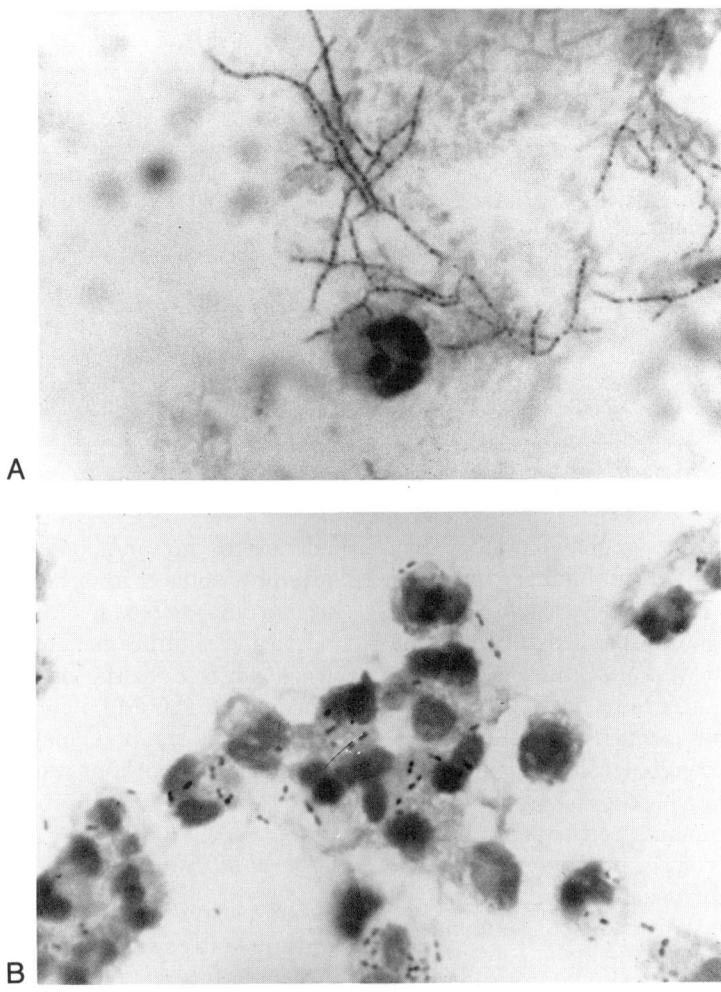

Fig. 22-1. Sputum. **(A)** *Streptococcus pneumoniae*. **(B)** *Norcardia* spp.

personnel. The laboratory diagnosis is best made by serologic testing or by identification of the organism in tissues or exudates by immunofluorescent staining.

Yersinia pestis. Pneumonic plague is rare in the United States, usually occurring as a secondary infection in bubonic disease. Infections are associated with a productive, purulent, bloody sputum, generally containing abundant organisms on smear. The bacterium has a distinctive bipolar (safety-pin) staining appearance. Although *Y. pestis* grows on ordinary blood containing media, colonies are not visible for 2 or 3 days. It is essential to notify the laboratory when this diagnosis is suspected, as specimens and cultures containing *Y. pestis* are hazardous and must be handled with extreme care.

Fungi. *Candida albicans* and other *Candida* spp. may be isolated from lower respiratory tract specimens in as many as one-half of all specimens submitted. These are generally part of the normal upper respiratory tract flora. The diagnosis of genuine infection requires proof by examination of biopsy material. *Geotrichum candidum* rarely causes disease. The organism is occasionally recovered from patients with bronchiectasis, cystic, or cavitary lung disease. Repeated isolation, especially in patients having tuberculosis, chronic cough, gelatinous sputum, or symptoms of allergic bronchopulmonary aspergillosis may be significant. Invasive diagnostic procedures are necessary to confirm the etiologic diagnosis. *Cryptococcus neoformans* is rarely detected in sputum and usually only in the immunocompromised host. Antigen detection in urine, serum, and other sites (e.g., blood and cerebrospinal fluid) is a necessary adjunct to interpreting culture results.

Aspergillus spp. may cause serious disease in compromised patients. Repeated isolations and microscopic examination of lower respiratory tract secretions re-

Table 22-17. Laboratory Features Associated With Pleural Effusions in Pneumonia

Cell Count (/μL)	Primary Cell Type	Glucose (gm/dL)	Interpretation
<3000	Mononuclear	Normal	Sterile effusion or viral infection
<5000	Mononuclear and neutrophils	Normal	Mycoplasma or viral infection
5000–10,000	Neutrophils	Normal	Legionella
5000–10,000	Lymphocytes and decreased mesothelial cells	Decreased	*Mycobacterium tuberculosis*
>10,000	Neutrophils	Decreased	*Staphylococcus aureus*, *Streptococcus* spp., *Haemophilus influenzae*, Enterobacteriaceae, anaerobes

vealing hyphae are important for the laboratory diagnosis. Three types of aspergillus pulmonary infections may occur: allergic, colonizing, and invasive. The allergic condition signifies exposure to heavy contamination with conidia. "Malt-worker's lung" is found in brewery workers handling moldy barley, grain mill workers, silo workers, and farmers susceptible to the allergic form of the disorder. The colonizing condition is recognized when aspirated spores of *Aspergillus* germinate in pre-existing pulmonary cavities produced by other diseases like tuberculosis, emphysema, and sarcoidosis. Invasive infection usually occurs in immunocompromised patients. *Aspergillus* spp. are ubiquitous making the diagnosis of disease involvement difficult. Repeated isolations are imperative and biopsy specimens are more convincing. Invasive *Aspergillus* infection of the lung occurs almost exclusively in the compromised host.

Penicillium spp. require biopsy confirmation before a causal relationship between isolation from sputum and disease can be established. The zygomycete genera, *Mucor*, *Rhizopus*, *Absidia*, and *Cunninghamella*, may cause opportunistic infections in patients with altered host defenses (Table 22-1). Zygomycetes are rarely encountered as contaminants of the upper respiratory tract, and their isolation in the compromised host should be considered significant. Cultures of a lung biopsy, however, are often negative even when zygomycetes are prevalent on histologic examination.

Virus and Chlamydia. In the presence of signs and symptoms of lower respiratory tract infection, the demonstration of influenza, parainfluenza, or respiratory syncytial virus by direct immunofluorescence or culture is always significant. However, the presence of adenovirus may not be significant, as this virus can often be isolated from healthy individuals. In the immunocompromised host, isolation of any virus is diagnostically significant. The significance of isolating *C. trachomatis* from the nasopharynx of an infant with pneumonia should be confirmed by serologic testing, because this organism may be shed from the upper respiratory tract without causing infection.

Pleural Effusion[11,12]

Examination of parapneumonic effusions helps differentiate between infected exudates (empyema), sterile, inflammatory exudates, and transudates (noninflammatory fluid accumulation) (Table 22-19). Exudates generally have a pleural fluid to serum ratio of greater than 0.5 for protein and greater than 0.6 for lactate dehydrogenase (LD). Sterile effusions and those associated with *Legionella* spp., viral, and mycoplasma infections are characterized by glucose concentrations greater than 60 mg/dL (>60 mmol/L) and total white blood cell (WBC) counts less than 10,000/μL. Exudates caused by other bacteria, including anaerobes, generally have pH values below 7.2, contain elevated LD (more than 200 U/L), and low glucose concentrations as well as high leukocyte counts (more than 10,000/μL) with neutrophils predominating. Conversely, transudates have few WBCs, normal glucose and LD levels, and low specific gravity (less than 1.016). Infected parapneumonic effusions with pH values below 7.2 and glucose below 40 mg/dL (<2.2 mmol/L), generally require chest tube drainage, whereas others are successfully treated with antibiotics alone. Lymphocytes predominate in exudates associated with *M. tuberculosis* infections and the pleural fluid is noteworthy for containing high protein concentrations and few or absent mesothelial cells.

Table 22-18. Testing and Interpretation of Respiratory Specimen Isolates

Result	Preferred Procedure	Interpretation and Associated Findings
Acinetobacter spp.	c	Contaminant, nosocomial pneumonia
Actinomyces israelii and other species	C	Commensal of oropharynx, chronic pneumonia, "sulfur granules"
Adenovirus	C, D, S	Commensal of oropharynx, bronchiolitis, pertussis-like syndrome, atypical pneumonia
Aspergillus spp.	c, C, D, S	Contaminant, allergic bronchopulmonary disease (associated with eosinophilia), colonizing aspergilloma in cavitated lung, invasive necrotizing pneumonia in immunocompromised host
Bacillus anthracis	c	Anthrax with acute hemorrhagic pneumonitis associated with wool contact and high mortality (exceedingly rare infection)
Bacillus spp.	c	Contaminant
Bacteroides spp.	C	Commensal of oropharynx aspiration pneumonia (polymicrobic), subacute necrotizing pneumonia, periodontal disease, lung abscess, empyema, septic pulmonary emboli
Blastomyces dermatitidis	C, D, S	Blastomycosis, with potential for skin, bone, prostate, and epididymis involvement
Moraxella catarrhalis	c	Commensal of oropharynx, community-acquired pneumonia (may be mixed with *Haemophilus influenzae* or *Streptococcus pneumoniae*), often associated with preexisting pulmonary disease
Bordetella pertussis	C, D	Whooping cough, lymphocytosis
Candida albicans, other *Candida* spp.	c, C, d, D	Commensal of oropharynx (isolation from sputum generally not significant), pneumonia, invasive disease, or hematogenous infection in immunocompromised host
Chlamydia pneumoniae	C, S	Atypical pneumonia in young adults
Chlamydia psittaci	S	Acute, atypical pneumonia after avian exposure
Chlamydia trachomatis	C, S	Colonization, interstitial pneumonia in vaginally delivered infant or immunocompromised host
Coccidioides immitis	C, D, S	Chronic pneumonia (usually self-limited) with potential to involve bone, skin, and CNS
Coxiella burnetii (Q-fever)	S	Acute pneumonia with headache and hepatitis, zoonosis involving domestic animals (cattle, sheep, and goats)
Cryptococcus neoformans	C	Saprophyte, asymptomatic pulmonary infection (yeast is rarely recovered from sputum), meningitis, disseminated infection
Cytomegalovirus	C, D, S	Infection in immunocompromised host, asymptomatic shedding, pneumonia in neonate and immunocompromised host, may coinfect with *Pneumocystis carinii*
Enterobacteriaceae	c	Colonization in hospitalized patient, tracheobronchitis, nosocomial infection, community-acquired pneumonia with *Klebsiella pneumoniae* in alcoholic or diabetic
Fusobacterium nucleatum	C	Commensal of oropharynx, aspiration pneumonia (polymicrobic), subacute necrotizing pneumonia, periodontal disease, lung abscess, empyema septic pulmonary emboli
Francisella tularensis	D, S	Secondary infection in ulceroglandular or typhoidal tularemia, primary pneumonia in exposed laboratory workers
Geotricum candidum	c, C, D	Commensal flora (isolation from sputum generally not significant), pneumonia, invasive disease, or hematogenous infection in immunocompromised host

(Continued)

Table 22-18. Testing and Interpretation of Respiratory Specimen Isolates (Continued)

Result	Preferred Procedure	Interpretation and Associated Findings
Haemophilus influenzae	c, d	Commensal of oropharynx, community-acquired pneumonia
Herpes simplex	C, D	Pneumonia in neonate and immunocompromised host
Histoplasma capsulatum	C, S	Pneumonia (usually self-limited) with potential to involve bone marrow, CNS, GI tract, nose and throat
Influenza virus A and B	C, D, S	Community acquired bronchitis, bronchiolitis, pneumonia; associated with pharyngitis, secondary bacterial pneumonia, Reye's syndrome (influenza B)
Legionella spp.	C, D, S	Community or nosocomial pneumonia associated with contaminated water systems
Mycobacterium kansasii, M. avium complex, *M. fortuitum*	C, D	Chronic pneumonia (usually self-limited) associated with preexisting pulmonary disease, potential for dissemination (*M. avium* complex) in immunocompromised host (AIDS)
Mycobacterium tuberculosis	C, D	Pulmonary tuberculosis
Mycoplasma pneumoniae	C, S	Common cause of community-acquired atypical pneumonia, myringitis
Neisseria meningitidis	c	Commensal of oropharynx, community-acquired pneumonia
Neisseria sicca, N. flavescens, N. mucosa, and *N. subflava*	c	Commensal of oropharynx
Nocardia spp.	C, d, D	Commensal of oropharynx, chronic pneumonia, usually occurring in immunocompromised host, associated with brain abscess
Parainfluenza viruses especially type 3	C, D, S	Bronchitis, bronchiolitis, mild pneumonia occurring primarily in children
Peptostreptococcus magnus and other species	C	Commensal of oropharynx, aspiration pneumonia (polymicrobic), subacute necrotizing pneumonia associated with periodontal disease, lung abscess, empyema, septic pulmonary emboli
Penicillium spp.	C	Contaminant
Pseudomonas aeruginosa (also *P. fluorescens, P. cepacia, P. alcaligenes,* and *P. stuzeri*)	c	Colonization in hospitalized patient, tracheobronchitis, nosocomial pneumonia, cystic fibrosis (*P. aeruginosa*)
Pseudomonas mallei	c, S	Glanders, contact with infected horses, pneumonia, pulmonary or cutaneous abscess
Pseudomonas pseudomallei	c, S	Melioidosis, bronchitis, necrotizing pneumonia, endemic to Southeast Asia
Respiratory syncytial virus	C, D	Bronchitis, bronchiolitis, pneumonia occurring primarily in children
Rubeola (measles)	S	Pneumonia in children associated with rash and conjunctivitis, atypical measles, interstitial pneumonia in immunocompromised host
Staphylococcus aureus	c	Nosocomial infection, secondary superinfection, cystic fibrosis, septic pulmonary emboli, infections associated with pneumothorax, lung abscess, and high mortality
Staphylococcus epidermidis	c	Commensal of oropharynx
Streptococcus agalactiae (group B)	c	Neonatal pneumonia associated with sepsis and respiratory distress syndrome, adult pneumonia

(Continued)

Table 22-18. Testing and Interpretation of Respiratory Specimen Isolates (Continued)

Result	Preferred Procedure	Interpretation and Associated Findings
Streptococcus pneumoniae	c	Commensal of oropharynx, common cause of community-acquired pneumonia
Streptococcus pyogenes (group A)	c	Interstitial or lobar pneumonia usually occurring in children associated with pharyngitis and empyema, secondary superinfection in adults
Varicella-Zoster	C, D, S	Pneumonia associated with rash and disseminated infection in immunocompromised host
Yersinia pestis	c, d, D, S	Secondary pneumonia in bubonic plague, primary pneumonia in exposed laboratory workers
Zygomycetes (*Rhizopus, Absidia, Cunninghamella* and *Mucor*)	c, C, D	Invasive necrotizing pneumonia in immunocompromised host and diabetic

Abbreviations: c, routine culture; C, special culture; d, routine direct examination; D, special direct examination (i.e., special stains, immunofluorescence, etc.), S, serology; CNS, central nervous system; GI, gastrointestinal.

TEST GROUP: SOLUBLE ANTIGENS

Antigens of pneumococcus and *H. influenzae* may be detected in the urine, pleural fluid, and blood of some patients with pneumonia caused by these pathogens. However, the tests are not very sensitive and are rarely indicated for the laboratory diagnosis. Antigen testing may be considered when the etiologic diagnosis is suspected but cannot be confirmed because of prior antimicrobial therapy. Detection of antigen directly in sputum is not appropriate, because the test cannot differentiate infection from colonization. Methods for detecting some *Legionella pneumophila* serogroup antigens and *H. capsulatum* antigen in urine have been developed, but their sensitivity for localized pulmonary infections and clinical application is under study.

Test: Direct Examination of Respiratory Specimens for Parasites[13,14]

Background

In addition to the usual respiratory tract pathogens, the lungs also may be infected with a variety of protozoa and helminths, which may occur either as a primary

Table 22-19. Morphologic Characteristics of Pathogens That May be Identified by Microscopic Examination of KOH Wet Mounted Sputum Sample

Pathogen	Morphologic Features
Actinomyces spp.	Thin branching filiments, often radiating out of central cluster (modified acid-fast negative)
Aspergillus spp.	Small, septated hyphae with bifurcated branching at 45 degree angles
Blastomyces dermatitidis	Medium to large thick, doubled wall yeast with broad-based single bud
Candida spp.	Round to oblong yeast with multiple buds (blastospores) and elongated buds joined by constricted attachment (pseudohyphae)
Coccidioides immitis	Large irregularly round, thick-walled spherules, which may be empty or contain tiny round endospores
Cryptococcus neoformans	Variably sized yeast with one or more buds; thick capsule may be seen; difficult to distinguish from other yeasts and rarely found in sufficient quantity for identification
Nocardia spp.	Thin branching filiments, often radiating out of central cluster (modified acid-fast positive)
Zygomyces spp.	Irregular branching hyphae without septa

Table 22-20. Parasitic Agents That May Cause Primary Pulmonary Disease, or May Infect the Lungs Secondarily as Part of Another Process

Parasite	Primary or Secondary Disease[a]
Protozoa	
Pneumocystis carinii	1°
Toxoplasma gondii	1° or 2°
Cryptosporidium spp.	2°
Entamoeba histolytica	2°
Helminths	
Nematodes	
Strongyloides stercoralis	2°
Ascaris lumbricoides	2°
Ancylostoma duodenalis	2°
Necator americanus	2°
Cestodes	
Taenia solium (cysticercosis)	1° or 2°
Echinococcus granulosus (hydatid disease)	1° or 2°
Trematode	
Paragonimus westermani	1°

[a] 1°, primary; 2°, secondary.

infection, transiently as part of a migratory phase, or as part of a systemic infection. Of the parasites that may localize in the lungs, protozoa usually produce the more fulminant disease because of their abilities to multiply within host tissues, unlike helminths, which, with the exception of *Strongyloides stercoralis*, are unable to do so.

Parasitic infections of the lower respiratory tract are usually diagnosed through the examination of sputum, BAL or tissue specimens. If lung involvement is part of a systemic infection, diagnosis may be made with other, more appropriate, specimens. The spectrum of parasitic diseases of the lungs may include those listed in Table 22-20.

Selection

The possibility of parasitic infections of the lungs should be considered in symptomatic individuals who (1) are immunosuppressed by reason of retroviral infection, malignancy, chemotherapy, or congenital immunodeficiency; or (2) have an appropriate history of travel or residency in areas of the world known to be endemic for parasitic diseases.

Immunosuppressed individuals are at particular risk for developing *P. carinii* pneumonia, but are also susceptible to *Toxoplasma gondii* pneumonitis and occasionally, pulmonary cryptosporidiosis. Pulmonary toxoplasmosis usually presents as part of a systemic infection and may accompany encephalitis or myocarditis. Cryptosporidiosis usually infects the small intestine, but has been reported from the lungs on several occasions. If an individual becomes immunosuppressed while carrying a latent *Strongyloides* infection, severe pulmonary disease may occur caused by dissemination of large numbers of larvae throughout the body. The remaining parasitic disease that may affect the lungs as either primary or secondary infections in otherwise immunocompetent hosts are acquired while traveling to endemic areas and being exposed to the various agents.

Logistics

Sputum

Examination of sputum is specifically recommended when the infections being considered include the lung fluke *Paragonimus*. Because of the presence of a transient migratory phase in the life cycle of some nematodes, including *Strongyloides* and *Ascaris,* and hookworms, sputum also may be examined for the presence of motile larvae. Stool examinations also should be performed when these infections are considered.

A first morning, deep sputum may offer the best material, which may be examined directly or after centrifugation or other traditional concentration techniques. Viscous specimens may be pretreated with sodium hydroxide. Preservation with formalin or polyvinyl alcohol fixative (for permanent stains) also may be performed. The latter may be useful for identifying the presence of *Entamoeba histolytica* from a pulmonary amebic abscess, if this possibility is being considered. Identification of the typical helminth eggs or larvae is made as for stool specimens.

Although examination of sputum or bronchial washings is not recommended for the diagnosis of *P. carinii* because of poor sensitivity, examination of a sputum specimen induced through the inhalation of nebulized saline offers increased yield when properly performed.[15] Performance of this technique may obviate the need to perform BAL or other more invasive procedures.

Bronchoalveolar Lavage

Bronchoalveolar lavage has been shown to be of particular value, especially in AIDS patients for the diagnosis of *P. carinii* pneumonia. This procedure compares well with transbronchial biopsy, although highest sensitivity is achieved when both are used. A variety of staining techniques are currently in use and include those staining the cyst wall (most silver stains, modified toluidine-blue, and Gram-Weigert), and those staining the trophozoites (primarily Giemsa and Wright stains). Papanicolaou stained smears are also useful, because of the characteristic cellular response present in *P. carinii*. More recently, immunofluorescence reagents have become commercially available and appear to offer the greatest specificity and sensitivity.

Tissue Specimens

Lung tissues acquired during thoracotomy or through transbronchial biopsy offer an excellent opportunity to examine the parasites listed in Table 22-20. Although routine hematoxylin and eosin stains are adequate for identifying most of these organisms, several exceptions are notable: silver stains are required to identify cysts of *Pneumocystis* and acid-fast stains are useful for recognizing the presence of *Cryptosporidium*. When transbronchial biopsies are taken, effort should be made to obtain multiple specimens to ensure adequate sampling.

Interpretation

Protozoa

Pneumocystis carinii was originally associated with interstitial plasma cell pneumonia in premature or chronically ill infants. Although this still occurs, it is now the most commonly recognized, recurring opportunistic pulmonary infection associated with AIDS. Long thought to be a protozoan, *Pneumocystis* recently has been shown to have stronger affinities to the fungi. The organism multiplies extracellularly in alveolar spaces by alternating between cystic and trophozoite forms. Both stages are usually present, but separate stains as described above are usually required to demonstrate each. Although dissemination from the lungs to a variety of other tissues has been reported, the mainstay of diagnosis relies on examination of pulmonary specimens. Seroepidemiologic surveys suggest that most individuals are exposed to the organism at a young age. Serologic tests have not proven to be of significant diagnostic help, because of the widespread occurrence of such antibodies.

Exclusive involvement of the lung by toxoplasmosis is atypical. Infections may be systemic with lymphadenopathy as a presenting sign, or more organ-specific with retinochoroiditis, encephalitis, myocarditis, or atypical pneumonia occurring. Its most severe form occurs as disseminated infection in neonates or the immunocompromised patient. Further discussion of this syndrome is found in the section on central nervous system disorders in Chapter 27.

Pulmonary infections with *Cryptosporidium* have been reported, but are rare events.[16] In most cases, the individuals have AIDS and suffer from intestinal cryptosporidiosis, concomitantly. Respiratory specimens, when examined with acid-fast stains, have revealed the typical oocytes, both from sputum and biopsies. The organisms appear to multiply on bronchial epithelium in the same fashion as in the intestine. Further discussion on cryptosporidiosis is found in the section on stool parasites.

Amebic abscesses of the lung occur occasionally and may result from direct extension of a liver abscess into the pleural space (pleuropulmonary infection) or via hematogenous spread from a primary intestinal source (pulmonary abscess.) The former event is thought to be more common and usually arises as an extension of an abscess in the upper level of the right lobe of the liver.[12] If a pulmonary abscess ruptures into a bronchus, contents may be expectorated and trophozoites of *E. histolytica* are subsequently seen in the sputum. Diagnosis of pulmonary amebiasis may be difficult, especially when the abscess is of hematogenous origin and when the often associated hepatic involvement is absent. Serologic tests are of value, especially in extraintestinal involvement and should be attempted in suspected cases. Further information about amebiasis is found in the stool and abdomen sections in Chapter 26.

Helminths

The presence of helminths in pulmonary tissues may result from the transient migration of nematode larvae, the permanent localization of larval cestodes (cysticerci and hydatid), or the permanent localization of adult trematodes *(Paragonimus)*.

All of the nematodes listed in Table 22-20 reside primarily within the gastrointestinal tract as adult worms. The pulmonary phase for each is generally of short duration and rarely associated with clinically significant disease. Heavy exposure over a short time period may, however, result in pneumonitis caused by tissue damage and sensitization. A specific condition produced by *Ascaris lumbricoides* infection that causes transient pulmonary infiltrates and peripheral eosinophilia is known as Löffler's syndrome. Hookworms typically do not cause as much tissue reaction in the lungs as does *Ascaris*. Pulmonary *Strongyloides* infections may mimic that of *Ascaris,* but may be more life-threatening, especially when hyperinfection occurs as a result of autoinfection. In such cases, larvae may be plentiful in sputum. Further details of the clinical significance of these nematodes is found in the stool section in Chapter 26.

Larvae of tapeworms that can localize in the lungs include those of *Taenia solium* (cysticercosis) and *Echinococcus granulosus* (hydatidosis). The presence of either cysticerci or hydatids in the lungs occurs as a result of the hematogenous spread of eggs following their ingestion, and other tissues and organs are likely to be infected concurrently. Although 60% of hydatids develop in the liver, approximately 20% are found in the lungs. Symptoms are usually related to the mechanical damage caused by the slowly enlarging cysts, but sensitization to cyst fluid may produce serious allergic reactions. When located in operable body sites, hydatids may be removed surgically; surgical removal of cysticerci is sometimes impaired by the smaller size and larger number of cysts. Severe inflammatory reactions may occur at the site of the dead cysts and appropriate medical care should be available to manage such reactions. Further information is present in Chapter 26.

Lung fluke infection, caused by the trematode *Paragonimus westermani* and related species, is found in many parts of Asia, Africa and South America, and occasionally cases have been described in North America. Transmission occurs when freshwater crayfish or crabs are eaten uncooked. The larval worms migrate from the intestine to the lungs where maturation and egg laying occur. The adult worms, often found paired in cysts, may cause significant tissue damage and inflammation from the accumulation of necrotic debris, metabolic wastes, and eggs. The cysts eventually rupture into bronchioles, releasing eggs into the respiratory tract. Eggs may then be recovered either from the sputum or stool. At onset, most infections are insidious but symptoms usually progress to include cough with blood-tinged sputum, chest pain, chronic bronchitis, and dyspnea. The larvae occasionally locate in a variety of ectopic sites, of which cerebral involvement is the most serious. Immunodiagnostic tests are available and may help confirm a clinical suspicion.[3]

REFERENCES

1. Reimann H: The Pneumonias. Philadelphia, WB Saunders, 1988.
2. Reynolds HY: Host defense inpairments that may lead to repiratory infections. Clin Chest Med 1987;8:339–358.
3. Winn WC: Symposium on respiratory infections. Clin Lab Med 1982;2:259–268.
4. Sodeman TM, Colmer J: Microbiology of the respiratory tract. Lab Med 1983; 14:96–101.
5. Tobin MJ: Diagnosis of pneumonia: techniques and problems. Clin Chest Med 1987;8:513–527.
6. de Viro F, Pond GD, Rhenman B et al: Transtracheal aspiration and fine needle aspiration biopsy for the diagnosis of pulmonary infection in heart transplant patients. J Thorac Cardiovasc Surg 1988;96:669–679.
7. Martin WJ, Smith TF, Sanderson DR et al: Role of bronchoalveolar lavage in the assessment of opportunistic pulmonary infections: utility and complications. Mayo Clin Proc 1987; 62:549–557.
8. Kim TC, Blackman RS, Heatwole KM et al.: Acid-fast bacilli in sputum smears of patients with pulmonary tuberculosis: prevalence and significance of negative smears pretreatment and positive smears post-treatment. Am Rev Respir Dis 1984; 129:264–268.
9. Winn WC: Legionnaires Disease: historical perspective. Clin Microbiol Rev 1988; 1:60–81.
10. Avila MM, Carballal G, Rovaletti H et al: Viral etiology in acute lower respiratory infections in children from a closed community. Am Rev Respir Dis 1989;140:634–637.
11. Varkey B: Pleural effusions caused by infection. Postgrad Med 1986; 80:213–223.
12. Houston MC: Pleural fluid pH. Diagnostic, therapeutic and prognostic value. Am J Surg 1987; 154:333–337.
13. Garcia LS, Bruckner DA: Diagnostic Medical Parasitology. Elsevier Science Publishing, New York, 1988.
14. Beaver PC, Jung RC, Cupp EW: Clinical Parasitology. 9th Ed. Philadelphia, Lea & Febiger, 1984.
15. Bigby TD, Margolskee D, Curtis JL, et al: The usefulness of induced sputum in the diagnosis of *Pneumocystis carinii* pneumonia in patients with the acquired immunodeficiency syndrome. Am Rev Respir Dis 1986; 133:515–518.
16. Ma P, Villaneuva TG, Kaufman D, Gillooley JF: Respiratory cryptosporidiosis in the acquired immune deficiency syndrome. Use of modified cold Kinyoun and hemacolor stains for rapid diagnosis. JAMA 1984; 252:1298–1301.

23 Skin, Wound, and Tissue Specimens

Leona Ayers Ales Pindur
Thomas R. Fritsche Steven Specter
Gerald Lancz

INTRODUCTION

The initial diagnosis of skin and soft tissue infections is made from the patient's history, signs, and symptoms. In many cases the etiologic diagnosis can be confirmed by culture and smear of an appropriate specimen. Exudates, drainage, fluids, and tissues from skin, soft tissues, and deep organs or cavities are among the most commonly tested and are usually submitted for "routine" general cultures for bacteria and fungi. In addition to the general culture, special procedures for identifying fastidious bacteria, mycobacteria, mycoplasma, fungi, parasites, and viruses as well as histochemical stains of biopsies can be obtained.

The challenge for the clinician is to select those tests that will most likely provide rapid confirmation of clinical impressions or will appropriately differentiate compatible diagnoses. Definitive inclusion or exclusion of an infectious disease often depends on confirmatory laboratory tests. The challenge for the laboratory is to recognize those instances when consultation with the clinician should be initiated for additional testing. Concordance should exist among the clinical history, physical findings, pathologic process, microbe identification, and the response to appropriate treatment or expected progression over time. Doubts about the diagnosis are eased for all participants when the identified microbe is a primary pathogen with a well defined pathologic behavior that matches the clinical appraisal. Interpretation requires caution when the identified organism has a variable history of disease production, is ubiquitous in the natural or hospital environment, or when the pathogen is rarely encountered in the patient's geographic region.

COMMONLY TESTED SPECIMENS

Specimen: Skin and Underlying Tissue

Background[1]

Normal Skin

Skin has a large resident microbial flora that ranges from thousands of organisms on the palms of the hands to over one million on the forehead. Concentrations are highest and most varied in the axillae, groin, and toe webs. Transient microbial populations are acquired from various contiguous body orifices, the skin and orifices of other humans, other animals or insects, and the inanimate environment. Intact skin is an efficient mechanical, chemical, microbial, and physiologic barrier to the movement of microbes into sterile subsurfaces. The rapid regeneration of the squamous epithelium, self-cleaning quality of desquamation, low pH, direct microbicidal quality of skin fatty acids, and rich microvascularity of skin all contribute to a naturally high resistance to infection.[2]

Initiation of Infection

Trauma. Tissue injury is one of the most important factors in the initiation of skin and soft tissue infections. Trauma inoculates organisms directly into the sterile soft tissue. The tissue injury compromises local and systemic defenses. A common presentation by secondary pathogens is the "polymicrobic infection," often presenting as an ulcer of the skin or mucosal surfaces. When taken individually, these organisms have low infection potential but in concert they can potentiate the development of capsule or slime protective coats in other microbes, combine exotoxins with possible synergistic action, as well as create low pH and highly anaerobic conditions that limit normal phagocytic and immune function and the action of many antibiotics. A spectrum from low grade indolent infection to rapidly progressive, necrotizing infection may be produced. In either case, treatment can proceed with the knowledge that the infection is not a single agent but is polymicrobic and probably originates in oropharyngeal, fecal, skin, or environmental flora. The direct specimen Gram stain examination helps assess the "mixed" quality of the isolated organisms that are often nothing more than contaminants. Commonly these are mixtures of aerobic and anaerobic bacteria but *Candida* species and other yeast may be admixed.

Foreign Bodies. If foreign bodies are associated with the trauma, infection can be initiated with much lower inocula of microbes. Dead tissue acts as a foreign body as does any implanted medical device. Minor trauma when associated with foreign body implantation or conditions of immunosuppression can also be associated with infection.[3]

Primary Pathogens

Viral. Viral infections of the skin and mucous membranes often result in a disturbed architecture with the production of discrete lesions. These disturbances are referred to as exanthems and enanthems, respectively, and their character together with the patient's findings are often sufficient for diagnoses.[4,5] The viral infections may be very mild and self-limiting infections (rubella) or may result in serious complications such as neoplastic transformation subsequent to papillomavirus infection of the cervix.

Parasitic. A variety of protozoa, helminths, and arthropods may be found on or in the skin and be responsible for serious disease. Definitive diagnosis of these parasitic infections requires the demonstration of responsible agent(s). The larger organisms, primarily arthropods, may be sent for directly examined, whereas the protozoa and helminths are usually detected in tissue specimens submitted for impression smears, histology, or culture.

Selection

General Approaches

History and Physical Examination. After the patient has been carefully examined and questioned concerning the present illness, a working diagnosis is developed based on the findings. The choice of tests to confirm the working diagnosis or explore a differential diagnosis flows from clinical interpretations. For example, general culture examination of decubitus ulcers should be reserved for only clinically infected ulcers because a culture cannot discriminate between contaminants and pathogens. Where the ulcer is clinically infected, a culture can be useful in defining the likely invasive pathogens for purposes of antibiotic therapy. Conversely, immunocompromised patients pose a special clinical difficulty because of the loss of the usual signs and symptoms of infection. All lesions occurring in these patients should be aggressively explored by direct smear and culture examinations because of the propensity for serious infections to occur "atypically."

Lesion Morphology. Possible diagnoses in skin and soft tissues keyed to the morphology of skin lesions with the etiologic agents and commonly used tests are presented in Table 23-1. For each morphologic lesion, the diagnostic possibilities are large. Prevalence and geographic distribution of diseases are critical in determining how a specific lesion should be evaluated. The pathologic processes that occur in response to microbial invasion direct attention toward specific diseases and suggest the tests required for confirmation.[2] These processes occur in all normal individuals in a predictable pattern. Routine bacterial culture and smear are usually sufficient to define those species likely to be aggressive or antibiotic resistant. Special procedures and cultures should be reserved for closed abscesses or unexplained antibiotic failures or where competent smear evaluation is unavailable. The Gram stained smear and general culture are adequate for evaluating most exudative lesions but proliferative lesions usually require that tissue be submitted for histology and/or special cultures, such as for fungi and mycobacteria.

Extent of Disease. In the patient with a skin or soft tissue lesion, the presence of fever and an abnormal

Table 23-1. Lesions, Organisms, and Tests for Cutaneous and Soft Tissue Infections

Disease	Etiologic Agent	Test
Petechiae/purpura/hemorrhage		
Bacillary angiomatosis	*Rickettsia* spp.	Clinical (AIDS), histology
Bed bug bite	*Cimex lectularius*	History (linear puncta)
Black widow spider bite	*Latrodectus mactans*	History
Bloodstream infections		
Meningococcemia	*Neisseria meningitidis*	Blood culture, skin biopsy
Gonococcemia	*Neisseria gonorrhoeae*	Blood culture, skin biopsy
Others	*Haemophilus influenzae*	Blood culture, skin biopsy
	Listeria monocytogenes	
	Pseudomonas aeruginosa	
	Streptococcus pneumoniae	
	Yersinia pestis	
Endocarditis	Viridans streptococci	Blood culture, skin biopsy
Fungemia, chronic	*Candida albicans*	Blood culture, skin biopsy
	Histoplasma capsulatum	
Dengue	Dengue, 1,2,3,4	Serology
Epidemic typhus	*Rickettsia prowazekii*	Serology
Exanthems	Enteroviruses (echo 9)	Serology, viral culture
	Coxsackie viruses (A5, A9)	
Hemorrhagic fevers	Togavirus, arenavirus, bunyaviruses	Serology
Measles, atypical	Rubella or rubeola	Serology
Rocky Mountain spotted fever	*Rickettsia rickettsii*	Biopsy (DFA), serology
Yellow fever	Arbovirus, group B	Liver biopsy, serology
Maculopapules (smooth or keratotic)/wheals (pale papule)		
Anthrax (papular stage)	*Bacillus anthracis*	Gram smear, culture
Body lice (pediculosis)	*Pediculus humanus*	Clinical
Boston exanthem	Echovirus 16	Serology
Chagas disease	*Trypanosoma cruzi*	Clinical, smear examination
Chigger bites	*Trombicula irritans*	Clinical, insect examination
Crabs		
Phthirus pubis		Clinical, insect examination
Cutaneous larva migrans (creeping eruptions)	Dog and cat hookworms (*Strongyloides stercoralis* larvae)	Clinical, serology
Endocarditis	Viridans streptococci	Blood culture, skin biopsy
Epidemic typhus	*Rickettsia prowazekii*	Serology
Erysipelas (early)	*Streptococcus pyogenes*	Culture (aspirate)
Erythema chronicum migrans (Lyme disease)	*Borrelia burgdorferi*	Serology, biopsy
Erythema infectiosum (fifth disease)	Parvovirus B19	Clinical, serology
Erythema marginatum	*Streptococcus pyogenes*	History, rheumatic fever
Erythrasma	*Corynebacterium minutissimum*	Wood's light, scales
Exanthema, nonspecific	Enteroviruses, adenovirus	Serology
Exanthema subitum	Human herpes virus 6	Clinical
Flea bites	*Pulex irritans*	Clinical, serology
German measles	Rubella	Clinical, serology
Hepatitis B	Hepatitis B virus	Clinical, serology
Hookworm (larvae)	*Necator americanus*	Clinical, stool examination
Infectious mononucleosis	Epstein-Barr virus	Clinical, serology
Pinta (1° papule, 2° macules)	*Treponema carateum*	Serology
Histoplasmosis, African	*Histoplasma duboisii*	Biopsy (GMS), culture

(Continued)

Table 23-1. Lesions, Organisms, and Tests for Cutaneous and Soft Tissue Infections (Continued)

Disease	Etiologic Agent	Test
Maculopapules (smooth or keratotic)/wheals (pale papule) (Continued)		
Histoplasmosis (vasculitis)	*Histoplasma capsulatum*	Biopsy (GMS), culture
Leprosy (tuberculoid)	*Mycobacterium leprae*	Biopsy (fite farraco stain)
Listeriosis	*Listeria monocytogenes*	Culture, skin and blood
Measles	Rubeola (paramyxovirus)	Clinical, serology
Prototheosis (scales)	*Prototheca* spp.	Punch biopsy, culture
Psittacosis	*Chlamydia psittaci*	Serology
Rat bite fever, bacillary	*Streptobacillus moniliformis*	Blood, smear and culture
Rat bite fever, spiral	*Spirillum minus*	Blood, smear, anaerobic culture
Relapsing fever	*Borrelia recurrentis*	Smear blood/spleen abscesses
Rocky Mountain spotted fever (early)	*Rickettsia rickettsii*	Biopsy (DFA), serology
Scabies (burrows)	*Sarcoptes scabiei*	Scrapings (KOH), skin biopsy
Scalded skin syndrome	*Staphylococcus aureus*	Culture
Scarlet fever	*Streptococcus pyogenes*	Culture, serology
Scrub typhus rash	*Rickettsia tsutsugamushi*	Serology
Syphilis (secondary)	*Treponema pallidum*	Serology, darkfield examination
Tineas (scaling)		
Tinea barbae	*Trichophyton verrucosum*	Calcofluor white smear, culture
	Trichophyton mentagrophytes	
Tinea capitis	*Microsporum audouinii*	
	Microsporum canis	
	Microsporum tonsurans	
	Trichophyton violaceum	
	Trichophyton schoenleinii	
Tinea corporis	*Microsporum canis*	
	Trichophyton mentagrophytes	
	Trichophyton rubrum	
Tinea cruris	*Epidermophyton floccosum*	
	Trichophyton rubrum	
	Candida albicans	
Tinea imbricata	*Trichophyton concentricum*	
Tinea nigra	*Exophialia werneckii*	
	Stenella arguata	
Tinea pedis	*Trichophyton violaceum*	
Tinea versicolor	*Malassezia furfur*	Wood's lamp, scales (calcofluor white, KOH, special culture)
Toxic shock syndrome	*Staphylococcus aureus*	Culture
Trench fever	*Rickettsia quintana*	Serology
Trichinosis	*Trichinella spiralis*	Biopsy (H&E), serology
Typhoid fever (Rose spots)	*Salmonella typhi*	Blood culture, serology
Vasculitis (sepsis)	*Pseudomonas aeruginosa*	Blood culture, biopsy
	Neisseria meningitidis	
Vesicles/bullae/pustules/crusts		
Acne	Coryneform bacteria	Clinical
Anthrax (vesicular stage)	*Bacillus anthracis*	Gram smear, culture
Cat-scratch disease	Gram-negative bacillus (fastidious)	Biopsy
Chickenpox	Varicella-zoster	Smear (Tzanck, FA), culture
Deep pustular ringworm	*Trichophyton rubrum*	Calcofluor white smear, culture
Furunculosis (boils)	*Staphylococcus aureus*	Gram smear, culture
Hand, foot, and mouth disease	Enterovirus	Clinical, culture

(Continued)

Table 23-1. Lesions, Organisms, and Tests for Cutaneous and Soft Tissue Infections (Continued)

Disease	Etiologic Agent	Test
Vesicles/bullae/pustules/crusts (Continued)		
Herpangina	Enteroviruses	Serology, culture
Herpes simplex	*Herpesvirus hominis*	Smear (Tzanck, FA), culture
Impetigo (bullous)	*Staphylococcus aureus*	Gram smear, culture
	Streptococcus pyogenes	
Kerion (scalp)	*Trichophyton violaceum*	Calcofluor white smear, culture
Listeriosis (cutaneous)	*Listeria monocytogenes*	Gram smear, culture
Rickettsia	*Rickettsia akari*	Serology
Scalded skin syndrome	*Staphylococcus aureus*	Gram smear, culture
	Trichophyton mentagrophytes	
Shingles	Varicella-zoster	History, serology
Smallpox/vaccinia	Variola group	Eradicated
Vesicular ringworm	Dermatophytes	Calcofluor white smear, culture
Vesicular stomatitis	Vesicular stomatitis virus	Culture
Ulcers		
Anthrax (black eschar)	*Bacillus anthracis*	Impression Gram smear, culture
Aspergillus infarct	*Aspergillus* species	Biopsy (GMS), culture
Bartonellosis	*Bartonella bacilliformis*	Blood culture, smear
Buruli ulcer	*Mycobacterium ulcerans*	Acid fast smear, biopsy, mycobacterial culture at 32°C
Candidosis, paronychia	*Candida albicans*	Gram smear, culture
Chronic burrowing ulcer	Microaerophilic streptococci	Gram smear, culture
Decubitus ulcer	Polymicrobial fecal or skin flora	Gram smear
	Antibiotic selected flora	
Dermal ulcer (granulomatous)	*Mycobacterium haemophilum*	Acid fast smear, biopsy mycobacterial culture
	Mycobacterium marinum	
	Mycobacterium chelonei	
Diphtheria (wound)	*Corynebacterium diphtheriae*	Gram smear, special culture
Ecthyma gangrenosum	*Pseudomonas aeruginosa*	Gram smear, culture
Granuloma inguinale	*Calymmatobacterium granulomatis*	Biopsy-smear
Leg ulcers	*Corynebacterium pyogenes*	Gram smear, culture
	Corynebacterium haemolyticum	
	Corynebacterium ulcerans	
Lymphogranuloma venereum	*Chlamydia trachomatis*, serogroup 1	Serology, biopsy
Paracoccidioidomycosis	*Paracoccidioides brasiliensis*	Biopsy (GMS), culture
Scrub typhus eschar (mite bite site)	*Richettsia tsutsugamushi*	Serology
Skin ulcer	*Streptococcus agalactiae* (group B)	Gram smear, culture
Sporotrichosis (linear)	*Sporothrix schenckii*	Biopsy (GMS), culture
Syphilis (chancre)	*Treponema pallidum*	Darkfield examination, serology
Tropical phagedenic	Fusobacteria, spirochetes	Gram smear, biopsy
Tularemia (ulceroglandular)	*Francisella tularensis*	Special culture, BCYE
Yaws	*Treponema pertenue*	Biopsy, serology
Cellulitis/wounds		
Bites	*Staphylococcus aureus*	Gram smear, culture
	Streptococcus pyogenes	
	Pasteurella multocida (animal)	
	CDC DF-2 group (animal)	
	Polymicrobic oral flora (human)	
Burns	*Staphylococcus aureus*	Gram smear, culture
	Pseudomonas aeruginosa	
	Enterics and *Candida* spp.	

(Continued)

Table 23-1. Lesions, Organisms, and Tests for Cutaneous and Soft Tissue Infections (Continued)

Disease	Etiologic Agent	Test
Cellulitis/wounds (Continued)		
Cellulitis, facial	*Streptococcus pyogenes* (group A) *Staphylococcus aureus* *Haemophilus influenzae* (children)	Gram smear, culture
Cellulitis, clostridial	*Clostridium perfringens*	Gram smear, culture
Erysipeloid, associated with contact with hides, raw sea food, uncooked meat	*Erysipelothrix rhusiopathiae*	Clinical, biopsy with culture
Hickman site infection	*Mycobacterium fortuitum*	Gram smear, acid fast smear, culture
Immunosuppression	Enterobacteriaceae, *Cryptococcus neoformans*	Gram stain, culture
Injection site granuloma	*Mycobacterium chelonei*	
Necrotizing fasciitis	Polymicrobic fecal flora	Gram smear, culture
Nosocomial infections	*Staphylococcus aureus* (MRSA) *Enterococcus faecium* *Pseudomonas aeruginosa* *Pseudomonas fluorescens-putida* *Pseudomonas alcaligenes* *Xanthomonas maltophilia* *Acinetobacter calcoaceticus*	Gram smear, culture
Protothecosis	*Prototheca* species	Smear, culture
Puncture wound	*Staphylococcus aureus* CDC Group Vd Polymicrobic skin flora Polymicrobic environmental flora	Gram smear, culture
Streptococcal gangrene	*Streptococcus pyogenes* (A)	Gram smear, culture
Synergistic gangrene	Polymicrobic fecal flora	Gram smear, culture
Surgical trauma/wounds	*Staphylococcus aureus* *Enterococcus faecalis* *Escherichia coli* *Mycobacterium chelonei* *Pseudomonas aeruginosa* Polymicrobic: oropharyngeal, skin, or fecal flora	Gram smear, culture
Wounds, other	*Corynebacterium bovis* *Corynebacterium xerosis* *M. fortuitum*	
Fresh water lakes	*Aeromonas hydrophilia*	Gram smear, wound and blood culture
Salt water exposure	*Vibrio vulnificus,* *Vibrio alginolyticus* *Vibrio parahaemolyticus*	Gram smear, wound and blood culture
Sinuses/fistulae		
Actinomycosis	*Actinomyces israelii* and other species *Arachnia propionica*	Gram smear "granule," culture
Botryomycosis	*Staphylococcus aureus* *Pseudomonas aeruginosa* *Actinobacillus* species	Gram smear, culture
Eumycetoma	*Microsporum audouinii*	Calcofluor white smear, "granule," culture
Pseudotuberculosis	*Corynebacterium tuberculosis*	Gram smear, culture
Scrofula (draining)	*Mycobacterium tuberculosis* *Mycobacterium scrofulaceum*	Acid fast smear, mycobacterial culture

(Continued)

Table 23-1. Lesions, Organisms, and Tests for Cutaneous and Soft Tissue Infections (Continued)

Disease	Etiologic Agent	Test
Nodules, ulceronodules, tumors, plaques, deep infiltrations		
Acne fulminans (cysts)	*Propionibacterium acnes*	Clinical, blood culture
Actinomycetoma	*Streptomyces somaliensis*	Culture of "grains"
	Actinomadura madurae	Biopsy with "grains"
	Nocardia brasiliensis and others	
Bartonellosis	*Bartonella bacilliformis*	Blood culture, peripheral, blood smears (direct examination)
Black piedra (hair shaft)	*Piedra hortae*	Calcofluor white smear, culture
Blastomycosis	*Blastomyces dermatitidis*	Biopsy (GMS), culture
Bovine papular stomatitis	Poxvirus	Clinical
Chromomycosis	*Fonsecaea pedrosoi*	Scraping, calcofluor white, or KOH smear
Coccidioidomycosis	*Coccidioides immitis*	Biopsy (GMS), culture, serology
Ecthyma infectiosum (Orf)	Orf	Clinical
Erysipelas (late)	*Streptococcus pyogenes*	Culture of aspirate
Erysipeloid	*Erysipelothrix insidiosa*	Biopsy leading edge, Gram stain, culture
Eumycetoma	*Madurella mycetomatis*	Biopsy with "grains"
	Madurella grisea	Culture of "grains"
	Exophiala jeanselmei	
Favus (scutulum crust)	*Trichophyton schoenleinii*	Calcofluor white smear, culture
	Trichophyton violaceum	
	Microsporum gypseum	
Filariasis	*Wuchereria bancrofti*	Serology, biopsy (H&E)
	Brugia malayi	
Injection site	*Mycobacterium chelonei*	Culture, routine mycobacterial culture
	Mycobacterium fortuitum	
Kerion (scalp)	*Trichophyton violaceum*	Calcofluor white smear, culture
	Trichophyton mentagrophytes	
Leishmaniasis (oriental sore)	*Leishmania tropica*	Smear, biopsy, special culture
(Kala-azar)	*Leishmania donovani*	
Lupus vulgaris	*Mycobacterium tuberculosis*	Biopsy, mycobacterial culture
Phaeohyphomycosis	16 different genera	Biopsy (GMS), culture
Milker's nodule	Poxvirus	Clinical, biopsy (H&E)
Molluscum contagiosum	Poxvirus	Clinical, biopsy (H&E)
Myiasis	Human bot fly	Morphology of larvae
Nodular folliculitis	*Trichophyton rubrum*	Biopsy (GMS), culture
Protothecosis (scales)	*Prototheca* spp.	Punch biopsy, culture
Rhinoscleroma	*Klebsiella rhinoscleromatis*	Culture, biopsy
Sporotrichosis	*Sporothrix schenckii*	Calcofluor white smear on aspirate, biopsy (GMS), culture
Streptococcal myositis	Anaerobic streptococci	Gram smear, culture
Swimming pool granuloma	*Mycobacterium marinum*	Biopsy, mycobacterial culture at 32°C
Tularemia (ulceroglandular)	*Francisella tularensis*	Special culture, BCYE
Verrucosa cutis	*Mycobacterium tuberculosis*	Biopsy, mycobacterial culture
Warts	Papillomavirus	Clinical, in situ hybridization
White piedra (hair shaft)	*Trichosporon beigelii*	Calcofluor white smear, culture
Yaws (papillomatous)	*Treponema pertenue*	Serology

Abbreviations: AIDS, acquired immunodeficiency syndrome; DFA, direct fluorescence antibody (test); GMS, Gomori's methenamine silver; BYCE, buffered charcoal yeast extract; KOH, potassium hydroxide; H&E, hematoxylin and eosin (stain); FA, fluorescent antibody (test).

peripheral blood leukocyte count suggest that the process may be generalized, disseminated, or metastasized from a deep source. When these conditions are met, blood cultures and other related site cultures should be obtained before beginning empiric antibiotic therapy. If the suspected agent can only be identified by a rising antibody titer or change in immune status, serum should be obtained and stored for comparison with a convalescence serum sample. A stool sample for *Clostridium difficile* toxin assay might be useful for evaluating a patient with the unusual symptoms of diarrhea and nonhealing perianal ulcers with negative viral (herpes) cultures. The individual patient with disseminated infection, complicated infection, or unusual infection with secondary or primary skin involvement may generate extensive testing of a variety of body systems and test types before the nature and extent of the infection are defined.

Suspected Pathogens. *Primary.* Single virulent agents or primary pathogens are the best recognized causes of clinical infectious disease and are frequently confirmed by narrowly directed laboratory examinations. For example, if mycobacterial acid fast bacilli (AFB) are suspected, a smear and culture examination of appropriate specimens should be performed. If a differential among several primary pathogens exists, then multiple special examinations must be considered. General bacterial cultures are also done at the same time in clinically ill patients because such infections may be caused or complicated by secondary pathogens whose identity may be hard to predict on clinical grounds. In patients with acquired immunodeficiency syndrome (AIDS) or organ transplant immunosuppression, for example, multiple studies such as batteries of special stains for tissue biopsies, multiple smear stains, and general and special cultures are initiated at the first sign of infection.

Unusual. The history may provide important clues to the etiology. For example, infection with *Aeromonas hydrophila* might be expected from a fresh water-associated traumatic wound infection, and *Vibrio parahaemolyticus* or other *Vibrio* species occurs with wounds exposed to salt water.[6] These organisms can cause particularly virulent infections and the asplenic patient is at high risk for sepsis. Erysipeloid (from *Erysipelothrix rhusiopathiae* infection) should be considered in the patient with a nonulcerated, painful, spreading skin lesion with raised borders; this is seen in workers who have contact with seafood, poultry, meat, or hides. The diagnosis of this uncommon infection is made clinically or by culture of biopsy from the advancing border of the lesion. A variety of other special procedures including cultures for fastidious bacteria such as *Francisella tularensis* (rabbit or other animal bite or exposure), parasites (amebae, leishmania), or any other organism group suggested by the patient history, lesion, or direct examination can be ordered for unusual cases.

Specific Diagnostic Approaches

Direct Examination. An important side benefit of direct examination is that a "catch net" is provided for unusual circumstances or unexpected findings. Direct examination gives the laboratory the opportunity to define the process, to view the organism and probable contaminates, and to use this information for diagnosis as well as a guide to subsequent culture interpretations or additional testing.

Examination by direct microscopy examination should be performed for exudative processes with scaly or crusted lesions, exudates, drainages, fluids, or tissues that can be scraped, smeared, sedimented, or crushed. Bacteria proliferate greatly by the time clinical infection is present and detection by microscopy becomes reliable at this concentration if the specimen is representative. For practical applications, the examination of exudates, fluids, and drainages by Gram stained smears allows the presumptive diagnosis of the most common, localized bacterial and selected fungal infections. This is particularly true for immunocompromised individuals in whom infecting organisms proliferate to very high numbers, or in polymicrobic infections for which culture isolation of all species is impractical and untimely. Direct fluorescent antibody staining from vesicular lesions is available for herpes simplex virus, but is typically reserved for testing on other affected sites, such as the throat and nasopharynx. Direct examination of smears made from scrapings may also reveal giant cells or intranuclear inclusions associated with herpes simplex infection.

Biopsy. For proliferative or chronic processes producing solid lesions, examination of a biopsy specimen is usually the best approach. The exact nature of the tissue reaction producing the lesion and the relationship of that reaction to the presence of organisms can be quickly ascertained. The quantity of organisms is usually scant. With the assistance of special stains, organisms can be effectively sought in the most highly suspect tissue locations. In immunocompromised patients, organisms are frequently abundant and direct examination is likely to be successful in defining the nature of many infectious and noninfectious diseases.

When the tissue pathologic process is defined but organisms are not visualized, rational therapy can proceed while more sensitive culture isolation and organism identification procedures are completed.

Routine Culture. The general or "routine" bacterial culture may differ among laboratories. The clinician must know the organisms that are and are not isolated by the general culture, the special cultures that are necessary, and the types of cultures that are available. Requests should reflect the specific lesion and differential diagnoses (Table 23-2). Random surveillance cultures of the skin surface to detect carriers of specific pathogen (such as methicillin resistant *Staphylococcus aureus*) is generally futile for resolving nosocomial infection problems unless there is strong epidemiologic evidence to accompany the culture results. Surface cultures are also not worthwhile for predicting the etiologic agent of neonatal sepsis.[7] Indications and selection of tests for other specimens from specific types of lesions such as burns, bites, trauma, etc., are reviewed separately below.

Diagnosis of Suspected Viral Lesions. Viral infec-

Table 23-2. Association of Pathologic Processes With Infectious Diseases

Process	Organisms/Diseases
Acute inflammation	
Exudative (purulent)	Extracellular pathogens: pyodermas with staphylococci, streptococci, enterics, pseudomonads, anaerobes, candida, and rapid growing mycobacteria. Cell necrosis: herpesviruses and adenovirus
Hemorrhagic	Vessel wall invasion: Rocky Mountain spotted fever, epidemic typhus, falciparum malaria, meningococcemia, hemorrhagic fevers. Toxin production: anthrax, plague, clostridial myonecrosis
Serous	Low protein fluid loss: *Streptococcus pyogenes* cellulitis
Fibrinous	Deposition of fibrin on serous membranes: viral pericarditis—pleuritis, rheumatic carditis, lobar pneumococcal pneumonia with pleuritis
Ulcerative	Lytic destruction of tissue: amebiasis Intense cellulitis with surface necrosis: anthrax, spider bites, chancroid, ecthyma
Acellular	Absence of migrating phagocytic cells: burn eschar infection; disseminated aspergillosis, zygomycosis, cryptococcosis in immunocompromised patients
Chronic nonspecific inflammation	Lymphocytic: viral infection, rickettsial infection, and chronic tissue injuries Eosinophilic: parasitic infestations: trichinosis (muscle) Plasmocytic: primary/secondary syphilis, trypanosomiasis, deep cutaneous fungal infections Macrophage: lymph node hyperplasia; infectious mononucleosis, typhoid fever, brucellosis, toxoplasmosis
Chronic granulomatous inflammation	Caseating: tuberculosis, histoplasmosis. Noncaseating: swimming pool granuloma, injection site granuloma *(Mycobacterium chelonei)* Necrobiotic: brucellosis, cat-scratch disease, lymphogranuloma venereum, tularemia, listeriosis, melioidosis, *Yersinia enterocolitica* adenitis Histiocytic: lepromatous leprosy, *Mycobacterium avium* complex (associated with acquired immunodeficiency syndrome), rhinoscleroma, anergic leishmaniasis
Necrosis	Individual cell death: lytic viruses (herpes simplex virus, varicella-zoster virus), cytomegalovirus, adenovirus Vasculitis/thrombosis: ecthyma gangrenosus, embolic aspergillus Toxic: histotoxic clostridial gas gangrene, streptococcal gangrene
Hyperplasia	Epithelial cell: molluscum contagiosum (pox virus), Milker's nodule (paravaccinia virus), verrucae, condyloma acuminata (papillomaviruses), condyloma lata (secondary syphilis) Capillary hyperplasia: cytomegalovirus?, human immunodeficiency virus?
Neoplasia	Squamous cell: papilloma virus, chronic infection, Transitional cell: bladder carcinoma *(Schistosoma hematobium).* Lymphoid cell: Burkitt's lymphoma (Ebstein-Barr virus)

tions account for a large proportion of acute skin lesions and their presentation often suggests the identity of the etiologic agent (Table 23-1).

Rashes. Most common among the viral exanthemata are maculopapular rashes, most of which are associated with self-limiting infections that occur in epidemics. In this setting, viral culture is seldom necessary when a local epidemic is ongoing. Although scraping a maculopapular exanthem may yield viruses such as rubella, rubeola, adenoviruses, and enteroviruses, when a specific etiologic diagnosis is attempted, these agents are more readily isolated from the oropharynx or stool. Complications involving visceral organs may have severe consequences and in this circumstance determination of the specific viral etiology by culture or serologic means becomes important (as discussed below).

Identification of parvovirus B19 is also important in a circumstance where a pregnant woman may be exposed to an infected patient. This is especially important since the clinical picture of parvovirus infection can be similar to other viral infections.[8] The significance of detection of enteroviruses in infections involving rashes is twofold. First, it is necessary to distinguish them from rubella rashes in females to insure that there is not a false history of rubella that could lead to a subsequent exposure of a susceptible individual during pregnancy. Second, some systemic enterovirus infections, most notably coxsackievirus type B viruses, can lead to carditis and pancreatitis. Viral diagnosis alerts the physician to such possibilities and therefore may prevent severe consequences if precautionary measures are taken to limit infection.

Papular Lesions. Papular lesions such as Milker's nodules or molluscum contagiosum are self-limiting and generally are diagnosed on the basis of clinical history and presentation; culture is rarely performed.[4] Milker's nodules are usually seen on the hands of individuals who work with cows. An erythematous papule develops 5–7 days after exposure, then becomes firm, elastic, and purplish with a central depression. Regional lymphadenopathy may occur. Healing takes place within 4–6 weeks. Molluscum contagiosum begins as a pimple that forms an umbilicated white papule, which lasts for months to years. Lesions on the face, trunk, and limbs usually occur by direct contact or fomites. The virus may also be transmitted by sexual contact causing lesions to appear on the lower abdomen, pubis, genitalia, and inner thighs. The infection is usually self-limiting, although it may cause severe disease in immunocompromised (AIDS) patients. Bovine papular stomatitis is another, less common papular infection obtained from handling calves with stomatitis.

Vesicular Lesions. Herpes simplex virus (HSV) types 1 and 2 and varicella-zoster virus (VZV) are the most common causes of vesicular lesions. This is perhaps the most common dermal lesions cultured for virus, and is done to establish a positive diagnosis of HSV and to distinguish HSV from VZV. In addition, culture of the cervix for HSV late in pregnancy for women with a history of recurrent genital lesions is performed even in the absence of visible lesions. About 3% of women without clinical evidence of lesions are culture positive. In this setting, vaginal delivery should be avoided to prevent neonatal infection (see Ch. 25). The most common sites of HSV skin lesions are the mouth and genitalia; however, vesicular lesions on the fingers (Whitlow), especially in physicians or dentists, and on the body (gladitorium), which are common in wrestlers, are seen. Varicella (chickenpox) does not usually require laboratory confirmation when the clinical diagnosis is obvious. However, in immunocompromised individuals, especially leukemic children, confirmation of varicella is important because of the severity of illness in these persons. Similarly, zoster (shingles) is usually diagnosed clinically, on the basis of a unilateral rash along a dermatome. In cases of more extensive lesions or a vesicular ophthalmic infection, viral culture can be used to distinguish VZV from HSV. Enterovirus 71 and coxsackievirus types A viruses 4, 5, 10, 16 can also cause vesicular exanthemata, most notably hand, foot, and mouth disease, characterized by ulcerating vesicles. While the diagnosis is usually made on clinical grounds, the virus can often be isolated from throat, feces, or even from the vesicular lesions.

Pustular Lesions. Pustular virus infections are not commonly seen since smallpox has been eradicated and vaccination with vaccinia is no longer a routine procedure. However, cowpox and orf are uncommonly encountered pustular diseases most frequently seen on the hands of those who handle cows or sheep, respectively. Clinical history rather than viral culture is usually the basis for diagnosis.

Miscellaneous. Positive diagnosis of papillomaviruses is also important, especially for virus strains that have been associated with malignant transformation of cells (Table 23-3). For lesions suspected of harboring these viruses (chiefly cervical dysplasia), a piece of the hyperplastic lesion is obtained by biopsy or by surgical removal of the growth. It is especially important to detect laryngeal papillomas since they may be effectively treated with surgical removal and/or interferon therapy. These viruses can be detected by in situ hybridization, although this is usually not needed for diagnosis.

Table 23-3. Dermal Lesions Caused by Papillomaviruses

Strain	Body Site	Lesion Description	Alternative Name
2, 4, 7	Skin	Common warts	Verrucae vulgaris
5, 8, 9, 12, 14, 15, 17, also 19–25	Skin	Epidermodysplasia verruciformis[a]	
3, 10	Skin	Flat warts	Verrucae plana
13	Mouth	Focal epithelial hyperplasia	
6, 11, 16, 18, 31	Genitalia	Genital warts	Condyloma acuminata
6, 11	Larynx	Laryngeal papillomatosis[a]	
1, 4	Palm	Palmar warts	Myrmecia
1, 4	Sole	Plantar warts	Myrmecia

[a] Can be associated with neoplastic change.

Diagnosis of Suspected Parasitic Infections. In the United States, skin manifestations from parasitic infections are much less common than from viral or bacterial etiologies, but must be considered when the patient presents with a suspicious lesion or consistent travel or immigration history. The laboratory assists by identifying specific organisms morphologically, or by performing serologic tests.

Ulcers. Several species of protozoa may be responsible for causing cutaneous ulcers, including *Leishmania* spp., *Acanthamoeba* spp., and *Entamoeba histolytica*. Cutaneous leishmaniasis first manifests itself as a painless papule occurring weeks to months after the bite of an infected sandfly. The papule eventually becomes necrotic and ulcerates, forming a crater with thickened edges. The lesion may produce an exudate (wet sore) or remain dry (dry sore) depending on the species of infecting *Leishmania*. Secondary lesions may form, and healing usually occurs spontaneously, although disfiguring scars may remain. Occasionally, multiple lesions may appear or the disease may progress to a diffuse form resembling lepromatous leprosy, which does not heal spontaneously. Cutaneous ulcers caused by species of *Acanthamoeba* occur rarely and may progress to central nervous system dissemination. The lesions first appear as pruritic pustules, which then ulcerate and increase in size, becoming indurated and painful. Cutaneous amebiasis caused by *E. histolytica* is usually a secondary manifestation of an internal amebic abscess, although primary cutaneous foci have been described from several body sites. Skin lesions usually present as a slowly developing ulcer with well demarcated borders, which may become secondarily infected. Aspiration of cutaneous ulcers may be useful in recognizing infections caused by amebae or leishmania.[9] Stained preparations may be prepared from smears, or alternatively, cultivation may be performed. Care should be taken to aspirate material through uninvolved skin and from below the ulcer bed to prevent bacterial and fungal contamination when submitting material for culture. In addition to culture and smears, skin biopsies may be obtained for histology.

Nodules, Papules, and Other Lesions. Onchocerciasis is caused by the filarial nematode *Onchocerca volvulus*, which often resides in palpable subcutaneous nodules. Adult worms release microfilariae, which migrate continuously through the dermis causing dermatitis and lymphadenitis. Ocular lesions develop in long-standing infections and may result in blindness. A geographic history is helpful when considering this diagnosis because the helminth is only found in regions of west central Africa and Central America. Skin snips should be examined for microfilariae when this diagnosis is considered. Another filarial nematode, *Loa loa*, migrates continuously through subcutaneous tissues as an adult worm, and produces localized angioedema known as "Calabar" or "fugitive" swellings. Such migratory swellings are suggestive of loiasis, given an appropriate travel history to west or central Africa. Occasional appearance of the adult worm migrating under the conjunctiva has given rise to the name "African eyeworm." The microfilariae of *Loa loa* appear with a diurnal pattern in the blood, which is best sampled around noon.

Cutaneous larva migrans or "creeping eruption" results from the penetration and migration through the skin of larval cat or dog hookworms (*Ancylostoma braziliense* or *Ancylostoma caninum*). Any part of the body that comes in contact with contaminated soil may be infected. Initial penetration by the larvae results in pruritic papules, which later develop into linear tracks. These tracts are erythematous and raised and ultimately become vesicular. Secondary infections may result from intense itching. Biopsy is usually not indicated because the larvae are hard to identify, therefore the diagnosis must be made clinically.

Individuals who have been previously infected with *Strongyloides stercoralis* may also develop a cutaneous form of larva migrans known as "larva currens" when re-exposed to infectious filariform larvae.[10] Penetration of skin by filariform larvae autoinfection produces urticaria and a linear cutaneous lesion that is often found in the anal area. Stool examination for the rhabditiform larvae is indicated for diagnosis.

Insect Bites and Stings. A large variety of arthropods cause skin lesions from their bites, stings, or transmission of infectious agents. A smaller number may actually live in or on the body for varying periods of time causing clinically apparent infections, and be identified from specimens sent to the clinical laboratory. Ticks, lice, and fleas are blood feeders that live on the body for variable time periods. Ticks and fleas remain on the skin only while feeding, whereas lice attach themselves to body hair and exist semipermanently on the skin surface. Bites from all these arthropods are irritating, resulting in local inflammation, pruritus, and occasionally, secondary infections. In addition, ticks may be responsible for an ascending flaccid paralysis (tick paralysis) that occurs in some persons. Myiasis, or human infestation with fly larvae (maggots), is a common occurrence in some parts of the world. Depending on the species of infecting fly, maggots may invade necrotic tissue associated with body wounds or healthy tissues. When present in wounds, these larvae may be seen actively crawling about. Larvae that will invade healthy tissues often appear as boil-like lesions in dermal and subdermal tissues. Itching and irritation of the tissues is common, and secondary bacterial infection may occur. More serious tissue invasion, including involvement of the nasopharynx, has been reported and may be life-threatening. All of these organisms may serve as vectors for serious viral, bacterial, rickettsial, or protozoal pathogens. The ectoparasitic arthropods, including fly maggots, should be removed intact from the skin, skin surface, hair shafts, or wounds and submitted in their entirety for examination and identification. It is not appropriate to submit the organisms for routine histologic sectioning, because key characteristics needed for identification will be lost.

The itch or mange mite *Sarcoptes scabiei* is transmitted directly from close contact with infected individuals and infects superficial layers of the skin causing intense itching. Repeated scratching results in further irritation, weeping, and spread of the lesion with possible secondary infection. Small reddish and slightly elevated tracks may be seen on the skin surface. The hands, elbows, axillae, groin, and breasts, among other areas, are most commonly infected. When characteristic skin lesions are seen, the diagnosis may be confirmed by examining skin scrapings or skin biopsy for infestation by the itch mite *(Sarcoptes)*. The use of mineral oil is preferred over potassium hydroxide because skin scales will mix better and mites will be more readily visible.

Terminology

General

Two levels of terminology apply when characterizing skin and soft tissue infections. At initial patient presentation, the terminology is descriptive. Included are the morphology and location of the lesion modified by complicating patient factors. A differential diagnosis usually accompanies the description. The many lesions and locations must be described using correct terminology if the considerable variety of diseases are to be efficiently pursued. Correct morphologic and pathologic terminology are of specific importance if consultation from specialists or the scientific literature is sought. Once primary pathogens are confirmed, the disease name and the location of the lesion are applied. For example, "erythematous macules" on the chest becomes "disseminated histoplasmosis with cutaneous vasculitis" once the causative organism and the nature of the lesion are identified by biopsy and culture results. If the etiologic agent is not a primary pathogen, the lesion description may be retained and the secondary pathogens or opportunistic pathogens appended. A "subcutaneous abscess" might be modified to "polymicrobic bacterial subcutaneous abscess" when the smear shows polymicrobic fecal flora in conjunction with culture isolation of *Escherichia coli, Enterococcus faecalis, Clostridium perfringens,* and *Bacteroides fragilis.*

Specific

Typical superficial cutaneous lesions are demonstrated in Figure 23-1. Each of these lesions is associated with differential considerations of etiology. Fluid filled vesi-

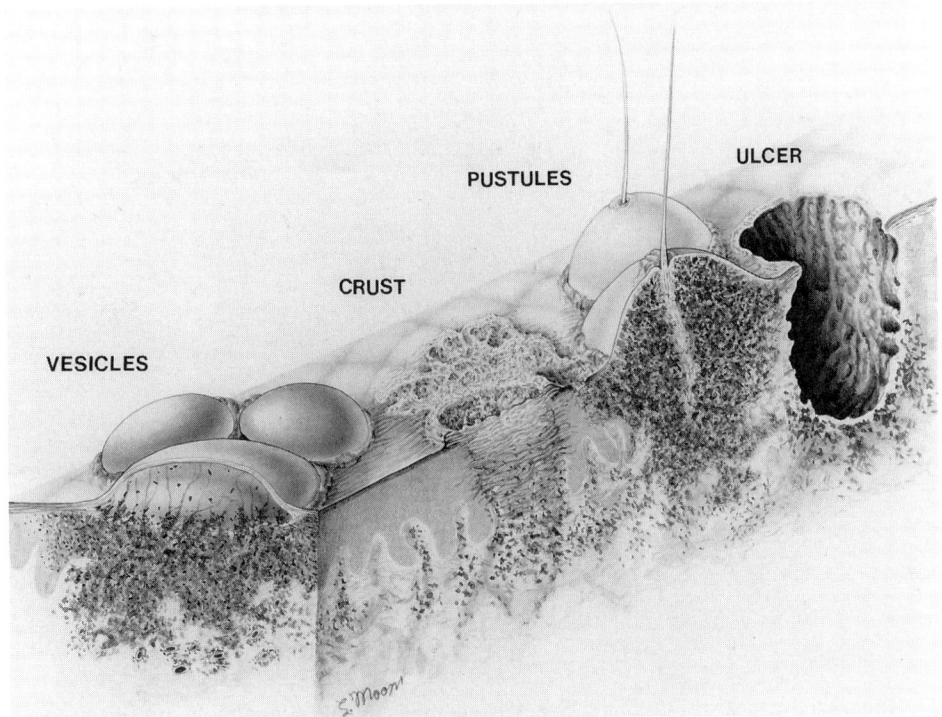

Fig. 23-1. Common superficial cutaneous primary (vesicles and pustules) and secondary (crust and ulcer) inflammatory lesions. *Staphylococcus aureus, Streptococcus pyogenes,* and herpes simplex infections are associated with these lesions.

cles (0.5 cm or less) and cell-rich exudate filled pustules (both primary lesions) can result in erosions, ulcers, and crusts (secondary lesions). Patients should be encouraged to accurately describe the time of onset and the evolution of these lesions. Lesions produced in the deeper or subsurface tissues result in surface changes or can be palpated through the surface tissues (Fig. 23-2). Macules that are flat, circumscribed areas (2.0 cm or less) of altered coloration may result from changes in pigment or alterations in the integrity of the superficial vascular bed. Lesions that are larger (more than 2.0 cm) are called patches. A small circumscribed addition of fluid forms a wheal; if the addition is solid, a papule is formed. Similar expansion of tissue causing a circumscribed, flat topped lesion larger than 1.0 cm is called a plaque. Plaques may be formed by epidermal or dermal exudates or infiltrates. Swellings with indistinct borders can result from edema or cellulitis. When the lesion is in the vascular bed, the damage may range from petechiae (small, focal areas of red blood cell leakage) to larger areas of blood extravasation called purpura. If the process in the blood vessel leads to thrombosis, the result is infarction of the skin with the formation of bloody vesicles, bullae, or gangrenous ulcers. The recognition of gangrene depends on the relationship of the process to the skin surface. Cutaneous gangrene is usually highly visible with a well demarcated advancing edge of erythema followed by blackened necrotic tissue or bloody bullae. Dermal compartment and/or muscle gangrene are less obvious. Pain and palpable tenderness are the important early clues with erythema, cyanosis, and blackening of the skin occurring late.

Surgical procedures create a variety of dermal lesions after incision or puncture of the skin (Fig. 23-3). Wound cellulitis with or without abscess formation (circumscribed areas of total tissue destruction and exudate accumulation) is a common complication. Special procedures such as central vascular line insertion, subcutaneous medication wells, breast implants, orthopedic devices, and pacemaker pockets all represent surgical intrusions regularly complicated by cellulitis and abscess formation.

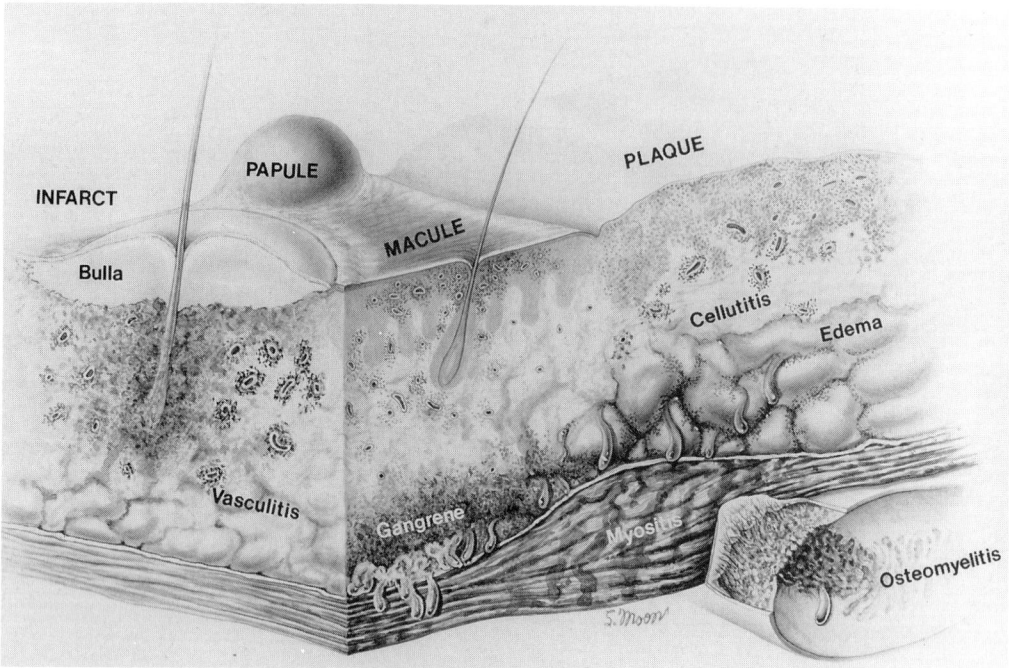

Fig. 23-2. Superficial cutaneous lesions of macules, papules, plaques, and bullae reflect deeper processes such as pigmentation, edema, cellulitis, vasculitis, and gangrene. Deep lesions require invasive techniques to sample infected materials.

Solid lesions such as those shown in Figure 23-4 usually reflect proliferative processes such as hyperplasia, chronic nonspecific inflammation, chronic granulomatous inflammation, or repair. These processes are seen as vegetative or verrucous protrusions from the skin surface or embedded nodules (1.0 cm or less), tumors (1.0 cm or more), or diffuse firm infiltrates. Superficial nodules and tumors may become confluent and cover large areas of skin. Necrosis of these lesions with ulcerations may occur producing a variety of appearances. Lesions may range from small ulceronodules or ulceropapillomas to large plaques of confluent nodules and tumors with disfiguring ulceration. The clinical and laboratory considerations of specific specimen examinations related to these lesions are described below.

Logistics

Specimen Collection

Equipment and Supplies. Collection of diagnostic materials determines whether a laboratory test result will be rewarding or confusing and misleading. Failure to obtain a sufficient quantity of representative material for the tests is a serious clinical error. The equipment and supplies for collection and transportation of specimens are relatively simple. The following should be available: glass microscope slides, nasopharyngeal swabs (Fig. 23-5), swabs with transport media (Fig. 23-6), anaerobic transport devices, tongue depressor blades, sticky transparent tape, surgical blades, cutaneous punch (2.0 and 4.0 mm) biopsy kits, syringes, needles, and sterile screw cap tubes and wide mouthed, sterile screw cap cups.

Techniques. *Scrapings.* Scraping for the collection of dry scales, for example, may be accomplished efficiently by using the sharp edge of a "twist" broken wooden tongue blade (Fig. 23-7). This tool has the advantage over a surgical blade in that it will cut neither the patient nor the operator and can be discarded into a regular trash container. If the lesion is "wet," collection for direct examination of scrapings is best accomplished using a surgical blade to avoid absorption of fluid by the porous wooden tongue blade. Fluid facilitates the spread and adhesion of cells onto the glass slide. Wet/moist lesions for culture should be aspirated

Skin, Wound, and Tissue Specimens • 689

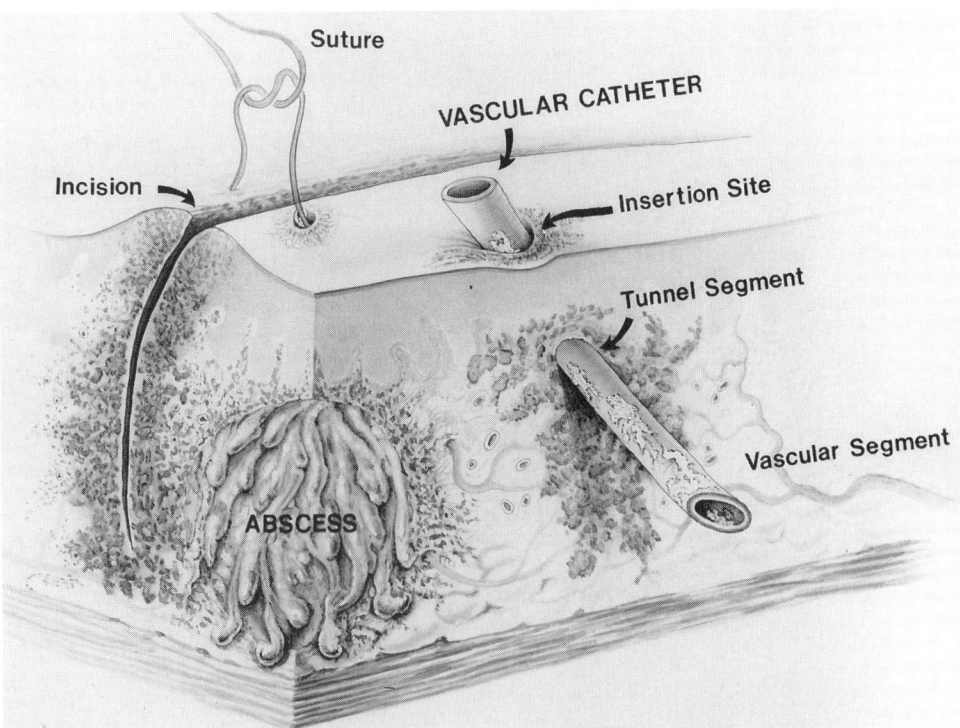

Fig. 23-3. Surgical procedures with incisions, sutures, and tunnel cellulitis and abscess formation. These lesions can be underestimated or inaccurately designated by surface inspection and surface sampling. Infectious material expands and accumulates below the surface and on the internal and external surfaces of foreign objects such as vascular catheters.

if closed and abraded with a swab after unroofing (Fig. 23-8). When obtaining material from cutaneous ulcers to examine for protoza, care should be taken to aspirate material through uninvolved skin and from below the ulcer bed to prevent bacterial and fungal contamination. Dry lesions should be scraped or wet before being swabbed.

Aspiration. Closed abscesses can be sampled by aspiration (Fig. 23-9). Following incision and drainage, purulence from the abscess center and from the viable tissue surface should be sampled for smear and culture. Organisms may not be spread evenly through the purulent debris. For example, important pathogens such as *E. histolytica* may be located at the viable tissue-abscess interface. In other infections, such as actinomycotic abscesses, the organisms are not at the edge but are within the purulence and within "granules." For successful capture of all pathogens, therefore, samples should be routinely taken from both areas (see Specimen: Fluids, Aspirates, and Tissues below).

Surgical lesions require special attention because the specimen can be easily contaminated by wound colonizing microbes (Fig. 23-10). Organisms proliferate at different rates and contaminants picked up by careless culture collection can overgrow or directly inhibit growth of the true pathogen. The wound should be cleaned, but not decontaminated, before samples are collected. When possible, the surgical wound should be opened, foreign material or medical devices removed, and material for smear and culture taken from the viable tissue interface or deep within the wound.

Specimens from skin lesions for viral studies may be collected by swabbing the lesion or, more preferably, by scraping the lesion with the dull side of a #10 scalpel blade. In the case of an open lesion it is best to obtain cells from the outer margin of the lesions where the tissues are most likely to be in a state of active infection. In the case of a closed lesion it is best to open the lesion and scrape cells from its base. Such cells are ideal

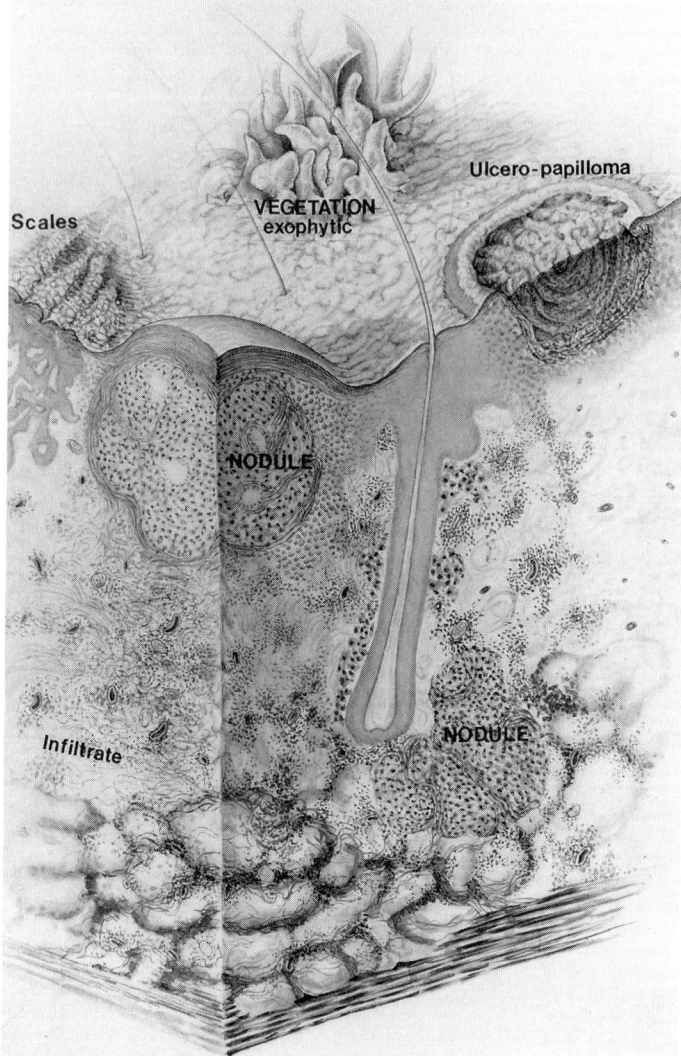

Fig. 23-4. Scales, vegetations, and nodules are formed from proliferation of host cells. Diffuse infiltrates may occur rather than the discrete accumulations that form the above lesions. Necrosis or degeneration of the proliferating cells leads to secondary ulcers with complex lesions such as the ulceropapilloma shown.

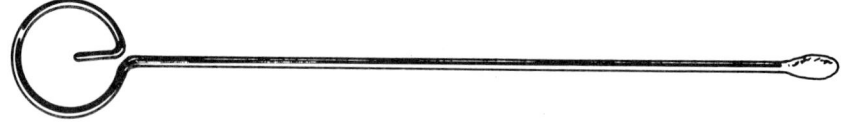

Fig. 23-5. Nasopharyngeal swab with flexible metal shaft. This tool is useful for exploration and specimen collection from narrow channels such as sinus tracts. Regular swabs should not be forced into narrow channels because contaminants are picked up from the tract and trauma to the tract may occur.

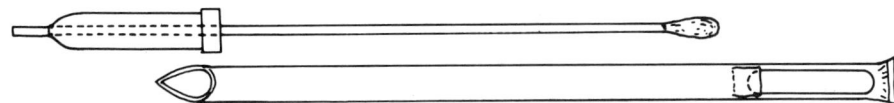

Fig. 23-6. Aerobic/anaerobic swab with transport media. No swab culture should be collected for transport to a distant laboratory without a "holding" media to prevent sample desiccation. Two swabs must be provided so that a smear and general culture can be performed. Additional swabs must be submitted for each additional test ordered. Swabs should only be used when material cannot be collected in sufficient volume to partially fill a culture tube.

for both viral isolation studies and direct examination for virus by electron microscopy or immunologic procedures. Vesicular fluid may be collected with a tuberculin syringe and small gauge (25 or 26) needle. A small amount of fluid, which can be obtained from the needle tip by rinsing with sterile medium, is adequate for inoculation into cell culture. Exudates for viral culture are collected using a sterile cotton or Dacron swab that is placed into 1–2 mL of viral transport medium.

Analysis

Appropriate examinations for selected sample types are presented in Tables 23-4 and 23-5. If care is taken in sampling and the tests are performed with care, the results can provide prompt confirmation of a diagnosis or indicate whether a diagnosis will be forthcoming. Infected materials from skin and soft tissue are routinely submitted for Gram stained smear, general culture, and antibiotic susceptibility testing. Culture ex-

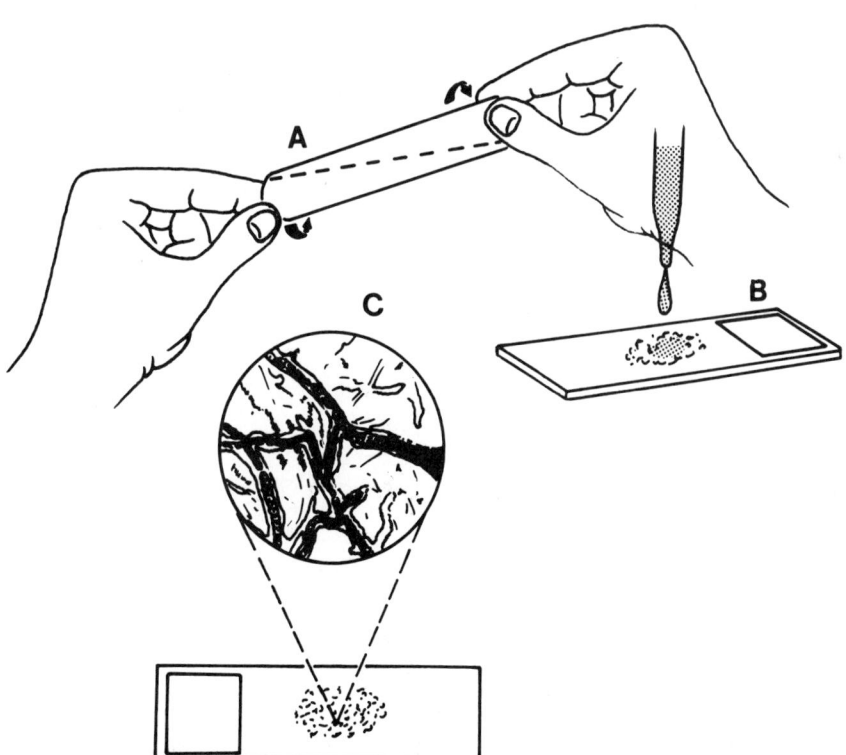

Fig. 23-7. Collection of scales for direct examination. The scaly lesion should be cleaned with 70% isopropanol. **(A)** Wooden tongue blade "twist" broken to provide a sharp scraping edge; **(B)** scales gently scraped onto a glass slide and mixed with calcofluor white and KOH (3 min); and **(C)** viewed with a fluorescent microscope for fungal hyphae and yeast.

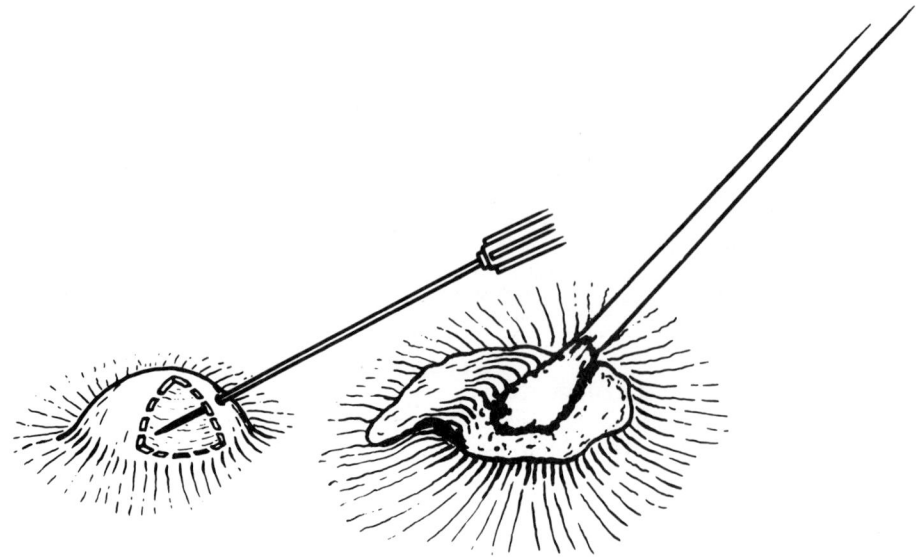

Fig. 23-8. Collection of samples from vesicles, bullae, and pustules. Each can be sampled by needle aspiration but unroofing of the lesion and vigorous swabbing of the lesion base to remove cells may provide a better sample, particularly for viral lesions.

amination should be performed for isolation and identification of common, rapidly growing bacterial and fungal pathogens.

General cultures are not designed to isolate all species present but to survey for rapidly growing organisms.

For example, if *S. auerus*, *Streptococcus pyogenes* *Pseudomonas aeruginosa*, or *Candida albicans* are present in significant numbers as pathogens or contaminants, other species cannot grow in culture because of inhibitors produced. *Nocardia* spp., *Neisseria gonorrhoeae*, and *Mucor* spp., are only a few of the impor-

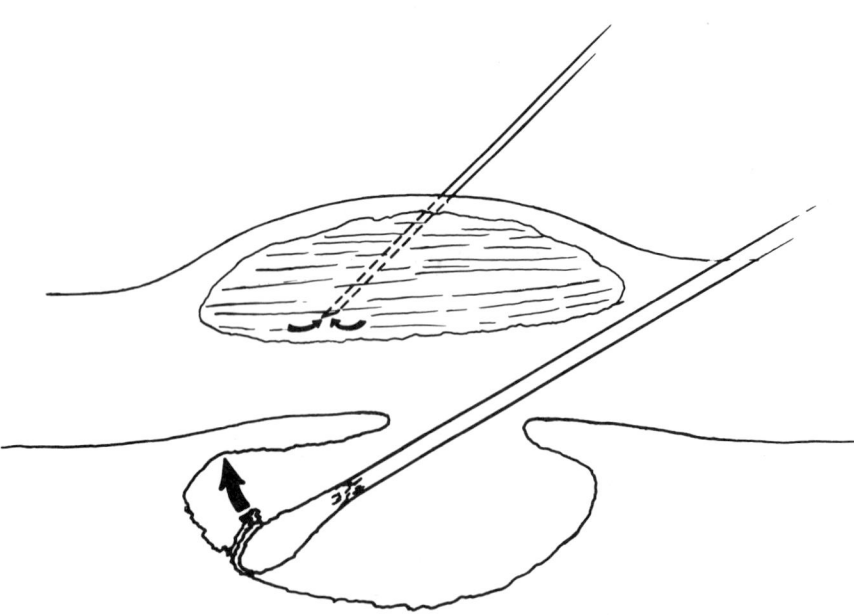

Fig. 23-9. Collection of samples from closed abscesses. Closed abscesses should be sampled by needle aspiration of the liquid debris and complemented by a sample of the abscess wall following incision and drainage.

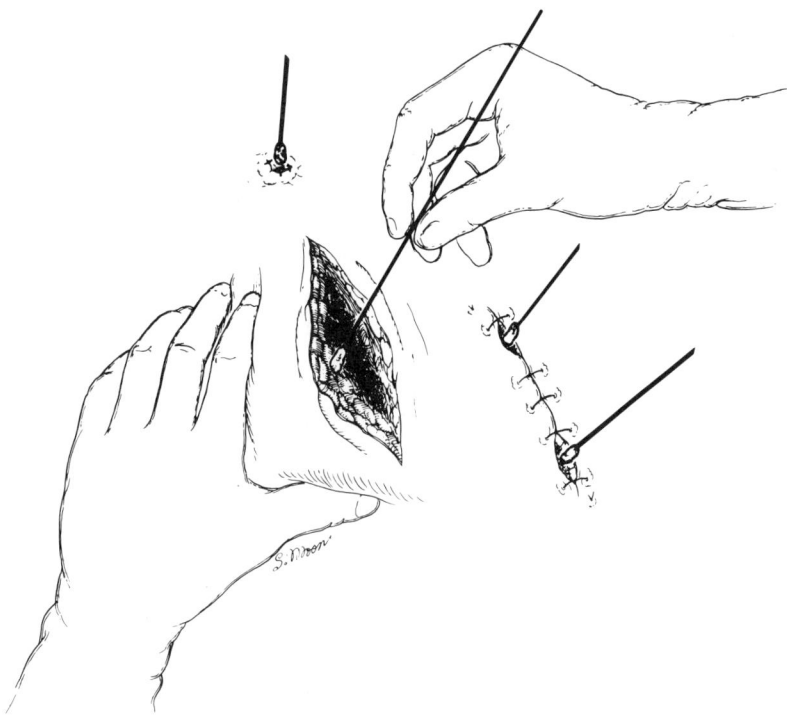

Fig. 23-10. Collection of samples from surgical wounds. Clean the surface of the inflamed wound and then sample the depth of the wound. Exudate should never be collected from the wound surface, bandages, or drains (chronic) for primary diagnosis.

tant pathogens that can be inhibited in culture by contaminating organisms.

Sufficient reference material should be available to support the diagnosis of unusual or rare cutaneous and soft tissue infections. This reference material should include lesion descriptions as well as the description of routine and special laboratory methods. Most trained medical personnel are able to effectively use reference materials and reference laboratories when advanced planning and practice have made both available.

Interpretation

Direct Examination

Infection-related processes and some of the prominently associated microbes and diseases are reviewed in Table 23-6. Acute purulent or exudative inflammation with or without fever and leukocytosis is the most frequently encountered process and is reliably associated with commonly isolated extracellular pathogens such as *S. aureus, S. pyogenes, E. coli, P. aeruginosa, E. faecalis,* and *C. albicans*. The clinician identifies this process by erythema, heat, swelling, and pain in the affected part. The laboratory identifies this process by finding polymorphonuclear cells, fluid protein, and necrotic debris in smears. Interpretation of culture and smear results must always be patient and disease based. Geographic and social considerations must be at the center of the evaluation. Most bacteria commonly isolated from skin lesions can be pathogens or contaminants depending on the clinical circumstances. The common exudative skin and soft tissue infections regularly sampled for general culture can best be managed by *always* evaluating a direct smear of the specimen. This examination should not be a "quick look" but should proceed in an orderly fashion as described below.

The background material provides valuable information. A properly collected purulent exudate will usually show polymorphonuclear leukocytes and few contaminating elements such as squamous epithelial cells. The exception is an infected epidermal cyst in which the epithelial cells would normally comprise part of the infected contents. Exudate or damaged tissue can disintegrate and result in a necrotic background. Next, a search for microorganisms should begin to determine if a single or several types of organisms are present and if the morphology is compatible with an expected pathogen or infectious process. In Figure 23-11, for example,

694 • Laboratory Medicine

Table 23-4. Direct Specimen Examinations for Selected Diagnoses

Specimen/Lesion	Direct Tests	Observation	Diagnosis
Clippings			
Hair/nails	Calcofluor white 10% potassium hydroxide (KOH) Lactophenol cotton blue	Thin hyphae, yeast	Dermatophytes, candida
Tape preparation	Lactophenol cotton blue Press to glass slide	Short hyphae, yeast Hyaline ova	*Tinea versicolor* *Enterobius vermicularis*
Scrapings			
Scales	Calcofluor white 10% KOH Lactophenol cotton blue	Thin hyphae, yeast Yeast & short hyphae	Dermatophytes, candida *Tinea versicolor*
Burrow	10% KOH	Mites, ova	Scabies
Patch	Calcofluor white	Oval budding or Gram-positive yeasts	Candida, *Torulopsis*
	10% KOH Gram stain	Thin hyphae Gram-positive bacilli	Dermatophyte Erythrasma
Vesicle	Tzanck preparation (Giemsa/Wright)	Multinucleated cells	Herpes simplex Varicella-zoster
Smears, imprints, wet preparations			
Ulcer	Dark-field examination Gram stained smear	Spirochetes "School of fish" Gram-negative bacilli Bacteria/yeast	Syphilis Chancroid Infection or contamination/colonization
	Aspirate	Amastigotes Trophozoites	*Leishmania* spp. *Entamoeba histolytica*
Cellulitis	Gram stained smear	Bacteria, yeast	Bacterial, fungal, or mixed
Pustules	Calcofluor white smear		Infection
Abscess			Contamination/colonization
Biopsy			
Skin snips	Placed in saline	Microfilariae	*Onchocerca volvulus*
Shave	Tissue sections	Pathologic process	Bacteria, fungi
Punch	Histochemical stains	Organism morphology	Mycobacteria, selected
Incisional	Immunologic stains	Viral inclusions	Viruses
Excisional	DNA probes, polymerase chain reaction		

a beaded gram-positive filamentous branching organisms is consistent with *Nocardia* spp. and the identification can be preliminarily confirmed by demonstrating modified acid fast staining. Furthermore, the interpretation takes into account that *Nocardia* is rarely seen as a contaminant and is presumed to be an etiologic agent when seen in smears with necrotic or purulent backgrounds. This presumption of pathogenicity cannot be presumed for the sole agent seen in Figure 23-12. *Candida* spp. can be identified in direct examination as a strongly gram-positive budding yeast, sometimes with pseudohyphae. Because this organism contaminates surface cultures, its evaluation in relationship with the background becomes important for

Table 23-5. Specimen Culture Selections for Diagnosis

Screening cultures	
Amoeba	McQuay modified charcoal agar diphasic medium (rarely used)
Bacteria	
Pyogenic cocci	5% Sheep blood agar for β-hemolytic *Streptococcus* groups A, B, C, D, F, G; *Staphylococcus aureus*
Legionella spp.	Buffered charcoal yeast extract with/without antibiotics
Others	Special media/growth conditions for *Brucella, Nocardia* spp., *Francisella tularensis*
Chlamydia	McCoy cell monolayers with cycloheximide for *Chlamydia trachomatis* (rarely used)
Fungi	
Dermatophytes	Dermatophyte test medium—dermatophytes (office-clinic use)
Malassezia	Olive oil overlay or special lipid media for *Malassezia furfur*
Leishmania	Novy McNeal-Nicolle media (rarely used)
Mycoplasma	H and U agars; *Mycoplasma hominis* (rarely used)
Viruses	
Herpes	Human diploid or primary human cells for Herpes simplex virus
Cytomegalovirus	Human diploid or primary human cells for cytomegalovirus
General cultures	
Anaerobe	Reduced blood medium with or without antibiotics, reduced anaerobic broth for *Clostridum perfringens, Bacteroides fragilis* group, anaerobic cocci, oral *Bacteroides* spp., *Fusobacteria* spp., most other pathogenic species
Fungal	Fungal media with or without cycloheximide antibiotics, with or without NH_4OH on Smith's yeast extract medium for dermatophytes, rapid and slowly growing fungi, aerobic actinomycetes
Bacterial	5% Sheep blood agar, chocolate agar, selective gram-negative agar, selective gram-positive agar, selective fungal and anaerobic media for staphylococci, streptococci, diphtheroids, haemophili, enterics, pseudomonads, yeasts, rapid growing fungi, some nocardiae, some rapid growing mycobacteria, aerotolerant anaerobes
Mycobacterial	Egg media (Lowenstein-Jensen), blood agar and 7H11 selective, 7H12 broth (at 32°C for skin and soft tissue infections, 35°C for slow and rapid mycobacteria including *Mycobacterium marinum* and *Mycobacterium haemophilum*
Viral	Primary rhesus monkey kidney, heteroploid line, human fibroblast cells for adenovirus, cytomegalovirus, enterovirus, Herpes simplex virus, varicella-zoster virus

interpretation. In this case (Fig. 23-12) the background is purulent without contamination and strongly suggests that *Candida* is the etiologic agent.

Routine Culture

Preliminary smear results should be confirmed by culture. False negative culture results may occur if the organism is fastidious or requires special growth conditions. The culture result should help confirm or clarify preliminary results obtained by interpretation of the smear morphology, along with sample site and clinical circumstance. The accuracy of these interpretations depends on the predictable participation of prevalent organisms at the site of infection (Table 23-6). For example, an infection in the skin and soft tissue with a purulent exudate showing gram-positive cocci in groups has a predictable etiology. When culture isolation does not confirm *S. aureus* in the rare individual case, the array of smear look-alikes is known and therapy is rarely altered. Gram-positive cocci in pairs and chains have culture isolation expectations and *S. pyogenes* is the pathogen of greatest concern. Anticipation of *S. pyogenes* isolation by culture will not alter therapy of other streptococcal infections at risk except for enterococcal infection. The change in prevalence of streptococci with the anatomic site is used to modify interpretations. For example, streptococcal morphotypes in the body zone influenced by fecal flora would be presumed to be enterococci, and streptococci involved in genital tract-related infections would be presumed to be group B until culture confirmation.

Species of gram-positive bacilli can also be interpreted based on lesion and anatomic location. Large gram-positive bacilli associated with polymicrobic fecal flora

Table 23-6. Smear and Culture Interpretation

Culture Result	Frequency	Interpretation/Associated Lesions or Diseases
Gram stain: gram-positive cocci in pairs, tetrads, and groups		
Staphylococci (rarely speciated by laboratory except for *S. aureus*)		
S. aureus	Common	Pyoderma: furuncles, carbuncles, abscesses, wound infections, polymicrobic skin flora infections, osteomyelitis, congenital or acquired hypogammaglobulinemia, toxic shock syndrome, contaminant
S. epidermidis	Common	Wound infection, vascular catheter insertion site, bacteremia (vascular line associated), mediastinitis (immunocompromised), contaminant
S. haemolyticus	Occasional	Nosocomial wounds, vascular catheter insertion site, antibiotic therapy, bacteremia (immunocompromised)
S. capitis	Uncommon	Postsurgical eye infections, central nervous system shunt infections, medication reservoirs
S. "others"	Uncommon	*S. cohnii* 1 and 2, *S. saprophyticus*, *S. caprae*, *S. intermedius*, *S. simulans*, *S. warneri*, *S. lugdunensis*: polymicrobic skin flora wound infections
Micrococcus		
Micrococcus spp.		Contamination, polymicrobic skin flora, cellulitis, vascular catheter insertion site tunnel infection
Peptostreptococcus		
P. magnus	Common	Polymicrobic infections, treated mixed wound infection
Leuconostoc	Rare	Vancomycin resistant opportunist
Gram stain: gram-positive cocci in pairs, clusters, and chains		
Streptococcus		
S. pyogenes, group A	Common	Pyoderma: cellulitis, erysipelas, impetigo, skin ulcers (ecthyma), abscesses, myositis, osteomyelitis, scarlatiniform rash (toxin), surgical wounds, minor trauma (insect bites), infants and young children, poor hygiene, diabetes, acute glomerulonephritis
S. agalactiae, group B	Common	Cellulitis, cutaneous ulcers, osteomyelitis, diabetes, myometritis
S. equisimilis, group C	Common	Cellulitis, cutaneous ulcers, lymphangitis, surgical wounds
S. anginosus, group F	Uncommon	Cellulitis, abscesses, wound infections, osteomyelitis
Streptococcus, group G	Uncommon	Polymicrobic oropharyngeal flora infections, wounds
Enterococcus		
E. faecalis	Common	Polymicrobic fecal flora, ischemic wounds, decubitus ulcers, surgical wounds
E. faecium	Occasional	Polymicrobic fecal flora, antibiotic treated mixed surgical/traumatic wound infections
E. durans	Occasional	Polymicrobic fecal flora, antibiotic treated wound infections
E. avium	Occasional	Polymicrobic fecal flora, antibiotic treated wound infections
Peptostreptococcus		
P. magnus	Common	Polymicrobic skin flora wound infections
Gram stain: gram-positive bacilli, pleomorphic, or beaded		
Corynebacterium jeikeium	Occasional	Nosocomial wounds (immunocompromised)
Nocardia spp. (branching, positive modified acid fast)	Occasional	Indolent wound, sinus drainage, Madura foot
Actinomyces israelii (branching, difficult to culture)	Rare	Indolent wound, sinus drainage, Madura foot
Others		
Propionibacterium acnes, Corynebacterium diphtheria, Arachnia propionica, Rothia dentocariosa, Kurthia spp., *Erysipelothrix rhusiopathiae*	Rare	Skin infection

(Continued)

Table 23-6. Smear and Culture Interpretation *(Continued)*

Culture Result	Frequency	Interpretation/Associated Lesions or Diseases
Gram stain: gram-positive bacilli, large, with or without spores		
Bacillus		
B. cereus	Occasional	Contaminant
Others	Rare	*B. anthracis,* malignant pustule, wounds
Clostridia		
C. perfringens	Common	Polymicrobial fecal flora infections, cellulitis myonecrosis
Others	Occasional	*C. bifermentans, C. innocuum, C. histolyticum, C. ramosum, C. septicum, C. sordellii:* polymicrobial fecal or environmental flora infections
Gram stain: gram-negative bacilli, small, pleomorphic		
Bacteroides		
B. fragilis	Common	Polymicrobic fecal flora wound infections
Others	Occasional	*B. thetaiotaomicron, B. ovatus, B. distasonis, B. uniformis, B. vulgatus:* polymicrobic fecal flora wound infections, undrained-antibiotic treated abscesses
	Occasional	*B. melaninogenicus:* polymicrobic oropharyngeal flora infections
	Occasional	*B. bivius, B. disiens:* polymicrobic abscesses of genital area
	Occasional	*Haemophilus influenzae, Eikenella* spp: cellulitis, bites polymicrobic oropharyngeal infection
	Occasional to rare	*Pasteurella multocida,* CDC Group EF4, CDC Group M5: zoonotic wounds from cat and dog bites
Gram stain: gram-negative bacilli, medium, regular-sized		
Escherichia coli	Common	Polymicrobic fecal flora wound infections
Pseudomonas aeruginosa	Common	Wounds and abscesses, antibiotic selected
Proteus mirabilis	Common	Polymicrobic fecal flora infections
Klebsiella pneumoniae	Common	Altered polymicrobic oropharyngeal and fecal flora wounds and abscesses.
Others	Occasional	*Enterobacter cloacae, Enterobacter* spp., *Serratia marcescens, Proteus vulgaris, Morganella morganii, Citrobacter* spp., *Providencia* spp: nosocomial wound infection
Gram stain: gram-positive yeast and (pseudo)hyphae		
Candida		
C. albicans	Common	Antibiotic selected cutaneous infections, vascular catheter sites
Others	Occasional	*Torulopsis candida, C. krusei, C. parapsilosis, C. tropicalis:* Antibiotic selected wound infections, vascular catheter site
Malassezia		
M. furfur	Occasional	Tinea versicolor, perifollicular and dermal abscesses, vascular line infection
Gram stain: gram-negative yeast (speckled gram-positive)		
Cryptococcus neoformans	Occasional	Cutaneous cellulitis, nodules, ulcers (immunocompromised)
Others	Occasional to rare	Dermatophytes, *Blastomyces dermatitidis, Histoplasma capsulatum,* chromoblastomycosis
Gram stain: gram-negative hyphae		
Aspergillus		
A. fumigatus	Occasional	Skin infarcts, burn wound infections (immunocompromised)
A. flavus		
Dermatophytes	Rare (invasive)	Can create a negative staining outline
Zygomycetes		
Mucor spp.	Occasional	Skin infarcts, burn wound infections (immunocompromised)
Rhizopus		

698 • Laboratory Medicine

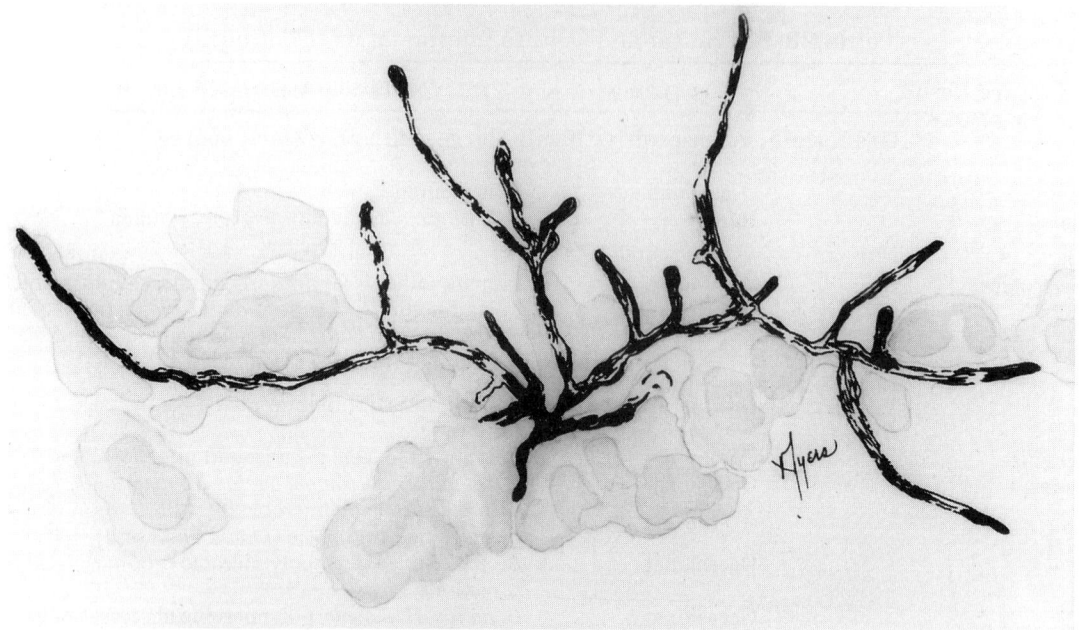

Fig. 23-11. Single agent infection, aerobic actinomycete. *Nocardia* spp. was presumptively confirmed by a positive partial acid fast stain. *Nocardia asteroides* was isolated in culture.

infections or necrotizing lesions are clostridia. *Bacillus* species have a similar morphologic appearance but only rarely cause infections.

The medium-sized gram-positive, pleomorphic, diphtheroid, or beaded gram-positive bacilli form a more heterogeneous array of considerations (Table 23-6). The critical element is to recognize their importance in the smear and then pursue their identification in culture. The presence of beaded gram-positive bacilli may represent rapid growing mycobacteria or diphtheroids. There is a tendency for colonies of "diphtheroids" in culture to be ignored as contaminants. All "diphtheroid-like" organisms should not be speciated but those that appear important in direct smears should be characterized following culture isolation. A culture report of

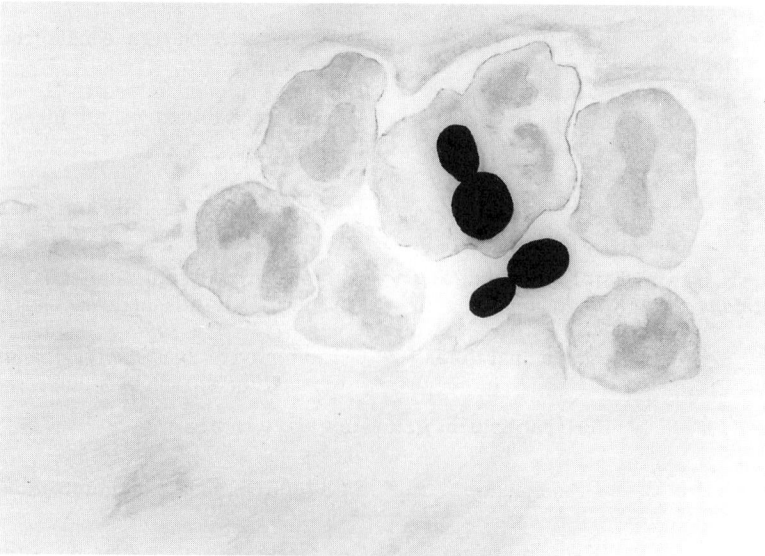

Fig. 23-12. Single agent infection, *Candida albicans*. The presence of an inflammatory exudate and the absence of contaminating materials support a presumption of this candida as pathogen in this infection.

"diphtheroids" will almost always be interpreted as a "contaminant," while a report of *"Mycobacterium fortuitum"* from culture of a subcutaneous abscess is always significant. The interpretation of gram-negative organisms can be correlated in culture with a Gram stained smear by dividing organisms into regular gram-negative bacilli and small gram-negative bacilli.

Fungal, Viral, and Parasitic Infections

Fungi in infections are also limited to a few morphologically distinct species. *Candida* spp. represents the most difficult culture isolate to interpret and again the direct smear is very helpful in separating pathogens from contaminants. Since fungi usually produce solid lesions and are isolated in special cultures, deep fungal infections are only occasionally recognized in "routine" smears.

Detection of any virus associated with a dermal lesion, exudate, or tissue is indicative of an etiologic role for the virus. Likewise, identification of any parasite in skin or tissue is diagnostic.

Contamination

Misinterpretation or failure to detect the etiologic agent can occur if the pathogen is overgrown by contaminating flora in a poorly collected specimen. When multiple organism morphotypes are present the type of background may help resolve whether they are infecting organisms (exudative background) or contaminants (epithelial cell background). Morphology of the polymicrobic mix may provide information about the type of organisms. Figure 23-13 shows a mixture of gram-positive cocci. This is consistent with polymicrobic skin flora infection, presumptively *S. aureus*, and/or *S. pyogenes*. A variety of other organisms such as viridans streptococci, micrococci, coagulase negative staphylococci, and cutaneous coryneforms are other possibilities. *S. aureus* or *S. pyogenes* has the greatest clinical significance and both will commonly inhibit many of the other organisms in general culture so that they will appear single or predominant. The less virulent members of the skin polymicrobic mix will on occasion be selected by chance or by antibiotic therapy and become the sole agents of infection. *Staphylococcus epidermidis, Corynebacterium jeikeium* (formally, group JK) or *Peptostreptococcus magnus* will appear in abscesses or wounds as sole or predominant pathogens when selected by antibiotic therapy.

Polymicrobic oropharyngeal flora infection (Fig. 23-14) presents an impressive array of different morphotypes. Most of these are fastidious anaerobic species and will not be seen in general bacterial culture. Viridans streptococci and *Neisseria* spp. may be the extent of the aerobic culture isolations. Polymicrobic infections with oropharyngeal flora are best handled by smear interpretation and empiric antibiotic therapy directed toward a mixed aerobic/anaerobic infection.

Polymicrobic fecal flora infection (Fig. 23-15) is distinctive for the presence of *C. perfringens, E. coli, B. fragilis* group, and *E. faecalis*, which can all be characterized in general culture. There are, however, many other species that may be involved in polymicrobial fecal flora infections. Presumptive therapy based on smear is useful because broad rather than narrow spectrum antibiotic treatment is required for the fecal polymicrobic infections regardless of culture results. Finally, smear examination may identify agents of infection that are not anticipated. Figure 23-16 shows a smear of *E. histolytica* from a cutaneous ulcer. Direct smear examination anticipates the occurrence of these types of unexpected infections. The major drawback to direct examination as a rapid means of diagnosis is that in most cases, interpretations of morphologic observations are subjective.

Interpretation of routine bacterial cultures from superficial skin lesions or wounds is particularly challenging because it is necessary to distinguish between the large variety of microbes known to produce disease and the indigenous or contaminating local microbial flora whose significance is not always clear.[11] The clinical setting will often provide important information for interpretation. Infection generally requires breaks in

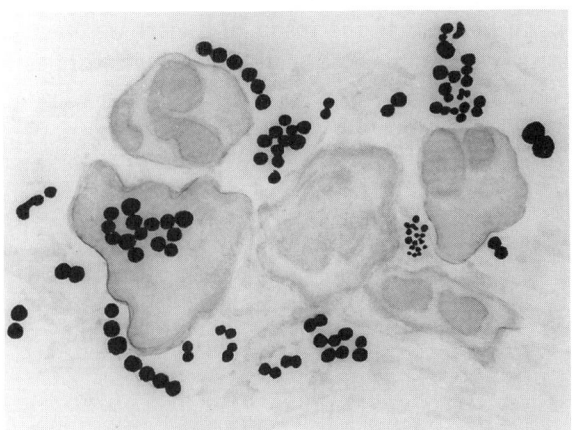

Fig. 23-13. Polymicrobic skin flora infection, exudate from cutaneous abscess. Precise aerobic/anaerobic culture isolated *Streptococcus pyogenes* (group A), *Staphylococcus aureus, S. lugdunensis,* anaerobic diphtheroids, and *Peptostreptococcus magnus*. General culture isolated and characterized only *S. pyogenes* and *S. aureus*.

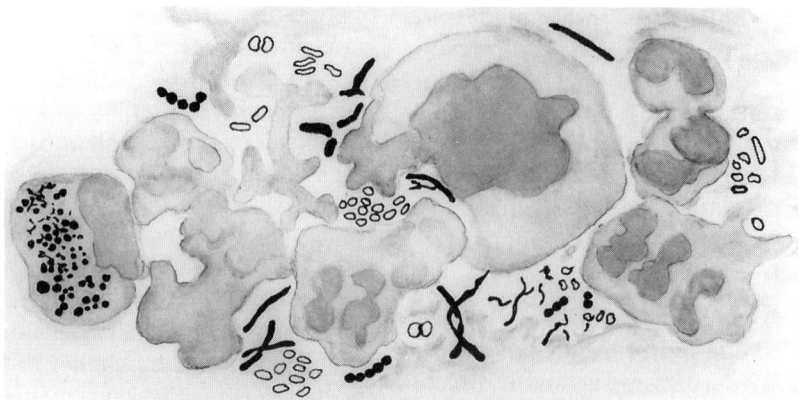

Fig. 23-14. Polymicrobic oropharyngeal flora infection, buccal space abscess. Aerobic and anaerobic culture isolated *Streptococcus sanguis*, *Neisseria* spp., *Staphylococcus epidermidis*, *Haemophilus parainfluenzae*, and anaerobic diphtheroids/actinomycetes. General culture reported "α streptococcus," *Neisseria* spp., *Staphylococcus* spp. (coagulase negative), and *Haemophilus parainfluenzae*.

the host's defenses or inocula with high numbers. Opportunistic pathogens occur in antibiotic treated or immunocompromised patients. Any isolated microbe must be interpreted with concern when poor nutrition, compromise in phagocytic cell populations, diminished immune functions, diminished microvascularity, severely traumatized surfaces, or indigenous microbial populations altered by antibiotic therapy occur.

Consultations

Good communications should exist among the patient's physician, microbiologist, and pathologist. Consultation is particularly important for serious or unusual cases in which the clues to diagnosis may be suggested in some but not all of the materials submitted for testing. For example, tissue submitted for histopathology may be positive for an important finding, while tissue from the same case submitted for culture can be negative or inappropriately cultured. An unusual finding in the culture may require knowledge about tissue pathologic processes for correct laboratory management of cultured organisms. Experts in infectious disease are invaluable consultants in unusual clinical presentations.

Specimen: Fluids, Aspirates, and Tissues

Background

Peritonitis

Bacterial infection in the abdominal cavity (peritonitis) can develop as the result of underlying vascular, obstructive, traumatic, infective, neoplastic, or postop-

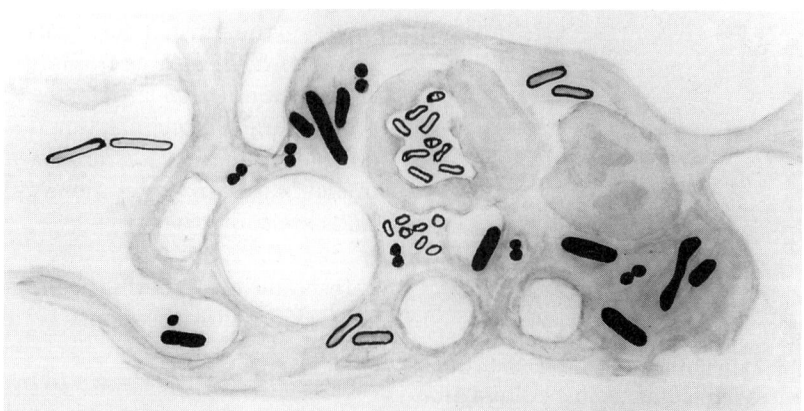

Fig. 23-15. Polymicrobic fecal flora infection and abdominal wall abscess. Aerobic and anaerobic culture isolated *Escherichia coli*, *Streptococcus faecalis*, *Clostridium perfringens*, and *Bacteroides fragilis*. General culture reported the same species isolated.

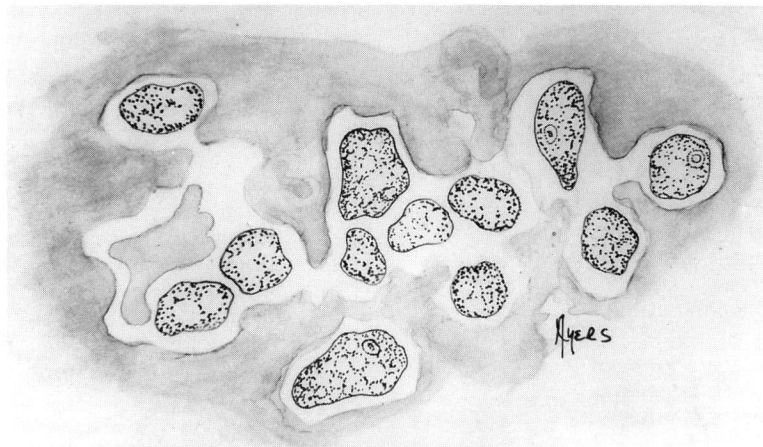

Fig. 23-16. Unexpected smear observation, cutaneous ulcer. Necrotic debris with foamy phagocytic cells. Special stains/culture confirmed *Entamoeba histolytica*.

erative conditions affecting the abdomen or adjacent areas. The infection is commonly polymicrobic including aerobic (Enterobacteriaceae, *P. aeruginosa*) and anaerobic gram-negative bacilli (*Bacteroides* spp.), as well as gram-positive cocci (enterococcus), *Clostridium* spp., and *Candida* spp. from the gastrointestinal or female genital tracts. Gonococcal peritonitis may also occur in females from infection in the fallopian tubes causing acute or chronic pelvic inflammatory disease. With expanded use of continuous ambulatory peritoneal dialysis (CAPD), the incidence of peritonitis as a complication from breaks in sterility has increased substantially.[12] *Staphylococcus epidermidis* is the most common etiologic agent followed by other organisms from the skin and environment (such as *S. aureus* and diphtheroids). Primary or spontaneous bacterial peritonitis is the least common type. This infection develops in patients with advanced, decompensated cirrhosis with ascites. *Escherichia coli* and other enteric organisms are most common, followed by pneumococci and *S. pyogenes*.[13] Microbiologic examination of peritoneal fluid is performed to identify the specific etiologic agent and to differentiate infection from nonbacterial peritonitis caused by introduction into the peritoneal cavity of irritants such as blood, bile, pancreatic juice, gastroduodenal juices, or meconium.

Abscesses

Liver and spleen abscesses are other important intra-abdominal infections.[14,15] Pylephlebitis of a portal vein tributary is produced by suppurative disease in tissues drained by the vessel, or from suppuration in contiguous structures, such as occurs in acute appendicitis or biliary tract infections. This may lead to pyogenic bacterial liver abscess. Multiple embolic abscesses may originate from foci anywhere in the body by way of the hepatic artery. Extension of infection directly, or by way of lymphatics, may develop from a perforated gallbladder, duodenal ulcer, or intra-abdominal abscess. Uncommon causes of liver abscesses are retrograde infection through the hepatic vein and infections secondary to penetrating wounds or foreign bodies. In many cases, the underlying cause of a liver abscess is unknown. Bowel flora (anaerobes, Enterobacteriaceae, *P. aeruginosa*, and *Enterococcus* spp.) predominate in pylephlebitis. Anaerobes are involved in at least 50% of cases of pyogenic liver abscess. Those most prevalent include streptococci, *Fusobacterium nucleatum*, and *B. fragilis*.

Splenic abscesses are rare. They usually arise as a result of hematogenous dissemination of microorganisms. The original focus of infection may be in the skin, respiratory tract, bone, endometrium, endocardium, or other organ. Occasionally, the infection spreads from contiguous organs or direct inoculation related to surgery or trauma.

Pelvic Infections

The etiologic agents causing soft tissue infections of the female pelvis (myometritis), as a postpartum or abortion complication, are similar to intra-abdominal infections, but may also include genital tract flora such as group B or group A *Streptococcus*, *S. aureus*, or even *Chlamydia trachomatis*. *Clostridium perfringens* infection is particularly severe and may require hysterectomy for cure. A pelvic abscess may complicate salpingo-oophoritis. Sometimes associated with intrauterine device use, the infection usually involves an-

Table 23-7. Acute Viruses That May Cause Hepatitis

Coxsackieviruses A4,9;B5
Herpesviruses
    Cytomegalovirus[a]
    Epstein-Barr virus[a]
    Herpes simplex virus
Togaviruses
    Dengue
    Yellow fever virus
Hepatitis virus
    Hepatitis A virus
    Hepatitis B virus
    Hepatitis C virus

[a] Often associated with concurrent mononucleosis

Table 23-8. Predominant Organ Parasites Causing Disease Syndromes Within the Liver, Spleen, Intestinal Wall, and Heart

Liver parenchyma
    Entamoeba histolytica
    Toxoplasma gondii
    Schistosoma mansoni
    Schistosoma japonicum
    Schistosoma mekongi
    Echinococcus granulosus (hydatidosis)
    Echinococcus multilocularis (alveolar hydatidosis)
    Taenia solium (cysticercosis)
    Toxocara spp.
Biliary system
    Clonorchis sinensis
    Opisthorchis viverrini
    Fasciola hepatica
Reticuloendothelial system (Kupffer cells)
    Leishmania donovani
    Toxoplasma gondii
Spleen
    Leishmania donovani
    Trypanosoma cruzi
Intestinal wall
    Schistosoma mansoni
    Schistosoma japonicum
    Schistosoma mekongi
    Trypanosoma cruzi
Heart
    Trypanosoma cruzi
    Toxoplasma gondii
    Taenia solium (cysticercosis)

aerobic bacteria, occasionally including *Actinomyces* spp.

Suspected Viral Infections

A limited number of viruses may infect the liver, either as a primary infection (hepatitis A, B, C, and delta viruses), or as a manifestation of more widespread disease (Table 23-7). Infection is typically more severe in the immunocompromised patient. Transmission of hepatitis A often occurs by the fecal-oral route and is associated with epidemics. Infected young children are commonly asymptomatic but can easily pass on the disease to adults. Chronic infection does not occur. Hepatitis B and C are transmitted by exposure to blood or by sexual contact. In some cases, infection progresses to a chronic stage with significant compromise of liver function and risk of secondary neoplasia (hepatoma). However, in most cases a diagnostic and protective serologic response is produced, and the infection resolves within a few weeks to months.

Suspected Parasitic Disease

A variety of protozoal and helminthic parasites may localize within internal organs and be responsible for significant disease (Table 23-8). Among the protozoa, *E. histolytica* is one of the most common parasitic infections and a well known cause of hepatic abscess in the United States. Infection occurs by ingesting cysts in contaminated food or water, or by fecal-oral contact. Although the organism is usually confined to the intestine, invasive extraintestinal disease occurs in a small proportion of patients for reasons that are not clear (see Ch. 28). Complications include rupture into the pleural space, extension into the peritoneum and through the skin, and secondary hematogenous spread to the lung or brain.

Leishmania donovani is responsible for visceral leishmaniasis, a disease of the reticuloendothelial system of the liver and spleen. *Toxoplasma gondii*, as part of a disseminated infection, may cause encephalitis, pneumonitis, myocarditis, or even hepatitis in susceptible individuals. It is also an important cause of congenital infection (see Ch. 29). Infection is usually acquired from ingesting raw meat (especially lamb) or by being exposed to infectious oocysts excreted in the feces of an infected pet cat. Less common means of transmission include blood transfusion and organ transplantation.

Among the helminths, a variety of flukes have a preference for the biliary system and are responsible for both acute and chronic disease. *Fasciola hepatica*, largest of the liver flukes (larger than 1 in.), resides primarily in the large bile ducts and gallbladder, and is acquired from eating freshwater plants such as watercress. *Clonorchis sinensis* and *Opisthorchis viverrini* are more slender worms, localizing in the smaller distal bile ducts, and are acquired from eating raw freshwater fish. Significant irritation to the bile ducts occurs with chronic worm infection, which may progress to fibrosis, obstruction, and abscess formation. *Clonorchis* is typically found in China, Taiwan, Japan, Korea, and Vietnam, whereas *Opisthorchis* is commonly found in Thailand, and *Fasciola* has a cosmopolitan distribution.

Serious hepatic and intestinal fibrosis results from infection with the blood flukes *Schistosoma mansoni*, *Schistosoma japonicum*, and *Schistosoma mekongi*. Disease syndromes include cercarial dermatitis, and acute (Katayama fever) and chronic schistosomiasis. Chronic disease occurs months to years after the initial infection and results from the continuous deposition and entrapment of worm eggs both in the intestinal wall and liver. Granulomas produced by host reaction to egg antigens ultimately lead to extensive fibrosis of both organs. With the development of portal hypertension, collateral circulation develops and ascites may become prominent. *Schistosoma mansoni* infections are found primarily in Egypt, western and central Africa, the West Indies, and portions of South America. *Schistosoma japonicum* occurs in the Far East and tends to cause the most severe disease because of increased egg production. *Schistosoma mekongi* is found in Indochina and causes a disease similar to that of *S. japonicum*.

Cysticercosis results from the accidental ingestion of *Taenia solium* eggs either in contaminated food or from self-infection via the oral-fecal route. It is endemic to Mexico and parts of Africa and South America. Cysticerci may appear in any of the internal organs as part of a systemic dissemination, but most commonly cause symptomatic disease either in the central nervous system or eye, and only rarely in the liver. Subcutaneous cysts may also be evident on physical examination, underlying the systemic nature of the infection. Hydatid cysts of the tapeworm *Echinococcus granulosus* commonly present as space occupying lesions in the liver. Hydatid disease occurs wherever sheep and cattle raising are prominent occupations, hence this syndrome is seen worldwide. Any member of the dog family may serve as definitive host for the adult tapeworms. Eggs shed in the feces of the dog are immediately infectious for the next host when ingested, including humans. Children are at highest risk for acquiring this infection because of their close attachment with pet dogs. Larval tapeworms most commonly develop in the liver (60–70%) and remain asymptomatic until their size affects adjacent organs.

The syndrome of visceral larval migrans caused by the cat or dog roundworm *Toxocara* is most commonly seen in children, and may affect the liver, lungs, central nervous system, and eyes.[16] Following accidental ingestion of *Toxocara canis* or *Toxocara cati* eggs by humans, larvae hatch in the small intestine and migrate to the liver, lungs, and other organs, including the eyes. The larvae do not mature, and continue their migrations until they are encapsulated and destroyed, which may take 1 year or more. A high level of eosinophilia is characteristic of this infection. Recognition of the disease syndrome is becoming more commonplace and use of serologic tests has shown it to be much more widespread than previously thought.

Selection

Peritonitis

Signs and Symptoms. The mode of onset of peritonitis varies according to the precipitating cause. Typical findings are pain, abdominal distension, absence of abdominal respiratory movement, diffuse muscle spasm, tenderness and rebound tenderness, decreased or absent peristalsis, rigidity of the abdominal wall, and fever. Pain and muscle spasm may be deceptively absent in the very old or young and in patients with shock. Signs of peritonitis may be overshadowed by manifestations of the primary process such as trauma to the abdomen. In primary bacterial peritonitis, there is often marked fever and leukocytosis, with typical abdominal findings. However, in patients with cirrhosis, the disease may be quite insidious. Radiographs of the abdomen or computed tomography (CT) scans may reveal free gas in the peritoneal cavity, features of ileus or obstruction, or evidence of peritoneal fluid. The presentation of salpingitis should not be confused with peritonitis unless it is complicated by abscess formation.

Specimen Collection and Examination. Collection of CAPD fluid, or in other cases, needle aspiration of the peritoneal cavity (paracentesis) is indicated whenever signs and symptoms suggest peritonitis.[17] Culdocentesis may be attempted to obtain infected fluid or abscess specimens in the pelvic region. The specimen should be examined microscopically with Gram stained smears for bacteria and fungi, and cultured under aerobic and anaerobic conditions. A cell count and amylase determination (to exclude pancreatitis) should be performed. Endocervical culture for *N. gonorrhoeae* should be performed whenever symptoms of pelvic inflammatory disease are present.

Abscesses

Hepatic. Patients with liver abscess frequently present with abdominal pain, nausea, vomiting, ascites, enlargement and tenderness of the liver, and sometimes splenomegaly. Fever is almost always present and frequently accompanied by chills and sweats. Right upper quadrant pain over the liver or epigastrium is common with painful percussion of the liver. Sometimes the course is quite indolent, although weight loss and jaundice indicate a poorer prognosis. A number of different radiographic and imaging studies are helpful in the diagnosis including ultrasonography, CT, liver scans, hepatic arteriography, splenoportography, and T-tube cholangiography. When bacterial infection is suspected, percutaneous aspiration may be undertaken for diagnostic purposes; however, surgical drainage is preferred.[18] It is during the surgical procedure that an aspirate of pus or tissue is obtained for microbiology cultures. Occasionally, medical therapy with antimicrobial agents with or without percutaneous aspiration drainage of the abscess is successful. This approach is used for patients who are poor surgical candidates.

Amebic liver abscess is suggested by the presence of upper right abdominal pain, fever, hepatomegaly, leukocytosis, and roentgenographic evidence of a fluid filled cavity. A history of residence or travel to Mexico is common. Patients who present with an amebic liver abscess often have no evidence of prior intestinal infection, and stool examinations may be negative. Serologic testing is always indicated because of its high sensitivity and specificity. In many cases, this infection can be diagnosed and treated without aspiration. This is fortunate because the procedure carries the risk of amebic peritonitis from leakage into the peritoneal cavity. In addition, when an aspirate is obtained, microscopic examination for bacteria and amoebae is always indicated, but the results are often negative.

Splenic. Splenic abscess often presents with sudden onset of chills, fever, and left upper quadrant pain. With the upper pole involvement, there is common left pleuritic pain radiating to the left shoulder, elevated left diaphragm, and left pleural effusion. Abscess in the lower pole gives rise to signs of peritoneal inflammation. The spleen is frequently palpable and tender. The helpful diagnostic procedure is CT scanning. Splenic arteriography may show displacement or splenic vessels. Splenectomy is often required for treating splenic abscess. The specimen obtained should be examined microscopically and cultured both aerobically and anaerobically. With smaller abscesses, antimicrobial therapy with close follow-up by CT scanning can be attempted.

Suspected Viral Disease

Previously healthy patients with viral hepatitis usually have characteristic findings of malaise, weakness, nausea, vomiting, and mild right upper quadrant pain. This is followed by the onset of jaundice and dark urine from bile obstruction. Fever, rash, and arthritis are variable findings. Various degrees of illness occur, from a common mild asymptomatic infection to a rare form of acute fulminate hepatitis. Laboratory findings are similarly characteristic with elevated serum transaminase and bilirubin levels. Serologic testing for the most likely viral agents based on the clinical and epidemiologic presentation is indicated for the diagnosis, as described in Chapter 29. Liver biopsy is sometimes necessary to evaluate immunocompromised patients with hepatic failure presumed to be caused by a viral agent. Viral culture and examination for inclusion bodies should be performed on these specimens.

Suspected Parasitic Disease

Visceral leishmaniasis is suspected in an individual with fever, anorexia, hepatosplenomegaly, anemia, leukopenia, hypergammaglobulinemia, and a history of travel or residence in an endemic area. Analysis of bone marrow, splenic or hepatic aspirates or biopsies, and buffy coat smears for the typical amastigotes are indicated. Although splenic puncture appears to be most sensitive, this technique poses significant risk to the patient. Culture should also be performed on these specimens. Serologic tests, if available, may be helpful if parasites are not detected by other means.

Clinical disease caused by *Toxoplasma* may take a variety of forms in the newborn or in the immunocompromised patient, and the diagnosis may be problematic. Although immunocompetent persons rarely appear symptomatic, those with AIDS or an other underlying immunodeficiency (such as organ transplant, cancer, or chemotherapy patients) may develop life-threatening disease following reactivation of latent infection in one or more organ systems. Serologic studies will usually provide evidence of acute disease. The use of histologic procedures including immunoperoxidase staining on biopsy specimens is a valuable adjunct, and may be performed along with attempts to isolate the organism in tissue culture or laboratory animals.

Symptoms of liver fluke infection relate to obstruction of the biliary tract and cholangitis, in addition to epigastric pain, fever, jaundice, hepatomegaly, and eosinophilia, depending on the intensity of infection. Chronic schistosomiasis may present with hepatosplenomegaly, portal hypertension, and ascites following the chronic deposition of eggs in the liver with continuous fibrosis. A variety of other presentations are also seen with schistosomiasis, and are reviewed elsewhere (see Ch. 26). When suspected, diagnosis of both liver and blood fluke infections is made predominantly with stool examination and in the case of fascioliasis, bile examination for characteristic ova and parasites.[19] In addition, liver or rectal biopsies may reveal evidence of schistosomiasis. Serologic studies are available for help in diagnosing possible occult schistosome infections, although cross-reactions with other helminths limit their usefulness.

Definitive diagnosis of cysticercosis depends on the surgical removal of a cyst and histologic examination for the presence of the suckers and hooks of the *T. solium* scolex. Computed tomography or magnetic resonance imaging (MRI) scans may reveal the presence of cysticerci in various organs, and calcified larvae may be readily seen on radiographs. Presentation of hydatid disease is dependent on the anatomic location and size of the cyst. Small cysts in a vital area may cause severe damage whereas some large cysts may remain undetected for many years. Hydatids may thus be detected as either symptomatic or asymptomatic space occupying lesions on radiograph or scan. Surgical removal remains the treatment of choice. If this intervention is selected, cyst fluid may be aspirated and examined for the presence of hydatid sand (protoscolices and hooklets of the larval tapeworms) to confirm the diagnosis. Accidental spillage of cyst contents during this procedure may, however, place the patient at risk for anaphylactic shock or dissemination of the disease. Serologic testing should be performed whenever cysticercosis or hydated disease is suspected. *Echinococcus multilocularis* is responsible for a related disease, alveolar hydatidosis. This infection is more insidious, mimicking a slow growing invasive carcinoma of the liver. Because protoscolices do not develop in humans infected with alveolar hydatidosis, the correct diagnosis may be difficult to make, and relies instead on identifying, by histology, laminated membranes typical for the species.

Visual larva migrans is often first suspected when high peripheral eosinophilia (up to 90%) is noted in children with fever, hepatomegaly, neurologic disturbances, pulmonary infiltrates, or endophthalmitis. Although larvae of *Toxocara* may occasionally be seen on biopsy specimens, sociologic testing for diagnosis is the best approach for diagnosing visceral larval migrans (*T. canis* or *T. cati* infection). Biopsy material is rarely of value. Children found to have *Ascaris* or *Trichuris* infection may be suspected of having toxocariasis as well, because of similar modes of transmission.

Logistics

Specimen Collection

Paracentesis is a procedure in which peritoneal fluid is aspirated from a needle sterilely inserted through the abdominal wall into the peritoneal cavity. Peritoneal lavage may be required if fluid cannot be obtained by needle aspiration. Similarly, dialysate fluid should be collected in a sterile manner through the intra-abdominal catheter. Fluid in the pelvic region can be collected by inserting a needle through the vaginal wall (culdocentesis). Contamination with normal flora from skin, rectum, vagina, or other body surfaces must be avoided. For percutaneous liver biopsy or aspiration, the overlying and adjacent areas must be carefully prepared to eliminate isolation of potentially contaminating anaerobes that colonize the skin surface. During surgery, fluid and pus should be aspirated and tissue collected for microbiologic examination. The use of swabs should be avoided. Anaerobic transport systems should be employed. All air should be expelled from a syringe after the specimen is collected. Every attempt should be made to deliver the specimen to the laboratory immediately.

Tissues for viral culture, whether biopsy or autopsy, should be collected aseptically and placed into a sterile container. A pea-sized piece of tissue or small punch biopsy is sufficient for study. When possible, a lesion in the tissue should be evaluated, taking care to avoid contamination of the specimen with blood if possible. Recent advances in in situ hybridization have made it possible to detect some viruses in tissue directly rather than using isolation in cell culture. Thus, the nature of the method used for detection may dictate the manner in which the specimen is submitted. Moreover, specimens submitted for cytologic examination to the pathology laboratory also may be used for in situ hybridization. These factors make it important to coordinate procedures between the clinician and laboratory to get a complete and efficient evaluation.

Analysis

Routine. The quantity of microorganisms in paracentesis fluid can vary markedly. In some cases, particularly CAPD associated infections, but also, other types of peritonitis, the concentration of organisms may be less than 1/mL of fluid. It is therefore important to apply methods that will increase sensitivity by culturing as much fluid as practical.[20] Microscopic examination and culture of a only a few milliliters will result in an unacceptably large proportion of false negative results. Several techniques have been described for increasing the sensitivity of paracentesis and CAPD fluid cultures. A sediment of the fluid can be prepared by centrifugation. This has the advantage that a large volume of specimen can be easily processed. Likewise, the specimen can be concentrated by using sterile disposable membrane filters (0.45 μm). After filtration, the membrane filter, which retains microorganisms, can be placed directly onto agar media. While this method is very sensitive, it is the most labor intensive and the filter is easily clogged by inflammatory cells. Direct inoculation of the specimen into broth bottles at the bedside or in the laboratory has been recommended. This method is reliable if a sufficient volume can be cultured. Alternatively, broth can be added to a bag containing CAPD fluid and the entire bag incubated.

The fluid should be grossly examined and described. It may be turbid, purulent, or bloody. A Gram stained smear of the fluid's sediment should be examined microscopically for organisms and inflammatory cells. The specimen should be cultured aerobically and anaerobically using nonselective media such as 5% sheep blood agar. Chocolate agar media should be used to detect *N. gonorrhoeae* and other fastidious organisms. Since anaerobic infections rarely, if ever, occur in CAPD associated peritonitis, the anaerobic culture can be excluded for these specimens. Aspirates of pus and ground tissue specimens should be examined by Gram stained smear and cultured aerobically and anaerobically.

Mixed culture results are commonplace when infection is secondary to gastrointestinal tract trauma.[21] When multiple different organisms are found by smear and culture, it is important to recognize that there is usually little value in identifying everything present to the species level and performing susceptibility tests on all isolates.[11] In this circumstance, surgery and treatment with broad spectrum antimicrobial agents take precedent over attempting to "fine tune" the therapy based on supplying a long list of organisms from fecal flora discharged into the abdominal cavity. However, when a single organism or only a few different organisms are isolated, the likelihood that they are responsible for the infection is high. These should be fully identified. Special cultures should be performed only when *Mycobacterium tuberculosis* or fungi are suspected from the clinical history.

For Parasites. Examination of a presumed amebic abscess may include either aspirate or biopsy material. Unfortunately, most of the aspirated material will contain necrotic debris, and care must be taken to examine material from the abscess wall where organisms are more likely to be found. Histologic diagnosis may be made using routine hematoxylin and eosin and/or periodic acid-Schiff stains. Visceral leishmaniasis may be diagnosed definitively by finding the amastigote stages in Giemsa stained smears from splenic or bone marrow aspirates, or from buffy coat preparations. Biopsy material may be used for imprint smears and submitted for histology.[22] The medium of Novy, McNeal, and Nicolle (NNN) can be used to culture clinical specimens for leishmania, and is easily prepared.

Infections caused by either liver or blood flukes may be diagnosed using routine direct ova and parasite examinations of stool, including use of concentration techniques. The formalin ethyl acetate concentration method is recommended over the zinc sulfate flotation technique for recovery of most helminth eggs. Direct examination of rectal biopsies between two glass slides is a simple method of examining for light schistosome infections. Schistosome eggs with associated granulomas should be looked for on liver biopsies.

Interpretation

Evaluation of peritoneal fluid for its appearance, volume, and cell count with differential are valuable adjuncts to preliminary and differential diagnosis.[23] The normal appearance of peritoneal, ascites, and CAPD fluid is clear and colorless to pale yellow. The white blood cell count is less than 500/mm^3 with fewer than 25% neutrophils and the red blood cell count is less than 100,000/mm.^{3} A cloudy fluid with large numbers of inflammatory cells suggests infectious peritonitis but must be differentiated from noninfectious causes. Failure to obtain fluid does not exclude acute infection.

Under sterile conditions of collection and handling, any organism, even in small numbers, should be considered the causative agent of infection. The exception to this is the isolation of multiple aerobic and anaerobic organisms from a patient with traumatic leakage of gastrointestinal or female lower genital tract flora into the peritoneal cavity. In this condition, the presence of "mixed flora" is a valuable indicator of the underlying pathologic process, but has much less value for directing specific therapy, since it is impossible to determine which of the many organisms is significant, and whether all have been recovered by culture. Cultures of paracentesis fluid may be negative when the patient has been previously treated with antibiotics or the culture method is insufficiently sensitive, even when high numbers of inflammatory cells are present. In this case "culture negative" bacterial peritonitis should be presumed and treated empirically.

In patients with liver abscess, the leukocyte count and serum alkaline phosphatase are almost always elevated, while serum transaminases can be normal.[18] Blood cultures are positive in one-third to one-half of the patients. Any organism isolated or parasite seen on direct examination can be considered to be the etiologic agent. As discussed above, failure to observe amebae by microscopic examination of an aspirate does not exclude the diagnosis of amebic liver abscess (see Ch. 29 for interpretation of amebic serology tests).

Specimen: Synovial Fluid

Background

Acute bacterial (septic) arthritis is a serious medical problem requiring prompt recognition and appropriate treatment to avoid permanent joint damage. The infection can occur as a secondary complication of bacteremia with *N. gonorrhoeae, S. aureus,* and others. Because the synovium is vascular and lacks a limiting membrane, bacteria from the bloodstream can freely enter the joint cavity. Joint infection may also result from an intra-articular steroid injection, penetrating trauma, direct extension of adjacent osteomyelitis, arthroscopy, or surgery. An increased susceptibility to joint infection occurs in patients with diabetes, cancer, liver disease, chronic alcoholism, hypogammaglobulinemia, and in those receiving steroids or immunosuppressive drugs. In addition, joints previously damaged by trauma or chronic arthritis, especially rheumatoid arthritis, are more susceptible to infections.

Acute bacterial arthritis is caused by many different types of bacteria. The most frequent pathogens in children are *S. pyogenes* and in neonates, *Haemophilus influenzae.* The most common cause of septic arthritis in young adults (particularly women) is *N. gonorrhoeae. Neisseria meningitidis* may mimic gonococcal arthritis and can cause both polyarthralgias and monoarticular involvement. *Staphylococcus aureus* is the most common nongonococcal infecting agent in adults, followed by gram-negative bacilli, group A *S. pyogenes,* and in patients over 60 years, *S. pneumoniae.* Gram-negative bacilli (*E. coli, Salmonella* spp., *P. aeruginosa*) tend to occur in patients with underlying infection of the urinary, biliary, or intestinal tract, patients with impaired resistance to infection, and in intravenous drug abusers. Patients with arthritis caused by *Salmonella* spp. often have evidence of underlying osteomyelitis. *Salmonella* spp. bacteremia in patients with sickle cell anemia is occasionally followed by septic arthritis, however, most cases of *Salmonella* spp. arthritis are not associated with hemoglobinopathies. Infectious arthritis of the spine is most frequently caused by staphylococci. Brucellosis, tuberculosis, and *Salmonella* spp. also preferentially involve the spine. *Pseudomonas* spp. and *Serratia* spp. arthritis are frequently associated with parenteral drug abuse. Septic arthritis caused by anaerobic bacteria may occur as a complication of musculoskeletal surgeries and traumatic injuries. The most frequently involved microorganisms are *Peptococcus* spp. and *B. fragilis.*

Tuberculous arthritis has an insidious onset, is usually monoarticular, and most commonly involves the hip or knee joints. *Mycobacterium tuberculosis* is the usual pathogen and is often associated with osteomyelitis. Nontuberculous *Mycobacterium* spp. cause infectious arthritis from local trauma. All fungi associated with deep mycotic infections may cause infectious arthritis, including *Candida* spp., histoplasmosis, coccidioidomycosis, blastomycosis, aspergillosis, and sporotrichosis. *Actinomyces israelii* and *Nocardia* spp. may cause arthritis clinically similar to arthritis produced by mycobacteria and fungi. These infections often occur in joints damaged by osteoarthritis, neuropathic joint disease (Charcot's arthritis), or ankylosing spondylitis.

Arthritis may develop in the course of several types of viral infections either from primary involvement (rubella or mumps) or as a complication from circulating immune complexes (hepatitis B virus). Viral causes of arthritis are coxsackieviruses, hepatitis B virus, lymphocytic choriomeningitis virus, mumps, parvovirus (associated with rheumatoid arthritis), rubella and rubella vaccine (usually seen in women), and varicella.

Selection

The diagnosis of septic arthritis cannot be established without examination of the synovial fluid.[24] In most cases of infectious arthritis, the clinical presentation of the patient and radiographic findings substantially narrow the differential diagnosis and suggest both how to acquire and process the specimen. In bacterial arthritis, the affected joint is warm, erythematous, swollen, and painful; however, these signs may be less marked in elderly patients or patients receiving immunosuppressive drugs. It is worthwhile to note that the manifestations of an acute infection might be dampened by the previous administration of corticosteroids. Mycobacterial or fungal infections may present with only a low grade fever and night sweats without prominent constitutional symptoms. Although the affected peripheral joint is usually swollen and warm, with a decreased range of motion, erythema is minimal and pain is initially mild.

The diagnosis can be made by finding microorganisms on Gram stain of synovial fluid or in synovial tissue, and is confirmed by isolating an organism from culture. It is important to draw blood at the time of arthrocentesis for blood culture as well as for the valid comparison of synovial fluid and blood glucose concentrations. Cultures of the oropharynx, cervix, and rectum should also be performed when *N. gonorrhoeae* is suspected. Other forms of acute arthritis such as gout, pseudogout, Reiter syndrome, rheumatoid arthritis, or psoriatic arthritis must be differentiated from infectious etiologies.

Serologic studies are useful when brucellosis or coccidioidomycosis is suspected but not yet diagnosed from other clinical findings. Antigens of *S. pneumoniae, H. influenzae,* and *S. pyogenes* can be detected in synovial fluid when these organisms are the cause of infection. Although these tests can provide a rapid diagnosis in some cases, they rarely provide more information than can be obtained from the Gram smear. Furthermore, the patient with suspected septic arthritis must be treated with antibiotics regardless of the results of preliminary tests (antigen and microscopic examination). Antigen testing is best reserved for use in partially treated cases that fail to grow an organism from the synovial fluid specimen. The *Limulus* lysate assay for endotoxin has also been shown to be positive in infections caused by gram-negative bacteria, but this is not a widely applied test. Lactic acid is typically elevated in synovial fluid infected by bacteria, although this test rarely contributes any information that is not already, and more specifically, provided by the microscopic and culture examination. Viral cultures of synovial fluid are rarely, if ever, indicated.

Terminology

Septic arthritis defines the invasion of the synovial membrane by microorganisms, usually with extension into the joint space to produce a close space infection. Synonyms include suppurative arthritis, infectious arthritis, acute pyogenic arthritis, and pyarthrosis.

Logistics

Specimen Collection

Using aseptic techniques, synovial fluid is obtained by percutaneous aspiration of fluid through a needle placed in the joint space (arthrocentesis). The specimen is divided into three tubes as follows: (1) a sterile tube for cultures and serology; (2) a tube with anticoagulant, such as EDTA for cell examination; and (3) a tube for chemical determinations. A small amount of sterile heparin can be added to avoid clotting. Synovial fluid may be directly inoculated into liquid culture media at the bedside, but part of the sample must be saved for microscopic examination and culture onto agar media.

A synovial tissue biopsy should be placed in a dry sterile container with a secure lid or in a Petri dish, without preservative and transported immediately to the laboratory. A synovial biopsy specimen (if submitted for culture) should be separated from the portion submitted for histopathology by the surgeon or pathologist using sterile techniques. The laboratory should be informed of the specific source of the specimen, age of patient, current antibiotic therapy, and clinical diagnosis. Specimens should be transported to the laboratory immediately at room temperature.

Analysis

A clear or slightly cloudy specimen should be concentrated by centrifugation to prepare a sediment for microscopic examination and culture. A frankly purulent specimen can be processed directly. A Gram smear of the synovial fluid should be examined for microorganisms and inflammatory cells. Under appropriate clinical circumstances, special stains may be used to detect mycobacteria or fungi. A cell count, glucose, and protein determination should also be performed on the fluid. Synovial fluid is cultured aerobically with increased CO_2 (5%) on nonselective media, such as 5% sheep blood or brucella agar. Chocolate agar, which supports the growth of *N. gonorrhoeae* and *H. influenzae,* should always be used. Appropriate antimicrobial susceptibility studies should be performed on all isolates. Special cultures for anaerobes, mycobacteria, or fungi should be reserved for patients in which the clinical presentation suggests the possibility of infection with these organisms. In rare cases, the use of hyperosomolar culture medium may aid in the isolation of cell wall deficient bacteria from the synovial fluid of patients who have already received antimicrobial therapy.

Interpretation

The etiologic diagnosis is made by isolating the organism in culture. The Gram stained smear is positive in about one-half of culture confirmed cases. Negative smears are particularly common in patients with gonococcal arthritis and in patients who have received antibiotic therapy before arthrocentesis. Microscopic ex-

Table 23-9. Characteristics of Synovial Fluid in Septic Arthritis Compared with Synovial Fluid in Noninfectious Conditions

Characteristic	Infectious	Noninfectious Inflammation	Noninflammatory effusion
Color	Yellow to green	Yellow	Colorless to pale
Turbidity	Purulent, turbid	Turbid	Clear to slightly turbid
Mucin precipitate	Small, friable	Small, friable	Tight, ropy clump
Leukocytes/μL	>10,000	1000–5000	<1000
Predominant cell	Neutrophil	Neutrophil	Mononuclear leukocyte
Synovial fluid/blood glucose ratio	<0.6	0.6–0.8	0.8–1.0
Protein (g/dL)	3–7	3–7	1–5
Lactic acid (mg/dL)	>65	<65	<65

amination of a Gram stained smear or identification of bacterial antigen using immunologic techniques supports the diagnosis but should be confirmed by culture findings. The culture results should always be correlated with Gram stain, synovial fluid gross appearance, cell counts, glucose, blood culture results, and the patient's clinical condition and previous history, including antibiotic treatment.

Bacterial infection provokes a brisk inflammatory reaction in the synovial fluid (polymorphonuclear leukocyte count greater than 50,000/μL) and a decreased concentration of glucose (Table 23-9). It should be noted that low glucose concentrations are not a consistent finding and may also be present in active rheumatoid arthritis. Synovial fluid leukocytosis may be depressed by immunosuppression including malignancies, steroid use, and intravenous drug abuse.[25] Viral arthritis is usually associated with a predominance of mononuclear cells. The erythrocyte sedimentation rate is typically elevated and the peripheral blood leukocyte count may or may not be elevated.

Specimen: Bone[26,27]

Background

General

Infection of bone (osteomyelitis) is usually caused by bacteria. They reach the site of infection by hematogenous spread, extension from a contiguous site of infection, or by direct entry by trauma or surgery. In children, osteomyelitis usually involves the long bones. The metaphyseal sinusoidal veins, with sluggish blood flow and paucity of phagocytes, favor the growth of organisms. The most common site in adults is the vertebrae where cellular marrow and abundant vascular supply still exist. Osteomyelitis caused by extension from a contiguous site of infection may occur with soft tissue suppuration resulting from such causes as trauma, burns, cellulitis (especially in diabetic patients with vascular insufficiency), necrosis of a malignant tumor, or pressure sores. Direct introduction of organisms into bone may occur with open fractures or penetrating trauma by foreign bodies. Osteomyelitis may also occur from perioperative contamination of bone during surgery for nontraumatic orthopaedic disorders. Most infections of joint prosthesis arise in this way. Osteomyelitis associated with a prosthesis generally requires its removal, thorough debridement, and appropriate antimicrobial therapy. In osteomyelitis associated with advanced vascular insufficiency, cure is seldom possible without amputation.

The diagnosis of infection associated with a prosthetic joint may be difficult. In general, infections may be divided into early versus late postsurgical events, and superficial versus deep infections. Early joint infections are acquired during surgical procedure. In the early postoperative period, a superficial wound infection is usually easy to identify and may require only simple drainage and a short course of antibiotics. A deep infection in this early period is marked by pain, swelling, fever, and leukocytosis. The most common cause is *S. aureus*, and aggressive surgical debridement (without removal of the prosthesis) and prolonged parenteral antibacterial therapy may salvage the prosthetic joint. Late prosthetic infections sometimes occur as a consequence of bacteremia. These infections typically cause pain without fever, chills, or evidence of acute joint infection.

Causative Organisms

Age is an important determinant of the etiology of osteomyelitis. *Staphylococcus aureus* is the most common agent causing osteomyelitis in children. However, infants are very susceptible to infection with gram-negative enteric bacilli and group B streptococci.[28] In children younger than 6 months of age, it is axiomatic that bacteriemia with these organisms may be followed by osteomyelitis. From infancy to about 5 years of age, *H. influenzae* commonly causes bacteriemia but rarely osteomyelitis. *Staphylococcus aureus* most often follows bacteriemia in late childhood and at puberty. In adults, in about 50% of the patients with hematogenous *S. aureus* osteomyelitis, there is a recognizable, preceding focus of infection, often furunculosis. The common sources for bacteriemias that lead to osteomyelitis are infections involving the skin, respiratory tract, and genitourinary tract. Intravenous drug abusers are particularly prone to develop infections of the spine and sternoclavicular joint caused by *P. aeruginosa*. Patients with sickle cell disease and sickle cell trait are predisposed to *Salmonella* spp. osteomyelitis. Puncture wounds are often associated with pseudomonal osteomyelitis. Immunosuppression may predispose the patient to osteomyelitis. Unusual microorganisms that may be involved include *Listeria monocytogenes, Aspergillus* spp., and *Candida* spp. In diabetic patients with peripheral vascular disease, osteomyelitis may occur in the distal extremities. Although these infections are most often caused by *S. aureus,* there is also a high incidence of infection with the Enterobacteriaceae, particularly *Proteus* spp., and anaerobic bacteria. *Bacteroides melaninogenicus* and other anaerobes of the oropharynx may cause osteomyelitis of the mandible or other bones of the face or head, especially in association with oral or dental infections. Granulomatous osteomyelitis is typically caused by *M. tuberculosis* or fungi. When several bones are apparently involved simultaneously, a specific cause of the osteomyelitis such as *Salmonella* spp. or *Cryptococcus neoformans* should be suspected.

Selection

General

Early recognition of osteomyelitis is important to avoid progression to chronic disease caused by impairment of blood flow to the involved bone. Findings include bone pain, soft tissue swelling, and limited motion of the extremities. The diagnosis of osteomyelitis should be considered even when there is soft tissue infection or ulceration that in itself could be responsible for the clinical findings (pus, draining sinuses). Radiographic evidence of infection typically appears late and cannot be relied on to confirm the diagnosis without risking progression to chronic disease. While the clinical presentation and radiographic findings help to narrow the field of suspected etiologic pathogens and aid in judgments about empiric antimicrobial therapy, it is vital to make a specific etiologic diagnosis by isolating the etiologic agent from appropriate specimens. Until this is done the diagnosis of osteomyelitis is only presumptive. Precise bacteriologic identification is also necessary for appropriate antibiotic treatment. Antimicrobial therapy is an important adjunct in the treatment of chronic osteomyelitis in which surgical removal of all necrotic bone and tissue and the elimination of dead space is most important. Negative results may also be helpful for excluding the diagnosis when the findings are not definite, for example, after a traumatic bone fracture. In addition, some tumors (e.g., eosinophilic granuloma) may be difficult to differentiate from osteomyelitis at the time of surgery, illustrating the need for routine submission of portions of surgical specimen for both culture and histologic examination. Sources for recovering the infectious agent include blood, closed needle aspirate and biopsy of involved bone, open surgical biopsy, aspiration of joint fluid, and when present, sinus drainage. Routine antimicrobial susceptibility studies are always indicated, and special tests, such as minimum bacteriocidal concentrations, and serum bacteriocidal assays should be considered for selective cases (see Ch. 28).

Presence of Internal Devices

Management of infection in the presence of internal devices is difficult. If infection persists despite antimicrobial therapy, the hardware should be removed and surgical debridement performed. At this time, cultures and susceptibility testing of the debridement tissue is performed. Any pain, swelling, fever, leukocytosis, drainage associated with previous surgery, and prosthetic device placement in the bone, joint, or soft tissue should alert the physician to consider a prosthetic device associated infection. An arthrogram with arthrocentesis for culture may define the infectious agent. The fluid, if infected, will have cellular and chemical findings consistent with septic arthritis. However, because bacteria are embedded within the glycocalyx matrix on the prosthesis, cultures of the joint fluid are frequently negative. Hence, it may become necessary to make a histopathologic, rather than a microscopic diagnosis, until or unless specimens are obtained at the time of surgical revision. Several sites (bone, cement, capsule, synovial fluid) should be cultured at the time a prosthetic joint is revised. Synovial fluid, biopsy of synovium, capsule, bone, and cement are all appropriate specimens.

Logistics

Specimens for aerobic and anaerobic culture should be collected and submitted directly to the laboratory. The diagnostic procedure of choice is a needle aspirate or biopsy of the bone, or both, for culture and histopathology. Blood cultures should also be collected. Drainage from a sinus tract that is present in some patients with chronic infection can be examined in addition to, but not in place of, specimens obtained by bone biopsy and aspiration procedures. Several smears from the involved site should also be made at the time of collection. One of the smears should be Gram stained and examined immediately. Other smears can be held for special stains if warranted for identifying mycobacteria or fungi. Sufficient history should be provided to guide the choice of culture. As a minimum, nonselective media (such as 5% sheep blood agar) should be used and incubated aerobically and anaerobically. If acid fast bacilli, actinomycosis, fungi, or other special pathogens are suspected, the laboratory should be alerted to use special procedures and media as needed to recover these organisms. The microbiologist should also request that a blood culture be obtained if this has not already been done.

Interpretation

Bone and disc tissue are normally sterile and under sterile conditions of collection and handling of the specimen any organism isolated can be considered the causative agent, especially if it is recovered from multiple sites. In patients with chronic, recurrent osteomyelitis who develop sinus tracts, cultures of the drainage often yield bacteria that are not present in the bone and also may fail to yield all agents in mixed infections. In this setting, cultures of superficial drainage should be used only as a rough guideline for initial therapy, especially if *S. aureus* is present. The culture results should always be correlated with Gram stain, gross appearance, radiographic studies, and the patient's clinical condition and history. Culture negative results occur frequently (30–50%) suggesting a noninfectious, inflammatory condition. The specificity for excluding osteomyelitis depends on many factors including recent antimicrobial therapy, evidence for progression or healing, and consideration of other infectious agents that were not sought with the culture procedures used.

The bacteria most commonly involved in prosthetic joint infections are *S. epidermidis, Propionibacterium acnes,* and diphtheroids. Since these organisms may also represent skin contaminants, confirmation by culturing the same organism from another specimen increases diagnostic accuracy. For this reason, it is recommended that organisms recovered from bone and joint lesions be stored for comparison with possible future culture isolates from the same patient (see Ch. 20).

Specimen: Pericardial Fluid

Background

Inflammation of the pericardium (pericarditis) is an unusual complication of common infectious diseases. Its occurrence reflects the epidemiologic characteristics of the primary infection. Virtually any infectious agent that reaches the myocardium or pericardium is capable of causing pericarditis. This may occur via the blood or lymph, direct extension from pulmonary or myocardial infectious foci, or direct inoculation during surgery, or other invasive procedures or penetrating trauma.[29]

The intensity of the pericardial inflammatory reaction reflects the pathogenicity of the etiologic agent. Viral infections typically produce a relatively mild inflammatory reaction that is associated with focal damage to the adjacent myocardium. The response varies from a small amount of serous fluid with mononuclear cells and fibrinogen to a large, neutrophil-rich, bloody effusion. Bacterial pericarditis is usually acute, purulent, and rapidly progressive. The mortality rate exceeds 50% and is related to general sepsis, myocardial damage, and rapidly progressive cardiac tamponade. In patients who survive, healing is associated with extensive fibrosis that may progress to a chronic, constrictive pericarditis requiring pericardectomy.

Enteroviruses are the most common etiologic agents of acute serofibrinous pericarditis although many other viruses can be involved, including coxsackieviruses and echoviruses.[30] Occasional cases of acute serofibrinous pericarditis may be caused by potentially treatable infectious agents such as *Mycoplasma pneumoniae, Chlamydia psittaci,* and *Coxiella burnetii.* Acute purulent pericarditis is most often caused by common bacterial pathogens such as staphylococci, pneumococci, streptococci, *H. influenzae,* and meningococci. Pneumococci, or other primary pulmonary pathogens, usually infect the pericardium by extension from an adjacent pneumonitis. Infection by staphylococci, meningococci, and *H. influenzae* are more likely to reach the pericardium through the bloodstream. The endocardium or myocardium may serve as the initial source of bacteria in infections such as staphylococcal endocarditis. Less commonly, Enterobacteriaceae and even anaerobic bacteria may be etiologic agents. Fungi such as *Candida* spp. and *Aspergillus* spp. may cause acute purulent pericarditis. Amebic pericarditis is most often a benign serous pericarditis, however, if untreated it may progress to acute purulent pericarditis. Chronic pericarditis is classically caused by *M. tuberculosis* or by fungi such as *Coccidioides immitis* or *Histoplasma capsulatum*.[31]

Selection

Signs and Symptoms

Frequent symptoms and signs in perciarditis include chest pain, fever and chills, pericardial friction rub, abnormal heart sounds, pericardial effusion, pulsus paradoxus, conduction changes, and signs of developing cardiac tamponade (dyspnea, agitation, orthopnea, and cough). Chest pain in perciarditis is typically rapid in onset, persists for several hours to days, and is worse during inspiration and recumbency, but improves with leaning forward. Differentiation from myocardial infarction is difficult. Fever and malaise are usually present. Chills are prominent in acute bacterial pericarditis. Tuberculous pericarditis usually includes other signs of tuberculous infection including fever, night sweats, weight loss, and fatigue. Pericardial friction rub is one of the most helpful signs for diagnosing pericarditis. It is found in most patients with acute viral pericarditis; however, it may be absent in up to 50% of patients with acute purulent pericarditis and in most patients with constrictive pericarditis. Pericardial effusion can be detected on chest x-ray by increased cardiac silhouette. A decrease in systolic blood pressure of more than 10 mmHg on inspiration (pulsus paradoxus) is seen in most patients with pericarditis and tamponade, and in approximately 30% of patients with constrictive pericarditis. The cervical venous pressure may increase paradoxically with inspiration (Kussmaul's sign). Echocardiography is the most accurate noninvasive method for detecting and monitoring pericardial effusions.

Laboratory Diagnosis

Because infectious pericarditis is less common than noninfectious (such as from trauma, cardiotomy, irradiation, and autoimmune diseases), laboratory assistance is critical for differential diagnosis and treatment. Definitive diagnosis of an infectious etiology is obtained by the evaluation of pericardial fluid or biopsy of the pericardium. Pericardiocentesis is a procedure to obtain pericardial fluid or biopsy of the pericardium. The decision to perform this procedure should be made carefully because pericardiocentesis is associated with risk of epicardial tear and bleeding. When the manifestations and course of pericarditis are totally consistent with viral infection, or if there is an underlying myocardial infarction, rheumatic fever, or uremia, it is reasonable to observe the patient first. A more aggressive approach toward diagnosis should be considered whenever there is an atypical presentation. Specific etiologic diagnosis of viral or bacterial pericarditis is helpful in determining prognosis and choosing appropriate therapy. When the setting is classic for acute bacterial pericarditis, as in a patient with bacteriemia or bacterial pneumonia with high fever, leukocytosis, and rapidly progressive course, there should be no delay in obtaining pericardial fluid. Blood cultures should also be performed. Pericardial tissue obtained by open surgical biopsy is more likely to yield diagnosis of either tuberculosis, histoplasmosis, or coccidioidomycosis than is examination of pericardial fluid.

Logistics

Using aseptic techniques, the pericardial fluid is obtained by pericardiocentesis and divided into three tubes as follows: (1) a sterile tube for cultures and serology; (2) a tube with anticoagulant for cell examination; and (3) a tube for chemical determinations. The pericardial fluid specimen for cultures may be directly inoculated into broth media used for blood cultures, although some should be reserved for inoculation onto plated media. The specimen should be transported immediately to the laboratory. Gram smear and routine aerobic and anaerobic bacterial, and viral and, if indicated, mycobacterial and fungal cultures are performed as previously described above for other fluids and tissues.

Interpretation

Pericardial fluid and tissues are normally sterile and under sterile conditions of collection and handling the specimen any organism isolated can be considered causative agent. The culture results should always be correlated with Gram stain, pericardial fluid gross appearance, cell counts, histopathologic appearance of the biopsy (if obtained), and the patient's clinical condition and previous history. Leukocyte counts greater than 10,000/μL, a left shift, and decreased glucose (50% or less, compared to serum) suggests bacterial infection, although this is not a consistent finding.

Specimen: Muscle Biopsy

Background

Skeletal Muscle Disease

Bacteria occasionally invade skeletal muscle from trauma or spread from a hematogenous or contiguous source. Although many different organisms may be involved, some are associated with specific diseases. These include *S. aureus* pyomyositis, which occurs more frequently in topical regions, myonecrosis caused by *C. perfringens* (gas gangrene), or by a variety of other anaerobic bacteria (synergistic myonecrosis).[32] In addition, group A, *S. pyogenes* may cause a particular virulent form of infection with secondary bacteremia.

Two species of parasite, the coccidial protozoan *Sarcocystis lindemanni* (causing sarcocystosis) and the nematode worm *Trichinella spiralis* (causing trichinosis) infect skeletal muscle as the primary site of human infection. Other parasites that may develop in muscle and cause symptomatic disease as part of multiorgan system infections include *Trypanosoma cruzi* (causing Chagas disease), *T. gondii* (causing toxoplasmosis), and *T. solium* (causing cysticercosis).

Cardiac Muscle Disease

Cardiac muscle may be affected during systemic infections or it may be the primary focus of infection. In most cases an infectious process involves both the myocardium and pericardium simultaneously (myopericarditis). Clinically there may be predominantly myocarditis or pericarditis (see Specimen: Pericardial Fluid above). Major infectious agents causing myocarditis in the United States are enteroviruses, several pyogenic bacteria, *M. tuberculosis,* and a few fungi. Rarely do other organisms such as *M. pneumoniae, C. psittaci,* and *C. burnetii* cause acute myocarditis.

Selection, Analysis, and Interpretation

Skeletal Muscle Disease

Pyomyositis is suspected when there is pain, swelling, and tenderness localized to a specific muscle group, especially with a history of trauma to that area. A specimen is obtained for smear and culture examination at the time of surgical drainage of the abscess. Myonecrosis is associated with generalized toxicity that may progress quickly to shock. Localized findings vary greatly from mild tenderness and edema to rapidly progressive cutaneous blebs with necrosis. The discharge from affected areas is serosanguinous rather than purulent. Gram smear of necrotic tissue or fluid often shows a lack of inflammatory cells and numerous bacteria (large gram-positive rods with *C. perfringens* infection or mixed morphology with gram-negative bacilli in synergistic myonecrosis). Although culture can be performed, a clinical diagnosis must be made rapidly because the prognosis is poor even with prompt surgical and antimicrobial treatment. The presence of inflammatory cells and mixed organisms suggest cellulitis.

Cardiac Muscle Disease

Infections of the myocardium (as well as pericardium) often present clinically in young people as an acute illness with breathlessness or pain in the chest. In severely affected patients there may be clinical confusion with a myocardial infarction. Electrocardiogram and microbiologic investigation may help to differentiate between these possibilities. Irrespective of the infectious cause, symptoms and signs are similar, although findings of bacterial myocarditis are frequently more severe than with viral infections. Patients with viral disease usually show signs of chest pain, malaise, fever, preceding respiratory infection, cough, nausea, vomiting, and dyspnea. Patients with bacterial myocarditis (and frequently, associated pericarditis) are toxic and acutely ill with anorexia, fever, chills, and chest pain. Blood cultures are always indicated when bacterial myocarditis is suspected. In cases of associated pericarditis or pericardial effusion the examination of pericardial fluid or pericardial biopsy may be useful as described in the previous section. For culture negative myopericarditis, paired sera can be evaluated for changes in titers for possible causes such as leptospirosis, Q-fever, or toxoplasmosis. Culture of cardiac muscle for viral and bacterial agents from a biopsy or autopsy specimen may rarely be needed to arrive at an etiologic diagnosis when pericardial fluid or blood cultures are not productive and infection is strongly suggested from the clinical findings.

Parasitic Muscle Disease

Human infection with *Sarcocystis* is a rare occurrence most commonly found as an incidental finding on biopsy or at autopsy. The parasite forms cysts (known as sarcocysts) in both skeletal and cardiac muscle that contain numerous slowly multiplying trophozoites. Because of the parasite's rare occurrence, little clinical information is available on symptoms associated with acute muscle infection. The sarcocysts are easily recognized using routine histologic methods.

Trichinosis may be acquired from the meat of carnivores and omnivores other than pork, including bear and walrus. Each female worm ingested may produce up to 500 larvae during 1 month, which then invade a variety of muscles. These larvae are encapsulated by host responses, but remain viable for a number of years. Therapy is primarily supportive during the period of larval invasion and encapsulation, after which the symptoms subside spontaneously. Most cases reported in recent years are common-source outbreaks in which pork products have not been cooked thoroughly. Microwave cooking is also suspect because of the common occurrence of "cold spots" during preparation. Symptomatic trichinosis is characterized by two phases. An acute gastrointestinal syndrome, which occurs within the first 30 hours after exposure from the activity of the excysted larvae entering the intestinal mucosa, consists of nausea, vomiting, abdominal cramping, and diarrhea. Muscle invasion and encapsulation of larvae occur over the next 30 days and are characterized by fever, periorbital and facial edema, and muscle pain and weakness. Depending on the infectious dose, life-threatening myocarditis, encephalitis, or respiratory arrest may also develop. Peripheral eosinophilia is pronounced during the muscle invasive stage, and often reaches 50% or more. A history of ingestion of raw or rare pork, especially in homemade sausage, may often be elicited. Diagnosis is usually made by examination of muscle biopsies from the gastrocnemius, biceps, and deltoid. Muscle biopsies for trichinosis may be examined by either routine histology, or, more quickly, by compressing the tissues between two glass slides and examining under the low power lens of the microscope. Because numbers of larvae will vary tremendously depending on the infective dose, serologic studies should be undertaken when biopsies are negative.

Cysticercosis of the skeletal and cardiac muscles is a common event as part of systemic infection. While symptomatic cysticercosis often presents with central nervous system signs, asymptomatic disease is often recognized incidentally on radiograph of soft tissues that contain calcified larvae. Demonstration of larvae anywhere in the body indicates probable concurrent central nervous system infection. Diagnosis depends on the microscopic identification of a larva following surgical removal. In the absence of a tissue diagnosis, serologic studies are especially helpful when coupled with suggestive CT or MRI scans, although cross-reactions with hydatid infections may confuse the interpretation.

Trypomastigotes of *T. cruzi* may infect skeletal, smooth, and cardiac muscle as part of an acute systemic dissemination characterized by fever, myalgias, rash, lymphadenopathy, hepatosplenomegaly, acute myocarditis, and subcutaneous edema. Persistent infection often results in cardiomyopathy with cardiomegaly, conduction changes and gastrointestinal disease manifest by dysfunctional esophageal or colonic motility. Blood from a person with appropriate symptoms and history of residence in an endemic area should be examined for trypomastigotes and tissue biopsies for amastigotes. Specimens should also be cultured in NNN media to improve chances of detection, especially during chronic stages of the disease when fever organisms are present. Serologic tests are available and offer supportive evidence of infection.

Myocarditis caused by *T. gondii* may occur as part of a systemic infection, and is most likely to develop in immunocompromised patients, especially those with AIDS or following cardiac transplantation. Diagnosis of acute disease is routinely made with *Toxoplasma*-specific IgG and IgM serology studies. The presence of any IgM positive serology strongly suggests acute or recent infection. The use of histology and immunoperoxidase staining are helpful adjuncts to the diagnosis and may be performed along with attempts to isolate the organism in tissue culture or laboratory animals.

Specimen: Lymph Nodes

Background

Lymphadenitis is an acute or chronic inflammation of the lymph nodes. It may be generalized during a systemic infection or it may be restricted to a solitary node or to a localized group of lymph nodes draining an anatomic area. Palpable lymph nodes do not always indicate serious or ongoing disease, or even infection. Tumors (lymphoma), developmental abnormalities (cysts), or autoimmune diseases may produce lymph node reactions. The location of lymphadenopathy as well as local signs and symptoms help narrow the wide differential diagnosis.

The most common presentation of acute lymphadenitis occurs as cervical adenitis in children. One or more nodes are enlarged and accompanied by tenderness, warmth, and sometimes redness. Viral infection of the upper respiratory tract with secondary cervical lymphadenitis is common and almost always resolves rapidly. Bacterial causes of cervical adenitis include *S. aureus* or *S. pyogenes* infection from impetigo, other facial lesions, or mixtures of anaerobes (*Bacteroides* spp., *Peptostreptococcus* spp.) as a result of periodontal infection. Suppuration and abscess formation may develop if the infection is allowed to progress without antimicrobial treatment. Slower enlargement of tender lymph nodes occurring over weeks instead of days suggests mycobacterial, fungal (histoplasmosis, coccidioidomycosis), or cat-scratch disease.[33] With the exception of AIDS, an infectious etiology is unlikely when enlarged cervical lymph nodes are not tender. A number of other infectious etiologies must be considered when painful lymphadenopathy occurs in the inguinal region. Besides *S. aureus* and *S. pyogenes*, lymphadenopathy may be a manifestation of sexually transmitted diseases, lymphogranuloma venereum (LGV), chancroid *(Haemophilus ducreyi),* or genital herpes (see Ch. 25). Syphilis and sometimes LGV produce painless inguinal lymphadenopathy. Many other agents may cause infectious lymphadenitis such as *Yersinia pestis* (plague) or certain helminthics *(Loa loa, Onchocerca volvulus)* in the inguinal region, or brucellosis, leptospirosis, rickettsia, toxoplasmosis, and many viruses as a generalized form. The patient's age, dental problems, sexual history, genital lesions, travel history, knowledge about animal exposures, and the location, progression, and characteristics of lymphadenitis provide important clues to the diagnosis.

Selection

In most cases of infectious lymphadenitis, it is unnecessary to subject the lymph node to laboratory examination. Either the underlying cause of infection is known from other clinical and laboratory (such as serology) manifestations, or the patient is given empiric antimicrobial therapy (e.g., cervical adenitis suspected of being caused by *S. aureus*). When the patient does not respond to therapy or the diagnosis cannot be made by other means, it is sometimes necessary to obtain a lymph node specimen for laboratory examination by either needle aspiration or total excision. Aspiration should not be performed in patients with suspected *Mycobacterium* spp. or *Nocardia* spp. infections because this may lead to a chronic draining sinus. Needle aspiration of a lymph node is most appropriate when abscess formation is suspected. Collection of exudate on a swab from lymph nodes with suppuration and developing fistulous tracts may also be submitted to the laboratory.

Logistics

Specimen Collection

Aseptic preparation of the aspiration site is needed for lymph node biopsy or aspiration. If a specimen cannot be obtained, a small amount of sterile saline may be injected and aspirated. The portion of the biopsy specimen submitted for culture should be separated from the portion submitted for histopathology by the surgeon or pathologist using sterile techniques. Ideally, material obtained from a lymph node should be put directly into anaerobic transport media or transported directly to the laboratory. To obtain material from a secreting fistulous tract, two swabs should be collected; one for culture and one for Gram stain. Specimens collected in syringes should be transported to the laboratory within half an hour of collection.

Analysis

A Gram smear of the specimen should be examined microscopically for inflammatory cells and bacteria. Aerobic and anaerobic cultures should be performed using selective and nonselective media. Appropriate media to isolate fungi and mycobacterial pathogens should be part of the routine examination. Special cultures (chocolate agar with increased CO_2) should be used for inguinal nodes that may be infected with *N. gonorrhoeae* or *H. ducreyi*. Viral cultures are usually unnecessary.

Interpretation

Any organism isolated from a lymph node specimen should be considered the etiologic agent. Potential contamination with skin flora must be recognized as a possibility for results obtained from fistulous tract drainage, which is collected on a swab. The culture results should always be correlated with Gram stain, gross and microscopic appearance, clinical findings, appropriate history, and histologic examination. The latter is particularly important if it alerts the laboratory to a specific diagnosis by showing characteristic granulomatous inflammation with the presence of fungi or mycobacteria. Negative bacterial cultures are expected for viral diseases, noninfectious etiologies, and fastidious organisms such as *H. ducreyi*.

Specimen: From Bite Wounds

Background and Selection[34]

Bite wounds, both human and animal, are common injuries frequently treated in the emergency room. Infectious complications frequently occur, accounting for significant morbidity. There are approximately 1 million dog bites, 400,000 cat bites, and 45,000 snake bites in the United States annually. No exact estimate is known on human bites but they are quite frequent as well. Although most patients cleanse their wounds with soap and water and administer topical treatment, these measures do not prevent infection.

Bite wounds are injuries inoculated with normal oral flora of the biter, including both aerobic and anaerobic bacteria. Organisms typically associated with animal bite infections are *Pasteurella multocida* (cat bite) and CDC group DF-2 (dog bite), although polymicrobial (including anaerobes) infections are common. Group A *Streptococcus pyogenes* is perhaps the most important and serious pathogen associated with human bites, although many different organisms from mouth flora may be involved (e.g., *Eikenella corrodens*). *Salmonella arizona* is associated with infected snake bites. Patients with liver disease and splenectomy are at high risk for fatal sepsis with DF-2 after a dog bite. Other diseases transmitted by animal bites include brucellosis, blastomycosis, tularemia, cat-scratch disease, and rat bite fever.

The bite wound starts showing signs of inflammation including onset of gray malodorous discharge, localized pain, tenderness, and erythema about 8 hours after the injury. This can progress to cellulitis and less often, regional lymphadenopathy, lymphangiitis, and fever. Puncture wounds have the greatest tendency to become infected and an abscess may form with surrounding cellulitis. Asplenic patients may develop fulminant species. Most patients bitten by humans will have established infection if seen more than 24 hours after the injury.

Logistics

Bite wounds should be profusely irrigated, drained, and debrided, both for therapy and to remove superficial contaminants before a specimen is collected for microbiologic examination. Aseptic preparation of the aspiration site is needed. The overlying and adjacent areas must be carefully prepared to eliminate isolation of potentially contaminating anaerobes, which colonize the skin surface. Fluid or pus draining from the lesion should be aspirated or collected with a swab. Two swabs should be collected; one for culture and one for Gram stain. An anaerobic transport container should be used.

A Gram smear of the specimen should be examined microscopically for inflammatory cells and bacteria. Aerobic and anaerobic cultures should be performed using selective and nonselective media. Since results are unpredictable for individual cases, it is important to identify the predominant organisms present with special regard for *P. multocida*, CDC group DF-2, *S. aureus*, and *S. pyogenes*. DF-2 is slow growing and may require prolonged incubation to isolate it. Antimicrobial susceptibility tests should be performed according to the procedures described in Chapter 28. Special media and culture conditions are required when the history suggests atypical pathogens, such as tularemia (rabbit bite) or rat bite fever *(Streptobacillus moniliformis, Spirillum minor)*.

Interpretation

Culture results often showed mixed flora. Those organisms described in the background section (DF-2, *P. multocida*, and *S. pyogenes*) have special significance and should be specifically treated. The culture results should always be correlated with Gram stain, gross and microscopic appearance, patient's clinical condition, and type of bite. Cultures of bite wounds secondarily contaminated that have not been cleansed or debrided have a limited significance.

Specimen: From Burn Wounds

Background

Burn wound infections are a serious complication that may increase injury to already damaged skin and progress to life-threatening sepsis. Infection also stimulates hypertrophic scarring in the healing wound. The risk is lowered by early excision of the dead burn eschar, which is frequently the primary source of infection in full thickness burns. Other burn-related infections include pneumonia, suppurative thrombophlebitis, and viremia with herpesvirus. Combination of meticulous care of the wound and aggressive augmentation of the patient's immune defenses are of paramount importance.

For a short period after injury, the surface of the burn wound is sterile unless there is initial gross contamination. After the second day, bacterial colonization of the wound begins. At first, bacteria come from the patient's own endogenous flora. This may include *S. epidermidis* and *S. aureus* from the skin, as well as other gram-positive bacteria from the upper respiratory tract, and enteric bacteria from fecal flora. Later, gram-negative bacilli from the hospital environment begin to predominate. The most significant are *P. aeruginosa*, *Providencia* spp., and *Serratia marcescens*.[35] These organisms are frequently resistant to standard antimicrobial therapy. Yeasts and filamentous fungi may also colonize the burn wound and cause sepsis. *Candida* spp. are most common, while *Fusarium* spp., *Aspergillus* spp., and *Zygomycetes* are less frequent. Treatment of burn wound infections is difficult because the avascular eschar is an excellent culture medium and the patient's cell mediated immune defenses are usually deficient. A decrease in burn mortality in recent years is primarily because of more aggressive measures to prevent infection rather than improved treatment of established infections.

Selection

Fever and leukocytosis are universally present in the burn patient with or without additional evidence of infection. Early symptoms of infection are frequently subtle and may include anorexia or fatigue. Late symptoms include deterioration of mental status and hemodynamic instability, including impaired perfusion of vital organs, and signs of sepsis. A high suspicion is required to make a diagnosis of infection in the early stage. A change in wound appearance marked by bleeding, poor eschar formation, or discoloration suggest infection. Documenting the presence of bacteria in the wound surface is not diagnostic of burn wound infection because all burns are colonized on the surface. Biopsy of a full thickness burn wound is the most reliable diagnostic method. Because the signs and symptoms of infection may be easily missed, it is not unreasonable to perform this procedure for surveillance on a scheduled basis.

Logistics

The laboratory should be contacted before specimen collection to ascertain availability of the specific procedures required. A biopsy is obtained using a sterile scalpel or punch biopsy instrument. More than 0.1 g of eschar specimen (not viable tissue) should be submitted. The specimen is analyzed by quantitative bacteriology to determine the number of bacteria per specimen.[36] Another specimen should be sent for histologic examination. The specimen is weighed immediately after it is obtained and then processed promptly by maceration in a glass homogenizer, suspension in 0.9% NaCl solution, then serial dilution with trypticase soy broth followed by inoculation on nonselective platted media such as 5% sheep blood agar. Colony counts are done at 24 and 48 hours of incubation at 35°C with 5–10% CO_2. Results are reported as the number of bacteria per gram of burn tissue. A portion of the specimen should also be examined microscopically with Gram stain. When indicated by findings on histologic or microscopic examination, fungal cultures can be performed with Sabouraud agar held at 30°C for 2 or more weeks.

Interpretation

The principal value of quantitative burn wound biopsies is the demonstration of the predominant burn wound flora. There is high agreement between quantitative cultures of less than 100,000/g of tissue and the absence of histopathologic invasive infection. Quantitative burn cultures have less value for identifying patients with invasive infections and in differentiating those who are not likely to develop burn wound sepsis. Nevertheless, more than 100,000 colonies/g of tissue suggests ongoing or risk of infectious complication, and the need to consider systemic antimicrobial therapy. The organism most frequently recovered from burns wounds is *P. aeruginosa*. Other organisms to be expected include *Klebsiella pneumoniae, Pseudomonas fluorescens, Providencia stuartii, S. marcescens, S. aureus, Aspergillus* spp., *Fusarium* spp., and *Rhizopus* spp.

Specimen: From Traumatic Wounds

Background

The risk of infection following any traumatic wound relates inversely with the local blood supply and directly with the concentration of microorganisms introduced, the amount of foreign material, the extent of tissue damage, and associated factors such as formation of hematomas or extensive injury to muscles. A substantial amount of contamination can be introduced without overt infection, provided no foreign material remains and tissue injury is minimal. Hematomas provide a favorable culture medium for bacterial growth. Normal, well vascularized tissues are resistant to infection and only *S. pyogenes* is usually able to infect a relatively clean wound with minimal tissue damage. Other organisms require some tissue destruction, hematoma, or foreign material. Anaerobic bacterial infections are likely in dead or devitalized tissue. The organisms involved in penetrating wounds that do not involve hollow viscera are those introduced from the environment outside the host. When the penetrating object enters a hollow viscus a high probability exists that there will be continuous contamination of the tract of the wound. A single episode of contamination is usually handled by local defenses. Continued soiling of tissues with bacteria can progress to severe infection. Blunt injuries in themselves are not necessarily contaminated and therefore do not carry the same risk of infection as do penetrating injuries. Occasionally, however, disruption of loops of bowel and gross peritoneal and retroperitoneal contamination will result from abdominal trauma. Complex infections with both aerobic and anaerobic flora may result from ruptures of the gastrointestinal tract. Necrotizing fascitis is an uncommon, but severe infection of subcutaneous soft tissues caused by traumatic injury to the surface of the body or abdominal cavity. The infection is usually mixed with anaerobes and members of the Enterobacteriaceae family. Sometimes only Group A *S. pyogenes* is involved.[37] Blood cultures are often positive.

Selection

Manifestations of infection consist of evidence of inflammation including erythema with induration, pain, tenderness, decreased function, or increased temperature of the affected area. Minimal induration with fast spreading erythema is characteristic of group A streptococcal infection. Constitutional symptoms such as fever and leukocytosis may be present. External signs of inflammation may be lacking initially in deep injuries. Many wound infections (especially those caused by *S. pyogenes*) show early appearance of cellulitis and lymphangitis. Abscess formation is more often seen with *S. aureus*. When abdominal injuries with intra-abdominal infection is suspected, prompt surgery is required.

Blood cultures should be taken at the time of chill or ascent of fever. When the wound itself is involved, exudate should be obtained for examination by Gram stain and cultures. If there is evidence of injury to the chest or abdominal cavity, thoracentesis or paracentesis fluid, respectively, should be submitted.

Logistics

Sterile preparation of the wound site is required. Cultures of contaminated open wounds that have not been cleansed or debrided are not appropriate. Pus or other material should be aspirated from a wound site or abscess. The syringe should be transported to the laboratory after air is expelled to prevent loss of anaerobic bacterial viability. Collection of a specimen onto a swab is less suitable, especially for isolating anaerobes, but can be done if a deep aspirate is unobtainable. In this case, an anaerobic transport container with anaerobic transport medium should be used. The specimen should be transported to the laboratory as soon as possible after collection. Contamination with normal flora from skin, rectum, vaginal tract, or other body surfaces should be avoided. The specimen can be refrigerated if it cannot be promptly processed, although this may compromise the optimal yield from culture.

A Gram stain should be performed on a smeared preparation of the specimen. Since these specimens often grow mixed flora, media selective for gram-positive (i.e., azide agar) and gram-negative organisms (i.e., eosin methylene blue agar) should be used as well as nonselective media (i.e., 5% sheep blood agar). Anaerobic media and conditions to support anaerobic growth should also be employed. Fungal and mycobacterial pathogens should be considered and appropriate cultures requested if suspected, but not as part of the routine examination.

Interpretation

Interpretation of culture results is difficult when mixed flora is isolated because it is usually hard to know which of the many organisms isolated is responsible for infection and which are part of the superficial colonizing wound flora. Evaluation of the Gram stained smear results may help if only a few morphotypes predominate and correlate with culture results. In addition, β-hemolytic streptococci and *S. aureus* should always be noted. However, if a large assortment of different organisms are found on culture, full identification and susceptibility tests on every one is not useful for clarifying the etiology. Timely knowledge that mixed aerobic and anaerobic flora is present may be all the information needed to manage the infection. Species commonly recovered from wounds include, *E. coli*, *Proteus* spp., *Klebsiella* spp., *Pseudomonas* spp., *Enterobacter* spp., enterococci, streptococci, *Bacteroides* spp., *Clostridium* spp., *S. aureus*, and *S. epidermidis*.

REFERENCES

1. Feingold DS, Hirschmann JV, Leyden JJ: Bacterial infections of the skin. J Am Acad Dermatol 1989;20:469–475.
2. Roth RR, James WD: Microbiology of the skin: resident flora, ecology, infection. J Am Acad Dermatol 1989;20:367–390.
3. Weissmann A: Infectious diseases of the skin. Geriatrics 1989;44(suppl A):22–23.
4. Buxton PK: ABC of dermatology. Viral infections. Br Med J Clin Res 1988;296:257–261.
5. Buxton PK: ABC of dermatology. Bacterial infections. Br Med J Clin Res 1988;296:189–192.
6. Semel JD, Trenholme G: Aeromonas hydrophila water-associated traumatic wound infections: a review. J Trauma 1990;30:324–327.
7. Evans ME, Schaffner W, Federspiel CF et al: Sensitivity, specificity and predictive value of body surface cultures in a neonatal intensive care unit. JAMA 1988;259:248–252.
8. Feder HM Jr, Anderson I: Fifth disease. A brief review of infections in childhood, in adulthood, and pregnancy. Arch Intern Med 1989;149:2176–2178.
9. Navin TR, Arana FE, de-Merida AM et al: Cutaneous leishmaniasis in Guatemala: comparison of diagnostic methods. Am J Trop Med Hyg 1990;42:36–42.
10. von Kuster LC, Genta RM: Cutaneous manifestations of strongyloidiasis. Arch Dermatol 1988;124:1826–1830.
11. Elner PD: Microbiology of Wounds. pp. 158–168. In Lorian V (ed): Significance of Medical Microbiology in the Care of Patients. 2nd Ed. Baltimore, Williams & Wilkins, 1982.
12. Saklayen MG: CAPD peritonitis. Incidence, pathogens, diagnosis and management. Med Clin North Am 1990;74:997–1010.
13. Wilcox CM, Dismukes WE: Spontaneous bacterial peritonitis. A review of pathogenesis, diagnosis, and treatment. Medicine 1987;66:447–456.
14. Rustgi AK, Richter JM: Pyogenic and amebic liver abscess. Med Clin North Am 1989;73:847–858.
15. Frey CF, Zhu Y, Suzuki M, Isaji S: Liver abscesses. Surg Clin North Am 1989;69:259–271.

16. Schantz PM: Toxocara larva migrans now. Am J Trop Med Hyg 1989;41(suppl 3):21–34.
17. Hoefs JC: Diagnostic paracentesis. A potent clinical tool. Gastroenterology 1990;98:230–236.
18. Barnes PF, DeCock KM, Reynolds TN, Ralls PW: A comparison of amebic and pyogenic abscess of the liver. Medicine 1987;66:472–483.
19. Lin AC, Chapman SW, Turner HR: Clonorchiasis: an update. South Med J 1987;80:919–922.
20. Holley JL, Moss AH: A prospective evaluation of blood culture versus standard plate techniques for diagnosing peritonitis in continuous ambulatory peritoneal dialysis. Am J Kidney Dis 1989;13:184–188.
21. Brook I: A 12 year study of aerobic and anaerobic bacteria in intra-abdominal and postsurgical abdominal wound infections. Surg Gynecol Obstet 1989;169:387–392.
22. Berger RS, Perez-Figaredo RA, Spielvogel RL: Leishmaniasis: the touch preparation as a rapid mean of diagnosis. J Am Acad Dematol 1987;16:1096–1105.
23. Albillos A, Cuervas-Mons V, Millan I et al: Ascitic fluid polymorphonuclear cell count and serum to ascites albumin gradient in the diagnosis of bacterial peritonitis. Gastroenterology 1990;98:134–140.
24. Shmerling RH, Delbanco TL, Tosteson AN, Trentham DE: Synovial fluid tests. What should be ordered? JAMA 1990;264:1009–1014.
25. McCutchan HJ, Fisher RC: Synovial leukocytosis in infectious arthritis. Clin Orthop 1990;257:226–230.
26. Markus HS: Haematogenous osteomyelitis in the adult; a clinical and epidemiological study. Q J Med 1989;71:521–527.
27. Green NE, Edwards K: Bone and joint infections in children. Orthop Clin North Am 1987;18:555–576.
28. Baxter MP, Finnegan MA: Skeletal infection by group B beta-hemolytic streptococci in neonates. A case report and review of the literature. J Bone Joint Surg [Br] 1988;70:812–824.
29. Sinzobahamvya N, Ikeogu MO: Purulent pericarditis. Arch Dis Child 1987;62:696–699.
30. Montague TJ, Lopaschuk GD, Davies NJ: Viral heart disease. Chest 1990;98:190–199.
31. Sagrista-Sauleda J, Permanyer-Miralda G, Soler-Soler J: Tuberculous pericarditis: ten year experience with a prospective protocol for diagnosis and treatment. J Am Coll Cardiol 1988;11:724–728.
32. Kingston D, Seal DV: Current hypotheses on synergistic microbial gangrene. Br J Surg 1990;77:260–264.
33. Dandapat MC, Mishra BM, Dash SP, Kar PK: Peripheral lymph node tuberculosis: a review of 80 cases. Br J Surg 1990;77:911–912.
34. Brook I: Human and animal bite infections. J Fam Pract 1989;28:713–718.
35. McManus AT: Opportunistic infections in severely burned patients. Am J Med 1984;75:146–154.
36. McManus AT, Kim SH, McManus WF et al: Comparison of quantitative microbiology and histopathology in divided burn-wound biopsy specimens. Arch Surg 1987;122:74–76.
37. Umbert IJ, Winkelmann RK, Oliver GF, Peters MS: Necrotizing fasciitis: a clinical, microbiologic, and histopathologic study of 14 patients. J Am Acad Dermatol 1989;20:774–781.

24 Urine

Thomas R. Fritsche   Ron B. Schifman
Gerald Lancz   Steven Specter

INTRODUCTION

The diagnosis or exclusion of bacterial infection involving the urinary tract is accomplished by examining a properly collected urine specimen. Laboratory testing generally establishes an etiologic diagnosis in patients with cystitis or pyelonephritis and is important in selecting proper antimicrobial therapy to prevent permanent injury to the urinary tract system. Routine examination consists of examining a cleanly voided specimen by direct microscopic and chemical analysis as well as by culture. When indicated, special specimen collection and testing procedures can be conducted to localize infection. In special situations, the urine is an appropriate specimen for identifying *Neisseria gonorrhoeae, Mycobacterium tuberculosis, Leptospira, Schistosoma haematobium, Trichomonas vaginalis,* and *Onchocerca volvulus* infections. Examination of urine for virus is beneficial in only a few circumstances, such as cytomegalovirus.

TESTS FOR BACTERIAL INFECTION[1-3]

Test: Urine Culture (Bacterial)

Background

Urinary tract infections nearly always arise from invasion of microorganisms through the external urethral meatus. Ordinarily, urine sterility is maintained by its low pH, extremes of osmolality, high urea concentration, secretory antibodies, and the flushing mechanism of the bladder. The short female urethra and bacterial colonization of the vaginal introitus are important predisposing factors, accounting for the 10-fold or higher incidence of urinary tract infections among young women as compared with men. Fortunately, these are usually self-limited or asymptomatic infections.

Predisposing factors with greater potential for causing serious or recurrent disease include vesicoureteral reflux, bladder outlet obstruction, neurogenic dysfunction, polycystic kidney disease, diabetes mellitus in women, chronic bacterial prostatitis, pregnancy, and sexual transmission of pathogenic organisms. The onset of obstructive prostatic hypertrophy is one of the more important factors contributing to the increased rate of urinary tract infection in older men. Urinary tract infection is a common complication of indwelling catheters, accounting for about 40% of all nosocomial infections. Catheter-related infections are also more likely to be caused by antibiotic-resistant organisms and serve as a major source of bacteremia. Recovery of microorganisms from the urine as a result of hematogenous spread is unusual, except during the newborn period, and occasionally in adults with *Staphylococcus aureus* or *Salmonella* spp. bacteremia, disseminated or renal *M. tuberculosis* infections, or disseminated candidiasis.

A wide variety of aerobic bacteria, generally originating from gut or skin flora, may infect the urinary tract. The ability of bacteria to adhere to uroepithelial cells through the pili is an important virulence factor facilitating colonization of the periurethral region and spread into the bladder.[4] *Escherichia coli* and, to a lessor extent, *S. saprophyticus* account for most minor urinary tract infections in women. More serious nosocomial and recurrent infections also are caused by these organisms in addition to other Enterobacteriaceae, *Enterococcus, Pseudomonas aeruginosa,* and *Candida* spp.

Selection

Lower urinary tract infections (cystitis and urethritis) are associated with varying degrees of dysuria (difficulty urinating), frequency, odynuria (pain or burning during urination), urgency, and suprapubic pain. These symptoms also occur with upper urinary tract infection (pyelonephritis), but this infection is more obvious with the occurrence of acute onset of fever and chills, flank pain, and renal tenderness on palpation. Culture may not be required for infrequent episodes of uncomplicated lower urinary tract infections in women.[5] These infections are nearly always caused by *E. coli* or, less often, by *S. saprophyticus;* organisms that have predictable susceptibility to antibiotics. In nearly all other cases of symptomatic disease, microscopic examination and culture of urine should be performed to document the cause of infection and to confirm the appropriateness of empirical therapy by susceptibility testing. A repeat culture examination of 48–72 hours serves as an indicator of therapeutic response. In complicated cases, cultures may be performed after completion of therapy, to verify a cure.

Asymptomatic infection can only be detected by screening with urine cultures. This may be considered for patients at high risk (i.e. pregnancy, postrenal transplantation, diabetes mellitus, and urolithiasis). There is a particularly high occurrence of asymptomatic infection during pregnancy. Screening during the first antenatal visit will identify most infected patients. Periodic follow-up screening cultures are indicated for women who have bacteriuria any time during pregnancy. Other circumstances for screening include evaluation of fever in hospitalized patients, evaluation of neonates with failure to thrive, and detection of occult infection before performing a surgical procedure involving the urinary tract. Screening also has been used with limited success as a means to detect occult urinary tract abnormalities in children. Although the use of indwelling urinary catheters introduce a high risk of infection, screening cultures are not appropriate for the asymptomatic patient.

Chronic bacterial prostatitis is associated with lower back pain and perineal pain, dysuria, recurrent bacterial cystitis, and occasionally prostatic calculi. Evaluation of sequential voided bladder and expressed prostatic secretion specimens is indicated for the differential and etiologic diagnosis of this disorder. The organism responsible for chronic prostatitis is suggested by recovery of the same strain repeatedly from recurrent bladder infections. Semen culture may also be beneficial as an aid to diagnosing this infection. Acute prostatitis is a serious infection accompanied by fever, chills, and severe perineal pain. Secondary bacteremia, cystitis, and urethritis are frequent complications. Culture of urine, blood, and spontaneous prostatic secretions is appropriate for determining the etiologic diagnosis in this condition. The etiologic diagnosis of epididymitis can usually be made by culture of the urine or urethra. In men younger than age 35, sexually transmitted agents (*Chlamydia trachomatis* and *Neisseria gonorrhoeae*) should be sought, and in older men, aerobic gram-negative bacilli are the usual pathogens.

Terminology

Urinary tract infection may involve a number of anatomic sites ranging from the anterior urethra to the kidney and prostate. Upper tract infection refers to involvement of the renal pelvis and kidney parenchyma (pyelonephritis), whereas lower tract infection involves the urethra (urethritis), bladder (cystitis), and prostate (prostatitis). The acute urethral syndrome or dysuria-pyuria syndrome generally implies infection of the lower tract with *Chlamydia, Mycoplasma,* or early bacterial infection, the latter, having propensity to evolve to cystitis. Nonspecific or nongonococcal urethritis are terms used for men with urethritis but no evidence by microscopy or culture of *N. gonorrhoeae* infection. These infections are frequently caused by *C. trachomatis.* Uncomplicated (or medical) urinary tract infection indicates that no abnormal anatomic lesion is present, in contrast to complicated (surgical) infection, which implies an obstructive lesion that impedes normal urine outflow.

Logistics

Specimen Requirements

Urine specimens have the potential to be contaminated by resident flora of the anterior urethra, vagina, labia, and periurethral area. Urine must therefore be collected using a midstream clean-voided technique. In women, the periurethral region, and in men, the glans penis, is washed with soap and dried before voiding. Patients must be carefully instructed about the collection procedure, including the importance of spreading labia apart or retracting foreskin during cleaning and voiding. Improper preparation and collection by a poorly instructed patient is the most important cause for misleading results. The first morning specimen provides maximum sensitivity. Generally, a single specimen is sufficient, but repeat examination may be necessary to reconcile nondiagnostic results or to increase sensitivity when screening asymptomatic patients.

Urine collection through the wall of a disinfected catheter and from suprapubic aspiration in infants are alternative methods. Catheterization performed exclusively for urine sampling should be avoided, because of the risk of introducing bacteria into the bladder and because of trauma to the meatus or urethra. Catheter tips and urine from drainage bags are not representative of bladder contents and should not be examined. The surface and interior of urinary calculi should be cultured, because each may harbor different organisms.

Processing should commence as soon as possible to prevent proliferation of organisms. Holding a urine specimen at ambient temperature for more than 1 hour can compromise the examination with false positive results. Refrigeration or use of transport media is an acceptable alternative when processing delays are unavoidable.

Analysis

Quantitative urine culture is required to properly interpret results. This is generally performed by the streak plate method. A 0.001-mL sample of urine is delivered to plated media with a calibrated inoculating loop, followed by streaking for isolation. With this method, each colony will approximate 100,000 organisms/mL. To achieve greater sensitivity, larger quantities of urine may be inoculated: this is appropriate for high quality specimens such as those obtained by suprapubic aspiration. Sheep blood agar, selective media for gram-negative bacilli (e.g. MacConkey, eosin-methylene blue), and selective media for gram-positive organisms (colistin-nalidixic acid agar) are preferred for urine culture.[6]

Several automated methods detect bacteriuria by measuring turbidity produced in broth during incubation. The procedure has limited value because specimens must be incubated 5 hours before negative results are verified. The AutoMicrobic system uses special lyophilized media having the ability to provide both semiquantitative enumeration and bacterial identification results on direct urine specimens, although this may require up to 13 hours of incubation. The accuracy of the method is comparable to that with standard quantitative culture methods, even with polymicrobic bacteriuria, but requires a large capital equipment expenditure and costly supplies.

Simplified methods, oriented toward the physician office laboratory, are commercially available. One of the most widely used is the dip slide procedure. A specially prepared agar slide is dipped into urine, removed, and incubated. The density of growth observed on the slide after 18 hours of incubation provides a semiquantitative estimate of bacteriuria. This method has limitations when heavy growth impedes isolation for bacterial identification and standardized susceptibility results. The test should only be used for testing patients with asymptomatic or uncomplicated infections.

Interpretation[7]

Of urine samples submitted to the hospital laboratory for culture examination, 20–40% yield an etiologic diagnosis. Likewise, cultures performed with adequate sensitivity that show no growth reliably exclude bacterial infections. Although urine is generally sterile, it is common, particularly in women, to recover a few contaminating organisms. Proper interpretation of urine culture results depends on the quantity, purity, and identification of microorganisms, in addition to the associated finding of pyuria.

Count

The presence of more than 10^5 organisms/mL is the classic, quantitative definition of significant bacteriuria. Although this serves as a dependable guideline under most circumstances, there is no quantitative measure of bacteriuria that will conclusively define the presence or absence of infection. Numerous variables affect the urine bacterial count. Among some of the more important factors are how carefully the specimen was collected, how rapidly it was processed, the site of infection, and type of organism.[8]

A urine bacterial count below 10^5/mL in the absence of pyuria has questionable diagnostic significance, unless the specimen was collected by catheter or suprapubic aspiration. Pyuria with low level bacteriuria of pure or predominant growth generally indicates cystitis, urethritis, or prostatitis. Low level bacteriuria is distinctly unusual with symptoms of acute pyelonephritis and suggests an obstructive lesion or perinephric abcess. It

Table 24-1. Causes of Pyuria Associated with Sterile Routine Bacterial and Fungal Cultures

Infectious Etiology	Noninfectious Etiology
Adenovirus	Contamination by vaginal contents
Anaerobes	Interstitial renal disease
Antibiotic therapy	Immunocomplex glomerulonephritis
Blastomycosis (prostatitis)	Malignancy of urinary tract
Campylobacter spp.	Renal stones
Chlamydia	Urethral trauma
Coccidiomycosis	
Gardnerella vaginalis[a]	
Haemophilus spp.	
Leptospira	
Legionella spp.	
Mycobacterium tuberculosis or other species	
Neisseria gonorrhoeae	
Prostatitis (nonbacterial)	
Trichomonas vaginalis (vaginitis, urethritis)	
Ureaplasma[a]	

[a] Questionable significance.

is important to recognize that bacteriuria is an expected consequence of indwelling catheter use. This finding does not necessarily imply infection unless symptoms are present.

A bacterial count greater than 10^5/mL in a properly collected and processed specimen usually implies urinary tract infection. Confirmation on a repeat specimen is generally recommended for making the diagnosis in asymptomatic patients. Occasionally, urinary tract symptoms and pyuria are present without growth on culture media. Termed *sterile pyuria*, this may be associated with a number of infectious and noninfectious causes (Table 24-1). In this situation, special procedures for identifying pathogens not detected by routine culture and evaluation of immunologic and neoplastic disorders of the urinary tract are warranted. A Gram stain examination of the urine is helpful in this circumstance. The presence of organisms on smear without culture confirmation suggests a fastidious organism, such as *H. influenzae*, *N. gonorrhoeae*, or an anaerobe that can not be isolated with routine culture procedures.

Organisms

Lactobacillus, microaerophilic *Streptococcus*, *Staphylococcus epidermidis*, and *Corynebacterium* are normal members of the vaginal and periurethral flora, and their recovery from women, even in large numbers, suggests contamination. The microbiologic etiology is obvious when a solitary pathogen is isolated. The significance of polymicrobic bacteriuria, however, can be problematic. Organisms that predominate on culture and have greater pathogenicity (e.g., *Pseudomonas aeruginosa* versus *Staphylococcus epidermidis*) are clues for evaluating the significance of results. Genuine polymicrobic infections tend to recur because of the underlying disorder. This finding ordinarily occurs in the setting of chronic obstruction, neurogenic bladder, long-term use of indwelling catheters, or urolithiasis. Mixed bacteriuria is usually caused by contamination from an improperly collected specimen or delay in transport. When the etiologic diagnosis is not obvious by recovery of a predominant pathogen, the test should be repeated with assurance that the specimen is obtained correctly.[9] Mixed bacteriuria associated with chronic catheter use may indicate colonization of the bladder and not necessarily active infection unless the patient is symptomatic. When infection is suspected, it is important to verify that the collection procedure was appropriate (e.g., the specimen was not taken from drainage reservoir) and to consider repeating the culture examination for confirmation. In many cases, another specimen will contain a different mixture of organisms. Thus, it is often difficult to evaluate the contribution of each organism to infection when the patient has an indwelling urinary catheter.

Follow-up Evaluation

Symptoms may subside with treatment even when bacteriuria remains. This may be caused by an unidentified resistant strain, poor compliance, or seeding from sequestered infection (e.g., prostatitis, pyelonephritis, perinephric abscess). A repeat culture at 48 hours showing persistent bacteriuria is considered a therapeutic failure. A repeat culture 2 weeks after completion of therapy indicates relapse (same infection) or recurrence (new infection).

Test: Reagent Strip (Dipstick)

Chemical analysis of urine is generally performed in conjunction with the microscopic examination. For infection, the two most important tests are the leukocyte esterase and nitrite tests.[10] These tests are usually performed together as components of the reagent strip dipstick method (see urinalysis, Ch. 3).

The detection of esterase activity from primary granules of neutrophils by reduction of a diazonium salt in buffered indoxyl carboxylic acid is the basis for chemical detection of pyuria. This test has the advantage of not being affected by leukocyte lysis but may be negative with relatively low numbers of leukocytes. False positive results may occur from interference of the reaction by high levels of urine albumin or ascorbic acid.

The nitrite test is capable of detecting bacteria that convert urine nitrate to nitrite. Although nitrate is reduced by common urinary tract pathogens (e.g., *E. coli, Staphylococcus*) the test will not detect other microorganisms, such as *Enterococcus* spp., many strains of *P. aeruginosa,* and fungi that do not reduce urine nitrate. First morning urine specimens that have remained in the bladder for an extended time provide the best sensitivity. A low dietary nitrate intake, which comes primarily from vegetables, may produce false negative results. In general, a positive nitrite result is highly sensitive for bacteriuria, whereas a negative test is unreliable for excluding infection.

Hematuria and albuminuria occur with bacterial urinary tract infection, but are inconsistent findings. *Proteus, Providencia, Klebsiella,* and some *Pseudomonas* species metabolize urea to ammonia, producing an alkaline urine (pH 8 or above) during infection, thereby providing a clue to the possible etiologic agent. However, this is not a specific finding; vegetarians and patients ingesting large quantities of antacids may have alkaline urine.

Test: Screening for Bacteriuria/Pyuria[11]

Background and Selection

A substantial amount of work is performed in the microbiology laboratory to process urine specimens, most of which are sterile. As a means of reducing costs and saving time, screening methods have been developed to identify specimens that presumably contain no bacteria or fungi, hence do not need to be cultured. Leukocyte esterase/nitrite (described above), filtration/staining, and bioluminescence are the leading screening tests. These procedures have in common the ability to provide rapid information in a convenient and economical way.

Logistics

The filtration staining test is performed by adding acetic acid or other lysate to urine to disrupt leukocytes and red blood cells. The mixture is passed through a filter by suction or gravity, stained with safranin, and then decolorized. The presence of sufficient quantities of bacteria, fungi, or cellular debris retained by the filter is identified by the intensity of staining.

Bacteriuria may be detected by measuring bacterial adenosine triphosphate (ATP) in urine. First, somatic ATP is removed from leukocytes and red blood cells by adding a lysing reagent and ATPase to a urine sample. After a short incubation period, releasing reagent is added to liberate bacterial ATP, which is measured in a luminometer by the bioluminescent luciferin-luciferase reaction.

Other bacteriuria screening methods have been developed, including tetrazolium reduction, catalase, subnormal glucose, and a proprietary method (Lypho-Qick, RUS) that claims to detect enzymes unique to urinary tract infections. None of these are widely used.

Interpretation

Screening tests are used almost exclusively to identify specimens not requiring culture. Sensitivity of all methods declines substantially with bacteriuria counts below 10^5/mL. The proportion of false positive results tends to be high and unfortunately, about 10% or more of specimens showing negative results contain a significant number of bacteria when cultured. Table 24-2 shows the relative sensitivity and specificity of these tests for detecting bacteriuria and pyuria. The procedures may perform well for screening asymptomatic patients or those with a low prevalence of infection, but negative results should be interpreted with caution, particularly in the symptomatic patient.

Test: Antigen Detection[12]

Latex agglutination and counter immunoelectrophoresis methods for detecting microbial antigens in urine are used primarily as rapid, preliminary tests in sus-

Table 24-2. Relative Sensitivity of Urine Screening Methods

Method	Bacteriuria[a] (>10^5/mL) Sensitivity	Specificity	Pyuria Sensitivity	Specificity
Microscopic examination	+++	++	+++	++
Filtration/staining	+++	+	+++	+
Leukocyte esterase	++	+	+++	+++
Nitrite	+	+++		
Bioluminescence	++	++		

[a] All methods have poor sensitivity and specificity below 5×10^4 organisms/mL.

pected cases of bacterial meningitis with negative cerebrospinal fluid Gram smear and culture results. These methods are used in identifying pneumococcal capsular polysaccharide, group B streptococcus, *N. meningitidis,* and *H. influenzae* (polyribophosphate polysaccharide) antigens. Testing a concentrated urine specimen in addition to cerebrospinal fluid may increase sensitivity. Antigen detection in urine but not in cerebrospinal fluid should be interpreted cautiously, because this combination of findings also is seen with bacteremia in the absence of meningitis. Antigenuria in the absence of infection may be present for 1 week or longer after administration of *H. influenzae* capsular vaccine. Antigenuria detection for identifying the etiologic agent in *S. pneumoniae* and *Legionella* pneumonia generally have poor sensitivity and are not routinely performed. The detection of *Histoplasmosis capsulatum* antigen in urine is a sensitive marker of disseminated disease, but the assay is not readily available.

TESTS TO LOCALIZE INFECTION

Test: Urine Culture of Specially Collected Specimens

In special cases, it may be desirable to know whether infection is confined to the bladder or involves the kidney. This differentation may have therapeutic implications, because upper tract infections tend to require longer therapy and closer follow-up. In most cases, the distinction can be made on clinical grounds. Furthermore, none of the noninvasive methods provide sufficient reliability or practicality to be employed as routine tests. With lower urinary tract infections, differential diagnosis by segmental sampling and culture of urine and prostate secretions helps differentiate between urethritis, cystitis, and prostatitis as discussed under Test: Urine Culture (Bacterial).

The method by which urine is collected can be helpful in identifying infection in specific anatomic regions of the urinary tract. Collecting a series of the first 10 mL voided urine (VB_1), midstream urine (VB_2), postmassage prostatic secretions (EPS), and postmassage urine (VB_3) is of value in discriminating among urethritis, cystitis, and prostatitis.

Differential diagnosis of the infection site using segmental sampling of urine and prostate secretion specimens is made by comparing relative and absolute differences in colony counts (Table 24-3). This is most useful for establishing the diagnosis and identifying the etiologic agent in chronic bacterial prostatitis. Infection is usually caused by Enterobacteriaceae and less often by *S. aureus, Enterococcus, P. aeruginosa,* and *N. gonorrhoeae.* Occasionally, *S. epidermidis,* diphtheroids, and other organisms ordinarily considered to be contaminants may cause prostatitis.

The bladder washout method helps differentiate between upper and lower tract infections with about 80% accuracy. This is done by collecting a series of three urine specimens over 30 minutes after the bladder has been irrigated with a disinfectant. The presence of increasing numbers of bacteria isolated from each sample indicates seeding from an upper tract source, whereas sterile cultures imply localized bladder infection.

Test: Antibody Coated Bacteriuria

Bacteria causing upper urinary tract infections tend to be coated with immunoglobulins, which can be detected by direct immunofluorescence staining of urine with polyspecific or monospecific antihuman immunoglobulin.[13] The antibody coated bacteriuria test is not standardized, nor is it commonly performed in clinical laboratories. It has been used as a parameter to localize and differentiate infection: antibody coated bacteriuria are present with pyelonephritis and absent with cysti-

Table 24-3. Differential Diagnosis by Segmental Sampling of Urine and Prostate Secretions

Interpretation	VB$_1$	VB$_2$	EPS	VB$_3$
Normal	<200[a]	<100	<100	<100
Urethritis	10^3–10^4	<10^3	<100	10^3–10^4
Cystitis	10^3–10^4	10^4–10^6	<10^3	10^4–10^5
Prostatitis	10^2–10^3	10^2–10^3	10^3–10^4	10^3–10^4

[a] Organisms/mL.
Abbreviations: VB$_1$, urethral urine specimen (10 mL); VB$_2$, midstream urine; EPS, secretions expressed after prostate massage, or ejaculate; VB$_3$, urine voided after prostate massage.

tis, but results are not specific. Positive staining is observed in patients with bacterial prostatitis, chronic indwelling catheters, diabetes mellitus, bladder tumors, and about 15% of patients with cystitis. Although the test lacks specificity for the site of infection, patients with antibody coated bacteriuria tend to require longer therapy to cure infection.

Other Tests

Elevated urine concentrations of lactate dehydrogenase isoenzyme 5, glucuronidase, and β_2-microglobulin may be found in association with upper urinary tract infection. These tests do not have sufficient sensitivity and specificity, however, to localize infection reliably to the upper urinary tract. Urine specific gravity below 1.020 found on a first morning collection from a patient not receiving fluids the evening before indicates a concentrating deficiency. Patients with pyelonephritis, but not cystitis, generally have such a defect.

Although infrequently done because of the invasiveness and risk of the procedure, analysis of specimens selectively obtained from ureteral catheterization is the most reliable method for localizing infection. Finally, a simple and functional test for localization is the therapeutic trial. Patients with uncomplicated lower tract infections usually respond to single dose treatment, in contrast to those with renal infection who relapse.

ADDITIONAL TYPES OF URINE CULTURES

Test: Anaerobic Culture

Routine anaerobic culture of urine is not indicated, because anaerobic organisms are rarely implicated as pathologic agents in urinary tract infections. Furthermore, anaerobes commonly inhabit the urethra, providing a likely source of culture contamination that makes it difficult to judge the significance of culture results. Consequently, in the rare instance that anaerobic culture is necessary, specimens should be collected via suprapubic aspiration. There are a few circumstances, such as chronic urolithiasis, renal abscess, necrotizing genital lesions (Fournier's disease), and sterile pyuria, in which anaerobic urine culture may be considered.

Test: Fungal Culture[14]

Background and Selection

There are two principal indications for performing fungal culture; symptoms and signs of urinary tract infection in the immunosuppressed patient and suspected disseminated infection with *Histoplasma, Blastomyces, Coccidioides, Aspergillus, Cryptococcus,* or *Candida.* The use of broad spectrum antibiotics or corticosteriods, hematologic malignancy, and diabetes mellitius constitutes predisposing conditions for ascending lower urinary tract infection with *Candida,* especially when an indwelling catheter is present. Primary or opportunistic disseminated fungal infections may spread to the kidney through the bloodstream and progress to the lower urinary tract.

Logistics

Candida generally grows into observable colonies on blood or gram-negative selective media within 2–3 days. Sabouraud agar, incubated at 30°C, is recommended when fungi are suspected from microscopic examination or in association with a predisposing condition. Enriched blood-containing media should be used for isolating dimorphic fungi in suspected cases of disseminated infection. Prolonged incubation is usually necessary to recover *Histoplasma* and *Blastomyces*.

Interpretation

Candiduria in uncomplicated infections generally indicates vaginitis or contamination from the vagina or gastrointestinal tract. Serious *Candida* and other fungal infections are nearly always associated with predisposing factors. Prolonged antibiotic therapy, chronic indwelling catheter usage, and diabetes mellitus are associated with primary (ascending) infections, whereas immunosuppression and hyperalimentation are conditions favoring hematogenously spread disseminated infection. In these infections, a colony count below 10,000/mL is typical. Recovery of *Rhodotorula* or *Saccharomyces* nearly always indicates contamination. The presence of *Histoplasma, Coccidioides, Cryptococcus,* or *Aspergillus* is significant and signifies systemic disease. *Aspergillus* urinary tract infection is generally associated with asymptomatic hematuria. *Blastomyces dermatitidis,* and less often *Coccidioides immitis,* isolated from the urine may indicate localized prostate infection.

Test: Leptospira Culture

Background and Selection

Leptospira spp. is a spirochete transmitted by contact with water or soil contaminated with infected urine of domestic and wild animals. Infection is generally subclinical but may present as a severe, relapsing, febrile illness with meningitis or hepatocellular injury. The diagnosis, which requires special urine culture procedures, should be considered in the patient having any of these symptoms and a history of occupational risk or animal exposure (e.g., veterinarians).

Logistics

Leptospiras appear in the urine during the second week of disease and, without therapy, may persist for months. Because organisms are shed intermittently, multiple urine specimens should be obtained when examination for this spirochete is warranted. To maintain organism viability, it is also helpful to alkalinize the urine before collection. Direct dark-field microscopic examination of urine has poor diagnostic sensitivity for identifying *Leptospira* and is complicated by artifacts.

A variety of special semisolid culture media (e.g., Fletcher's) are used for *Leptospira* culture. Before inoculation, urine is adjusted to neutral pH and diluted 1000-fold with 1% bovine serum albumin (BSA). Isolation also can be performed by intraperitoneal inoculation of urine into weanling hamsters. Because the process of culturing *Leptospira* is hazardous and relatively demanding for the clinical laboratory, serologic testing is a suitable alternative method for diagnosis.

Interpretation

Recovery of *Leptospira* from urine is diagnostic.

Test: Mycobacterial Culture

Background and Selection

Renal infection by *M. tuberculosis* should be considered with persistent pyuria, hematuria, and negative bacterial cultures. Most patients have a positive tuberculin skin test and abnormal chest x-ray.

Logistics

Three consecutive, clean-catch, midstream, first morning urine specimens are recommended for *M. tuberculosis* culture. *Mycobacteria* spp. are recovered by culturing urine sediment on Lowenstein-Jensen and Middlebrook 7H-11 media. Although urine specimens do not ordinarily require decontamination, cultures may be quickly overgrown by contaminating flora if a poorly collected specimen is processed.

Interpretation

When renal infection by *M. tuberculosis* is suspected, examination of an acid-fast smear of urine sediment can provide a preliminary diagnosis, if substantial numbers of organisms are observed, but does not preclude culture, because the urine sediment may contain nonpathogenic, commensal acid-fast bacilli. Numerous acid-fast bacilli in the urine sediment of patients with acquired immunodeficiency syndrome (AIDS) suggest disseminated *M. avium* complex infection. The isolation of *M. tuberculosis* indicates disseminated or renal infection, and it is common for patients with renal infection to have positive urine cultures. Isolation of other mycobacteria is distinctly unusual and its significance must be correlated with clinical manifestations of disease.

Test: Neisseria Gonorrhoeae Culture

Neisseria gonorrhoeae can be recovered using an appropriate medium (Thayer-Martin agar) from the urine sediment or an unspun first voided urine specimen. A urine specimen is nearly as good as the urethral swab in men, but has less sensitivity than the cervical specimen in women. Urine culture for *N. gonorrhoeae* has been applied to screening asymptomatic men.

Test: Viral Culture

Background and Selection

Urine is the specimen of choice for virus isolation in only a few viral diseases. In some instances, virus is present in urine before the onset of clinical symptoms but disappears before the infection is apparent. The list of viral agents that may be isolated from urine is short and limited primarily to cytomegalovirus (CMV), adenovirus, and mumps virus.

Cytomegalovirus is readily isolated from urine during acute infections. Culture is indicated for newborns with jaundice, petechial rash, lethargy, respiratory distress syndrome, and neurologic defects; and immunocompromised hosts, most notably transplant recipients and AIDS patients having fever, mononucleosis, interstitial pneumonitis, chorioretinitis, and hepatitis. Identification of CMV in symptomatic patients receiving immunosuppressive agents for a transplanted organ may be warranted as an indicator to modify immunosuppressive therapy to permit recovery from infections without endangering the transplant. Cytomegalovirus infection in the AIDS patients is often fatal, and its identification may be grounds for experimental therapy.

Acute hemorrhagic cystitis, often denoted by dysuria and blood in the urine, may be caused by adenovirus types 2, 11, and 21. This infection occurs more commonly in children than in adults. The diagnosis requires urine culture.

Mumps has been isolated from urine on some occasions when all other specimens failed to yield infectious virus. The virus may be isolated from urine for up to 2 weeks after the onset of clinical illness. This finding may be of critical importance for diagnosis of mumps virus meningitis. Viral cultures are not routinely indicated for self-limited infections with mumps virus and adenoviruses.

Herpes simplex virus may be recovered from the urine in disseminated infection of the newborn. The infant appears normal at birth, but within a few days, lethargy, irritability, and loss of suck and gag reflexes develop. Vesicular skin lesions, hepatitis, thrombocytopenia, and encephalitis follow with disease progression. Identification of herpes simplex virus (HSV) in this circumstance is important, because acyclovir (Zovirax) therapy may lessen the severity of infection and decrease viral shedding.

Although other viruses may be transiently present in urine during the course of infection, there is little indication for attempting to recover them. Consultation between the physician and laboratory is advisable before examining urine in order to determine availability of testing procedures and to provide specific information that may aid in viral identification.

Logistics

Specimen Requirements

A first morning, clean-catch, midstream specimen is recommended. Cytomegalovirus is excreted only sporadically during infection, requiring collection and analysis of three specimens on successive days to achieve optimal sensitivity. Urine should be kept cold (on an ice slurry), not frozen. Specimens for viral culture requiring storage for more than 48 hours should be frozen at $-70°C$. Dry Ice is used when transported to a distant laboratory.

Method

Urine for viral culture is inoculated onto the appropriate cell cultures directly, or it may be diluted 1:2 in phosphate-buffered saline (PBS) or a balanced salt solution to reduce inherent toxicity in urine. Cells are observed daily for cytopathogenic effect. In the case of suspected CMV disease, inoculated cells should be observed for 3 weeks before being considered negative for virus. Other viruses, such as HSV or adenovirus, are detected from 1 day to 2 weeks after inoculation. The identity of the virus isolate is confirmed by immunologic analysis.

Interpretation

In association with clinical symptoms, isolation of any of the viruses listed in Table 24-4 is significant and indicative of an etiologic role of the virus. It should be noted that in some instances CMV can be cultured from the urine in asymptomatic patients, especially

Table 24-4. Viruses isolated from urine

Result	Interpretation, Associated Disease
Adenovirus: types 2, 11, or 21	Hemorrhagic cystitis, dysuria
Cytomegalovirus	Congenital infection, immunosuppression with pneumonitis, mononucleosis, hepatitis, systemic disease
Mumps virus	Parotitis, meningitis, orchitis
Virus infrequently isolated from or identified in urine	
Arbovirus	Hemorrhagic fevers
Hepatitis B virus	Hepatitis (acute, chronic), nephritis, glomerulonephritis
Herpes simplex virus	AIDS, disseminated congenital infection
Papovavirus	
BK polyomavirus	No disease association
JC polyomavirus	Progressive multifocal leukoencephalopathy
Rubeola	Measles

during late pregnancy, in children under 1 year of age, and for prolonged periods after a primary infection. Recovery of CMV from the urine of a newborn indicates congenital infection.

Urine specimens may also contain JC or BK polyomaviruses (Table 24-4), which are periodically shed throughout the life of infected persons. BK virus is not associated with disease, whereas JC virus causes progressive multifocal leukoencephalopathy in immunocompromised patients.

DIRECT MICROSCOPIC EXAMINATION

Test: Microscopic Examination of Urine for Bacteria and Fungi[15]

Background and Selection

When bacterial or fungal infection of the urinary tract is suspected, direct microscopic analysis of the urine sediment may provide a presumptive diagnosis and serve as an ancillary test to culture.

Terminology

Pyuria indicates the appearance of leukocytes in the urine. Bacteriuria or bladder bacteriuria refers to the presence of bacteria in the urinary bladder.

Logistics

A wet-mounted urine specimen for microscopic examination is prepared by first centrifuging a 10-mL sample for 5 minutes at 1200g. After pouring off the supernatant, the remaining sediment is placed on a glass slide, stained with methylene blue or left unstained, protected with a glass coverslip, and microscopically examined under reduced light at 400×. Alternatively, a heat-fixed smear of unspun urine or its centrifuged sediment is gram stained and inspected at 1000×. At this magnification, one organism seen per field approximates 10^5 organisms/mL.

Interpretation

The presence of more than 10 bacteria or more than 5 white blood cells per field observed in clean-catch specimens indicates possible infection, but any number is significant from catheter or suprapubic aspiration samples (Fig. 24-1). A small number of leukocytes or bacteria in asymptomatic women has dubious significance because of the likelihood of vaginal contamination. Identification of white blood cell casts (Fig. 24-1) is a key diagnostic finding, indicative of pyelonephritis. Diuresis can affect the interpretation of results by reducing the quantity of cells observed per specimen aliquot. White blood cell enumeration also may be falsely decreased by lysis in hypotonic or alkaline urine when specimen examination is delayed, even if for only a few hours.

The number of white blood cells observed in urine sediment is variable and dependent on methodologic differences in preparing and examining the specimen. A more precise quantitation of pyuria is obtained by examining an unspun urine specimen with the hematocytometer. Urine containing more than 10 leukocytes/mm^3 indicates significant pyuria. Pyuria is such an important finding associated with urinary tract infections that its absence in a properly collected and ana-

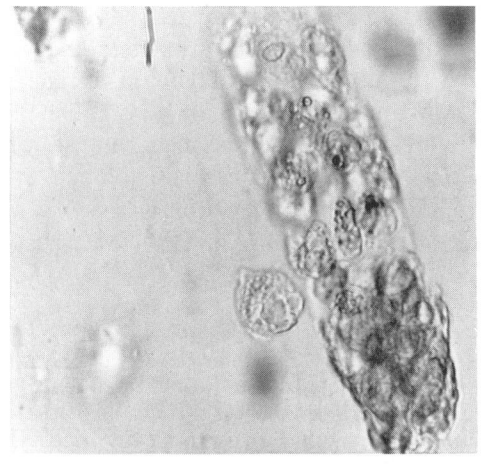
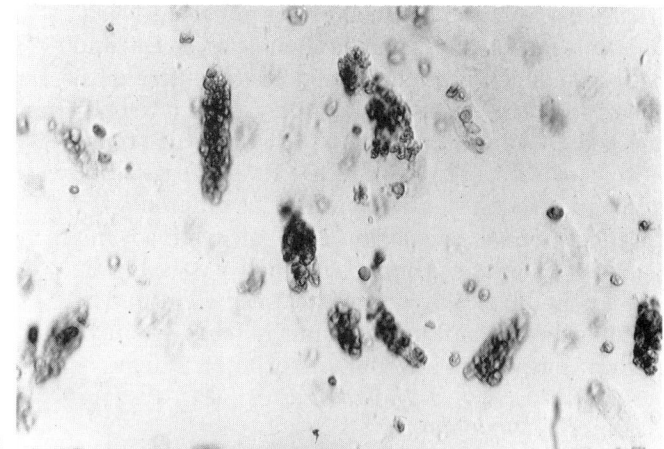

Fig. 24-1. (A&B) Wet mount of urine sediment. Pyuria with white blood cell casts. (Fig. A, 100×; Fig. B, 400×.)

lyzed specimen helps exclude the diagnosis. Pyuria is not specific, however. White blood cells may come from the vagina or be associated with noninfectious inflammatory conditions of the urinary tract.

The Gram stain procedure has some advantages over the wet-mount examination by contributing more information about organism morphology and identity, providing more reproducible results, having slightly greater sensitivity, and requiring less technical skill to read. These benefits are achieved at the cost of being more labor intensive, a factor accounting for why the urine Gram smear and hematocytometer methods are not generally performed as routine laboratory examinations.

Test: Direct Examination for Protozoa and Helminths

Background and Selection

When indicated, examination of urine is useful for diagnosing *Schistosoma haematobium*, *Trichomonas vaginalis*, or *Onchocerca volvulus* infection. Some form of concentration technique such as simple sedimentation or centrifugation, or both, is used. Direct examination of the sediment is done to identify the diagnostic stage of the parasite.

Interpretation

Urinary Schistosomiasis

Schistosoma haematobium, a trematode common in parts of Africa (along the Nile river) and western Asia, is acquired after exposure to cercaria-infested waters. Adult worms live in the venous plexuses of the urinary bladder, rectum, pelvis, and are occasionally found in ectopic sites. Because of the close proximity of these flukes to the bladder during oviposition, eggs break free of the vessel, cross the mucosa, and rupture into the lumen, accompanied by extravasated blood. Acute infection is usually asymptomatic, although eosinophilia is common. Frequency, terminal dysuria, proteinuria, and elevated levels of IgG and IgE occur with chronic infection and large worm load. Hematuria is one of the earliest symptoms to appear and is usually noted at the end of micturition. Urinary schistosomiasis should be considered in patients with appropriate exposure history and eosinophilia, proteinuria, hematuria, obstructive uropathy, or urinary tract infection. Diagnosis is made by identifying the parasite in a urine or tissue biopsy specimen.

Pathologic effects from *S. haematobium* infection occur as a result of the infiltration and accumulation of eggs in the bladder wall and tissues of adjacent pelvic structures. Exuberant tissue reaction occurs with marked granulomatous inflammation. With continuous exposure to the parasites and concurrent egg deposition, marked fibrosis of the bladder wall and adjacent structures occurs, leading to obstruction of the urinary tract and hydronephrosis. Recurrent secondary bacterial infections eventually result in damage to the upper urinary tract. The development of squamous cell carcinoma of the bladder has long been associated with this infection, but no direct cause and effect relationship has been demonstrated.

Eggs of this species measure 112–170 μm by 40–70 μm and have a terminal spine. Either single urine specimens or 24-hour collections may be used to recover the eggs of this species. If single specimens are to be submitted, early afternoon collections are preferred. Negative results on a single specimen should be suspect, and a patient should not be considered infection free until three to four specimens over as many days have been examined. In addition, eggs may be discharged in seminal fluid or recovered from feces. Rarely, eggs of *S. mansoni* are seen in urine and must be differentiated from those of *S. haematobium*. Serologic testing is not reliable for diagnosis. Enumeration of live eggs may be useful for monitoring efficacy of treatment. This can be accomplished by counting miracidia hatched after ova have been suspended in water and exposed to light.

Trichomonas Vaginalis

Examination of the urine in females suspected of harboring *T. vaginalis* is of little value compared with evaluation of vaginal and urethral discharges. In males, however, urine examination may be useful in attempting to diagnose occult infections and serves as an adjunct to the examination of urethral discharges or prostate secretions. Ideally a fresh urine sediment is examined for the presence of typical motile trophozoites. The organism rapidly loses motility and begins to degenerate on standing at room temperature. Culture offers additional sensitivity, as does direct examination using fluorescent monoclonal antibody reagents. Indications for, and interpretation of, this test are described in Chapter 25.

Onchocerca Volvulus

Microfilarieae of *O. volvulus* are found in the urine sediment of infected patients. If microfilarieae are detected on wet mount, smears of the sediment should be stained with Giemsa to confirm the diagnosis. Indications for and interpretation of this test are described in Chapter 20.

Test: Direct Examination for Virus[16]

Direct examination of cells in the urine sediment for CMV or HSV by immunofluorescence is a rapid ancillary test to culture. Caution must be used in interpreting negative results, because the sensitivity of direct examination is consistently lower than with culture. A portion of the original specimen from patients for whom there is a high suspicion of a viral infection should be retained for viral culture if direct testing is negative. False positive results are generally not a complication with these examinations. Viral antigen detection of CMV and HSV is usually accomplished using immunofluorescence or immunoenzyme staining of cells after concentration by centrifugation.

REFERENCES

1. Lipsky BA: Urinary tract infections in men. Epidemiology, pathophysiology, diagnosis and treatment. Ann Intern Med 1989;110:138–150.
2. Stamm WE, Hooton TM, Johnson JR, et al: Urinary tract infections: from pathogenesis to treatment. J Infect Dis 1989;159:400–406.
3. Kunin CM: Detection, Prevention and Management of Urinary Tract Infections. 4th Ed. Philadelphia; Lea & Febiger, 1987.
4. Harber MJ, Asscher AW: Virulence of urinary pathogens. Kidney Int 1985;28:717–721.
5. Komaroff AL: Urinalysis and urine culture in women with dysuria. Ann Intern Med 1986;104:212–218.
6. Fung, JC, Lucia B, Clark E, et al: Primary culture media for routine urine processing. J Clin Microbiol 1982; 16:632–636.
7. Kellogg JA, Manzella JP, Shaffer SN, Schwartz BB: Clinical relevance of culture versus screens for the detection of microbial pathogens in urine specimens. Am J Med 1987;83:739–745.
8. Platt R: Quantitative definition of bacteriuria. Am J Med 1983;75(1B):44–52.
9. Bartlett RC, Treiber N: Clinical significance of mixed bacterial cultures of urine. Am J Clin Pathol 1984; 82:319–322.
10. Pfaller MA, Koontz FP: Laboratory evaluation of leukocyte esterase and nitrite tests for the detection of bacteriuria. J Clin Microbiol 1985;21:840–842.
11. Murray PR, Smith TB, McKinney TC: Clinical evaluation of three urine screening tests. J Clin Microbiol 1987; 25:467–470.
12. Coonrod JD: Urine as an antigen reservoir for diagnosis of infectious disease. Am J Med 1983;75(1B):85–92.
13. Thomas V, Shelokow A, Forland M: Antibody coated bacteria in the urine and the site of urinary-tract infection. N Engl J Med 1974;290:588–590.
14. Frangos DN, Nyberg LM: Genitourinary fungal infections. South Med J 1988;79:455–559.
15. Jenkins RD, Fenn JP, Matsen JM: Review of urine microscopy for bacteriuria. JAMA 1986;255:3397–3403.
16. Minnich LL, Smith TF, Ray CG: Cumitech 24, Rapid detection of Viruses by Immunofluorescence. S. Specter (coord ed). Washington DC, American Society for Microbiology, 1988.

25 Genital Tract

George P. Schmid
Robert C. Barnes
Thomas R. Fritsche

INTRODUCTION

Sexually transmitted diseases (STDs) are extremely common in all social strata of society. Although some diseases occur with more frequency than others in varying social strata, the transmission of one or more of the approximately 30 organisms known to be sexually transmitted is possible whenever a person has sexual intercourse (Table 25-1). Although gonorrhea is the most common nationally reportable disease in the United States, with 734,485 cases reported in 1989, most cases are probably not reported, and additional STDs that are not reported nationally total a far greater number of infections. It is estimated that (1) as many as 40 million Americans have had genital herpes, with as many as 500,000 new cases occurring annually; (2) four million Americans develop a chlamydial genital tract infection each year; and (3) up to 750,000 Americans are infected annually with human papillomavirus (HPV) (the cause of genital warts and perhaps important in the development of cervical cancer). These figures, and evidence from research studies, suggest that STDs are easily transmitted. Although the skin offers relative protection against penetration by STD agents, the mucosal surfaces of the cervix in women and the urethra in men offer portals of entry, as do minor abrasions acquired during intercourse. For example, it has been estimated that the minimal infecting dose (ID_{50}) for *Treponema pallidum* is 57 organisms or fewer and that during a single act of intercourse with an infected patient, transmission will occur in one-third of cases. Similarly, men have about a 20% chance of acquiring gonorrhea from an infected female partner during a single act of intercourse.

The significance of STDs and the recent awareness that certain STDs, particularly those associated with genital ulceration, enhance the transmission of human immunodeficiency virus (HIV) have led to renewed emphasis on the diagnosis and treatment of STDs. New diagnostic tests for many STDs are appearing, although the time-honored methods of microscopy and culture remain benchmark tests.

BASIC TESTS

Test: Urethral Exudate Examination

Background

Both men and women can have urethral infections with any of several STD agents. Most urethral infections in women, however, are inapparent and occur concomitant to cervical or vaginal infection. Similarly, in men, many urethral infections occur without obvious symptoms.

Table 25-1. Sexually Transmitted Disease: Clinical Syndromes and Associated Pathogens

Syndrome	Pathogen
Urethritis	Neisseria gonorrhoeae
	Chlamydia trachomatis
	Ureaplasma urealyticum
	Herpes simplex virus
	Trichomonas vaginalis
	Mycoplasma genitalium
Genital ulcer	Treponema pallidum
	Haemophilus ducreyi
	Herpes simplex virus
	Calymmatobacterium granulomatis
Cervicitis	Neisseria gonorrhoeae
	Chlamydia trachomatis
	Herpes simplex virus
Rectal discharge	Herpes simplex virus
	Campylobacter spp.
	Neisseria gonorrhoeae
	Chlamydia trachomatis
Vaginitis	Bacterial vaginosis (Gardnerella vaginalis, Mobiluncus spp., Bacteroides spp., Mycoplasma hominis)
	Trichomonas vaginalis
	Candida spp.

The most commonly identified causes of urethritis are *Neisseria gonorrhoeae* and *Chlamydia trachomatis*. Nongonococcal urethritis (NGU), which is urethritis not caused by *N. gonorrhoeae*, is twice as common as urethritis caused by *N. gonorrhoeae*,[1] and about one-half are caused by *C. trachomatis*. Simultaneous involvement with *N. gonorrhoeae* and *C. trachomatis* occur in about 30% of urethral infections in women. *Ureaplasma urealyticum* may be responsible for as many as 10% of NGU cases, although most men with a urethral infection by *U. urealyticum* do not develop symptoms. *Trichomonas vaginalis* occasionally causes urethritis. Infection in the male is usually manifest by recurring urethritis and rarely prostatitis and may even result in reversible sterility. Males are often symptomless, however, and may serve as reservoirs for their sexual partners.

The etiologic diagnosis of approximately one-half of NGU infections is not obtained by laboratory testing. Although the pathogenic role of other agents is not well defined, candidates include uropathogenic *Escherichia coli*, anaerobic bacteria, *Mycoplasma genitalium*, and herpes simplex virus (HSV). Urethritis can be a prominent finding in HSV infection of the genitalia, particularly during primary episodes of infection. Painful regional lymphadenopathy and cutaneous ulcerations are helpful in suggesting this etiology; however, isolated urethritis in the absence of skin lesions is unusual.

Selection

Dysuria and/or urethral discharge in a sexually active man is the most common clinical presentation for which a urethral specimen is obtained to identify *N. gonorrhoeae* or *C. trachomatis*. Examination of specimens from the throat and anus is also indicated if there is a history of homosexual contact. *Trichomonas vaginalis, U. urealyticum,* or HSV should be considered as potential causes of urethritis in men with persistent objective evidence of urethritis, that is, visible discharge or Gram stain showing white blood cells (WBCs), after treatment with antimicrobial agents generally indicated for urethritis (tetracycline, doxycycline, or erythromycin). Because up to 10% of *U. urealyticum* strains may be resistant to tetracycline, continued objective signs of urethritis after tetracycline therapy in the absence of potential reinfection is one of the few indications for laboratory isolation of genital mycoplasmas. Asymptomatic infection, especially with *C. trachomatis*, is common and plays an important role in the transmission of disease. Laboratory evaluation should be considered in the asymptomatic man who has an infected or new sexual partner, is in a high risk group, or has unexplained pyuria. Specimens for the laboratory diagnosis of urethritis in women also are obtained from other sites, such as the cervix and urine.

Logistics

Specimen Requirements

Many agents associated with urethritis are fastidious, and sensitivity of isolation may fail if improper techniques or materials are used in specimen collection. Specimens for microscopic examination by Gram stain or by antigen detection methods should be obtained with a urethral swab. A metallic wire shaft with a fiber tip is the standard collection device. The tip may be cotton, Dacron, or alginate material. If similar swabs are to be used for cultivation of organisms, they must be evaluated for toxicity or growth inhibition of the organisms to be isolated, because materials in some lots of swabs may be inhibitory or may produce a cytopathic effect in cell culture monolayers. In general, cotton and Dacron are superior to alginate for cultivation of *C.*

trachomatis.[2] Calcium alginate swabs are preferred for recovery of *N. gonorrhoeae*.

If the urethral discharge is spontaneous and profuse, the clinician may be tempted to use material freely expressed at the urethral meatus. Material at the urethral meatus or material obtained by stripping the urethra is generally sufficient for Gram staining, for the diagnosis of urethritis and *N. gonorrhoeae* infection. If specimens for the culture of *N. gonorrhoeae* and *C. trachomatis* are to be obtained, however, this is not the best approach. For these tests, the swab should be inserted 2–4 cm into the urethra and rotated for several seconds. This technique provides specimens that are not exposed to the highly oxygenated environment outside the urethra and samples sufficient urethral epithelial cells to isolate intracellular *(C. trachomatis)* or cell-associated *(U. urealyticum)* organisms.

Specimen Transport. Transport systems for cultivation of *N. gonorrhoeae* and *C. trachomatis* are critical for sensitive identification of these pathogens. The most effective culture system for *N. gonorrhoeae* is immediate ("bedside") inoculation of the specimen onto selective medium and immediate incubation in a moist 3–10% CO_2 chamber. In general, nutrient transport media, such as the Transgrow, Jembec, and Bio-bag systems, which use CO_2 and selective media, are superior to "holding media" designed to permit survival of organisms without promoting growth. Holding media (culturettes containing buffered media, e.g., Amies' or Stuart's) must be plated within 6 hours of collection to avoid loss of organism viability.

Culture of *C. trachomatis* is dependent on maintaining a satisfactory cold chain to maintain organism viability for cell culture isolation. Few studies have systematically compared available transport media for *C. trachomatis*. The media that appear satisfactory are SPG, 2-SP, and 4-SP, each of which contains sodium in excess of potassium.[3] The addition of bovine serum albumin (BSA) to *C. trachomatis* transport medium may provide stability if specimens are to be stored for more than a few hours before inoculation into cell culture.

Analysis

Smears for microscopic examination should be applied to slides immediately upon collection. The swab should be rolled gently and evenly over the slide surface to obtain a thin layer of exudate for examination. Urethral smears usually contain sufficient proteinaceous material to ensure adequate fixation of material to a glass slide. Gentle heat fixation of the slide before Gram staining may be applied, but if slides are overheated, cellular morphology will be distorted.

Neisseria Gonorrhoeae. Specimens for primary isolation of *N. gonorrhoeae* should be streaked heavily onto a selective medium and incubated for 48 hours in a 3–10% CO_2 atmosphere in high humidity at 35°C. A Z pattern is often used, with all sides of the swab—the laboratory then streaks the entire surface of the plate. Nonselective medium is occasionally recommended simultaneously, because 2–30% of strains of *N. gonorrhoeae*, which are sensitive to the concentration of vancomycin in selective media, will be inhibited. Colonies of *N. gonorrhoeae* appear as light-colored, mucoid colonies, 1–3 mm in diameter, that may be transparent or opaque. Presumptive identification of *Neisseriaceae* can be made on the basis of colony morphology, Gram stain demonstration of gram-negative diplococci, and a positive oxidase reaction. Further identification is based on biochemical testing or antigen detection of culture results. In cases of medicolegal importance, such as in alleged sexual abuse, absolute confirmation requires the use of two tests based on different methodologies: biochemical, immunologic, or enzymatic profile. A test for β-lactamase production should also be performed on all *N. gonorrhoeae* isolates.

Chlamydia Trachomatis. Various cell culture procedures are available for isolation of *C. trachomatis*. The most sensitive method is generally accepted to be the shell vial method of growth in McCoy or HeLa-229 cells, in which the clinical specimen is centrifuged onto cells and incubated in a culture medium containing supplementary glucose, 1-glutamine, and fetal bovine serum. Cycloheximide in the medium increases the size and number of chlamydial inclusions. The microtiter plate method of Yoder et al.[4] is more convenient for processing large sample volumes but may require one or more blind passages to achieve comparable sensitivity to the shell vial method. The use of monoclonal fluorescent antibody has improved the sensitivity and timeliness of in vitro detection methods. It is important to realize that specimen collection and transport are critical to optimal cell culture sensitivity. Even under optimal conditions, no method of chlamydial detection is currently accepted as having an adequate sensitivity to rule out infection with a single specimen.

Nonculture methods currently available for the diagnosis of *C. trachomatis* include direct fluorescent antibody (DFA), enzyme-linked immunoassay (ELISA), and nucleic acid probes. As these methods do not require viable chlamydial particles, specimens are generally easier to transport than are specimens for cell culture. Comparative testing has demonstrated that both

Table 25-2. Diagnostic Value of Direct Antigen Detection for the Diagnosis of *Chlamydia trachomatis* Infection

| | Sensitivity | | Specificity | | Predictive Value of | | | |
| | | | | | Positive | | Negative | |
Group	ELISA	DFA	ELISA	DFA	ELISA	DFA	ELISA	DFA
Men								
Symptomatic	79	92	97	97	93	87	90	98
Asymptomatic	49	—	95	—	85	—	88	—
Women								
Symptomatic	89	90	95	95	80	90	98	98
Asymptomatic	85	77	97	97	70	79	98	98

Abbreviations: DFA, direct fluorescent antibody; ELISA, enzyme-linked immunosorbent assay.
(Data from Stamm.[8])

DFA and ELISA tests are acceptable alternatives to culture for patient groups at high risk of chlamydial infection. Direct fluorescent antibody is more labor intensive (Table 25-2) than ELISA for analyzing large groups of specimens, but tends to be more sensitive and specific. Comparative studies of the performance of nucleic acid detection methods have not adequately defined the clinical role for these tests.

Other. When other pathogens are suspected, urethral exudate in broth medium (urea broth for *U. urealyticum* and Diamond's medium for *T. vaginalis*) or cell culture (for HSV) is indicated.

Interpretation

The presence of inflammatory cells in a smear from the distal urethra is diagnostic of urethritis, the most common STD syndrome occurring in men. A WBC count of at least 4 in each of five 1000× microscopic fields of a urethral exudate obtained by swab supports the diagnosis of urethritis.[5] In the absence of urinary tract infection in a male, pyuria observed in the first 10–15 mL of urine obtained at least 2 hours after the last void is also strong evidence of urethral inflammation. The low cost of rapid testing of first-void urine by leukocyte esterase dipsticks makes these tests an attractive screening tool for urethritis in asymptomatic men. There are, however, conflicting data regarding the sensitivity of these tests.

Neisseria Gonorrhoeae

Observation of intracellular gram-negative diplococci on a urethral smear from a symptomatic male is both sensitive (96%) and specific (nearly 100%) for gonorrhea. In asymptomatic men, sensitivity is reduced to only 70%, and specificity to around 85%.[6] Tests that detect antigens of *N. gonorrhoeae* by ELISA have not achieved sufficient sensitivity to be recommended for primary detection. Improvements in these and other rapid test methods will have little value over the inexpensive and rapid Gram stain for urethral specimens from symptomatic men.

Culture of a single urethral swab on selective *N. gonorrhoeae* medium has a sensitivity in excess of 95% and a specificity that depends on the confirmatory tests used for identification, but that approaches 100%. The presence of diphtheroids, *Staphylococcus epidermidis*, and α-hemolytic streptococci has no diagnostic significance. False positive results may occasionally be produced if the laboratory identification is insufficiently comprehensive to differentiate *N. gonorrhoeae* from other *Neisseria* spp., as well as other biochemically similar organisms, such as *Kingella denitrificans*, which will grow on selective media. False positive identifications caused by nonspecific reactions may occur with antigen detection methods.

Chlamydia Trachomatis

The sensitivity of a single urethral swab for isolation of *C. trachomatis* by cell culture methods is probably about 80%. Comparisons with cell culture have shown that ELISA for detecting *C. trachomatis* has a sensitivity of 67–92% and a specificity of 76–96%.[7] Direct fluorescent antibody detection methods have shown sensitivities that have depended on the number of elementary bodies used as a test cutoff, but which ranged from 49–100%, with test specificities of 73–98%.[8] In general, these tests have adequate performances for screening symptomatic, high risk men. Because of their high specificity, cell culture methods are the diagnostic method of choice in disputed or medicolegal cases.

Other

When appropriate laboratory tests do not suggest *C. trachomatis* or *N. gonorrhoeae* as the cause of urethritis, further laboratory testing may identify HSV, *T. vaginalis*, or *U. urealyticum*. Isolation of HSV or *T. vaginalis* strongly suggests that these agents are responsible for the symptoms. Although *U. urealyticum* has been associated with urethritis in epidemiologic and human volunteer studies, the ubiquitous nature of this agent makes interpretation of its pathogenicity difficult; nevertheless, treatment directed toward it is probably warranted.

Test: Examination of Vaginal Secretions

Background

Most vaginal secretions arise from mucus-secreting columnar epithelial cells in the cervix, with the remainder derived from epithelial cells in the vaginal mucosa. Infection with a pathogenic organism at either location can lead to an abnormal vaginal discharge. Normal vaginal secretions are thin or mucoid, white, and are without an unpleasant odor. The predominant flora are lactobacilli, which outnumber smaller numbers of diphtheroids, *S. epidermidis,* and anaerobic microorganisms. The production of lactic acid by the lactobacilli keeps the vaginal secretions relatively acid (pH less than 4.5), which inhibits the growth of other microorganisms and attachment of *Gardnerella vaginalis* to epithelial cells.

The three leading vaginal infections are trichomoniasis (caused by *T. vaginalis*), candidiasis (usually caused by *C. albicans*), and bacterial vaginosis (formerly called nonspecific vaginitis, caused by a replacement of the normal vaginal flora by *G. vaginalis,* anaerobes, *Mobiluncus* spp., and perhaps *Mycoplasma hominis*).

Bacterial vaginosis typically lacks clinical and laboratory findings of inflammation. The disease is marked by an increase in concentration as well as an alteration of normal vaginal flora. It is a common infection; as many as 50% of cases are asymptomatic. Infection may resolve spontaneously or be recalcitrant, even with metronidazole therapy. Although still not clear, there is evidence that this disease may increase the risk of upper genital tract infections (salpingitis, posthysterectomy fever) and may complicate pregnancy with endometritis, amnionitis, or premature ruptured membranes.[9]

Three species of trichomonads are known to infect humans: *T. tenax,* in the mouth; *T. hominis,* in the intestine; and *T. vaginalis,* in the urogenital tract. Only the latter has been associated with clinical disease. Occasionally, conjunctival *T. vaginalis* infections of the newborn are recognized; organisms also have been described from respiratory specimens in association with neonatal pneumonia.[10] Trichomoniasis usually occurs in the sexually active population and is transmitted during intercourse. It may be the most commonly acquired STD, with several million cases estimated yearly within the United States alone. Nonsexual spread of the organism appears to be limited because of the absence of a resistant cyst stage, although the trophozoites are known to survive in a moist environment for some time. Orally administered metronidazole remains the drug of choice for therapy, although strains resistant to this drug have been described. More often, however, the apparent resistance has resulted from reinfection by an infected, asymptomatic sexual partner. The need to treat both partners simultaneously should be emphasized.

The mechanism by which *C. albicans* and bacteria cause genital infection is poorly understood. Predisposing conditions include diabetes mellitus and acquired immunodeficiency syndrome (AIDS), whereas pregnancy and menstruation may intensify infections. Typically, a white "thrush" exudate is present on the epithelial surfaces, and the patient has itching or burning symptoms. Vulval involvement may also accompany the infection, sometimes with marked erythema and pustular lesions. Unfortunately, approximately 25% of infections do not respond to initial therapy, due in part to failure to make an accurate diagnosis. It should also be recognized that co-infections of trichomoniasis and *C. albicans* are not uncommon.

Selection

Complaints of lower abdominal pain, vaginal discharge, or disagreeable odor to the vaginal secretions (particularly noted after intercourse, when relatively alkaline semen may lead to volatilization of amines) should prompt an examination of vaginal secretions. During the examination, the cervix should be visually examined to determine whether it is inflamed and to ensure that it is not the source of secretions. Vaginal bleeding, lower abdominal pain, and uterine or adnexal tenderness are distinctly unusual for vaginal infections and suggest endometritis or pelvic inflammatory disease (PID). The cervix should be examined grossly for mucopus and microscopically for WBCs; tests for detecting *N. gonorrhoeae* and *C. trachomatis* should be performed. The large majority of women with an abnormal vaginal discharge, however, have vaginitis. In

Table 25-3. Differential Diagnosis of Vulvovaginal Infections

Infection	Diagnosis
Candida vulvovaginitis	*Candida* spp. present on wet preparation or culture, pH ≤ 4.5
Bacterial vaginosis	Three of four: pH > 4.5, positive whiff test, clue cells, abnormal discharge
Trichomonas vaginitis	Presence of *T. vaginalis* on wet preparation or culture, pH usually ≤ 4.5

these cases, examination of vaginal discharge by microscopic examination (wet mount and/or Gram stain), pH, and whiff test is indicated (Table 25-3). Culture of vaginal secretions can be performed for *Candida* spp. and *T. vaginalis* when the wet mount is negative.

Logistics

Specimen Requirements

When vaginal infection is suspected, secretions are best collected from the posterior vaginal pool. Cervical secretions should not be used because they are not representative of vaginal secretions. The speculum should not be lubricated with petroleum jelly. Specimens obtained from the speculum may be affected if water is used to lubricate the speculum. When making an appointment, the patient should be advised not to douche for at least 2 days and to avoid using vaginal medications or contraceptive creams or gels for at least 5 days before being examined.

Analysis

At the bedside, the pH and odor of vaginal secretions are determined. The pH value is determined by the use of narrow range pH paper (4.0–6.0) applied directly to the secretions. The odor is easily checked by smelling the withdrawn speculum for the presence of a pungent fishy, or amine, odor. If this method is aesthetically displeasing to the examiner, 1 or 2 drops of vaginal secretion can be mixed with 10% KOH on a slide and the slide immediately smelled for a characteristic amine odor (whiff test).

A wet mount of vaginal secretions is prepared by obtaining secretions with a cotton or Dacron-tipped swab and either by mixing the swab directly on a slide with a few drops of nonbacteriostatic saline or by placing it in a tube containing 0.5–1.0 mL of nonbacteriostatic saline, which is transported to the laboratory for examination. A Gram stain of vaginal secretions can be obtained by rolling the swab gently one time, to prevent distortion and provide an even film over an area about 1 × 2 cm. In performing wet mounts, it may be helpful to lower the condenser to provide more contrast; phase-contrast microscopy provides even more definition.

Although organisms remain viable outside the body for several hours, a wet-mount examination should be performed immediately to best observe the typical jerky motility of *T. vaginalis* trophozoites. The wet mount should be examined under low power (100×) for clue cells and motile trichomonads. Possible trichomonads should be confirmed by visualizing motile flagella under high power (400×). Material may be preserved with Polyvinyl alcohol (PVA) for permanent staining if immediate examination is not possible.

Clue cells are vaginal epithelial cells covered with coccobacillary bacteria (*G. vaginalis*), giving the cell a stippled appearance. A good rule is to identify a cell as a clue cell only if at least part of its border is fuzzy and indistinct (caused by adherent bacteria). Occasionally, other bacteria, particularly lactobacilli or *Mobiluncus* spp., may adhere to epithelial cells. The former are longer than *G. vaginalis,* and the latter are typically comma shaped. Thus, the morphology of the adherent bacteria must be considered in identifying a true clue cell. Yeast, occasionally with buds, can easily be identified by their size and morphology; *Mobiluncus* spp. may be recognized by their motility.

Acridine orange (a fluorescent stain) has been used to examine smears for *T. vaginalis* under low power. In addition, methods employing fluorescein- or immunoperoxidase-labeled antitrichomonal antibody are available and, although more cumbersome than the wet mount, may provide greater diagnostic sensitivity. The diagnosis of *T. vaginalis* in difficult cases may be aided with repeat examination or by culture of the vaginal or urethral exudate.[11] Cultivation is a sensitive procedure and is not particularly difficult with the use of Diamond's medium. An aliquot of the wet-mount tube (if used) or a swab of vaginal secretions can be used to inoculate the medium.[12] Careful attention must be paid to the proper collection, immediate inoculation, and incubation of such cultures, however, to prevent false negative results. Serologic tests have not been shown to be of value in the diagnosis of trichomoniasis. *Candida* spp. can be grown on any medium formulated for yeast or on blood agar.

Interpretation

The clinical diagnosis of bacterial vaginosis is made on the basis of three of four criteria: (1) an abnormal vaginal discharge consisting of thin, homogeneous secretions that cling to the vaginal walls; (2) pH greater than 4.5; (3) a typical amine odor to the vaginal secretions; or (4) the presence of clue cells.[13,14] Alternatively, some workers believe that bacterial vaginosis can best be diagnosed by Gram stain.[15] With this method, the diagnosis of bacterial vaginosis is made if the normally dominant lactobacilli is replaced by a background of gram-negative coccobacillary bacteria (*G. vaginalis*) and other organisms, often with accompanying gram-negative or gram-variable curved rods (*Mobiluncus* spp.).

A positive wet mount or culture for *T. vaginalis* is diagnostic of trichomoniasis. A positive wet mount for yeast is highly suggestive of the presence of *Candida* spp., but misinterpretation can be a problem. Puzzling or recurrent cases should be confirmed by culture. Because not all women with *Candida* spp. in vaginal secretions have clinical symptoms, the decision to treat should not be based solely on finding yeast in vaginal secretions.

Test: Examination of the Cervix

Background

Four organisms account for most infections of the cervix. The endocervix, which contains numerous mucus-secreting cells, is the site of infection for *N. gonorrhoeae* and *C. trachomatis*, whereas human papillomavirus preferentially infects the transformation zone. First-episode genital herpes often involves the entire cervix.

The endocervix can appear normal in spite of infection by *N. gonorrhoeae* or *C. trachomatis*. Alternatively, the endocervix can be inflamed with WBCs and friability (cervicitis) and often with pus exuding from the endocervix (mucopus). Infection may present with vaginal discharge and dysuria, whereas in many cases no symptoms are present. Why cervicitis develops in some infected women and not in others is not well understood. Vaginal bleeding, lower abdominal pain, and uterine or adnexal tenderness suggest upper genital tract infection. Herpes simplex virus also infects the cervix during the initial genital infection (first-episode genital herpes), often leading to inflammation of the cervix well beyond the endocervix. Herpes cervicitis should be suspected when cervical ulceration is noted. Subsequently, asymptomatic shedding of HSV may occur from the cervix in the absence of physical signs on either the cervix or vulva.

Infection of the cervix with HPV occurs commonly, in women with and without genital warts of the vulva; as many as 2–3% of Papanicoulaou (PAP) smears show infection with HPV.[16] Exophytic warts, typical of genital warts, are very uncommon on the cervix. Far more common are flat warts, best visualized by application of 3–5% acetic acid (acetowhitening) and, preferably, the aid of colposcopy. Human papillomavirus also can infect the vagina by producing acetowhite areas. In addition, HPV may produce either single or grouped, barely visible papillae (asperities) or totally subclinical diffuse disease seen only with acetic acid application and colposcopy.[17] Most vaginal disease is asymptomatic, although pruritus may occur.

Selection

Dysuria and pelvic pain are the major symptoms in *N. gonorrhoeae* and *C. trachomatis* infections in women, although many patients are asymptomatic. On examination, there may be a purulent discharge from the cervical crypts, Bartholin's gland ducts, and urethra. Microbiologic examination of the endocervix is warranted in the asymptomatic patient when there is suspicion of infection. Also culturing the urethra and rectum (and pharynx, if fellatio is practiced) will detect additional infections when the cervical culture is negative. Cervical culture for *N. gonorrhoeae* and *C. trachomatis* is always indicated when signs and symptoms of pelvic inflammatory disease are present.

Logistics

Specimen Requirements

The cervix should be wiped free of grossly adherent vaginal secretions. A cotton- or Dacron-tipped swab is introduced into the endocervix and rotated several times. To determine purulence, the color of the cervical secretions should be noted. A smear of cervical secretions for Gram stain diagnosis of gonorrhea or cervicitis can be obtained by gently rolling the swab over a 1 × 2 cm area on a slide, to preserve cellular morphology.

For a gonorrhea culture, a swab is introduced into the endocervix, where it should remain for about 10 seconds. Preferably, culture media should be inoculated at the bedside with the swab by forming a large Z on the surface of the plate, using all sides of the swab to form the Z. Alternatively, the swab can be placed into transport medium such as Stuart's, in which *N. gonorrhoeae* will survive well for 6 hours, although dilution may limit the recovery of small numbers of *N. gonorrhoeae* (see under Urethritis).

Infection by *C. trachomatis* can be diagnosed by culture or nonculture tests (immunofluorescence, ELISA, nucleic acid probe). For a *Chlamydia* culture, a plastic-handled swab is introduced into the endocervix, gently rotated, and placed into transport media (see under Urethritis); cytobrushing may increase the positive yield. Specimens for nonculture tests should be obtained according to the manufacturer's instructions.

An HSV culture is obtained with a cotton- or dacron-tipped plastic swab, which is then placed into transport medium. Nonculture tests should not be used to detect cervical infection in the absence of lesions because of low sensitivity, although amplification steps may increase the yield.[18]

Cervical HPV infection is diagnosed by cytology, biopsy, or in situ DNA hybridization tests. Of these, HPV infection is most commonly diagnosed by cytology using the PAP smear, in which cells characteristic of infection by HPV are found. These cells are of two types: koilocytes and dyskeratotic cells.[16] Commercial DNA hybridization tests are available to identify HPV DNA in cervical cells.

Analysis

Cultures for *N. gonorrhoeae* and *C. trachomatis* and nonculture tests for *C. trachomatis* are discussed under Test: Urethral Exudate Examination, whereas cultures for HSV are discussed under Test: Examination of Genital Ulcers.

Interpretation

The diagnosis of cervicitis is made by finding either (1) mucopus, (2) over 10 WBCs per oil immersion field on Gram stain of cervical secretions, or (3) friability (bleeding when the first swab culture is taken) and/or erythema or edema within a zone of cervical ectopy. Mucopurulent cervicitis, defined as the presence of either of the first two criteria, has been associated with *C. trachomatis*.[8,20] Mucopus is defined as yellow or green pus on the end of the cotton swab; normal cervical secretions are clear or white. The number of WBCs needed for a diagnosis of mucopurulent cervicitis was originally defined as 10 or more per oil immersion field,[20] although subsequent experience has found that many patients with this number of WBCs are not infected with *C. trachomatis*; for this reason, some investigators consider over 30 WBCs diagnostic. Cervicitis also may be caused by *N. gonorrhoeae*, and simultaneous infections by *N. gonorrhoeae* and *C. trachomatis* are common. Thus, the Gram stain of cervical secretions should be searched diligently for intracellular gram-negative diplococci, a finding diagnostic of infection by *N. gonorrhoeae*. Unfortunately, the endocervical Gram stain has a sensitivity of only 50–70% in the diagnosis of gonorrhea; nevertheless, the finding of intracellular organisms is highly specific.

A positive culture for *N. gonorrhoeae*, *C. trachomatis*, or HSV establishes a diagnosis by the respective organism. Identification of *C. trachomatis* by DFA or ELISA is slightly less sensitive than culture but is generally reliable in the symptomatic patient. The ELISA test may occasionally produce false positive results from cross-reactions with other bacterial antigens present within the endocervix.[8]

Human papillomavirus is usually diagnosed by PAP smear by the finding of characteristic cellular morphologic changes (either koilocytes or dyskeratotic cells) typical of infection by HPV, either of which suggests the presence of HPV in the cervix. Alternatively, DNA hybridization tests in which HPV DNA is found in cervical cells appear to be diagnostic. No one test, however, will detect all infections.[21] The sensitivity of DNA probes in detecting cervical infection will partly depend on the number of HPV types included in the probe. The cervix can be infected by many of the more than 50 types of HPV, although types 6, 11, 18, and 31 are the most common.

Test: Examination of Genital Ulcers

Background

Any break in the skin in the genital area, even if not appearing to be an ulcer, should initially be considered an STD, even if the patient provides a history of trauma to the area, for example, from a zipper. Three STDs are characterized by genital ulcers: genital herpes, syphilis, and chancroid (soft chancre). Two other infectious diseases—lymphogranuloma venereum (caused by *C. trachomatis*, types L_1, L_2, and L_3) and granuloma inguinale (presumed to be caused by *Calymmatobacterium granulomatis*)—are often listed as causing genital ulcers. The ulcer associated with the former, however, is transient and rarely seen, whereas ulcers associated with the latter are better characterized as chronic tissue destruction with secondary granulation.

In the United States, genital herpes is by far the most common of the genital ulcerative diseases, with an estimated 200,000–500,000 new cases occurring annually. This figure contrasts with only 39,673 cases of primary and secondary syphilis (about one-half of which are primary syphilis, the stage characterized by ulcers), and 5491 cases of chancroid, which occurred in 1988. It is believed that all of these infections are a risk factor for heterosexual spread of HIV-1.

Primary genital herpes is manifested by multiple painful vesicles on the genitalia that rapidly coalesce into pustular and ulcerative lesions and resolve within a few weeks. Recurrent episodes are common but are nearly always milder and shorter in duration. Asymptomatic recurrences frequently account for transmission of primary infection to the sexual partner.

Infection by *T. pallidum* is characterized by a painless papule that erodes and becomes an indurated ulcer with no exudate. The lesion disappears within 2–6 weeks, followed a few weeks later by signs of disseminated infection (secondary syphilis), characterized by skin rash and occasionally constitutional symptoms (fever, malaise, headache), and lesions in the mouth and genitals. Late complications (tertiary syphilis), occurring years later, primarily affect the central nervous and cardiovascular systems.

Chancroid occurs in focal outbreaks but is also endemic in certain large U.S. cities. The infection is heralded by one or more painful papules that quickly ulcerate; without therapy, these papules persist for weeks to months.

Granuloma inguinale is endemic in India, New Guinea, and the Caribbean but is rarely seen in the United States. The infection causes painless, indurated papules that erode into an ulcer and enlarge over several months. Lymphogranuloma venereum, endemic to Asia, Africa, and South America, is rarely seen in the United States. The first sign of infection is a small painless vesicle that heals quickly without scarring and often goes unnoticed. This is followed by painful regional (usually inguinal) lymphadenopathy, leukocytosis, and systemic symptoms (fever, myalgia). Late complications occurring in fewer than 10% of infections, include rectal and urethral strictures, fistulas, and lymphatic fibrosis with obstruction.

Selection

Sufficient overlap in clinical presentations between diseases exists such that diagnostic tests to distinguish them should be performed, whenever possible. Genital herpes typically shows multiple grouped vesicles surrounded by an erythematous base. After several days, the vesicles break and form shallow, tender ulcers; with coalescence, large ulcers may be formed. In women having their first attack, the cervix may be inflamed and have ulcerations. Primary syphilis usually occurs as a single nontender ulcer with indurated borders; squeezing elicits little pain. The ulcers of chancroid are few in number, appear ragged and inflamed, and are, particularly in men, extremely tender. In all three diseases, lymphadenopathy may occur. Lymph nodes are rubbery and nontender in syphilis and tender in genital herpes and chancroid. Only in chancroid (except rarely in genital herpes) do lymph nodes reach the status of buboes (tender, swollen, and fluctuant nodes in which pus is present). Although the presence of *T. pallidum*, HSV, and *Haemophilus ducreyi* may all be demonstrated in inflamed or noninflamed lymph nodes, examination of lymph node aspirates is generally reserved for patients with buboes. *Treponema denticola*, found at the gum margin, cannot be differentiated from *T. pallidum*, mitigating against dark-field microscopy of oral lesions.

Syphilis is most commonly diagnosed by serology. Serologic tests are of two types: nontreponemal tests include the rapid plasma reagin (RPR) and the Venereal Disease Research Laboratory (VDRL), and treponemal tests include fluorescent treponemal, absorbed (FTA-ABS) and microhemagglutination antibody, *T. pallidum* (MHA-TP). Nontreponemal tests detect reaginic antibody, which cross-reacts with *T. pallidum* and is formed as a result of infection with *T. pallidum*. Nontreponemal tests are considered screening tests because they are easy and inexpensive to perform, whereas treponemal tests are considered confirmatory tests, that is, tests that are more specific and used to confirm positive nontreponemal tests as truly indicating syphilis. When syphilis is suspected, it is appropriate to perform the nontreponemal screening test first and, if positive, to perform a confirmatory treponemal test (see Ch. 29).

Varied methods to diagnose etiologies of genital ulcers must be used because of the widely varying types of organisms that cause them. These methods can be roughly divided into two categories: direct detection methods and culture. Direct detection methods include the Gram stain (chancroid), Tzanck smear (genital herpes), dark-field microscopy (syphilis), fluorescent antibody (genital herpes, syphilis), and several additional immunologic assays for genital herpes. Culture can be used to diagnose chancroid and genital herpes.

Culture for HSV is most sensitive for vesicular lesions. In this infection, when blisters are unroofed and fluid and cells are obtained from the base of the ulcer, virus will be detected in nearly all specimens under optimal transport and culture conditions. Tzanck smears also are indicated during the vesicular stage of genital herpes, although they are less sensitive than culture.[22] The use of a Tzanck smear during the ulcerative stage is of less value because the sensitivity is lower; also, once lesions have crusted, the likelihood of a positive test is very low. Direct detection methods for HSV are being used with increasing frequency, and the merits of each test must be judged independently. Sensitivity compared with culture is slightly less, but it is highest during the vesicle stage.[23] As with any nonculture test, specificity is a concern and in any situation in which an absolute diagnosis is essential, culture should be performed.

Serology should not be used to diagnose genital herpes infection, because commercially available assays are cross-reactive to some degree between type 1 and type 2 viruses. In addition, finding a positive titer against type 2 virus, even if specific, does not necessarily indicate genital herpes, because up to 30% of primary genital herpes infections are caused by the type 1 virus and some cases of herpes labialis are caused by the type 2 virus.[24] Thus, although a single positive titer against HSV indicates infection, it should not be selected to make the diagnosis.

The diagnosis of granuloma inguinale is made by direct examination of a biopsy specimen or a crushed preparation from the lesion prepared with Wright or Giemsa stain. Diagnosis of lymphogranuloma venereum can be made by culture of *C. trachomatis* from a lesion but is only successful in about one-third of cases. Serology of acute and convalescent serum samples also should be done when this diagnosis is suspected.

Logistics

Specimen Requirements

Lesions that are fresh and clean, that is, not healing or filled with pus, are most likely to contain a pathogen that is easily demonstrated or cultured. When testing patients with ulcers for genital herpes, intact vesicles give the highest yield. Ulcers should be cleaned of gross contamination by gently rubbing them with dry sterile gauze. The Tzanck smear requires material from the base of the ulcer; the base should be thoroughly swabbed and the swab rolled over the surface of a clean slide, so that the cellular architecture is not disturbed. The smear is air dried, fixed with methanol for about 15 seconds, and then stained with Wright or Giemsa stain, to identify multinucleated giant cells. Gram stain of *H. ducreyi* should be made with material from the base or edge of the lesion. The material can be collected by rolling a cotton swab on the glass slide, although a wire loop may also be used.

Dark-field microscopy to identify *T. pallidum* requires examination of fluid from the base and margins of the ulcer. The ulcer is squeezed so that serum exudes from the margins. A clean glass slide of appropriate thickness (see manufacturer's instructions for the microscope being used) or coverslip (the latter is most useful in difficult-to-reach ulcer locations) is then pressed against the exudate. After sufficient material is obtained, a coverslip (or slide, if a coverslip was used to obtain material) is immediately placed over the exudate to prevent drying, and the slide is immediately taken to the laboratory. Examination requires a dark-field condenser, and most microscopes can be fitted with one. Dark-field, rather than light-field, microscopic examination is required because the thinness of *T. pallidum* prevents it from being seen with aniline dyes. The slide must be examined under oil immersion. *Treponema pallidum* is a tightly, regularly coiled spirochete that moves with slow translational (forward and backward) motion; if a spirochete is seen to move rapidly about or off the field, it is not *T. pallidum*. *Treponema pallidum* may flex but springs back to a straight, rigid position.

Immunofluorescent reagents now permit direct identification of *T. pallidum* and HSV; research conjugates against *H. ducreyi* are also available. Specimens should be taken from the base of the ulcer, unless otherwise directed by the manufacturer. Other immunologic assays, such as ELISA, are being increasingly developed for the diagnosis of genital herpes and may be useful where culture facilities are not available. These assays have not been widely evaluated but appear to be reliable when blisters or very fresh ulcers are tested. Direct fluorescent antibody testing also can be performed on tissue, as well as material that would be suitable for dark-field examination.

Culture. Culture for *H. ducreyi* requires special media that are not commercially available. Because strains of *H. ducreyi* appear to have varying nutritional requirements, the use of two different media is preferable to just one. A blood agar medium and a chocolate blood agar medium are usually chosen; if these media are not available, a commercial, enriched chocolate agar plate may be used.[25] All media for the growth of *H. ducreyi* are rich, often using fetal calf serum; all use vancomycin (3 μg/mL) to prevent the overgrowth of *H. ducreyi* by other microorganisms. The swab with material from the lesion should be applied to one corner of the plate and an inoculating loop used to cover the surface of the plate. Plates are best incubated at 33°C in a humid atmosphere containing CO_2. These conditions can be met by using a candle jar with a moist paper towel in the bottom.[26]

Herpes simplex virus is isolated in cell culture, using specimens obtained from the ulcer by the use of Dacron- or cotton-tipped plastic swabs; calcium alginate swabs bind virus and should be avoided. Swabs for culture or DFA detection of HSV should be moistened in transport medium and rubbed at the ulcer margins. Cultures should be stored at 4°C until cultured. If more than 72 hours (preferably no more than 24 hours) will elapse before specimens are inoculated, they should be stored at −70°C using a medium containing sorbitol or DMSO. Leibovitz-Emory medium containing agarose and charcoal will preserve HSV titer for several days.

Herpes simplex virus is cultured in human diploid fibroblast (WI-38, MRC-5) cell lines or in monkey kidney (Vero) cells. The characteristic cytopathic effect (CPE) consists of cytoplasmic granularity, followed by cellular ballooning and lysis. All CPE-positive specimens should be passed to new cell cultures. The CPE of HSV is rapid in onset, with 65% of cultures showing CPE within 5 days.[23] Detection of HSV-infected cells can be facilitated through the use of fluoresceinated monoclonal antibody culture confirmation reagents, although this adds significantly to the cost of isolation and identification. The use of fluoresceinated antibody allows the detection of positive specimens in tissue culture at 24 hours, well before CPE is apparent in most positive specimens.

Treponema pallidum can only be isolated in primary specimens by inoculation of material into immunosuppressed rabbits; this is impractical for clinical laboratories.

Interpretation

A positive dark-field examination for *T. pallidum* is confirmatory for syphilis. Previous antimicrobial therapy can render an ulcer temporarily negative, however, and dark-field microscopy must be carefully interpreted, because *T. denticola* can be found in oral lesions and *T. refringens* can be found in genital lesions. *Treponema refringens* is a more loosely coiled organism and moves rapidly and with a much more flexible bending than *T. pallidum*.

Spirochetes can be visualized in tissue or impression smears by silver impregnation stains, but spirochetes other than *T. pallidum* will be similarly stained. If numerous spirochetes with the characteristic morphology of *T. pallidum* are found in a lesion compatible with syphilis, the diagnosis is confirmed. Unfortunately, in some tissues, spirochetes are sparse; in these situations, it is difficult to differentiate tissue artifacts from actual organisms. This most often becomes a problem in late syphilis, when spirochetes are sparse (late benign syphilis) or are not present at all (tertiary syphilis). Because serology can remain positive for months to years after treatment, however, the finding of a positive titer is not as specific as a positive dark-field examination. Thus, the significance of a positive test must take into account the possibility of a past infection.

A positive nontreponemal test is found at the initial presentation in 59–87% of patients with primary syphilis, 100% of patients with secondary syphilis, and 37–94% of patients with tertiary syphilis.[27] Titers are highest in patients with secondary syphilis, commonly greater than 1:8, whereas titers less than this commonly occur in primary and tertiary syphilis. Titers in secondary syphilis can be so high, however, that a prozone phenomenon can occur. Thus diluted serum should be tested if an undiluted sample is negative in a patient suspected of having secondary syphilis. Patients with positive titers, but with no symptoms, have latent syphilis. If it can be determined that the duration of infection is less than 1 year, early latent syphilis is diagnosed. If it can be determined that the duration of infection is more than 1 year, or if the duration of infection cannot be determined, late latent syphilis is diagnosed. Biologic false positive (BFP) tests may occur in patients with autoimmune diseases or malaria, in intravenous drug users and possibly in pregnant women. In these instances, titers are generally 1:8 or less. (See Chapter 29 for additional discussion on the serologic diagnosis of syphilis.) A positive culture or Tzanck smear for HSV is diagnostic. The diagnosis of granuloma inguinale is made by finding characteristic clusters of dark blue, bipolar-staining organisms within macrophages, termed Donovan bodies.

Test: Proctorectal Exudate

Background and Selection

Sexual transmission of infectious agents through anogenital intercourse is facilitated by the proximity of the anus and rectum to the genitals. Infection of the rectum or more proximal large bowel is a common cause of symptomatic disease. The prevalence of anorectal infection has declined in recent years, because of the modification of homosexual practices precipitated by public awareness of HIV transmission.

Inflammation of the small or large bowel may produce clinical manifestations as a result of infection by numerous infecting agents. The site of infection generally varies for each agent, depending on the initial route of inoculation, tissue tropism, and host factors that define the anatomic environment. Thus, *N. gonorrhoeae* infection of the rectum is frequently asymptomatic; when symptomatic, it is generally caused by invasion of the rectal mucosa within several centimeters of the anal verge. By contrast, invasive *Campylobacter* spp. may become clinically apparent in various regions of the intestine; test sensitivity may vary, depending on the precise location of the infection and from where the specimen is collected.

Agents frequently identified in symptomatic anorectal infections include *Shigella* spp., enterohemorrhagic *E. coli*, *C. trachomatis* (both genital and LGV biovars), HSV, *Entamoeba histolytica*, *Campylobacter* spp., *Giardia lamblia*, *N. gonorrhoeae*, and *T. pallidum*. The species of *Campylobacter* most often associated with sexually transmitted proctorectal disease are *C. jejuni*, *C. cinaedi*, and *C. fennelliae*.[28] *Campylobacter hyointestinalis* also has been isolated in cases of proctitis.

The presence of commensal spirochetes within the gut lumen precludes the use of the dark-field microscopic examination of exudate from luminal ulcers for *T. pallidum*. Serologic detection of reactive syphilis tests should be used. Ulceration of the lower bowel by amebic infection is an infrequent presentation of sexually acquired infection that may be life threatening. Visual detection of crypt abscesses may be confirmed by rectal biopsy.

Noninfectious causes of proctorectal inflammation that may occur in sexually active patients include inflammatory bowel disease and antimicrobial-associated colitis (AAC). The latter may occur in patients recently treated for STDs and should be considered in the differential diagnosis of proctorectal inflammation. In instances of chronic or severe disease, biopsy for pathologic diagnosis of inflammatory bowel disease is indicated. In the setting of recent use of antimicrobial agents, AAC should be evaluated by *C. difficile* culture and/or toxin assay (see Ch. 26).

Logistics

Specimen Requirements

Culture for *N. gonorrhoeae* may be obtained without anoscopy. Because the most productive site for culture of *N. gonorrhoeae* is the crypts, 3–5 cm inside the anal verge, it suffices to insert a cotton swab blindly while asking the patient to bear down gently. The swab should be rotated for several seconds, withdrawn, and examined. If the swab is grossly contaminated with feces, another sample should be attempted, or a specimen should be obtained by anoscopy. In patients with symptoms of proctitis or colitis, anoscopic examination may provide the best sampling for focal infections. Specimens should be obtained from areas of localized inflammation, if such exist. Removal of excess mucus and pus followed by vigorous swabbing of a rectal ulceration may provide a superior specimen for cultivation or DFA testing for *C. trachomatis* or HSV. *Campylobacter jejuni* remains viable in bacterial transport medium, such as the commercial thioglycollate (Campythio) for several days after collection; however, other *Campylobacter* spp. are more fastidious, particularly *C. fennelliae* and *C. cinaedi*.

Analysis

Rectal swabs should be cultured as soon as possible after specimen collection. Culture on selective bacterial media for *Salmonella* spp., *Shigella* spp., *Campylobacter* spp., and *E. coli* 0157:H7 should be performed, in addition to chylamydial and appropriate viral studies.

Direct phase-contrast microscopy of stool may presumptively identify *Campylobacter* spp., which have darting motility. A Gram stain of rectal exudate may also reveal small, curved, gram-negative rods consistent with *Campylobacter* spp. Commercial media, which may contain cephalothin, are acceptable for primary isolation of *C. jejuni*. Cephalothin inhibits growth of *C. fennelliae* and *C. cinaedi* and should not be used in media for primary isolation of these agents. In addition, incubation of plates at both 37° and 42°C is recommended to distinguish *C. jejuni* (growth at both 37° and 42°C) from *C. fennelliae* and *C. cinaedi* (no growth at 42°C). All three of these *Campylobacter* spp. grow satisfactorily in a reduced microaerophilic environment, are motile, and produce oxidase and catalase. Further distinguishing tests are presented in Table 25-4. Isolation of *Chlamydia trachomatis* in cell culture may be improved and the yield increased by the use of specimen sonication to reduce bacterial contamination, but care must be taken because of the biohazard involved in this procedure. Direct fluorescent antibody tests also detect *C. trachomatis*; however, false positive tests are more common with specimens from the rectum than from the genitals.

Fresh colonic fluid should be examined within 30 minutes of collection, to avoid lysis of trophozoites. Trophozoites of *Entamoeba histolytica* may occasionally be

Table 25-4. Identification of Sexually Transmitted Enteric *Campylobacter* Species

	C. jejuni	*C. cinaedi*	*C. fennelliae*
Nitrate reduction	+	+	−
Hippurate hydrolysis	+	−	−
Cephalothin susceptible (30 μg)	−	+	+
Growth at 42°C	+	−	−

(Data from Cornick and Gorbach.[28])

seen in stained smears of ulcer exudate. Microscopic examination of a single specimen for *G. lamblia* or *E. histolytica* is insensitive. Multiple specimens or cultures are necessary to approach sensitivities of 80%. More often, however, diagnosis is dependent on serologic testing for *E. histolytica* in the presence of compatible clinical findings.

Interpretation

The finding of inflammatory cells in exudate specimens in the presence of mucosal abnormalities of the rectum suggest an infectious etiology or the presence of inflammatory bowel disease. Serologic tests for *T. pallidum*, nontreponemal (e.g., VDRL or RPR) and *E. histolytica* (latex agglutination or IHA) are particularly useful if substantially elevated. The detection of agents such as *Shigella* spp., *E. coli* 0157:H7, *C. trachomatis*, *N. gonorrhoeae*, or *Campylobacter* spp. is diagnostic.

Test: Examination for Pubic Lice

Background and Selection

Phthirus pubis, the cause of pubic lice, primarily infests the pubic region but may also be found in other body regions with hair, including the armpits, beard, eyelashes, and eyebrows. Infestation with these insects is termed pubic pediculosis. Pubic pediculosis is a very common sexually transmitted infection. Although no figures are readily available, it is known that many persons treat themselves with over-the-counter preparations. Fortunately, crab lice are not known to transmit the bacterial diseases of epidemic typhus, trench fever, or epidemic relapsing fever normally associated with body lice. When a case is discovered, close contacts and sexual partners also should be examined and treated as necessary to prevent reinfection.

Bites of pubic, body, and head lice are all extremely pruritic, and the recurring, persistent feeding activities of these insects result in oozing and crusting of serous fluids on the skin surface. Bite sites may become inflamed and papular with the onset of secondary bacterial infections. Both the lice and their eggs (nits) should be readily visible on inspection of the affected area.

Logistics and Interpretation

The diagnosis of pubic pediculosis is made by recovery and identification of the typical organism and/or their nits (eggs). The latter are found firmly attached to body hairs and appear as small ovoid protrusions. Adult lice as well as nits should be submitted for examination to differentiate between the body louse *(Pediculus humanus)* and the crab louse *(Phthirus pubis)*.

REFERENCES

1. Hooton TM, Barnes RC: Urethritis in men. Infect Dis Clin North Am 1987;1:165–178.
2. Mahony JB, Chernesky MA: Effect of swab type and storage temperature on the isolation of *Chlamydia trachomatis* from clinical specimens. J Clin Microbiol 1985;22:865–867.
3. Gordon FB, Harper IA, Quan AL et al: Detection of *Chlamydia* (Bedsonia) in certain infections of man. I. Laboratory procedures: comparison of yolk sac and cell culture for detection and isolation. J Infect Dis 1969;120:451–462.
4. Yoder BL, Stamm WE, Koester CM, Alexander ER: Microtest procedure for isolation of *Chlamydia trachomatis*. J Clin Microbiol 1981;13:1036–1039.
5. Bowie WR: Urethritis in males. pp. 644–645. In Holmes KK, Mardh PA, Sparling PF, Wiesner PJ (eds): Sexually Transmitted Diseases. New York, McGraw-Hill, 1984.
6. Judson FN: A clinic-based system for monitoring the quality of techniques for the diagnosis of gonorrhea. Sex Transm Dis 1978;5:141–145.
7. Barnes RC: Laboratory diagnosis of human chlamydial infections. Clin Microbiol Rev 1989;2:119–136.
8. Stamm WE: Diagnosis of *Chlamydia trachomatis* genitourinary infections. Ann Intern Med 1988;108:710–717.
9. Sobel JD: Bacterial vaginosis—an ecologic mystery. Ann Intern Med 1989;111:551–553.
10. McLaren L, Davis L, Healy G, James G: Isolation of *Trichomonas vaginalis* from the respiratory tract of infants with respiratory diseases. Pediatrics 1983;71:888–890.

11. Lossick JG: The diagnosis of vaginal trichomoniasis. JAMA 1988;259:1230.
12. Schmid GP, Matheny LC, Zaidi AA, Kraus SJ: Evaluation of six media for the growth of *Trichomonas vaginalis* from vaginal secretions. J Clin Microbiol 1989;27:1230–1233.
13. Amsel R, Totten PA, Spiegel CA et al: Nonspecific vaginitis: diagnostic criteria and microbial and epidemiologic associations. Am J Med 1983;74:14–22.
14. McCue JD: Evaluation and management of vaginitis. Arch Intern Med 1989;149:565–568.
15. Eschenbach DA, Hillier S, Critchlow C et al: Diagnosis and clinical manifestations of bacterial vaginosis. Am J Obstet Gynecol 1988;158:819–828.
16. Drake M, Medley G, Mitchell H: Cytologic detection of human papillomavirus infection. Obstet Gynecol Clin North Am 1987;14:431–450.
17. Campion MJ: Clinical manifestations and natural history of genital human papillomavirus infection. Obstet Gynecol Clin North Am 1987;14:363–388.
18. Warford AL, Chunmg JW, Drill AE, Steinberg E: Amplification techniques for detection of herpes simplex virus in neonatal and maternal genital specimens obtained at delivery. J Clin Microbiol 1989;27:1324–1328.
19. Martin DH: Chlamydial infections. Med Clin North Am 1990;74:1367–1388.
20. Brunham RC, Paavonen J, Stevens CE et al: Mucopurulent cervicitis—the ignored counterpart in women of urethritis in men. N Engl J Med 1984;311:1–6.
21. Kiviat NB, Koutsky LA, Paavonen JA et al: Prevalence of genital papillomavirus infection among women attending a college student health clinic or a sexually transmitted disease clinic. J Infect Dis 1989;159:293–302.
22. Solomon AR, Rasmussen JE, Varani J, Pierson CL: The Tzanck smear in the diagnosis of cutaneous herpes simplex. JAMA 1984;251:633–635.
23. Mertz GJ: Genital herpes simplex virus infections. Med Clin North Am 1990;74:1433–1454.
24. Corey L, Adams HG, Brown ZA et al: Genital herpes simplex virus infections: clinical manifestations, cause and complications. Ann Intern Med 1983;98:958–972.
25. Nsanze J, Plummer FA, Maggwa ABN et al: Comparison of media for the isolation of *Haemophilus ducreyi*. Sex Transm Dis 1984;11:6–9.
26. Schmid GP, Faur YC, Valu JA et al: Effect of temperature on the recovery of *Haemophilus ducreyi* from clinical specimens. Presented at the Twenty-ninth Interscience Conference of Antimicrobial Agents and Chemotherapy, September 18-20, 1989.
27. Jaffe HW: Management of the reactive serology. pp. 313–317. In Holmes KK, Mardh PA, Sparling PF, Wiesner PJ (eds): Sexually Transmitted Diseases. New York, McGraw-Hill, 1984.
28. Cornick NA, Gorbach SL: Campylobacter. Infect Dis Clin North Am 1988;2:643–654.

26 Gastrointestinal Tract

Joseph M. Campos Gerald Lancz
Thomas R. Fritsche Steven Specter

INTRODUCTION

Infections of the gastrointestinal tract are the most common cause of morbidity and mortality in developing nations, especially in young children. Although a less severe problem in the United States, the incidence of enteric infections is second only to infectious respiratory illnesses. A large variety of viral, bacterial, and parasitic agents may cause infection of the GI tract. However, in spite of sensitive and sophisticated techniques, the etiologic agent cannot be identified in up to 30% of these infections, many of which are presumed to be caused by viral agents.

Diverse mechanisms for protection against infection exist along the entire length of the GI tract.[1] Mucus produced by cells lining the GI tract deters adherence of exogenous microorganisms and helps neutralize endogenously produced and ingested toxins. Hydrochloric acid in the stomach kills almost all microorganisms that enter the stomach with food and water. Humoral and cell-mediated immunities protect the intestinal mucosa from the onslaught of bacteria residing in the lumen and from the microorganisms that survive passage through the stomach. The saprophytic bacteria of the large intestine, over 99% of which are obligate anaerobes, compete effectively with exogenous bacterial pathogens for the limited numbers of colonization sites present along the intestinal walls. The saprophytes also produce bacteriocins and toxic metabolites that impede the propagation of exogenous bacteria. Finally, intestinal peristalsis plays a key role by constantly forcing pathogenic microorganisms through and out of the lower GI tract, before they can cause infection.

A variety of mechanisms are involved in microbial pathogenicity. The common viral agents (rotavirus and Norwalk agent) localize to the small bowel and injure the villi at the tip of the epithelial cells, causing malabsorption. Bacterial pathogens, such as *Vibrio cholerae,* and some types of enterotoxigenic *Escherichia coli* produce toxins that interfere with normal GI function and cause massive amounts of watery diarrhea and severe dehydration. Other toxin-producing bacteria produce inflammatory cytotoxic reactions. Adherence factors that permit attachment and colonization of bacteria to the colonic mucosa is an additional pathogenic mechanism. Some bacterial species, such as *Salmonella typhi,* have the ability to directly invade gastric mucosa and enter the bloodstream and lymphatics.

The GI tract is the most common location for parasitic infections. A wide variety of serious parasitic infections are being seen with increasing frequency. Infected persons are usually immigrants from countries where such diseases are endemic, or travelers to these areas. While we often regard parasitic diseases as "exotic" by their nature, all of the intestinal protozoa and many of the intestinal nematodes and cestodes may be acquired in the more socioeconomically stable regions of the world, including Europe and North America. Persons who are immunosuppressed by reason of malignancy, chemotherapy, organ transplantation, or viral infection (human immunodeficiency virus [HIV]) are also at increased risk for acquiring intestinal parasitic infections, especially those with the biologic potential for unrestricted multiplication such as the protozoa and *Strongyloides*.

The laboratory tests to be considered for specific GI infections depend largely on the patient's history and suspected agents. In many cases, little, if any, testing is necessary to manage the patient, and if done, testing is often not productive. Specific indications for viral, bacterial, and ova and parasite examinations are described below.

ROUTINE TESTS

Test: Bacterial and Fungal Culture of the Esophagus

Background

The esophagus is an uncommon site of infection in the immunologically intact host. However, immunodeficient patients, in particular those with defects of cellular immunity (e.g., acquired immunodeficiency syndrome [AIDS], leukemia), are susceptible to viral and fungal infections of the esophagus. Members of the herpesvirus group and *Candida albicans* are the most frequent causes of infection.[2] The herpesviruses lay dormant in the cells of the reticuloendothelial and central nervous systems, and reactivate to cause clinically apparent infection in response to any of several stimuli. The source of *C. albicans* infection is the colonized/infected upper respiratory tract or mouth. Organisms reach the esophagus via swallowing of yeast-laden secretions and saliva, or by direct extension to the esophagus from a site of oral candidiasis ("thrush").

Selection

Infectious esophagitis is usually associated with oropharyngeal disease. Endoscopic biopsy of the upper GI tract should be considered for immunosuppressed patients with clinical (retrosternal pain and dysphagia) or radiologic evidence (by barium swallow) of esophagitis. Since most infections are caused by *C. albicans,* biopsy material should be examined microscopically for fungal elements and inoculated onto fungal culture media.

Logistics

Esophageal biopsy or blind brushing[3] can be performed for diagnosis. Biopsy material from the edge of the fungal plaque is the specimen of choice. Care should be taken not to contaminate the specimen with upper respiratory or mouth flora during removal from the esophagus, as *Candida* spp. are frequent colonizers of the oropharynx.

Microscopy

Bushings or small sliced fragments of an esophageal biopsy should be examined for yeast cells and hyphae after treatment for 5 minutes with 10–20% potassium hydroxide (KOH). Gentle heating of the KOH preparation hastens clarification of the specimen. An alternate approach is to examine tissue impression smears after staining with calcofluor white, methylene blue, or Gram reagents. A microscope equipped for ultraviolet illumination is necessary to read calcofluor white stained smears.

Culture

The most likely cause of esophagitis in the immunosuppressed patient, *C. albicans,* grows readily on bacterial and fungal culture media. Because of the possibility of contamination of the specimen with upper respiratory flora, the use of fungal culture media is recommended to suppress the growth of bacteria. In the unusual circumstance that bacterial esophagitis is a consideration, routine aerobic bacterial culture is sufficient.

Esophageal biopsies should be homogenized in sterile saline with a tissue grinder before culture. Homogenates for fungal culture should be inoculated to Sabouraud dextrose and brain heart infusion agars. Media containing cycloheximide should not be used without including nonselective fungal media. Cultures should be incubated at 25–30°C in an aerobic atmosphere for 21–28 days. Viral cultures of tissue specimen for herpes simplex virus (HSV) and cytomegalovirus (CMV) are performed by standard methods.[4]

Interpretation

Observation of yeast cells and/or hyphae in a properly collected esophageal biopsy from a symptomatic patient is presumptive evidence of candidal esophagitis. The presence of bacteria in a methylene blue or Gram stain suggests the specimen is contaminated with upper respiratory flora. Culture of large numbers of *C. albicans* from an uncontaminated specimen is definitive evidence of candidal esophagitis. In the event that only small numbers or no *C. albicans* are recovered, the possibilities of herpes viral esophagitis or that the specimen was collected from an uninfected section of the esophagus should be considered. A positive culture for HSV or CMV in the appropriate clinical setting is diagnostic.

Test: Stomach and Small Intestine Culture

Background

The stomach of normal hosts is an uncommon site of infection because the acidic environment is uninhabitable for most organisms. In fact, as specified earlier, the stomach is a crucial barrier to infection of the lower GI tract. Patients with decreased gastric acidity suffer from lower GI infections much more often than normal persons and are at increased risk of bacterial overgrowth of the small intestine and stomach. Patients receiving medications (β-adrenergic blockers) to decrease gastric acidity are also at higher risk for nosocomial bacterial pneumonias from aspiration of stomach contents. Decontamination of the upper GI tract has been attempted to prevent such infections.[5]

The most important pathogen involved with gastric infections is *Helicobacter (Campylobacter) pylori*.[6] This gram-negative, urease-producing spiral bacillus is associated with chronic gastritis. It is capable of destroying the mucus lining of the stomach causing acute inflammation and injury to gastric epithelial cells. A very high percentage of patients with chronic duodenal ulcers harbor this organism in the stomach, suggesting that hyperacidity is another manifestation of infection.[7] The mode of transmission, incidence in normal persons, and details of pathogenicity are under investigation.

Selection

A search for *H. pylori* may be considered in patients with symptoms of gastritis or peptic ulcer disease, especially when an endoscopic biopsy is obtained for histologic examination. However, because the association between histologic and microbiologic results is so high, specific testing for *H. pylori* may not be warranted as a routine examination, especially if the result would not affect the patient's treatment. Multiple gastric biopsies may be needed to detect gastritis histologically, while a single specimen is usually adequate for culture confirmation.[8] Attempts to detect *H. pylori* in asymptomatic patients has little benefit because the clinical implication of colonization is uncertain and treatment should not rest solely on this finding.

Patients with possible pulmonary tuberculosis who are unable to produce sputum on demand for laboratory examination (e.g., young children) should have gastric aspirates collected for acid-fast smears and cultures. Mycobacteria resist the destructive effects of stomach acidity for brief periods of time.

Diagnosis of bacterial overgrowth of the upper small intestine and stomach, sites that should harbor very few, if any, viable organisms, can be achieved by Gram stain and quantitative culture of gastric/duodenal aspirates. This may be considered in patients suspected of having blind loop syndrome.

Logistics

Gastric/duodenal aspirates should be collected in a manner that minimizes contamination with upper respiratory flora. If both aerobic and anaerobic cultures are ordered, aspirates should be brought to the laboratory in an anaerobic transport device or in a capped syringe with the needle removed. If specimens cannot be processed promptly, gastric acidity should be neutralized with a base (e.g., NaOH) or a neutral buffer to prevent killing of microorganisms during storage.

Gastric mucosal biopsies should be collected during direct visualization of the biopsy site during gastroscopy. Samples from the periphery of the lesion return the highest yield. Contamination of the biopsied tissue with upper respiratory flora should be averted. Tissue may be homogenized in sterile saline (preferably in a 20% glucose solution) with a tissue grinder before examination.

Microscopy

Impression smears from tissue biopsies and thin smears from tissue homogenates and gastric/duodenal aspirates should be prepared on glass microscope slides, air-dried, and Gram stained. Substitution of a 1:5 dilution of Kinyoun carbol-fuchsin for safranin provides a means to obtain darker staining of *H. pylori*. Smears should be examined under oil immersion magnification ($\times 1000$).

When Mycobacteria spp. are suspected, thin smears from gastric aspirates should be air-dried, stained by the auramine-rhodamine, Kinyoun, or Ziehl-Neelsen methods, and examined microscopically. Auramine-rhodamine stained smears must be read with a microscope equipped for ultraviolet illumination, preferably at high dry magnification ($\times 450$). Kinyoun and Ziehl-Neelsen stained smears should be read under oil immersion magnification ($\times 1000$).

Culture

Specimens for culture of *H. pylori* should be inoculated to nonselective enriched agar media (such as chocolate) and selective media (such as Skirrow *Campylobacter* agar). Culture plates should be incubated at 42°C in a microaerophilic atmosphere (ideally 85% N_2, 10% CO_2, 5% O_2) for 1 week. Tiny, weakly β-hemolytic colonies appear at 72 hours. Gastric or duodenal aspirates for routine bacterial culture should be inoculated to 5% sheep blood, chocolate and MacConkey, or eosin-methylene blue (EMB) agar plates. The chocolate agar plate should be inoculated with a calibrated loop and streaked for colony count. Cultures are incubated at 35°C in an aerobic atmosphere enriched with 5–10% CO_2 for 48–72 hours. Anaerobic culture of gastric or duodenal aspirates should be inoculated to nonselective, prereduced anaerobic blood agar enriched with vitamin K and hemin, and to media selective for gram-positive and gram-negative anaerobes. The enriched anaerobic blood agar plate should be inoculated with a calibrated loop and streaked for colony count. Cultures should be incubated at 35°C in an anaerobic atmosphere for 5–7 days.

Cultures of gastric aspirates for mycobacteria should be inoculated to Löwenstein-Jensen medium and Middlebrook 7H10 or 7H11 agar. Cultures should be incubated at 35°C in an aerobic atmosphere containing 5–10% CO_2 for 8–12 weeks.

Urease Activity in Gastric Specimens

Indirect evidence of the presence of *H. pylori* in the stomachs of patients with peptic ulcer disease can be obtained by demonstrating urease activity in gastric specimens. A popular approach among gastroenterologists is to monitor formation of radiolabeled NH_3 or CO_2 gas (the products of the urease reaction), following instillation of radiolabeled urea into the stomach.[9] Another more practical method involves the addition of urea to pH neutralized (not buffered) gastric biopsies or gastric aspirates, followed by monitoring of the pH. Hydrolysis of urea results in a pH increase as a result of NH_4OH formation from dissolved NH_3. Alternatively, a piece of the specimen can be placed directly into urea broth and monitored for urease production during the following 24 hours.[10] A positive reaction is usually evident within 1 hour.

Interpretation

Detection by culture or smear of curved gram-negative rods, or evidence of urease production by biochemical means in a gastric biopsy is evidence for the presence of *H. pylori*. These results must be correlated with histologic and clinical findings since this organism can occasionally be found in the absence of disease.

Gastric or duodenal aspirate cultures from patients with suspected bacterial overgrowth of the small bowel are suggestive of overgrowth if the colony count is more than 10^5 colony forming unit (cfu)/mL and comprised of aerobic and anaerobic gram-negative rods (predominately members of the Enterobacteriaceae family and the *Bacteroides fragilis* group).

Interpretation of positive acid-fast smears and cultures must be carried out with caution. Normal drinking water frequently contains saprophytic mycobacteria, which are indistinguishable from *Mycobacterium tuberculosis* by smear. Positive acid-fast cultures must be identified to the species level before making final judgment as to the clinical significance of the isolate (see Ch. 22).

Test: Stool Culture

Background[11,12]

The small and large intestines are sites for a large assortment of bacterial, parasitic, and viral infections. The acquisition of most intestinal infections occurs by one of three mechanisms.

1. Many infections are acquired via fecal-oral spread, and following ingestion of contaminated food or water harboring a sufficient number of organisms to cause infection. Similarly, direct contact with an infected or colonized person's feces (e.g., hand-to-mouth contact in children or institutionalized persons) also results in transmission of infection.
2. Ingestion of toxins produced during microbial growth in food may result in food poisoning. Disease-producing enterotoxins may retain activity in inadequately cooked food or may arise during improper storage of food contaminated after cooking.
3. Venereal transmission of enteric pathogens during anal sexual intercourse may occur. Although venereal transmission is a minor route of spread overall, within the male homosexual population, it is responsible for a significant percentage of infectious diarrheas.

Infectious diarrheas are categorized as noninflammatory, inflammatory, or related to food poisoning (Table 26-1).

Table 26-1. Etiologic Agents of Bacterial, Viral, and Protozoal Gastroenteritis[11,12]

Organism	Diarrhea	Clinical/Epidemiologic Manifestations
Adenovirus 40 and 41	Watery	Common cause of viral gastroenteritis in children younger than 2 years; tends to persist longer (1–2 weeks) than other GI viral (rotavirus) infections, but generally a milder disease; no seasonal variation in attack rates; virus may be shed in stool months after acute infection
Aeromonas hydrophila	Watery	Normal stool commensal, found in fresh water, isolation does not indicate pathogenic role[20]; enterotoxigenic strains may cause illness
Astrovirus	Watery	Accounts for only a small proportion of symptomatic viral gastroenteritis with variable degrees of vomiting and diarrhea; affects all age groups, although more common in children
Bacillus cereus	Watery	Cause of food poisoning (fried rice); preformed toxin causes nausea and vomiting within 6 hours of ingestion; may also present after longer incubation period (12 hours) as abdominal cramps and diarrhea when toxin produced in vivo
Balantidium coli	Inflammatory, hemorrhagic	Parasite of hogs and other wild and domestic animals; produces asymptomatic to invasive disease similar to *Entamoeba histolytica*
Blastocystis hominis	Watery	Questionable pathogenicity,[30] often found in conjunction with other protozoan parasites; has been associated with acute and chronic diarrhea. Commonly found in asymptomatic persons
Calicivirus	Watery	Similar to rotavirus infections, involving primarily children younger than 2 years; slight increased prevalence in winter; virus can be seen in stools of healthy persons (usually adults)
Campylobacter fetus, subsp. *jejuni*	Inflammatory	Most common cause of bacterial gastroenteritis in United States; zoonotic reservoirs (milk, poultry), water supplies, and person-to-person transmission
Campylobacter cinaedi, *Campylobacter fennelliae*	Inflammatory, watery	Proctitis or enteritis in homosexual men
Clostridium botulinum	Watery	Cause of food poisoning; associated with contaminated home-canned foods (preformed toxin); disease in infants occurs from in vivo toxin production (contaminated honey)[38]; nausea, vomiting, and diarrhea occur about 25 hours after ingestion followed by descending weakness or paralysis, and constipation
Clostridium difficile	Inflammatory	Associated with antibiotic use and overgrowth of toxin-producing strain[21]; causes pseudomembranous colitis
Clostridium perfringens	Watery	Cause of food poisoning (meats and gravies); about 12 hours after ingestion, presents as abdominal cramps and diarrhea from toxin produced in vivo
Coronavirus	Watery	Found in stools of normal persons and persons with symptoms of gastroenteritis (mostly infants and children); role of virus in causing disease has been questioned; high prevalence in Southwest United States, but uncommon elsewhere
Cryptosporidium spp.	Watery	Zoonotic infection, most common in AIDS patients (chronic, sometime severe, life-threatening diarrhea) and children younger than 2 years (acute, self-limited infection)

(Continued)

Table 26-1. Etiologic Agents of Bacterial, Viral, and Protozoal Gastroenteritis[11,12] (Continued)

Organism	Diarrhea	Clinical/Epidemiologic Manifestations
Dientamoeba fragilis	Watery	Associated with *Enterobius vermicularis* (pinworm) infections; children most commonly symptomatic with mild intermittent diarrhea and eosinophilia; symptoms are similar to *Giardia* infection
Escherichia coli	Inflammatory, hemorrhagic, watery	Numerous types and diseases: enterotoxic, invasive, adherent, hemorrhagic strains[18]; usually mild illness; common cause of "travelers diarrhea"; common cause of infantile diarrhea, may cause outbreaks in nurseries; enterohemorrhagic (O157:H7) strains may produce hemolytic uremic syndrome or thrombotic thrombocytopenic purpura[13,14]; most common in summer and in children
Entamoeba histolytica	Inflammatory, hemorrhagic	Common worldwide parasitic infection, most prevalent in developing countries. Asymptomatic to fulminant GI and extraintestinal disease[27]; highly associated with foreign travel (Mexico); fecal-oral transmission common and may cause institutional outbreaks; important cause of serious infection in AIDS patients; diagnosis may require multiple stool examination or endoscopy; serologic diagnosis is helpful for invasive disease
Giardia lamblia	Watery	Most common intestinal parasite in United States, and prevalent in developing countries; commonly acquired with foreign travel, person-to-person contact, or from contaminated food or water; outbreaks occur in day-care centers and infection is common among homosexuals; disease is often mild or asymptomatic; prolonged diarrhea with malabsorption, weight loss, and fatigue occur with symptomatic infections; examination of duodenal contents may be helpful when stool examination is negative
Isospora belli	Watery	Infection of immunocompromised (AIDS) patients; illness ranges from self-limited condition to persistent diarrhea with eosinophilia; diagnosis is important because antibiotic therapy is effective but may be difficult because of paucity of oocyst excretion; small bowel endoscopy may be required for diagnosis
Norwalk-like virus	Watery	Common cause of "intestinal flu"; usually affects older children and adults; outbreaks of infection are common; illness characterized by abrupt onset of nausea and vomiting, often with only mild diarrhea; transmitted by food and water; etiologic diagnosis is complicated by small numbers of viral particles present in stool during infection
Plesiomonas shigelloides	Inflammatory	Consumption of raw or undercooked shellfish, endemic in Mexico, not stool commensal; role in gastroenteritis is controversial
Rotavirus	Watery	Common cause of infectious diarrhea in children 6–24 months; transmitted by fecal-oral route; often begins as sudden onset of vomiting, followed by diarrhea; prevalent in winter months
Salmonella enteritidis	Inflammatory	Common cause of bacterial enteritis in United States (especially children younger than 5 years); transmitted person-to-person and by food (eggs, poultry); outbreaks common

(Continued)

Table 26-1. Etiologic Agents of Bacterial, Viral, and Protozoal Gastroenteritis[11,12] (Continued)

Organism	Diarrhea	Clinical/Epidemiologic Manifestations
Salmonella typhi	Inflammatory	Common in developing countries, rare in United States; invasive disease with spread to bloodstream, reticuloendothelial system, lymphatics, liver, and biliary tree; associated with prolonged febrile illness (enteric fever), chronic carrier state, and metastatic infectious foci (arteritis, osteomyelitis, and neonatal meningitis)
Sarcocystis	Watery	Coccidian protozoa may cause serious infection in immunocompromised (AIDS) patients
Shigella dysenteriae	Inflammatory, hemorrhagic	Severe, invasive, and often life-threatening infection; associated with sepsis; malnutrition is important risk factor for fatal invasive disease in children; rare in United States, endemic in Mexico and many other parts of the world
Shigella spp.	Inflammatory	Common cause of dysentery in children and adults; person-to-person and food borne transmission[19]; endemic in United States; usually mild disease
Staphylococcus aureus	Watery	Cause of food poisoning (meats, potato salad, cream pies); preformed toxin causes nausea and vomiting within 6 hours of ingestion; contamination occurs by transmission from *S. aureus* carrier during food preparation in conjunction with suboptimal food storage
Vibrio cholera	Watery	Consumption of raw or undercooked shellfish; endemic in Mexico, sporadic cases in Gulf coast states (Texas, Louisiana, Florida)[17]; peak incidence in summer/fall
Vibrio parahaemolyticus	Watery, inflammatory	Consumption of raw or undercooked shellfish; very common in Japan, rare in United States; suspect in seafood-related outbreaks[18]
Yersinia enterocolitica	Inflammatory	Tends to produce mild, but prolonged (>2 weeks) illness; asymptomatic excretion may occur after recovery; extraintestinal manifestations include mesenteric adenitis, arthritis, and erythema nodosum[16]

Abbreviations: GI, gastrointestinal; AIDS, acquired immunodeficiency syndrome.

Noninflammatory diarrheas are caused by viruses (e.g., rotavirus, Norwalk agent, enteric adenovirus), parasites (e.g., *Giardia lamblia, Strongyloides stercoralis, Cryptosporidium* spp.), and toxin-producing bacteria (e.g., *E. coli, V. cholerae*). They are watery, mucoid diarrheas, either a result of toxin-mediated disruption of the fluid balance between the lower GI tract and the body, or physical impairment of fluid absorption from the intestines into the circulatory system. Stool specimens are notable for their lack of inflammatory cells and blood.

Inflammatory diarrheas are caused by bacteria that invade the intestinal mucosa (e.g., enteroinvasive *E. coli*, *Shigella* spp., *Salmonella* spp., *Campylobacter jejuni*, *Campylobacter coli*, *Yersinia enterocolitica*, *Vibrio parahaemolyticus*) or produce tissue damaging cytotoxins *(Clostridium difficile*, enterohemorrhagic *E. coli*), and by certain tissue invading parasites *(Entamoeba histolytica, Balantidium coli)*. These diarrheas are characterized by dysenteric stools that are visibly bloody and contain many inflammatory cells.

Diarrheas associated with food poisoning occur within 72 hours of ingestion of contaminated food. Symptoms are caused by toxic metabolic products elaborated during bacterial growth in food *(Staphylococcus aureus, Bacillus cereus, Clostridium perfringens, Clostridium botulinum)* or by growth of microorganisms ingested with tainted food. Symptoms exhibited after food poisoning include diarrhea, nausea, vomiting, abdominal cramps, and in the unique case of botulism, paralysis.

The onset of the AIDS epidemic in the early 1980s was hallmarked by the frequent appearance of previously rare infectious diseases. One such disease was disseminated *Mycobacterium avium* complex infection. These bacteria are common inhabitants of soil and water and are probably acquired through ingestion. These intracellular organisms multiply uncontrollably in the immunologically unprotected lower GI tract of the AIDS patient, enter the circulatory system, and cause infection throughout the body. Large numbers are excreted in the stool and are readily detected by acid-fast smear and culture.

Hospital infection control personnel frequently call on the microbiology laboratory to assist in their investigation of problems. Cultural surveillance of patients or patient care personnel for rectal carriage of nosocomial pathogens may be requested. The laboratory should be prepared to inoculate surveillance specimens to whichever selective media facilitate detection of the pathogen in question.

Selection

The stool of patients with signs and symptoms of bacterial gastroenteritis can be evaluated by smear and culture examination of a stool specimen. The results have both therapeutic and epidemiologic purposes. Enteric bacterial pathogens usually begin with nausea and vomiting (hours to days after exposure) followed by crampy abdominal pain and diarrhea with tenesmus. Fever is common. When disease is associated with limited symptoms, patients may not seek medical attention for what is considered a "stomach flu." Stool cultures are typically reserved for patients with severe or persistent (more than 3–5 days) symptoms. Routine examination is usually done for *Shigella* spp., *Salmonella* spp., and *C. jejuni*. Enteropathogenic *E. coli*, *Y. enterocolitica*, *Vibrio* spp., *Aeromonas hydrophila*, *Plesiomonas shigelloides*, and other potential stool pathogens are not routinely pursued, although they can be searched for under special epidemiologic or clinical circumstances.

The type of diarrhea produced (watery, hemorrhagic, or inflammatory) may provide clues about the etiologic agent (Table 26-1). *Escherichia coli* 0157:H7 should be suspected in patients (especially in children during the summer months) with hemorrhagic colitis and little or no fever.[13] Infection with this organism is being recognized more commonly as being associated with microangiopathic hemolytic anemias (hemolytic uremic syndrome and thrombotic thrombocytopenic purpura).[14,15] Persistence of unexplained abdominal pain and fever may suggest *Y. enterocolitica*, especially if extraintestinal manifestations are evident.[16] A history of undercooked or raw seafood (especially from the Gulf coast) should prompt a search for *Vibrio* spp.[17] *Clostridium difficile* should be considered with a history of recent antibiotic use (see below). Although illness after recent travel to foreign destinations (travelers' diarrhea) should be investigated with routine bacterial cultures and ova and parasite examinations, the etiologic agent (often enterotoxigenic *E. coli*) will often not be detected by these studies. It is always important to notify the laboratory of any and all suspected agents.

Enteric fever (caused by *S. typhi*) is a distinctive infection that is usually more severe than other salmonella infections. Bloodstream invasion is common and metastatic foci may develop. Unlike other enteric infections, a chronic, asymptomatic carrier state with persistence of *S. typhi* in the stool for longer than 1 year may follow acute infection in up to 3% of those infected. This is defined as persistence of *S. typhi* for more than 1 year. Fortunately, infection is rare in the United States (two per 10^6 cases annually). *Salmonella paratyphi* A, B, or C, or *Salmonella choleraesuis* may resemble *S. typhi* infection although a chronic carrier state does not occur. *Shigella dysenteriae* (Shiga bacillus) is another rare (in the United States) but distinctively aggressive and potentially life-threatening infection. Whenever these infections are suspected on epidemiologic or clinical grounds, culture should be performed because the diagnosis has important management and prognostic implications.

Stool specimens are quite useful for detecting disseminated *M. avium* complex infections in patients with AIDS.

Laboratory investigation of food poisoning is rarely done, with the exception of an epidemiologic study of an outbreak, or when botulism is suspected.

Terminology

Dysentery: Lower GI tract infection characterized by bloody, mucoid diarrhea associated with abdominal pain

Gastroenteritis: Lower GI tract infection characterized by nausea, vomiting, and diarrhea

Pseudomembranous colitis: Lower GI tract infection characterized by abdominal pain, diarrhea, and the presence of pseudomembranous nodules or plaques on the walls lining the colon

Logistics

Specimen Requirements

Laboratory diagnosis of bacterial intestinal infection is performed by examination of stool or rectal swabs. Stool is preferred over rectal swabs for two reasons.

1. The quality of a stool specimen is likely to be better than a rectal swab. Too often, rectal swabs are improperly collected or allowed to dry before commencement of testing.
2. The quantity of a stool specimen permits selective examination of blood- or mucus-laden portions where intestinal pathogens are likely to be present at highest concentrations. Some patients (e.g., young children) are unable to produce stool on demand, and a carefully collected rectal swab or stool from a very recently soiled diaper is an acceptable substitute.

Stool/rectal swab specimens may be examined for polymorphonuclear leukocytes to distinguish inflammatory from noninflammatory diarrheas. This examination can be performed on Wright, methylene blue, or Gram-stained smears. Stool or rectal swabs from AIDS patients thought to be infected with *M. avium* complex organisms should be examined for acid-fast bacteria by acid-fast stain and culture.

Stool for culture should be delivered to the laboratory promptly after collection. Some bacterial pathogens (e.g., *Shigella* spp.) quickly lose viability in stool after defecation because fermentative waste products resulting from continued bacterial metabolism accumulate and lower the stool pH. A transport medium, such as buffered glycerolized saline, should be used to reduce loss of viability if specimens cannot be cultured immediately. *Campylobacter* spp., unfortunately, do not survive well in buffered glycerolized saline, and for this organism, a second transport medium (e.g., Cary-Blair) is recommended.

If rectal swabs are collected, a separate swab is necessary for each type of smear and culture ordered. Rectal swabs should be moistened with transport medium (e.g., modified Stuart's) to minimize drying and pH change in the specimen and processed immediately by the laboratory.

Stool for toxin studies should be brought to the laboratory immediately or frozen to prevent loss of heat-labile activity. Rectal swabs are not acceptable for toxin detection tests.

Rectal swabs for surveillance of hospital patients or patient care personnel for colonization with nosocomial pathogens should be accompanied with a specific indication for the organism(s) being sought.

Microscopy

Smears from stool or rectal swabs must be thin. If needed, a portion of the specimen may be diluted with sterile saline before preparation of the smear. Methylene blue may be used to quickly stain smears for detection of polymorphonuclear leukocytes. Smears should be heat or methanol-fixed, stained with aqueous methylene blue for 1 minute, and examined under high dry ($\times 450$) or oil immersion ($\times 1000$) magnification. Stool or rectal swab specimens may also be stained with Gram reagents for detection of polymorphonuclear leukocytes. In patients with possible *C. jejuni* enterocolitis, direct observation of the distinctive curved rod morphology of the organisms is presumptive evidence of infection. A 1:5 dilution of Kinyoun carbol-fuchsin may be substituted for the safranin counterstain to obtain darker staining of *Campylobacter*. Smears should be examined under oil immersion magnification ($\times 1000$).

Specimens from AIDS patients for acid-fast staining should be thinly smeared on glass microscope slides, heat-fixed, and stained with rhodamine-auramine, Kinyoun, or Ziehl-Neelsen reagents. Rhodamine-auramine stained smears should be examined microscopically with ultraviolet illumination at high dry magnification ($\times 450$). Kinyoun and Ziehl-Neelsen stained smears should be examined at oil immersion magnification ($\times 1000$) with a standard light microscope.

Culture

Culture for lower GI tract bacterial pathogens is complicated by the simultaneous presence of large numbers of saprophytes in the specimen. The use of selective, differential, and enrichment media is tremendously helpful in screening specimens for pathogens.

Specimens should be inoculated to 5% sheep blood, MacConkey or EMB, and *Salmonella-Shigella* (SS), hektoen enteric (HE), or xylose lysine deoxycholate (XLD) agars for detection of *Salmonella* spp., *Shigella* spp., *Aeromonas* spp., and *S. aureus*. Inoculation of selenite C, selenite F, or gram-negative enrichment broths improves detection rates in specimens with low numbers of *Salmonella*. Moderate to heavy growth of *Y. enterocolitica* is easily recognized by experienced microbiologists on MacConkey or SS agars, although inoculation of cefsulodin-irgasan-novobiocin (CIN) agar or preparation of a stool saline suspension for incubation at 4°C is recommended for detection of low numbers of the organism. When any of the *Vibrio* spp. are possible pathogens, inoculation of thiosulfate citrate bile sucrose (TCBS) agar should be performed.

All of the agar media mentioned above, with the exception of CIN agar, should be incubated aerobically at 35°C for 18–24 hours. Cefsulodin-irgasan-novobiocin agar, since it is solely for recovery of *Y. enterocolitica*, is best incubated aerobically for 24–48 hours at 25°C, a preferable temperature for growth of psychrophilic bacteria. Enrichment broth cultures for *Salmonella* should be incubated at 35°C for 4–24 hours, subcultured to MacConkey, EMB, SS, HE, or XLD agar, and the subculture plate incubated aerobically at 35°C for 18–24 hours. Over a 30-day interval, cold enrichment suspensions for *Y. enterocolitica* should be subcultured periodically to MacConkey agar and the subculture plate incubated aerobically at 25°C and examined after 24–48 hours.

All stool or rectal swab specimens submitted for bacterial culture should be tested for *C. jejuni*. Specimens should be inoculated to selective agar (e.g., *Campylobacter* BAP) and optionally a selective broth (e.g., *Campylobacter* thioglycolate). Agar and broth subcultures should be incubated in a microaerophilic atmosphere (85% N_2, 10% CO_2, 5% O_2) at 42°C for 48–72 hours. Broth cultures should be incubated at 42°C for 24 hours, and then subcultured to selective agar.

Specimens for culture of *E. coli* 0157:H7 should be inoculated to MacConkey-sorbitol agar. Culture plates should be incubated aerobically at 35°C for 18–24 hours. *Escherichia coli* 0157:H7 is unable to ferment sorbitol, whereas most other *E. coli* serotypes have this capability. Identification is performed by serologic typing for the somatic (O) and flagellar (H) antigens (tube agglutination method). Cultures for enteropathogenic, enterotoxigenic, enteroinvasive, enteroadherent, and enterohemorrhagic (other than serotype 0157:H7) *E. coli* are not available in routine clinical laboratories, because of the difficulty in demonstrating each group's pathogenic properties.

Specimens for culture of *M. avium* complex species from AIDS patients should first be decontaminated (digestion is not necessary) in the same manner as is sputum before culture, and then inoculated to Löwenstein-Jensen medium and Middlebrook 7H10 or 7H11 agar. Cultures should be incubated at 35°C in an aerobic atmosphere containing 5–10% CO_2 for 8–12 weeks.

Rectal swab surveillance cultures for nosocomial pathogens should be inoculated to relevant selective media and incubated accordingly. Positive culture results should be immediately reported to infection control personnel.

Interpretation

In patients with diarrhea, detection of large numbers of polymorphonuclear leukocytes in methylene blue or Gram stained smears of stool or rectal swab specimens is evidence of inflammatory diarrhea. However, a lack of leukocytes, particularly in rectal swab specimens, does not necessarily denote noninflammatory diarrhea. Seeing curved gram-negative rods in Gram stained smears of specimens from patients with bloody diarrhea suggests *C. jejuni* infection. Confirmed diagnosis of campylobacter enteritis, though, requires isolation of the organism in culture. Likewise, the presence of large quantities of acid-fast bacteria in specimens from AIDS patients points toward *M. avium* complex infection. The diagnosis is not established, however, until the organism is recovered in culture.

Cultural detection of *Salmonella* spp., *Shigella* spp., *C. jejuni*, *Y. enterocolitica*, *Vibrio* spp., or *E. coli* 0157:H7 in patients with diarrhea is solid evidence of infection.[18,19] Pathogens are usually present in very high numbers. When only low numbers are found, consideration should be given to simultaneous infection with nonbacterial agents (e.g., parasites, viruses). Infection by more than one bacterial pathogen simultaneously is not uncommon. The presence of *Aeromonas* spp. must be correlated with clinical findings (watery diarrhea).[20]

Growth of *M. avium* complex organisms in stool/rectal swab cultures from AIDS patients is significant when present in abundance or when stool smears are replete with acid-fast bacteria. Low numbers of *M. avium* complex organisms are present in drinking water, and are found occasionally in specimens from healthy persons.

Test: *Clostridium Difficile* Toxin Detection

Background

Examination for toxins produced by *C. difficile*, *C. botulinum*, enterotoxigenic *E. coli*, and a number of other enteric pathogens can be performed in stool. Only the assay for *C. difficile* toxin is commonly performed in the clinical laboratories. In special cases, other toxin assays can be obtained from state health, Centers for Disease Control (CDC), or reference laboratories.

Gastrointestinal illness caused by *C. difficile* is a relatively common GI infection.[21] Disease is often sporadic but outbreaks are known to occur in hospitals, nursing homes, and even day-care centers. The spectrum of severity ranges from self-limited diarrhea to life-threatening toxic megacolon. While first described as being associated with clindamycin therapy, a large number of other antibiotics can initiate the infection (especially β-lactam antibiotics). The patient commonly presents with a history of antibiotic or antineoplastic therapy, fever, abdominal pain, diarrhea (five or more loose stools per day) and if endoscopy is done, pseudomembranous colitis. Symptoms generally resolve without therapy, but when diarrhea persists for more than 2 days, metronidazole or vancomycin is indicated. Infection probably occurs by exogenous acquisition from the environment or from fecal-oral contact, although endogenous activation may be responsible for some infections. Even without infection, the stool of hospitalized patients is more likely to contain *C. difficile* than stool specimens from a nonhospitalized control group, and the prevalence may be as high as 20% in patients receiving antibiotics.

Selection

There are two key procedures for the laboratory diagnosis of *C. difficile* infection: (1) recovery of cytotoxin-producing organisms from the stool and (2) direct detection of one of its toxins (A or B) by immunoassay or specific neutralization (by *Clostridium sordellii* antitoxin) of cytopathic effect (CPE) in tissue culture. When these methods are not readily available, the clinical diagnosis can be made with fair reliability if symptoms are compatible with the infection and the patient responds to therapy. Searching for pseudomembranous colitis is also helpful for making the diagnosis, although this is not practical and is unpleasant for the patient.

Logistics

Detection of *C. difficile* toxin B, a cytotoxin whose presence correlates highly with that of disease producing toxin A, can be accomplished in stool extracts inoculated to one of several cell cultures lines. The cytotoxin assay requires a bacteria-free stool extract, a suitable cell culture line (e.g., WI-38 human diploid lung fibroblasts), and *C. difficile, C. sordellii,* or gas gangrene polyvalent antitoxin. The specimen extract and antitoxin are inoculated to individual cell culture tubes or microtiter tray wells, incubated at 35°C, and the cells examined microscopically for CPE after 4, 24, and 48 hours of incubation. A positive result is indicated by detection of CPE (rounding of the cells) in the tube without antitoxin combined with no change in the tube with antitoxin neutralization. A commercial latex particle agglutination assay for *C. difficile* toxin A also is available. Serious questions about the assay's specificity for toxin A have been raised (see under Interpretation). A commercial ELISA test is under development.

Stool or rectal swab specimens may be cultured for *C. difficile* by inoculation to selective agar (e.g., cycloserine-cefoxitin-egg yolk-fructose), and incubation anaerobically at 35°C for 48–72 hours.

Interpretation

The interpretation of laboratory tests to detect *C. difficile* infection can be problematic.[22] The presence of the organism or its toxin in a stool specimen is not definitive proof of infection and may indicate an asymptomatic carrier state. Unfortunately, the most convenient laboratory test (latex agglutination) is associated with false positive and false negative results and is not completely specific for the *C. difficile* toxin. However, the reference method for laboratory diagnosis (detection of cytotoxin-producing *C. difficile*) is more costly and labor intensive. There is controversy surrounding the indications for selecting and applying the latex agglutination test. Under the best circumstances the text is about 90% sensitive and specific when compared with the cytotoxic tissue culture method. However, testing for toxin by either the latex or tissue culture test is only about 50% sensitive for identifying asymptomatic carriers when compared with culture. The diagnostic utility of the latex cytotoxin detection test depends largely on the population tested and the circumstances under which the test is used. If the prevalence of disease is high then the predictive value will similarly be high. Use of toxin detection methods alone to identify carriers for epidemiologic investigation and control of outbreaks, of *C. difficile* is not recommended because of the relatively low prevalence of carriers. By contrast, a positive latex test in the patient with the appropriate clinical history, signs, and symptoms of *C. difficile* infection provides additional support for the diagnosis. A more conclusive diagnosis, made by culturing stool for cytotoxin-producing *C. difficile* is warranted if resources are available. A negative latex test result in a similar situation is fairly reliable for excluding the diagnosis and alternative etiologies should be considered to explain the patient's GI illness.

While positive *C. difficile* cytotoxin assays in adults correlate highly with sigmoidoscopic evidence of pseudomembranous enterocolitis, this does not hold when interpreting assay results in young children. It is not unusual for healthy patients in this age group to be both culture and cytotoxin positive for *C. difficile*. Diagnosis of disease in young children should be based on clinical and sigmoidoscopic findings only.

Test: Viral Detection in Gastrointestinal Specimens[23]

Background

Viral gastroenteritis is a common infection that affects all ages. The prevalence of this infection in the United States is second only to the common cold. These viruses usually infect the small intestine producing a self-limited illness with loose, watery diarrhea and variable degrees of nausea and vomiting. However, viral gastroenteritis can have severe morbidity and even mortality in infants, immunocompromised patients, and the elderly. Several viral agents have been observed in the stool of patients with GI illness, but not all have been established as genuine pathogens.

Rotavirus occurs as a sporadic infection during the winter months and primarily affects children between the ages of 6 and 24 months, while adults are usually asymptomatic. It is transmitted by the fecal-oral route. It usually has a gradual onset and fever is variably present. Symptoms may last up to 1 week. Dehydration, from numerous watery stools, is the most important consequence of infection. Treatment is simply to replace lost fluids.

Norwalk virus is more often associated with outbreaks of infections within family or community groups. Infection occurs with no seasonal tendency in older children and adults and is marked by sudden onset of abundant watery diarrhea, often accompanied by vomiting. Symptoms usually abate within a few days. The virus is transmitted by food or water, which accounts for the high prevalence of outbreaks.

Gastroenteritis causing adenoviruses (types 40 and 41) commonly produce diarrhea in young children. Clinical manifestations are similar to rotavirus infections.

Astroviruses, so named for their star-like appearance, have been isolated from the stools of children with diarrhea. The ability of cell-free filtrates of these stools to transmit disease to adults has not been demonstrated. Thus, their role as etiologic agents of gastroenteritis is still in doubt.

Coronaviruses are implicated in diarrheal disease in newborn animals. However, in humans these viruses may be isolated from stool of both asymptomatic adults as well as persons with diarrhea. Infants with necrotizing enterocolitis have yielded coronavirus in their stool as shown by electron microscopy. The lack of other agents suggested an etiologic role for this virus. Infection appears to be more prevalent in the southwest United States.

Cytomegalovirus infection is generally not associated with GI tract infection; however, in immunocompromised hosts with systemic infection, it can cause esophagitis or ulceration of the colon. In such cases the virus may be present in an esophageal biopsy or stool specimen, respectively.[24]

Selection

The clinical presentation of viral gastroenteritis is insufficiently distinctive to reliably make the diagnosis by clinical assessment alone. However, the precise diagnosis seldom has important implications for patient management, and even then, an etiologic diagnosis cannot be made by laboratory methods in as many as 50% of cases. Attempts to establish a diagnosis is most often indicated in severe or prolonged illnesses, or in immunosuppressed patients. In these cases a large array of viral, bacterial, and parasitic etiologies should be investigated.

Gastroenteritis caused by virus infection does not require antiviral therapy. Occasionally, in cases of severe dehydration, supportive therapy (electrolyte replacement) is required. Virus detection in GI tract infections can be useful for epidemiologic and public health purposes and to prevent unnecessary and inappropriate antibiotic therapy.

When other organ systems are involved, the viral agent is sometimes shed in the feces, which becomes the specimen of choice for its isolation and identification (Tables 26-2 and 26-3). These infections primarily enteroviruses) are discussed in chapters dealing with the specific organ system(s) involved.

Logistics

Many viruses causing gastroenteritis can be detected by electron microscopy.[25] A commercially available enzyme-linked immunosorbent assay (ELISA) procedure is available for rotavirus detection. Specimens to be evaluated by either procedure should be collected during the earliest stages of illness when viral shedding is highest.

Table 26-2. Clinical Conditions for Which a Stool Specimen or a Rectal Swab Should be Considered for Viral Diagnosis

Central nervous system
    Aseptic meningitis
    Encephalitis
    Myelitis
    Paralysis
Diarrheal disease
Hepatitis
Maculopapular exanthem[a]
Myocarditis/pericarditis
Orchitis[b]
Necrotizing enterocolitis (infants)
Respiratory infection[c]
Pleuritis
Ulcerative colitis
Vesicular exanthemata

[a] For consideration of adenovirus or enterovirus infections.
[b] In the absence of parotitis.
[c] Concomitant with diarrhea, herpangina, and/or pharyngoconjunctivitis.

Table 26-3. Viruses Isolated From Stool or Rectal Swabs That are not Primarily Associated With Gastroenteritis

Virus	Interpretation, Associated Disease(s)
Cytomegalovirus	Possible systemic infection in immunocompromised host with ulcerative colitis
Enteroviruses	
Poliovirus	Aseptic meningitis, paralysis
Coxsackievirus A	Aseptic meningitis, paralysis, pharyngitis, common cold, pneumonitis (infant), exanthem, hand, foot, and mouth disease, hepatitis
Coxsackievirus B	Aseptic meningitis, meningoencephalitis, paralysis, respiratory infection, pleurodynia, pneumonia, exanthem, pericarditis, myocarditis, myalgia, hepatitis, pancreatitis, diabetes, systemic infection
Echoviruses	Aseptic meningitis, encephalitis, paralysis, Guillain-Barré syndrome, common cold, exanthem, pericarditis, myocarditis, myalgia, hepatic disease
Enterovirus 68	Pneumonia and bronchitis
Enterovirus 70	Acute hemorrhagic conjunctivitis
Enterovirus 71	Aseptic meningitis, meningoencephalitis, hand, foot, and mouth disease

Interpretation

The presence of virus in stool or a rectal swab is indicative of the presence of that virus in the host, although it does not necessarily imply an etiologic relationship. Several viruses recovered from the GI tract (reoviruses, astroviruses, small round viruses, and coronaviruses) are still considered to be of uncertain medical importance and are often found in the stool of healthy people. In addition, some agents, such as adenoviruses, may be shed in the stool months or even years after acute infection. Failure to identify a viral (or other) etiologic agent does not necessarily exclude the diagnosis. Norwalk-like viruses, for example, are often present in only small amounts in stool and may be easily missed by electron microscopic examination. Furthermore, isolation of more than one virus from the GI tract has become more common, especially in immunocompromised hosts, so that the assumption that the isolation of a single organism during a clinical infection can be equated with identification of the etiologic agent may not be correct.

Test: Ova and Parasite

Background and Selection

Diagnosis of parasitic infections of the GI tract relies heavily on the direct detection of helminth eggs or larvae and protozoal trophozoites or cysts in fecal samples. Specimens may be submitted fresh or in preservatives, and examined using direct wet mounts, concentration techniques, and permanent stained smears. Special stains may be required for the detection of some parasites, such as *Cryptosporidium* or *Isospora*. The recent introduction of enzyme immunoassay (EIA) antigen detection tests for the diagnosis of giardiasis is an important adjunct to the traditional stool examination. Other parasite antigen detection tests will surely be available in the years ahead, but will not replace the need for a single test such as the "O&P" (ova and parasites) examination, which can rapidly screen for the entire spectrum of intestinal parasites.

Stool examination for ova and parasites is usually recommended when appropriate clinical and historical information suggest that parasitic infections be included in the differential diagnosis. This test is often ordered in addition to studies for other enteric pathogens that may present with similar symptoms. However, the "O&P" examination should not be performed unless the history and clinical finding are compatible. For example, gastroenteritis in hospitalized patients is rarely, if ever, caused by organisms that are detected by the stool "O&P" examination.[26] Specific characteristics of parasitic infections, which may suggest the need for stool examination, are as follows.

Protozoa[27]

The spectrum of protozoa most commonly known to infect the human GI tract is summarized in Table 26-4. In all cases of symptomatic infection with the pathogenic intestinal protozoa, abdominal pain and diarrhea are common clinical complaints. Simple diarrhea may progress to true dysentery (multiple bowel movements daily, streaked with blood-tinged mucus) with fever and dehydration when disease is caused by either *E. histolytica* or *B. coli*.

Diarrhea caused by *G. lamblia* tends to be episodic and occurs with epigastric pain, gaseousness and bloating, and weight loss. Stool is often characterized as having increased fat and mucus present, but no blood. When suspicion of giardiasis is high but the initial stool examination is negative, additional specimens on consecutive days may be submitted.[28] Other diagnostic techniques available include use of the "string" test for sampling duodenal contents or the *Giardia* antigen detection test, which offers help in identifying occult infections. They are best used as a follow-up to traditional stool examination when suspicion of disease remains high.[29]

Dientamoeba fragilis may cause a diarrheal syndrome similar to giardiasis with fatigue being a common compliant, and is most often seen in children. Infection with *Blastocystis hominis* has anecdotally been reported to cause a crampy disease with fever, nausea, and vomiting. However, this association and the pathogenicity of *B. hominis* is uncertain.[30]

Diarrheal disease caused by the coccidian protozoa *Cryptosporidium*, *Isospora*, and *Sarcocystis* tends to be mild and self-limited, although fever, abdominal cramps, and anorexia may occur in otherwise healthy persons. Immunocompromised patients (especially those with AIDS) may develop a persistent profuse, watery diarrhea with these protozoa that may prove fatal. Cryptosporidiosis is particularly common because large numbers of domestic animals may serve as reservoirs. Children are at high risk for acquiring *Cryptosporidium*, and numerous outbreaks in day-care settings have been described. This disease is seen less frequently in adults presumably because of acquired immunity. Infection with *Isospora* is seen less often than with *Cryptosporidium*, probably because humans are the only known host for the parasite. Isosporiasis is acquired from ingestion of infectious oocysts with contaminated food or water or from close personal contact with an infected person. Enteric sarcosporidiosis (caused by *Sarcocystis hominis*) is a rarely seen infection acquired from eating raw beef or pork, and results in a mild diarrheal disease similar to those caused by the other coccidia. Treatment for *Cryptosporidium* infection is only supportive at this time, whereas *Isospora* responds promptly to treatment with trimethoprim/sulfamethoxazole. Information on the treatment of *Sarcocystis* infection is lacking. Should infection with coccidia be considered, notation to this effect should be made when submitting a specimen, because special staining techniques are often required for their detection.

Table 26-4. Commonly Encountered Intestinal Protozoa and Their Degree of Known Pathogenicity in Humans

Degree of Pathogenicity	
Pathogenic	**Nonpathogenic**
Amoebae	
Entamoeba histolytica	*Entamoeba coli*
	Entamoeba hartmanni
	Entamoeba polecki
	Endolimax nana
	Iodamoeba beutschlii
Flagellates	
Giardia lamblia	*Chilomastix mesnili*
Dientamoeba fragilis[a]	*Enteromonas hominis*
	Retortamonas intestinalis
	Trichomonas hominis
Ciliates	
Balantidium coli	
Coccidia	
Cryptosporidium spp.	
Isospora belli	
Sarcocystis hominis	
Others	
Blastocystis hominis[a]	

[a] Possibly pathogenic.

Helminths

The severity of symptoms associated with enteric helminth infections is almost always dose-related. Infection with *Trichuris, Capillaria,* and *Ascaris* does not occur directly, as the eggs must embryonate for a period of time outside of the body before their ingestion. Eggs of hookworms (*Necator* and *Ancylostoma*) also embryonate outside the body, but hatch and molt to the infectious stage in the soil. *Strongyloides* eggs usually hatch within the intestine, and larvae are then passed in the feces, which subsequently molt to the infectious stage in the soil. Infectious larvae of both hookworms and *Strongyloides* can then penetrate the skin directly. Thus, with the sole exception of *S. stercoralis,* none of the other nematodes, cestodes, or trematodes have the biologic potential to multiply within their human host.

The spectrum of illness with intestinal infections caused by helminths is variable among different species; however when present, common clinical findings include abdominal pain, malabsorption syndrome, diarrhea, and peripheral eosinophilia. Anemia commonly occurs with the various nematode infections, especially hookworms *(Necator americanus* and *Ascaris duodenale),* but may also be seen with *Diphyllobothrium latum* infection. Bowel obstruction is a potentially fatal complication occasionally seen with the larger helminths, including *Ascaris, Taenia, Diphyllobothrium,* and *Fasciolopsis* infections. Urticaria, asthma, and other allergic manifestations may also be seen with these same infections.

Penetration and migration through the skin by hookworm and *Strongyloides* larvae cause a minimal to severe pruritus commonly known as "ground itch." Larvae of these same species also migrate through the lungs, and may be responsible for mild pneumonitis. Pulmonary migration of *Ascaris* larvae is a potentially more serious complication, and when associated with infiltrates and peripheral eosinophilia is known as Löffler syndrome (see Ch. 22).

Pinworm *(Enterobius vermicularis)* infection is usually transmitted directly from host to host, as the egg is fully embryonated when passed from the body. Pruritus ani is a common clinical complaint with this infection because of the female worm's habit of crawling onto the perianal skin at night to deposit eggs. Infection rarely causes intestinal symptoms. Diagnosis is not made by stool examination, but by examination of the perianal skin for typical eggs using the cellophane tape technique.

Trichostrongylus spp. are animal nematodes that humans usually acquire by ingesting infectious larvae with uncooked vegetables, as they are not able to penetrate skin directly. Other than for *Trichostrongylus* infections, children are at highest risk for all nematode infections because their potential for exposure is much greater than for adults.

Identification of *Hymenolepis nana* tapeworm infection is common in many parts of the world, especially in children, but rarely is it a cause of clinical disease. This is the most commonly reported cestode infection found in the United States, and is usually seen in the southeastern states. Children are at highest risk for infection because of the worm's ability to be transmitted directly from person to person, much the same way as pinworms, where the eggs are immediately infectious to the next host when passed. *Hymenolepis diminuta* and *Dipylidium caninum* are seen less frequently than *H. nana* as they require arthropod intermediate hosts such as beetles and fleas, respectively, in their life cycles. Like *H. nana,* infection with these species is rarely associated with symptoms.

Diphyllobothrium latum (broad fish tapeworm) is acquired from eating raw freshwater fish and may cause a vitamin B_{12} deficiency with pernicious anemia, especially in persons with marginal nutrition or those with a genetic predisposition to this type of anemia.

Taenia saginata (beef tapeworm) is acquired from eating raw beef, and infection is especially common in certain countries where this practice is customary. Of all cestodes infecting humans, *Taenia solium* (pork tapeworm) has the greatest disease-producing potential. The adult *T. solium* is acquired from eating raw pork, and is rarely a cause of clinical disease. Eggs passed in the feces are, however, immediately infectious and become a possible source of cysticercosis to the person carrying the adult worm as well as to close contacts.

All trematodes require a freshwater snail to serve as the first intermediate host. Free-swimming cercariae are released from the snail and swim about until contact is made with an appropriate second intermediate host, whereupon the larvae encyst as metacercariae. Humans are infected by incidental ingestion of the infectious metacercariae with uncooked foods. Only cercariae of schistosomes are able to directly penetrate the skin. Epidemiologic information on the most common trematodes infecting humans is summarized in Table 26-5.

Table 26-5. Epidemiology of Human Trematode Infections

Species	Endemic Areas	Source of Infection
Fasciolopsis buski	Far East	Aquatic vegetation
Heterophyes heterophyes	Far East, Middle East	Freshwater fish
Metagonimus yokogawai	Far East, Middle East, Spain, U.S.S.R.	Freshwater fish
Echinostoma ilocanum	Far East	Freshwater mollusks
Nanophyetus salmincola	Eastern Siberia, U.S. Pacific Northwest	Freshwater fish
Clonorchis sinensis	Far East	Freshwater fish
Opisthorchis viverrini	Far East	Freshwater fish
Fasciola hepatica	Worldwide	Aquatic vegetation
Paragonimus westermani	Far East, Africa	Crabs, crayfish
Paragonimus mexicanus	Central and South America	Crabs
Schistosoma mansoni	Africa, South America, West Indies	Freshwater
Schistosoma japonicum	Far East	Freshwater
Schistosoma mekongi	Indochina	Freshwater
Schistosoma haematobium	Africa, Middle East	Freshwater

Fasciolopsis buski is the largest intestinal fluke and one of the most important and pathogenic trematodes to infect humans. Infections are common in the Far East, and usually acquired from eating uncooked bamboo shoots or water calthrop, or from peeling water chestnuts with the teeth. Light infections may result in intestinal malabsorption, and allergic responses to worm metabolites are commonly referred to as "verminous intoxication." Obstruction and ileus may occur in heavy infections.

Heterophyes, Metagonimus, and *Nanophyetus* infections occur less frequently but are known causes of GI disease. These species are small compared with *Fasciolopsis,* and large numbers must be present for disease to be manifest. Popularity of eating raw fish is a known risk factor for acquiring these helminths. *Nanophyetus salmincola* is the only species documented from North America, and is acquired primarily from eating raw or smoked salmon or trout that originate in the Pacific Northwest.[31]

Estimates of nematode and trematode worm burdens may occasionally be desirable, especially to monitor response to therapy. Both the Kato and Stoll methodologies are well known, and provide adequate quantitation. Specialized recovery and culture techniques are also available to help detect light infection with hookworms or *Strongyloides,* which may be overlooked in the routine stool examination.

Extraintestinal Infections

Certain trematodes may infect the liver, lungs, and bloodstream, yet are diagnosed by examination of stool because eggs are able to pass into the feces from their extraintestinal location (Table 26-6). Several different species infect the biliary tract. *Clonorchis* and *Opisthorchis* liver fluke infections are common in the Far East, and may be suspected if a history of eating uncooked fish is elicited. As with other fish transmitted helminths, thorough cooking will kill any worm larvae present. Clinical findings may include fever, abdominal pain, hepatomegaly, jaundice, and peripheral eosinophilia. Infection may result in chronic inflammation, scarring, and obstruction of the biliary tract (see Ch. 23). Development of cholangiocarcinoma has been indirectly linked to infection with these trematodes.

Fasciola hepatica causes a widespread but rare infection acquired from eating uncooked water plants, such as watercress. *Fasciola* infection differs from that of the other liver flukes in being a true zoonosis, and is acquired from eating aquatic plants rather than fish. Also, larval worms of this species migrate through liver parenchyma directly, causing significant tissue damage before arriving in the bile ducts.

Paragonimiasis (lung fluke infection) usually presents with increasing cough, hemoptysis, and chest pain (see Ch. 22). Infections occurring in ectopic locations are not uncommon, however, and may mimic other diseases. The disease is most commonly acquired in the Far East, Africa, and Central and South America, and is associated with a history of eating uncooked crabs or crayfish. Paragonimiasis is a zoonotic disease, and occurs sporadically in various parts of the world where crabs or crayfish are eaten raw. While most worms are associated with lung disease, the migrating larvae may localize in a variety of ectopic sites. Cerebral paragonimiasis is a serious complication which may be life-threatening.[32]

Table 26-6. Commonly Encountered Human Helminthic Infections Which may be Diagnosed Upon Examination of Stool

Intestinal infections
  Nematoda
     Enterobius vermicularis
     Trichuris trichiura
     Capillaria philippinensis
     Ascaris lumbricoides
     Necator americanus
     Ancylostoma duodenale
     Trichostrongylus spp.
     Strongyloides stercoralis

  Cestoda
     Hymenolepis nana
     Hymenolepis diminuta
     Taenia solium
     Taenia saginata
     Diphyllobothrium latum
     Dipylidium caninum

  Trematoda
     Fasciolopsis buski
     Heterophyes heterophyes
     Metagonimus yokogawai
     Echinostoma ilocanum
     Nanophyetus salmincola

Extraintestinal infections
  Trematoda
     Clonorchis sinensis (liver)
     Opisthorchis viverrini (liver)
     Fasciola hepatica (liver)
     Paragonimus westermani (lung)
     Paragonimus mexicanus (lung)
     Schistosoma mansoni (inferior mesenteric venules)
     Schistosoma japonicum (superior mesenteric venules)
     Schistosoma mekongi (superior mesenteric venules)

Schistosome (blood fluke) infections are among the most common and most serious of all helminthic infections, and epitomize the chronicity often accorded to parasitic infections. Because the free-swimming cercariae are immediately infectious to humans, the intensity of infection is partially related to the amount of time spent in infested freshwaters. The worms are long lived, however, and continue to produce thousands of eggs for many years after infection. Hepatic fibrosis with all its potential complications is a common consequence of long-standing infection and reinfection with all the *Schistosoma* spp. except *Schistosoma haematobium*. Infections by *Schistosoma japonicum* and *Schistosoma mekongi* are potentially more serious than infection by *Schistosoma mansoni* because of a much larger number of eggs shed by the female worm of those species. Occasionally worms may be found in ectopic locations, and eggs may be carried to distant sites including the lungs, brain, spinal cord, spleen, and myocardium.

Intestinal schistosomiasis may be caused by several different species, but disease presentation is similar in all. Symptoms of acute schistosomiasis occur as the worms initiate egg laying, and may mimic serum sickness. This usually occurs several weeks after exposure and is typically seen only in persons infected for the first time. As egg deposition progresses the person experiences continued fever, malaise, abdominal pain, liver tenderness, and hepatosplenomegaly, and may have blood and mucus in diarrheic stools. Chronic schistosomiasis can result in hepatosplenomegaly and portal hypertension with the development of varices and ascites. Other complications may include progressive nephrosclerosis and recurrent *Salmonella* bacteremia. In all cases, persons are exposed to schistosome cercariae by swimming, bathing, or wading in freshwater in endemic areas of the West Indies, South America, Africa, and the Far East. *Schistosoma haematobium* usually infects venules surrounding the bladder and is diagnosed by examining urine (see Ch. 24). Tests useful in the diagnosis and management of schistosomiasis other than the routine stool examination include rectal biopsy and the egg hatching test.

Logistics

Specimen Requirements

For routine evaluation, 20–40 g of formed stool or 5 to 6 T of watery stool are submitted in a clean container free of water or foreign debris. If specimens cannot be delivered to the laboratory within the hour (ideally within the half hour), patients should submit material that has been preserved both in formalin and polyvinyl alcohol (PVA), merthiolate-iodine-formalin (MIF), or other recommended fixatives. Patients are instructed to mix a small portion of specimen into each vial provided, in the ratio of 1 part specimen to 2 parts preservative. For certain procedures entire fecal specimens may be required.

Some infections, such as giardiasis and amoebiasis, are notoriously difficult to detect, and may require the submission of multiple specimens. If such a series is desired, three stools collected on three consecutive mornings should be submitted, and repeated at weekly intervals.[28] Specimens collected after administration of a purgative such as sodium biphosphate/sodium phosphate may increase the sensitivity of the examinations. Use of a 1-vial (MIF) or 2-vial (formalin and PVA) preservation method is usually adequate and saves the patient multiple trips to the hospital. When a patient has recently ingested barium sulfate, pepto-Bismol, oily substances such as Castor oil, or antibiotics (specifically tetracycline), stools are usually unsatisfactory for parasitic examination and must be resubmitted at a later time.

Direct sampling of duodenal contents using either duodenal aspiration or the "string" test may be of use in diagnosing giardiasis or strongyloidiasis when stool examinations have remained negative, but the index of suspicion remains high. To collect a specimen using the "string" test, the patient swallows a small gelatin capsule that is attached to a nylon string secured at the proximal end. The capsule dissolves in the stomach and the string is allowed to pass into the small intestine. After 6–8 hours the string is removed and bile stained mucus from its distal end is placed on a glass slide and immediately examined for motile larvae or trophozoites.

Analysis

Gross Examination. Gross examination of fresh and preserved fecal material is performed initially to detect the presence of blood, mucus, evidence of fat malabsorption, and tapeworm proglottids or roundworms. Loose or diarrheic stools are more likely to contain protozoal trophozoites, whereas formed stools would more likely contain cysts.

Direct Wet Mount. The microscopic examination is usually conducted in three parts: direct wet mount preparations; wet mount preparations after a concentration procedure; and permanent stained preparations. Direct wet mount preparations of fresh material are useful for the detection of motile protozoa and helminth larvae. A second wet mount made with a drop of iodine is performed to identify protozoal cysts. Direct wet mounts are also made from formalin-fixed material as for fresh stool.

Concentration Techniques. Concentration procedures are usually of the flotation or sedimentation type, and may be performed on either fresh or preserved specimens. Effectiveness, however, varies significantly depending on the parasites present and the techniques used.

Flotation using zinc sulfate at a specific gravity of 1.18 (for fresh material) or 1.20 (for formalin preserved material) assists in the recovery and recognition of most protozoal cysts and some nematode eggs. The heavier eggs of trematodes and cestodes do not concentrate as well with this method, and the remaining sediment should also be examined for their presence. The formalin-ether or formalin-ethyl acetate sedimentation technique is probably the most common concentration procedure in use by clinical laboratories for the detection of both protozoal and helminthic intestinal parasites. This procedure may be adapted for use with fresh material or material preserved by a variety of methods including formalin, PVA, MIF, and sodium acetate-acetic acid-formaldehyde (SAF) among others. In practice both saline and iodine wet mounts are prepared from the sediment and examined as for the direct wet mount. Other described techniques are aimed at the enhanced recovery of particular parasites, such as Sheather's sugar flotation technique for *Cryptosporidium*. Simple gravity sedimentation alone is an effective concentration procedure, especially when the glassware, reagents, and centrifuge needed for these other techniques are unavailable.[33]

Permanently Stained Smears.[34] The use of permanently stained smears is an extremely important adjunct in recognizing the presence of intestinal protozoa, and may be performed on both fresh feces and feces preserved in PVA. The two most commonly used stains include Wheatley's modification of Gomori's trichrome stain and the Heidenhain's iron hematoxylin stain. Use of permanent stains is important for both the recovery and proper identification of intestinal protozoa, and provides a permanent record of the infecting organisms for later review or further consultation. Smears from fresh material should be prepared and fixed in Schaudinn's fixative as soon after passage as possible, and certainly within the hour. Material preserved in PVA should be allowed to fix for at least 30 minutes before the preparation of smears. While both staining methods produce excellent results, the trichrome stain has slowly replaced the time-honored iron hematoxylin stain primarily because of the shorter time required for its performance.

Special Procedures

Acid-Fast or Immunofluorescence Staining for *Cryptosporidium*. Small size and lack of staining by iodine or trichrome make *Cryptosporidium* difficult to detect without the aid of special techniques. The organisms are known to be acid-fast and use of such techniques, especially the cold carbol fuchsin (Kinyoun) method or the fluorochrome auramine-O, is especially effective. The recent introduction of immunofluorescence reagents for *Cryptosporidium* detection is also helpful, and provides a high level of specificity.[35]

Cellophane Tape Swab. Clear cellophane tape is useful for sampling the perianal skin for eggs of the pinworm *E. vermicularis,* and perhaps the whipworm *Trichuris trichiura* as well. After removal from the perianal skin, the tape is applied to a microscope slide and examined directly.

Egg Quantitation. The Kato thick smear technique allows for the examination of a larger quantity of fecal material than would be possible in the direct examination, and is performed without the need for concentration methods. This procedure is used to determine worm burdens in persons and for epidemiologic studies of *Ascaris, Trichuris,* and hookworms. Quantitative response to therapy may also be followed with this technique. The Stoll egg quantitation technique provides a numerical value for helminth eggs (number of eggs per gram of feces), and is also used to determine worm burdens, follow response to therapy, and estimate rates of reinfection in endemic areas.

Culture for Nematodes. The Harada-Mori technique is performed by smearing fecal material on a filter paper strip and incubating it in a tube with the bottom of the strip in contact with distilled water. As larvae hatch, they collect in the water in the bottom of the tube and may be recovered. This procedure and its variants are useful in detecting primarily hookworms and *Strongyloides.* Alternatively, fecal material may be mixed with granulated charcoal and incubated in a moist, dark container. After several days, infective larvae may be seen actively crawling about on the surface of the fecal suspension. Use of the Baermann funnel technique is effective for the recovery of *Strongyloides* larvae, and is based on the migration of larvae from the fecal material suspended in gauze and into the water beneath. This procedure is especially useful in detecting possible latent infections.

Rectal Biopsy. The submission of rectal biopsies is often useful in the diagnosis of suspected *S. mansoni* and occasionally *S. haematobium* infections. While the biopsies may be submitted for routine histology, pressing the sample between two glass slides and examining for the presence of typical eggs is a simple and effective way to detect infection.

Hatching of Schistosome Eggs. Determining the viability of schistosome eggs may help in deciding whether treatment is necessary for an infection acquired in the past. Eggs from stool or urine may be examined directly for excretory or "flame" cells. Alternatively, a homogenized stool specimen may be repeatedly washed with saline and allowed to settle. Dechlorinated water is then added to the sediment, which stimulates viable eggs to hatch, usually within several hours. When held in a side-arm flask with only the side-arm exposed to light, the newly hatched miracidia are attracted to the light and may be seen actively swimming about when examined with a hand lens. This procedure may also be used with *S. haematobium* eggs recovered from urine.

Interpretation

Intestinal Protozoal Infections

Entamoeba histolytica is the only intestinal amoeba of the six recognized species in humans known to be associated with significant disease. While dysentery is the most common serious sequelae to this infection, hematogenous spread to the liver or other sites may also occur, often from an asymptomatic intestinal infection (see Ch. 23). Infection by any of the intestinal amoebae, pathogenic or nonpathogenic, does imply that fecal-oral contamination has occurred, and that consideration should be given to the possible presence of other fecally transmitted pathogens.

Giardia lamblia is a well known cause of recalcitrant diarrhea, although infection may produce few or no obvious symptoms. Infectious cysts can be transmitted from contaminated food, water, or from intimate contact with an infected person. Numerous outbreaks have been documented in children attending day-care facilities. Persons who drink untreated stream or lake water are also at risk, possibly from animal sources.

Despite its name, *D. fragilis* is actually a flagellate protozoan related to *Trichomonas.* Incidence is highest in pediatric populations in which symptoms of infection appear to be more common. Although the status of this organism as a pathogen is ill defined, specific treatment does provide relief when symptoms are present. The remaining species of intestinal flagellates that infect humans (Table 26-4) have not been associated with apparent disease. Their presence is, however, as significant as that of the nonpathogenic amoebae in serving as markers of oral-fecal contamination.

Balantidium coli is the only pathogenic ciliate to infect humans, and may cause a serious dysentery similar to that of *E. histolytica.* The organisms rarely spread to distant sites, however. Hogs are an important reservoir for *B. coli,* and may place pig farmers and slaughterhouse workers at particular risk. Patient history may suggest such exposure. *Balantidium coli* is rarely encountered in the United States, but is prevalent in certain areas of the tropics.

Blastocystis hominis is a common protozoan inhabitant of the human intestinal tract that alternates between cystic and amoeboid forms in its life cycle. Although this organism has been associated with clinical disease, questions remain as to its true pathogenic potential because of its high prevalence in persons without obvious disease.[30] When symptoms are present however, *B. hominis* is often found in large numbers with the amoeboid form predominating. Specific therapy may be warranted in such circumstances, especially when the presence of other etiologic agents has been carefully ruled out.[36] Identification of any of the enteric coccidia *Cryptosporidium, Isospora,* and *Sacrocystis* confirms their role as etiologic agents of diarrheal disease in individual patients.

Helminthic Infections

Most nematode, cestode, and trematode infections of the GI tract may be diagnosed on finding the typical morphologic stage (egg, larva, or adult) of the parasite in the stool. Certain extraintestinal infections caused by trematodes infecting the liver, lung, or bloodstream may also be diagnosed by the presence of typical eggs in feces. Disease caused by any of the intestinal helminths listed in Table 26-6 is dose related, being dependent on the number of eggs or larvae to which the infected person is exposed. The one exception is *S. stercoralis,* which has the potential to reproduce within the host by autoinfection, which may persist for decades. Identification of this parasite in the immunosuppressed patient is especially serious because of the potential to develop a disseminated potentially fatal hyperinfection syndrome.

Infection by the large intestinal tapeworms is rarely associated with serious disease but can cause considerable consternation when a length of strobila is passed per rectum. Because eggs of the two Taenia species are indistinguishable, infected persons should be treated to eradicate the adult worms and prevent the possibility of cysticercosis. Caution should be exercised, however, in administering praziquantel, as this drug is active against both adult and larval stages. Inadvertent treatment of pre-existing asymptomatic cysticercosis may result in serious sequelae as the larval forms die.[37] Further discussion on cysticercosis may be found in Chapter 27.

A number of intestinal trematode infections have been described, which may result in symptomatic disease when worms are present in large numbers. The presence of eggs from these parasites should cause concern about extraintestinal infection (Table 26-6).

REFERENCES

1. Abrams, GD: Pathogenesis of gastrointestinal infections. Am J Surg Pathol 1988;12:76–81.
2. Alexander JA, Brouillette De, Chien MC et al: Infectious esophagitis following liver and renal transplantation. Dig Dis Sci 1988;33:1121–1126.
3. Bonacini M, Laine L, Gal AA et al: Prospective evaluation of blind brushing of the esophagus for *Candida* esophagitis in patients with human immunodeficiency virus infection. Am J Gastroenterol 1990;85:385–389.
4. Wilcox CM, Diehl DL, Cello JP et al: Cytomegalovirus esophagitis in patients with AIDS. A clinical, endoscopic, and pathologic correlation. Ann Intern Med 1990; 113:589–593.
5. Meijer K, van-Saene HK, Hill JC: Infection control in patients undergoing mechanical ventilation: traditional approach versus a new development—selective decontamination of the digestive tract. Heart Lung 1990; 19:11–20.
6. Maddocks AC: *Helicobacter pylori* (formerly *Campylobacter pyloridis/pylori*) 1986–89: a review. J Clin Pathol 1990;43:353–356.
7. Graham DY: *Campylobacter pylori* and peptic ulcer disease. Gastroenterology 1989;96:615–625.
8. Nedenskov-Sorensen P, Aase S, Bjorneklett A et al: Sampling efficiency in the diagnosis of *Helicobacter pylori* infection and chronic gastritis. J Clin Microbiol 1991;29:672–675.
9. Rauws EA, Royen EA, Langenberg W et al: ^{14}C-urea breath test in *C. pylori* gastritis. Gut 1989;30:798–803.
10. McNulty CA, Dent JC, Uff JS et al: Detection of *Campylobacter pylori* by the biopsy urease test: an assessment in 1445 patients. Gut 1989;30:1058–1062.
11. Bishop WP, Ulshen MH: Bacterial gastroenteritis. Pediatr Clin North Am 1988;35:69–87.
12. Gorbach SL: Infectious diarrhea. Infect Dis Clin North Am 1988;2:(3)557–778.
13. Marshall WF, McLimans CA, Yu PK et al: Results of a 6-month survey of stool cultures for *Escherichia coli* 0157:H7. Mayo Clin Proc 1990;65:787–792.
14. Griffin PM, Ostroff SM, Tauxe RV et al: Illnesses associated with *Escherichia coli* 0157:H7 infections. A broad clinical spectrum. Ann Intern Med 1988;109:705–712.
15. Karmali MA: Infection by verocytotoxin-producing *Escherichia coli.* Clin Microbiol Rev 1989;2:15–38.
16. Cover TL, Aber RC: *Yersinia enterocolitica.* N Engl J Med 1989;321:16–24.
17. Lowry PW, Pavia AT, McFarland LM et al: Cholera in Louisiana. Widening spectrum of seafood vehicles. Arch Intern Med 1989;149:2079–2084.
18. Doyle MP: Pathogenic *Escherichia coli, Yersinia enterocolitica,* and *Vibrio parahaemolyticus.* Lancet 1990; 336:1111–1115.
19. Halpern Z, Dan M, Giladi M et al: Shigellosis in adults:

epidemiologic, clinical, and laboratory features. Medicine 1989;68:210-217.
20. Golik A, Modai D, Gluskin I, et al: Aeromonas in adult diarrhea: an enteropathogen or an innocent bystander? J Clin Gastroenterol 1990;12:148-152.
21. Gerding DN: Disease associated with *Clostridium difficile* infection. Ann Intern Med 1989;110:255-257.
22. Biddle WL, Harms JL, Greenberger NJ, Miner PB Jr: Evaluation of antibiotic-associated diarrhea with a latex agglutination test and cell culture cytotoxicity assay for *Clostridium difficile*. Am J Gastroenterol 1989;84:379-382.
23. Christensen ML: Human viral gastroenteritis. Clin Microbiol Rev 1989;2:51-89.
24. Rene E, Marche C, Chevalier T et al: Cytomegalovirus colitis in patients with acquired immunodeficiency syndrome. Dig Dis Sci 1988;33:741-750.
25. Fong CK: Electron microscopy for the rapid detection and identification of viruses form clinical specimens. Yale J Biol Med 1989;62:115-130.
26. Siegel DL, Edelstein PH, Nachamkin I: Inappropriate testing for diarrheal diseases in the hospital. JAMA 1990;263:979-982.
27. Tanowitz HB, Weiss LM, Wittner M: Diagnosis and treatment of protozoan diarrheas. Am J Gastroenterol 1988;83:339-350.
28. Senay H, MacPherson D: Parasitology: diagnostic yield of stool examination. Can Med Assoc J 1989;140:1329-1331.
29. Rosoff JD, Sanders CA, Sonnad SS et al: Stool diagnosis of giardiasis using a commercially available enzyme immunoassay to detect Giardia-specific Antigen 65 (GSA 65). J Clin Microbiol 1989;27:1997-2002.
30. Sun T, Katz S, Tanenbaum B, Schenone C: Questionable clinical significance of *Blastocystis hominis* infection. Am J Gastroenterol 1989;84:1543-1547.
31. Fritsche TR, Eastburn RL, Wiggins LH, Terhune CA Jr: Praziquantel for treatment of human Nanophyetus salmincola (Triglotrema salmincola) infection. J Infect Dis 1989;160:896-899.
32. Johnson RJ, Jong EC, Dunning SB et al: Paragonimiasis: diagnosis and the use of praziquantel in treatment. Rev Infect Dis 1985;7:200-206.
33. Shidham VB: A rapid, economical, and simple method for concentration of *Schistosoma mansoni* ova in feces. Am J Clin Pathol 1991;95:91-95.
34. Shetty N, Prabhu T: Evaluation of faecal preservation and staining methods in the diagnosis of acute amoebiasis and giardiasis. J Clin Pathol 1988;41:694-699.
35. Garcia LS, Brewer TC, Bruckner DA: Fluorescent detection of Cryptosporidium oocysts in fecal specimens by using monoclonal antibodies. J Clin Microbiol 1987;25:119-121.
36. Zierdt CH: Blastocystis hominis-past and future. Clin Microbiol Rev 1991;4:61-79.
37. Nash TE, Neva FA: Recent advances in the diagnosis and treatment of cerebral cysticercosis. N Engl J Med 1984;311:1492-1496.
38. Smith GE, Hinde F, Westmoreland D et al: Infantile botulism. Arch Dis Child 1989;64:871-872.

27 Central Nervous System

Joseph M. Campos
Thomas R. Fritsche
Gerald Lancz
Steven Specter

INTRODUCTION[1]

Acute infection of the central nervous system (CNS) is a medical emergency requiring rapid diagnostic and therapeutic intervention. In a busy microbiology laboratory, where specimens typically are processed in batches for greatest efficiency, the arrival of a CNS specimen immediately shifts the laboratory into an emergency mode. Although test results are usually not available until after empirical administration of antimicrobial therapy, critical decisions regarding further diagnostic tests, hospitalization of the patient, alteration of antimicrobial therapy, and prophylaxis of the patient's family members and close contacts may hinge on laboratory findings.

Several categories of CNS infection exist, including meningitis, abscess, and encephalitis. Bacteria cause meningitis and nearly all forms of CNS abscesses. Viruses also cause meningitis and are responsible for most cases of encephalitis. Occasional CNS infections are fungal (coccidioidomycosis, *Cryptococcus* meningitis) or parasitic in origin (toxoplasmosis cerebritis, amebic brain abscess). In most cases, serious infection is limited to the CNS, although some, such as Lyme disease, neurosyphilis, or acquired immunodeficiency syndrome (AIDS), are manifestations of a disseminated infectious process.

Bacteria and fungi enter the CNS through several routes: (1) from a distant infectious site by breaching of the barriers between the bloodstream and the CNS, and (2) from a neighboring infectious focus, by means of (a) direct extension through the barriers protecting the CNS (traumatic fracture, osteomyelitis), (b) along normal anatomic pathways (perineural lymphatics of olfactory nerve), or (c) along anatomic defects in skull or spinal column (defect in cribriform plate).

BASIC TESTS

Test: Cerebrospinal Fluid

Background

The human brain and spinal cord are surrounded by three membranous layers (meninges): the pia mater, the arachnoid, and the dura mater. The pia mater is immediately adjacent to the brain and spinal cord. The area between the pia mater and the arachnoid membranes is termed the subarachnoid space and is filled with cerebrospinal fluid (CSF). Cerebrospinal fluid is manufactured by the choroid plexus in the center of the brain and is stored in the ventricles, from which it is distributed to the cisterna magna and subarachnoid space. The subdural space is located between the arachnoid and the dura mater, and the epidural space is found between the dura mater and the skull. Leptomeningitis is an infection of the CSF and of the membranes lining the subarachnoid space. The etiologic diagnosis of these infections are primarily determined by examining a CSF specimen.

Bacterial and Fungal Infections[2,3]

Acute bacterial meningitis is predominantly a disease of childhood, with *Haemophilus influenzae, Streptococcus pneumoniae,* and *Neisseria meningitidis* (in order of prevalence) serving as the leading causes of infection. Meningitis in children younger than 6 months of age is caused by the same bacteria, as well as other agents (group B *streptococcus, Escherichia coli, Citrobacter diversus,* or *Listeria monocytogenes*), which are acquired from the mother at birth. *Neisseria meningitidis* is the most frequent pathogen in patients aged 6–60 years. It may occur in epidemics (serogroups A and C) or sporadically (serogroups B and Y). Infection can be rapidly fatal and is frequently accompanied by petechiae and shock. *Streptococcus pneumoniae* and *L. monocytogenes* prevail in the elderly population, with the latter pathogen an important cause of CNS infection in the immunosuppressed, particularly renal transplant patients.

Neisseria meningitidis colonizes the respiratory tract, enters the bloodstream, and reaches the CNS by hematogenous spread. *Streptococcus pneumoniae* infection of the CSF is more often a secondary complication from involvement at another site (ears, sinuses, or lower respiratory tract). Initial symptoms of bacterial meningitis may include fever, headache, neck stiffness, vomiting, nausea, and an altered state of consciousness. A peripheral blood leukocytosis is common. These findings may be absent in the elderly, and infection in a young infant may be suspected only from a bulging fontanelle. The patient's course may proceed rapidly to lethargy, ataxia, seizures, stupor, paralysis, and coma. Without treatment, death often ensues. Residual deficits are common and include hearing loss, seizure disorders, or hemiparesis.

Chronic meningitis is a rare infection in which patients manifest symptoms and abnormal CSF findings for at least 4 weeks.[4] Causative agents include *Brucella* spp., *Mycobacterium tuberculosis,* and *Treponema pallidum, Cryptococcus neoformans, Coccidioides immitis,* and rarely, *Histoplasma capsulatum* or *Candida* spp. Chronic meningitis also may occur from an incompletely treated bacterial infection. Patients usually present with a low grade fever, malaise, and mild headache, but neck stiffness is typically absent during the early stages of disease. Symptoms become progressively worse. The initial presentation may be seizures, somnolence, or change in behavior. Cranial nerve palsies are common, for example, occurring in about 25% of tuberculous meningitis.

Recurrent meningitis, in which patients experience multiple bouts of infection because of structural abnormalities (e.g., CSF leak, dermal sinus), is usually caused by *S. pneumoniae* or members of the Enterobacteriaceae family. The clinical findings may be subtle; early detection requires a high degree of suspicion (usually from history of trauma) and the willingness to obtain a CSF sample to evaluate the patient.

Nosocomial meningitis and/or ventriculitis is an important complication of neurosurgery. In particular, placement of ventricular shunts to relieve intracranial pressure in patients with hydrocephalus leads to infection in 10–30% of cases. The main causes of infection are cutaneous and enteric flora, with coagulase negative staphylococci, *S. aureus, Corynebacterium* spp. (diphtheroids), *Propionibacterium acnes,* and *Candida* spp.

Viral Infection[5,6]

A variety of disease conditions and postinfection syndromes are associated with viral infection of the central and peripheral nervous systems (Tables 27-1 to 27-3). These include encephalitis and encephalopathies, meningitis, meningoencephalitis, paralysis, paraparesis, neuritis, and mental disorders. Encephalitis is the most devastating type of viral infection and is often associated with high morbidity in the form of permanent neurologic deficits. Clinical manifestations may initially appear similar to bacterial meningitis, but neurologic symptoms become progressively worse, and there is no response to antibiotics. Infection can be fatal; for those who survive, the outcome may be mental retardation, paralysis, loss of sight and/or hearing, or epilepsy.

Viral meningitis is often referred to as *aseptic meningitis,* because of the failure to recover a bacterium. This infection is relatively mild by comparison with encephalitis. Symptoms include fever, headache, nausea, and vomiting, with occasional alterations in consciousness. Disease is generally self-limiting with full recovery.

Viral meningoencephalitis affects both the meninges and the brain, although it is generally associated with more limited brain involvement than is encephalitis.

Table 27-1. Viral Diseases of the Nervous System

Disease Entity	Cause
Encephalitis/encephalopathies	Many viruses (see Table 27-2)
Meningitis	Enteroviruses, HSV, lymphocytic choriomeningitis virus, mumps
Paralysis	Poliovirus, enterovirus 70 and 71, coxsackievirus A7
Postinfectious syndrome	Several viruses (see Table 27-3)
Progressive multifocal leukoencephalopathy (PML)	JC polyomavirus
Spongiform encephalopathy Creutzfeldt-Jakob disease, kuru	Unconventional virus (prion)
Tropical spastic paraparesis	HTLV-I

Abbreviations: HSV, herpes simplex virus; HTLV, human T-lymphotropic virus, type I.

Fatalities are also less common. Damage to motor neurons is one of the most frequent complications that can persist or eventually cause death from the development of cardiopulmonary insufficiency. However, patients typically have partial or complete recovery from paralysis.

A large diversity of viruses infect the CNS (Tables 27-1 to 27-3). Adenoviruses cause meningoencephalitis in infants and in immunocompromised persons and can be fatal. Adenoviruses 7, 34, and 35 have most commonly been implicated in these infections. Less frequently, cytomegalovirus (CMV), Epstein-Barr virus (EBV), and varicella-zoster virus (VZV) cause meningoencephalitis in this category of patients.

Arenaviruses include four agents that infect humans. Only lymphocytic choriomeningitis (LCM) virus is widespread in Europe and North America. Spread occurs through contact with infected wild or laboratory mice. Lymphocytic choriomeningitis virus infection of the CNS may result in a meningitis or, more rarely, meningoencephalitis, which is a more serious infection. Lassa virus is endemic to West Africa and causes lassa fever, which can result in encephalopathy, in severe cases. Fatalities occur in about 2% of all cases, but 20% of infections for which hospitalization is required result in deaths. In the West, the only known cases have resulted from laboratory transmission. Junin and Machupo viruses produce occasional outbreaks of hemorrhagic fever in Argentina and Bolivia, respectively. Although encephalitis may occur in these patients, the predominant symptom is hemorrhage.

Bunyaviruses are found in Asia, Africa, and the United States. In the United States, the California group of encephalitis viruses is responsible for a relatively mild encephalitis transmitted to humans by *Aedes* mosquitoes. Most cases caused by California encephalitis viruses are caused by LaCrosse virus and occur in children and forestry works. Rift Valley fever is a disease of animals in East and South Africa that results in periodic epizootic outbreaks. This virus causes a mild encephalitis that usually resolves without sequelae. Crimean-Congo hemorrhagic fever is seen in Central Asia and Zaire; the disease presents as an encephalitis and may progress to a hemorrhagic fever. Case fatality rates are 5–50%, depending on the ability of available medical care to support shock resulting from hemorrhage.

Enteroviruses are a leading cause of CNS viral infection. The most notable members of the group are the polioviruses, which produce poliomyelitis, the name of which reflects the CNS involvement associated with the disease. Fortunately, effective vaccines against the three poliovirus serotypes have drastically reduced the number of infections and the accompanying CNS infection. The paralytic disease occurred in approximately 1% of poliovirus infections, often resulting in bulbar poliomyelitis, with death resulting from respiratory or cardiac failure.

More commonly, aseptic meningitis results from infection with other enteroviruses. This virus group is the most common cause of meningitis but, in comparison with bacterial meningitis, the patient usually recovers fully without therapy. The more common strains isolated from cases of meningitis include echoviruses 3, 4, 6, 9, 11, 14, 16, 18, 19, 30, 33; coxsackieviruses A7, 9, and B 1–6; enterovirus 71; and polioviruses 1–3 (in developing countries). Neurologic complications after infection with some of these viruses may result. Coxsackievirus A7 has, on rare occasion, been implicated in paralysis. Enterovirus 71 outbreaks have resulted in encephalitis, paralysis, and, in some cases, death. In a pandemic caused by enterovirus 70, some patients exhibited a radiculomyelitis that resulted in acute, flaccid lower motor neuron paralysis similar to polio, which was usually reversible.

Neurologic disease caused by CMV, EBV, and VZV infections is most frequently seen in immunocompromised persons and neonates. Cytomegalovirus infec-

Table 27-2. Viruses That Cause Encephalitis

Virus	Geographic Distribution
Adenoviruses	Worldwide
Arenaviruses	
Junin	Argentina
Lassa fever	Africa
Machupo	Bolivia
Bunyaviruses	
California group	
Encephalitis viruses	United States
LaCrosse	United States
Congo-Crimean hemorrhagic fever	Africa, Asia
Rift Valley fever	Africa
Enteroviruses	
Enterovirus 71	Worldwide
Herpesviruses	
B virus	Africa
Herpes simplex virus (HSV)	Worldwide
Cytomegalovirus (CMV)	Worldwide
Epstein-Barr virus (EBV)	Worldwide
Varicella-zoster virus (VZV)	Worldwide
Human T-lymphotropic viruses	
HTLV-I	Tropics
Human immunodeficiency virus (HIV)	Worldwide
Paramyxoviruses	
Mumps	Worldwide
Reoviruses	
Colorado tick fever	Western United States
Rhabdoviruses	
Rabies virus	Worldwide
Togaviruses	
Alphaviruses	
Eastern equine encephalitis (EEE)	Americas
Western equine encephalitis (WEE)	Americas
Venezuelan equine encephalitis (VEE)	Americas
Flaviviruses	
Japanese B encephalitis	East and Southeast Asia
Kyasanur Forest disease	India
Louping ill	Britain
Murray Valley encephalitis	Australia, New Guinea
Omsk hemorrhagic fever	Russia
Powassan	North America, Russia
Rocio	Brazil
St. Louis encephalitis	Americas
Tick-borne encephalitis	
Central European	Europe
Russian Spring Summer encephalitis	Europe, USSR
West Nile fever	Africa, Europe, Middle East
Unconventional viruses	
Creutzfeldt-Jakob (rare)	Americas

Table 27-3. Postinfectious Viral Syndromes of the Nervous System

Syndrome	Associated Viral Agent
Guillain-Barré syndrome (idiopathic polyneuritis)	Influenza (and vaccine), cytomegalovirus, Epstein-Barr virus, others rare
Panencephalitis	
Subacute sclerosing panencephalitis (SSPE)	Measles
Progressive rubella panencephalitis	Rubella
Postinfectious encephalomyelitis	Measles, rubella, vaccinia, varicella, others rare
Reye syndrome	Influenza, varicella

tion occurs in 1 of 200 births, with 1 in 10 of those infected developing cytoplasmic inclusion disease (CID). The latter frequently produces encephalitis and microcephaly, which may lead to mental retardation, cerebral palsy, and/or sensory deficits. Encephalitis occurs in about 1 of 1000 cases of varicella, often with severe morbidity and a relatively high mortality. As with CMV and EBV, VZV may result in Guillain-Barré syndrome (GBS), an acute inflammatory demyelinating polyradiculoneuropathy. Varicella infection, in addition to influenza, has been associated with the development of Reye syndrome, most often in patients receiving antipyretic salicylates. This sequela usually occurs within 1–4 weeks postinfection in adolescents, resulting in encephalopathy and fatty degeneration of the liver. The fatality rate is approximately 25%.

Herpes simplex virus (HSV) is the most common viral cause of encephalitis, although this is an infrequent complication of primary HSV infection. Before effective chemotherapy was introduced, it was a devastating illness with up to 70% mortality and severe sequelae in 25–50% of those who survived. With the development of a number of antiherpetic drugs, morbidity and mortality have been substantially reduced. Infection is most commonly due to HSV type 1 (HSV-1), except in neonates, in whom HSV type 2 (HSV-2), acquired at birth, predominates. The virus, spread to the brain during either primary or recurrent infection, is generally limited to the temporal lobes.

Influenza viruses are not associated with CNS infection during acute infection, although they are the cause of two postinfection syndromes. Guillain-Barré syndrome has been reported after influenza infection and was seen in 1 in 100,000 patients given the swine flu vaccine in 1976. No other incidents of GBS are recognized from previous or subsequent influenza vaccinations. Reye syndrome is a more severe consequence associated with a prior influenza virus infection, influenza B more commonly than influenza A. Because of the late onset of symptoms, virus is not generally recovered in these cases, and diagnosis rests on clinical history and serologic evidence of a recent infection.

Mumps and rubeola (measles) are the only viruses in the paramyxovirus group that are associated with CNS disease. Rubeola may rarely cause a postinfectious panencephalitis years after acute infection. Meningitis may occur in 10% of mumps infections. Before the development of a vaccine, this virus was the most common cause of aseptic meningitis. The infection usually resolves without sequelae. Less frequently, mumps virus infection produces an encephalitis that may have more severe consequences. Rare complications include chronic mumps encephalomyelitis and unilateral nerve deafness.

Encephalomyelitis arises in about 1 in 1000 measles infections. About 15% of those developing this CNS complication die. The introduction of an effective measles vaccine in developed countries has made this an extremely rare complication. Subacute sclerosing panencephalitis (SSPE) is a sequela of acute measles infection that usually occurs in children infected before 2 years of age, typically occurring 4–13 years after the primary infection. Again, because of an effective vaccine, SSPE has become rare.

Progressive multifocal leukoencephalopathy (PML) is a rare disease caused by JC virus, a papovavirus. Infection occurs only in immunocompromised persons. Progressive multifocal leukoencephalopathy is characterized by demyelination of neurons and proliferation of abnormally large astrocytes. Patients exhibit loss of mental acuity and motor function, with disease progressing to death in all cases.

Rabies is one of the most feared CNS infections that follows an animal bite, usually from a dog. Disease occurs in only a few bite cases and, until recently, was believed to be universally fatal. However, extensive supportive therapy has resulted in full recovery in a few cases. The virus travels from the wound to the CNS by means of a nerve, primarily infecting the neurons of the limbic system and cerebellum.

Colorado tick fever (CTF) virus is transmitted by the wood tick, *Dermacentor andersoni*. Infection is usually limited to persons who have a recent history of camping in the western United States. Colorado tick fever has a sudden onset, 3–6 days after infection. Encephalitis does occur, but infection is usually mild and resolves within a few days.

Both alphaviruses and flaviviruses (of the Togavirus family) can cause encephalitis. The most notable of these are the equine encephalitides and St. Louis encephalitis. The other togaviruses are not usually seen in the United States. Encephalitis caused by this group has a case fatality rate of 10–20%, with greater morbidity and mortality associated with Eastern equine encephalitis virus.

Creutzfeldt-Jakob disease and kuru in New Guinea are the result of infection by a transmissible agent that does not have the form of a classic virus. These have been classified as unconventional or slow viruses and more recently have been termed *prions*, because they are reported to contain protein without detectable nucleic acid. These diseases are characterized by an insidious onset and progressive neurologic symptoms, with the development of a spongiform encephalopathy.

Human T-lymphotropic viruses are a recently discovered cause of neurologic infections. Human T-lymphotropic virus type I (HTLV-I) is implicated in tropical spastic paraparesis. Involvement of the human immunodeficiency virus (HIV), the etiologic agent of AIDS, in neurologic disease occurs at two levels. The first is encephalopathy caused by HIV, per se. The second is caused by opportunistic infection with other microorganisms resulting from HIV depression of immunity. Human immunodeficiency virus-induced encephalopathy is not associated with mass lesions in the brain. The infection is most often noted as a result of behavioral changes in the patient, commonly seen as a form of dementia. It is estimated that more than 60% of patients with AIDS exhibit these symptoms.

Parasitic Infection[7,8]

Invasion of the CNS may be caused by parasitic organisms either as a primary event or as part of a systemic infection. *Toxoplasma gondii* is a coccidian parasite found worldwide that completes its life cycle only in the intestinal mucosa of members of the cat family. Many warm-blooded vertebrates are susceptible to infection by parasites in asexual stages. Humans become infected after exposure to the infective oocysts in cat feces, through ingestion of undercooked meats, by placental transfer, and through organ transplantation or blood transfusions. After primary exposure, immunocompetent hosts are usually asymptomatic or may suffer from mild flu-like symptoms and transient lymphadenopathy. The large number of persons with antibodies to *Toxoplasma* suggests that this is a common infection. Persons at risk of the development of acute toxoplasmosis include (1) seronegative transplant recipients who receive organs from seropositive donor; (2) seronegative patients who are immunosuppressed and exposed to the organism by any of the mechanisms described above; (3) seropositive patients who are at risk of reactivation, if immunosuppressed; and (4) neonates infected in utero. When immunocompromised hosts are exposed to the organism acutely or by reactivation of latent infection, serious systemic disease may result, including encephalitis, myocarditis, or pneumonitis. Transplacental infection is a serious event that may result in congenital ocular or CNS disease, spontaneous abortion, or stillbirth.

Free-living water and soil amebae of the general *Naegleria* and *Acanthamoeba* may be responsible for the CNS infections referred to as primary amebic meningoencephalitis (PAM) and granulomatous amebic encephalitis (GAE), respectively. The infections differ significantly in the progression of clinical disease and epidemiology. Primary amebic meningoencephalitis is a fulminant, suppurative infection that cannot usually be differentiated from pyogenic meningitis clinically. The disease is often associated with exposure to contaminated water through swimming or bathing activities and is thought to be transmitted through the olfactory neuroepithelium. Most cases have been described in previously healthy children and young adults. Granulomatous amebic encephalitis usually presents as a more chronic or indolent brain infection. It is thought to enter through traumatized skin, corneal epithelium, or perhaps the lungs. Presenting symptoms include the gradual onset of altered mental status, with progression to diplopia, seizures, hemiparesis, coma, and death. Many affected people have a preexisting disease, such as diabetes, or are immunocompromised. There is usually no previous history of bathing or swimming exposure.

African sleeping sickness caused by *T. b. gambiense* and *T. b. rhodesiense* is similar, except that the Gambian form of the disease has a prolonged, chronic course, whereas the Rhodesian infection causes a more fulminant, acute course that is usually fatal within weeks to months. After multiplying at the site of a tsetse fly bite, trypanosomes disseminate through the lymphatics to lymph nodes and the bloodstream, causing systemic symptoms. A variety of systemic symptoms appear with African trypanosomiasis before invasion of the CNS occurs and include fever, cervical lymphadenopathy (Winterbottom sign), decreased pain sensation, and skin rash. Because of the rapidity with which Rhodesian sleeping sickness progresses, death may occur before the development of meningoencephalitis. (See Ch. 20, Blood and Bone Marrow.)

Angiostrongyliasis or parasitic eosinophilic meningitis is caused by the meningeal inhabiting nematode *Angiostrongylus cantonensis*. In the definitive rat host, the helminths mature in the meninges and subsequently migrate to the lungs, where oviposition takes place. The eggs hatch, and larvae are then expelled through the digestive tract in the feces. The larvae are ingested by intermediate hosts, including land snails and slugs, molting to the infective stage. Human infections are usually acquired from the accidental or intentional ingestion of snails or slugs containing infective larvae. The severity of human disease is dose related, and most cases are probably subclinical, although deaths have been reported. Symptoms are related to the damage caused by the migratory activities of developing larvae in the CNS. Although therapy is mostly supportive and symptomatic, anthelminthic therapy may be beneficial when started early.

Cerebral malaria is one of the life-threatening complications of *P. falciparum* infection. Parasites of this species are able to infect erythrocytes of all ages, resulting in parasitemias that may involve more than 50% of the red blood cells. Other malarial species rarely infect more than 5% of red blood cells. Organ damage that occurs with falciparum malaria is a result of the sticking of infected erythrocytes to capillary endothelium, with subsequent infarction and tissue necrosis. Because of the high morbidity and mortality associated with falciparum malaria, the disease should be treated as a medical emergency. (See Ch. 20.)

Selection[9]

Routine Tests

Laboratory diagnosis of meningitis is best accomplished by direct CSF examination. If the results of the patient's history and physical examination warrant a lumbar puncture, enough fluid should be obtained to perform the following tests: (1) CSF cell and differential count; (2) CSF protein, glucose, and lactate; (3) CSF Gram stain or acridine orange (AO) smear; and (4) CSF culture. Routine ordering of additional CSF tests (e.g., acid-fast smear, India ink preparation, microbial antigen detection, *Limulus* lysate test, lactate level, C-reactive protein level) should be discouraged, because the results benefit the average patient very little, yet add significantly to the patient's laboratory bill.

Tests for Bacterial and Fungal Infections

Blood culture is indicated when bacterial infection is suspected.

Manufacturers of commercially available antigen detection kits promote their products as essential for the rapid diagnosis of meningitis. What they neglect to mention is the lack of clinical impact of test results in most situations. By the time testing is completed, meningitic patients should already be receiving broad spectrum empirical antimicrobial therapy. A negative test result does not rule out bacterial meningitis, because the test is far from 100% sensitive. A positive test result confirms the diagnosis, but adjustment of antimicrobial therapy for patients with *H. influenzae* or *S. pneumoniae* infection must await results of antimicrobial susceptibility testing of the culture isolate many hours later. In short, there are only a limited number of situations in which bacterial antigen detection results affect the course of patient management. Bacterial antigen detection tests of CSF provide relevant information and are indicated in the following situations:

1. *Partial treatment with antimicrobial agents before an etiologic diagnosis has been made:* Since the CSF Gram stain and culture from such a patient are likely to be negative, a positive antigen detection result may be the only indication of the cause of infection. Such information can be used for decision-making regarding prophylaxis of the patient's family and close contacts.
2. *Borderline age between the neonatal period and infancy (approximately 2 months of age):* A positive result dictates selection between choices of empirical antimicrobial therapy for neonatal or childhood meningitis.
3. *Compelling evidence of meningitis with a negative CSF Gram stain and other household members younger than 6 years of age not immunized against H. influenzae type b:* The antigen detection results can govern decision making regarding prophylaxis of the patient's family unit.

4. *Clinical evidence of meningococcal infection with a negative CSF Gram stain:* A positive *N. meningitidis* antigen detection result documents the need for prophylaxis of the patient's close contacts.

The tuberculin skin test should be done when *M. tuberculosis* meningitis is considered. Culture of the CSF for mycobacteria should always be done in suspected cases of tuberculous meningitis. However the predictive value of doing acid-fast smears from CSF is so poor that the wisdom of even doing the test should be questioned. CSF chloride is of no value for tuberculous meningitis.

By contrast, the results of the cryptococcal antigen test are universally useful. The test is both highly sensitive and specific. Furthermore, CSF antigen titers can be monitored over time in positive patients to assess the clinical response to the selected antifungal therapy. The cryptococcal antigen detection test is a very useful diagnostic tool and a great deal more sensitive than the India ink preparation. The test should be ordered on CSF specimens collected from all patients manifesting symptoms consistent with *C. neoformans* meningitis.

Tests for Suspected Viral Infections

Cerebrospinal fluid is the specimen most commonly submitted for virus isolation in suspected cases of *aseptic meningitis*[10] (Table 27-4); however, CSF does not yield virus at a high rate. The estimated positivity rate is only 4%, although in some studies, up to 80% of CSF specimens examined for *Enterovirus* were positive. Nonpolio enteroviruses and mumps virus are the most common isolates from CSF. In most cases of enteroviral meningitis, the agent is more readily isolated from stool. Likewise, although mumps virus also can be recovered from CSF during meningitis, it is more readily detected in the throat (Table 27-5). Herpes simplex virus type 2 is occasionally detected in the CSF during bouts of meningitis. Less frequently, adenoviruses, CMV, and VZV have been isolated from CSF obtained

Table 27-4. Viruses That May Be Isolated from Cerebrospinal Fluid

Arenavirus[a] (rarely encountered)
Bunyavirus (isolation not commonly performed)
Enteroviruses
Herpesviruses (HSV-2, HSV-1, CMV, EBV rarely)
Human immunodeficiency virus
Paramyxoviruses
Mumps
Togaviruses (virus present but rarely isolated)

[a] Should only be attempted by an experienced reference laboratory under P3 or P4 conditions.
Abbreviations: HSV-1, -2, herpes simplex virus types 1 and 2; CMV, cytomegalovirus; EBV, Esptein-Barr virus

from immunocompromised patients. Other viruses, including the alphaviruses and flaviviruses, can also be isolated from CSF but represent a small percentage of cases annually in the United States. However, because of the risk to laboratory workers, arboviruses isolation should only be attempted in specially equipped laboratories.

It is rare to isolate a virus from the CSF of patients with encephalitis. Diagnostic confirmation of the etiologic agent usually depends on serology by monitoring for a rise in antibody titer to a particular virus. Serodiagnosis should be considered for echovirus, coxsackievirus, polio-virus, mumps, HSV and arbovirus infections. A history of travel to an endemic area is an indication for consideration of serologic testing for specific arboviruses. In the absence of the isolation of a virus, useful information can be obtained from CSF by examination for antiviral antibodies. A presumptive diagnosis is made by the finding of a disproportionately high antiviral antibody titer in CSF relative to serum.

The recovery rate of HSV from CSF is higher in cases of meningitis compared to encephalitis. Because it is possible to intervene in HSV encephalitis with acyclovir or adenine arabinoside (ara-A) and clinical distinction

Table 27-5. Appropriate Specimens to Test for Laboratory Diagnosis of Viral Central Nervous System Infections

Agent	Throat	Stool	CSF	Urine	Other
Enterovirus (coxsackie, echo, polio)	++	+++	+	−	Autopsy tissue
Mumps virus	+++	−	++	+/−	
Herpes simplex virus	+/−	−	+/−	−	Brain biopsy
Arboviruses	−	−	+/−	−	Blood (low yield), autopsy tissue

Abbreviation: CSF, cerebrospinal fluid.

Table 27-6. Viruses Isolated from, or Identified in, Brain Tissue

Viruses
    Enteroviruses
    Herpesviruses (HSV, EBV, CMV)
    Paramyxoviruses
    Rhabdoviruses
    Papovavirus
        JC virus
    Togaviruses
        Alphaviruses
        Flaviviruses
    Human T-lymphotropic virus
        HTLV-I
        HIV
    Arenaviruses
        LCM
Unconventional viruses (prions?)
    Creutzfeldt-Jakob disease (worldwide)
    Kuru (New Guinea)

Abbreviations: HSV, herpes simplex virus; EBV, Epstein-Barr virus; CMV, cytomegalovirus; HTLV-I, human T-lymphotropic virus; HIV, human immunodeficiency virus; LCM, lymphocytic choriomeningitis.

from other infections is not apparent, biopsy of the temporal lobe can be performed to obtain an appropriate specimen for isolation of the virus. A punch biopsy of the temporal lobe is performed. Because infection can form discrete foci that are often missed on biopsy, there is the potential for great variability in successful isolation of virus. Thus, isolation of virus from alternate sites, most commonly the oropharynx, should be attempted. Brain tissue may also be used for virus isolation (Table 27-6). This tissue is most frequently obtained at autopsy, although biopsy specimens are used for the diagnosis of acute encephalitis. Isolation of CMV, EBV, or VZV from the CSF is quite rare and should not be attempted unless this rare form of encephalomyelitis is suspected in the immunocompromised host and there is failure to obtain virus from other sources to establish an etiology of infection.

Laboratory diagnosis of rabies should only be performed by experienced reference laboratory personnel. The usual specimen used for rabies diagnosis is the brain of the animal that inflicted the bite. Finding cytoplasmic inclusion in neurons (Negri bodies) is diagnostic. Corneal impression smears collected from the patient either pre- or postmortem can be examined, and serologic testing should be considered (see Ch. 29).

The diagnosis of Creutzfeldt-Jakob disease or kuru infection is based on clinical symptoms and brain pathology.

Although HIV can be isolated from the CSF or brain tissue, the cause of AIDS encephalopathy is inferred in patients with appropriate clinical and serologic findings. Serologic testing for HTLV-I is indicated in patients with suspected tropical spastic paraparesis.

The diagnosis of CNS parasitic infections often relies on direct specimen examination and/or serologic studies. Those parasitic organisms most commonly causing disease of the CNS are summarized in Table 27-7.

Tests for Suspected Parasitic Infections

Toxoplasma encephalitis is suspected when local neurologic deficits are present and multiple enhancing lesions are seen on computed tomography (CT) scan in the immunocompromised host. Initial symptoms may include headache, altered mental status, and seizures. Patients with AIDS are at particular risk, especially if preexisting antibody titers suggest latent infection. When these manifestations are present, specific IgM and IgG serologies should be requested. When avail-

Table 27-7. Parasitic Disease Entities Occurring Within the Central Nervous System

Disease	Responsible Organism(s)
Abscess	*Entamoeba histolytica*
Encephalitis	*Toxoplasma gondii*
Meningoencephalitis	*Naegleria fowleri*
	Acanthamoeba spp.
	Trypanosoma brucei rhodesiense
	T. b. gambiense
	Angiostrongylus cantonensis
Cerebral malaria	*Plasmodium falciparum*
Mass lesions	*Echinococcus granulosus* (hydatidosis)
	Taenia solium (cysticercosis)

able, specimens taken 2–4 weeks apart should be tested simultaneously to detect changes in titers. Occasionally, specimens from certain patients (e.g., those with AIDS) remain nonreactive or weakly reactive in serologic tests despite acute infection. In such patients, for whom serologies are nondiagnostic but clinical suspicion is high, biopsies may be considered.

Diagnosis of primary amebic meningoencephalitis and granulomatous amebic encephalitis is made by demonstrating and/or culturing amebae from CSF or other clinical sources. Histologic examination of tissues and use of immunofluorescence staining also may help.

The onset of severe headaches and other neurologic signs in Gambian trypanosomiasis signals invasion of the CNS, which occurs late in the infection and is usually a poor prognostic indicator. Diagnosis is made upon examination of blood, CSF, and lymph node aspirates for trypomastigotes. The parasitemia in Gambian trypanosomiasis may be undetectable, and serologic studies may be necessary for confirmation of suspected cases.[7,8]

Infection with the meningeal worm *Angiostrongylus cantonensis* usually presents with severe headache and other symptoms, including neck stiffness, fever, and paresthesias. Travel and food histories should be taken into consideration, as the helminth is primarily found in the Pacific region and the Far East and is associated with the ingestion of snails and slugs. Blood and CSF should be examined for eosinophilia; occasionally, a larval worm will be observed in the CSF. Serologic tests may be helpful if available.

The signs and symptoms of cerebral malaria (disorientation, severe headaches, convulsions, coma) usually appear after the onset of the primary malaria attack. The diagnosis is made on clinical grounds. *Plasmodium falciparum* is the species most commonly responsible for this condition. Infection with any of the malarial species, however, may cause symptoms of meningoencephalitis. In most cases, the initial diagnosis will have already been made using the techniques described elsewhere. Serologic studies are available but are used chiefly for epidemiologic purposes.

Logistics

Specimen Requirements

Collection of CSF should be performed using aseptic technique, either by lumbar puncture or, in patients with neurosurgical shunt infections, by aspiration from a Ommaya (or similar) reservoir. When lumbar puncture CSF fails to yield diagnostic information and there is lack of clinical response to empirical antimicrobial therapy, removal of CSF from the cisterna magna (cisternal puncture) should be considered.

Cerebrospinal fluid should be placed in three separate sterile, leakproof tubes for the hematology, chemistry, and microbiology sections of the clinical laboratory. At least 1 mL of CSF should be collected in each tube. A fourth tube may be collected if any additional CSF tests are needed. When mycobacterial or fungal meningitis is likely, 5–10 mL of CSF should be submitted to the microbiology laboratory for analysis. Examination of a high volume of spinal fluid (5–10 mL) is recommended for detecting acid-fast bacilli microscopically; multiple samples are sometimes required to obtain a positive result. Less volume (1 mL) is sufficient for bacterial culture, virus isolation, and serologic or antigen studies. Cerebrospinal fluid has the highest probability of containing infectious virus if collected within 2–3 days of the onset of illness, before CSF pleocytosis occurs. Bacterial cultures should be obtained before antimicrobial therapy, if possible.

Rules as to which laboratory should receive which tube are often a concern. In general, when the tap is traumatic, the first tube should not go to the hematology or chemistry sections, because peripheral blood contamination of CSF markedly affects the cell/differential count and the glucose/protein levels. When the tap is not traumatic, the first tube should not go to the microbiology laboratory for culture, because the initial fluid is most likely to be contaminated with cutaneous flora.

When more than 1 mL of CSF is submitted for Gram/AO stain and culture, the specimen should be centrifuged at 1500g for 15 minutes. After centrifugation, the sediment should be resuspended in 200 μL of supernatant and used to prepare smears, wet mounts, and to inoculate cultures. The remainder of the supernatant should be saved for additional tests. When 1 mL or less of CSF is received, the advantages afforded by centrifugation are too small to risk tube breakage in the centrifuge.

Analysis

Microscopy

Microscopic examination of CSF in the microbiology laboratory is rapid, inexpensive, and very informative. Every specimen should be examined by Gram stain.

Smears of CSF or its sediment should be prepared on glass microscope slides and allowed to air dry. The use of a cytocentrifuge for preparation of CSF smears for Gram/AO staining is appropriate. Alternatively, the addition of more drops of CSF to previously dried drops increases the sensitivity of the Gram stain examination. The smears should be heat- or methanol-fixed and then stained. The standard Gram staining procedure should be followed. Smears are examined under oil immersion magnification (1000×). The focal plane of a smear can be difficult to find when a specimen lacks inflammatory cells. Focusing the microscope on a wax pencil mark on the slide surface next to the smear facilitates the examination.

Acridine orange stain offers the advantage of higher contrast between stained organisms and background material. This stain is of greatest value in aiding detection of *H. influenzae* and other gram-negative bacteria in specimens containing high concentrations of protein. Protein strands and fibrils appear gram negative, making recognition of bacteria very difficult. Acridine orange smears should be prepared in the same manner as Gram stain smears. Smears should be methanol-fixed for 1 minute and then stained with AO solution for 1 minute. Smears are examined with a microscope equipped for ultraviolet (UV) illumination. Microorganisms appear bright orange against a greenish black background. Positive AO smears should be Gram stained to discern the gram reaction of the microorganisms present.

Smears examined for mycobacteria should be prepared from CSF sediment, heat-fixed and stained by the standard auramine-rhodamine (fluorochrome) method. As an alternative, smears may be stained directly with Ziehl-Neelsen or Kinyoun reagents, but specimens prepared with these staining methods take longer to examine and may be less sensitive than the fluorochrome method. However, a microscope equipped for UV illumination is not needed. Mycobacteria in specimens stained with the fluorochrome method are identified as golden yellow bacilli against a black background. The mechanical stage coordinates of organisms on a positive fluorochrome smear should be recorded so that the smear can be restained with Ziehl-Neelsen or Kinyoun reagents and the organisms confirmed as acid-fast bacilli. Ziehl-Neelsen or Kinyoun-stained positive smears should display red organisms against a blue or green background, depending on the counterstain used.

The India ink preparation is a negative stain for encapsulated yeasts. The most common application of the test is to examine CSF specimens for *C. neoformans*. Wet mounts are prepared by mixing a small drop of India ink with a large drop of resuspended CSF sediment and applying a coverslip. The wet mount is examined at 450× magnification for yeast cells surrounded by a clear halo. The examiner must be careful not to confuse inflammatory cells with yeast cells, since some inflammatory cells may display the semblance of a narrow halo. The best advice is to search for haloed cells displaying buds. Inflammatory cells never form buds. While examining the India ink preparation, one should also be on the lookout for motile amebae. Occasional cases of amebic meningoencephalitis have been diagnosed by India ink preparation.

Naegleriosis (PAM) can be identified by examining the CSF for motile trophozoites. These forms actively produce round pseudopods in wet preparations. Unfortunately, amebae may be misidentified as unusual white blood cells or macrophages. More commonly, the causative agents of PAM and GAE are diagnosed histologically, often at autopsy. The organisms are relatively easy to culture when placed on non-nutrient agar plates to which a lawn of *E. coli* has been plated. The culture technique is described in Chapter 21.

Examination of Wright- or Giemsa-stained peripheral blood smears, CSF, or lymph node aspirates for the presence of typical trypomastigotes is the usual technique available for the diagnosis of African trypanosomiasis. In addition to thin and thick smears, other concentration techniques, such as centrifugation of blood or CSF, should be used. The number of parasites in the bloodstream may fluctuate widely. Multiple examinations should be performed before the diagnosis is excluded. Organisms are typically most numerous during febrile episodes.

Examination of CSF for trophozoites of *Toxoplasma* can be diagnostic but has poor sensitivity. Histologic diagnosis of *Toxoplasma* in brain tissue may also be confirmatory and has been made more sensitive with the introduction of the immunoperoxidase staining technique. In addition to serologic and histologic methods, tissue culture and animal inoculation of clinical specimens may be used to demonstrate the presence of the organisms.

Angiostrongyliasis is usually not detectable by laboratory means, although a peripheral eosinophilia is often noted, and the CSF may display eosinophilic pleocytosis. Young adult worms are found in the CSF in about 10% of cases. Serologic assays have been described and may be of value in the appropriate clinical setting, if available.

Antigen and Antibody Detection

Immunologic detection of microbial antigens in CSF has been practiced since the early 1970s. The earliest tests used counterimmunoelectrophoresis (CIE), a 45–60 minute procedure that was quite effective but that required specialized equipment. During the late 1970s, 5–10 minute particle agglutination immunoassays were developed that were more sensitive than CIE and did not require special equipment. Today, particle agglutination for antigen detection in CSF and other body fluids is most widely used.

Several particle agglutination bacterial antigen detection immunoassays are commercially available. The assays depend on agglutination of antibody coated microscopic latex particles or coagglutination of antibody coated *S. aureus* cells. Antigens for which detection reagents are available include *H. influenzae*, *S. pneumoniae* (83 different serotypes), *N. meningitidis* (serogroups A, B, C, D, X, Y, Z, and W135), *E. coli* (KI), and group B streptococcus. The assays are performed by mixing small amounts of CSF with antibody coated particles. Some assays call for pretreatment of specimens with heat or sorbent to inactivate or remove interfering substances. The mixture is rotated for a few minutes and examined for macroscopic agglutination. A negative control using a nonspecific IgG antibody coated particle suspension is also tested with each specimen to detect substances in CSF (e.g., rheumatoid factor), which nonspecifically agglutinate antibody coated particles. Agglutination of the test particle suspension coupled with lack of agglutination of the control particle suspension indicates the presence of antigen. If both particle suspensions agglutinate, the test results are not interpretable.

Several commercially available assays for detection of *C. neoformans* antigen are available. The procedure is done by latex particle agglutination. The results are interpreted in the manner described above for bacterial antigens. If the qualitative test for antigen is positive, the specimen should be serially diluted, retested, and reported as a titer (the highest dilution yielding a positive result). When both test and control latex suspensions agglutinate in the presence of CSF, the specimen should be serially diluted and retested with both suspensions. If the agglutination end points for both suspensions are within one dilution of each other, the test results should be reported as "not interpretable." However, if the test latex agglutination end point is two or more dilutions higher than the control latex, the results should be reported as positive for cryptococcal antigen at the indicated titer.

A variety of specific and sensitive serologic tests for the diagnosis of parasitic diseases is described in Chapter 29. Many of these tests are available only from reference laboratories and are not well standardized. However, serologic tests for toxoplasmosis are commercially available, including radioimmunoassay (RIA), enzyme immunoassay (EIA), and fluorometric assays, among others.

Bacterial and Fungal Culture[9]

Almost all bacterial and fungal agents that cause meningitis can be recovered on laboratory media without difficulty. Cerebrospinal fluid sediment for routine bacterial culture should be inoculated to nonselective 5% sheep blood and chocolate agars, as well as to a nonselective enrichment broth (e.g., Fildes broth). Inoculation of selective media (e.g., MacConkey agar) ordinarily is not recommended. Agar media should be incubated at 35°C in an aerobic atmosphere supplemented with 5–10% CO_2 for 48–72 hours. Broth cultures should be incubated at 35°C for 3–7 days.

Cultures for *M. tuberculosis* should be inoculated to Lowenstein-Jensen medium, Middlebrook 7H10 or 7H11 agar, and to 7H9 or Dubos Tween 80 broth. Cultures should be incubated at 35°C in an aerobic atmosphere containing 5–10% CO_2 for 8–12 weeks. Cloudy broth cultures should be acid-fast stained and subcultured to mycobacterial solid media.

The most common fungal cause of meningitis, *C. neoformans*, grows quite well on culture media used for routine bacterial culture. However, because some fungi grow too slowly to form visible colonies during the 48–72 hours that routine bacterial cultures are incubated, additional cultures for fungal pathogens (inoculated to Sabouraud dextrose and brain heart infusion agars) should be set up when indicated. Media containing cycloheximide, which inhibits the growth of *C. neoformans*, should not be used without including a nonselective fungal media. Cultures should be incubated at 25–30°C in an aerobic atmosphere for 21–28 days.

Viral Culture

Viral cultures are performed on CSF, feces, throat, and urine. Appropriate cell lines are used to isolate mumps, enteroviruses, and when indicated, HSV (Table 27-4).

Interpretation

Table 27-8 displays the differential diagnosis using chemical and cellular findings in CSF.

Table 27-8. Differential Diagnosis of CNS Infections

	WBC Count (μL)	Differential PMN (%)	Mono (%)	Protein (mg/dL)	Glucose % of Blood
Bacterial meningitis					
Early	50–1000	>75	<25	50–200	Variable
Late	300–10,000	>95	<5	50–200	<60
Fungal and tuberculous meningitis	50–1000	<50	>50	100–1000	<60
Viral meningitis	0–1000	<50[a]	>50	50–200	>60[b]
Brain abscess	0–200	<50	>50	50–200	>60
Subdural/epidural abscess[c]	0–200	>50	<50	50–200	>60

[a] PMNs may predominate in early infection.
[b] CSF glucose concentration may be low relative to serum in mumps, lymphocytic choriomeningitis, herpes simplex virus, and enterovirus infections.
[c] Lumbar puncture contraindicated.
Abbreviations: CNS, central nervous system; WBC, white blood cell; PMN, polymorphonuclear; Mono, monocyte; CSF, cerebrospinal fluid.

Bacterial and Fungal Infections

Gram and AO stains of CSF smears can be expected to detect organisms in approximately 90% of cases of culture-proven bacterial meningitis. When present, bacteria are usually found in abundant numbers, leaving little doubt in the microscopist's mind that the smear is positive. Occasionally, specimens are encountered in which no organisms can be found, despite the presence of large numbers of segmented neutrophils. In such situations, it is important not to over-read the smear and mistake artifacts for organisms. A false negative report does no harm to the patient already on empirical broad spectrum antimicrobial therapy. A false positive report may induce an inappropriate change in antimicrobial therapy with disastrous consequences. Once the CSF Gram/AO stain examination is completed, the laboratory personnel have the responsibility of immediately notifying the physician of the results.

The most persuasive laboratory evidence of bacterial meningitis is the demonstration of the infecting organisms by culture. Recovery of organisms from CSF culture is always significant from the laboratory's perspective and should be reported promptly to the physician. Undoubtedly, a significant percentage of positive cultures reflect contamination of CSF with cutaneous organisms during specimen collection, but the laboratory is in no position to make that judgment.

Very few organisms are present in the CSF of patients with tuberculous meningitis. Even when 5–10 mL of CSF is collected, centrifuged, and the sediment stained and examined, most culture positive specimens reveal negative acid fast smears. Because the incidence of positive culture results is quite low, patient history, physical examination, and skin test results, should be the basis for diagnosis of tuberculous meningitis.

The India ink preparation detects no more than 50% of culture-proven cases of *C. neoformans* meningitis. Although the sensitivity of the test is low, the specificity is quite high, if the examiner is experienced in distinguishing encapsulated yeasts from inflammatory cells. When the index of suspicion for cryptococcal meningitis is high and the India ink preparation is negative, the latex particle agglutination test for cryptococcal antigen should be ordered. The cryptococcal antigen test is both more sensitive and specific than the India ink preparation. Laboratories sufficiently staffed to perform cryptococcal antigen tests on specimens as they are received should consider whether India ink testing is warranted.

The sensitivity of the particle agglutination assays for detecting bacterial antigens in CSF vary from antigen to antigen. The assays for *H. influenzae* type b and group B streptococcus appear to be the most sensitive (more than 90%), followed by *S. pneumoniae* (~80%) and by *N. meningitidis* and *E. coli* (~60%). All the assays are very specific; cross-reactions with other bacteria are very rare.

Viral Infections

The cerebrospinal fluid is generally clear in viral meningitis and the white blood cell count is usually less than 300 cells/mm, with a predominance of lymphocytes. This is in contrast to bacterial infection in which the CSF is turbid and there is a predominance of poly-

Table 27-9.	Changes in CSF in Viral Infections of the CNS

Possible increased levels of antiviral antibody relative to serum
Clear (not turbid) CSF
WBCs present are predominantly lymphocytes
Glucose normal or near normal (except lymphocytic choriomeningitis virus)
Protein normal to increased

Abbreviations: CSF, cerebrospinal fluid; CNS, central nervous system; WBCs, white blood cells.

morphonuclear neutrophils. In addition, glucose and protein levels tend to be near normal in viral meningitis as compared to bacterial meningitis. In encephalitis, glucose tends to be normal and protein increased. The presence of virus in the CSF or brain tissue is indicative of an etiologic role for that agent in the associated clinical condition in most instances. In this regard, viruses have occasionally been isolated from brain tissue in patients with neurologic disease of unknown etiology (e.g., measles in multiple sclerosis patients). In these instances, it has not yet been possible to establish an etiologic role for the virus. When virus isolation is not possible in CNS infection, it is often possible to determine etiology on the basis of appropriate serologic testing (see Ch. 29).

In most cases, isolation of a virus from CSF or other appropriate site will help guide the physician in patient management and confirm a diagnosis in the absence of isolating bacterial, fungal, or parasitic agents. In most cases, there is little the physician can do to treat the infection. An important exception is HSV infection, as noted earlier. In the absence of the isolation of a virus, other useful information can be obtained from CSF (Table 27-9).

The ratio of viral antibody titers in the CSF and serum is usually 1:300–1:500. In CNS infections, there is often a disproportionate rise in CSF antiviral antibodies. This finding may be indicative of infection with a particular virus, but results must be interpreted with caution. For example, a disproportionate increase in CSF antibodies to measles virus in patients with multiple sclerosis has led to speculation that this virus has an etiologic role in the disease. However, this could also be caused by reactivation of latent virus and be unrelated to etiology (see Ch. 29).

Parasitic Infections

Identification of a parasite in brain tissue (*E. histolytica, Toxoplasma gondii, Taenia solium, Echinococcus*), CSF (trypomastigotes, *Naegleria, Acanthamoeba, Angiostrongylus*), or other sites with associated CNS symptoms provides a definite diagnosis. As with many helminthic diseases, peripheral eosinophilia is often present, and examination of CSF may also demonstrate the presence of eosinophils.

Meningoencephalitis caused by infection with one of the free-living amebae is obvious when the organism is found, but the diagnosis is difficult to make, and often not considered because of the rarity of the conditions. The lack of effective diagnostic and therapeutic modalities when dealing with *Naegleria* or *Acanthamoeba* meningoencephalitis is demonstrated by the high mortality associated with these infections.

The presence of trypomastigotes in the CSF occurs late in African trypanosomiasis infection and is a poor prognostic indicator. Other CSF findings include increased protein, total IgM levels, and lymphocytosis. The presence in CSF of mulberry-shaped plasma cells known as morular cells of Mott, are considered pathognomonic for this disease. Serologic tests must be interpreted cautiously because of poor specificity (see Ch. 29).

The diagnosis of cerebral malaria is made from clinical symptoms and the presence of parasitemia, although the degree of parasitemia does not necessarily correlate with the severity of symptoms. Severe anemia, jaundice, fluid and electrolyte disturbances, hypoglycemia, and renal failure may also be present.

Chapter 29 describes the serologic diagnosis of specific parasitic infections. Only the interpretation of serologic tests for *Toxoplasma* infection is described here. Although the presence of anti-*Toxoplasma* IgG antibodies in a single random serum specimen are not diagnostic of acute infection, the presence of specific IgM antibodies and rising IgG antibodies over several weeks is strongly suggestive of such an infection. Unfortunately, in AIDS patients, acute *Toxoplasma* encephalitis is not always characterized by rising titers; in fact, titers may be low or negative. In such circumstances, strong clinical suspicion often warrants empirical anti-*Toxoplasma* therapy. Congenital infections are documented by finding persistent or rising anti-*Toxoplasma* IgG titers and/or any titer positive for anti-*Toxoplasma* IgM. Definitive diagnosis is made by demonstrating the presence of the organisms in brain tissue or by isolating them in culture. *Toxoplasma* encephalitis rarely occurs in immunocompetent hosts and, when present, suggests previously undiagnosed immunodeficiency syndrome. (Further information on eye specimens is presented in Ch. 21.)

Test: Brain Abscess and Other CNS Specimens

Background

Central nervous system abscesses usually result from spread from an adjacent site of infection. Pressure that mounts during infectious sinusitis, mastoiditis, or otitis media, for example, leads to rupture and spillage of purulent material into the epidural or subdural spaces—or even into the brain itself—resulting in secondary infection.[11] Central nervous system abscesses also occur subsequent to trauma and after infarction caused by hematogenously spread septic emboli.

Epidural, subdural, and brain abscesses are most often caused by upper respiratory bacteria. Microaerophilic streptococci (e.g., *S. intermedius*, *S. constellatus*, *S. milleri*), miscellaneous anaerobes (e.g., *Bacteroides* spp., *Fusobacterium* spp., *Actinomyces* spp.), *Haemophilus aphrophilus,* and members of the Enterobacteriaceae family participate in what are often polymicrobial infections. When abscesses are secondary to head trauma, the leading cause of infection is *S. aureus.* Gram-negative rod meningitis in neonates may progress to brain abscess, especially when *C. diversus* is the etiologic agent.

Parasitic infection may involve the brain, but are uncommon in the United States. Amebic abscess of the brain caused by *E. histolytica* is a rare event. It is usually thought to be hematogenous in origin but often occurs concomitant with the development of liver or lung abscesses. When present, the infection usually occurs in the cerebral hemispheres and is often fulminant. Although most amebic abscesses are bacteriologically sterile, a small percentage are secondarily infected and display a more intense acute inflammatory response.

Hydatid disease, caused by the larval tapeworm of *Echinococcus granulosus,* most commonly involves the liver (50–75%) or the lungs (25%), with a smaller percentage of cysts developing in other organs including the CNS. The definitive hosts include members of the dog family. Human infection results from accidental ingestion of the infectious eggs after exposure to dog feces. The eggs hatch in the intestine and spread to the various organs hematogenously, where they develop slowly over a period of years. Dogs acquire intestinal infection with adult worms from feeding on the offal of domestic animals, usually sheep. Depending on anatomic location, the cysts may remain asymptomatic. The mass effect caused by a growing cerebral cyst may cause focal epileptic seizures and raised intracranial pressure. Rupture or leakage of cyst fluid may also cause acute allergic reactions.

Humans may be infected with either the adult *Taenia solium* tapeworm or the larvae known as cysticerci, or both. The adult tapeworm is acquired from eating incompletely cooked pork containing cysticerci. The eggs shed from gravid proglottids of adult tapeworms in human feces serve as the source of infection for human cysticercosis. The eggs hatch in the intestine and spread hematogenously to many sites. Clinically apparent CNS disease results either from obstruction to CSF flow or, more commonly, from inflammatory reactions to dead or dying worms. The cysts may remain viable for 4–5 years. Management of neurocysticercosis is difficult, because anthelminthic therapy may result in severe inflammatory reactions at the site of dead cysts.

Selection and Interpretation

Focal neurologic deficits are the hallmark of the brain abscess but are present in only about one-half of cases. The patient typically has headache and low grade fever. Seizures may be the initial presenting finding. A probable epidural, subdural, or parenchymal brain abscess constitutes a true medical emergency. First and foremost, it is critical for the examining physician to determine quickly whether the patient's problem is caused by an abscess or by meningitis/encephalitis. Even though obtaining CSF by lumbar puncture would be the first step in evaluating a patient with suspected meningitis/encephalitis, it is contraindicated when an abscess is present, because of the likelihood of herniation.

If the history and physical examination point toward an abscess, the next order of business is to determine its location radiologically. The CT scan is usually the diagnostic procedure of choice. Once pinpointed, the abscess must be surgically drained, both for therapeutic reasons and to obtain specimens for microbiologic testing. Material obtained at the time of neurosurgical removal of the abscess should be submitted to the laboratory for examination. Gram stain, aerobic/anaerobic bacterial cultures and, in rare situations, fungal smears and cultures, should be ordered.

Entamoeba histolytica abscess of the brain is usually associated with an intestinal source, although the intestinal infection may be asymptomatic and missed on stool examination. Hepatic or pulmonary abscesses may also be present and tend to occur more frequently than brain lesions. Most extraintestinal amebic abscesses present with fever and symptoms related to a mass lesion. Direct examination of the abscess may be required unless the history, symptoms, and other clinical information, including serologic studies, are unequivocal. Serologic methods, if available, offer a noninvasive approach to assist in diagnosis and are particularly useful for extra-intestinal infections.

Symptoms of CNS infection with *Echinococcus granulosus* are usually those of an expanding mass lesion, mimicking a tumor. The presence of positive radiographic findings and history of residence or travel to an endemic area may suggest the diagnosis. Definitive diagnosis is made upon examination of the cyst and its contents obtained at surgery. The disease tends to predominate in sheep-raising countries and is found in many parts of the world. Screening serologic tests are particularly useful when cerebral infection with *E. granulosus* is considered and may be confirmed with the examination for *Echinococcus* antigen 5 in immunodiffusion studies.

Laboratory evaluation of mass lesions suspected of being larval tapeworms relies on either serologic procedures or direct morphologic examination following aspiration, biopsy, or surgical removal. Serologic tests are available and may be of significant help in some cases, although cross-reactions between these two tapeworm infections are known to occur. Although the hydatid cysts may occur anywhere in the body, liver, lung, and brain are common sites in descending order.

Symptoms of neurocysticercosis (larval *Taenia solium* infection) may result from active invasion of brain tissue or from the death of a cyst with resultant tissue reaction. Epileptiform seizures are an especially common complication of this infection and may be the presenting symptom. Other symptoms may include hydrocephalus, headaches, visual impairment, and nausea. The CSF may contain eosinophils along with reactive lymphoid cells; peripheral eosinophilia may also be noted. Routine radiographs may reveal calcified cysts in other parts of the body, and CT scans may demonstrate brain lesions. Even though serologic tests may be helpful, the definitive diagnosis requires surgical removal and microscopic examination of the lesion.

Logistics

Aspirates of abscess fluid are preferred over swab specimens. Aspirates should be brought to the laboratory in an anaerobic transport device or in a capped syringe with the needle removed. In the latter case, specimens must be delivered without delay. All the required smears and cultures may be set up from anaerobically transported specimens. If swabs are submitted, there should be a separate swab for each test ordered, and the swab for anaerobic culture must be conveyed in an anaerobic transport device.

Thin smears should be prepared from abscess aspirates or swabs. If the specimen is particularly thick, it may be diluted with sterile saline before smear preparation. Smears should be air-dried, heat- or methanol-fixed, and Gram-stained by the standard method. Smears should be examined under oil immersion magnification (1000×) for microorganisms and inflammatory cells. Calcofluor white or methylene blue stain can be used to detect fungi that are not stained well with Gram reagents. A microscope equipped for UV illumination is necessary to read calcofluor white-stained smears.

Aspirates or swabs for aerobic bacterial culture should be inoculated to 5% sheep blood, chocolate, and MacConkey or eosin-methylene blue (EMB) agar plates. In addition, a tube of nonselective nutrient-rich broth should be inoculated. Blood and chocolate agar plates should be incubated at 35°C in an aerobic atmosphere enriched with 5–10% CO_2 for 48–72 hours. MacConkey or EMB agar plates should be incubated at 35°C in an aerobic atmosphere for 24 hours. Broth cultures should be incubated at 35°C for 3–7 days. Specimens for anaerobic culture should be inoculated to nonselective, prereduced anaerobic blood agar enriched with vitamin K and hemin, media selective for gram-positive anaerobes (e.g., prereduced CNA agar) and gram-negative anaerobes (e.g., prereduced laked blood agar with kanamycin and vancomycin), and to a tube of prereduced chopped meat glucose broth. Cultures should be incubated at 35°C in an anaerobic atmosphere for 5–7 days. Turbid broth cultures should be Gram-stained and subcultured aerobically and anaerobically. Specimens for fungal culture should be inoculated to Sabouraud dextrose and brain heart infusion agars. Media containing cycloheximide should not be used without including a nonselective fungal media. The growth of some opportunistic fungi capable of causing CNS abscesses is inhibited by cycloheximide. Cultures should be incubated at 25–30°C in an aerobic atmosphere for 21–28 days.

Virus isolation from brain tissue is usually achieved at autopsy. A few grams of tissue are aseptically obtained, placed in a sterile container, and immediately transported to the laboratory or kept on ice. Caution must be practiced when obtaining infected brain tissue, especially for rabies, Creutzfeldt-Jakob disease, and AIDS, because virus may be transmitted during the course of sampling.

As with the diagnosis of amebic liver abscess caused by *E. histolytica,* the diagnosis of suspected amebic brain abscess may be made from aspirate or biopsy material taken from the margin of the abscess pocket. Material taken from the center of such lesions is usually necrotic and is of little value. Smears from aspirated material are usually stained with trichrome, whereas routine hematoxylin and eosin (H&E) stains are adequate for biopsies.

Aspiration of cyst fluid may reveal the hooklets or scolices (hydatid sand) of *E. granulosus.* The individual cysticerci of *Taenia solium* may be readily recognized on histologic examination following surgical removal. The presence of cysticerci in other tissues of the body would indicate with high probability that brain lesions are also present.

MISCELLANEOUS TESTS

Test: CSF *Limulus* Lysate

The *Limulus* amebocyte lysate (LAL) assay is an exquisitely sensitive assay for gram-negative endotoxin. The presence of endotoxin in the CSF is demonstrated by causing a clot to form from a protein extracted from amoebocytes of the *Limulus polyphemus* horseshoe crab. The test is performed by mixing CSF with LAL reagent and incubating at 37°C for 2 hours. Visible clot formation indicates the presence of endotoxin in the specimen.

Only rarely do LAL assay results have clinical value. Although extraordinarily sensitive, it is fraught with specificity problems. Infinitesimal contamination of reagents, tubes, or pipettes with endotoxin produces false positive results. A negative result effectively rules out gram-negative meningitis and obviates the need for prophylaxis of family members and close contacts. However, a negative result does not rule out gram-positive meningitis. A positive LAL result cannot differentiate between *H. influenzae* type b, *N. meningitidis,* or *E. coli* infection. All are important causes of meningitis, and each demands specific management of patients and patient-contacts.

Test: CSF Lactate (See Ch. 6)

Measurement of CSF lactate helps differentiate bacterial meningitis from aseptic meningitis. Assays are usually performed in the chemistry laboratory by gas-liquid chromatography (GLC) or by a spectrophotometric enzymatic method. The results of the CSF lactate test are useful when the CSF differential cell count, CSF glucose, and CSF protein tests show equivocal results. The CSF lactate test can help sway the interpretation of initial results by helping to differentiate between bacterial or aseptic meningitis before culture results are available. An elevated CSF lactate level (more than 35 mg/dL) points toward bacterial meningitis. The reliability of the test in young children is still in question.

Test: CSF C-Reactive Protein

C-reactive protein (CRP) is an acute-phase reactant that, when present in the CSF, serves as a nonspecific signal of bacterial infection. This protein is readily detected immunologically, either by qualitative latex particle agglutination or by quantitative rate nephelometry. The latex particle agglutination assays are carried out by mixing 1 drop of CSF with 1 drop of antibody-coated latex particles. The mixture is rotated for 2 minutes and examined for agglutination. Performance of the rate nephelometric assay requires instrumentation, usually found in chemistry or immunology sections of the clinical laboratory. The assay is started by mixing diluted CSF with CRP antibody reagent. The resultant formation of immune complexes is monitored over time with a nephelometer.

Results of the CSF CRP test are useful in the same context as the CSF lactate test. Furthermore, because the qualitative test is inexpensive and the negative predictive value of the results high (~99%), the qualitative test has been advocated for screening CSF specimens before testing for bacterial antigens. The absence of CSF CRP appears to rule out bacterial meningitis. The presence of CSF CRP in patients with other evidence of meningitis is suggestive, but not diagnostic, of bacterial infection.

REFERENCES

1. Molavi A, LeFrock JL (ed): Infections of the central nervous system. Med Clin North Am 1985;69:217–435.
2. Salaki JS, Louria DB, Chmel H: Fungal and yeast infections of the central nervous system: a clinical review. Medicine (Baltimore) 1984;63:108–132.
3. Tunkel AR, Wispelwey B, Scheld WM: Bacterial meningitis: recent advances in pathophysiology and treatment. Ann Intern Med 1990;112:610–610.
4. Wilhelm C, Ellner JJ: Chronic meningitis. Neurol Clin 1986;4:115–141.
5. Johnson RT: Viral Infections of the Nervous System. New York, Raven Press, 1982.
6. Whitley RJ: Viral encephalitis. N Engl J Med 1990;323:242–250.
7. Beaver PC, Jung RC, Cupp EW: Clinical Parasitology. 9th Ed. Philadelphia, Lea & Febiger, 1984.
8. Gascia LS, Bruckner DA: Diagnostic Medical Parasitology. New York, Elsevier, 1988.
9. Scheld WM, Wispelwey B: Meningitis. Infect Dis Clin North Am 1990;4:555–854.
10. Chohmaitree T, Menegus M, Powell K: The clinical relevance of CSF viral culture. JAMA 1982;247:1843.
11. Maniglia AJ, Goodwin WJ, Arnold JE, Ganze E: Intracranial abscesses secondary to nasal, sinus, and orbital infections in adults and children. Arch Otolaryngol Head Neck Surg 1989;115:1424–1429.

28 Antimicrobial Therapy

Peter C. Fuchs
Joseph Rindone
William Jones

Part I In Vitro Susceptibility

Peter C. Fuchs

INTRODUCTION

The antimicrobial susceptibility tests are in vitro methods that determine the susceptibility of microorganisms to antimicrobial agents under specific standard laboratory conditions. The aim of such testing is to predict in vivo response of specific infections in patients to therapy with specific antimicrobial agents and thereby provide a guide to appropriate drug selection by the clinician. Unfortunately, the achievement of this goal has been extremely difficult to assess.

Some of the recognized and theoretical causes of discrepancies between in vitro susceptibility test results and clinical response are listed in Table 28-1. Obviously, if a contaminant or colonizer, rather than the true pathogen, is cultured and tested for susceptibility, the clinical response is totally independent of the test results. Thus, the importance of appropriate and careful specimen procurement by qualified persons cannot be overemphasized. This is particularly true of specimens that are commonly contaminated or colonized by potential pathogens but are considered easy to obtain and are often relegated to less qualified personnel (e.g., sputum, wounds).

The failure to culture and test all pathogens from a mixed infection may also account for poor in vitro/in vivo correlation. This may be caused by a failure to detect a resistant pathogen in the infection or by protection of a susceptible pathogen by the presence of another organism. For example, the β-lactamase of *Moraxella* (formerly, *Branhamella*) *catarrhalis* from a bronchial specimen (which was either not cultured or ignored) could conceivably protect the cultured *Streptococcus pneumoniae* during penicillin therapy.

If we assume that the in vitro test conditions that might affect the activity of an antibiotic are the same as those that occur in vivo, the correlation between in vitro test results and clinical response would be determined by the concentration of the antibiotic at the site of the infection. Because the usual concentration of an antimicrobial agent in plasma is the basis for susceptibility criteria of in vitro tests and because the pharmacokinetics of different antimicrobial agents vary considerably, the concentration of drugs at sites of infection outside the vascular compartment may differ significantly from the susceptibility breakpoint in test conditions. For example, cephalothin does not cross the blood-brain barrier; therefore, a meningitis caused by *Escherichia coli* susceptible to cephalothin by in vitro testing would not be expected to respond to cephalothin therapy. By contrast, a cystitis, caused by *E. coli* resistant to cephalothin by in vitro testing might very well respond to cephalothin therapy, because of the very high concentration achieved in urine.

Another potential cause of in vitro/in vivo discrepancy is the so-called *inoculum effect* observed in laboratory testing. The standard inoculum concentration of organisms in susceptibility testing is 5×10^5 colony forming units (CFU)/mL. For many antimicrobial agents, increasing or decreasing the concentration of inoculum 1 or 2 logs will significantly increase or decrease the minimum inhibitory concentration (MIC) for some or-

Table 28-1. Causes of Poor Correlation Between In Vitro Susceptibility Test Results and In Vivo Responses

In vitro susceptibility with clinical failure
    Wrong organism isolated and tested
    Mixed infection
    Antibiotic unable to reach site of infection
        Pharmacokinetically
        Abscesses
    Inoculum effect—organism concentration in vivo greater than in vitro test conditions
    Bacterial tolerance
    Suprainfection
    Protein binding of the antibiotic
In vitro resistance with clinical success
    Wrong organism isolated and tested
    Antibiotic concentrated at site of infection
    Patient's defenses adequate without antibiotic

ganisms. For infections in which the concentration of pathogens is significantly greater than the 5×10^5 CFU/mL used for in vitro testing, a theoretical potential for failure exists for antibiotics that exhibit a pronounced inoculum effect.

The results of standard in vitro susceptibility tests refer to the inhibitory activity of an antimicrobial agent. For some infections, bactericidal activity is necessary for clinical cure (e.g., endocarditis). For most commonly used antimicrobial agents, such as the β-lactams, aminoglycosides, and fluoroquinolones, the minimum bactericidal concentration (MBC) is usually the same as, or, at most, one doubling concentration higher than, the MIC. Occasionally, a microorganism is encountered for which the MBC of a usually bactericidal antibiotic is up to 32-fold higher than the MIC, a phenomenon referred to as *bacterial tolerance*. In vitro demonstration of tolerance is very method dependent. The concept of tolerance, although somewhat controversial, has been invoked increasingly in recent years as an explanation for clinical failures in the face of susceptibility by standard in vitro methods.

Suprainfection is increasingly a cause of clinical failure or relapse despite appropriate antimicrobial therapy, particularly in the hospital setting in patients with decreased host defenses. Resistant microorganisms, such as pseudomonads, enterococci, and fungi, may colonize and subsequently infect the site previously infected by a susceptible organism against which therapy was directed. This is an example of bacteriologic response but clinical therapeutic failure. Also some infecting organisms may develop resistance to an antimicrobial agent during therapy, particularly when concentrations of the drug are not well above the MIC.

Finally, clinical therapeutic success has often been attributed to antimicrobial agents to which the pathogen is resistant, when in fact the patient's normal defenses were responsible for the cure. For example, abscesses are often cured by adequate drainage alone. Antibiotics are commonly used in conjunction with drainage but, even if an inappropriate drug (based on in vitro testing) is used, clinical success is a common outcome.

From the foregoing comments, it is apparent that the in vitro antimicrobial susceptibility test results, taken in isolation, may not be good predictors of clinical outcome of specific antimicrobial therapy. Nevertheless, when considered in the light of the many variable factors mentioned above (and subsequently), the susceptibility test can be a valuable adjuvant in the choice of appropriate antimicrobial therapy.

Table 28-2 lists some of the factors to be considered by the clinician in selecting an antimicrobial agent for therapy. Any of these, if inadequately considered, may lead to an unsatisfactory outcome, particularly in serious infections. The antimicrobial susceptibility test is just one of those factors. Because therapy often must be initiated before the results of the susceptibility test are available, the antimicrobial susceptibility test is often not a consideration in the initial choice of antibiotics. This is not to say that the susceptibility test is not important, but rather indicates its broader role in medicine today.

Table 28-2. Factors to Consider in Choice of Antimicrobial Agents

Patient factors
    Acuity and seriousness of infection
    Site of infection
    Underlying diseases
        Immunosuppressed
        Diseases prone to drug toxicity
    Allergies
Organism factors
    Virulence
    Usual susceptibility pattern
    Susceptibility test results
Antimicrobial agent factors
    Pharmacokinetics
    Toxicity
    Interaction with other drugs
    Antimicrobial spectrum
Past experience

The primary roles of the susceptibility test are (1) to provide data for the choice of a more appropriate antimicrobial agent in the event the initial drug is not successful, (2) to provide data for the choice of a more specific and narrow-spectrum agent when a broad-spectrum drug was initiated, to reduce the likelihood of suprainfection; (3) to provide data for the choice of a more economical drug when a costly drug was initiated and long-term therapy is anticipated; and (4) to confirm that the initial agent selected was appropriate. Important by-products of the susceptibility test are data on the susceptibility profiles of nosocomial pathogens. Because profiles change with time (dependent, at least in part, on the selective pressures of prevalent antimicrobial usage) and are unique with each institution, they should be tabulated and made available to the medical staff in a routine and timely fashion — at least annually.

BASIC TESTS

Test: Antimicrobial Testing

Background and Selection

There is no point in performing a test if the results are known beforehand. Similarly, susceptibility testing is useful only when the information gained is not predictable from knowing the identity of the organism. For instance, in a case in which *Streptococcus pyogenes* is isolated from a wound, the drug of choice is penicillin. There is no value in conducting a susceptibility test for penicillin because all *S. pyogenes* known to date are susceptible to this drug. By contrast, if the patient with the *S. pyogenes* wound infection is allergic to penicillin and a tetracycline or erythromycin is being considered, susceptibility testing would be appropriate because up to 25% of *S. pyogenes* isolates are resistant to these drugs.

Unfortunately, the list of organisms with 100% susceptibility to specific drugs is diminishing. For example, the incidence of ampicillin-resistant *Haemophilus influenzae*, penicillin-resistant *Neisseria gonorrhoeae*, and penicillin-resistant pneumococci (or pneumococci that are only moderately susceptible to penicillin) is increasing, indicating the need for susceptibility testing of these isolates, particularly in serious infections and in endemic areas. With these factors in mind, the major indications for the antimicrobial susceptibility test are listed in Table 28-3.

Table 28-3. Indications for the Antimicrobial Susceptibility Test

Problem	Reason for AST
Patient not responding as expected to initial therapy	To find a more effective drug
Patient on broad-spectrum drug	To find a more narrow-spectrum drug
Patient on costly drug with anticipated long-term therapy	To find a more economical drug
Patient not yet on treatment	To choose initial drug therapy
Drug of choice is contraindicated	To find alternate drug effective against particular organism

Logistics

An understanding of the principles of susceptibility testing is necessary to understand the limits not only of the testing itself but the test results as well. Many methods of testing can be found in the United States (Table 28-4), but the great majority of laboratories use either the disk diffusion or broth microdilution method.

Dilution Methods[1,2]

In dilution susceptibility tests, the test organism is inoculated into a series of media containing varying concentrations of antibiotic. After 18–24 hours of appropriate incubation, they are observed for the presence or absence of growth. The lowest concentration of an antimicrobial agent that inhibits growth is the minimal inhibitory concentration. The concentrations of drugs

Table 28-4. Antimicrobial Susceptibility Test Methods

Disk diffusion method
  Bauer-Kirby method
  Agar overlay method
Dilution methods
  Agar dilution
  Broth dilution
    Macrodilution
    Microdilution
Disk elution method
Automated methods

tested are usually in twofold dilutions and range from 1 or more concentrations above what is considered the resistant breakpoint to 1 or more concentrations below what is considered the susceptible breakpoint. In some cases, particularly with agar dilution, only breakpoint concentrations may be tested. Regarding dilution methods, the following points should be remembered:

1. Numerous variables in the procedure affect the results. To ensure that the results reflect the susceptibility of the test organism to the drug, it is essential that the procedure be rigidly standardized, preferably according to the recommendations of the National Committee for Clinical Laboratory Standards (NCCLS).[2]
2. Even when rigidly standardized, the MIC end point will vary somewhat on repeated testing. An acceptable MIC range is when, on repetitive testing, at least 95% of end points fall within the mode ± 1 twofold concentration. Thus, in the clinical situation, when an ampicillin MIC of 8 μg/mL for an *E. coli* is reported, one must think in terms of 4–16 μg/mL.

Disk Diffusion Test[3,4]

In this procedure the test organism is swab-inoculated onto the surface of an agar medium, after which antimicrobial agent-impregnated paper disks are applied to the surface. During the subsequent incubating period (16–18 hour), the antibiotics radially diffuse into the agar and inhibit the growth of susceptible isolates, producing a circular zone of growth inhibition around the disks. The diameter of the inhibitory zone is roughly proportional to the degree of susceptibility. The inhibitory zone diameter that is considered susceptible varies with each antibiotic and is determined by the diffusibility of the antibiotic in the agar and the MIC-susceptible breakpoint. There are several points to remember about the disk diffusion test:

1. Even more variables in this test than in dilution testing affect the results. The importance of standardization of the procedure cannot be overemphasized. Again, the NCCLS method is highly recommended.[4]
2. When carefully standardized, repeat tests with the same organism and antibiotic will usually produce inhibitory zone diameters within a range of 4–6 mm of each other. When these are at or near the susceptible breakpoint diameter, the same organism may be susceptible or not susceptible on different tests. To ameliorate this situation, a buffer zone, indeterminate (I), of 3 or 4 mm is often inserted between the susceptible and resistant breakpoints.
3. Although the inhibitory zone diameters exhibit a rough inverse correlation with MICs, there is sufficient variation in zone sizes above and below the MIC breakpoint correlates to make attempts at correlating specific zone diameters with MICs very unreliable.

Anaerobic Susceptibility Test

For testing the susceptibility of anaerobic bacteria, the agar dilution method is currently considered the standard method.[5] Because agar dilution is not practical unless large numbers of isolates are being tested, most laboratories use either a broth microdilution system (as described above) or a disk elution method. Although the broth microdilution method is well outlined by the NCCLS, the disk elution method is no longer considered acceptable by this agency.[5]

Interpretation

Regardless of the method of testing, the results of such tests are reported in some categorical manner. Commonly used categories are susceptible (S, very susceptible, category I), intermediate (I, indeterminate), moderately susceptible (MS, category II), susceptible to urine levels (U, category III), and resistant (R, category IV). There are a number of variations on this theme. It is important to understand the definition and limitations of the category system in use. The usual definitions of the aforementioned categories are listed in Table 28-5.

In the case of dilution susceptibility testing, MICs may also be provided. For many infections, this adds little useful information. However, for a few infections, usually serious ones, MIC data may be valuable in selecting the most appropriate drug and the necessary dosage. This assumes knowledge of the pharmacokinetics of the drugs in question. For example, if one is treating endocarditis and wishes to provide antibiotic levels such that the trough level is still severalfold higher than the MIC, knowing the MIC is important. If the level of the drug being selected is known to be substantially lower at the site of infection (e.g., meninges) than in serum, knowing the MIC may dictate a higher dosage schedule.

Table 28-5. Definitions of Interpretive Designations of Antimicrobial Agent Susceptibility Test Results

Common Designations	Definition
I, S, VS	The organism is susceptible to the drug at serum levels readily achieved by standard dosage regimens recommended for mild to moderate infections
II, MS	The organism is susceptible to the drug at serum levels that are achieved by higher than standard dosages, although the levels are still below toxic levels
III, U	The organism is susceptible to the drug at levels achieved by physiologic concentration (e.g., in urine)
I,—	The susceptibility of the organism to this drug is indeterminate (intermediate); used in disk diffusion and some automated systems
IV, R	The organism is resistant to the drug

It is important to remember that the laboratory testing of antibiotic susceptibility is performed in isolation (i.e., in vitro, outside the patient). Clinical interpretation of the results require placing them in perspective within the overall clinical picture. The factors listed in Table 28-1 must always be considered along with the susceptibility test results.

For each pathogen a select few antibiotics are usually recognized as highly effective therapeutic agents clinically. Knowledge of the drugs of choice for a particular pathogen or suspected pathogen is important in drug selection before availability of antimicrobial susceptibility results. Ideally, the laboratory would only test and/or report those antibiotics appropriate for each pathogen. However, there are many practical reasons, both technical and clinical, why this is not the rule. Technically, for example, this would require identification of the organism before susceptibility testing, which could further delay the results. Clinically, many infections involve two or more organisms. If a single antimicrobial agent is desirable, it may be necessary to select an agent that is not the drug of choice for one or more pathogens, but to which they all are still susceptible.

In interpreting laboratory susceptibility reports, it is useful to have some notion of typical susceptibility patterns for the organisms in question (Table 28-6). One should be particularly wary of reports indicating susceptibility to an antimicrobial agent to which the organism in question is nearly always resistant. Ideally, the laboratory will either not report such results or will verify them before reporting. Examples of some susceptibility test results that can be very misleading if the discrepancy is not recognized are presented in Table 28-6. Although laboratories should not report such results, clinicians should be sufficiently aware of the problems to recognize them in the event such results are inadvertently reported.

RELATED TESTS

Test: β-Lactamase

There are three tests in common use for the detection of β-lactamase production by bacteria: chromogenic cephalosporin (Nitrocefin),[6] acidometric,[7] and iodometric.[8] The significance of these tests is that they are performed quickly (in less than 1 hour) and thus can provide the clinician with information useful in selecting therapy before susceptibility test results are available for certain pathogens.

β-Lactamase testing is indicated for the following organisms:

1. *Haemophilus influenzae:* β-Lactamase production in this species is increasing in prevalence and occurs in greater than 25% in many parts of the United States. The enzyme renders *H. influenzae* resistant to ampicillin—the drug of choice for β-lactamase negative strains.
2. *Neisseria gonorrhoeae:* The incidence of β-lactamase producing *N. gonorrhoeae* in the United States is also increasing, although not to the degree of *H. influenzae*, but the high incidence still tends to be somewhat focal geographically. Where β-lactamase-positive *N. gonorrhoeae* are known to occur, routine β-lactamase testing is prudent, because β-lactamase producers are resistant to penicillin therapy.
3. *Staphylococcus species:* Laboratories that test the antibiotic susceptibility of staphylococci by the broth dilution method may encounter strains that are falsely susceptible to penicillin (i.e., inhibited by up to

Table 28-6. Examples of Susceptibility Test Results With Poor Clinical Correlation

Organisms	Test Result	Comment
Oxacillin-resistant *Staphylococcus* spp.	Susceptible to Cephalothin	Oxacillin-resistant staphylococci do not respond to cephalosporins
Cerebrospinal fluid (CSF) isolates	Susceptible to Cephalothin Aminoglycosides	Such drugs do not penetrate CSF
Nonurinary tract isolates	Susceptible to Nitrofurantoin Nalidixic acid	Such drugs attain effective concentrations only in urine
Pseudomonas aeruginosa	Susceptible to Tetracycline Chloramphenicol	*P. aeruginosa* only rarely susceptible; consider possible laboratory error

0.12 μg/ml of penicillin) but are β-lactamase producers. To avoid reporting false susceptibility to penicillin, β-lactamase tests should be performed on all isolates that appear susceptible to penicillin. Such tests should be performed after induction, that is, by first growing the organism in subinhibitory concentrations of a β-lactam such as oxacillin.

4. *Anaerobic gram-negative bacilli:* Most strains of the *Bacteroides fragilis* group and increasing numbers of *B. melaninogenicus* and other gram-negative anaerobes produce β-lactamase. The rapid β-lactamase test can provide a valuable therapeutic guide well before the isolate is identified or susceptibility tests are performed. A positive test would direct therapy away from enzyme-susceptible drugs such as penicillin, which might otherwise be preferable.

5. *Moraxella catarrhalis:* The role of *M. catarrhalis* as a pathogen is becoming increasingly apparent. Most strains today produce β-lactamase. Because many infections with this agent are treated with aminopenicillins, the β-lactamase test can provide quick guidance to more appropriate therapy.

Test: Minimum Bactericidal Concentration (MBC) and Serum Bactericidal Test (SBT)

Background and Selection

Tests for bactericidal activity of antimicrobial agents have been poorly standardized. A standardized method for both the MBC and SBT was recently proposed by the NCCLS.[9,10] As intimated earlier, there may be instances in which the bactericidal activity of an antibiotic against a specific organism may be useful information. This has most often been suggested for endocarditis, osteomyelitis, and possibly other infections in immunocompromised patients. The validity of this concept remains controversial, however. This is due in large part to the conflicting reports of investigators attempting to correlate in vitro bactericidal activity with clinical results, which in turn may be attributed in part to the variation in methods used by different investigators.[11,12] The proposed NCCLS standardized method has not been used sufficiently long enough to resolve the controversy. In any event, these tests are used by a number of infectious disease specialists but are not universally accepted.

Logistics and Interpretation

Bactericidal activity is usually determined by one of two methods. The most common of these is a modification of the broth dilution test for determining MICs. The principle is as follows. Those tubes or wells in the broth dilution test that inhibited growth (i.e., no turbidity) may still contain viable organisms. Thus, a measured quantity of the broth from these is subcultured onto nonselective plated media and the number of colonies counted after 24-hour incubation. The MBC is the lowest concentration of drug that produces a 99.9% reduction in viable bacterial counts. This requires careful determination of bacterial counts in the inoculum prior to inoculation.[13] There are numerous variables and vagaries in this test; and thus, before contemplating performance of the tests, the NCCLS proposed standard on bactericidal testing should be consulted.[9]

The other method of bactericidal testing, usually performed in research and specialty laboratories, is the time-kill method. In this method, broths containing an antibiotic in concentrations at and/or above the MIC are inoculated with a standardized inoculum of the microorganisms in question. Colony counts are performed at time 0 and at specified intervals thereafter. From these counts, curves are prepared graphically that depict the rate of reduction of bacterial counts. This method also is not standardized, and many variations have been published.

The SBT, often referred to as the Schlicter test, is a modification of the method for determining MBCs.[10] Instead of preparing a standard concentration of antibiotic from which doubling dilutions are prepared, the serum of a patient on antibiotics (usually peak and/or trough levels) is serially diluted with a 50:50 mixture of serum and Muller-Hinton broth. The remainder of the test is essentially the same as the test for MBCs. The results are reported as the highest dilution of serum that produces a 99.9% reduction of viable bacteria. The organism tested should be the patient's own infecting pathogen. The interpretation of the test results remains somewhat controversial. For example, it appears that endocarditis trough levels of 1:8 or higher are highly predictive of a successful outcome but that levels as low as 1:2 are not highly predictive of failure.[14]

Part II: Therapeutic Monitoring of Antibiotics

Joseph Rindone
William Jones

INTRODUCTION

During the past 25 years, a great deal of knowledge has accumulated regarding pharmacokinetics and therapeutic drug monitoring. With this knowledge, it has been possible to tailor drug regimens to patients' needs. The use of serum concentration data should be applied to drugs with narrow therapeutic indices. Drugs such as the penicillins and cephalosporins rarely need serum concentration monitoring because the margins of safety are wide. Applied pharmacokinetics may be considered the integration of laboratory examination, pharmacokinetic concepts, and clinical responses. Integration of these parameters permits drug regimens to be tailored to the individual patient. In the areas of immunology and microbiology, there are a limited number of agents for which therapeutic drug monitoring appears clinically useful. The use of serum drug concentration data may be useful in avoiding toxicity or for improving efficacy of individual drugs.

BASIC TESTS

Test: Aminoglycoside Antibiotics

Background and Selection

Within the aminoglycoside antibiotics are streptomycin, neomycin, kanamycin, paromomycin, gentamicin, tobramycin, amikacin, netilmicin. The most commonly used of these agents are gentamicin, tobramycin, and amikacin.

The purpose of monitoring aminoglycoside serum concentrations is to maximize efficacy while minimizing toxicity. Serum levels should be monitored in most patients receiving aminoglycosides for systemic infections. A possible exception would be patients with uncomplicated lower urinary tract infection who are receiving low doses of an aminoglycoside. From published studies, it is not clear how often aminoglycoside assays should be performed. For patients with changing renal function, assays may need to be performed on a daily basis. For patients with stable renal function, it is important to establish that therapeutic levels have been obtained. Serial predose levels may be useful in monitoring for toxicity because a rise in trough levels may be an early indicator of nephrotoxicity. It is unclear how often this needs to be done, but measurement of a trough level every 3–4 days of therapy (or possibly more often, if therapy is prolonged beyond 14 days) is reasonable. Repeat levels (both trough and peak) should be considered when a change in dose is made.

Logistics

There are no special requirements for specimen preparation except to note the exact timing of collection. Some authorities recommend obtaining serum levels after the initial dose to provide data that can permit forecasting of maintenance doses.[15] An alternative approach is to estimate the aminoglycoside dose using a nomogram and to measure serum concentrations 30 minutes before and after a dose (i.e., 30 minutes after the end of the infusion).[16] Trough and peak levels should be drawn when serum levels reach a steady-state condition, which usually takes about 6–12 hours of therapy in patients with normal renal function. The time to reach steady-state is dependent on the patient's renal function; it can be nearly 1 week for patients with end-stage renal disease. The drugs are stable in serum unless high concentrations of pencillins are present.

Amikacin is the most stable and tobramycin the least stable drug in the presence of such drugs as carbenicillin, ticarcillin, ampicillin, and piperacillin.[17,19] The physical inactivation of the aminoglycosides is dependent on the concentration of the penicillin, the contact time, and the temperature.[19] If aminoglycoside assays are done in a batch, serum specimens should be frozen until shortly before assay to avoid degradation of the aminoglycoside by the penicillin.

Interpretation

Interpretation of aminoglycoside serum levels requires evaluation of both peak and trough serum levels. In general peak levels are more predictive of efficacy than of toxicity.[21–23] Conversely, trough levels are associated more with nephrotoxicity than with efficacy. Target aminoglycoside serum levels are outlined in Table 28-7. As with any serum level determination, aminoglycoside serum levels are best interpreted in the context of the patient's clinical condition. Doses of an aminoglycoside should always be adjusted to give a trough level within the desired range (Table 28-7), to minimize the risk of nephrotoxicity.[20] However, maintaining a desired peak level may depend on how the patient is responding to antibiotic therapy. Doses may not have to be adjusted upward to maintain a therapeutic peak in patients who are apparently responding to the aminoglycoside regimen. It is unclear what a toxic aminoglycoside peak level is, because there are few data correlating peak serum levels with side effects.

Test: Vancomycin

Background and Selection

Vancomycin is a glycopeptide antibiotic useful in the treatment of gram-positive infections. The use of vancomycin has increased substantially over the last decade, chiefly because of the emergence of methicillin-resistant *S. aureus* and coagulase-negative staphylococcal species. Monitoring serum level determinations to assist in tailoring dosing regimens is increasing with the widespread use of vancomycin.

The routine use of vancomycin serum level is controversial. Some investigators have suggested that routine measurement of levels increases efficacy, minimizes toxicity, and potentially reduces the overall cost of vancomycin therapy.[24] Others have suggested that routine monitoring cannot be justified. They recommend obtaining levels in patients with a poor response to treatment or severe renal impairment or those in whom an unusually high MIC value against the infecting organism is documented.[25] Repeated measurements of vancomycin levels are not needed unless renal function changes significantly.

Logistics

Timing of the serum specimen is important for proper interpretation of the results. Usually two specimens are drawn: one just before a dose and the other 2 hours after infusion ends. Vancomycin is usually infused over 60

Table 28-7. Reference Range for Aminoglycoside Antibiotics

	Peak (µg/mL)		Trough (µg/mL)
	Soft Tissue[a] or Bacteremia	Pneumonia	
Gentamicin Tobramycin Netilmicin	5–7	8–10	<2
Amikacin Kanamycin	20–40	20–40	<10

[a] Subtherapeutic peak levels may be adequate for lower urinary tract infections.
(Data from Moore et al.[21,23] and Noone et al.[22])

minutes. Drawing a peak level before the 2-hour window may result in a spuriously high value. Generally levels are drawn on the second or third day of therapy, so that vancomycin concentrations can reach steady-state. Vancomycin is stable in serum.

Interpretation

The therapeutic range for serum vancomycin levels is not known with certainty, because there are few data correlating serum levels with either efficacy or toxicity. Some authorities recommend maintaining a peak concentration of 30–40 μg/mL and a trough concentration of 5–10 μg/mL.[26] Others have recommended lower peak values of 20–30 μg/mL.[27] These levels should be more than sufficient to treat *S. aureus* infections, because the MIC of vancomycin for this organism is usually less than 3 μg/mL.[28] Toxic serum levels of vancomycin are poorly described: toxicity has been reported in patients with peak serum concentrations of 80–100 μg/mL.[29] Nephrotoxicity has been associated in patients with trough serum levels in excess of 10 μg/mL.[30] There are no data correlating other toxicities of vancomycin with serum concentration.

Test: Chloramphenicol

Background and Selection

Chloramphenicol is a broad spectrum antibiotic used to treat many infections, including those caused by ampicillin resistant *H. influenzae*. Because of dose-related toxicities, chloramphenicol serum level monitoring has been advocated to tailor dosing regimens.

Chloramphenicol serum levels should be monitored in selected patients to minimize the risk of potential toxicity. Serum level determinations should be considered in patients with life-threatening infections (e.g., meningitis), in infants, and in patients with hepatic insufficiency. Repeated measurements of chloramphenicol levels are not indicated unless hepatic function changes while on therapy, a dosing change is made, or possible dose-related toxicities are occurring.

Logistics

Only peak serum levels are needed. Levels should be drawn 1 hour after the end of a 30-minute intravenous infusion. When administered orally, a level should be drawn 2 hours after a given dose. Usually, levels are drawn after 1–2 days of therapy to permit a steady-state condition.

Interpretation

There are few concentration response data for chloramphenicol. Peak serum levels of 10–20 μg/ml are generally considered therapeutic.[31] Reversible bone marrow suppression (reticulocytopenia, anemia, neutropenia, thrombocytopenia) may occur if levels exceed 25 μg/mL. Cardiovascular collapse may occur (especially in neonates) if serum levels exceed 40 μg/mL.

Test: Sulfonamide

Background and Selection

Sulfonamide serum assays are indicated when used to treat serious infections caused by *Nocardia asteroides*, because of their long-term use and the importance of reaching adequate therapeutic concentrations. Monitoring this antibiotic for other infections (e.g., urinary tract infection) is seldom indicated.

Logistics

The sulfonamides used most commonly for nocardia are sulfamethoxazole (with trimethoprim) and sulfisoxazole. Peak serum levels should be used and are generally attained about 2–4 hours after an oral dose. Levels should be drawn after 3–4 days of therapy to permit a steady-state condition.

Interpretation

The optimal therapeutic range for sulfonamide in *Nocardia* infections is not well defined. Generally serum levels of 80–160 μg/mL are recommended for both sulfisoxazole and sulfamethoxazole (with trimethoprim).[32,33] A correlation between serum concentration and toxicity has not been established for these drugs.

Test: Flucytosine

Background and Selection

Flucytosine is an oral antifungal agent used to treat certain fungal infections, such as candiasis and cryptococcal meningitis. Flucytosine has dose-related toxicities that may be minimized by monitoring the serum concentration. Flucytosine levels should be considered in any patient who is receiving a full therapeutic dose for systemic fungal infections. Flucytosine levels should be repeated in patients with changing renal function or in patients with suspected dose-related toxicities to the drug.

Logistics

Peak serum levels of flucytosine should be monitored by collecting a blood specimen approximately 2–3 hours after a dose. Levels should be measured on the second or third day of therapy to allow the serum concentration to reach steady-state.

Interpretation

The optimal therapeutic range of flucytosine is unknown, although some authorities recommend maintaining peak serum levels of 50–100 μg/mL.[34] The major reason to avoid high concentrations is that reversible bone marrow suppression may occur if serum levels exceed 125 μg/mL.[35]

REFERENCES

1. Gavan TL, Town MA: A microdilution method for antibiotic susceptibility testing: an evaluation. Am J Clin Pathol 1970;53:880–885.
2. National Committee for Clinical Laboratory Standards: Methods for Dilution Antimicrobial Susceptibility Tests for Bacteria That Grow Aerobically. Approved Standard M7-A2. Villanova, PA, NCCLS, 1990.
3. Bauer AW, Kirby WMM, Sherris JC, Turck M: Antibiotic susceptibility testing by a standardized single disc method. Am J Clin Pathol 1966;45:493–496.
4. National Committee for Clinical Laboratory Standards: Performance Standards for Antimicrobial Disk Susceptibility Tests. Approved Standard M2-A4. Villanova, PA, NCCLS, 1990.
5. National Committee for Clinical Laboratory Standards: Methods for Antimicrobial Susceptibility Testing of Anaerobic Bacteria. Approved Standard M11-A2, Villanova, PA, NCCLS, 1990.
6. O'Callaghan CH, Morris A, Kirby SM, Shingler AH: Novel method of detection of β-lactamase by using a chromogenic cephalosporin substrate. Antimicrob Agents Chemother 1972;1:283–288.
7. Thornsberry C, Kirven LA: Ampicillin resistance in *Haemophilus influenzae* as determined by a rapid test for beta-lactamase production. Antimicrob Agents Chemother 1974;6:653–654.
8. Catlin BW: Iodometric detection of *Haemophilus influenzae* beta-lactamase: rapid presumptive test for ampicillin resistance. Antimicrob Agents Chemother 1975;7:265–270.
9. National Committee for Clinical Laboratory Standards: Methods for Determining Bactericidal Activity of Antimicrobial Agents. Proposed Standard M26-P. Villanova, PA, NCCLS, 1987.
10. National Committee for Clinical Laboratory Standards: Methodology for the Serum Bactericidal Test. Proposed Standard M21-P. Villanova, PA, NCCLS, 1987.
11. Pien FD, Vosti KL: Variation in performance of the serum bactericidal test. Antimicrob Agents Chemother 1974;6:330–333.
12. Weinstein MP, Stratton CW, Ackley A et al: Multicenter collaborative evaluation of a standard serum bactericidal test as a prognostic indicator in infective endocarditis. Am J Med 1985;78:262–269.
13. Pearson RD, Steigbigel RT, Davis HT, Chapman SW: Method for reliable determination of minimal lethal antibiotic concentrations. Antimicrob Agents Chemother 1980;18:699–708.
14. Drake TA, Sanda MA: Studies of the chemotherapy of endocarditis. Correlation of in vitro, animal model and clinical studies. Rev Infect Dis 1983;5, suppl 2:345–355.
15. Lesar TS, Rotchafer JC, Strand LM et al: Gentamicin dosing errors with four commonly used nomograms. JAMA 1982;248:1190–1193.
16. Sarubbi FA, Hull JH: Amikacin serum concentrations: prediction of levels and dosage guidelines. Ann Intern Med 1978;89:612–618.
17. Pickering LK, Gearhart P: Effect of time and concentration upon interaction between gentamicin, tobramycin, netlimicin, or amikacin and carbenicillin or ticarcillin. Antimicrob Agent Chemother 1979;15:592–596.
18. Konishi H, Mitsuyoshi G, Yoshinori N et al: Tobramycin inactivation by carbenicillin, ticarcillin, and piperacillin. Antimicrob Agent Chemother 1983;23:653–657.
19. O'Bey KA, Jim LK, Gee JP et al: Temperature dependence of the stability of tobramycin mixed with penicillins in human serum. Am J Hosp Pharm 1982;39:1005–1008.
20. Matzke GR, Lucarotti RL, Shapiro HS: Controlled comparison of gentamicin and tobramycin nephrotoxicity. Am J Nephrol 1983;3:11–17.
21. Moore RD, Smith GR, Lietman PS: The association of aminoglycoside plasma levels with mortality in patients with gram-negative bacteremia. J Infect Dis 1984;149:443–448.
22. Noone P, Parsons TM, Pattison JR et al: Experience in monitoring gentamicin therapy during treatment of serious gram-negative sepsis. Br Med J 1974;1:477–478.
23. Moore RD, Smith CR, Lietman PS: Association of aminoglycoside plasma levels with therapeutic outcome in gram-negative pneumonia. Am J Med 1984;77:657–662.
24. Rodrold KA, Zokufa H, Rotschafer JC: Routine monitoring of serum vancomycin concentrations: can waiting be justified? Clin Pharm 1987;6:855–858.
25. Edwards DJ, Pancorbo S: Routine monitoring of serum vancomycin concentrations: waiting for proof of its value. Clin Pharm 1987;6:652–654.
26. Hermans PE, Wilhelm MP: Vancomycin. Mayo Clin Proc 1987;62:901–905.
27. Lake KD, Peterson CD: A simplified dosing method for initiating vancomycin therapy. Pharmacotherapy 1985;5:340–344.
28. Cunhya BA, Ristuccia AM: Clinical usefulness of vancomycin. Clin Pharm 1983;2:417–424.
29. Geraci JE, Heilman FR, Nichols DR et al: Antibiotic therapy of bacterial endocarditis. VI. Vancomycin for acute micrococcal endocarditis. Mayo Clin Proc 1958;33:172–181.

30. Cimino MA, Rotstein C, Slaughter RL et al: Relationship of serum antibiotic concentrations to nephrotoxicity in cancer patients receiving concurrent aminoglycoside and vancomycin therapy. Am J Med 1987;83:1091–1097.
31. Marks MI, Laferriere C: Chloramphenicol: recent developments and clinical indications. Clin Pharm 1982; 1:315–320.
32. Simego RA, Moeller MB, Gallis HA: Tirmethoprim-sulfamethoxazole therapy for nocardia infections. Arch Intern Med 1983;143:711–718.
33. Lerner PI: Nocardia species. pp. 1926–1932. In Mandell GL, Douglas RG Jr., Bennett JE (eds): Principles and Practice of Infectious Diseases. 3rd Ed. New York, Churchill Livingstone, 1990.
34. Stam AM, Diasio RB, Dismukes WE et al: Toxicity of amphotercin B plus flucytosine in 194 patients with cryptococcal meningitis. Am J Med 1987;83:236–242.
35. Kauffman CA, Frame PT: Bone marrow toxicity associated with 5-fluorocytosine therapy. Antimicrobial Agent Chemother 1977;11:244–247.

29 Serodiagnosis of Infectious Disease

Thomas R. Fritsche
Gerald Lancz
Ron B. Schifman

Steven Specter
Michael A. Saubolle
Raymond Widen

OVERVIEW

The detection of specific antibodies in serum and other body fluids is an important adjunct to the laboratory evaluation of various infections, and in certain cases is the principal test for confirming the diagnosis. In general, serologic testing is most helpful for infectious agents that are difficult or dangerous to culture, that cause chronic infections, or that are associated with prolonged incubation periods. Serology also can be used to demonstrate protective immunity in an individual or as an epidemiologic tool for studying the exposure of one or many persons to a specific pathogen.

Specificity of serologic testing depends on finding a rise or fall in antibody titers on paired serum samples, or in some cases detecting a single IgM class or very high serum antibody titer in a single specimen. The significance of titers or other values generated by any serologic test is dependent on a number of variables including test methodology, manufacturer's recommendations, and some threshold that is empirically determined to provide the most reliable interpretation. In some situations, quantitative tests can be used to gauge the severity of infection and provide prognostic information. Serial examinations may be useful for following disease activity or response to therapy. Qualitative tests, which provide only positive or negative results, cannot be used for these purposes. Serodiagnosis of certain infections such as viral hepatitis B or infectious mononucleosis is often accomplished by examining serum with a panel of different tests. Although not yet widely applied, new techniques in molecular biology show promise for direct identification by detecting specific microbial DNA or RNA in blood or other body fluids.

Unfortunately, serologic diagnosis has a number of drawbacks that restrict its clinical usefulness. Unlike culture, in which a few procedures will identify diverse pathogens, separate serologic tests must be chosen for each specific etiologic agent under consideration. Serodiagnosis of acute infections is often retrospective because a specific humoral response is normally produced days or sometimes weeks after symptoms first appear. Analysis of acute and convalescent sera necessitates waiting up to 3–4 weeks after the onset of disease and precludes using results to assist in managing the patient during the acute infection. Immunosuppression or antimicrobial therapy may blunt the immune response, and nonspecific reactions to cross-reacting epitopes limit the specificity of many serologic assays. Nevertheless, when properly correlated with clinical findings, serologic testing can be nearly as reliable as isolating the specific etiologic agent.

GENERAL TESTING INFORMATION

Background and Selection

Indications for performing serologic tests are described below for each specific test. It is always important to match the chosen test(s) with the expected etiologic agent. In some conditions, serology is the only method of choice, whereas in other circumstances it should be attempted only if the diagnosis cannot be made by culture. An impulsive selection of numerous serologic examinations in patients with fever, rash, or other nonspecific findings has little benefit and may produce misleading results. For example, testing for the "Torch" agents (toxoplasma, rubella, cytomegalovirus, [CMV] and herpes simplex virus [HSV]) was recommended at one time for pregnant women to determine their immune status. As it has turned out, interpretation of these results is often unclear, and this practice has been largely discontinued. However, testing for one or more of these agents when a specific illness is suspected, is of value, particularly when attempting to diagnose a primary infection in the neonate. Another example is the use of a "febrile agglutinin" panel for evaluating patients with fever of unknown origin. This collection of tests usually consists of assays for *Brucella* spp., *Francisella tularensis,* and *Salmonella typhi* antibodies. However, as discussed below, each has limitations in sensitivity and specificity. Reflexive use of these or other serologic tests without corroborating history, clinical findings, and a high index of suspicion can lead to a perplexing or deceptive interpretation and should be avoided.

Appropriate selection of any serologic test depends on the sensitivity and specificity of the test being offered, characteristics of the patient population being tested, and the predictive value of positive and negative results. Because of this, no single serologic methodology is appropriate for all possible cases. In addition, known differences exist in the ability of the various infectious agents to elicit immune responses. Specific test characteristics also vary significantly depending on the test methodology, techniques used in the preparation of test antigens and other reagents, as well as known reactivity of control sera.

Logistics

Specimen Collection

A single tube of blood of approximately 2–5 mL without anticoagulant is usually sufficient for most assays, although viral neutralization tests require that the specimen be collected aseptically to avoid contamination of the cell culture. When congenital infection is suspected, a specimen of cord blood may be analyzed, although direct sampling of the newborn's peripheral blood is preferred. In many circumstances, the timing of specimen collections is important for accurate diagnosis. When results must be interpreted by determining if there is a rising or falling titer, collection of both acute and convalescent phase serum specimens is required. The acute serum specimen is collected as soon as possible after the onset of infection. The convalescent specimen is collected between 2 and 4 weeks later. It may be necessary to collect a specimen at 7 days or longer after onset of infection to permit a specific IgM antibody response to develop. However, delaying collection for longer than 1 month risks missing the diagnosis because by this time, IgM antibody titers may no longer be detectable. A test for immunity to an infectious agent, which relies on detection of IgG antibodies, does not have any time limitation relative to the disease state.

Although serum antibodies are quite stable in sterile serum, it is best to freeze samples if the analysis is delayed for more than 2 days after collection. For nonrefrigerated transportation by mail, specimens can be preserved by adding Merthiolate to a final concentration of 1:10,000.

When serologic testing on cerebrospinal fluid (CSF) is performed, care must be taken to avoid traumatic contamination of the specimen with blood, which may cause misinterpretation of results from the presence of serum antibodies or antigens. Direct comparison between CSF and serum titers may be helpful for pointing to central nervous system (CNS) involvement by a specific agent. This can be done by comparing ratios of specific IgG titers to total IgG levels in both serum and CSF as follows:

$$\frac{\text{CSF antibody titer} \times \text{IgG serum concentration}}{\text{Serum antibody titer} \times \text{IgG CSF concentration}}$$

A ratio that is higher in the CSF specimen compared to the serum measurement indicates localization of infection to the CNS. Comparison of CSF and serum titers can be used to demonstrate CNS involvement in some infections, including neuroborreliosis (Lyme disease), chronic neurosyphilis, herpes encephalitis, toxoplasmosis, and cerebral cysticercosis.

Analysis[1]

A variety of immunologic methods are available for detecting specific serum antibodies. Results usually are given as a specific titer determined from a twofold serial dilution, which provides an approximation of the concentration or strength of the antibody reaction. Tests on paired serum specimens should be assayed together to enhance reliability and reproducibility of the results. Concentration of serum four- to eightfold may increase sensitivity of some procedures, but is not routinely performed.

Procedures for monitoring the performance of serologic tests with positive and negative controls are similar to quality control procedures used for other reagents. However, these materials tend to be more labile and susceptible to contamination. Exposure to room temperature for prolonged periods should be avoided. Antisera should be grossly inspected before tests are performed and contamination suspected when a clear solution becomes turbid. It is usually necessary for reagents to be monitored each time a test is performed. Controls not only ensure proper reactivity but also aid in the interpretation of agglutination and precipitation reactions. Before a new lot is placed into service, its reactivity should be tested in parallel with the expiring lot to check for consistency in reactivity.

A variety of immunoassays can be employed to detect and quantitate specific antibodies in serum. A brief description of common procedures follows. Special variations or alternative methods will be described as they pertain to specific tests.

Specific Methods

Immunodiffusion (ID). Antibodies capable of forming precipitating complexes with an antigen can be detected in gels (usually agarose) as an immobilized precipitin line. Immunoprecipitation between two separate wells of diffusing antigen and antibody is termed *double diffusion* (Ouchterlony method) and is the least sensitive. Other methods in which antibody is incorporated into the gel (such as radial ID) are primarily used to detect antigen rather than antibody. Diffusion assays can achieve greater sensitivity by driving the reaction with electrical current (counterimmunoelectrophoresis [CIE] and electroimmunoassay). Because of the ease of performance and higher specificity, ID assays are frequently used as screening tests or for confirmation of the specificity of reactions observed with other methods.

Agglutination Reactions. Specific serum antibodies may be identified by their ability to react with and directly agglutinate killed bacterial cells. These tests include detection of antibody against *S. typhi* (Widal test), *Brucella* spp., *F. tularensis*, *Bordetella pertussis*, and cross-reacting antibodies to *Proteus vulgaris* strains OX-2, OX-19, and OX-K associated with various Rickettsial infections (Weil-Felix test).

Particle-Enhanced Immunoassay. Serum antibodies can be detected by their ability to agglutinate antigen coated particles such as latex beads. These methods are relatively sensitive for detecting IgM class antibodies although nonspecific cross-reactions are a common source of error that limit their reliability. This method is also plagued by nonspecific agglutination of particles caused by immune complexes (associated with rheumatoid factor) or by the presence of high protein concentrations.

Complement Fixation Test (CF). Serum antibody can be detected by its ability to bind (fix) complement to red blood cells in the presence of a specific antigen. The amount of complement-induced hemolysis under appropriately controlled conditions is proportional to the concentration of complement fixing antibody present in the test sample. Although still used, the assay is cumbersome and requires careful technique to obtain reliable results.

Serum Neutralization Test (NT). The etiology of a large variety of viral infections can be identified on the basis of detecting serum antibody that inhibits (neutralizes) infectivity of the specific virus in cell culture. A rise or fall in neutralizing antibody implies acute infection, while a stable titer indicates past infection. Neutralizing antitoxin antibodies also can be used to identify exotoxin-producing bacterial infections. Detection of *Clostridium difficile* toxin is one of the most common applications of this test (see Ch. 26).

Enzyme Immunoassay (EIA). This test uses the principle that specific serum antibodies will bind to immobilized antigen attached to a solid phase (such as beads) or the bottom of plastic microtiter wells (enzyme-linked immunosorbent assay [ELISA]). After excess serum is washed away, immunoglobulin captured on the solid phase is detected by its reaction with enzyme labeled antihuman globulin plus enzyme substrate. The color reaction produced by the enzyme reagent system is proportional to the antibody concentration. This assay has a number of advantages including high sensitivity, quantitative results, ability to identify the presence of specific immunoglobulin classes, and stability of reagents and conjugates.

BACTERIAL AND RICKETTSIAL SEROLOGY

BACTERIAL SEROLOGY

Serologic diagnosis of bacterial infections is limited to a few special situations in which the etiologic agent cannot be readily isolated from the site of infection (Table 29-1).

Test: Anti-O

See under Test: *Salmonella Typhi.*

Test: Anti-Streptolysin O

See under Test: *Streptococcus Pyogenes.*

Test: Anti-Teichoic Acid

See under Test: *Staphylococcus Aureus.*

Test: Anti-Vi Agglutinins

See under Test: *Salmonella Typhi.*

Test: *Brucella* Spp. (Brucellosis)[2]

Although blood culture should always be performed, serology is an important adjunct to the diagnosis of brucellosis, especially if chronic infection is suspected. A description of the disease manifestations are reviewed in Chapter 20. Antibody to *Brucella* spp. is detected by tube agglutination using commercially available *Brucella abortus* antigen. A fourfold rise in paired sera or a single titer of 160 or more (IgG) is evidence for infection with *B. abortus, Brucella melitensis,* or *Brucella suis.* Rising titers are also present in disease relapses. False negative results are rare when paired sera are analyzed, but may sometimes occur if the patient produces only nonagglutinating antibodies. Negative tests should be confirmed with dilution to exclude false negative results from a prozone effect. False positive cross-reactions occur rarely with antibody responses to *F. tularensis, Yersinia enterocolitica,* and *Vibrio cholerae* infections. Brucella-specific antibodies can be detected in the CSF of most patients with neurobrucellosis. An EIA test that measures only IgM antibodies and is specific for acute infection has also been evaluated. The standard agglutination test will not detect the extremely rare case caused by *Brucella canis,* which requires specific testing with an EIA (ELISA) method.

Test: *Helicobacter Pylori*[3]

Helicobacter pylori causes dyspepsia, gastritis, and ulcers of the stomach and duodenum. The presence of this organism can be detected by biopsy, culture, or rapid urease tests (see Ch. 26). Various serologic assays (CF, hemagglutination inhibition, and EIA) have been used successfully to measure antibody responses to infection with this organism. The tests have high sensitivity and specificity and are convenient for the patient and physician. Furthermore, unlike other diagnostic methods, serologic testing is not affected by therapy. However, serologic testing for this infection is relatively new, not yet widely available, and the value of its routine use in clinical practice for the diagnosis and management of gastritis or ulcers of the upper gastrointestinal tract has not been determined.

Test: *Legionella* Spp. (Legionnaire's Disease)

Legionella spp. can be difficult to isolate because of its special growth requirements and the difficulty in obtaining, by noninvasive means, an adequate specimen from the site of infection (see Ch. 22). Serologic tests can be used for retrospective confirmation of the diagnosis when culture results are negative. However, except for very serious infections and for epidemiologic investigations, serologic diagnosis rarely has any clinical value.

Specific antibody is detected by indirect immunofluorescence assay using killed suspensions of various serogroups of *Legionella pneumophilia.* Alternatively, antibody can be detected by an ELISA method. A measurable serologic response is usually first detected within 2 weeks of the onset of infection. A fourfold rise in paired sera or single titer of 1:128 or more suggests acute infection. Test sensitivity and specificity is high in patients with pneumonia; however, false positive results from cross-reacting antibodies are known to occur, notably in patients with cystic fibrosis.

Table 29-1. Infectious Diseases in Which Serologic Diagnosis is Indicated

Primary Diagnostic Test	Ancillary Test
Amebiasis (invasive)	Adenovirus
Arbovirus encephalitis	Blastomycosis
Arenaviruses	Borrelia
Aspergillosis[a]	Brucellosis
(allergic bronchopulmonary and aspergilloma)	*Chlamydia trachomatis* pneumonia
Chagas disease (chronic)	Coxsackie virus (myocarditis)
CMV congenital infection	Cysticercosis
Coccidiomycosis[a]	Enterovirus
Echinococcosis	Filariasis
Ehrlichiosis	Glanders
HIV-1	Herpes virus
HTLV-1	Histoplasmosis
Infectious mononucleosis	Influenza virus
Leptospirosis	*Legionella* spp. pneumonia
Lyme disease	Leishmaniasis
Lymphogranuloma venereum[a]	Malaria
Measles	Melioidosis
Mycoplasma pneumonia	Mumps
Parvovirus (aplastic anemia)	Paragonimiasis
Psittacosis	Plague (*Yersinia pestis*)
Q fever	Polio
Rabies[b]	Rat bite fever (*Spirillum minor*)
Rheumatic fever	Schistosomiasis
Rocky mountain spotted fever[b]	Strongyloidiasis
Rubella	**Limited Diagnostic Value**
Syphilis	Candidiasis (invasive)
Toxocariasis (visceral larva migrans)	*Salmonella typhi*
Toxoplasmosis	*Staphylococcus aureus* endocarditis
Trichinosis	
Tularemia[a]	
Typhus	
Viral hepatitis (A, B, C, and delta)	

Abbreviations: CMV, cytomegalovirus; HIV-1, human immunodeficiency virus type 1; HTLV-1, human T-cell lymphotropic virus type 1.
[a] Culture indicated.
[b] Direct examination indicated.

Test: *Leptospira* Spp. (Leptospirosis)

Leptospira spp. is difficult to isolate because of its special growth requirements and the diagnosis is often entertained only after the organism is no longer present in the blood or urine (see Chs. 20 and 24). For these reasons, serologic diagnosis is the primary method for laboratory diagnosis. Slide agglutination or microscopic agglutination tests using formalin fixed or live organisms and EIA methods are available. Because antibody production to different *Leptospira* spp. serovars is specific, as many as 15 different strains must be tested. Serum antibodies appear between 1 and 2 weeks after infection, which is often when the diagnosis is first considered.[4] The antibody response will be blunted by therapy but once present, tends to persist for years. False negative reactions may occur if the infecting *Leptospira* spp. serotype is not included in the test battery.

Test: *Borrelia Burgdorferi* (Lyme disease)

Although only first described in the early 1970s, Lyme disease has become recognized as an important and often serious infection caused by *B. burgdorferi*. The organism is transmitted to humans from the bite of an infected deer tick *(Ixodes dammini)*. Blood and lymphatic dissemination occurs commonly. In as many as 75% of adults and 45% of children, infection is marked by a characteristic skin eruption (erythema migrans) that appears about 1 week after the bite. It begins as one or more small maculopapular lesions that expand with a distinctive circular border and fading center. This is often accompanied by systemic symptoms including fatigue, chills, low grade fever, headache, arthralgias, and myalgias. After a latent period lasting several weeks to months, patients may experience mild to serious neurologic, cardiac, or ocular derangements. A persistent infection is marked 6–12 months later by development of intermittent or chronic arthritis of the large joints and various CNS and cardiac manifestations.

Although the spirochete can sometimes be isolated from the skin, blood, spinal fluid, or other sites, cultures are typically not positive. The diagnosis therefore depends on clinical criteria combined with serologic testing. Enzyme-linked immunosorbent assay and other varieties of EIA procedures are the most commonly used.[5] Because positive results are typically not observed within the first 3–6 weeks of the primary infection, nonreactive or borderline results during this period do not exclude the diagnosis and repeat studies are indicated. Serially rising antibody levels or an abnormally high IgM titer suggest acute infection. Caution must be used in interpreting the IgM test alone however, because it is detected in only about 50% of individuals with acute infections, and elevations are occasionally observed during exacerbations of chronic Lyme disease. Elevated titers of IgG antibody are not typically detected until 8–12 weeks after infection, but persist once present. Highest titers are seen with carditis, neuritis, and arthritis complications. Measurement of antibody in CSF is useful as a confirmatory test when Lyme neuroborreliosis is suspected and is highly sensitive (90%).[6]

False negative results occur when testing is done before a specific serologic response has occurred. In suspected cases of seronegative acute Lyme disease, it is important to retest (sometimes multiple times) before concluding that the test is truly negative. If sufficient time has elapsed for a serologic response, the test is nearly always positive if performed correctly. False positive results occur from cross-reactions with other spirochetal infections (syphilis, relapsing fever) and infectious mononucleosis.[7] In these cases, an immunoblot test can be performed by a reference laboratory to confirm or exclude the suspected false positive result. A highly specific and sensitive polymerase chain reaction (PCR) test for amplifying and detecting *B. burgdorferi* DNA has been developed and may prove to be the most sensitive test for the earliest stage of Lyme disease.

Test: *Staphylococcus Aureus* (Anti-Teichoic Acid Antibody)

Commercial radial and counter ID kits are available for detecting anti-teichoic acid antibodies. Anti-teichoic antibody is present in the sera of almost all adults when sensitive methods are employed. Higher than normal titers are present with serious infections, and when combined with a positive blood culture for *S. aureus*, support the diagnosis of endocarditis or metastatic infection. Increased titers are usually absent in uncomplicated, localized infections. A normal titer does not exclude serious focal infections of bone or soft tissue, but is rarely seen with endocarditis. The test has only limited indications. It aids interpretation when the significance of a positive culture for *S. aureus* (from the blood or other site) is unclear and may help suggest the etiology when a *S. aureus* infection is suspected at a site in which specimen collection is difficult, such as osteomyelitis. When initial results are negative, and diagnostic confirmation is required, the test should be repeated after 1 or 2 weeks to allow time for antibody production. False positive cross-reactions occur with *Haemophilus influenzae* infection.

Test: *Streptococcus Pyogenes* (Anti-Streptolysin O [ASO], Anti-DNAase B, Anti-Hyaluronidase, and Streptozyme)[8]

Evidence for recent infection with group A β-hemolytic *Streptococcus* is important in any patient suspected of having postinfectious, nonsuppurative complications of rheumatic fever (RF) or acute glomerulonephritis (AGN) because by the time these diseases occur, the throat culture is negative. Although rarely indicated and of questionable reliability, the test has been used to differentiate invasive disease from carrier states in patients with persistence of *S. pyogenes* in the throat (see Ch. 21). The streptozyme method is used as a rapid screening test but negative results in suspected cases of RF or AGN should be confirmed by measuring specific antibodies. Anti-DNAase is the most reliable and reproducible single test, although ASO and anti-hyaluronidase tests also should be done when nonsuppurative streptococcal complications are suspected because none are 100% sensitive.

The streptozyme test measures the highest titer of serum that agglutinates erythrocytes coated with a mixture of streptococcal antigens (streptolysin O, DNAase B, hyaluronidase, and others). The ASO assay measures the highest serum dilution that neutralizes red blood cell hemolysis by streptolysin O. The anti-DNAase B assay measures the highest dilution of serum inhibiting DNA digestion by streptococcal DNAase B enzyme. The antihyaluronidase measures the highest dilution of serum that inhibits streptococcal hyaluronidase digestion of hyaluronic acid as indicated by failure of hyaluronic acid to form a clot when precipitated by 2 N acetic acid.

A rising, falling, or single ASO titer of greater than 200 Todd U/mL suggests invasive disease, but will be negative in about 15% of patients with acute RF. The ASO test is unreliable for diagnosis of poststreptococcal AGN after skin infection, and titers rise and fall faster than antibodies against DNAase. For this reason, the anti-DNAase test is more reliable, especially for documenting the postinfectious complications of carditis or Sydenham's chorea, which may occur after a relatively long quiescent period. It is important to recognize that serologic confirmation of recent streptococcal infection is not diagnostic for RF or AGN and must be interpreted in association with appropriate clinical and laboratory findings.

Test: *Salmonella Typhi* (Anti-O and Anti-Vi Agglutinins)

Serologic diagnosis of *S. typhi* infection (typhoid fever) with anti-O agglutinins is not normally indicated except for epidemiologic evaluations in locations in which this organism is endemic. The test is not appropriate for the evaluation of other *Salmonella* spp. infections or for fever of unknown origin. The presence of specific flagellar antibodies (anti-Vi) can identify chronic typhoid carriers with about 75% sensitivity. The test may be considered when this diagnosis is suspected and stool cultures for *S. typhi* are negative. Antibody to *S. typhi* O antigen is detected by agglutination of killed suspensions of the organism (Widal test). Antibody to Vi antigen is performed in reference laboratories by ELISA, or passive hemagglutination.

The anti-O agglutination test not only has poor sensitivity (below 50%) and specificity but assay methods are not well standardized and results can vary widely between laboratories. This makes interpretation of the test treacherous, especially when disease prevalence is low. The test, however, has been successfully applied in developing countries where the capacity to perform cultures is lacking. Interpretation of anti-Vi antibodies for detecting a chronic carrier should be done in consultation with the reference laboratory that performs the test.

Test: *Treponema Pallidum* (Syphilis)[9]

Syphilis is most commonly diagnosed by serology. The clinical manifestations and indications for serologic diagnosis of syphilis are described in Chapter 25. Serologic tests are of two types: nontreponemal tests (rapid plasma reagin [RPR] and Venereal Disease Research Laboratory test [VDRL]) and treponemal tests (fluorescent treponemal test, absorbed [FTA-ABS] and microhemagglutination antibody, *T. pallidum* [MHA-TP]). Nontreponemal tests are used for screening because they are easy and inexpensive to perform and are diagnostically sensitive. Nontreponemal tests also are indicated for following response to therapy after the diagnosis is made. Treponemal tests are confirmatory tests and are more specific than the RPR or VDRL tests. When syphilis is suspected, the nontreponemal screening test is done first and if positive, a confirmatory treponemal test is performed.

Nontreponemal Tests (RPR, VDRL)

Nontreponemal tests detect anticardiolipin antibody that cross-reacts with *T. pallidum* lipid antigens as well as antigenic material released from infected host cells. A positive test is identified as a flocculation reaction when serum is added to a suspension of the antigen. Quantitative results are obtained by testing serial dilutions of serum. VDRL and RPR tests are reactive (positive) in about 75% of patients with primary syphilis, 99% with secondary syphilis, and variably reactive (about 70%) in untreated late syphilis. A rising serum titer in an infant indicates congenital syphilis. Persistence of reactivity depends on the interval between onset of infection and treatment. Nonreactive serology is expected within 1 year after therapy for primary syphilis, 2 years after therapy for secondary syphilis, and 2–5 years after therapy for late syphilis—the latter being a function of the length and severity of infection. However, low titer reactivity may persist for very long periods in as many as 10% of treated (and not reinfected) cases. Nontreponemal tests are useful for following the response to therapy. A fourfold decline in titer is expected within 3 months of treatment in primary or secondary syphilis. Persistence of reactivity during treatment suggests reinfection or a biologic false positive reaction.

False positive reactions, which almost always have a titer of 1:8 or less, occur in about 1% of the general population, but may be as high as 10% in intravenous drug abusers. False positive reactions may be transiently associated with acute febrile illness or immunizations or they may be long lasting with autoimmune and chronic infectious diseases. False negative tests are rare but may occur as a "prozone" effect if the titer is very high. Therefore, it is important to repeat the test on diluted nonreactive sera, especially when a negative result is unexpected. Reinfection in the patient with prior reactive results can be diagnosed serologically by demonstrating a rising titer.

Specific Treponemal Tests

The FTA-ABS is an indirect fluorescent antibody (IFA) test using whole killed *T. pallidum* as the antigen. The patient's serum is added to antigen preparations, which are fixed on a glass slide. This is followed by washing excess serum from the slide, after which rhodamine labeled antihuman globulin is added. After a second wash to remove unreacted antihuman globulin reagent, the slide is examined with a fluorescent microscope for attachment of antibody to the spirochetes. Counterstaining with fluorescein labeled antitreponemal conjugate helps locate treponemal organisms in a nonreactive test. The hemagglutination assay is performed by mixing serum with treponeme coated red blood cells. A positive reaction is detected by agglutination of the cells. All treponemal tests employ a serum absorption procedure to eliminate cross-reactivity to nonpathogenic treponemes.

Specific treponemal tests are 75–85% sensitive in primary syphilis, 100% sensitive in secondary syphilis, and 95% sensitive in late syphilis with specificities of 98% or more. A positive test indicates active or past infection. Reactivity generally persists for life, although the test becomes nonreactive after several years in about 10% of patients treated for primary syphilis. The test is also positive in congenital syphilis although FTA-ABS IgM measurements improve specificity. False negative treponemal tests have been noted in acquired immunodeficiency syndrome (AIDS) patients with treated syphilis.[10] False positive reactions are associated with the same conditions (but usually not the same patients) as seen with false positive nontreponemal tests (see above). False positive reactions also occur with other spirochetal infections such as Lyme disease, leptospirosis, and *Borrelia* spp. relapsing fever.[7] The interpretation of syphilis serology tests is reviewed in Table 29-2. Serologic tests for syphilis can be used for the diagnosis of other treponemal diseases such as Yaws, Pinta, and Bejel although these disorders are not endemic to the United States.

Treponima pallidum has been documented to invade the CNS in about 30–40% of patients during the early stages of infection.[11] Clinical manifestations may be minimal, although the CSF leukocyte count, protein concentration, and VDRL titer are often abnormal if tested during this period. A chronic form of neurosyphilis develops in as many as one-half of patients who are not treated. Central nervous system involvement may be asymptomatic or be associated with various clinical manifestations, the most specific being pupillary disturbances (Argyll Robertson pupil) and tabes dorsalis. Patients found to have latent syphilis (asymptomatic with reactive VDRL or RPR confirmed by a specific treponemal test) or late syphilis (cardiovascular or gummatous findings) must be evaluated for chronic neurosyphilis, regardless of whether neurologic

Table 29-2. Interpretation of Serologic Tests for Syphilis

Signs/Symptoms	VDRL/RPR	FTA-ABS/MHA-TP	Interpretation
+	+	+	Primary, secondary, or late syphilis
+	+	−	Primary syphilis
+	−	+	Reinfection, late infection
+	−	−	Primary syphilis
−	+	+	Primary, secondary, or late syphilis (recently treated or untreated); VDRL titer should decline with treatment if infection is active
−	+	−	Biologic false positive result, unrecognized primary syphilis
−	−	+	Biologic false positive result, treated syphilis, untreated late syphilis

Abbreviations: VDRL, Venereal Disease Research Laboratory; RPR, rapid plasma reagin; FTA-ABS, fluorescent treponemal test, absorbed; MHA-TP, microhemagglutination antibody, *Treponema pallidum*.

symptoms are present or absent.[12] This is accomplished by measuring VDRL and either FTA-ABS or MHA-TP titers in CSF. The RPR is not reliable for testing CSF specimens. The VDRL is variably reactive (25–50%), whereas the treponemal test is positive in most patients (80–95%) with neurosyphilis. At least 50% of patients also will have elevated CSF protein concentration or lymphocytes or both.

Test: *Francisella Tularensis* (Tularemia Serology)

Serologic testing is the primary means for the laboratory diagnosis of tularemia because recovering the organism by culture is both difficult and dangerous. Antibodies are first detected within 2–3 weeks after infection and remain positive for years. Acute and convalescent serum specimens should be tested. See Chapter 20 for description of the infection. Antibody to *F. tularensis* in dilutions of the patient's serum is detected by agglutination of killed suspensions of whole organisms. The removal of cross-reacting antibodies can be accomplished by serum pretreatment with dithiothreitol. A fourfold rise in titer on paired sera indicates acute infection, while any single titer of 1:40 or more indicates acute or past infection. Because titers may be elevated for years after infection, it is important to always measure serial specimens to differentiate acute from past infection. False positive tests may rarely be caused by cross-reactions with *Brucella* spp. antigens.

RICKETTSIAL SEROLOGY

Test: Rocky Mountain Spotted Fever

Rocky Mountain spotted fever *(Rickettsia rickettsii)* is the most common and serious rickettsial infection in North America. The infection is transmitted by ticks and is more prevalent in the southeastern and south central United States. Clinical manifestations include fever, a centrally spreading peripheral maculopapular rash (often including the palms), myalgia, photophobia, thrombocytopenia, and sometimes meningoencephalitis or shock. Early diagnosis is important, because there is substantial mortality without appropriate therapy. Rapid and definitive diagnosis is made by demonstrating *R. rickettsii* in skin biopsy tissue by immunofluorescence staining. Blood culture is hazardous to laboratory workers and not usually available. Serologic testing is used to confirm the diagnosis.

Nonspecific cross-reacting agglutinating antibodies to *P. vulgaris* OX-K, OX-19, and OX-2 agglutinins (Weil-Felix test) have largely been superseded by more specific tests because of their poor sensitivity and specificity. In particular, the use of these tests for evaluating fever of unknown origin is nearly always unrewarding and inappropriate. The most sensitive and specific assays for confirming suspected rickettsial infections are the indirect hemagglutination (IHA) and microimmunofluorescence tests (MIF). The MIF is performed by adding serum to microscopic glass slides containing one or more fixed suspensions of the organism. Specific antibody is detected by further addition of fluorescein-conjugated antihuman globulin (either polyspecific or anti-IgM). Agglutination by the patient's serum of erythrocytes coated with rickettsial antigen forms the basis of the IHA test. Serum should first be absorbed with nonsensitized erythrocytes to avoid nonspecific reactions. Other tests include ELISA, latex agglutination (LA), and CF. A fourfold or single CF titer of 1:16 or more, IHA titer of 1:128 or more, MIF titer of 64 or more, or the presence of any IgM reacting antibody indicates acute infection. Indirect hemagglutination and MIF are the most sensitive and specific. Unfortunately, antibodies to *R. rickettsii* are typically not present in the early stages of infection when the diagnosis is first suspected and antibiotic therapy may further delay the serologic response.

Test: Q Fever

Q fever *(Coxiella burnetii)* is an infection associated with fever, headache, and interstitial pneumonia. It is transmitted by contact with farm animals such as sheep and cattle. Serologic testing is most valuable when searching for etiologies of culture negative endocarditis and occasionally in rapidly progressive atypical pneumonia when the differential diagnosis includes *C. burnetii* (see Chs. 20 and 22). A fourfold rise in CF titer or single titer of 1:200 or more is diagnostic. The presence of IgM antibody by MIF is also consistent with Q fever under appropriate clinical circumstances.

Test: Ehrlichiosis

Ehrlichia canis, another member of the Rickettsiaceae family, has the dog as its natural host. The organism is occasionally transmitted to humans by ticks and perhaps other vectors. Infection with *E. canis* causes mild to severe symptoms that include sudden onset of fever, rigors, headache, anorexia, and malaise. Lymphopenia,

Table 29-3. Rickettsial Infections: Serodiagnosis, Transmission Vector, and Geographic Domain

Organism	Infection	Proteus Vulgaris Strains			Preferred Test	Transmission	Geography
		OX-K	OX-2	OX-19			
Rickettsia rickettsii	Rocky Mountain spotted fever	– –	+	+	MIF	Tick	United States, worldwide
Coxiella burnetii	Q fever	– –	– –	– –	CF, MIF	Aerosol, contact with farm animals	United States, worldwide
Rickettsia typhi	Murine typhus	– –	+/–	++	MIF	Fleas	United States (Texas), worldwide
Rickettsia akari	Rickettsialpox	– –	– –	– –	MIF	Mite	North America, United States (very rare)
Rickettsia prowazekii	Epidemic typhus	– –	+/–	++	MIF	Louse	Worldwide, United States (very rare)
Rickettsia tsutsugamushi	Scrub typhus	++	– –	– –	CF	Mite	India, Asia, Pacific islands

Abbreviations: MIF, microimmunofluorescence; CF, complement fixation.

thrombocytopenia, and elevated serum transaminase levels are common. In many respects, the infection is similar to Rocky Mountain spotted fever or Lyme disease, except for the absence of a rash. Sporadic cases and outbreaks of ehrlichiosis have only recently been recognized, and although probably uncommon, the incidence of infection is unknown.[13] Most cases in the United States have been identified in the southern states. The diagnosis is made by serologic testing. An elevated or rising titer of serum antibodies to *E. canis* antigen measured by the indirect fluorescent antibody assay test is evidence of infection. The test should be considered when the patient has systemic illness after tick exposure in the southern United States, and the diagnosis of Lyme disease and Rocky Mountain spotted fever have been excluded.

Test: Other Rickettsial Infections

Other rickettsial infections are rarely seen in the United States and are nearly always associated with history of travel to the endemic area (Table 29-3). Antigen-specific MIF (IgG and IgM) helps differentiate the various pathogenic rickettsial species, *Rickettsia akari* (rickettsialpox), *Rickettsia prowazekii*, *Rickettsia typhi*, and *Rickettsia tsutsugamushi* (typhus). The interpretation and limitations of testing are similar to those described for Rocky Mountain spotted fever.

CHLAMYDIAL, MYCOPLASMAL, AND VIRAL SEROLOGY[14]

INTRODUCTION

Diagnosis of viral, chlamydial and mycoplasmal infections, is often accomplished with serologic tests in lieu of isolation procedures because of two major factors: (1) many serologic procedures are readily available and less costly than culture; and (2) culture systems are not available for certain viruses. The development of sensitive techniques such as radioimmunoassay (RIA), EIA, and immunofluorescence, as well as commercially available reagents have led to a significant expansion in the number of clinical laboratories able to offer extensive viral diagnostic services.

Serologic procedures for the detection or confirmation of viral infections are available for most pathogenic viruses that are commonly encountered. However, the clinical utility of serologic procedures varies considerably with the particular virus and to a lesser extent, the individual patient. The clinical importance of perform-

Table 29-4. Factors Influencing the Selection and Interpretation of Serologic Tests for Diagnosis of Viral Infections

Distribution of virus in the population	A positive serologic result on a single serum sample has little diagnostic value if a virus (such as herpes simplex virus) is widely distributed in the general population, while a single serologic result is significant if the virus is only narrowly distributed to a select population (such as human immunodeficiency virus).
Persistence of viral agent in the host	Lifelong and relatively strong seropositivity is typically associated with viruses causing latent or chronic infections (such as the herpes group viruses), while viral infections that do not persist may or may not lead to prolonged seropositivity and titers tend to decline with time.
Nature of the in vitro test used to detect antibody to the particular virus	Antibodies detected by complement fixation or neutralization test generally decline more rapidly than do antibody titers obtained by more sensitive methods such as enzyme immunoassay or immunofluorescence. Detection of antibodies by less sensitive tests may be more suggestive of recent infection than positive results by more highly sensitive procedures.
Isotype of the antibody being tested	Detection of IgM antibody to a given viral agent is more likely to be of clinical significance than detection of IgG class antibodies to the same virus, since presence of IgM antibodies usually indicates recent primary or reactivated infection. This assumes importance in serologic diagnosis of newborn viral infections when the presence of maternal antibody precludes the use of IgG-specific tests, while detection of IgM, which does not cross the placenta, indicates antibody production by the infant.

ing serologic testing for viral diagnosis ranges from being the method of choice for instituting therapy to being performed primarily for seroepidemiologic purposes with little direct impact on individual patients. Additionally, serologic studies are used to determine a person's immune status against a particular virus, such as screening women of child bearing age for immunity to rubella virus. Factors that determine the clinical utility of serodiagnosis for viral infections are listed in Table 29-4.

Diseases, syndromes, or circumstances in which viral etiologies are considered in the differential diagnosis are an indication that serum should be collected for serologic studies. Because the serum can be stored frozen until the need for testing is specifically indicated, specimens should be collected at the earliest opportunity. Viral infection such as the common cold, mild gastroenteritis, or rashes of obvious origin generally do not require laboratory diagnosis by serologic means. Conversely, the laboratory diagnosis of lower respiratory tract infections, meningoencephalitis, most exanthemata, severe gastrointestinal infection, hepatitis, and systemic infections may be aided by serologic testing. Specific serologic tests are described below.

CHLAMYDIAL SEROLOGY

Test: *Chlamydia* Spp.

Chlamydiae infections include respiratory, ocular, and genital diseases. Serologic tests are of greatest value for the diagnosis of lymphogranuloma venereum (LGV) and *Chlamydia psittaci* or *Chlamydia trachomatis* respiratory infections. Serodiagnosis is not sensitive or specific enough for evaluating *C. trachomatis* urethritis. The background rate of seropositive persons varies with the group tested. However, it is sufficiently high in sexually active adults to necessitate running acute and convalescent sera to confirm the serodiagnosis of recent infection. A fourfold rise in CF titer on paired sera or single titer of 32 or more with appropriate clinical findings for the specific illness, indicates acute infection with either LGV or psittacosis, and is about 80% sensitive. Other *C. trachomatis* infections, such as inclusion conjunctivitis (trachoma), cervicitis, and urethritis, produce little if any antibody response.

The MIF test is more sensitive and specific than CF, especially for the diagnosis of LGV. A fourfold rise in titer to a specific serovar (L_1, L_2, or L_3) or single titer of 512 or more in the appropriate clinical setting is strong evidence for LGV. High titers may sometimes be seen with other *C. trachomatis* infections including proctitis and salpingitis, but these are usually more reactive with the non-LGV serovars. The IgM MIF test is particularly helpful for confirming the diagnosis of *C. trachomatis* pneumonia in neonates when the titer is 32 or more. The measurement of antibody in tear specimens has been used to diagnose chronic ocular infections.

Serologic diagnosis is the method of choice for psittacosis (culture is hazardous), and is of value to support the diagnosis of LGV since culture of buboes is positive for *C. trachomatis* in fewer than one-half of patients with this infection. Serologic testing is usually not helpful for neonatal conjunctivitis because of the presence of maternal antibody and failure of the immature immune system to respond. However, the presence of IgM antibody in infants with or without inclusion conjunctivitis suggests progression to pulmonary infection. Diagnosis of adult pulmonary infections by *C. trachomatis* and *Chlamydia pneumoniae* (TWAR agent) can be made by specific serologic tests.[15] This is especially useful for *C. pneumoniae*, which is difficult to culture. The advent of improved techniques for chlamydia culture and the widespread use of direct methods for chlamydia antigen detection have relegated serologic testing for genital tract infections to primarily an epidemiologic role or as a method to attempt to establish a diagnosis of infection in an individual who has already begun antimicrobial chemotherapy.

MYCOPLASMAL SEROLOGY

Test: *Mycoplasma* Spp.

Mycoplasma pneumoniae is one of the leading causes of community acquired "atypical pneumonia" (see Ch. 22). The diagnosis can usually be made clinically, especially if respiratory and constitutional symptoms are mild. In more serious infections, when positive confirmation and differentiation of mycoplasmal pneumonia from other etiologic agents (such as Q fever, psittacosis, or legionnaire's disease) is desired, culture and serologic tests can be used. Because many clinical laboratories are not equipped for or have experience with mycoplasma cultures, serologic diagnosis is usually selected. In addition, culture of expectorated sputum or throat swabs for *M. pneumoniae* is relatively insensitive. A recently developed molecular probe for mycoplasma RNA in clinical specimens may circumvent some of the limitations of culture and serology tests.

Two types of serologic responses can be measured: a nonspecific (cold agglutinin) test and an antigen-specific test (CF, IFA, or EIA). The cold agglutinin procedure is the simplest to do, but also the least specific. Dilutions of the patient's serum are mixed with red blood cells and incubated for a short time at 4°C. The cells are observed for microscopic agglutination that disappears with warming. Cold agglutinin titers are elevated in 34–68% of patients with *M. pneumoniae* respiratory infections, but the test is not specific for the infection unless the titer is relatively high (1:64–1:128). Antibody to the streptococcus MG or a false positive serologic test for syphilis also may be observed occasionally as "nonspecific" serologic responses to acute infection.

Detection of specific serum antibodies to *M. pneumoniae* antigens by EIA or IFA is the serologic method of choice.[16] These tests are commercially available and configured to detect either IgG or IgM antibody. The likelihood of seropositivity in the general population mandates the collection of acute and convalescent sera when testing for IgG antibody. Because *M. pneumoniae* infections have a relatively long incubation period, the antibody response may be peaking when the first specimen is collected, which obviates detection of a rising titer. Although fourfold rises in IgG titer are necessary to achieve the highest level of confidence for the serodiagnosis of recent *M. pneumoniae* infection, some of the commercial kits available have threshold levels for single measurements that are strongly suggestive of recent infection. Additionally, IFA and EIA procedures for mycoplasma, which are specific for detecting the IgM class antibodies to the bacterium, offer the ability to make a rapid serologic diagnosis from a single specimen. It is important to note however, that IgM antibodies may persist for many months, therefore results must be interpreted in the appropriate clinical context. The CF test for antibodies to *M. pneumoniae* will evince a fourfold rise in titer in approximately 60% of individuals with culture positive pneumonia, whereas the remainder will fail to show a rising titer but have titers of 1:16 or more. False positive results from cross-reactions have been reported with other *Mycoplasma* spp., pancreatitis, and other inflammatory conditions.

VIRAL SEROLOGY

Test: Adenovirus

See under Test: Respiratory Infections.

Test: Arboviruses (Viral Encephalitis)

The clinical and microbiologic features as well as tests available for viral encephalitis are reviewed in Chapter 27. In general, a specific serologic diagnosis is not attempted unless there is a high index of suspicion for a specific agent, such as failure to culture the virus in suspected herpes encephalitis or a distinctive clinical syndrome.

Serodiagnosis is the method of choice for detecting arboviruses. The procedures available for the serologic confirmation of infection include CF, hemagglutination inhibition (HAI), NT, IFA, and EIA. As with other serologic tests, collection of acute and convalescent sera is required for serologic diagnosis of arbovirus infection regardless of the method of testing. Because of the diversity of viruses in this general group, it is important to focus the serologic testing to a subgroup of viruses most likely to be associated with the clinical presentation of the patient, taking into consideration travel history and other pertinent information relating to the patient. In the absence of a local epidemic caused by one particular virus, it is necessary to test for a panel of viruses. The HAI and IgM EIA tests become positive earlier than other tests. A single serum specimen that is reactive for one of the arboviruses by the IgM EIA or HAI test can be followed up with either CF, NT, or HAI tests using acute and convalescent sera. A fourfold or greater rise in titer confirms the diagnosis. The presence of stable antibody titers in the absence of a rise in titer indicates a previous infection with the particular virus but no relationship to the patient's current illness. An additional complication of serology for detection of arbovirus infection is the problem of heterotypic responses, particularly in individuals previously infected or vaccinated with another virus that is antigenically cross-reactive with the currently infecting agent.

Test: Cytomegalovirus

Cytomegalovirus is associated with a variety of infectious processes. Most are asymptomatic, although life-threatening pulmonary or systemic illnesses occur relatively often in immunocompromised individuals. In addition, congenital CMV infections may cause a variety of developmental abnormalities and neurologic deficits.

Serologic prevalence studies have demonstrated that 60–90% of adults in the United States, depending on socioeconomic level, are positive for antibody to CMV. A single serum sample tested for the IgG class of anti-CMV will tell only whether an individual has been infected. This type of testing provides no reliable information concerning the timing (recent or past) of the infection. IgM-specific testing for CMV antibodies is used to detect acute infection in neonates. When this test is positive, viral cultures (urine, blood) are indicated to help determine if there is continued virus shedding, indicating persistent infection. Antibody testing to check for CMV immune status should be done on all organ transplant candidates before surgery. Seronegative recipients of an organ from a seropositive donor are at much higher risk for acquisition of CMV disease and graft failure. In addition, blood for transfusion to seronegative transplant patients and all premature neonates should be obtained from donors who lack CMV antibodies.

In order to confirm acute infection in an adult, serologic testing for CMV infection requires collection of acute and convalescent sera to demonstrate the obligatory fourfold rise in IgG titer. An alternative is to use an IgM-specific antibody test, which if positive, is highly suggestive of recent CMV infection. Reactivated CMV infections may not be detected reliably using serologic procedures in all cases, regardless of whether IgG or IgM-specific serologies are performed, because antibody titers may not change. Cytomegalovirus antibody titers are of little value in determining the presence of CMV infection in an immunocompromised adult, because of the high incidence of CMV seropositive individuals in the general population. Virus isolation is required for the diagnosis.

Test: Encephalitis

See under Test: Arboviruses.

Test: Enteroviruses and Other Gastrointestinal Viruses

Serodiagnosis of gastrointestinal viral infections is not routinely performed. Rotavirus infections are generally diagnosed by direct detection of virus in stool with immunoassays. Tests for reovirus infections are not performed. Enterovirus infections require extensive serologic testing owing to the large number of serotypes involved (more than 70) and are usually not performed unless virus has been isolated. In certain circumstances in which only a limited number of serotypes are involved (e.g., cardiomyopathy and Coxsackie B viruses) testing may be indicated in the absence of virus isolation. Demonstration of a specific antibody response (neutralization assay) to a virus isolated from the patient provides evidence of an etiologic role, when, for whatever reason, this is in doubt. Finally, NT and EIA tests for antibodies to poliovirus are helpful in suspected cases of polio when the virus cannot be isolated.

Test: Epstein-Barr Virus (EBV) (Infectious Mononucleosis)

Infectious mononucleosis caused by EBV is characterized by fever, sore throat, cervical lymphadenopathy, splenomegaly, hepatitis, and peripheral atypical lymphocytis. Splenic rupture is a potential serious complication, as are rare occurrences of nervous system, lung, or kidney infection. The virus remains dormant in lymphocytes after the acute infection subsides.

The definitive diagnosis of infectious mononucleosis is made by serologic testing. This includes both heterophile antibody tests as well as specific viral antibody tests. The classic heterophile test (Paul-Bunnell) measures the titer of serum antibodies that agglutinate sheep erythrocytes after serum has been absorbed with guinea pig kidney antigens. Modifications of this test with horse erythrocytes has improved sensitivity. These are commercially available as slide agglutination tests that use either formalinized or papain treated horse erythrocytes and can be performed with only a single dilution of serum. The most reliable of these assays use a pretreatment guinea pig absorption step before testing. The heterophile test should be viewed as a screening test. Although false positive results are unusual, negative results must be confirmed by specific viral antibody tests. In general these tests are quite dependable in young adults (85–90% sensitive), but are usually negative in young children with EBV infection.

Three major classes of specific EBV antibody are used in combination for serologic testing. They are usually performed by indirect immunofluorescence. The viral capsid antigen (VCA) IgM antibody and early antigen appear during the acute infection. Viral capsid antigen IgM is the most sensitive and specific test; it is present in nearly 100% of cases during the acute infection, but disappears within 1–2 months. Antibody to Epstein-Barr nuclear antigen (EBNA) appears later, indicates past infection, and measurable levels remain for life. Table 29-5 summarizes the various patterns used to interpret these tests.[17]

In the presence of typical clinical findings of infectious mononucleosis but with negative heterophile and specific viral antibody tests, primary CMV infections should be considered.

It has been observed that patients with nasopharyngeal carcinoma (NPC) or other head and neck tumors often present with elevated IgA antibody titers to EBV VCA and with elevated IgG titers to early antigen (EA), sug-

Table 29-5. Serologic Testing for Infectious Mononucleosis (Epstein-Barr Virus)

		Antibody Tested				
		VCA		EA-D	EA-R	EBNA
Disease	Heterophile	IgM	IgG	(IgG)	(IgG)	(IgG)
Uninfected (nonimmune)	−	−	−	−	−	−
Subclinical primary infection	+/−	+	+	+/−	+/−	−
Acute infectious mononucleosis	+	+	++	+	+/−	−
Previous infection	−	−	+	+/−	−	+
Reactivated infection	+/−	+/−	++	++	+/−	+/−[a]
Burkitt's lymphoma	−	−	++	+/−	++	+
Nasopharyngeal carcinoma	−	−	++	++	−	+

Abbreviations: VCA, virus capsid antigen; EA-D or EA-R, early antigen (diffuse or restricted); EBNA, Epstein-Barr nuclear antigen; +/−, variable reactivity; ++, elevated or rising titers.

[a] May be low or lacking in immunosuppressed individuals.

gesting a role of this virus in the disease. Additionally, many patients with chronic fatigue syndrome present with high titers of IgG antibody to EA and VCA, although elevations of these antibodies are inconsistently observed and may be unrelated to disease etiology.[18]

Test: German Measles

See under Test: Rubella Virus.

Test: Hemorrhagic Fever Viruses (Arenaviruses and Filoviruses)

The arenaviruses include Lassa fever virus and Junín and Machupo viruses; the former is seen primarily in Africa or associated with laboratory accidents, and the latter two are seen in Argentina and Bolivia, respectively. The filoviruses include Marburg and Ebola viruses. All of these viruses are associated with hemorrhagic fevers and relatively high mortality rates. Laboratory tests, whether culture or serologic testing, are available only in maximal containment facilities such as state laboratories or the Centers for Disease Control (CDC).

The IFA test is the method of choice for these agents, because it provides the earliest seropositive results and may be used to detect IgM class antibodies for early serodiagnosis. The presence of a positive IFA result for Junín, Marburg, and Ebola infections coincides with the waning of viremia and is predictive of recovery. In Lassa fever, there is no absolute correlation between appearance of a positive IFA result and recovery as some patients succumb to infection even after seroconversion. Positive IFA results for Machupo are detectable later in the course of disease, after the critical stage of the illness has passed.

Test: Hepatitis Virus A, B, C, and Delta (Hepatitis)[19]

Because suitable tissue culture systems for virus isolation are not available, serologic testing is the principal means of establishing the etiologic diagnosis when infection with hepatitis A (HAV), B (HBV), C (HCV), or delta (HDV), when viral disease is suspected (see Ch. 23).

Hepatitis A Virus

Hepatitis A tends to occur in epidemics and common source outbreaks associated with contaminated food or food handlers. There is also an increase risk of infection for travelers to areas with poor sanitation conditions. Young children infected by fecal-oral transmission often have asymptomatic infection that is easily spread to household members. Infections are typically mild, sometimes debilitating, but invariably self-limited. A chronic carrier state does not occur. Approximately 30–40% of adults in the United States have evidence of past infection, although this prevalence varies widely by region and socioeconomic group. In hepatitis outbreaks, or in the previously healthy patient without a history of blood exposure (transfusion, intravenous

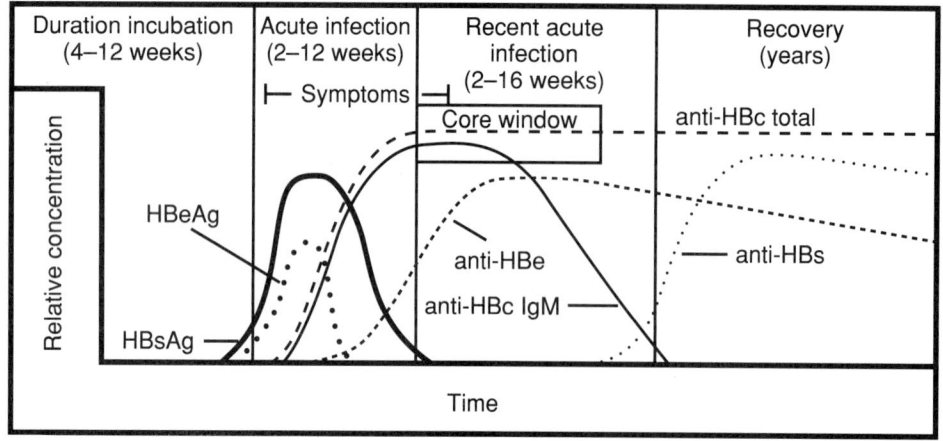

Fig. 29-1. Serologic response to viral hepatitis B infection with development of immunity.

drug abuser) serologic testing for acute HAV (IgM anti-HAV) is indicated. A positive result confirms the diagnosis, although other etiologies must be considered when the test is negative. Testing for anti-HAV IgG may be done to assess immunity in exposed individuals or for epidemiologic studies.

Hepatitis B Virus

Hepatitis B has become a preventable disease with the development of a highly effective vaccine. Transmission occurs by contact with blood or body fluids of a patient with acute or chronic infection. This can occur during birth when the mother is infected, by sexual contact with an infected partner, by exposure from medical procedures, or by parenteral drug use.

The serodiagnosis of HBV infection is complex (Figs. 29-1 to 29-3; Table 29-6). The best approach for evaluating acute viral hepatitis B is to test for the presence of IgM-specific antibody to the hepatitis B core antigen (anti-HBcAg) in serum. The presence of IgM-specific anti-HBcAg, with or without hepatitis B surface antigen (HBsAg), indicates acute HBV infection. Recovery and developing immunity is heralded by rising titers of anti-HBsAg and total anti-HBcAg antibodies along with the disappearance of HBsAg. These antibodies will often remain for life, although titers of anti-HBsAg may decline and sometimes even disappear after many years.

Chronic hepatitis is evaluated by testing for HBsAg. A chronic carrier state is distinguished by persistence of HBsAg for longer than 6 months. Anti-HBcAg titers

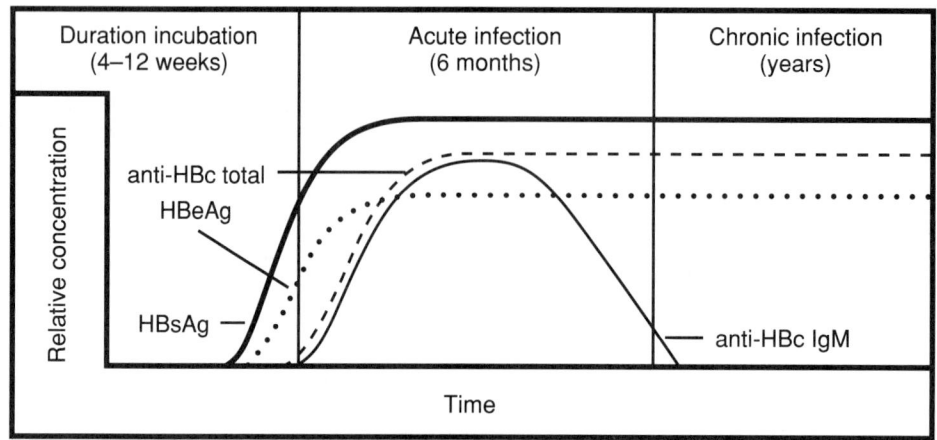

Fig. 29-2. Serologic response in chronic viral hepatitis B infection.

Table 29-6. Serodiagnosis of Hepatitis B Viral Infection

Anti-HBcAg IgM	Total	HBsAg	Anti-HBsAg	Interpretation
−	−	−	−	Uninfected (nonimmune)
−	−	−	+	Vaccine immunity
−	−	+	−	Very early infection
−	+	−	−	False positive result, natural immunity, or chronic infection
−	+	−	+	Natural immunity
−	+	+	−	Chronic infection[a]
+	+	−	−	Acute infection (core window period)
+	+	−	+	Resolving infection
+	+	+	−	Acute infection

Abbreviations: Anti-HBcAg, antibody to hepatitis B core antigen; Anti-HBsAg, antibody to hepatitis B surface antigen; HBsAg, hepatitis B surface antigen.
[a] Anti-HBsAg may be detected in some patients.

are high and anti-HBsAg is usually absent (Fig. 29-2), although there is little value in performing these tests to confirm a chronic carrier state when there is persistence of HBsAg. However, testing for the presence in serum of viral hepatitis B e antigen (HBeAg) may be helpful. The presence of HBeAg indicates a stage of disease in which there is ongoing viral replication. These patients are more infective than chronic carriers who are HBeAg negative. About 10% per year of HBeAg positive chronic carriers eventually develop a "late" seroconversion with disappearance of HBeAg and rising anti-HBeAg titers (Fig. 29-3). This indicates transformation from a viral replicative phase to a more quiescent stage of disease. HBeAg also may be used to follow patients which chronic infection who are treated with interferon-α. Disappearance of the e antigen indicates effective response to treatment. Finally, this test is of value in evaluating risk of infection in neonates. The presence of both HBsAg and HBeAg during pregnancy indicates a higher risk for perinatal HBV infection, than when only HBsAg is present. Hepatitis B virus DNA in serum can be measured in a few specialized reference laboratories. Its significance is similar to that of HBeAg, although it is a more sensitive marker of active viral replication.

Hepatitis B serology is performed in special circumstances to screen asymptomatic patients for chronic

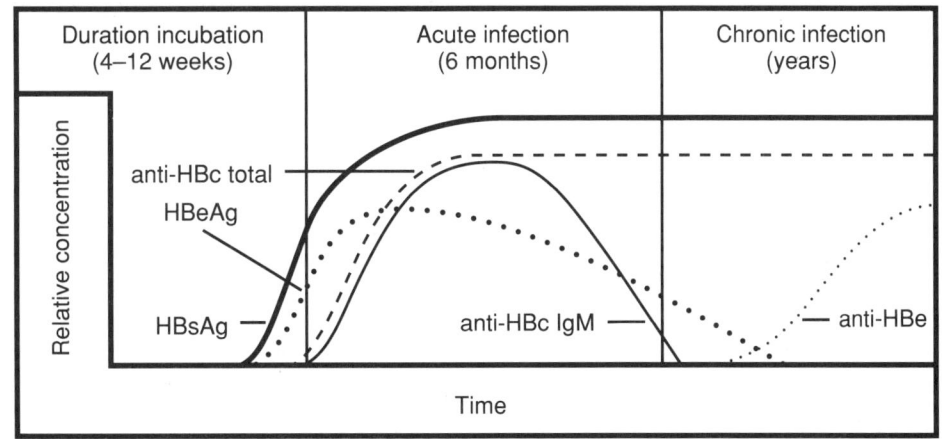

Fig. 29-3. Serologic response in chronic hepatitis B infection with late seroconversion.

infection. It is common practice to test for chronic HBV infection with HBsAg during pregnancy, and blood donors are routinely tested for HBsAg and anti-HBcAg. When the prevalence of natural immunity to HBV is relatively high (8–12%), it may be cost-effective to screen candidates for vaccine with anti-HBsAg to avoid unnecessary vaccination of individuals who are already immune. Those who receive HBV vaccine and who have not previously been infected, produce only anti-HBsAg. Titers of this antibody tend to decline several years after vaccination although the significance of this finding and the need to periodically measure anti-HBsAg to evaluate ongoing protective immunity is unclear.

Hepatitis C Virus

Hepatitis C virus should be considered as a cause of chronic hepatitis when HBV has been excluded. A test for antibody to HCV is now available and can be used for documenting this infection in patients with chronic hepatitis. The interpretation requires that the clinical findings be consistent with viral hepatitis, because a very high rate of false positive results are present in patients with autoimmune hepatitis, presumably caused by cross-reacting antibodies. The disappearance of anti-HCV during disease remission suggests an initial false positive result. A radioimmunoblot assay can be performed in reference laboratories to improve the test's specificity when the interpretation is uncertain. In acute HCV infection, the anti-HCV test may be negative in the early stages. Serial testing and rising titers of anti-HCV help establish the correct diagnosis. The presence of anti-HCV in an otherwise healthy adult is being seen with greater frequency as this test is used to screen blood donors. The finding is not specific and diagnostic possibilities include subclinical acute or chronic infection, immunity, or a false positive result.

Hepatitis Delta Virus

Hepatitis delta virus is a defective virus that infects only patients who are also infected with HBV. It may be transmitted simultaneously with HBV as a coinfection or separately as a superinfection in patients already infected with HBV. The infection is confined primarily to parenteral drug users, in persons from geographic areas with high endemic rates of HBV infection, or in households where one member is infected with HDV. Evidence for HDV infection is found in one-third to one-half of fulminant viral HBV cases. It is therefore appropriate to test for HDV infection in this circumstance.

Diagnosis of HDV infection involves detection of the δ antigen (HDAg) or antibody to the δ antigen in the patient's serum. Coinfection of HBV and HDV may be differentiated from HDV superinfection of a chronic HBV infected individual by using the anti-HBcAg IgM antibody test; in coinfection, the IgM anti-HBcAg will be positive whereas it will be negative in cases of HDV superinfection.

In some instances of acute infectious hepatitis, it may be necessary to extend the differential diagnosis to consider serologic testing for other etiologic agents including EBV, CMV, or nonviral etiologies (Q fever, syphilis, leptospirosis, toxoplasmosis). Acute hepatitis caused by EBV or CMV is frequently associated with symptoms of infectious mononucleosis and splenomegaly.

Test: Herpes Simplex Virus

Infections with HSV type 1 or type 2 are relatively common worldwide. Serologic studies indicate that most persons have been infected with HSV by the time they are 20 years old. Therefore, a single positive test for IgG antibody against HSV is of no value in diagnosing a current infection; however, it may be used to establish immune status. Only paired, acute, and convalescent sera to demonstrate seroconversion provide evidence of primary acute HSV infection. Many different types of tests are available including EIA, NT, CF, and passive hemagglutination.

Infection with either HSV type 1 or 2 leads to production of IgG and IgM antibodies to the heterologous virus type as well as to the specific infecting serotype. Procedures using purified antigens (gG1 and gG2) are available for differentiating between HSV types 1 and 2. Indications for distinguishing between HSV type 1 or 2 include genital infection where recurrence is more likely to occur with HSV-2 and perhaps in neonatal infections. In most other circumstances, knowledge of the specific serotype is of little clinical consequence and confirmation of HSV infection by culture or direct examination without establishing serotype is sufficient. Latent infection with either HSV-1 or HSV-2 occurs in most persons after primary infection and may lead to recurrent disease. Recurrences, especially when they occur as multiple episodes, may not lead to rising IgG antibody levels or to detectable production of an IgM-specific antibody response. Cross-reactions between HSV and varicella-zoster virus (VZV) have been reported. Persons previously infected with HSV who subsequently become infected with VZV may demonstrate a rise in antibody titer to HSV as well as to VZV.

The reciprocal also is true. A more pronounced rise in antibody titer is generally associated with the current infectious agent.

In cases in which a clinical impression of a vesicular rash suggests HSV infection, direct examination and culture of the specimen is the most rewarding diagnostic test (see Ch. 25). Serologic testing has a limited role in the diagnosis. Even though a rising titer suggests primary infection, this finding also may be present in early recurrences. Tests for IgM-specific antibody are available, but are likewise not always reliable for separating acute from recurrent infections. Testing for IgM specific anti-HSV, however, is useful for the diagnosis of infection in the neonatal period.

Test: Human Immunodeficiency Virus (HIV)[20,21]

Infection with HIV-1 causes the acquired immunodeficiency syndrome (AIDS). The mode of transmission, via contact with blood and body fluids from infected individuals, is similar to that of HBV, although the virus is not as highly infectious. HIV-1 infection is relatively prevalent in homosexual men, parenteral drug abusers, and hemophiliacs. Initially, HIV-1 infection may be occult or may present with acute, but transient illness, characterized by fever, malaise, anorexia, pharyngitis, and rash. Infection usually progresses slowly during which there is an asymptomatic (but infective) carrier period that may last for many years. Common findings of early disease include a persistent generalized lymphadenopathy and constitutional ailments such as weight loss, diarrhea, fatigue, and intermittent low grade fevers. Eventually the patient develops manifestations of the syndrome that are related to worsening immunosuppression caused by a selective depletion of T-helper/inducer lymphocytes and neuropsychiatric disorders from brain involvement. Opportunistic infections such as oral candidiasis and *Pneumocystis carinii* pneumonia may be the first manifestation of disease.

The patient often seeks medical attention when there is suspicion of HIV-1 exposure or when early symptoms develop. A sensitive test (EIA or particle agglutination assay) to detect antibodies to the virus is the initial procedure to evaluate patients suspected of having HIV-1 infection. When positive, results must be confirmed by a second, more specific test (Western blot), because the implications of this diagnosis demand verification with a high degree of specificity. T-helper and T-suppressor cell lymphocytes should be serially enumerated in patients with confirmed HIV-1 infection to assess the degree of immunosuppression and as a prognostic indicator (see Ch. 30). Viral cultures and tests for viral proteins or nucleic acids are generally not helpful except for special cases. Human immunodeficiency virus DNA by PCR or HIV-1 core antigen p24 can be detected in patients with early infections. A few weeks to months after infection the core antigen disappears while antibodies (anti-p24 and anti-gp41) rise. In the latter stages of disease, the p24 antigen rises and its antibody declines (Fig. 29-4). This development generally portends a poor prognosis. Procedures to detect p24 antigen or HIV-1 DNA may be useful for the diagnosis of perinatal infections, additional evaluation of an indeterminate confirmatory test, or confirmation of a negative result in the patient with an impaired humoral immunity. In particular, the use of PCR technology to detect HIV-1 DNA in circulating white blood cells is the most effective procedure for the diagnosis of HIV-1 infection in infants born to infected mothers, because maternal antibodies may be present in the blood of a noninfected infant for at least 1 year. The value of using PCR or HIV-1 antigen tests in routine clinical practice for other reasons, such as early diagnosis (before seroconversion), is yet to be determined.

Enzyme immunoassays and particle agglutination assays for HIV-1 antibody detection use either whole viral lysates or specific recombinant or synthetic peptide antigens. Although the specificity of these assays is extremely high (more than 99.8%), the predictive value may nevertheless be very low when used for screening populations with a low prevalence of infection. For ex-

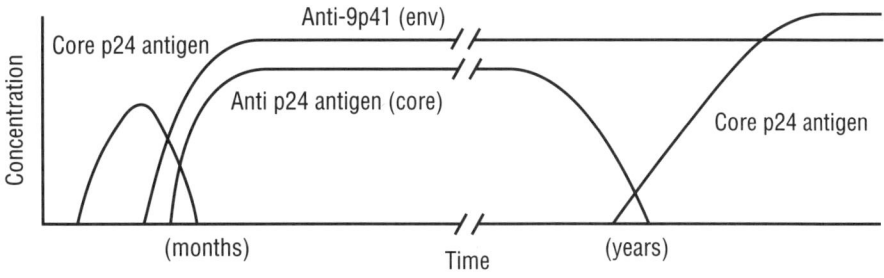

Fig. 29-4. Serologic response in human immunodeficiency virus type 1 infection.

ample, less than 10% of blood donors who test positive with the immunoassay test are truly infected with HIV-1. The Western blot test is used to identify which specific anti-HIV-1 antibodies (if any) reacted with the screening test's antigens. This test is performed by adding the patient's serum to a partially purified whole viral lysate that has been separated by electrophoresis and transferred by electroblotting to nitrocellulose paper. The presence of specific antibody combining with any of the separated viral proteins is detected by addition of an enzyme-conjugated antihuman immunoglobulin reagent. Up to 10 different bands may be seen. The most important ones include those corresponding to the envelope (gp41, gp120, gp160) and core (gp24) proteins. The gp120 and gp160 bands tend to migrate together and are difficult to differentiate. They must therefore be considered as one band (gp120/160) when interpreting the test. A positive test result requires two or three of the proteins to react with the patient's serum. A single positive band is interpreted as indeterminate, and a negative result requires the absence of any reactivity. This interpretation is recommended by the CDC, although slightly different criteria have been used by others. Two other confirmatory methods (indirect immunofluorescence and radioimmunoprecipitation) have been described, which compare well with the Western blot, but are not commercially available.

Test: Human T-Cell Lymphotropic Virus Type 1 (HTLV-1)

Infection with HTLV-1 is common in Southern Japan and the Caribbean, but at this time it is rarely seen in the United States, except among intravenous drug abusers. As with HIV, this retrovirus is transmitted by exposure to infected blood and body fluids. Although usually benign and asymptomatic, a small proportion (1–2%) of patients will develop T-cell leukemia/lymphoma (ATL) or tropical spastic paraparesis (TSP) myelopathy several decades after infection. The neurologic illness is characterized by gait disturbances, spasticity, hyperreflexia, and urinary incontinence. An EIA is available to detect antibody to HTLV-1. The test may be used for differentiating ATL from other overlapping T-cell lymphoproliferative disorders or when symptoms of TSP HTLV-1 associated myelopathy is suspected. The test also is used to screen blood donors for HTLV-1 infection. Positive results should be confirmed by a Western immunoblot assay. This procedure cannot distinguish HTLV-1 from HTLV-2 specific antibodies, although this can be done by a recently developed PCR method. The clinical significance (if any) of HTLV-2 infection is unclear at this time.

Test: Infectious Mononucleosis

See under Test: Epstein-Barr Virus.

Test: Influenza

See under Test: Respiratory Infections.

Test: Measles

See under Test: Rubeola Virus.

Test: Mumps Virus

Because of the distinct clinical features of mumps, serologic diagnosis is usually not required. Fortunately, mumps has become a relatively rare infection with development of an effective vaccine. A sensitive EIA method for detecting IgM mumps antibodies is available. Nearly all patients will have detectable antibodies during the first week of infection, which tend to persist for months. This test is preferred over CF and NT procedures. Use of nucleocapsid antigen also eliminates cross-reaction with parainfluenza antibodies. Mumps antibodies can be detected in the CSF of patients with mumps meningoencephalitis. This can be a valuable diagnostic test when mumps is considered in the differential diagnosis of encephalitis etiologies.

Test: Parainfluenza

See under Test: Respiratory Infections.

Test: Parvovirus[22]

Parvovirus B19 infection is the cause of erythema infectiosum (fifth disease) in children and a flu-like illness in adults. The infection is nearly always benign and self-limited although a transient arthroplasty sometimes follows the acute illness. More importantly, parvovirus infection is associated with substantial injury to marrow erythroid precursors. Perinatal infections lead to fetal death in about 10% of cases. Parvovirus infection may induce red blood cell aplasia in patients with hemolytic anemia or other causes of increased erythropoiesis.[23] Chronic infection developing in the immunodeficient patient may cause a severe and long lasting anemia. The diagnosis is made by detecting a specific IgM response during the acute illness. More recently, a PCR method has been developed for detecting parvovirus DNA in serum, urine, or amniotic fluid. The test should be considered to document infection and rule out other etiologies in patients with unexplained acute red blood cell aplasia. The test is not needed in otherwise healthy adults or children with self-limited illnesses.

Test: Polio Virus

See under Test: Enteroviruses.

Test: Rabies Virus

Rabies is discussed in Chapter 27. The diagnosis is made by examining the brain of the suspect animal (when possible), and the patient's tissues (skin biopsy), and saliva for the virus. These services are available at the CDC and many state health laboratories. Serologic testing also should be done on suspected cases. Antibodies to the rabies virus, measured by IFA, can usually be demonstrated (in both serum and CSF) within 1–2 weeks after the appearance of neurologic symptoms. The test also can be used to test for protective immunity after vaccination of persons with exposure risks, although confirmation is rarely needed unless the vaccine recipient has a known immunodeficiency.

Test: Reovirus

See under Test: Enteroviruses.

Test: Respiratory Infections

Viral infections involving the upper respiratory tract do not usually require serologic testing to identify the etiologic agent. However, when infection progresses to the lower respiratory tract and other organ systems, or if infection occurs in a setting where persons are at high risk (e.g., respiratory syncytial virus [RSV] in a hospital nursery), serodiagnosis may be indicated as an ancillary test to direct examination and culture. In addition, testing for adenoviruses, influenza viruses, and paramyxoviruses may occasionally be used for epidemiologic purposes. In the midst of an epidemic, patients exhibiting characteristic symptoms of a particular virus are seldom tested. However, when the causative agent of the outbreak needs to be identified, it may be convenient to test acute and convalescent serum specimens against a panel of tests of specific viral etiologies.

Adenovirus

The human adenoviruses consist of a group of 41 antigenically related viruses associated with a variety of human illnesses including upper respiratory, gastrointestinal, and ocular infections. The CF and EIA procedures measure antibody responses to group-specific antigens common to all of the adenovirus antigenic types. The HAI and NT tests are specific for each individual serotype. Because of the high degree of cross-reactivity and ubiquity of these viruses, it is essential that both acute and convalescent sera be collected in order to observe the necessary fourfold rise in antibody titer to confirm recent adenovirus infection. Rising antibody titers to a specific adenovirus serotype other than an outbreak strain may occur in as many as 25% of adults. Therefore, isolation of the virus is the preferred method for accurate identification. Another problem encountered when performing serology for adenoviruses results from the persistence of these viruses. Infection with an unrelated virus may cause adenovirus to reactivate or directly stimulate the host to produce antibodies to adenovirus. Serologic tests may falsely implicate adenovirus as a cause of the patient's disease to the exclusion of other etiologic agents. This demonstrates the need to consider the overall clinical presentation of the patient when interpreting serologic tests for adenoviruses.

Influenza Virus

The group of influenza viruses consists of three major serotypes (A, B, and C) defined by their nucleoprotein or matrix antigenic types. Numerous subtypes, based on the hemagglutinin and neuraminidase components of the virus, provide further diversity. Serologic tests for influenza virus infection include CF and EIA for type-specific responses and HAI for detection of the specific subtype of virus. Because of anamnestic responses, HAI titer against more than one antigenic subtype may be detected, with the response to the previously infecting subtype rising faster than the response to the currently infecting virus. Even though acute and convalescent sera are necessary for serodiagnosis of influenza virus infections, the results of these tests will have little impact on management of the patient. Culture is the preferred method when a specific diagnosis is sought.

Respiratory Syncytial Virus and Parainfluenza Viruses

Serologic diagnosis of RSV and parainfluenza virus infections are most useful for epidemiologic studies. The tests should not be done in patients less than 6 months of age because of the presence of maternal antibody and failure of the patient's immature immune system to mount an antibody response. In addition, parainfluenza virus serotypes share some antigenic specificities with each other and with mumps virus, which may lead to heterotypic rises in antibody responses. The most reliable tests for diagnosis of these infections is either by viral isolation or antigen detection with immunofluorescence or EIA methods.

Test: Respiratory Syncytial Virus

See under Test: Respiratory Infections.

Test: Rotavirus

See under Enteroviruses and Other Gastrointestinal Viruses.

Test: Rubella Virus (German Measles)

Rubella is ordinarily a subclinical or mild infection, marked by lymphadenopathy and rash, unless it occurs during pregnancy. Infection of the fetus can be devastating, leading to multiple congenital defects (such as deafness, heart defects, and mental retardation) or intrauterine death. The primary applications of rubella virus serology are in determining the immune status of women of childbearing age, in the diagnosis of rubella infection in pregnant women, and in the diagnosis of congenital rubella in neonates whose mothers were infected during the first trimester of pregnancy. Procedures available for rubella serology include hemagglutination, LA, HAI, EIA, IFA, and CF. All of the tests are sensitive, and some are capable of specifically detecting IgM class antibodies.

The presence of antibody indicates prior infection with rubella or immunization and suggests the patient is probably resistant to subsequent rubella infection and risk of congenital infection during pregnancy. The serologic evidence of conversion from a previously seronegative to seropositive state or observation of a fourfold rise in antibody titer is diagnostic for a recent rubella infection. Immunoglobulin M serology for rubella may be positive as early as 4 days after the onset of the rash. This test is particularly useful for rapid serologic confirmation of infection in the newborn, as IgM antibodies do not cross the placenta. Another approach to serologic diagnosis of congenital rubella is the use of serial measurements of IgG antibodies during the first 6–12 months of life. A persistence of antibody or a rise in titer is expected in congenital rubella infection, while in the absence of infection, the levels of maternal IgG antibodies will decline over this period. Serologic testing is also important to distinguish between rubelliform exanthems that may be caused by other viral infections such as enterovirus.

Test: Rubeola Virus (Measles)

As with mumps, the incidence of measles is declining because of widespread vaccination. Although the diagnosis can usually be made reliably by characteristic clinical findings (cough, coryza, conjunctivitis, Koplik's spots, and distinctive maculopapular rash), serologic testing is required for confirmation. Verification of infection by serologic means is important because measles is a reportable disease and clinical laboratories are not equipped to culture the virus. Also, because the incidence of measles is low, it may be confused with other exanthems. Measles serology is also helpful in making an accurate diagnosis of atypical measles (caused by suboptimal immunity from use of killed vaccine), for distinguishing measles from rubella in pregnant women, and for evaluating the etiology of pneumonitis or encephalitis in the patient with compromised cellular immunity (AIDS, transplant immunosuppression). HAI and EIA (IgM-specific) tests are most reliable. Measles virus serologic response is not subject to heterotypic responses to other common human pathogens. Serologic testing on both serum and CSF is also of value for confirming suspected cases of subacute sclerosing panencephalitis, a chronic and progressive degenerative neurologic disease affecting children and young adults.

Test: Varicella Zoster Virus

Primary VZV infection causes chickenpox in children. Reactivation of latent VZV in adults is responsible for zoster infection (shingles). Most adults (90%) are seropositive for VZV, at the onset of symptoms (neuralgia followed by a unilateral vesicular skin lesions localized to one or more dermatomes), indicating previous exposure to this virus. This effectively limits the utility of a single serum specimen for serodiagnosis of recent VZV infection, unless IgM-specific antibody is measured. In situations in which one is interested only in determining the patient's immune status, a single serum sample is sufficient. The diagnosis of VZV infections is usually made clinically. Although uncommon, HSV and coxsackie virus infection may clinically resemble VZV infection. Serology is indicated as an ancillary procedure to culture and direct examination of lesions when the diagnosis is unclear in adult or neonatal infections.

The tests available for serodiagnosis of VZV include EIA, IFA, and CF. Antibodies detected by the CF test may decline to undetectable levels within 1 year after acute infection. This test is therefore unreliable for assessing a person's immune status. Specific antibodies detected with the IFA and EIA tests remain positive for long periods, potentially for the life of the patient. As noted above for HSV, cross-reactions between HSV and VZV have been reported. Interpretation of antibody responses to both viruses simultaneously helps account for false elevations caused by cross-reactivity.

FUNGAL SEROLOGY[24,25]

INTRODUCTION

Serologic documentation of systemic fungal infections has normally been less successful than cultural or histologic studies combined with clinical or epidemiologic evaluations in suspected cases. Reliability of serologic testing for fungal infections is predicated on availability of sensitive and specific reagents, as well as on timely humoral antibody production by the patient. Unfortunately, only crude fungal antigenic preparations have been historically available, and patients with immunodeficiencies may initiate delayed or poor antibody responses. Together, these characteristics have hampered serologic techniques in gaining widespread acceptance and have obfuscated their clinical efficacy for diagnosis of many systemic fungal infections.

A variety of methods exist for measurement of antifungal antibodies in body fluids. These range from the least sensitive ID and CF tests to the more sensitive LA, RIA, and ELISA methods (Table 29-7). Although less sensitive, ID and CF methods are usually more specific, whereas the LA, RIA, and ELISA tests lack adequate specificity and do not routinely contribute to clinical diagnosis of fungal infections. Decreased specificity is augmented by the availability of only crude fungal derivatives for antigens that cause enhanced cross-reactivity between antigenic components often shared by several fungal or even bacterial genera (e.g., the mycobacteria). The LA test method also is plagued by nonspecific agglutination of particles caused by large immune complexes (e.g., rheumatoid factor) or by the presence of high protein concentrations. Because of ease of performance and higher specificity, ID tests are frequently used for screening and positive results are confirmed by other, more specific methods.

Serologic diagnosis of nonopportunistic fungal infections (coccidioidomycosis, histoplasmosis, and blastomycosis) is more reliable than for opportunistic fungal infections (aspergillosis, candidiasis). Fortunately, an excellent antigen-detecting LA test exists for diagnosis of cryptococcosis and is discussed in Chapter 27. However, antigen detection systems are still either inadequate or to controversial for routine use in evaluation of other fungal infections including candidiasis. Serologic studies should be initiated only after ascertaining adequate reliability of the tests for suspected agents. Suspicion of etiologies should be based on clinical, epidemiologic, as well as historic data (Table 29-8). Specific tests are described below (Table 29-9 and 29-10). See also Chapter 22.

Test: Aspergillosis[26]

Precipitin antibodies against aspergillus are most frequently detected by microimmunodiffusion (MID) methods. Antibodies are detectable in less than 1% of

Table 29-7. Comparative Sensitivity and Specificity of Fungal Serologic Techniques

Test Method	Sensitivity	Specificity
Immunodiffusion	+(+)	+++
Counterimmunoelectrophoresis	++	+++
Complement fixation	++	++
Latex agglutination	+++	+
Radioimmunoassay	++++	+(+)
Enzyme immunoassay (ELISA)	++++	+(+)

Abbreviations: ELISA, enzyme-linked immunoabsorbent assay; +, least sensitive; ++++, most sensitive.

Table 29-8. Epidemiology and Description of Fungi Causing Potentially Severe Disease for Which Serologic Studies are Available

Fungus	Description and Predisposing Factors
Aspergillus spp.	Mycelial (mold) fungi; ubiquitous; opportunistic pathogen: nosocomial, generally immunocompromised host, chronic pulmonary disease
Blastomyces dermatitidis	Dimorphic soil fungus; in United States restricted geographically to southeast and central regions, especially associated with river and lake shore soils
Candida spp. yeasts	Ubiquitous on mucous membranes, some species found on fruit, etc; opportunistic pathogens: nosocomial, generally immunocompromised host, diabetes, broad spectrum antimicrobic therapy, indwelling catheters
Coccidioides immitis	Dimorphic soil fungus; New World distribution; in United States restricted to southwest regions, especially in arid lower Sonoran life zone
Cryptococcus neoformans (*Filobasidiella neoformans*)	Yeast; ubiquitous in soil, but often associated with bird and especially pigeon droppings; often considered opportunistic pathogen: various malignancies, predilection for central nervous system
Histoplasma capsulatum	Dimorphic soil fungus; worldwide distribution; in United States restricted geographically to east central regions, especially Ohio and Mississippi river valleys; often associated with bird droppings, and chicken, starling, or bat roosting areas

[a] Exclusive of fungi geographically restricted to areas outside of the United States (e.g., *Paracoccidioides braziliensis*).

the normal population, in up to 70% of patients with allergic bronchopulmonary aspergillosis, and in over 90% of those with aspergillomas. Unfortunately, precipitins are less frequently detectable in patients with invasive aspergillosis (especially in the immunocompromised host) and serologic studies in such patients are usually inadequate. Two or more precipitin lines of identity may be detected with any clinical form of aspergillosis; however, multiple lines are most frequently associated with pulmonary aspergillomas or systemic aspergillosis. Sensitivity is enhanced by testing multiple aspergillus antigens separately (including *Aspergillus fumigatus, Aspergillus flavus, Aspergillus niger,* and *Aspergillus terreus*). Nonspecific reactions may occur between a polysaccharide (C-substance) present in some aspergillus reference antigens and C-reactive protein that may be present in patients with certain inflammatory diseases. Such nonspecific reac-

Table 29-9. General Status of Serologic Tests for the Diagnosis of Fungal Infections

Clinical Disease	Serologic Test(s)/Comments
Aspergillosis	Serologies inadequate in invasive disease or in immunocompromised patients; immunodiffusion tests often positive in allergic bronchopulmonary disease and aspergilloma
Blastomycosis	Direct visualization and culture more helpful than serologies; complement fixation and immunodiffusion tests available but lack sensitivity and/or specificity
Candidiasis	Immunodiffusion test available but not reliable for differentiation of invasive disease in compromised patients; reliability of antigen detection studies controversial
Coccidioidomycosis	Early (IgM): latex agglutination, very sensitive, not specific; immunodiffusion, specific (replaces tube precipitins) Late (IgG): immunodiffusion, primarily qualitative; complement fixation, quantitative titers useful for prognosis and monitoring
Cryptococcosis	Antigen detection by latex agglutination more useful than detection of antibody
Histoplasmosis	Serologies most useful in chronic cavitary disease and least in primary or disseminated disease Complement fixation: more sensitive, but less specific Immunodiffusion: less sensitive, but more specific Skin testing may elicit seroconversion

Table 29-10. Sensitivities, Specificities, and Interpretations of Primary Serologic Tests for Fungal Infections

Clinical Disease	Test (Sensitivity)	Interpretation and Comments
Aspergillosis		
Allergic bronchopulmonary	ID (70%)	Precipitins in <1% of normal population
Pulmonary aspergilloma	ID (90%)	Increased (3 or more) lines of identity associated with aspergilloma or invasive disease
Invasive (systemic)	ID (poor)	
Candidiasis		
Normal host	ID (90%)	Sensitivity: 17–100%
		Specificity: 61–100%
Immunocompromised host	ID (poor)	Serologic conversion suggestive of invasive disease
Cryptococcus	Agglutination (poor)	Killed cell agglutination, not available commercially; antibody present in only 30% of patients with meningitis
Blastomycosis		
Acute pulmonary	ID (30%); CF (10%)	ID specific; CF titers ≥1:32 significant, titers 1:8 and 1:16 suggestive but not confirmatory
Chronic pulmonary	ID (60%); CF (40%)	
Disseminated	ID (80%); CF (50%)	
Coccidioidomycosis	LA/ID (IgM) (50% 1st week, 80–90% 3rd week)	LA lacks specificity; precipitins disappear in 2 months (10% positive by 5th month)
	CF/ID (IgG) (10% 1st week, 60% 4th week, 80–90% 8th week)	CF titers ≥1:2 significant; rising titers 1:16 and 1:32 suggestive of dissemination
Histoplasmosis		
Primary (acute pulmonary)	ID (<25% 2 weeks)	M + H bands adds specificity
	CF (60% 2 weeks)	Fourfold titer increase or titer ≥32 significant with compatible picture; many patients may have equivocal titers of 1:8 or 1:16 in endemic areas
Chronic cavitary	ID (75%)	Specificity of both tests best in areas not endemic for histoplasma or blastomyces
	CF (90%)	
Disseminated	ID (30%)	Only about 50% of patients are serologically reactive
	CF (50%)	Sensitivity is poor in immunocompromised patients

Abbreviations: ID, immunodiffusion; CF, complement fixation; LA, latex agglutination.

tions are eliminated by treatment with sodium citrate; however, lines of nonidentity also may occur in cases of aspergillosis. The latter situations are not diagnostic but suspicious enough to warrant further evaluation using batteries of aspergillus antigens as clinically warranted.

Test: Blastomycosis

In most instances (except a few cases of chronic pulmonary disease) the diagnosis of blastomycosis is readily made by direct visualization or culture of the organisms from tissue or sputum, with serodiagnosis playing only a small role. Although CF, ID, RIA, and ELISA methods have all been described, only CF and ID are routinely available and are more widely used, yet neither is overly reliable.

The CF test lacks both sensitivity (50% using mechanically disrupted yeast phase antigens) and specificity (cross-reactions occur against histoplasma and coccidioides). Use of a chromatographically purified A antigen increases sensitivity to about 70%.[27] Titers of 1:8 or higher are diagnostic if using yeast phase antigens, but only suggestive if using the general blastomyces pool antigen alone. The CF test may have prognostic value where increasing titers are associated with progressive disease.

The ID test is both more sensitive (70–80%) and more specific (100%) than the CF test if only lines of identity with the A antigen are considered as being positive in the former. Thus, positive ID tests are diagnostic of blastomycosis and may be used to confirm questionable CF studies. Negative ID tests do not, however, eliminate possibility of infection. Studies using RIA methods have been shown to be quite sensitive (90%), but have poor specificity and are not readily adaptable to routine clinical laboratories. Recently, ELISA was found comparable to RIA (good sensitivity, but poor specificity).[28]

Test: Candidiasis (*Candida* Spp.)

Several agglutination methods directed at detection of anti-*Candida* spp. antibodies have been described, including ID, LA, CF, and CIE. Of these, only the ID test is readily available.[26] Because sensitivity and specificity of serologic techniques in most reports have been inadequate, their value in diagnosis or management of deep infections is controversial. *Candida* spp. is often present as normal flora of human skin and mucous membranes; therefore, the significance of reactive serologies is difficult to interpret in an immunologically competent host when attempting to separate systemic invasion from colonization. In such patients, agglutination and CF tests are of little value, whereas the ID, CIE, and quantitative LA tests may occasionally be helpful in the immunosuppressed patient. Serologic evaluation for candida, however, is least reliable in the immunologically incompetent host.

Production of one or more precipitin lines in the ID procedure constitutes a positive reaction, with serologic conversion from negative to positive being suggestive of invasive disease. Candida serologies remain only adjunct tests for evaluation of febrile patients at risk for this infection. Their interpretation should be guided by other clinical and laboratory data. Recently, greater impetus has been given to diagnosis of systemic candidiasis by detection of antigenemia or other candida products in body fluids, rather than by detection of antibodies.

Test: Coccidioidomycosis

Serologies have been more useful for the diagnosis and prognosis of coccidioidomycosis than of blastomycosis. The most useful tests have included tube precipitins (TP) and CF tests. The TP test measures early antibody (probably IgM), whereas the CF test measures antibody corresponding with later appearing IgG. The more cumbersome TP test has been replaced by an ID test for IgM (IDTP). A sensitive LA test is also commercially available as a rapid screen for IgM; however, it lacks specificity and should be confirmed by IDTP or TP tests. A simplified ID test for IgG has been introduced as a screen for CF antibody. Normally, such screening studies are limited to qualitative evaluation, although quantitative studies have been described. In areas endemic for coccidioides, the CF test is usually reserved for quantitating the IgG levels for management, prognosis, and follow-up of patients in whom antibody has been detected by a combination of ID screening tests. Cross-reactions may be seen in up to 20% of CF studies when using mycelial antigens (coccidioidin) and in up to 50% when using spherule antigens (spherulin), but usually are at low titer. Such cross-reactions may cause interpretative problems in areas that are endemic for histoplasma and blastomyces, but rarely cause problems in areas endemic for coccidioides.

Precipitins detected by LA and/or IDTP screening tests appear in approximately 50% and 80–90% of patients (inclusive of asymptomatic or minimally symptomatic cases) during the first and second to third weeks of infection, respectively. They normally disappear after 2 months and only 10% of patients still have detectable levels by the fifth month. Complement fixing antibodies are detectable by both ID and CF in only 10% of symptomatic patients during the first week, in 60% by the fourth week, and in 80–90% by the eighth week of illness. Seroconversion may occur as late as the third month and asymptomatic cases may never seroconvert. In cases of minimal disease activity and localized involvement, CF titers remain at less than 1:8. Titers of 1:32 are encountered in less than 5% of self-limited disease, but in 60% of disseminated infection. Therefore, rising titers between 1:16 and 1:32 are suggestive of disease extension and potential dissemination. In disseminated disease, CF titers are a useful indicator for following disease activity during therapy. Quantitative CF tests also can be performed on CSF and cord blood, as well as on pleural, peritoneal, and synovial fluids. Studies performed on CSF are diagnostic of meningitis (when compatible with other CSF values) in 75–95% of cases.

Test: Cryptococcosis

The LA test for cryptococcal polysaccharide antigen is sensitive as well as specific and therefore the most reliable for diagnosis of systemic cryptococcal disease. In contrast, serologic studies for antibody are rarely helpful because only one-third of patients with meningitis have detectable IgG. Killed cryptococcal yeast cell agglutination tests have been described, although commercial reagents are not available. The test may be used in certain cases in which antigen detection studies remain negative but for which suspicion for cryptococcal involvement is very high. Use of the test for prognosis of clinical outcome has also been described. In this circumstance, antigen and antibody levels are measured simultaneously. Increasing antibody titers in conjunction with decreasing antigenic load are indicators of a favorable clinical response.

Test: Histoplasmosis

As with blastomycosis, serologic evaluation of histoplasmosis remains problematic. Cultural and/or histologic support of serologic results are in many instances necessary for confirmation and diagnosis. Reliability of serologic diagnosis of histoplasmosis depends on the clinical stage of illness (i.e., primary acute, chronic cavitary, or disseminated). Serodiagnosis is most useful in chronic cavitary disease (because of its less rapid progress) and least helpful in acute primary or disseminated disease. The most common serologic procedure used for diagnosis of histoplasmosis is the CF test using either yeast or mycelial antigens and an ID test that detects precipitin M and H bands. Recently, RIA and ELISA tests have been introduced, but are not yet readily available.

The CF test has the greatest sensitivity (70–95%) but the poorest specificity. A significant degree of cross-reactivity occurs with other fungal as well as bacterial antigens and a high degree of background reactions may occur in endemic areas. Complement fixation antibody titers greater than 1:16 may occur in cases caused by etiologies other than histoplasma and may even be elicited by recent skin test applications, usually within 7–15 days. Normally, fourfold CF titer increases or titers of 1:32 or greater are considered diagnostic of histoplasmosis in patients with clinically compatible disease. In the early stages of acute pulmonary histoplasmosis, the sensitivity of the CF test (with yeast antigen) is 20% after the first week of infection, 60% after the second week, and 80% by the fourth week. Test sensitivity is highest (90%) in the chronic cavitary form. Complement fixation antibodies against the mycelial antigens (histoplasmin) appear not only later but at lower titers. A CF antibody titer in the CSF of 1:8 or higher is evidence for histoplasmosis meningitis.

The ID test is less sensitive but more specific than the CF test. Comparatively, sensitivity and specificity for ID range from only 1–5% and 75%, respectively, and for RIA range from 50–90% and 95%, respectively. Conversely, in patients with other infectious pulmonary diseases, false positive rates for CF, ID, and RIA have been reported to be 15–25%, 2–5%, and 45%, respectively. Studies in areas endemic for histoplasmosis normally report lower test specificities than do those from nonendemic areas. Antibody levels detectable by ID rise more slowly after primary infection, with fewer than 25% of clinically symptomatic cases having positive titers after the first 2 weeks. However, the ID test may be useful in determining the specificity of a CF titer or in cases of anticomplementary serum activity. Precipitin lines of identity to the M antigen alone may indicate present or past disease or even a seroconversion to skin testing. Precipitin lines to the M antigen in combination with the H antigen (10–20% of time) is suggestive of active disease. Tests such as RIA and ELISA have been reported to be very sensitive (90–95 percent) but lack specificity (55% in endemic areas), thus significantly decreasing their usefulness.

The most promising new test for histoplasmosis is direct detection of the polysaccharide antigen in urine by RIA or EIA. This test is reported to be over 90% sensitive and appears at the earliest stages of infection. It is particularly valuable in immunocompromised patients with disseminated disease who may be unable to mount an adequate humoral response.

PARASITIC SEROLOGY

INTRODUCTION

Serologic studies are an important adjunct in the clinical evaluation for certain parasitic infections, especially when routine examination of stool or blood would be ineffective or more invasive techniques are required.[29] Some of the more common parasitic infections for which routine parasitologic examination of stool or blood would fail to make the diagnosis are shown in Table 29-11 and include extraintestinal amebiasis, toxoplasmosis, cysticercosis, toxocariasis, trichinosis, leishmaniasis, and echinococcosis. Other parasitic diseases that may be undetectable by standard techniques either because of light infection or lim-

Table 29-11. Parasitic Diseases for Which Serologies Have Demonstrated Clinical Utility and are Available From Public Health, Hospital, or Commercial Laboratories

	Common Methodologies
Protozoan diseases	
Amebiasis	DD, EIA, IHA
Chagas disease	CF, EIA, IFA, IHA
Leishmaniasis	CF, DA, IFA
Malaria	IFA
Toxoplasmosis	DA, EIA, IHA
Helminthic Diseases	
Trichinosis	BF, EIA, IHA
Toxocariasis	EIA
Strongyloidiasis	EIA, IHA
Filariasis	IHA
Cysticercosis	EIA, IHA
Echinococcosis	IHA, IEP or DD (arc-5)
Schistosomiasis	EIA, IFA
Paragonimiasis	CF, EIA

Abbreviations: DA, direct agglutination; DD, double diffusion; EIA, enzyme immunoassay; IHA, indirect hemagglutination; CF, complement fixation; IFA, indirect fluorescent antibody; BF, bentonite flocculation; IEP, immunoelectrophoresis.

ited infection in partially immune patients include Chagas disease, filariasis, malaria, strongyloidiasis, schistosomiasis, and paragonimiasis.

Many of the antigen separations used in parasitic serology tests are crude homogenates of whole organisms, and significant cross-reactivities may occur with other diseases, parasitic or otherwise. This is especially problematic when testing for a specific helminthic disease in areas where a number of parasites are endemic and patients are commonly infected with several. Because of these drawbacks, the ordering physician must remain aware of potential pitfalls when requesting such studies and view results in light of the overall clinical evaluation.

Test: Amebiasis[30,31]

The diagnosis of intestinal amebiasis is usually made by demonstrating trophozoites or cysts in feces, and serologic studies are usually of little help. Serology is particularly helpful, however, in cases of invasive disease of the bowel, liver, and other sites, especially when symptoms of dysentery are lacking and stools are negative for the parasite (see Ch. 23).

Use of the IHA or EIA tests provide high sensitivity and specificity for diagnosis of invasive amebiasis (such as liver abscess). Ninety-five percent or more of cases of invasive amebiasis will have positive IHA titers (1:32 or higher) compared with 70% of individuals with active intestinal disease alone. Only 10% of asymptomatic cyst passers will be seropositive. Indirect hemagglutination antibodies may persist for several years or more after successful treatment, although IgM-specific antibody responses are helpful for distinguishing acute from past infection. Immunoglobulin M antibodies decline with successful treatment and can be used for monitoring purposes.

Test: Cysticercosis

Serologic evaluation for cysticercosis is usually performed as an adjunct to the clinical history and radiologic studies. Invasion of many different tissues and organs may occur, creating diagnostic difficulties. Both IHA and EIA studies are available and may be performed on CSF as well as serum, especially in cases of possible neurocysticercosis.

Serologic reactivity to cysticercosis is dependent on the disease activity and locations of the cysticerci. Both EIA and IHA are useful and are highly sensitive when there is evidence of meningitis or increase intracranial pressure. Testing of CSF as well as serum may increase sensitivity, with a positive CSF result being highly suggestive of neurocysticercosis. Although occasional false positive reactions may occur with either hydatid disease or *Taenia saginata* infection, positive test results are highly indicative of infection when radiologic or computed tomography (CT) scan findings fit the diagnosis.

Test: Echinococcosis (Hydatid)[32]

Routine noninvasive parasitologic evaluation cannot identify hydatid infection (echinococcosis) and serologic screening tests including IHA and EIA are very helpful. Detection of antibodies to a specific antigen known as "arc-5" increases specificity and is used in either double diffusion or immunoelectrophoresis tests on specimens that test positive with one of the screening tests. Aspiration of cyst contents should not be attempted for diagnostic purposes because of the danger of rupture and spillage of contents.

Hydatid cysts occurring in the liver tend to produce stronger serologic responses (up to 90% sensitive) than those in the lung or other sites (up to 30% sensitive). Once calcified, however, responses tend to diminish regardless of the site. Indirect hemagglutination remains as one of the more sensitive tests commonly used for screening. Positive IHA results require confirmation with the more specific immunoelectrophoresis or double diffusion tests that use the specific arc-5 antigen. Although cross-reactions may occur with cysticercosis, disease presentations differ widely. Cyst removal does not dramatically lower antibody titers, which may persist for years. The skin "Casoni" test, which has been used for many years, is nonspecific and lacks sensitivity.

Test: Filariasis

Filariasis is usually diagnosed from blood smears, skin snips, or from biopsy (depending on the species) where the typical microfilariae may be found. Serologic tests are of value primarily for individuals who do not reside in endemic areas, but who may have been exposed during travels. Difficulty in detecting filarial infections in humans has long been recognized and has stimulated the search for more useful serologic tests. Unfortunately, antigen preparations to date have been highly cross-reactive between filariae, other nematodes, and trematodes, which have lessened their clinical usefulness. The tests currently in use, including IHA, are unable to distinguish between the various species infecting humans nor can they determine the age of the infection.

Test: Leishmaniasis

Cutaneous or visceral leishmaniasis may be diagnosed by demonstrating organisms in stained smears, tissue sections, or in cultures. Serologic studies should be included when these methods fail to make the diagnosis in suspected cases or when more invasive procedures, such as splenic puncture, would be considered. Use of the Montenegro skin test has largely been replaced with serologic tests. Serologic testing is an important adjunct in the evaluation of leishmaniasis, especially visceral disease caused by *Leishmania donovani,* because it avoids the difficulties associated with biopsy. Unfortunately, antibodies may not always be produced and a negative result therefore may not be predictive. Cross-reactivity may also be a problem, especially in areas where *Trypanosoma cruzi* is endemic, and in areas where leprosy, malaria, and schistosomiasis occur.

Test: Malaria

The analysis of both thick and thin smears remains the method of choice for the diagnosis of all malaria species and should be pursued to best direct specific therapy. Serologic tests for the detection of malaria are available and may be of value in identifying cases of occult (smear negative) disease in presumed partially immune individuals from endemic areas. Most malaria serology testing has been used for epidemiologic surveys in endemic areas. Specific antibodies can be detected up to 6 months after curative therapy and may persist in persons with prolonged exposures and disease relapses.

The laboratory diagnosis and subsequent clinical management of malaria should always rely on species identification using blood smear evaluation. The serologic tests available are primarily used in epidemiologic screening and for identifying persons from endemic areas who may be smear negative (occult malaria). Species-specific IFA tests are available and help distinguish between *Plasmodium falciparum, Plasmodium vivax, Plasmodium malariae,* and *Plasmodium ovale.*

Test: Paragonimiasis (Lung Fluke)

Serologic testing may be of value for possible paragonimiasis (lung fluke infection) when either sputum or stool specimens are negative for the eggs, and clinical suspicion remains high. Both ELISA and CF tests have been described as being of use and are available. Sensitivity is quite high and titers are known to decrease with effective treatment. Cross-reactions may occur with schistosomiasis and clonorchiasis.

Test: Schistosomiasis

The diagnosis of schistosomiasis is routinely made on stool or urine examination, depending on the species. Frequently, eggs are shed in small numbers and may not be detected. Serologic tests may be of help and can avoid more invasive procedures such as rectal or hepatic biopsy. ELISA tests are most commonly available, although some sources offer IFA tests. A variety of antigen preparations have been used in serologic assays, which have varying degrees of sensitivity and specificity. Most tests available use either the IFA or EIA technique and offer high sensitivity. Specificity tends to be low, however, because of cross-reactions with other helminths, including nematodes. Intensity of serologic responses does not correlate with severity of disease and chronically infected individuals may be seronegative.

Test: Strongyloidiasis

The diagnosis of strongyloidiasis is usually made by stool examination and culture, duodenal aspiration, or string test. Unfortunately, light infections may not always be detected by these methods and serologic tests, usually EIA, may be of help.[33] Testing is especially appropriate for persons who will undergo immunosuppression for any reason and have a relevant geographic and/or clinical history. Enzyme immunoassay and IHA methods are commonly used with good results, although sensitivity of the test is partially dependent on the extent of tissue invasion. Cross-reactions with other nematode infections may occasionally occur giving false positive results.

Test: Toxocariasis

The diagnosis of toxocariasis (visceral larva migrans) is often made with great difficulty and requires careful examination of clinical and laboratory data, including serology (see Ch. 23).[34] The EIA procedure, which uses excretory-secretory products harvested from cultured *Toxocara* larvae for the antigen, is the method of choice for diagnosing visceral larva migrans. Because the clinical syndrome is often vague, a combination of laboratory studies are used to assist in the diagnosis. Interpretation of positive serologies must be carefully considered as asymptomatic *Toxocara* infection is felt to be quite common. Up to 10% of normal persons have increased antibody titers. Sensitivity of serologies for ocular larva migrans is usually less than for visceral larva migrans and probably reflects a decrease in titers because of a longer interval between exposure and testing.

Test: Toxoplasmosis

Serologic studies provide the clinician with excellent support in the diagnosis of toxoplasmosis and remains the test of choice given the impracticality of direct examination or isolation of the parasite (see Ch. 27). In nearly all circumstances, tests should be requested for both toxoplasma IgG and IgM determinations to provide the optimal information for determining disease activity. Measurement of toxoplasma-specific IgG alone is of value primarily when screening for evidence of prior exposure, such as in prepregnancy or pretransplant screening.

Serologic studies for toxoplasmosis are usually the only useful way to establish a diagnosis. A number of different methodologies to detect toxoplasma-specific antibodies are available. The double-sandwich EIA IgM assay (also known as antibody-capture EIA) is recommended for susceptible pregnant women and newborns, because of its increased sensitivity and specificity. This test and the immunosorbent agglutination assay have largely replaced the older Sabin-Feldman dye test.

Tests that differentiate between IgG and IgM antibody responses have proven diagnostic utility and are especially useful in detecting both early and congenital infection. The presence of IgG alone usually indicates that exposure has occurred in the past. The presence of IgM and IgG or IgM alone suggests that the infection is of recent origin or acute. However, when interpreting these tests it is important to note that IgM titers may not appear in the early stages (first 4 weeks) of infection and may persist for up to 1 year after infection. Any IgM titer in a newborn suggests acute infection. Difficulties occur in interpreting results with immunocompromised patients, especially those with AIDS, because of altered immune responsiveness or the frequent absence of IgM response during reactivation of latent disease. Presence of rheumatoid factor may cause false positive IgM test results. Interpretation of toxoplasma serology results may be complex, and false positive results do occur, especially with the indirect IgM EIA. Careful consultation between the clinician and laboratory staff may be required to correctly interpret positive results.

Test: Trichinosis

Trichinella spiralis remains an endemic disease in most parts of the world where pork is eaten. Serologic studies are usually performed to confirm the characteristic clinical symptoms and not to diagnose acute disease. The bentonite flocculation test has been used for this purpose for many years and is highly specific. The use of IHA and EIA is now becoming more common and offers increased sensitivity as well as specificity. All of these tests are more sensitive than muscle biopsy.

Muscle biopsy remains the test of choice for the rapid diagnosis of presumed trichinosis. Unfortunately, sensitivity with this technique is dependent on the inoculating dose of larvae and amount of muscle sampled and is positive in only slightly more than one-half of patients. Serologies, including the bentonite flocculation test, EIA, or IHA, become positive early in the infection and are quite specific, making them important adjuncts in the diagnosis of the disease. When trichinosis infection is highly suspected and initial serologic results are negative, another examination should be performed after 1 or 2 weeks to detect a delayed response.

Test: Trypanosomiasis (Chagas Disease)

Serologic testing for Chagas disease (American trypanosomiasis) may be of significant help when suspicion of infection persists despite repeated negative blood smears. Trypomastigotes may often be detected in the bloodstream by direct examination during acute infection, but become scarce during chronic disease when either serology or xenodiagnosis is most helpful. The latter technique, although extremely sensitive, is generally unavailable except in endemic areas. This test is also used to screen blood donors in areas of the world in which Chagas disease is endemic. After infection, antibodies tend to persist for life. A positive result suggests that the individual is at risk for developing symptoms of chronic Chagas disease. Results must be interpreted, however, in light of the strong cross-reactivity, which may occur with syphilis, leishmaniasis, and *Trypanosoma rangeli* infection, three diseases known to occur in areas endemic for Chagas disease.

REFERENCES

1. James K: Immunoserology of infectious diseases. Clin Microbiol Rev 1990;132–152.
2. Gazapo E, Gonzales-Lahoz J, Subiza JL et al: Changes in IgM and IgG antibody concentration in brucellosis over time: importance for diagnosis and follow-up. J Infect Dis 1989;159:219–225.
3. Evans DJ Jr, Evans DG, Graham DY, Klein PD: A sensitive and specific serologic test for detection of *Campylobacter pylori* infection. Gastroenterology 1989;96:1004–1008.
4. Watt G, Alquiza LM, Padre LP et al: The rapid diagnosis of leptospirosis: a prospective comparison of the dot enzyme-linked immunosorbent assay and the genus-specific microscopic agglutination test at different stages of illness. J Infect Dis 1988;157:840–842.
5. Berardi VP, Weeks KE, Steere AC: Serodiagnosis of early Lyme disease: analysis of IgM and IgG antibody responses by using an antibody-capture enzyme immunoassay. J Infect Dis 1988;158:754–760.
6. Steere AC, Berardi VP, Weeks KE et al: Evaluation of the intrathecal antibody response to *Borrelia burgdorferi* as a diagnostic test for Lyme neuroborreliosis. J Infect Dis 1990;161:1203–1209.
7. Magnarelli LA, Anderson JF, Johnson RC: Cross-reactivity in serological tests for Lyme disease and other spirochetal infections. J Infect Dis 1987;156:183–188.
8. Gerber MA, Wright LL, Randolph MF: Streptozyme test for antibodies to group A streptococcal antigens. Pediatr Infect Dis J 1987;6:36–40.
9. Larsen SA: Syphilis. Clin Lab Med 1989;9:545–557.
10. Haas JS, Bolan G, Larsen SA et al: Sensitivity of treponemal tests for detecting prior treated syphilis during human immunodeficiency virus infection. J Infect Dis 1990;162:862–866.
11. Lukehasrt SA, Hook EW III, Baker-Zander SA et al: Invasion of the central nervous system by *Treponema pallidum*: implications for diagnosis and treatment. Ann Intern Med 1988;109:855–862.
12. Smikle MF, James OB, Prabhakar P: Diagnosis of neurosyphilis: a critical assessment of current methods. South Med J 1988;81:452–454.
13. Fishbein DB, Kemp A, Dawsen JE et al: Human ehrlichiosis: prospective active surveillance in febrile hospitalized patients. J Infect Dis 1989;160:803–809.
14. Bryan JA: The serologic diagnosis of viral infection. An update. Arch Pathol Lab Med 1987;111:1015–1023.
15. Grayston JT: *Chlamydia pneumoniae*, strain TWAR. Chest 1989;95:664–669.
16. Lee SH, Charoenying S, Brennan T et al: Comparative studies of three serologic methods for the measurement of *Mycoplasma pneumoniae* antibodies. Am J Clin Pathol 1989;92:342–347.
17. Pochedly C: Laboratory testing for infectious mononucleosis. Cautions to observe in interpreting the test. Postgrad Med 1987;81:335–342.
18. Holmes GP, Kaplan JE, Gantz NM et al: Chronic fatigue syndrome: a working case definition. Ann Intern Med 1988;108:387–389.
19. Lee HS, Vyas GN: Diagnosis of viral hepatitis. Clin Lab Med 1987;7:741–757.
20. Schindzielorz A: HIV-1 serology and AIDS testing: a practical approach to understanding. South Med J 1989;82:1529–1533.
21. Burke DS: Laboratory diagnosis of human immunodeficiency virus infection. Clin Lab Med 1989;9:369–392.
22. Anderson LJ: Human parvoviruses. J Infect Dis 1990;161:603–608.
23. Kurtzman G, Ozawa K, Cohen B et al: Chronic bone marrow failure due to persistent B19 parvovirus infection. N Engl J Med 1987;317:287–294.
24. Penn RL, Lambert RS, George RB: Invasive fungal infections: the use of serologic tests in diagnosis and management. Arch Intern Med 143:1215–1220, 1983.
25. Davies SF, Sarosi GA: Role of serodiagnostic tests and skin tests in the diagnosis of fungal disease. Clin Chest Med 1987;8:135–146.
26. de Repentigny L, Reiss E: Current trends in immunodiagnosis of candidiasis and aspergillosis. Rev Infect Dis 1984;6:301–312.
27. Klein BS, Juritsky JN, Chappell WA et al: Comparison of the enzyme immunoassay, immunodiffusion and complement fixation tests in detecting antibody in human serum to the A antigen of *Blastomyces dermatitidis*. Am Rev Respir Dis 1986;133:144–148.
28. Lo CY, Notenboom RH: A new enzyme immunoassay specific for blastomycosis. Am Rev Respir Dis 1990;141:84–88.
29. Walls KW, Wilson M: Immunoserology of parasitic infections. pp. 191–214. In Aloisi RM, Hyum J (eds): Immunodiagnostics. Alan R Liss, New York, 1983.
30. Shetty N, Das P, Pal SC, Prabhu T: Observations on the interpretation of amoebic serology in endemic areas. J Trop Med Hyg 1988;91:222–227.
31. Healy GR: Immunologic tools in the diagnosis of amebiasis: epidemiology in the United States. Rev Infect Dis 1986;8:239–246.
32. Moir IL, Ho-Yen DO: The use of serology in patients with suspected hydatid disease. Scott Med J 1989;34:466–468.
33. Genta RM: Predictive value of an enzyme linked immunosorbent assay (ELISA) for the serodiagnosis of strongyloidiasis. Am J Clin Pathol 1988;89:391–394.
34. Shantz PM: Toxocara larva migrans now. Am J Trop Med Hyg 1989;41:21–34.

30 Diagnostic Immunology

Ernest S. Tucker III
Robert M. Nakamura
Mary Jane Hicks

Part I Humoral Immunology

Ernest S. Tucker III
Robert M. Nakamura

INTRODUCTION

The selection of appropriate clinical laboratory tests in evaluating antibody-dependent immunologic disorders necessitates a review of basic concepts of immune response and immune competence. Since the classic description early in this century by Maurice Arthus of the induction of an ulcerative skin reaction by injection of antigen into a sensitized animal, it has been apparent that immunoreactions can cause destructive tissue injury.[1] In recent decades, there have been many reports by investigators showing the role of antibody in experimental and human immunologic diseases. Such disorders range from allergic dermatitis to disseminated vasculitis. Many human disorders have been studied so extensively that identification of the specific immunoreactants involved in the disease process is now easily accomplished.[1] This chapter discusses an approach to the laboratory assessment of the integrity of immune function and specific tests to identify immunoreactants in human disease.

Review of Basic Concepts of Immune Function

Normal development of the immune system begins late in fetal life, continuing through childhood until full maturity is reached around the time of puberty. In the mature adult, the numbers of peripheral lymphocytes in the circulation and lymphatic tissues constitute the active cell populations of the immune system.[2] In the healthy individual, the most abundant cells are T lymphocytes, comprising about 80–85% of total cells, whereas B cells constitute about 15–20%.[2,3] The absolute (total) lymphocyte count in peripheral blood can range as high as 3000–4000/mm^3 during childhood, but in the adult the average is around 2500 lymphocytes/mm^3, with a lower limit of about 1000/mm^3.

A schema showing the major components of the immune system is illustrated in Figure 30-1. It can be seen from Figure 30-1 that the immune system functions as a servoregulated system with a negative feedback loop.[2] The initiating or input signal of the immune system is designated *immunogen* or *antigen*. This input signal prompts activation of the central processor (the lymphatic tissues), stimulating the proliferation of specific populations of lymphocytes that further differentiate into effector lymphocytes or antibody secreting cells. The lymphocytes that comprise the two major populations are the T cells that have matured through development in the thymus and the B cells that have matured in the bone marrow (bursal equivalent) tissue. These different populations of lymphocytes exhibit varied functions.[2,3] There is a notable diversity of function in immunoregulation exhibited by various subpopulations of T lymphocytes.[3] B lymphocytes are destined to differentiate into immunoglobulin-secreting plasma cells after antigen exposure.

Figure 30-2 shows the usual course of an immune response.[2,4] After initial exposure, antigen in the tissues of the host is phagocytosed by macrophages or reticu-

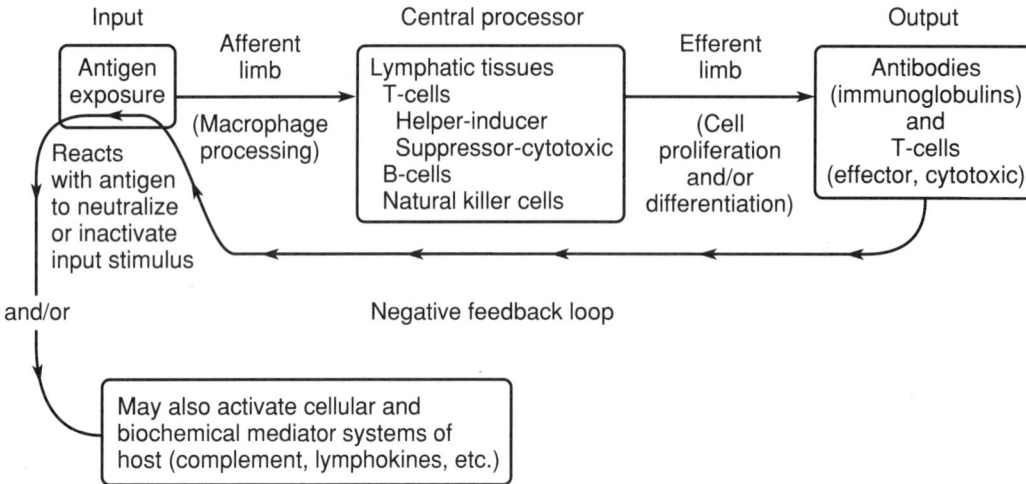

Fig. 30-1. Interrelationships of the major components of the immune system.

loendothelial cells. In these phagocytic cells, the antigen undergoes intracellular breakdown by enzymatic hydrolysis. After hydrolysis, the smaller fragments of antigen move to the surface of the phagocytic cell and are presented to specific T and B lymphocytes.[4,5] This presentation to T or B lymphocytes necessitates that antigen bind to specific receptors as well as matching class II histocompatibility antigens on the lymphocyte cell membrane.[4] Once antigen contact has occurred, cell membrane receptors on the specific lymphocytes are bridged, causing the individual T or B lymphocyte to undergo a proliferative response.[2-4] This proliferation leads to clonal expansion of the specifically activated lymphocytes.[4,5] Clonal expansion yields notable increases in the numbers of T and B lymphocytes reactive for the specific antigen. Subsequent exposure to the same antigen thereafter produces a heightened specific immune response. The immune response may be either increased secretion of antibody and/or proliferation of specific populations of T lymphocytes. The specific antibody that is formed can combine with the initiating antigen, which may be neutralized or inactivated as a result. If increased numbers of cytotoxic effector T cells result, they can contact antigen-laden target cells and result in either destruction of the target cells or granulomatous tissue response.

In these ways, antigen binding by antibody or effector T lymphocytes can initiate a chain of events that leads to cell damage, producing the tissue lesions found in the different immunologic diseases.[1] These lesions of immune reactions are largely caused by activation of cellular and biochemical systems of the host, such as complement and cells in the peripheral blood.[1] They play a major role in the pathogenesis of the tissue injury. This chapter focuses on those clinical laboratory assays that measure the specific immunoreactants of critical significance in major immunologic disorders.

BASIC TESTS

Test: Total Lymphocyte Count (Absolute Lymphocyte Count)

Background and Selection

There is normal extensive circulation of the various populations of lymphocytes through the blood and tissues of the body.[6] At any time, the total number of lymphocytes in the blood is in direct relationship to the total numbers throughout the body. The determination of total numbers of lymphocytes in the blood thus provides a direct assessment of the cellular immune system. A total lymphocyte count is used to ascertain whether there is a normal number and turnover of lymphocytes or an increase or decrease associated with a particular clinical disorder.[7] A total lymphocyte count should be ordered when clinical questions arise regarding immunocompetence and/or maturation of the immune system.[1,2]

Terminology

The universally recognized designation for this assay is total lymphocyte count or absolute lymphocyte count.

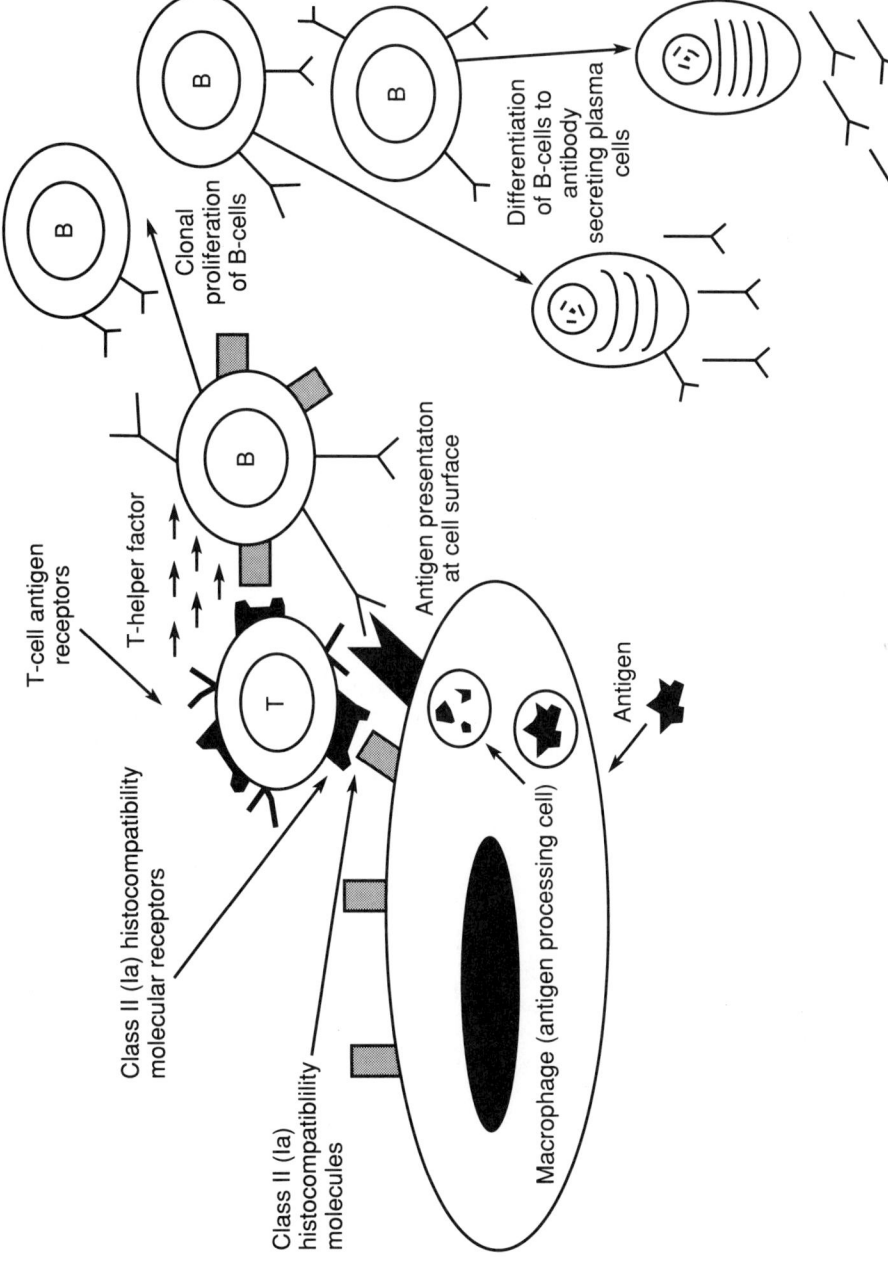

Fig. 30-2. Cellular events during the course of B-cell immune response. T, mature T cell; B, mature B cell.

Logistics

This assay does not have specific patient preparation or specimen timing requirements. The specimen procured for study is anticoagulated peripheral blood from either venipuncture or fingerstick and is stable for 4–8 hours at room temperature.

In the analytic procedure, the use of an automated cell counter is the common format for a total white blood cell (WBC) count and, in many laboratories, the newer cytometers can provide differential counts that separate the mononuclear cells from other types, giving an approximation of the total lymphocyte count.[7] Otherwise, it is necessary to do a manual differential count to determine percentages and calculate the total lymphocyte count from the total number of WBCs.[7] A manual count can be readily obtained by using a microscope and counting chambers, but the number of cells counted is substantially lower than in an automated procedure.[7]

Interpretation

The reference range depends on the age of the patient under study.[8] The total lymphocyte count in peripheral blood may range up to 3000–4000 cells/mm^3 during childhood, but in the adult the average is around 2500 cells/mm^3.[7,8] Deficiencies become suspect in childhood when the count drops below a level of 2000/mm^3 and in the adult when counts drop below 1000 cells/mm^3.[6-8] By contrast, disorders associated with immunologic stimulation may exhibit substantial increases in total lymphocyte count. When there is neoplastic proliferation of lymphocytes, the counts may be very high as in lymphatic leukemia and other lymphoproliferative disorders.[6,7]

Abnormalities in total lymphocyte count should be further evaluated to determine the lymphocyte subpopulations affected.[6,7] This can be done by techniques of specific lymphocyte marker studies, discussed in the following section.

Test: Lymphocyte Marker Studies (Lymphocyte Subpopulations, Specific Lymphocyte Quantitation)

Background and Selection

Studies of lymphocytes by detection of cell surface markers are used to determine the number of specific T and B lymphocytes in the total population.[9,10] Such studies aid in clarifying the nature of a decrease or increase in lymphocyte count by determining whether single or multiple clones of individual lymphocytes are involved in a disorder.[3,6,9] In immunodeficiencies, such as agammaglobulinemia, an associated lack of B lymphocytes may be found in addition to the deficiency of immunoglobulins. In combined immunodeficiencies, both T- and B-cell deficiencies occur. Other clinical disorders, such as a human immunodeficiency virus (HIV) infection, may be associated with clinical immunodeficiency caused by a selective decrease in T-helper cells (CD4). In autoimmune disease, increases in numbers of T-helper cells have been reported. This finding is helpful in evaluating a suspected autoimmune disease. Lymphocyte marker studies should not be used indiscriminately. The significance of the assay results must always be evaluated within the clinical context along with other laboratory findings (see Part II of this chapter).

Terminology

Until recently, various terms were applied to lymphocyte markers based on the antibodies designated by individual manufacturers for their detection. Recently, there has been a consensus among investigators to use designations based on the cell cluster of differentiation (CD) to identify a particular cell marker reactive with certain monoclonal antibodies.[3,9,10] In this way, common patterns of cell reactivity with different manufacturers' reagents can be expressed in the CD nomenclature that is now widely used. Table 30-1 summarizes the major lymphocyte populations by their CD designations and their relative numbers and percentages in peripheral blood.

Logistics

There is no specific patient preparation requirement for lymphocyte marker studies, but a number of factors relate to proper specimen collection and processing. Blood specimens should be collected in sufficient volume (usually 10–15 mL whole blood) into heparin, gently but thoroughly mixed, and rapidly transported to the laboratory for separation of the mononuclear cells from the other cells in the blood.[10] After the mononuclear cells are separated, they can be stabilized with certain reagents and reacted with fluorescein-labeled specific monoclonal antibodies.[9,10,11] They can then be stored satisfactorily for a number of days at 4°C before being counted either by fluorescence microscopy or in a flow cytometer.[12,13]

The preferred analytic method is to use a flow cytometer, because large numbers of cells (at least 10,000)

Table 30-1. Human Lymphocyte Populations by Cell Marker Designations

Cell Type	Cluster of Differentiation	Monoclonal Markers(s)	Normal Peripheral Blood % Lymphocytes	Cells/mm³ (Cells × 10⁹/L)
T lymphocyte markers				
Total T cells	CD3	OKT3, T3, Leu-4	56–78	660–2640 (0.660–2.640)
Helper T cells	CD4	OKT4, T4, Leu-3	32–50	410–1640 (0.410–1.640)
Suppressor T cells	CD8	OKT8, T8, Leu-2	13–38	250–1000 (0.250–1.000)
T and null cells	CD7	Leu-9	66–86	757–3028 (0.757–3.028)
B lymphocyte markers				
Total B cells	CD20	B1, Leu-16	8–17	120–480 (0.120–0.480)

can be rapidly analyzed, in contrast to the smaller number of cells (1–200 cells) analyzed in the more tedious manual method.[10,11] Reference ranges used must be appropriate to the techniques and reagents[9–11]; interpretation of the assay results should always be in relationship to such reference ranges. General reference ranges for the numbers of cells in specific lymphocyte subpopulations are found in Table 30-1.

Interpretation

Deficiencies of certain lymphocyte subpopulations may be found in association with specific defects in immune function.[3,6] Deficiencies of B cells are often associated with clinical agammaglobulinemia, hypoplasia of the thymus, and severe combined immunodeficiency also exhibiting deficiencies in numbers of T cells. An imbalance among different regulatory T-cell subpopulations (i.e., the T-helper cells [CD4] and T-suppressor cells [CD8]) has been described in various autoimmune diseases (e.g., systemic lupus erythematosus [SLE]) and in other disorders such as active progressive multiple sclerosis.[3,9,10,12] Abnormalities in the ratio of helper to suppressor cells (CD4/CD8) are associated with viral infections, most notably in infections with HIV, where there may be a striking decrease in numbers of T-helper cells (CD4) with normal numbers of suppressor T cells (CD8). In HIV infection, there is an abnormal ratio of helper to suppressor cells. The usual ratio ranges between 1 and 2.[10,12] These subpopulations of T lymphocytes are involved in immune regulation. Increased T-helper cell activity is often associated with an increase in the helper to suppressor ratio accompanied by either increased immunologic activity involving T-cell proliferative responses and/or increased immunoglobulin production.[3,10,12] By contrast, an increased population of T-suppressor cells with a decrease in the helper to suppressor ratio is commonly associated with decreased immune function in disorders such as acquired immunodeficiency syndrome (AIDS).

Lymphoproliferative disorders (lymphomas, leukemias) may be accompanied by an increase in certain lymphocyte subpopulations.[3,9,10] An increase in numbers of specific lymphocytes can be an important aid in the specific clinical diagnosis of leukemia. For example, in acute T-cell leukemias, total numbers of T cells may be significantly increased, whereas in B-cell leukemias, there is significant increase in B cells.[9]

Information from lymphocyte cell marker studies can often aid in the clarification of a problem diagnosis and is useful in following therapy after a specific diagnosis has been established.[6,9,10] The use of lymphocyte cell markers as a routine in the practice of clinical medicine is becoming commonplace.

Test: Immunoglobulin Quantitation (IgM, IgA, IgG, IgD, and IgE Quantitations), Quantitation of Immunoglobulins (QIgs)

Background and Selection

Quantitative measurement of immunoglobulins is useful in a variety of clinical situations that involve the assessment of immunocompetence and function, acute or chronic immunologic stimulation, response to immunization, abnormalities in immune responsiveness, and neoplastic proliferations of lymphocytes.[13–15] Increases in one or more classes of immunoglobulins can be helpful in the differential diagnosis of acute and chronic inflammatory, infectious, or autoimmune disorders.[18] As noted in the Introduction, immunoglobulins are one of the major products of the activated immune system.[5,17] Usual levels reflect normal functional relationships of T and B cells in the course of immune function. Quantitative measurements of the major serum immunoglobulins can be used to make a rapid and inexpensive assessment of the status of immune function in a patient.[13,14]

Terminology

The common terminology for these assays is *specific immunoglobulin quantitation,* or *quantitation of immunoglobulins* (QIgs), which usually refers to quantitative measure of the three major immunoglobulins, IgG, IgA, and IgM.[18] Occasionally, the tests may be referred to as *measurement of gammaglobulin levels* or as *globulin content of plasma* or commonly as *immunoglobulin levels.* These differences in nomenclature relate to the evolution of understanding immunoglobulins and their functional significance over the past four decades. Measurements of each class of immunoglobulin can answer certain specific clinical questions about immune function in a patient.

Logistics

Blood specimens for immunoglobulin measurements can be obtained at any time and do not require any special type of patient preparation or special timing for procurement. Assays may be performed on either serum or plasma.[18] The analytes are relatively stable at room temperature for 6–8 hours or for days to weeks at 4°C. They are readily preserved by freezing of serum or plasma at −20°C and can be preserved for very long periods at −70°C. Specimens heated at temperatures above 55°C will aggregate. The analytes will become denatured, losing considerable reactivity in analytic procedures.

The assay techniques in common use are based on specific immunoprecipitin reactions either in gel diffusion or in fluid phase nephelometry.[16] These are rapid and accurate techniques for measuring IgG, IgA, and IgM. Measurements of IgE are performed by radioimmunoassay (RIA) or by an enzyme-linked immunosorbent assay (ELISA), because IgE is present in only nanogram amounts.[18] In the nephelometric assay, substances such as lipids and microaggregates of protein can interfere with end point determinations but do not affect kinetic nephelometric measurements. In immunodiffusion gel assays, there are no interfering substances of major concern.

Interpretation

Table 30-2 shows the general reference range for each of the major classes of immunoglobulins. It will be noted that there is an important age variation for each.[13,14,16] The transfer of IgG from the mother to the infant accounts for a high IgG level at birth that rapidly decreases during the first 6–8 months of life. IgA and IgM are at very low or unmeasurable levels at birth, progressively increasing over the first decade of life until adult levels are reached. An adult profile is then maintained. Assay results of immunoglobulin quantitation should always be interpreted in relationship to the reference ranges of the laboratory performing the assays. There are sufficient variations in techniques and reagents to require each laboratory to establish its own reference range for these measurements.

Measurements of IgG, IgA, and IgM are used to determine whether there is a normal state of immune development and immune function in a patient evaluation.[13,14] Measurement of IgG is usually sufficient for such an assessment, because both IgA and IgM may fluctuate significantly over time in relationship to varied antigen exposure.[6] IgA tends to increase when there are infections along mucous membranes in the respiratory and gastrointestinal tracts. IgM levels increase with active acute stimulation of the immune system, such as in acute viral infections or recent immunization. IgG tends to increase over longer periods of time because of chronic immunologic stimulation. When the reference values of IgG are exceeded, the possibility of a chronic disease such as a chronic infection, inflammation, autoimmune disease, or neoplasm should be considered. Substantial decreases are found in a variety of immunodeficiencies,[13,14] most notably hypogammaglobulinemia (agammaglobulinemia), which can occur as inherited or acquired disorders. Adult levels of IgG below 300 mg/dL (3.0 g/L) are regarded as clear evidence of deficient B-cell function.[6,16] Levels of IgA and IgM below the lower limits of the reference range are also indicative of a deficiency in the adult. In a child, low levels should be interpreted cautiously, because of the variable delay in maturation of these components of the immune system during childhood development.[6,13,14]

Selective abnormal increases in any individual immunoglobulin should suggest the possibility of a neoplastic proliferation. Additional studies by electrophoresis are

Table 30-2. Quantitative Immunoglobulin Serum Level Reference Ranges by Age

Immuno-globulin	Infant Newborn	Infant 4–6 mo	Infant 12 mo	Child 2–3 yr	Child 5–8 yr	Child 10–16 yr	Adult
IgG mg/dL[a] (g/L)	1031 ± 200 (10.31 ± 2.00)	427 ± 186 (4.27 ± 1.86)	661 ± 219 (6.61 ± 2.19)	762 ± 209 (7.62 ± 2.09)	923 ± 256 (9.23 ± 2.56)	946 ± 124 (9.46 ± 1.24)	1158 ± 305 (11.58 ± 3.05)
IgM mg/dL[a] (g/L)	11 ± 5 (0.11 ± 0.05)	43 ± 17 (0.43 ± 0.17)	54 ± 23 (0.54 ± 0.23)	58 ± 23 (0.58 ± 0.23)	65 ± 25 (0.65 ± 0.25)	59 ± 20 (0.59 ± 0.20)	99 ± 27 (0.99 ± 0.27)
IgA mg/dL[a] (g/L)	2 ± 3 (0.02 ± 0.03)	28 ± 18 (0.28 ± 0.18)	37 ± 18 (0.37 ± 0.18)	50 ± 24 (0.05 ± 0.24)	124 ± 45 (1.24 ± 0.45)	148 ± 63 (1.48 ± 0.63)	200 ± 61 (2.00 ± 0.61)
IgE IU/mL[b] (mIU/L)	0.2 ± 1.3 (0.2 ± 1.3)	0.7 ± 5.5 (0.7 ± 5.5)	3.3 ± 15 (3.3 ± 15)	3.1 ± 16 (3.1 ± 16)	8.5 ± 145 (8.5 ± 145)	24 ± 370 (24 ± 370)	20 ± 190 (20 ± 190)

[a] Data from Stiehm and Fudenberg.[53]
[b] Data from Asser and Hamburger.[21]

necessary to determine whether such increases are polyclonal or monoclonal.[15] Monoclonal increases are characteristically associated with either multiple myeloma or Waldenström's macroglobulinemia.[15] If such diagnoses are suspected, studies of bone marrow, renal function, peripheral blood, and bone are indicated. In addition to deficiencies, immunoglobulin levels may be low because of either altered metabolism or pathologic loss of immunoglobulins, in clinical disorders such as protein-losing enteropathy or nephrotic syndrome.[6]

Measurement of IgD is of rare clinical import only in situations in which it is suspected that a lymphoproliferative disorder such as multiple myeloma is producing a monoclonal protein of the IgD type. Quantitative measurement of IgE can be helpful in the clinical assessment of allergic conditions of the hay fever type commonly associated with asthma, rhinitis, hives, or eczema.[18] At birth, levels of IgE are low or undetectable, as indicated in Table 30-2. Suspected allergic disorders in children are often detected by finding elevated levels of IgE during the first year of life that continue throughout childhood.[18] The measurement of IgE is usually reported in international units (IU) (1 IU = 2.4 ng of IgE). Children who have elevations of IgE during the first year of life at or above 60 IU are considered to be at extremely high risk (almost 100%) of exhibiting a major allergic disorder.[18] In adults, levels at 200–400 IU are associated with a risk of about 35% of severe allergic disease; persons whose IgE levels are above 450 IU commonly have one or more major allergic disorders.[18] Elevated levels of IgE must always be evaluated in relationship to the environmental and ethnic status of a patient, because individuals from countries in which there are problems in public health and poor hygiene frequently may have parasitic infestations that cause elevations of IgE.[18] Among certain ethnic population groups from Southeast Asia, usual levels of IgE are substantially higher than those found in the U.S. population.[18]

Test: Autoantibody

Background and Selection

Tests for specific autoantibodies are indicated in clinical disorders in which an autoimmune etiology is suspected.[19,20] Table 30-3 lists the many clinical disorders in which autoantibodies are implicated and in which their detection aids in clarification of the diagnosis. Autoimmune disease may be directed toward either a specific organ (organ-specific autoimmune disorder) or a constituent of tissue. That is, it may be more widely distributed through the body, such as antigens in cell nucleii in SLE, where there are numerous autoantibodies against the various nuclear antigens found in every tissue throughout the body.[19] Such disorders are known as *systemic*, or *non-organ specific, autoimmune disorders*. An assay for an autoantibody may be requested as a screening procedure in the course of evaluating a patient with nonspecific complaints. Caution must be used, however, to avoid inappropriate test selection or an indiscriminate request without adequate clinical suspicion of an underlying autoimmune disorder. These tests also can be helpful after a diagnosis has been established, because they can be used to monitor the effects of therapy, which often causes the level of autoantibody to decline.

Terminology

Specific autoantibodies are usually named by the reactive tissue target antigen (e.g., thyroglobulin antibody reacts with thyroglobulin; nuclear antibody reacts with nuclear structures, acetylcholine receptor antibody reacts with the specific acetylcholine receptor.[19,20] A list of the major autoantibodies is given in Table 30-3. In common usage, the autoantibody is named by first stating the tissue or constituent, followed by the term *antibody* (e.g., thyroid antibody). In some instances, however, *anti* may precede the name of the tissue, followed by the word *antibody;* thus, occasionally an assay will be listed as *antinuclear antibody* or *antithyroid antibody*, and so forth. Such differences in usage have arisen from common laboratory parlance over recent years, since autoantibodies first attracted investigative study. Only recently has there been an attempt to standardize designations using the tissue name first, followed by the term *antibody*. Increased levels of autoantibodies are generally associated with more severe tissue injury. Assay results are usually quantitatively expressed in titers or units of antibody.

Logistics

Autoantibody assays do not require specific patient preparation. Specimens of serum or plasma can be obtained and have the stability characteristics similar to those of immunoglobulins discussed earlier.[21] Specimens are stable at room temperature for 6–8 hours and in the refrigerator at 4°C for 2–3 days, frozen at −20°C for a few months, and stable for a number of years at −70°C.

The analytic techniques for measuring specific autoantibodies range from indirect immunofluorescent study of serum or plasma on selected target tissue to specialized RIA or ELISA using purified antigens.[20-22] Most autoantibodies are not species specific; therefore, tar-

Table 30-3. Essential Data on Human Serum Autoantibodies

Autoantibody	Reference Range	Assay Technique	Associated Clinical Disorders
Acetylcholine receptor	<0.5 nmol/L	Radioassay	Myasthenia gravis
Adrenal	None detected	IIF	Addison's disease (38–60%), adrenal atrophy
Nuclear antigens	Titer <1:40	IIF	Multiple systemic rheumatic disorders
Centromere	None detected	IIF	CREST Syndrome
DNA	<11 U	ELISA	SLE (high titers); other rheumatic disorders (low titers)
Epidermal	None detected	IIF	Pemphigus, bullous pemphigoid
Glomerular basement membrane (GBM)	None detected	IIF	Acute progressive glomerulonephritis
Histone	None detected	ELISA	Drug induced SLE
Intrinsic factor	None detected	Radioassay	Pernicious anemia
Microsomal (liver kidney)	None detected	IIF	Chronic active hepatitis with hepatitis B virus (HBsAg+)
Mitochondrial	None detected	IIF	Primary biliary cirrhosis (high titers)
Myocardial	None detected	IIF	Acute and chronic myocardial injury
Islet cells (pancreas)	None detected	IIF	Type I diabetes mellitus (prediabetic and early)
Parietal cells	Titer <1:20	IIF	Pernicious anemia, atrophic gastritis
Platelets	None detected	IIF	Thrombocytopenia, SLE, Post-transfusion
Reticulin	None detected	IIF	Childhood celiac disease (90%), dermatitis herpetiformis
Rheumatoid arthritis precipitin (RAP)	None detected	ID	Rheumatoid arthritis with Sjögren syndrome (20%)
Rheumatoid factors (RF)	Titer <1:20	Latex	Rheumatoid arthritis (80%), other rheumatic disorders (60%)
Scleroderma (Scl-70)	None detected	ID	Scleroderma (progressive systemic sclerosis) (20–30%)
Sjögren's antigens (SS-A/SS-B)	None detected	ID	Sjögren syndrome
Skeletal muscle (striational)	None detected	IIF	Myasthenia gravis with thymoma (95%), connective tissue disorders (low titers)
Sm antigen	None detected	CIE	SLE (when present, is diagnostic)
RNP (ribonucleoprotein)	None detected	CIE	Mixed connective tissue disease (high titers), other rheumatic disorders (low titers)
Smooth muscle (SMA)	None detected	IIF	Chronic active hepatitis (high titers), other liver disease and malignancies (low titers)
Thyroid microsomal thyroglobulin	None detected Titer <1:10	IIF IHA	Chronic thyroiditis (Hashimoto's thyroiditis, high titers); SLE, pernicous anemia, rheumatoid arthritis, and other rheumatic disorders (low titers)

Abbreviations: IIF, indirect immunofluorescence; ELISA, enzyme-linked immunoassay; SLE, systemic lupus erythematosus; ID, immunodiffusion; latex, latex agglutination; CIE, counter immunoelectrophoresis; IHA, indirect hemagglutination.

get tissue from a variety of animal sources can be used in indirect immunofluorescent assays.[19–21]

Interfering substances, such as nonspecific heterophil antibodies that react with components of animal tissue, may cause increased background in some immunofluorescence assays and there may be variability in the fluorescein labeling of specific antibody reagents used in the assay. Interpretation of patterns of immunofluorescent staining in specific target tissues requires special training, expertise, and appropriate controls.[21]

Interpretation

In general, the titer of a specific autoantibody will bear a direct relationship to tissue injury in the clinical disorder associated with the autoantibody.[23] In indirect immunofluorescence studies, results are usually expressed as a titer proceeding in twofold dilutions, a result is given as the highest titer at which a positive reaction is observed or as positive at one titer and negative at the next higher titer.[20,21] In ELISA and RIA, the results may be quantitatively expressed as amounts of antibody or units of reactivity. In most instances, reference ranges among a healthy unaffected population should be low or "none detected." [19-21,24] When autoantibodies are present, the suspicion of a particular autoimmune disorder increases when titers are elevated.[19,20,22,24] Careful clinical and laboratory studies should be undertaken to assess the extent of tissue damage by the disease. For example, in a case of high titers of thyroid antibodies, it would be appropriate to study patient thyroid function to determine the extent of impairment. Autoantibodies may be unexpectedly encountered with various clinical presentations, as it is not uncommon for autoimmune disease to remain clinically silent for a long period before it emerges with sufficient tissue damage to produce clinical signs and symptoms.[19,20]

Test: Complement Activation (Hemolytic Activity, Total Complement, Complement Split Products)

Background and Selection

A number of antibody-mediated immunologic disorders are associated with immune complex formation and complement activation.[25] These include rheumatologic diseases, gram-negative sepsis, glomerulonephritis, dermatologic disorders (bullous pemphigoid), and immune hemolytic anemia. Assays to determine complement activation are useful in diagnosing suspected complement-dependent disorders as well as in monitoring disease activity and therapeutic response. Confusion in selecting the appropriate assay for evaluating complement activation can be reduced by understanding the molecular events involved in complement activation, as illustrated in Figure 30-3. The most useful assays are those that measure activation of the classical (immunologic) pathway as well as the alternative pathway and/or activation of terminal complement components.[26] The availability of new assays for complement split products unique to specific pathways now permits a more precise approach to complement evaluation in a wide range of clinical disorders in which complement is suspected to be an important biochemical mediator.

Used correctly, complement assays can yield considerable information, whereas inappropriate selection can lead to increased confusion. For example, total hemolytic complement is often requested inappropriately to evaluate complement activation, but this test is best used to assess the functional integrity of the complement components of the classical pathway leading to hemolysis.[25,26] Total hemolytic complement is relatively insensitive to minor component changes that would indicate activation. The preferred assays for activation are those that measure molecular split fragments of individual components cleaved from the parent molecule during the course of activation. In assessing activation of the classical (immunologic) pathway, a sensitive assay is the measure of the ratio of the split fragment C4d to the amount of parent molecule C4, thereby gaining an index of activation.[27] Likewise, alternative pathway activation can be determined by measuring the amount of the molecular split fragment Ba from factor B as a sensitive indicator.[28] The activation of C3 can be determined by the amount of the split fragment iC3b in the circulation.[29] When split fragment determinations are not readily available, less sensitive information regarding complement activation may be obtained by quantitative measure of key components of the two major pathways. In the classical pathway, quantitative measurement of C1q and C4 may provide useful information.[26] In the evaluation of the alternative pathway, quantitative measurement of factor B may be helpful, whereas C3 quantitation may provide useful information regarding activation of one or both pathways. The quantitative component assays are most useful when there has been substantial complement activation with reduction of individual components below the level of synthesis. In such instances, the serum values will be near or below the lower end of the reference range for each component.

Terminology

The names applied to the various complement assays have evolved with improved understanding of molecular structure and functional aspects of the complement system. There is now uniform agreement on the nomenclature for individual complement components as well as the assays for specific component activation and/or function. Measurement of total hemolytic complement is often referred to as *total complement* or *complement by CH_{50}*, or simply as *hemolytic complement*. A request for quantitation of individual complement components is usually designated by the individual component, such as C3, C4, and C1q. In the case of the components of the alternative pathway, older designations may occasionally be used; for example, factor B may

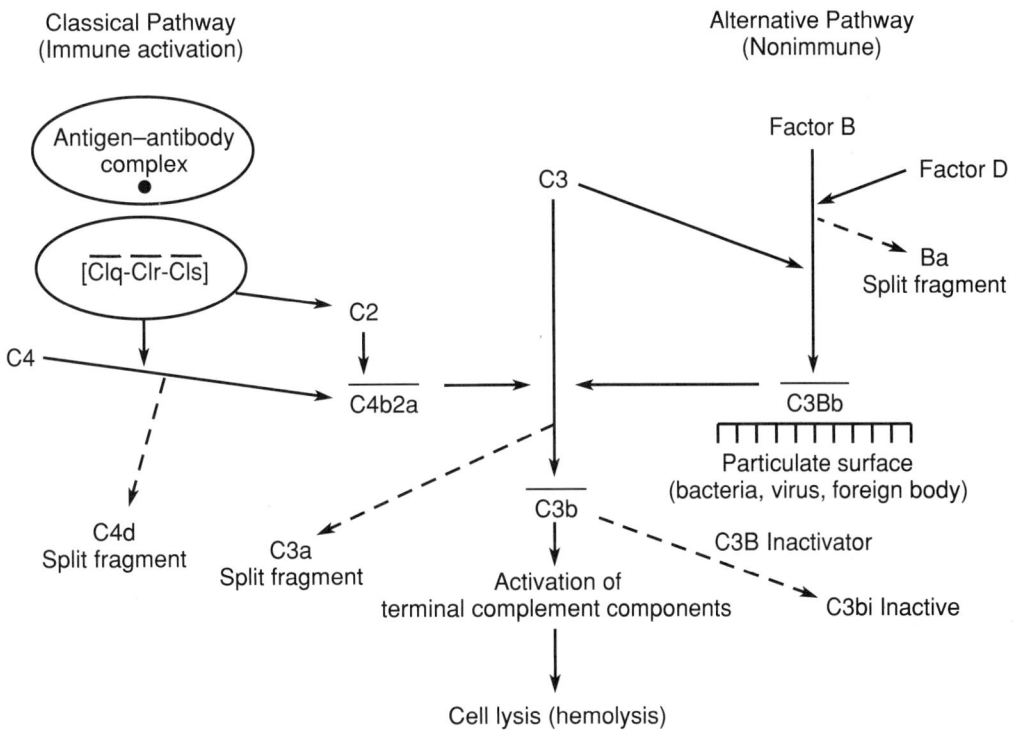

Fig. 30-3. Pathways of complement activation. Bar above symbol denotes activation (e.g., $\overline{C3b}$).

occasionally be requested as *C3 proactivator* or as *C3PA*. Recent assays for measuring split fragments are designated either by measurement of the split product (i.e., C4d) or as the ratio of split product to parent molecule (i.e., C4d/C4 ratio). Occasionally, these split fragment assays may be requested by the general term, *complement activation studies*.

Logistics

For complement assays, the most important consideration is an awareness of the state of clinical activity at the time a specimen is obtained for analysis. Other than this consideration, no special patient preparation is required. The blood specimen is collected into EDTA anticoagulant, and the plasma is separated within 2–3 hours after the specimen is obtained. Specimens can be refrigerated at 4°C or frozen at −20°C for short periods in order to ensure the stability of the complement components. Serum can be used in complement component assays if collected, rapidly separated, and assayed within 2–3 hours after procurement. Otherwise, there is considerable hydrolytic cleavage by proteases in serum activated during clotting. This may produce artifacts in the measurement of individual complement components as well as artifactual production of split products in the serum specimen. Plasma EDTA specimens can be stored for longer terms at −70°C in sealed containers, to avoid dehydration.

The total hemolytic complement method is based on the classic method of Kabat and Mayer, in which lysis of a standardized number of sensitized sheep erythrocytes by dilutions of the patient's serum is determined and the units of activity calculated.[30] The optimum point in the assay is at 50% hemolysis; the assay is therefore known as CH_{50}, to designate the units used in the assay. There have been modifications of the assay to simplify the measurement of total hemolytic complement activity. One such modification is the CH_{100} assay, an end point hemolytic assay usually performed in a gel containing sensitized sheep erythrocytes. The techniques for quantitation for individual complement components are immunoassays using specific antisera in either an immunodiffusion technique or nephelometric assay.[30] Measurement of split fragments has developed using highly specific antibodies, either monoclonal or those specifically prepared by immunosorbent techniques.[26-29] The assays are commonly performed in gel by immunodiffusion or by ELISA. Reference ranges for the various complement assays are given in Table 30-4. Generally, there are no major interfering substances in the techniques for complement component quantitation other than those related to limited specificity and/or increased cross-reactivity of antibody.

Interpretation

The measurement of total hemolytic complement activity provides a quantitative assessment of the functional activity of the complement components in the classical pathway.[30] When CH_{50} values are below the lower limit of reference range or at 0, the patient should be thoroughly evaluated for the possibility of an inherited or acquired deficiency in one or more of the components of the classical pathway.[31] Severe liver disease or malnutrition may depress complement levels by decreased synthesis. Increased catabolism of complement often occurs with diseases that produce circulating immune complexes (SLE, rheumatoid arthritis, viral hepatitis B infection, bacterial endocardicity, gram-negative sepsis, certain viremias, and cryoglobulinemia). Congenital deficiency may lead to agioedema (C1 inhibitory deficiency), which is associated with recurrent swelling of subepithelial tissues of skin, upper respiratory tract, and gastrointestinal tract or various manifestations of impaired host defenses, such as recurrent meningicoccal sepsis (C5 through C9 deficiency). A hemolytic level just at or below the lower limits of the reference range may indicate either increased consumption of complement components caused by activation or diminished synthesis.[26] In order to evaluate the individual components, specific quantitation should be done. The hemolytic assay is most sensitive to decreases in components C2, C4, and/or C5. In the evaluation of suspected complement activation, quantitation of individual components may be helpful: low C4 levels reflect classical pathway activity, factor B decreases reflect alternative pathway activity, and C3 may be reduced by activation of either pathway.[30] Decreases in the levels of individual components usually indicate activation when they fall to or below the lower reference range values. However, component blood levels may vary depending on the rate of synthesis and degradation of the individual component.

The most sensitive assays for measuring complement activation are those that determine the amount of specific split fragments arising in the course of activation.[26-29] These fragments are C4d cleaved during classical pathway activation of C4 and the Bb cleavage fragment from alternative pathway activation. C3 activation can be determined by the plasma level of iC3b, which is the inactivation product of C3b. Increases in iC3b fragment occur with either classical or alternative pathway activation of C3. A useful maneuver for evaluation of classical pathway activation is to determine the ratio of the split fragment C4d to the parent molecule C4.[3] A number of clinical studies have shown that this is a sensitive and useful technique with which to follow activation of the classical pathway.[27] The usual C4d/C4 ratio has a reference range of less than 1.1. Clinical disorders with significant activation may show elevations of 2–4; in severe cases, the ratio may rise to 7 or higher. Table 30-5 summarizes the directional changes in complement components and split fragments encountered in the differential clinical laboratory assessment of suspected complement activation.

Table 30-4. Reference Ranges for Complement Assays

Component Quantitation	Reference Range
CH_{50} (hemolytic)	60–195 CH_{50} units
C1q	14–20 mg/dL
C4	15–45 mg/dL
C4d	<8 µg/mL
C4d/C4	Ratio <1.1
C3	75–175 mg/dL
iC3b	<12 µg/mL
Factor B	12–30 mg/dL
Bb	<1.3 µg/mL

Test: Immune Complex (Raji Cell Assay, Immune Complexes by C1q Binding, Circulating Immune Complexes)

Background and Selection

The clinical indications for selecting serum immune complex assays are initially to determine whether they are present in excessive amounts in a patient with a suspected immunologic disorder or chronic infectious disease (see previous section, under Interpretation).[32-34] As with complement determinates, these assays can aid in monitoring the activity of a disease and response to therapy. They are not indicated as primary diagnostic tests but should be used as adjunctive measures in determining the severity of an immunologic disorder. Because many physiologic conditions are associated with transient elevations of serum immune complexes, it is necessary to confirm the presence of high levels by retesting 5–7 days after the initial assay.

Terminology

Many techniques have been developed for measuring immune complexes during the past two decades.[35,36] As a result, many of the currently used assays differ considerably in methodology and differ by name, but all are

Table 30-5. Changes in Complement Assay Results with Activation

		Complement Assay Component Quantitations						
	CH$_{50}$ (hemolysis)	C1q	C4	C4d/C4	C3	iC3b	Factor B	Bb
Classical pathway								
Activation	±↓	↓	↓	↑(>1.1)	↓	↑	N	N
Total function	N	N	N	N(<1.1)	N	N	N	N
Alternative pathway								
Activation	±↓	N	N	N(<1.1)	↓	↑	↓	↑
Hereditary angioedema (inherited C1 inhibitor deficiency)	±↓	N	↓↓	↑(>1.1)	N	N	N	N
Acquired C1 inhibitor deficiency	±↓	↓	↓	↑(>1.1)	N	N	N	N

Abbreviations: N, normal; ↑, significant increase; ↓, significant decrease.

directed at determining the quantitative levels of immune complexes in the blood.[4,5] The two assays most commonly used and suggested by the World Health Organization (WHO) are the Raji cell assay and immune complexes by C1q binding.[35,36] In the Raji cell assay, a lymphoblastoid B-cell line is used as a reagent to bind immune complexes through receptors for various forms of complement component C3 on their cell membrane surfaces. The C1q binding assay is based on interaction of antibody molecules in the immune complex with purified radiolabeled C1q, where the amount of binding is directly proportional to the quantity of immune complexes in the specimen. A finding of elevated levels of immune complexes by either of these assays, when confirmed by repeat testing, is regarded as a precondition for the systemic deposition of complexes in tissues throughout the body. Clinical disorders such as disseminated vasculitis, glomerulonephritis, myositis, and serositis commonly exhibit persistence of elevated immune complexes.[32-34]

Logistics

In preanalytic considerations, no specific patient preparation is required, but the timing of blood specimen collection should be when clinical symptoms and signs are most severe.[35,36] The specimen required for these assays is serum collected and separated as soon as possible from the cells of the blood to avoid artifactual binding of immune complexes to receptors on blood cell surfaces. It is also important to proceed to assay the serum specimen promptly within 4–6 hours; otherwise, it should be immediately frozen and preserved at −70°C, until it can be assayed directly after thawing. Freezing and thawing of a serum specimen will produce artifactual changes that alter the validity of the assay. The reference value for these assays will vary among laboratories, but the values in Table 30-6 serve as a general guide.

A number of factors can interfere with these assays and limit the validity of the results. These include improper specimen collection and processing as well as the presence of cryoglobulins, cold agglutinins, rheumatoid factors, and monoclonal proteins in the patient.[35,36] In the Raji cell assay, the presence of antilymphocyte antibodies and antinuclear antibodies can produce false positive results.[35,36]

Interpretation

The formation of immune complexes in the blood is part of a normal physiologic process of clearing foreign antigenic material from the tissues and blood. Such antigens may be infectious agents, breakdown products of tissue proteins, and/or foreign substances, including drugs. However, there are many conditions in which elevated levels of immune complexes may persist in the circulation for prolonged periods, especially in chronic infectious diseases and autoimmune disorders.[32-34] In such situations, prolonged high levels of immune complexes can lead to widespread dissemination and deposition of complexes in tissues around postcapillary venules.[32-34] This may happen especially in those organs in which there is a high degree of permeability in the vascular bed, permitting deposition of the pathogenic immune complexes. Such tissue deposits of immune complexes activate complement and are a focus of inflammation caused by an influx of neutrophils with their hydrolytic enzymes. Almost any organ or tissue may be involved by this disseminated vasculitis.[33] The kidney is often affected with deposition of complexes in glomeruli causing either acute or chronic glomerulonephritis, or both.

Because of the foregoing considerations, it is imperative that the results of immune complex assays be interpreted cautiously and always within the context of the patient's clinical condition.[32-34] The finding of an elevated value for immune complexes in a patient who has only minor clinical complaints or who is otherwise healthy should probably be viewed as a physiologic response to a transient unrecognized antigenic stimulation. However, continued high levels of immune complexes in a patient with evidence of a systemic disorder such as arthritis, myositis, serositis, or renal disease should be regarded as serious.[32-34] Additional clinical and laboratory studies would be indicated to evaluate the extent of tissue injury in such a case, especially in the kidneys, which are common target organs in immune complex disease.

Table 30-6. Reference Values for Immune Complex Assays

Assay	Reference Value[a]
C1q binding	
Normal	<13%
Borderline	13–16%
Abnormal	>16%
Raji cell	
Normal	<50 μg AHG Eq/mL
Borderline	50–100 μg AHG Eq/mL
Abnormal	>100 μg AHG Eq/mL

[a] Conventional units for the Raji cell assay are μgAHG Eq/mL; SI units are mg AHG Eq/L; the number remains the same as the conversion factor is 1.
Abbreviation: AGH, aggregated human gammaglobulin.

Part II Cellular Immunology

Mary Jane Hicks

INTRODUCTION

The usual immune response is a polyclonal event. Multiple antigens are generally involved in an immune response; hence the activation of multiple specific and cross-reacting lymphocyte clones, that is, B cells bearing diverse immunoglobulin heavy and light chains. B cells mediate the humoral immune response by differentiating into plasma cells, which then secrete immunoglobulins of the same class as the B-cell surface immunoglobulin (SIg). Thymus-dependent T cells mediate the cellular immune response (CMI).

The T-cell system is composed of effector T cells (e.g., killer T cells—not to be confused with natural killer [NK] cells) and regulatory T cells (T-helper and T-suppressor cells). The regulatory T-cell system is functionally heterogeneous and quite complex. As their names imply, the helper cells facilitate or induce T- and B-cell immune functions, and the suppressor cells down-regulate or suppress these immune functions. In addition there are T-helper cells that induce or "help" other helper cells and those that induce or "help" suppressor cells. Therefore, normal T-helper function is necessary for both facilitation and suppression of the immune response. Regulatory T cells exert a more general influence on many clones of lymphoid cells, whereas other regulatory T cells are antigen or class specific. These regulatory influences are mediated primarily by soluble proteins called *lymphokines*. Some lymphokines recruit, inhibit migration, and activate monocytes or macrophages, which then function as important effector cells of the CMI response. T4 (CD4) cells primarily mediate helper functions, and T8 (CD8) cells primarily mediate suppressor-cytotoxic functions (see Table 30-7 for explanation of terminology). However, there is no precise concordance between phenotype and function; that is, some CD4 cells exhibit cytotoxic function, and some CD8 cells function as helpers. The characteristic that most strongly discriminates between T4 (CD4) and T8 (CD8) cells is their differing interactions with class I and class II major histocompatibility antigens. The antigen receptor of T4 cells interacts with foreign antigen, which is closely associated with class II (HLA-Dr) molecules (on the surface of the antigen-presenting cells, e.g., macrophages). The antigen receptor of T8 cells interacts with foreign antigen that is closely associated with class I (HLA-A, -B, -C) molecules (on the surface of target cells, e.g., virus-infected cell). In many instances, lymphocyte testing sits on the border between proven clinical value (e.g., monitoring the progression of HIV infection in an AIDS patient) and clinical investigation (e.g., monitoring autoimmune disease).

Test: Lymphocyte Typing

Background

Primary disorders of the immune system fall into three major categories: (1) malignancies (lymphomas or leukemias); (2) immunodeficiencies (congenital or acquired); and (3) abnormalities or imbalances of immune regulation (autoimmune disease, hypersensitivity reactions). In general, lymphocyte typing is useful for differentiating between benign, reactive lymphocytosis and a well-differentiated lymphoid

Table 30-7. Definitions of Representative Monoclonal Antibodies and Their Respective Antigen Cluster Designations[a]

Antigen Cluster Designation	Predominant Reactivity	Monoclonal Antibodies
CD1	Thymocytes	Leu 6, OKT6, T6
CD2	E-rosette receptor	Leu 5b, OKT11, T11
CD3	T cells (mitogenic)	Leu 4, OKT3, T3
CD4	T-helper/inducer cells	Leu 3a, OKT4, T4
—	T-"helper" of inducers	4B4
—	T-"helper" of suppressors	2H4
CD5	T cells	Leu 1, OKT1, T1
CD7	T cells and natural killer cells	Leu 9
CD8	T-cytotoxic-suppressor cells	Leu 2a, Leu 2b, OKT8, T8, OKT5
CD10	Common acute lymphoblastic leukemia antigen	Anti-CD10 (CALLA), J5
CD11	T-suppressor cells, natural killer cells, monocytes, granulocytes	Leu 15 (anti-CR3), OKM1, Mo. 1
CD14	Monocytes, granulocytes	Leu M3
CD15	Monocytes, granulocytes	My 1, Leu M1
CD16	Fc IgG receptor on natural killer cells and neutrophils	Leu 11a,b,c
—	T-cell and natural killer cell subsets	Leu 7, HNK-1
CD19	B cells	Leu 12, B4
CD20	B cells	Leu 16, B1
CD21	B cells	B2 (anti-CR2)
CD22	B cells	Leu 14

[a] The Leu series of mAb is produced by Becton-Dickinson (Mountain View, CA). The OKT series of mAb is produced by Ortho Diagnostics (Raritan, NJ). The T series and B1, B2, B4, HNK-1, 4B4, 2H4, MY1, and J5 are produced by Coulter Immunology (Hialeah, FL). Additional myeloid mAb markers include My7 (Coulter Immunology) and Leu-M5 (Becton Dickinson).

malignancy. Either of the following findings supports the diagnosis of a lymphoid malignancy: (1) a predominance of one cell type (e.g., IgM-, κ-bearing B lymphocytes); (2) an alteration in the usual proportions or populations of lymphocyte subsets in the peripheral blood; or (3) the expression of an aberrant phenotype (e.g., T-cell marker on a B cell or variable expression of usual T-cell markers on a malignant T-cell clone). Lymphocyte typing is frequently necessary for the diagnosis and classification of immunodeficiency states, including the classification of congenital immunodeficiency states; for assessment of allograft rejection status or adequacy of immunosuppressive therapy after organ transplantation; and for detection of the selective decrease in T-helper cells in HIV infection. Finally, activation of an autoimmune disease (e.g., SLE) may be associated with a decrease in T-suppressor cells, resulting in an elevated helper to suppressor ratio.

Selection

The selection of immunologic tests depends on the clinical situation (Table 30-8). In addition to staining with monoclonal antibodies, staining for SIg is useful for detecting a monoclonal B-cell population. Also, terminal deoxynucleotidyl transferase (TdT), a nuclear enzyme found in immature lymphoid cells of both T- and B-cell lineage, is a useful marker for acute lymphocytic leukemia (ALL). However, about 5% of cases of acute myelocytic leukemia (AML) will express TdT in varying proportions of the leukemic cells. Staining for CD10 (or, common acute lymphoblastic leukemia antigen, CALLA) is a useful marker for common ALL (an immature B-cell form of ALL).

Logistics

Specimen Requirements

Peripheral blood can be collected in heparin, or EDTA can be used. Lymphocyte suspensions prepared from lymphoid organs (e.g., lymph nodes, spleen) can be stained by direct or indirect fluorescent antibody (FA) and analyzed by fluorescence microscopy or flow cytometry (see below). Similarly, lymphocytes from any body fluid containing a significant lymphoid population can be phenotypically analyzed.

Table 30-8. Suggested Lymphocyte Testing Batteries in Different Clinical Circumstances[a]

Clinical Category	Test Battery
Lymphoproliferative disorders	Surface Ig, CD19, CD20, CD22 CD1, CD2, CD3, CD4, CD8, CD7 TdT, CD10 (CALLA) CD15, Leu M3, Leu M5 CD16
Immunodeficiency states congenital or acquired	CD19, CD20 CD1, CD3, CD5, CD4,[b] CD8[c] CD16, Leu-7 Mitogen stimulation (PHA, ConA, PWM)
Immune regulatory abnormalities and miscellaneous conditions	CD19 CD2, CD3, CD4, CD8 CD16 Anti-HLA-Dr (Ia)

[a] The actual test battery used depends on each laboratory's experience with individual mAb, patient population, and potential research interests.

[b] 4B4 and 2H4 mAb can also be used if there is a clinical or research need to evaluate the numbers of "helpers" of inducer or suppressor cells, respectively.

[c] Leu 15 mAb can be used if there is a clinical or research need to evaluate the number of specific T-suppressor cells. This needs to be done in dual-labeling techniques with a CD8 marker because of the nonspecificity of Leu 15.

Abbreviations: TdT, terminal deoxynucleotidyl transferase; PHA, phytohemagglutinin; ConA, concanavalin A; PWM, pokeweed mitogen.

The stability of both the initial unstained specimen and the stained specimen must be considered. If there is to be any delay in processing a peripheral blood sample for lymphocyte typing, the whole blood specimen should be kept at room temperature in the initial collection tube and placed on a flat surface. Specimens can be kept this way for 24–48 hours before staining by whole blood methods for flow cytometric analysis. This allows for the transport of specimens to regional laboratories for testing. If mononuclear cell suspensions are to be made, the specimen should be processed within about 6 hours. After this time, increased granulocyte and monocyte contamination leads to a proportionately lower lymphocyte yield. A freshly prepared lymphocyte suspension in tissue culture medium (e.g., RPMI-1640) containing neonatal calf serum (10–15%) can be stored overnight at 4°C for lymphocyte phenotyping by manual methods.

The volume of blood needed to perform lymphocyte phenotyping varies with the method. For each monoclonal antibody (mAb) (or dual-label combination) used in the phenotyping battery for whole blood staining (either indirect or direct methods) and flow cytometric analysis, 0.1–0.2 mL of blood is needed. However, if manual staining methods on mononuclear cell suspensions are used, 15–30 mL of blood or more may be required, depending on the lymphocyte count. This poses obvious difficulties in the lymphopenic newborn or child.

Specimen stability may vary for different mAb reagents and for different methods. For example, specimen stability for subsequent indirect FA staining is usually greater than that for direct FA methods. The stability of the stained material is dependent on both specimen type (whole blood versus mononuclear cell suspension) and method of staining (indirect FA versus single or dual-label direct FA). Mononuclear cell suspensions and whole blood stained by indirect FA methods, including a final fixation step (2% paraformaldehyde) can be stored at 4°C for up to 1 week for flow cytometric analysis. Slides prepared for fluorescence microscopy and differential counting can be held for at least 2 weeks, but some markers may be stable for longer periods. Direct FA methods inherently result in weaker fluorescent staining than do indirect FA methods, resulting in reduced stability in the stained samples. Specimens stained by direct FA can be evaluated by flow cytometry (FCM) up to 48 hours after staining, if the direct tag is fluorescence isothicyanate and the surface marker (e.g., CD4, CD8, CD19) is intrinsically bright (high density). However, analysis is more difficult at 48 hours if the marker is intrinsically less bright (e.g., CD3) or if the fluorescent tag is less stable (e.g., phycerythrin). Either manual or automated dual staining or two-color staining (simultaneous staining with two mAb bearing different tags) results in the least specimen stability. These specimens should be analyzed within 24 hours for accurate results. Specimens held longer show less differentiation between positive and negative populations, resulting in less accurate results.

Reagents

Several commercial sources of mouse mAb against lymphoid surface antigens are available, among them Becton Dickinson (Mountain View, CA), Coulter Immunology (Hialeah, FL), and Ortho Diagnostics (Raritan, NJ). Each manufacturer has its own term for mAb reactive with the various lymphoid surface molecules. The Annual International Workshop and Conference on Human Leukocyte Differentiation Antigens has reduced the confusion created by these multiple systems of nomenclature since 1984. Authorities at these conferences have devised an antigen cluster designation (CD) nomenclature and have designated each commercially available mAb by a CD name. Table 30-7 illustrates the commonly used CD groups with their predominant reactivity and other corresponding monoclonal antibodies.

Methods

During the past decade, manual FA staining of mononuclear cell suspensions and fluorescence microscopy differential counting have been replaced in many laboratories by manual or automated staining of whole blood and analysis by laser powered FCM. All the following approaches to typing of peripheral blood lymphocytes give clinically useful results: (1) whole blood staining (by manual or automated methods) and analysis by flow cytometric techniques; (2) density gradient separation of mononuclear cells (containing about 80% lymphocytes and 20% monocytes) from blood and staining by manual methods (direct or indirect FA, with preparation of slides read by fluorescence microscopy; or (3) flow cytometric analysis of manually stained mononuclear cells.

Some important mAb nonspecificities warrant discussion. The CD4 molecule on T-helper cells is also on monocytes. Electronic gating by FCM can usually exclude most monocytes from the lymphocyte population, especially in whole blood analysis methods. However, staining for monocytes is crucial for determining whether there is any significant monocyte contamination within the "lymphocyte" population defined by the gates. The CD8 molecule is expressed as bright staining on true CD3+ T-suppressor-cytotoxic cells and weaker staining by NK cells (CD3−, CD16+, Leu-11+), respectively. Despite the differences in these populations, it is still common practice to include both populations in calculating total T-suppressor-cytotoxic cells.

Various software packages are available for calculating results by flow cytometric analysis. The method of calculating results depends on the staining characteristics of the mAb (strong versus weak intensity) and method of staining (e.g., single versus two color).

Surface Immunoglobulin Staining. Many lymphoid cell types have SIg, but only B cells have SIg that is endogenously synthesized and incorporated into the cell membrane as an integral component. Other cells have immunoglobulin attached by Fc receptors. Incubation at 37°C will elute off Fc-receptor-attached Ig so that subsequent staining for B-cell-specific SIg can be performed. The most sensitive method of SIg staining remains a manual direct FA stain read by fluorescence microscopy. Surface immunoglobulin is used primarily in the assessment of a lymphoid malignancy of the peripheral blood. Chronic lymphocytic leukemia (CLL) is the most common clinical entity studied and SIg staining is frequently very faint in this condition. With whole blood staining techniques and flow cytometric analysis, weak SIg staining is often difficult to distinguish from the background staining caused by Fc-receptor-attached Ig. This difficulty persists whether mononuclear cell suspensions are made from peripheral blood or from lymphoid organs. Only B-cell neoplasms that show SIg of very bright intensity can be easily stained and analyzed by flow cytometry (e.g., circulating cells of a poorly differentiated lymphoma). Because CLL is usually considered in the differential diagnosis of an atypical lymphocytosis, manual direct FA staining of a mononuclear cell suspension with examination by fluorescence microscopy, as well as cytologic assessment of a Wright-stained cytocentrifuged smear of a mononuclear cell suspension and of a peripheral blood smear are advisable.

Another characteristic of the B cells of CLL is their affinity for mouse erythrocytes, resulting in the formation of mouse erythrocyte rosettes.[37] The erythrocytes of BALB/c mice can be used for this rosetting technique. The mouse rosette assay is useful for distinguishing between the B cells of CLL and those of well differentiated (B cell) lymphocytic lymphoma (WDLL) in the peripheral blood. Fifty percent or more of the CLL B cells form mouse rosettes, whereas the B cells of WDLL form fewer rosettes (usually less than 20%).[37]

Blast Transformation. In addition to the enumeration and phenotyping of lymphocyte subsets, lymphocyte function tests can be performed, such as mitogen-induced polyclonal blast transformation. Mitogens are substances that nonspecifically activate lymphocyte blast transformation in a polyclonal fashion. Blast transformation assays are based on the phenomenon that lymphocytes, when activated by a stimulus, undergo cytologic and functional dedifferentiation, that is, cellular enlargement, development of a more immature nuclear chromatin pattern, DNA synthesis, cell division, and lymphokine production. After 3 days of mitogen or 5 days of antigen stimulation, the in vitro culture system is pulse-labeled with tritiated thymidine. The degree of lymphocyte functional capability is directly related to the counts per minute (CPM) measured in a β-scintillation counter.

Three commonly used mitogens include phytohemagglutinin (PHA), concanavalin A (ConA), and pokeweed mitogen (PWM). Phytohemagglutinin is the most potent general stimulator of polyclonal lymphocyte transformation. Concanavalin A is another potent lymphocyte stimulator that induces the production of lymphokines that mediate suppressor functions. The supernatant from ConA stimulated lymphocytes can be used in assays of suppressor function. Pokeweed mitogen is a less potent stimulator and induces T-cell-dependent B-cell activation and immunoglobulin (Ig) production. Microbial antigens can also be used to stimulate specific in vitro blast transformation. Skin test antigens, dialyzed to remove preservatives, can be used to assess specific CMI capability in the assessment of suspected immunodeficiency states. Tetanus toxoid is a good antigen to use because it is a potent stimulator of antigen-specific blast transformation, and tetanus immunization during infancy induces strong in vitro responsiveness to the antigen in infants with an intact CMI system. The tetanus skin test antigen is readily available and easily dialyzed for use in the blast transformation assay. Other microbial and mineral antigens have been used in blast transformation assays. The microbial antigen used in these assays is often related to local research interests or to regional incidence of infectious diseases, for example, coccidioidomycosis in the southwestern United States.

Interpretation

Normal percentages of lymphocyte subsets in adults are approximately as follows: (1) T cells (CD2) 72–92% and (CD3) 62–82%; (2) T-helper/inducers (CD4) 36–64%; (3) T-suppressor-cytotoxic cells (CD8) 13–37%; (4) B cells (CD19) 1–12%; (5) T-helper/suppressor cytotoxic ratio 0.9–3.5. Reference ranges for relative and absolute numbers of lymphocyte subsets must be established in each laboratory and for each method used, because there are minor method-dependent differences in lymphocyte typing results. In addition, lymphocyte counts as well as the percentages of B and T cells change with age, for example, during infancy and early childhood.[8]

Lymphoproliferative Disorders

An extensive phenotyping battery may be necessary for assessment of lymphoid malignancy (multiple mAb, surface immunoglobulin, TdT). The immunologic approach to the classification of non-Hodgkin's lymphomas is extensively and excellently reviewed elsewhere.[38] Figures 30-4 and 30-5 illustrate the usual immunotypic profile of various B- and T-cell leukemias or lymphomas related to their state of B- or T-cell differentiation.

A mature B-cell malignancy (chronic lymphocyte leukemia) will demonstrate an increase in B-cell numbers and will usually show a monoclonal pattern of SIg staining. In about 15% of cases of CLL, the cells have such sparse SIg that it is undetectable. However, the cells of CLL and those of well to intermediately differentiated B cell lymphomas may paradoxically express a pan-T-cell surface marker (i.e., Leu-1). The intensity of this Leu-1 staining on CLL B cells is characteristically weaker than that seen for normal T cells, making intensity of expression a useful diagnostic tool. There are rare cases of T-cell CLL. One clinically and phenotypically unique entity primarily affects younger men (20–40 years of age) and is associated with neutropenia and an indolent course. Phenotypically, the T cells have Fc receptors for IgG and are called Tγ cells. Most express the CD8 molecule. The neutropenia may relate to suppressive influences from the tumor cells. Because of the indolent course, there is some controversy about whether this represents a true neoplasm. The cells are morphologically larger and contain azurophilic cytoplasmic granules.

Most cases of ALL belong to an immature B-cell lineage (pre-pre-B) and express TdT and CD10 and mark with pan-B cell markers (e.g., B1, B4). Immature B cells may express cytoplasmic IgM (pre-B) but do not express SIg. T-cell ALL will mark with pan-T markers. Most cases of T-cell ALL involve a proliferation of immature T cells, which express TdT and markers for thymocytes (CD1, e.g., Leu-6) and usually have both helper (CD4) and suppressor-cytotoxic (CD8) surface molecules. Approximately one-third of cases of chronic myelocytic leukemia (CML) transform into ALL during blast transformation. A TdT stain in conjunction with histochemical staining is valuable for differentiating lymphoblastic (TdT-positive) transformation from myeloblastic. TdT staining should not be used as the only test for differentiating ALL from AML be-

856 • Laboratory Medicine

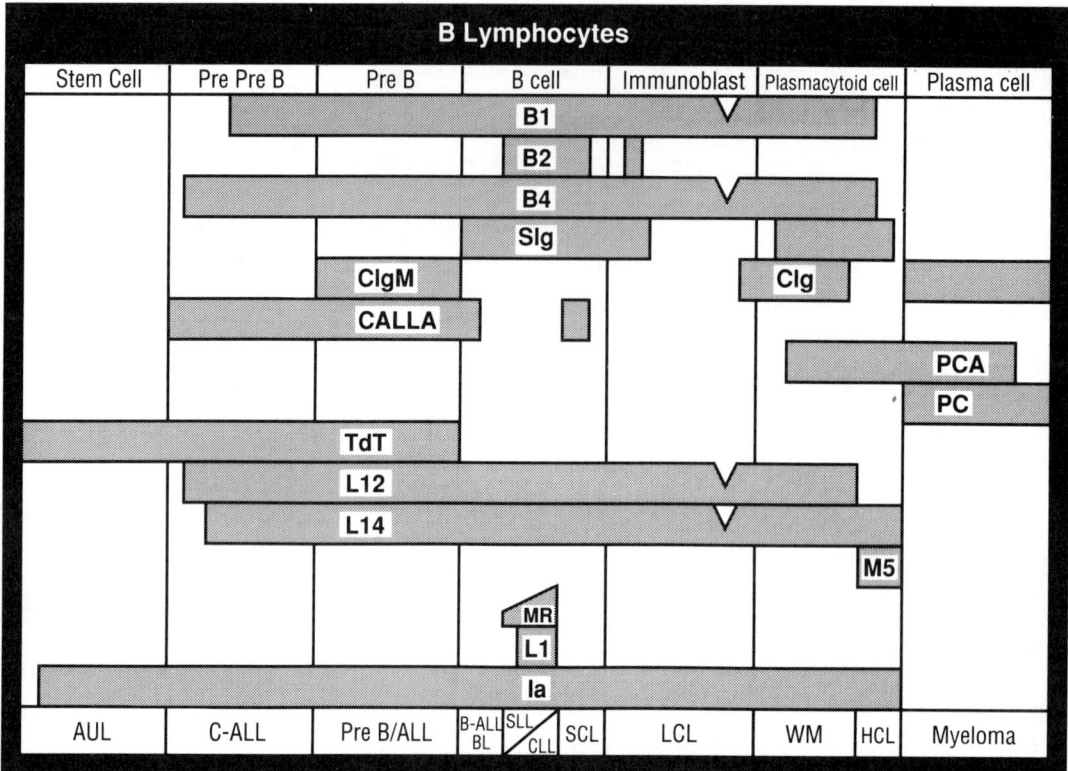

Fig. 30-4. B-cell phenotypes. Diagrammatic representation of the range of B-cell antigenic expression in both normal B-cell development (ontogeny) and the B-cell neoplasms derived from each stage of ontogeny. SIg, surface immunoglobulin; CIg, cytoplasmic immunoglobulin; PCA, plasma cell antigen; PC, plasma cell (marker); TdT, terminal deoxynucleotidyl transferase; AUL, acute undifferentiated leukemia; C-all, common acute lymphocytic leukemia; pre-B all, pre-B-cell acute lymphocytic leukemia; B-all, B-cell acute lymphocytic leukemia; BL, Burkitt's/Burkitt's-like leukemia/lymphoma; SLL, small cell lymphocytic lymphoma; CLL, chronic lymphocytic leukemia; SCL, small cleaved cell lymphoma; LCL, large cell lymphoma; WM, Waldenström's macroglobulinemia; HCL, hairy cell leukemia; myeloma, multiple myeloma; MR, mouse rosette. See Tables 30-7 and 30-8 for descriptions of antibodies or tests. (From Grogan et al.,[38] with permission.)

cause there are biphenotypic acute leukemias, expressing both lymphoid and myeloid markers.

There are cases of more mature T-cell leukemias/lymphomas, which may or may not have immature markers (e.g., TdT, CD1), but they usually express either CD4 or CD8 surface molecules in a mutually exclusive fashion. These T-cell malignancies frequently show aberrant expression of pan-T-cell markers; that is, they fail to express all the usual T-cell surface antigens. Therefore, aberrant T-cell marker expression may be the only phenotypic evidence that a leukemia or lymphoma is of T-cell lineage. A few mature T-cell leukemias (often called *peripheral* because these neoplasms phenotypically resemble normal, circulating or peripheral T cells) warrant specific mention because of their unique clinical presentation. In Sézary syndrome (circulating mycosis fungoides), the malignant cells usu-

ally express the CD4 molecule and have a typical cerebriform nuclear shape. In human T-cell lymphotropic virus type I (HTLV-I) associated T-cell leukemia, the cells usually express the CD4 surface molecule and often have a convoluted or cloverleaf-shaped nucleus. There are also phenotypically similar leukemia cells not associated with HTLV-I. These examples illustrate the extreme importance of cytologic and histologic examination in the workup of a suspected lymphoid malignancy. Lymphocyte phenotyping should never be used alone to classify a lymphoid malignancy.

Immunodeficiency

Various congenital or acquired deficiencies or functional abnormalities of lymphocytes result in immunodeficiency syndromes. Lymphocyte phenotyping and function testing are often insensitive indicators of im-

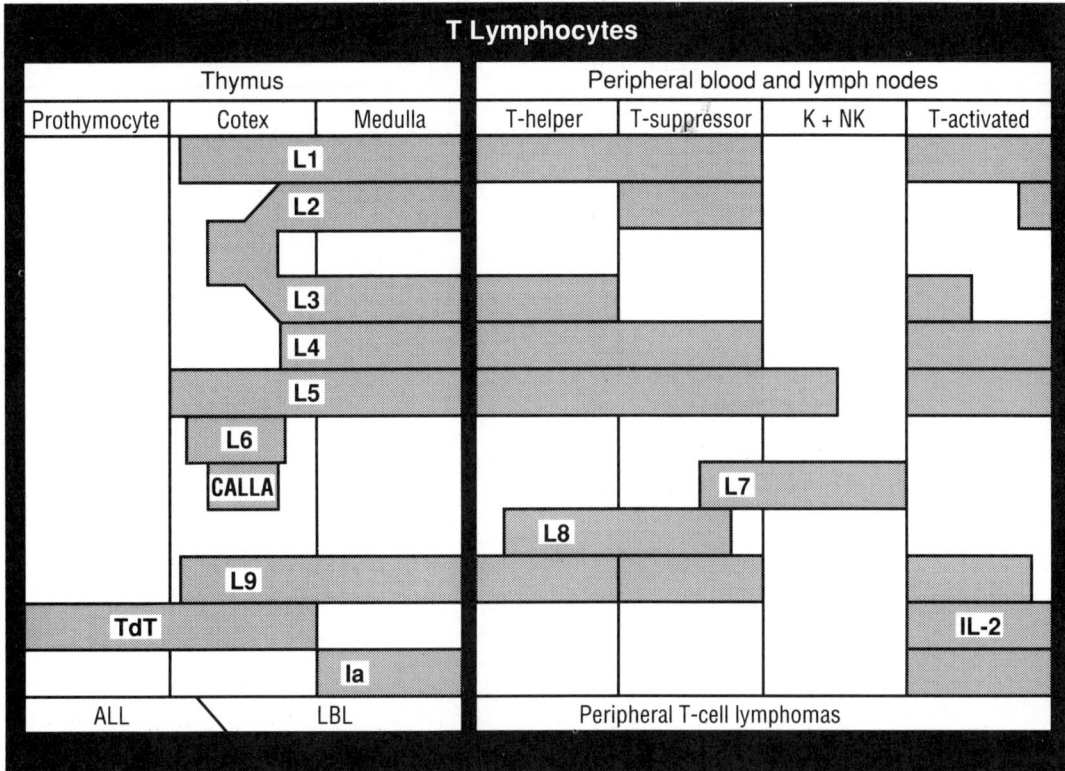

Fig. 30-5. T-cell phenotypes. Diagrammatic representation of the range of T-cell antigenic expression in both normal T-cell ontogeny and the T-cell neoplasms derived from the developmental phases. ALL, acute lymphocytic leukemia; LBL, lymphoblastic lymphoma; K + NK, Killer plus natural killer (cell); TdT, terminal deoxynucleotidyl transferase. See Tables 30-7 and 30-8 for descriptions of antibodies or tests. (From Grogan et al.,[38] with permission.)

munodeficiency because specific functional abnormalities may not be detectable by the methods routinely performed in the clinical laboratory. For example, immunodeficiency states (e.g., acquired hypo- or agammaglobulinemia) may result from inadequate functioning of T-helper cells or excessive T-supressor cell function. Autoimmune disease and immunodeficiency states (e.g., selective IgA deficiency) often coexist because both circumstances may result from immune regulatory abnormalities. Overall, the inherited, congenital forms of immunodeficiency are rare or unusual.

Primary Immunodeficiency States

The three major categories of primary or congenital immunodeficiency states are (1) predominant humoral defects, (2) predominant T-cell (CMI) defects, and (3) immunodeficiency states associated with other defects or conditions. Each of the above categories contains several subtypes (Tables 30-9 and 30-10). This classification differs from previous classification schemes by defining *combined* immunodeficiency as a predominant T-cell defect, reflecting greater understanding of the role of the T cell in the pathogenesis of combined immunodeficiency. Many of these syndromes are so rare that their pathophysiology is poorly understood. The primary immunodeficiency states have been reviewed elsewhere.[14]

Humoral Defects

X-linked agammaglobulinemia is characterized by very few or absent mature B cells. The bone marrow contains normal numbers of pre-B cells; the defect therefore appears to be a maturation block in B-cell development. The number and function of circulating T cells and T-cell subsets are normal. The defect in autosomal recessive agammaglobulinemia (which varies only in that female patients are also affected) is presumed to be the same. Another humoral deficiency, immunoglobulin deficiency with increased IgM, appears to be caused by an intrinsic defect in the immunoglobulin class "switch" mechanism. Normally, IgM is produced first during a humoral immune response, which later

Table 30-9. Classification of Predominantly Humoral Primary Immunodeficiency States

Predominant antibody defects
    X-linked panhypo- or agammaglobulinemia[a] (with or without growth hormone deficiency)
    Autosomal recessive agammaglobulinemia[a]
    Immunoglobulin (e.g., IgG or IgA) deficiency with increased IgM[b,c]
    Selective IgA deficiency[b-d]
    Selective deficiency of other immunoglobulin isotypes (e.g., IgM) or subclasses (e.g., IgG, IgG$_2$[b-d]
    Transient hypogammaglobulinemia of infancy[b,e]
    Hypogammaglobulinemia associated with thymoma[a]
    Common variable immunodeficiency (CVID)[f] with
        Normal B-cell numbers[c]
        Low B-cell numbers[c]
        Increased B-cell numbers[c]
        "Nonsecretory" B cells and plasma cells[c]
        Defective T-helper cells
        Activated T-suppressor cells
        Autoantibodies to B or T cells

[a] Mature B cells are severely decreased or absent in the circulation. T cells are normal in number and function.
[b] B and T cells are usually present in normal numbers for age.
[c] B cells are present but may exhibit inherent functional defects in experimental procedures.
[d] "Selective" IgA deficiency may occur in association with IgG subclass deficiency or IgE deficiency.
[e] This may represent a delay in the normal functional maturation of B cells.
[f] T-cell function in CVID often deteriorates over time. There may be decreased in vitro responsiveness to individual or multiple mitogens.

switches to IgG, IgA or IgE production. Again, the cellular immune system is quantitatively and qualitatively normal.

Selective IgA deficiency is one of the more common humoral immunodeficiency states. Approximately 1 of 600–700 people have decreased levels of this antibody class. Most affected persons appear to be entirely well, but IgA deficiency has been associated with recurrent infections and autoimmune disease. There have been reports of IgG subclass and IgE deficiencies in association with IgA deficiency. Therefore, this disorder may not be an isolated IgA defect but rather a more general abnormality in the terminal differentiation of the B cell. Lymphocyte typing results are usually normal.

Transient hypogammaglobulinemia of infancy may represent delayed maturation of the normal ontogeny of the humoral immune response; patients recover by the first or second year of life. The numbers of circulating T and B cells are normal, but there may be inadequate T-helper cell function in inducing B-cell responses. Intrinsic B-cell function appears to be normal.

Common variable immunodeficiency (CVID) can result from three different causes: (1) intrinsic B-cell defects, (2) immunoregulatory T-cell imbalance, or (3) autoantibodies to T or B cells. The latter two categories are rare. B-cell numbers may be low, normal, or high, but they may be functionally abnormal and fail to respond to antigens or mitogens. The T-helper/suppressor-cytotoxic ratio is often low or reversed. In some cases, however, there is an absence of T-helper cells or the presence of excessively activated suppressor T cells that prevent B-cell function.

T-Cell Defects

Severe combined immunodeficiency (SCID) is usually associated with a profound lymphopenia. The number of mature T cells is consistently low, but the number of B cells may be low or normal. The circulating B cells may function normally in the presence of normal T cells. In some cases, a normal number of immature T cells is present in the circulation. If mature T cells are present, they may be of maternal origin and may mediate graft-versus-host disease (GVHD). Many patients have an eosinophilia, but a small subgroup have congenital aleukocytosis, that is, reticular dysgenesis. Severe combined immunodeficiency can be an autosomal recessive or X-linked disease. About one-half of the autosomal recessive forms have an associated deficiency of adenosine deaminase. In some SCID cases, T cells do not express HLA antigens; this is called the *bare-lymphocyte syndrome*. These cells are not functionally normal, because HLA antigens are essential for normal activation and effector T-cell function. Purine-nucleoside phosphorylase and adenosine deaminase deficiencies are associated with T-cell deficiency with normal antibody formation and normal immunoglobulin levels. Deoxyguanosine and deoxyadenosine triphosphates are incriminated as the toxic metabo-

Table 30-10. Classification of Predominantly Cellular Primary Immunodeficiency States and Those Associated with Other Defects

Predominant T-cell defects
    Severe combined immunodeficiency (SCID) (with or without adenosine deaminase or purine-nucleoside phosphorylase deficiency)[a]
        Reticular dysgenesis (aleukocytosis)
        Low T- and B-cell numbers
        Low T- and normal B-cell numbers
    Nezelof syndrome[b] (cellular immunodeficiency with immunoglobulins)
    Immunodeficiency with unusual susceptibility to Epstein-Barr virus[c]

Immunodeficiency associated with other defects
    Wiscott-Aldrich syndrome[d] (immunodeficiency with eczema and thrombocytopenia)
    Ataxia telangiectasia[e]
    DiGeorge syndrome[f] (third- and fourth-pouch syndrome)

[a] The number of T cells is severely decreased. Correlating with this is usually a depressed responsiveness to mitogens. In some cases, the few T cells present may fail to express HLA surface molecules (i.e., bare lymphocyte syndrome). Immunoglobulin levels are markedly decreased.

[b] Nezelof syndrome usually has a later onset than that of SCID. T-cell counts, although usually decreased, may be higher than in infants with SCID. Responsiveness to mitogens usually is depressed. There may be normal levels of one or more classes of immunoglobulins.

[c] Epstein-Barr virus infection in these patients may result in B-cell lymphomas, marrow aplasia, fatal infectious mononucleosis, or agammaglobulinemia.

[d] There is a progressive decrease in T-cell numbers and responsiveness to specific antigen. Responsiveness to mitogens is variable and may require higher stimulating doses.

[e] The number and mitogen responsiveness of T cells are normal or decreased. Mitogen responsiveness may be decreased even with normal T-cell numbers. The immunoglobulin deficiency is variable (IgE and IgA are usually decreased). Most have normal IgG levels. The syndrome is dominated by progressive neurologic deterioration. About 10% develop a lymphoma (a central nervous system primary tumor is not uncommon).

[f] The T-cell defect is variable (i.e., ranging from complete aplasia to partial degrees of thymus dysplasia). This is reflected by correspondingly decreased T-cell numbers and functional capability (mitogen responsiveness). B cells are normal in number and function.

lites, respectively. The number of T cells is extremely low, but the number of B cells is within the reference range. The greater immunodeficiency usually associated with adenosine deaminase deficiency, compared with purine-nucleoside phosphorylase deficiency, is attributed to the fact that resting T cells are readily killed by deoxyadenosine triphosphate, whereas deoxyguanosine triphosphate affects only dividing cells.

There is a group of patients in whom Epstein-Barr virus (EBV) infection is followed by B-cell lymphoma, marrow aplasia, fatal infectious mononucleosis, or agammaglobulinemia. After the infection, B-cell numbers and immunoglobulin levels are decreased. The cause for this disastrous complication of EBV infection is unknown.

Immunodeficiency Associated with Other Defects

Wiscott-Aldrich syndrome is characterized by severe eczema, thrombocytopenia, and susceptibility to opportunistic infection. It is inherited as an X-linked recessive trait. Elevated concentrations of IgA and IgE, decreased IgM levels, and normal IgG levels are usually seen. Also isohemagglutinins are usually absent. The number and function of T cells show a progressive decline. A profound lymphopenia may occur by middle childhood.

Ataxia telangiectasia is a complex syndrome, including progressive cerebellar ataxia, telangiectasia formation (dilatation of small blood vessels), as well as an immunologic defect. Variable numbers of patients have low or undetectable levels of total IgG, of IgG subclasses, and/or IgA. T-helper function is usually defective, whereas T-suppressor function remains intact.

Defects in the third and fourth embryonic pharyngeal pouches (DiGeorge syndrome) affect development of the thymus and parathyroid glands. Other congenital anomalies frequently coexist (e.g., cardiac, midline facial clefts, low-set ears, hypertelorism). There is a profound lymphopenia of T cells, leading eventually to a general lymphopenia, but B cells are normal. There can be variable degrees of defective thymic development leading to correspondingly variable degrees of T-cell immunodeficiency (partial expression of the syndrome). With increasing age, there may be a gradual increase in T-cell immune function.

Acquired Immunodeficiency Syndrome

Currently, the major "acquired" form of immunodeficiency is associated with HIV infection. This human lymphotropic retrovirus was formerly also known as the human T-cell lymphotropic virus type III (HTLV-III) and lymphadenopathy-associated virus (LAV). Human immunodeficiency virus infection and its immune effects have been extensively reviewed elsewhere.[39-44] The Centers of Disease Control (CDC) definition of AIDS, revised in August, 1986, is as follows: a disease, at least moderately predictive of a defect in cell-mediated immunity, occurring in a person with no known cause of diminished resistance to that disease. Such diseases must be reliably diagnosed (i.e., histology or culture) and include Kaposi sarcoma (KS), *Pneumocystis carinii* pneumonia (PCP), and other serious opportunistic infections. These other infections include candidiasis, cryptococcosis, cytomegalovirus (CMV), nocardiosis, strongyloidosis, toxoplasmosis, or atypical mycobacteriosis (other than tuberculosis or lepra). The following specific infections also qualify: esophagitis caused by candidiasis, CMV, or herpes simplex virus (HSV); progressive multifocal leukocephalopathy; chronic enterocolitis (more than 4 weeks) caused by cryptosporidiosis; or unusually severe mucocutaneous HSV infection of more than 5 weeks duration. In adults with HIV seropositivity, additional diseases (reliably diagnosed, e.g., culture, histology, microscopy, antigen detection) qualify, including disseminated histoplasmosis; isosporiasis, causing chronic diarrhea; bronchial or pulmonary candidiasis; non-Hodgkin's lymphoma of high-grade pathologic type; and histologically confirmed KS in patients aged 60 years or older. Lymphoreticular malignancies, diagnosed more than 3 months after any of the above diagnoses, are no longer excluded as AIDS cases.

The hallmark of HIV infection is severe depletion of T-helper cells. The virus primarily infects CD4-bearing cells (e.g., T-helper cells and monocytes). The CD4 molecule appears to be the receptor for viral infection. After penetrating of the cell, viral RNA is transcribed into DNA by reverse transcriptase, producing a *provirus* that may be integrated into the host cell DNA. Infection of a T-helper cell may remain silent or latent for 2-10 years before some event triggers activation of the lymphocyte, resulting in transcription and translation of the integrated viral genome (productive infection).

Because only about 0.01% of the circulating lymphocytes are actually infected with the HIV virus, mechanisms in addition to actual cytolytic infection must be operative in order to cause the profound loss of T-helper cells seen with HIV infection. Interaction between the HIV envelope glycoprotein on the surface of an infected cell and the CD4 molecule of uninfected cells can lead to fusion of 100-150 T-helper cells, resulting in destruction of uninfected cells by syncytium formation. Envelope glycoprotein may also diffuse from infected cells and bind to the CD4 molecule of uninfected cells leading to cytotoxic effects.

The immunologic findings in HIV-infected individuals vary with the stage of infection (Table 30-11). During the acute infection there may be a transient decrease in number of CD4-bearing lymphocytes and an increase in number of CD8-bearing cells (frequently coexpressing Leu-7), which may persist. During the latent stage of infection, a variety of immunologic patterns may be seen, including (1) quantitatively normal lymphocyte subset numbers with normal or decreased functional responses to antigen or mitogen stimulation; (2) decreased numbers of CD4-bearing cells with normal or increased numbers of CD8-bearing cells; or (3) normal numbers of CD4-bearing cells with increased numbers of CD8-bearing cells. Human immunodeficiency virus-seropositive persons, asymptomatic except for lymphadenopathy, may show increased CD8 cells with variable numbers of CD4 cells. When double-staining techniques are used, these patients frequently show a depletion of the helper-inducer cells (CD4+4B4+) and an increase in cytotoxic cells (CD8+Leu-15−).

The most striking result of these immunologic changes is a decreased CD4/CD8 ratio. However, a decreased ratio may occur nonspecifically when the number of CD8 cells is increased, after many types of infectious processes, including hepatitis B, infectious mononucleosis, CMV, and syphilis. Therefore, it is imperative to quantitate absolute numbers of both CD4- and CD8-bearing cells in order to determine why a CD4/CD8 ratio is decreased.

Functional responses to mitogens (PHA, ConA, PWM) are variable but are usually reduced when the number of CD4 cells is decreased. Responses may be decreased to all mitogens or to any combination of mitogens, or responses may be surprisingly normal with very low numbers of CD4-bearing cells. Table 30-11 outlines in more detail the immunologic findings in HIV infection.

The major immunologic finding correlating with progression of HIV infection is decreasing numbers of CD4 cells. Depending on the method used, the number of CD4 cells decreases as the intensity of staining decreases. Therefore, serial determinations are useful for the assessment of disease progression. In addition, the

Table 30-11. Lymphocyte Testing Results in Various Stages of HIV Infection

Stage of Infection	Results
Initial[a]	Decreased numbers of CD4 cells Normal or increased numbers of CD8 cells
Asymptomatic HIV-seropositive	Decreased or normal numbers of CD4 cells Normal or increased CD8 cells In vitro mitogen (PHA, ConA, PWM) responsiveness usually normal, but may be depressed In vitro microbial antigen responsiveness often depressed
Symptomatic[b] Generalized lymphadenopathy	Decreased or normal numbers of CD4 cells Normal or increased CD8 cells[c] In vitro responsiveness as above
Constitutional or neurologic manifestations[d]	Usually decreased numbers of CD4 cells Normal or increased CD8 cells In vitro mitogen responsiveness variable[e] In vitro microbial antigen responsiveness usually depressed
Opportunistic infection or secondary cancers[f]	Decreased numbers of CD4 cells (usually <200 πl) Normal, decreased, or increased numbers of CD8 cells In vitro mitogen responsiveness variable[e] In vitro microbial responsiveness as above

[a] The initial infection may be asymptomatic or may produce a mononucleosis-like syndrome, aseptic meningitis, rash, or musculoskeletal complaints.
[b] AIDS-related complex (ARC) is usually diagnosed at this time.
[c] Some patients with generalized lymphadenopathy have very high numbers of CD8 cells (>1500–4000/μL).
[d] Constitutional symptoms may include any of the following: fever >1 month, involuntary weight loss of >10% of baseline weight or diarrhea of >1 month duration, or any combination of these. Neurologic disorders include dementia, acute atypical meningitis, myelopathy, sensory neuropathy, or demyelinating polyneuropathy.
[e] Responses to all mitogens (PHA, ConA, PWM) may be normal or response(s) to any single mitogen or combination of any two mitogens may be depressed. Conversely, mitogen responsiveness may be surprisingly intact with extremely low numbers of CD4 cells.
[f] AIDS is designated when serious opportunistic infections occur that are at least moderately predictive of a defect in CMI in a person with no other known cause for diminished resistance to disease (e.g., PCP or Kaposi's, disease).
Abbreviations: HIV, human immunodeficiency virus; PHA, phytohemagglutination; ConA, concanavalin A; PWM, pokeweed mitogen; AIDS, acquired immunodeficiency syndrome; CMI, cellular immune response; PCP, *Pneumocystis carinii* pneumonia.

following immunologic findings have been associated with more rapid initial or subsequent disease progression: (1) lower initial CD4 levels, (2) higher initial CD8 levels, (3) late decrease in previously normal or increased CD8 levels, and (4) decreased responsiveness to at least one mitogen.

Immunoregulatory Abnormalities

A functional or quantitative imbalance in T-helper and T-suppressor cell influences has been implicated in many presumed autoimmune diseases.[45-48] For example, a decrease in CD8 cells occurs in acute or chronically active polymyositis, dermatomyositis, multiple sclerosis (MS), SLE (spontaneous and drug-induced), severe atopic eczema, hyper-IgE syndrome, Kawasaki disease, warm hemolytic anemia, and acute GVHD. An increase in CD8 cells has been associated with chronic GVHD. Decreased numbers of total T cells and CD4 cells have been observed during acute primary biliary cirrhosis. Increased proportions of activated (Ia or HLA-Dr antigen expression) CD8 cells have been described after viral infection, including herpesviruses and rubeola. Increased numbers of activated T cells also have been demonstrated during recently diagnosed insulin-dependent diabetes mellitus.

Therapy-Associated Changes in Lymphocyte Subpopulations

Cytotoxic drugs and radiation therapy can cause total lymphopenia variably affecting the T-cell subsets with subsequently variable CD4/CD8 ratios. Cyclosporine treatment causes a lymphopenia primarily affecting the CD4 subset, frequently resulting in a decreased

CD4/CD8 ratio. After renal transplantation and immunosuppressive therapy, the patient is at risk of infectious complications or rejection. The T-helper/suppressor-cytotoxic ratio may be useful in making this distinction between rejection and infection. A normal or increased ratio indicates a relatively high risk of rejection (unless the total T-cell count is less than 150/μL [<150 × 10⁻⁶/L]). Conversely, a low ratio (less than 1.3) indicates a decreased risk of rejection but an increased risk of infection. This ratio may vary depending on the lymphocyte phenotyping methods used. Antithymocyte globulin therapy causes a profound T-cell lymphopenia and a corresponding relative increase in B cells. Steroid treatment is associated with a relatively selective lymphopenia, that is, absolute sparing of the subsets bearing the γ-Fc receptor (e.g., T γ cells).[49]

Miscellaneous Conditions

Lymphocyte subsets have been studied in a variety of conditions empirically associated with immunodeficiency.[50-52] For example, protein malnutrition is accompanied by a decrease in total T cells with a relatively greater decrease in T-helper cells. In iron deficiency anemia, there is a slight increase in total T cells and a decrease in functional responsiveness to mitogens. Critically ill surgical or post-trauma patients have been studied extensively with conflicting results, but decreased functional responsiveness to mitogens and to specific antigen (e.g., streptokinase/streptodornase) has been described. A decrease in relative number of T-helper cells has been described during pregnancy.

Summary

Variations in relative and absolute numbers of CD4 and CD8 cells are nonspecific findings that must be interpreted within the context of a specific clinical situation, for example, HIV infection, workup of a newborn with suspected immunodeficiency, or flareup of MS. Also, the cause of a decreased CD4/CD8 ratio can be either a decrease in number of CD4 cells (as in HIV infection) or an increase in number of CD8 cells (as in infectious mononucleosis or other infection), or both. Therefore, a decreased ratio is a nonspecific finding with different implications, depending on the cause of the decrease. When classifying a lymphoproliferative disorder, the workup should include a phenotyping battery large enough to distinguish unusual myeloid (TdT positive) from lymphoid disease and to demonstrate proliferation of a specific T-cell subset or an aberrant or "novel" T-cell phenotype. It is also imperative that any workup of a lymphoproliferative disorder include careful cytologic or histologic assessment.

REFERENCES

1. Nakamura RM, Tucker ES III: Mechanisms of immunologic disease and autoimmunity. pp 146–168. In Sodeman WA, Sodeman TM (eds): Pathologic Physiology. 6th Ed. Philadelphia, WB Saunders, 1979.
2. Tucker ES III, Nakamura RM: Dynamics of immune response, immunocompetence, immunodeficiency and tumor immunology. In Sodeman WM, Sodeman TM (eds): Pathologic Physiology. 6th Ed. Philadelphia, WB Saunders, 1979.
3. Paul WE (ed): Fundamental Immunology. New York, Raven Press, 1984.
4. Claman HN: The biology of the immune response. JAMA 1987;258:2834–2840.
5. Miedema F, Melief CJR: T-cell regulation of human B-cell activation. Immunol Today 1985;6:258–259.
6. Twomey JJ (ed): The Pathophysiology of Human Immunologic Disorders. Baltimore, Urban and Schwarzenberg, 1982.
7. Nelson DA, Davey FR: Leukocytic Disorders. pp. 1036–1100. In Henry JB (ed): Todd-Sanford-Davidsohn Clinical Diagnosis by Laboratory Methods. 16th Ed. Philadelphia, WB Saunders, 1979.
8. Hicks MJ, Jones JF, Minnich LM et al: Age-related changes in T- and B-lymphocyte subpopulations in the peripheral blood. Arch Pathol Lab Med 1983;107:518–523.
9. Ault K: Flow cytometric evaluation of normal and neoplastic B cells. pp. 247–273. In Rose NR, Freidman H, Fahey JL (eds): Manual of Clinical Laboratory Immunology. 3rd Ed. Washington, DC, American Society for Microbiology, 1986.
10. Jackson AL, Warner NW: Preparation, staining, and analysis by flow cytometry of peripheral blood leukocytes. pp. 226–235. In Rose NR, Freidman H, Fahey JL (eds): Manual of Clinical Laboratory Immunology. 3rd Ed. Washington, DC, American Society for Microbiology, 1986.
11. Braylan RC: Flow cytometry. Arch Pathol Lab Med 1983;107:1–6.
12. Young M, Geha RS: Human regulatory T-cell subsets. Annu Rev Med 1986;37:165–172.
13. Buckley RH: Immunodeficiency diseases. JAMA 1987;258:2841–2850.
14. Rosen RS, Cooper MD, Wedgwood RJP: The primary immunodeficiencies. N Engl J Med 1984;311:235–242, 300–310.
15. Osserman EF, Merlino G, Butler VP Jr: Multiple myeloma and related plasma cell dyscrasias. JAMA 1987;258:2930–2937.
16. Check IJ, Piper M: Quantitation of immunoglobulins. pp. 138–151. In Rose NR, Friedman H, Fahey JL (eds): Manual of Clinical Laboratory Immunology. Washington, DC, American Society for Microbiology, 1986.
17. Hamaoka T, Ono S: Regulation of B-cell differentiation: interactions of factors and corresponding receptors. Annu Rev Immunol 1986;4:167–204.
18. Asser S, Hamburger RN: The use of the laboratory in the diagnosis of allergic disease. Schumpert Med Q 1986;4:272–280.
19. Rose NR, Mackay IR (eds): The Autoimmune Disease. San Diego, Academic Press, 1985.
20. Condemi JJ: The autoimmune diseases. JAMA 1987;258:2920–2929.

21. Bigazzi PE, Burek CL, Rose NR: Antibodies to tissue-specific endocrine, gastrointestinal, and neurological antigens. pp. 762–770. In Rose NR, Friedman H, Fahey JL (eds): Manual of Clinical Laboratory Immunology. Washington, DC, American Society for Microbiology, 1986.
22. Deodhar S (ed): Autoimmune diseases: clinical considerations and laboratory testing. Clin Lab Med 1988;8:253–414.
23. Adorini L: Antigen presentation and self-nonself discrimination. Clin Immunol Immunopathol 1990;54:327–336.
24. Nakamura RM, Peebles CL, Rubin RL et al: Autoantibodies to Nuclear Antigens (ANA). Chicago, American Society of Clinical Pathologists, 1985.
25. Schar PH: Complement studies of sera and other biologic fluids. Hum Pathol 1983;14:338–342.
26. Tucker ES III: Complement activation in autoimmune disease. J Clin Immunoassay 1984;7:310–320.
27. Nitsche JF, Tucker ES III, Sugimoto S et al: Rocket immunoelectrophoresis of C4 and C4d. A simple sensitive method for detecting complement activation in plasma. Am J Clin Pathol 1981;76:679–684.
28. Pangburn MK, Müller-Eberhard HJ: The Alternative Pathway of Complement. pp. 185–191. In Müller-Eberhard HJ, Miescher PA (eds): Complement. Berlin, Springer-Verlag, 1984.
29. Tamerius JD, Pangburn MK, Müller-Eberhard HJ: Detection of a neoantigen on human C3bi and C3d by monoclonal antibody. J Immunol 1985;135:2015–2019.
30. Ruddy S: Complement. pp. 175–184. In Rose NR, Friedman H, Fahey JL (eds): Manual of Clinical Laboratory Immunology. Washington, DC, American Society for Microbiology, 1986.
31. Colten HR: Molecular basis of complement deficiency syndromes. Lab Invest 1985;52:468–473.
32. Nakamura RM, Tucker ES III: Immune complex diseases. pp. 295–330. In Ritzmann SE, Daniels JC (eds): Serum Protein Abnormalities: Diagnostic and Clinical Aspects. Boston, Little Brown, 1975.
33. McCluskey RT, Fienberg R: Vasculitis in primary vasculitidies, granulomatoses and connective tissue diseases. Hum Pathol 1983;14:305–315.
34. Barba L, Pawlowski I et al: Diagnostic immunopathology of the kidney biopsy in rheumatic diseases. Hum Pathol 1983;14:290–304.
35. Agnello V: Immune complex assays in rheumatic diseases. Hum Pathol 1983;14:343–349.
36. Dougal JS, Hubbard M, Strobel PL et al: Comparison of five assays for immune complexes in rheumatic diseases. J Lab Clin Med 1982;100:705–719.
37. Hicks MJ, Grogan TM, Fielder K, Spier CM: Differentiation of chronic lymphoproliferative disorders by the human mouse rosette assay. Diagn Immunol 1986;4:1–6.
38. Grogan TM, Spier CM, Richter LC, Rangel CS: Immunologic approaches to the classification of non-Hodgkin's lymphomas. pp. 31–148. In Bennett JM, Foon KA (eds): Immunologic Approaches to the Classification and Management of Lymphomas and Leukemias. Boston, Kluwer Academic Publishers, 1988.
39. Broder S, Gallo RC: A pathogenic retrovirus (HTLV-III) linked to AIDS. N Engl J Med 1984;311:1292–1297.
40. Ho DD, Pomeranz RG, Kaplan JC: Pathogenesis of infection with human immunodeficiency virus. N Engl J Med 1987;317:278–286.
41. Rosenberg ZF, Fauci AS: Immunopathogenesis of human immunodeficiency virus infection. Clin Immunol Newsl 1988;9:1–4.
42. Fauci AS: The human immunodeficiency virus: infectivity and mechanisms of pathogenesis. Science 1988;239:617–622.
43. Seligman M, Chess L, Fahey JL et al: AIDS: an immunologic reevaluation. N Engl J Med 1984;311:1286–1292.
44. Lane HC, Depper JM, Greene G et al: Qualitative analysis of immune function in patients with acquired immunodeficiency syndrome: evidence for a selective defect in soluble antigen recognition. N Engl J Med 1984;313:79–84.
45. Reinherz EL, Weiner HL, Hauser SL et al: Loss of suppressor cells in active multiple sclerosis: analysis with monoclonal antibodies. N Engl J Med 1980;303:125–129.
46. Morimoto C, Reinberg EL, Steinberg AD et al: Alterations in immunoregularity T cell subsets in active SLE. J Clin Invest 1980:66–1171.
47. Reinherz EL, Schlossman SF: Regulation of the immune response: inducer and suppressor T lymphocyte subsets in man. N Engl J Med 1980;303:370–373.
48. Reinherz EL, Parkman R, Rappaport J et al: Abberations of supressor T cells in human graft-versus-host disease. N Engl J Med 1979;300:1061–1068.
49. Glasser L, Hicks MJ, Lindberg R, Jones J: The effects of *in vivo* dexamethasone on lymphocyte subpopulations: differential response of EAhu rosette-forming cells. Clin Immunol Immunopathol 1981;18:22–31.
50. Chandra RK: Nutrition, immunity and infection: present knowledge and future directions. Lancet 1983;1:688–691.
51. McIrvine AJ, Mannick JA: Lymphocyte function in the critically ill surgical patient. Surg Clin North Am 1983;63:245–261.
52. Sridama V, Pacini F, Yang SL et al: Decreased levels of T helper cells: a possible cause of immunodeficiency in pregnancy. N Engl J Med 1982;307:352–356.
53. Stiehm ER, Fudenberg HH: Pediatrics 1966;37:715–727.

31 Blood Bank and Transfusion Service

Lawrence D. Petz

INTRODUCTION

Appropriate blood transfusion practice requires the use of numerous blood products for various clinical needs. Table 31-1 provides a list of components that are available as part of modern transfusion practice and also summarizes some laboratory aspects of storage, time to expiration, dosage, and handling requirements.

Laboratory testing prior to transfusion is required to ensure the safety of the product to be transfused. This chapter reviews the principles and techniques regarding pretransfusion testing of red blood cell (RBC) components, platelets, granulocytes, plasma, and plasma derivatives. In addition, special immunohematologic problems that are appropriately resolved in the blood bank are reviewed, including the diagnosis of autoimmune hemolytic anemias and drug-induced immune hemolytic anemias.

The purpose of pretransfusion testing is to select, for each recipient, blood products that, when transfused, will have acceptable survival and will not cause clinically significant destruction of the recipient's own RBCs.

The following procedures must be part of pretransfusion compatibility testing[1]:

1. Positive identification of recipient and blood specimen
2. Review of transfusion service records for results of previous testing on specimens from the recipient
3. ABO and Rh group tests
4. Selection of blood products of appropriate ABO and Rh groups
5. Antibody detection tests using the recipient's serum or plasma
6. Tests with the recipient's serum or plasma and donor's RBCs (i.e., the major crossmatch)
7. Labeling and issue of the blood products

If performed properly, pretransfusion tests will

1. Ensure that a patient is issued the designated blood products
2. In most cases, verify that blood products are ABO compatible
3. Detect most of the commonly encountered antibodies in the recipient's serum
4. Detect most antibodies in the recipient's serum directed against antigens on the donor's RBCs

One must keep in mind that RBC compatibility cannot be ensured even with appropriately performed compatibility tests, because hemolytic transfusion reactions may occur on rare occasions even in the absence of demonstrable RBC antibodies. Furthermore, if low concentrations of RBC alloantibodies are present prior to transfusion, antibody production may be stimulated as a result of the transfusion, causing an anamnestic reaction; the result is a high concentration of antibody and hemolysis of the transfused cells, known as a delayed hemolytic transfusion reaction.

Table 31-1. Blood Component Summary

Product	Description	Storage (°C)	Expiration	Indications	Dose	Handling Comments
Whole blood	All the components of 450 mL donor blood plus the anticoagulant	1–6	ACD, CPD—21 days CPDA-1—35 days	Symptomatic anemia with acute volume deficits; massive transfusions/exchange transfusions	As needed for replacement: Adults: 1 unit will increase Hct 3% Infants: 3 mL/kg will increase Hgb 1 g/dL	Neonates may require whole blood <1 wk old with the Hct adjusted to 50%; can be infused as fast as patient tolerates
Whole blood, platelets/cryoprecipitate removed	Whole blood with platelets or cryoprecipitate removed; may have less plasma and 30–40% less fibrinogen	1–6	Closed system—see whole blood Open system—24 h	Same as whole blood	Same as whole blood	—
Red blood cells	CPD, CPDA-1: whole blood with 200–250 mL plasma removed; final volume is ~300 mL, Hct <80% AS: whole blood with most plasma removed and 100 mL preservative added; final volume is ~350 mL, Hct 55–65%	1–6	Closed system—see whole blood AS additive—42 d Open system—24 h	Symptomatic anemia not treatable with diet/medication; decreased plasma volume ideal for patients with chronic anemia, volume change intolerance, and renal and liver disease	Same as whole blood	Allow 10-min preparation time if packed just before issue; neonates may require RBCs <1 wk old; infuse within 4 h or as patient tolerates
Red blood cells, WBCs removed	RBCs modified by centrifugation, washing, or filtration to remove >70% WBCs while retaining >70% of the original RBCs	1–6	Closed system—see RBCs Open system—24 h	Symptomatic anemia plus history of repeated nonhemolytic febrile transfusion reactions; filtered products may prevent HLA alloimmunization	Same as whole blood	Allow 15–60 min if prepared just before issue; if prepared at bedside, use special designated filter

Red blood cells, washed	RBCs washed with normal saline to remove non-RBC elements; RBC loss (often 20%), plasma removal (≤99%), WBC reduction (≤85%) varies with methodology	1–6	24 h	Symptomatic anemia plus history of repeated allergic or febrile transfusion reactions; paroxysmal nocturnal hemoglobinuria	Same as whole blood	Allow 20–30 min preparation time
Red blood cells, frozen-deglycerolized	RBCs frozen with cryoprotectant glycerol, which is washed away before transfusion; final product contains >80% original RBCs, 1–10 × 10^7 WBCs, and minimal plasma and platelets, and is resuspended in normal saline; a trace of glycerol may remain	Frozen <−65 (high glycerol) <−120 (low glycerol) Deglycerolized 1–6	10 y 3 y 24 h	Prolonged storage for rare or autologous units; see also indications for RBCs, washed	Same as whole blood	Allow ~1 h to thaw and deglycerolize
Platelets	>5.5 × 10^{10} platelets in 40–70 mL plasma (20–24°C storage) or 20–30 mL plasma (1–6°C storage); may contain trace—0.5 mL RBCs, ~10^8 WBCs, and hemostatic levels of coagulation factors	1–6 with no agitation 20–24 with agitation	3 or 5 d, depending on storage bag, 4 h after pooling	Bleeding related to thrombocytopenia or platelet dysfunction, low or rapidly dropping platelet counts	Hemostatic dose: 1 bag/10 kg body weight Adults: 1 bag will increase platelet count 5000–10,000/µL Infants: 1 bag will increase platelet count 75,000–100,000/µL	Allow 10–20 min to pool, 10–60 min to prepare as leukocyte-poor or volume-reduced; infuse 5 mL/min or as patient tolerates

(Continued)

Table 31-1. Blood Component Summary (Continued)

Product	Description	Storage (°C)	Expiration	Indications	Dose	Handling Comments
Platelets, pheresis	>30 × 10¹⁰ platelets in 200–500 mL plasma; may contain trace–20 mL RBCs, 0.3–6 × 10⁹ WBCs, and hemostatic levels of coagulation factors depending on collection method	20–24 with agitation	24 h or 5 d, depending on method and storage bag	See platelets; when HLA-matched or crossmatch-compatible donors are needed for refractory patients; may help reduce donor exposures	Hemostatic dose: 1 U	—
Granulocytes	About 1 × 10¹⁰ granulocytes in 200–400 mL plasma; may contain 5–50 mL RBCs, 10⁹ other WBCs, 20–100 × 10¹⁰ platelets, and hemostatic levels of coagulation factors, depending on collection method; 6–12% of volume may be HES, if used	20–24 without agitation	24 h	Severe neutropenia with infection unresponsive to antibiotic therapy	Adults: 1 U/d for 4–6 days or until patient recovers or granulocyte count returns to 500/µL Infants: 0.5–1 × 10⁹ granulocytes as needed	Do not infuse with depth microaggregate filter; infuse slowly over 2–4 h
Fresh frozen plasma (FFP)	200–250 mL plasma plus anticoagulant frozen within 6 h of collection; contains ~200 U of all plasma clotting factors and 200–400 mg fibrinogen	Frozen: <−18 Thawed: 1–6	1 y 24 h (AABB) 6 h (FDA)	Bleeding related to coagulation factor deficiencies where specific concentrates are not available or are contraindicated; coumarin drug reversal; TTP	Hemostatic dose: 10 mL/kg body weight; 15 mL/kg may be indicated for initial loading dose	Allow 15–30 min to thaw; infuse 5–10 mL/min or as patient tolerates

Plasma; liquid plasma	180–300 mL plasma plus anticoagulant that does not meet FFP rigid requirements; contains ~200 U of stable clotting factors; depending on method of preparation, may contain reduced factor V, VIII, fibrinogen	Plasma: <−18 Liquid plasma: 1–6	5 y 5 d after whole blood expiration	See FFP; not indicated with known factor V and VIII deficiencies	Same as FFP	Same as FFP
Cryoprecipitated AHF	A concentration of 80–120 U factor VIII, 40–70% von Willebrand factor, and 20–30% factor XIII present in original unit; 150–250 mg fibrinogen, ~55 mg fibronectin in <15 mL plasma	Frozen: <−18 Thawed: 20–24	1 y 6 h 4 h after pooling	To control bleeding associated with hemophilia A, von Willebrand's disease, uremia, and factor XIII and fibrinogen deficiencies; fibronectin replacement; fibrin glue to stop topical bleeding or to remove renal calculi	Dose is calculated on plasma volume; 8–10 bags supply 2 g fibrinogen (hemostatic dose)	Consider alternative therapies; allow 5–10 min to thaw, 15 min to pool; transfuse 5–10 mL/min or as patient tolerates
Albumin; Plasma Protein Fraction (PPF)	Albumin: 5% or 25% protein solution; ~96% albumin and 4% globulins PPF: 5% solution; 83% albumin, 17% α/β globulins All 3 products have sodium content ~145 mEq/L	2–8 Room temperature	5 y 3 y ~4 h after opening	Large, acute colloid losses occurring with severe burns or hypovolemic shock; blood pressure support during hypotensive episodes; not indicated for nutritional hypoproteinemia	Shock: determined by patient's condition and response Burns: as needed to maintain protein level of 5.2 g/dL	No filter required; PPF infusion can precipitate severe hypotensive episodes; do not infuse intra-arterially or >10 mL/min; PPF has been reported to cause hemolysis when mixed with older RBCs

(Continued)

869

Table 31-1. Blood Component Summary *(Continued)*

Product	Description	Storage (°C)	Expiration	Indications	Dose	Handling Comments
Immune serum globulin (ISG)	ISG: concentrated solution containing 16 g/dL protein (95–98% IgG, 1–2% IgM and IgA) IVIG: 5 g/dL protein solution	2–8	1–3 y, depending on specific product	ISG: prophylactic passive immunity for immunoincompetent patients or those at risk of disease IVIG: same as above, for patients requiring high-dose therapy or those who cannot tolerate IM injection	Congenital deficiencies: ISG—0.7 mL/kg/mo IVIG—100 mg/kg/mo Hyperimmune products for specific diseases: as manufacturer recommends ITP: 1–2 g IVIG/kg as needed	No filter required; must be given via proper route: ISG — IM IVIG — IV
Rh immunoglobulin	Special ISG: standard vial: 300 µg anti-D "Mini" vial: 50 µg anti-D	2–8	6 mo	To prevent Rh-negative individual from becoming sensitized to D antigen after being exposed to RH-positive RBCs through pregnancy or transfusion	20 µg/1 mL RBCs, Termination of pregnancy within 1st 12 wk: 1 minivial All other situations: 1 standard vial or as indicated	No filter required; give IM
Factor VIII concentrate	Lyophilized concentration of factor VIII, activity units are on label; may also contain some fibrinogen and von Willebrand factor	2–8 Room temperature	1 y ≤3 mo, consult manufacturer; ~3 h after reconstituting for infusion	To control bleeding in severe hemophilia A	As needed: 1 U/kg will increase activity level 2%; larger loading dose required	Must be filtered; reconstitute per manufacturer's directions; give IV and use plastic syringe
Factor IX concentrate (prothrombin complex)	Lyophilized concentration of factors II, VII, IX, X, plus minimal amounts of other proteins; activity units are stated on label	2–8 Room temperature	1 y Up to 1 mo, consult manufacturer; ~3 h after reconstituting for infusion	To control bleeding in severe hemophilia B or specific factor deficiencies	As needed: 1 U/kg will increase activity level 1%; larger loading dose required	Must be filtered; reconstitute per manufacturer's directions; give IV

Abbreviations: AABB, American Association of Blood Banks; FDA, Food and Drug Administration; Hct, hematocrit; Hgb, hemoglobin; RBCs, red blood cells; WBCs, white blood cells; HES, hydroxyethyl starch; ITP, idiopathic thrombocytopenia purpura; ISG, immune serum globulin; IVIG, intravenous immunoglobulin; TTP, thrombotic thrombocytopenic purpura; IV, intravenous; IM, intramuscular; ACD, acid citrate dextrose; CPD, citrate phosphate dextrose; CPDA, CPD adenine; AS, adenine saline.
(From Calhoun,[37] with permission.)

PRETRANSFUSION TESTING

Transfusion Request Forms

Blood request forms must contain sufficient information for positive identification of the patient. The Standards for Blood Banks and Transfusion Services of the American Association of Blood Banks[2] (AABB) requires that at least the first and last names of the patient and the patient's unique hospital identification number be on the form. Additional information, such as sex and age of the patient, diagnosis, previous transfusion history, pregnancy history, and the name of the requesting physician, may be helpful in resolving problems, should they occur. Blood request forms lacking the required information or containing illegible information must not be accepted by laboratory personnel.

Specimen Collection and Handling

Patient Identification

Critical to safe transfusion is collecting a properly identified and labeled blood specimen from the correct patient for pretransfusion testing.[1] The person who draws the blood specimen must positively identify the patient by comparing identifying data with the information on the wristband. A specimen should not be collected if there is a discrepancy between the two. It is inappropriate to rely on a bed tag or on charts or records placed on the bed or on nearby tables or equipment.

If the patient does not have a wristband, the patient should be asked to state his or her full name. The patient should not be offered a name and asked to confirm that it is correct. In addition, the patient's identity must be confirmed by someone who knows the patient; the name of the person who made the identification should be noted on the request form. The phlebotomist should follow up with the staff to ensure that the patient is properly identified with a wristband. This will facilitate identification of the patient at the time of transfusion.

If the patient's identity is unknown, the emergency identification attached to a patient may be used. This emergency identification should be cross-referenced with the patient's name and identification number, when they are known.

Specimen Requirements

It is permissible to collect a blood specimen from an infusion line if the patient is receiving intravenous fluids. The tubing should be flushed with saline solution; approximately the first 5 mL of blood withdrawn should be discarded because residual fluid in the line could interfere with serologic testing.

Serum or plasma may be used for pretransfusion testing. Serum is preferable to plasma because, with plasma, small fibrin clots sometimes form that are occasionally difficult to distinguish from agglutination. Fibrin can be a problem in specimens that fail to clot; this usually is caused by heparin therapy. In this situation, thrombin or protamine sulfate can be added to the specimen.

Rarely, antibodies are demonstrable only through complement activation and cannot be detected if plasma is used. Anticoagulants such as EDTA or citrate chelate calcium and prevent complement activation.

Specimen Labeling

The blood specimen must be drawn into a stoppered tube. Before the phlebotomist leaves the bedside, the blood collection tubes must be labeled with the patient's first and last names and identification number, as well as the date. Imprinted labels may be used if the information on the label is identical to that on the wristband and request form. In addition, there must be a way to identify the phlebotomist. This can be done by having the phlebotomist initial or sign either the tube label or the transfusion request form. Because the request form is a permanent record and the tube is discarded, signing the request form records the information in a more permanent fashion.

Age of Specimen

For patients who have been pregnant or who have received transfusions within the preceding 3 months, the specimen used for compatibility testing must be no more than 3 days old at the time of the transfusion. Recent transfusion or pregnancy may stimulate the appearance of unexpected antibodies. Because it is not possible to predict when such an antibody will be demonstrable, a 3-day limit has been somewhat arbitrarily selected. Many laboratory directors prefer to set a 3-day limit on all specimens used for pretransfusion testing, to avoid problems that might occur because of record-keeping errors or inaccurate history. If a fresh specimen from a patient who has not been recently pregnant or transfused is unavailable, the director may approve an exception.

Confirming Identification

When a specimen is received in the laboratory, a qualified member of the staff must confirm that the information on the label and on the transfusion request form is identical. If there is any discrepancy or any doubt about the identity of the patient, a new specimen must be obtained. It is unacceptable for anyone to correct an incorrectly labeled specimen.

Retaining and Storing Blood Specimens

The recipient's blood specimen and a sample of the donor's RBCs must be sealed or stoppered and kept at 1–6°C for at least 7 days after each transfusion. The sample from the donor may be the remainder of the segment actually used in the crossmatch or a segment removed just before issuing the blood. If the original segment is saved, it must be placed in a sealed or stoppered tube; an intact segment removed before issuing is already sealed. Keeping the patient's and donor's samples makes it possible to do repeat or additional testing if the patient experiences an unfavorable response to the blood transfusion.

Previous Records

Compatibility testing must include checking previous transfusion service records for information on the recipient's past serologic history. If the patient has been previously tested, results of current testing must be compared with interpretation of previous testing. Discrepancies must be resolved before blood is issued.

The specificity of previously detected antibodies should be compared with currently detectable antibodies. Even if the current antibody detection test is negative, the antiglobulin phase of the crossmatch is required for such patients. Blood lacking that particular antigen should be selected for transfusion even though RBCs possessing the antigen may now be serologically compatible.

Specimens from Infants

The requirements for specimens from neonatal recipients (less than 4 months old) are different.[1]

1. If there are no unexpected antibodies detected by initial tests and the infant receives no blood products containing clinically significant antibodies, antibody detection and crossmatching tests can be omitted throughout the 4-month neonatal period. The serum or plasma of either the mother or infant may be used for initial testing.
2. After the baby's ABO and Rh groups have been determined, ABO and Rh grouping tests may be omitted, provided the baby receives only RBCs that are of the baby's ABO group or group O and are either the baby's Rh group or Rh-negative.

TRANSFUSION OF RED BLOOD CELL PRODUCTS

Indications

Red blood cell products may be ordered for the indications briefly outlined in Table 31-1. The principles of appropriate transfusion of RBCs are as follows.[3] Red blood cell transfusions increase oxygen-carrying capacity in anemic patients. Transfusing 1 U of RBC will usually increase the hemoglobin by 1 g/dL and the hematocrit by 2–3% in the average 70-kg adult.

Adequate oxygen-carrying capacity can be met by a hemoglobin of 7 g/dL (a hematocrit value of approximately 21%) or even less when the intravascular volume is adequate for perfusion. In deciding whether to transfuse a specific patient, the physician should consider the person's age; the etiology and degree of anemia; hemodynamic stability; and the presence of coexisting cardiac, pulmonary, or vascular conditions. To meet oxygen needs, some patients may require RBC transfusions at higher hemoglobin levels.

When a treatable cause of anemia can be identified, specific replacement therapy (e.g., vitamin B_{12}, iron, folate) should always be used before transfusion is considered. If volume expanders are indicated, fluids such as crystalloid or nonblood colloid solutions should be administered. Red blood cell transfusions are often used inappropriately as volume expanders. Red blood cells should not be transfused for volume expansion, in place of a hematinic, to enhance wound healing or to improve the patient's general well-being.

Compatibility Testing

Serologic testing must be performed prior to transfusion to determine compatibility of the product to be transfused. The ABO and Rh groups of the intended recipient must be determined; in addition, if the patient is to receive whole blood, RBCs, platelet, or granulocyte concentrates containing 5 mL or more of RBCs, the recipient's serum must be tested for unexpected antibodies and for serologic compatibility with the donor's RBCs.[2]

Tests for RBC compatibility serve to prevent hemolytic transfusion reactions. Compatibility testing includes (1) verification of the groups of the donor blood, (2) tests on the recipient's blood to include ABO and Rh and screening for unexpected antibodies; and (3) a major crossmatch between donor RBCs and recipient serum.[2] It should be noted that the terms *compatibility test* and *crossmatch* are not synonymous but that the crossmatch is a component of compatibility testing.

The most appropriate means of performing compatibility test procedures are not mandated in detail by regulatory agencies; many alternative approaches are possible. Numerous procedures with varying degrees of cost-effectiveness have been suggested by workers in the field, and concepts continue to evolve.

Blood Group Tests

To determine the ABO group of the recipient, the RBCs must be tested with anti-A and anti-B and the serum with A_1 and B RBCs. As indicated in Table 31-2, such testing will determine the person's ABO blood group as O, A, B, or AB. Any discrepancy in test results should be resolved before blood is given.[2,4] If the problem cannot be defined with certainty before transfusion, the patient should receive group O RBCs, which are safest in an emergency situation.

The terms Rh-positive and Rh-negative refer to the presence or absence of the RBC antigen called D. The D antigen is, after A and B, the most important RBC antigen in transfusion practice. Unlike the situation with A and B, persons whose RBCs lack the D antigen do not regularly have anti-D in their serum. Formation of the antibody results from exposure to immunizing RBCs possessing the D antigen as a result of transfusion or pregnancy.

The patient's RBCs must be tested with anti-D, but routine testing for other Rh antigens is not recommended. Tests with anti-D must be controlled to avoid incorrectly concluding that an Rh-negative person is Rh-positive.

The best way to detect possibly invalid reactions in anti-D testing is to use as the immunologically inert control reagent the actual diluents used for manufacturing the particular anti-D reagent. This material contains the same additives present in the anti-D serum except for the antibody component and can therefore be expected to potentiate spurious agglutination to the same degree as the anti-D reagent itself. Manufacturers offer their own high protein diluents as control reagents. If there is a problem in interpreting tests for D, the patient should be given Rh-negative blood until the problem is resolved.

D^u Test

Not all D+ RBC samples react equally well with every anti-D blood grouping serum. Most D+ cells show clear-cut macroscopic agglutination after centrifugation of cells with serum and can readily be classified as D+. Cells that are not immediately agglutinated cannot as easily be classified as D− because some D+ cells that react with anti-D are not directly agglutinated. The cells are D+ because the D antigen is present, but additional testing may be required to demonstrate the presence of a weakly expressed D antigen.

Cells classified as D^u possess the D antigen but express it so weakly that they are not directly agglutinated by most anti-D sera. D^u can be recognized most reliably by the indirect antiglobulin test after the test cells have been incubated with anti-D serum. Not every anti-D serum is suitable for the D^u test, either because testing by the manufacturer has not shown reliable reactions with D^u cells or because the antiserum contains other antibodies reactive by the antiglobulin test. The manufacturer's package insert will state whether the reagent may be used for D^u testing.[1]

Table 31-2. Results Obtained in Blood Group Tests and Their Interpretation

RBCs			Serum			RBCs			Serum		
−A	−B	−D	A_1	B	Interpretation	−A	−B	−D	A_1	B	Interpretation
0	0	0	4+	4+	O Rh−	0	0	4+	4+	4+	O Rh+
4+	0	0	0	4+	A Rh−	4+	0	4+	0	4+	A Rh+
0	4+	0	4+	0	B Rh−	0	4+	4+	4+	0	B Rh+
4+	4+	0	0	0	AB Rh−	4+	4+	4+	0	0	AB Rh[a]

[a] Rh type cannot be determined because of absence of a negative control test; the AB Rh+ conclusion can only be made after the RBCs have been tested with an appropriate Rh control reagent and found to be nonreactive.
(From Judd,[4] with permission.)

Either a diluent control test or a direct antiglobulin test must accompany the D^u test procedure. Agglutination in the anti-D tube and none in the control tube constitutes a positive test result. The blood must be classified as D+. It is incorrect to report D^u cells as being D-negative, D^u-positive. A negative result is absence of agglutination in the test with anti-D. This means that the cells do not have D activity and are to be classified as D−. If the control test is positive, no valid interpretation of the D^u test can be made. In this situation, Rh-negative blood should be given if the test cells are from a patient; if the cells are from a donor, the cells should not be used for transfusion.[1]

It is not necessary to determine whether a recipient's RBCs are of the D^u phenotype because no harm results from giving these patients Rh-negative RBCs. In some laboratories, the test for the weaker expression of D, the D^u test, is done. Patients of the D^u phenotype can receive Rh-positive blood and only rarely make anti-D. Rh-negative blood can thus be reserved for recipients whose cells lack the D antigen. Performing the D^u test routinely and then giving Rh-negative blood to patients of the D^u phenotype accomplishes no useful purpose.[1]

Donor RBCs giving positive reactions in D^u tests should be regarded as Rh-positive. In perinatal testing of maternal blood, a weakly reactive D^u test may be associated with a large fetal-maternal hemorrhage. Infants with reactive D^u tests should be regarded as Rh-positive when making decisions related to Rh immunoglobulin therapy for Rh-negative mothers.

Antibody Detection (Screening) Tests

American Association of Blood Banks Standards[2] require testing of the serum or plasma of a recipient against suspensions of group O RBCs from individual donors. The cells are selected on the basis of whether they possess the relevant blood group antigens for detection of clinically significant unexpected antibodies. Unexpected antibodies in the sera of potential transfusion recipients are those other than anti-A or anti-B. It is difficult to define "clinically significant," because the significance may depend on the specific clinical situation and on the condition of the patient. In general terms, an antibody is clinically significant if antibody with that specificity has caused overt hemolytic transfusion reactions or unacceptably short survival of transfused RBCs. The antiglobulin phase of testing is required by AABB Standards. It must be performed as part of antibody detection (screening) tests, or in the crossmatch, or both.

Crossmatch

Unless the situation is urgent, the recipient's serum or plasma must be tested with the donor's RBCs before whole blood and RBC components are given; that is, a major crossmatch must be done. The methods used must include those that will demonstrate ABO incompatibility and detect clinically significant unexpected antibodies and include an antiglobulin test unless both of the following conditions are met:

1. No clinically significant antibodies are detected in antibody screening tests.
2. There is no record that a clinically significant antibody has at any time been detected.

When these two requirements are met, an antiglobulin test is not required as part of the crossmatch test; instead, ABO blood group compatibility may be verified by an *immediate spin crossmatch*. This is acceptable because only rarely is a clinically significant unexpected antibody detected by the antiglobulin test phase of the crossmatch when the antibody screening test is negative.

The immediate spin crossmatch is performed by simply adding 1 drop of 2–4% saline suspended donor RBCs to 2 drops of the recipient's serum, centrifuging, and reading for agglutination. An immediate spin test is acceptable, but a 5-minute incubation improves the sensitivity of the test if the recipient has a weakly reactive anti-A or -B or if the donor's RBCs have a weak expression of an antigen, for example, the A antigen on A_2 RBCs.

IDENTIFICATION OF UNEXPECTED ALLOANTIBODIES

Procedures described in this section are those used to evaluate blood specimens that contain unexpected antibodies as determined by the antibody screening tests or crossmatch. They also may be used for antibody screening and crossmatching.

Unexpected alloantibodies are antibodies, other than naturally occurring anti-A or -B, that react with antigens not present on the RBCs of the antibody producer. Immunization to RBC antigens occurs through pregnancy or transfusion or after deliberate injection with immunogenic material. In unusual instances, the immunizing event is unknown.

The selection of any given procedure for antibody identification should be influenced by the antibody detection method used; initially, it is advisable to use those techniques by which the reactive pretransfusion tests were first encountered. Furthermore, many workers advocate routine use of an enzyme technique in antibody identification studies. This recommendation is made because enzyme techniques do not detect certain antibody specificities, whereas the reactivity of other specificities is enhanced. Thus, results of enzyme tests can provide important clues to the specificity of antibodies under investigation.[4]

General Procedures

Blood Specimens

A sample of 10 mL of clotted blood usually supplies sufficient serum for identifying simple antibody specificities, but complex problems may require additional serum. To avoid the possibility of complement attaching to the RBCs, blood anticoagulated with EDTA is preferred for studies on autologous RBCs. Antibody studies can be performed on serum or plasma.

Medical History

It is useful to know a patient's clinical diagnosis, transfusion history, obstetric history, and drug therapy.

Reagent Red Blood Cells

The serum under investigation is ordinarily tested against a panel of eight or more group O RBC samples of known antigen composition that may be obtained from commercial sources. An example of an RBC panel for alloantibody identification is given in Table 31-3. A list is provided with each commercially prepared panel that shows, in moderate detail, the phenotype of each RBC sample. A well-constituted reagent RBC panel permits confident identification of those clinically significant alloantibodies that are most frequently encountered, such as anti-D, -E, -K, and -Fy^a. A distinct pattern of reactivity should be apparent for each of the commonly encountered alloantibodies; for example, the K+ samples should not be the only ones that are also E+. There must be sufficient numbers of informative RBCs to exclude chance alone as the cause for seemingly definitive patterns associated with most of the antigens listed in Table 31-3.

Autologous Control

It is important to know how the serum under investigation reacts with the autologous RBCs. This helps determine whether alloantibody or autoantibody, or both, are present. Serum that reacts only with reagent RBCs usually contains only alloantibody; reactivity with both reagent and autologous RBCs suggests the presence of an autoantibody or of both auto- and alloantibodies. A patient with alloantibodies directed against recently transfused RBCs may have a positive autologous control, because circulating donor RBCs are coated with alloantibodies. This may be misinterpreted as being caused by autoantibody. A detailed transfusion history is especially important in patients whose RBCs are coated with antibody.

Methods

A number of serologic techniques have been developed for antibody identification that vary in their sensitivity and specificity. Serum should be tested at all test phases at which antibody activity was initially detected. The use of different test phases and additional procedures, such as extended incubation periods, cold

Table 31-3. Reagent Red Blood Cell Panel for Alloantibody Identification

Sample #	Rh Phenotype	C	C^w	c	D	E	e	K	Fy^a	Fy^b	Jk^a	Jk^b	P$_1$	Le^a	Le^b	M	N	S	s
1	r'r	+	0	+	0	0	+	0	+	0	+	+	+	0	+	+	+	0	+
2	R$_1^w$R$_1$	+	+	0	+	0	+	+	+	+	0	+	+	+	0	+	+	+	+
3	R$_1$R$_1$	+	0	0	+	0	+	0	+	+	+	+	0	0	+	+	0	+	0
4	R$_2$R$_2$	0	0	+	+	+	0	0	0	+	0	+	+	+	0	0	+	0	+
5	r''r	0	0	+	0	+	+	0	+	0	+	0	0	+	+	+	+	+	0
6	rr	0	0	+	0	0	+	0	0	+	+	0	+	0	0	+	+	0	+
7	rr	0	0	+	0	0	+	+	0	+	+	0	+	0	+	+	0	+	0
8	rr	0	0	+	0	0	+	0	+	0	0	+	+	0	0	+	0	+	0
9	rr	0	0	+	0	0	+	0	0	+	0	0	+	0	+	0	+	+	0
10	R$_o$r	0	0	+	+	0	+	0	0	0	+	+	+	0	0	+	+	+	+

+, presence of antigen; 0, absence of antigen.
(From Walker,[1] with permission.)

temperatures, or enhancement methods, may uncover additional antibodies or enhance the reactivity of the antibody initially detected. Several methods have been used for antibody identification.

Saline Test

The simplest serologic method is the saline technique. The recipient's serum is mixed with saline-suspended cells. The tube may be centrifuged immediately or incubated at room temperature before centrifugation. ABO incompatibilities and antibodies reactive at room temperature (e.g., anti-M, anti-P_1, and anti-Le^a) are most often detected at this phase.

The serum-cell mixture is usually incubated only at 37°C. Some antibodies, such as anti-K and anti-D, directly agglutinate or lyse antigen-positive cells (e.g., anti-Le^a, anti-PP$_1$P^k) after incubation at 37°C. Most often, however, antibodies bind to the RBCs during incubation but are not demonstrable unless the antiglobulin test or other more sensitive methods are used.

Antiglobulin Test

Incomplete antibodies, by definition, sensitize RBCs but do not cause their agglutination or lysis. When such antibody sensitized RBCs are washed and incubated with antiglobulin serum, agglutination occurs. Either anti-IgG or a polyspecific antiglobulin reagent that contains anti-IgG and anti-C3d may be used for the antiglobulin phase of antibody detection and crossmatching tests.[1]

There have been numerous reports of RBC alloantibodies that were not detectable with anti-IgG antiglobulin serum but that were detected with the anticomplement component of antiglobulin serum. These antibodies may cause shortened RBC survival.[5] Also, there have been reports indicating that complement-fixing blood group antibodies are frequently detected at a higher dilution and/or with stronger reactions when a polyspecific antiglobulin serum is used rather than a monospecific anti-IgG. This occurs even though the concentration of anti-IgG is the same in the monospecific antiserum as in the polyspecific antiserum, as determined by titration tests.[5]

Unfortunately, however, positive reactions may be obtained with anticomplement antiglobulin serum in some instances not caused by a clinically significant RBC alloantibody. Most of these false positive reactions are only very weakly positive and are caused by the presence of clinically insignificant cold antibodies. Thus, the frequency of this problem is higher in laboratories that (misguidedly) retain incubation at room temperature as a phase of compatibility testing. The use of low ionic strength solutions (LISS) also will affect the number of clinically insignificant reactions obtained when using antiglobulin serum containing anticomplement.[5]

Therefore, one must balance the advantage of detecting a small number of clinically significant alloantibodies that would not be detected with anti-IgG antiglobulin serum with the disadvantages that result from using an antiglobulin serum containing anticomplement. One recommended method is to use polyspecific antiglobulin serum with albumin techniques but not in association with LISS; room temperature incubation should be omitted.[5] An alternative approach is to use anti-IgG antiglobulin serum in association with LISS.

Enzyme Techniques

Treatment of RBCs with proteolytic enzymes enhances the serologic reactivity of some blood group antibodies, yet destroys or denatures a variety of RBC antigens, including, notably, M, N, S, Fy^a, and Fy^b. At least in part, serologic enhancement is caused by removal of glycoproteins carrying *N*-acetylneuraminic acid, a sialic acid with a negatively charged COOH group contributing significantly to RBC surface charge. Because like charges repel, normal RBCs are kept apart at a distance too great for IgG molecules to span.

Enhancement of serologic reactivity is not the sole purpose of using proteases. Their usefulness in antibody identification occurs because loss of serologic reactivity after protease treatment is often an indication of antibody specificity. Similarly, the ability to hemolyze protease-treated RBCs is a characteristic of certain complement-binding antibodies. Thus, reaction patterns with enzyme-treated RBCs provide important clues to antibody identification.[4]

Several proteolytic enzymes (papain, bromelin, trypsin, ficin) are suitable for blood bank use. Papain and bromelin are usually added directly to a serum-cell mixture, in a one-stage technique; papain, ficin, and trypsin are used in a two-stage technique to treat the RBCs before serum is added. The one-stage technique is less sensitive than the two-stage method because serum proteins serve as substrate in addition to RBC membrane proteins. Although there is less modification of the membrane, the one-stage technique is a more convenient procedure. In addition to being more sensitive, the two-stage method has the advantage that the enzyme-modified cells can be tested before use, to ensure that optimal modification has been achieved. Enzyme solutions and reagent RBCs pretreated with enzymes are commercially available. It is important to follow the designated methods carefully.[1]

Low-Ionic Strength Solutions

In 1964, two groups of investigators reported on the significance of suspending RBCs used for antibody detection media with a salt solution of low ionic strength. In detecting a wide variety of blood group antibodies by the indirect antiglobulin test, the use of a low ionic strength solution permitted the incubation time to be reduced from 1 hour to 5 minutes. Also, the titer of a wide range of antibodies was increased. However, some false positive results also were noted and LISS techniques were not applied to routine compatibility testing, even by the blood bankers who published the original reports.

Interest in this methodology was suddenly awakened in 1974 by the report of Low and Messeter,[6] who reported that LISS methods had been used for more than 100,000 consecutive crossmatches. Further reports followed quickly; the current view is that the use of LISS permits detection of RBC antibodies in the antiglobulin test after only 10 minutes incubation. The sensitivity is somewhat greater than incubation in albumin media for 15–30 minutes. Also, somewhat stronger reactions than with albumin-suspended cells are obtained with a significant percentage of sera. Although false positive or nonspecific reactions and the detection of clinically insignificant cold antibodies occur somewhat more frequently with LISS than with saline or albumin techniques, they may not be a significant problem if the room temperature incubation phase of the crossmatch is omitted.[5]

Albumin

Since 1945, bovine serum albumin solutions have been used to enhance direct agglutination of RBCs by antibodies of the IgG class.[1] Albumin can be used as an additive to the serum-cell mixture or can be layered on the cell button. The addition technique is more frequently used in the United States, but the layering method is probably the more sensitive method for detecting direct agglutination by Rh antibodies and by occasional examples of anti-Fy^a and anti-D.

Interpreting Serologic Results

Alloantibodies of certain blood group specificities often display consistent serologic characteristics (Table 31-4). In interpreting the results of serum studies, it is important to look for these characteristics and to examine the phenotypes of both reactive and nonreactive RBC samples. Several factors should be considered:

1. What is the effect of temperature, suspending medium, or proteolytic enzymes on the reactions of individual RBC samples?
2. Does the strength of agglutination vary among reactive RBC samples?
3. Is hemolysis present?
4. Are the autologous RBCs reactive or nonreactive?

With these data and the results of tests against a reagent RBC panel, it usually is possible to identify an antibody or to select additional reagent RBCs or procedures that can be used for conclusive identification. The following is an approach to interpreting the results of alloantibody identification tests and selecting additional tests for confirmation:

1. Eliminate from initial consideration antibodies to antigens present on nonreactive reagent RBCs
2. Examine the phenotypes, especially M, N, S, Fy^a, and Fy^b antigens, of samples that react with untreated RBCs but not with enzyme-treated RBCs
3. Eliminate from consideration antibodies, especially Rh antibodies, that should react with antigens present on nonreactive enzyme-treated RBCs
4. Eliminate from consideration antibodies to antigens present on the autologous RBCs
5. Examine the reaction patterns at each test phase: evaluate possible specificities with regard to test phase and manner of reactivity
6. Test sufficient RBCs of appropriate phenotypes to obtain a probability of less than 0.05 (1 of 20) for each suspected specificity; this is accomplished by testing six reagent RBC samples and finding three antigen-positive samples to react and three antigen-negative samples to be nonreactive (see under Probability)
7. Test serum against RBCs carrying a double-dose expression of common antigens of

Table 31-4. Serologic Behavior of the Principal Antibodies of the Different Blood Group Systems[a]

Antibody	In Vitro Hemolysis	Saline 4°C	Saline 22°C	Saline 37°C	Albumin AGT	Enzyme 37°C	Enzyme AGT	Associated with HDN	Associated with HTR
Anti-M	0	Most	Some	Few	Few	0	0	Few	Few
Anti-N	0	Most	Few	Occ.	Occ.	0	0	Rare	?
Anti-S	0	Few	Some	Some	Most	see text		Yes	Yes
Anti-s	0	0	Few	Few	Most	see text		Yes	Yes
Anti-U	0	0	Occ.	Some	Most	Most	Most	Yes	Rare
Anti-P₁	Occ.	Most	Some	Occ.	Rare	Some	Few	No	?
Anti-P	Some	Most	Some	Some	Some	Some	Some	No	?
Anti-PP₁Pₓ	Some	Most	Some	Some	Some	Some	Some	Rare	?
Anti-Luᵃ	0	Some	Most	Few	Few	Few	Few	No	Yes
Anti-Luᵇ	0	Few	Few	Few	Most	Some	Most	Mild	Yes
Anti-K	0		Few	Some	Most	Some	Most	Yes	Yes
Anti-k	0		Few	Few	Most	Some	Most	Yes	Yes
Atni-Kpᵃ	0		Some	Some	Most	Some	Some	Yes	?
Anti-Kpᵇ	0		Few	Few	Most	Some	Some	Yes	Yes
Anti-Jsᵃ	0		Few	Few	Most	Few	Few	Yes	?
Anti-Jsᵇ	0		0	0	Most	Few	Few	Yes	?
Anti-Leᵃ	Some	Most	Most	Some	Many	Most	Most	No	Few
Anti-Leᵇ	Occ.	Most	Most	Few	Some	Some	Some	No	No
Anti-Fyᵃ	0		Rare	Rare	Most	0	0	Yes	Yes
Anti-Fyᵇ	0		Rare	Rare	Most	0	0	Yes	Yes
Anti-Jkᵃ	Some		Few	Few	Most	Some	Yes	Yes	Yes
Anti-Jkᵇ	Some		Few	Few	Most	Some	Most	Yes	Yes
Anti-Xgᵃ	0		Few	0	Most	0	0	No	Yes
Anti-Diᵃ	0		Some	Some	Most	Some	Some	Yes	Yes
Anti-Diᵇ	0				Most	Some	Some	Yes	Yes
Anti-Ytᵃ	0		0	0	All	0	Some	No	?
Anti-Ytᵇ	0							No report	No report
Anti-Doᵃ	0		0	0	Some	Some	Most	?	Yes
Anti-Doᵇ	0				All		All		
Anti-Coᵃ	0		0	0	Some	Some	Most	Yes	No report
Anti-Coᵇ	0		0	0	Some	Some	Most		?
Anti-Sc1	0				All			No report	No report
Anti-Sc2	0		Some	Some	Most	Most	Most	No report	No report

Abbreviations: AGT, antiglobulin test; HDN, hemolytic disease of the newborn; HTR, hemolytic transfusion reactions.

[a] The reactivity shown is based on the tube methods in common use. If tests are carried out by more sensitive test procedures, such as in capillary tubes, in microtiter plates or by the albumin layering method, direct agglutination (prior to the antiglobulin phase) may be observed more often with some antibodies. Blank spaces indicate a lack of sufficient data for generalization about antibody behavior. (From Walker,[1] with permission.)

the major blood groups, if these were not among the original nonreactive samples: for example, Fy (a+, b−) RBCs should be used to exclude anti-Fy[a]
8. Test the autologous RBCs with reagent antisera for absence of the antigen against which the test serum manifests specificity; absence of the antigen on the patient's own RBCs indicates that the antigen in question is foreign to the patient's immune system and confirms that the antibody is an alloantibody that developed as a result of prior transfusion or pregnancy

Probability

Conclusive antibody identification requires testing the serum against sufficient reagent RBC samples that lack, and sufficient that carry, the relevant antigens to ensure that an observed pattern of reactivity does not result from chance alone.[1] Table 31-5 shows the probabilities of various combinations of reactive and nonreactive tests, as calculated by Fisher's exact method for estimating probabilities.

The probability (P) values shown in Table 31-5 are the result of statistical tests that show the likelihood that a given set of results is due to chance alone. A P value of 1/20 means that an identical set of results would be obtained by chance once in 20 similar studies. For example, if a serum agglutinates three reagent RBC samples that are D+ and fails to agglutinate three that are D−, P is 1 of 20; therefore, there is a 19 to 1 probability that the antibody is anti-D.

Most reagent RBC panels are limited in their ability to provide statistically conclusive identification of some blood group antibodies. It is important to bear these unavoidable limitations in mind when only one panel of reagent RBCs is available for testing. It is often necessary to test additional RBC samples before assigning conclusive specificity to an antibody.

Clinical Significance of Various RBC Alloantibodies

In consultation with the physician director of the blood transfusion service, clinicians must determine the appropriate course in the face of in vitro incompatibility. Some RBC alloantibodies cause life-threatening hemolysis, whereas others are benign and cause no shortening of survival of transfused RBCs. Thus, one factor in decision-making is an understanding of which RBC alloantibodies are likely to cause severe hemolysis and which are not. In each case of incompatibility, the clinician expects the director of the transfusion medicine service to provide as accurate an assessment as possible of the risk of a hemolytic transfusion reaction. The clinician, in turn, should have an adequate understanding of compatibility testing to allow for meaningful communication with the blood bank director; the clinician must incorporate information regarding the risks of blood transfusion into the decision-making process concerning management of the patient.

For example, for patients who have RBC alloantibodies in their serum that are likely to cause hemolysis of transfused RBCs containing the corresponding antigen, the course of least risk is usually to delay transfusion. This approach is recommended even if it means delaying a surgical procedure for the amount of time necessary to provide compatible blood. Most incompatibility problems can be resolved within a few hours. In other instances of serologic incompatibility, it may be inappropriate to delay transfusion, because the transfusion is an extreme emergency, or because the antibody is one that can be expected to be benign.

Many factors may influence whether a RBC antibody is clinically significant, that is, will cause hemolysis in vivo. Unfortunately, there are as yet no recognized in vitro characteristics or group of characteristics that can be used to indicate the in vivo significance of all RBC antibodies. Serologic characteristics of an antibody and information regarding previous experiences

Table 31-5. Probability of Identification for Combinations of Reactive and Nonreactive Tests

No. Tested	No. Reactive	No. Nonreactive	P
6	4	2	1/15
6	3	3	1/20
7	5	2	1/21
7	4	3	1/35
8	7	1	1/8
8	6	2	1/28
8	5	3	1/56
8	4	4	1/70
9	8	1	1/9
9	7	2	1/36
9	6	3	1/84
10	9	1	1/10
10	8	2	1/45
10	7	3	1/120
10	6	4	1/210
10	5	5	1/252

(From Walker,[1] with permission.)

Table 31-6. Clinical Significance of Some Red Blood Cell Alloantibodies
Group I — clinically significant antibodies
ABO
Rh
Kell
Duffy
Kidd
SsU
Group II — benign antibodies
Chido/Rodgers (Ch^a/Rg^a)
Xg^a
Bg
"HTLA" (high titer, low avidity)
Cs^a
Kn^a
McC^a
JMH
Group III — clinically insignificant if not reactive at 37°C; possibly significant when reacting at 37°C
Lewis (Le^a/Le^b)
M, N
P$_1$
Lutheran (Lu^a/Lu^b)
A$_1$
Group IV — antibodies that are sometimes clinically significant
Yt^a
Vel
Ge
Gy^a
Hy
Sd^a
York (Yk^a)

(From Petz,[5] with permission.)

have provided most of our present knowledge. In addition, RBC survival studies have contributed significantly. The two serologic characteristics that have been found most helpful in predicting the in vivo significance are the specificity of an antibody and its ability to react in vitro at 37°C. Red blood cell antibodies may be divided into four groups on the basis of clinical significance, as in Table 31-6.[5]

Antibodies that react at 37°C and that cause a large majority of hemolytic transfusion reactions are antibodies of the ABO, Rh, Kell, Kidd, Duffy, and SsU blood group systems (Table 31-6, group I). When antibodies of group I are found or if the patient's record indicates that these antibodies have been present in the past, every effort should be made to supply antigen-negative blood, unless extraordinary circumstances require transfusion of incompatible blood.

Other antibodies are "benign" or cause only minimal RBC destruction, even though they may react at 37°C; some of these are listed in group II. Hemolytic transfusion reactions caused by antibodies of group II have not been reported. It is therefore an appropriate policy to transfuse RBCs having the pertinent antigen, regardless of in vitro incompatibility, in patients who have group II antibodies.

Group III antibodies are those that are clinically insignificant if not reactive at 37°C and are only sometimes clinically significant when reactive at 37°C. Antibodies of such specificities that do not react at 37°C can safely be ignored. When reacting at 37°C, their in vivo significance is uncertain, but they should be considered to have potential clinical significance. Antigen-negative blood or crossmatch compatible blood should be transfused.

Group IV antibodies are inconsistent in regard to in vivo significance. When an antibody of one of these specificities is detected, an effort should be made to obtain antigen-negative blood, although in some instances such blood will only be available through rare donor files. Consideration should be given to autologous transfusion, including freezing of the patient's RBCs for long-term storage. If antigen-negative RBCs cannot be obtained, an in vivo survival study may be performed. If this study demonstrates acceptable survival of an aliquot of incompatible RBCs, blood may be transfused with a low probability of an immediate symptomatic hemolytic transfusion reaction.

If the in vivo survival study involving group IV antibodies demonstrates short survival or cannot be performed, and there is no time to obtain antigen-negative blood, a clinical decision is required. This should be based on the primary physician's assessment of the urgency of the transfusion and on the transfusion medicine specialist's assessment of the probability of a serious hemolytic transfusion reaction. If the urgency of the clinical situation truly requires emergency transfusion, it is necessary to proceed. If practical, one begins with slow administration of a small volume of RBCs (15–20 mL of packed RBCs over 30 minutes), carefully monitoring the patient for symptoms, and obtaining a blood specimen from the patient after 30 minutes to determine whether hemoglobinemia is present. Continued clinical observation and follow-up blood specimens for hemoglobinemia, perhaps after each unit, will allow for repeat assessment of the results of the transfusions. Even if transfusion is tolerated well, the volume of RBCs transfused should be kept as small as possible because of the possibility of an anamnestic reaction that may lead to a delayed hemolytic transfusion reaction. Certain very urgent clinical situations may necessitate less detailed monitoring.

Summary of Clinical Decision-Making When a Patient with Unexpected RBC Alloantibodies Requires Transfusion

When a RBC alloantibody is present that reacts at 37°C, the following approach is recommended.[5]

Group I antibodies: If the antibody is expected to be clinically significant, that is, has a specificity listed in group I of Table 31-6, antigen-negative blood should be transfused, except in an extreme emergency.

Group II Antibodies: If the antibody reacts at 37°C but is an antibody listed in group II of Table 31-6, antigen-positive blood may be transfused, even though it is incompatible in vitro.

Group III Antibodies: For antibodies of group III, crossmatch-negative blood may be issued without the necessity of ensuring that the blood is negative for the antigen in question.

Group IV Antibodies: For antibodies in group IV, an effort should be made to obtain antigen-negative blood from rare donor files (through reference laboratories) and/or typing of family members. Consideration should be given to autologous transfusion, including freezing of the patient's RBCs for long-term storage. If antigen-negative blood cannot be obtained, an in vivo survival study may be performed. If this study indicates acceptable survival of an aliquot of incompatible RBCs, blood may be transfused with a low probability of an immediate symptomatic hemolytic transfusion reaction. If the in vivo compatibility test indicates shortened survival, cautious transfusion may nevertheless be necessary in emergencies.

AUTOLOGOUS BLOOD TRANSFUSION

Background

Autologous blood transfusion eliminates the risk of most adverse effects associated with blood transfusion.[7] Thus, autologous blood transfusion minimizes the probability of transmission of infectious diseases, such as hepatitis B, hepatitis C, acquired immunodeficiency syndrome (AIDS), cytomegalovirus infection, HTLV-I infection, malaria, and Chagas disease. In addition, immunologically mediated transfusion reactions, such as hemolysis, chills, fever, rashes, noncardiogenic pulmonary edema, anaphylaxis, and alloimmunization (to RBC, human leukocyte antigen [HLA], and platelet antigens), should not occur. However, risks, such as adverse results caused by volume overload and clerical errors that lead to transfusion of the wrong unit of blood, are the same regardless of the source of the donation.

Indications

Patients should be considered candidates for autologous blood transfusion if they are scheduled for elective surgery and if there is good reason to expect blood transfusion. Donors of blood for autologous transfusion do not necessarily have to meet all the criteria established for normal volunteer blood donors. As compared with the general volunteer donor minimal criteria for hemoglobin and hematocrit are lower for the autologous donor and are 11 g/dL and 34%, respectively. There is no minimum weight, but for underweight donors proportionately smaller units may be withdrawn. Guidelines regarding autologous transfusion do not exclude anyone solely on the basis of age. Children as young as 8 years of age and weighing as little as 27 kg have donated prior to elective surgery.[8] Similarly, elderly persons are not excluded from donating. Haugen and Hill[9] reported 1672 patients who donated 6615 U of autologous blood during a 10-year period. In this study, 91% of the donors were older than 50 years of age, 81.6% were older than 60 years of age, and there were 162 donors aged 80–91 years. Many patients with coronary artery disease and in need of coronary artery bypass graft surgery may donate.

Patients who should be excluded from donating include those who have unstable angina or angina at rest, marked hypertension (greater than 180/100), congestive heart failure, myocardial infarction within the past 3 months, aortic stenosis, sustained ventricular tachycardia, severe left main stem coronary artery stenosis, transient ischemic attacks, and current bacteremia or infection.

Logistics

Patients can enter into predeposit autologous blood donation programs only at the request of a physician, usually the patient's surgeon or anesthesiologist. Autologous donors must sign an informed consent form as a prerequisite to donating blood. The consent form should outline the advantages, nature, and purposes of autologous transfusion; the risks involved; and the possibility of complications. If blood that is unused by the patient is to be released for transfusion to others, specific permission for release of the unused blood should be obtained from the patient.

An important aspect of patient management is iron replacement. With oral iron administration, the marrow can increase production after multiple phlebotomies to two or three times its usual levels, about 8–10 days after the initial phlebotomy.

The most practical schedule is to obtain 1 U of blood at weekly intervals, with the last unit withdrawn no later than 72 hours before surgery. The patient's hematocrit can be expected to fall initially and then stabilize with continued donations. For example, Finch et al.[10] reported that weekly phlebotomy over an 8-week period resulted in a decrease in the hematocrit from 44% to 37% during the first 5 weeks. Thereafter, the hematocrit stabilized and subsequently increased slightly to 38% by the eighth week, in those subjects who received iron therapy. In unusual circumstances, patients can tolerate a more intense donation schedule, for example, every 3 or 4 days, but this is rarely necessary if appropriate attention is given in advance to optimal scheduling.

Freezing of RBCs, allowing for storage up to 10 years, has an important but limited role in predeposit autologous transfusion programs. One application is for the donor who will need more units than can be collected within the shelf life of liquid blood. Another application is for the patient whose surgery is postponed beyond what would be the normal expiration date of the predonate units. However, freezing results in added expense (approximately two- to threefold the cost of liquid-stored units) and should therefore be done only when necessary. Some investigators have suggested that it is appropriate to freeze blood cells even for people who do not have a scheduled need for transfusion, in the event that they may be needed in the future. However, the cost of long-term storage is a strong disincentive to such programs; furthermore, it is impossible to guarantee that the frozen units could be processed and transported quickly enough to be of use when needed.

Use

Clinical Aspects of Transfusion of Autologous Blood

Because autologous blood is safer than homologous blood, it is appropriate to adopt somewhat more liberal indications for transfusion in patients who have predeposited autologous units. However, no transfusion should be given without a reasonable indication. This is because of the risks of clerical errors resulting in the transfusion of the wrong unit of blood and because of the possibility of volume overload. Transfusion of autologous units simply because they are available is unacceptable.

Red blood cells are the component prepared for the overwhelming majority of patients participating in predeposit autologous transfusion programs. It is also possible to harvest and store other components, such as fresh frozen plasma, cryoprecipitate, and platelets. These components are, however, rarely required for elective surgical procedures unless massive transfusion leading to dilutional coagulation factor and platelet deficiencies is anticipated.

Because not all blood that is donated as part of an autologous predeposit program is used by the donors, an additional advantage of these programs would seem to be the generation of additional blood from a group of participants who are not normally part of the donor pool. If the donor/patient qualifies as a usual blood donor on the basis of medical history, and all test results on the donated units are negative, the blood may be used for other patients. However, crossover of unused units of autologous blood is controversial, because some physicians suggest that autologous donors are not truly "volunteer" donors and may falsify their histories in order not to be excluded from donating.

Accomplishments of Autologous Transfusion Programs

The aim of autologous transfusion programs should be to eliminate or markedly diminish the use of homologous blood transfusion for patients who can participate in an autologous program. A number of published reports indicate various degrees of success in attaining this goal.[9, 11-14] For example, in one report, 1672 patients donated 6615 U of autologous blood during a 10-year period. The autologous units were used in 1938 surgical procedures. Intraoperative blood salvage also was used to supplement the predeposited autologous blood. In 91% of cases, surgical procedures were performed without the use of homologous blood.

INTRAOPERATIVE BLOOD SALVAGE AND PERIOPERATIVE HEMODILUTION

Several types of apparatus are now available for intraoperative blood salvage. This procedure has been used chiefly in cardiac and vascular surgery and in orthopaedic surgery. Optimal blood salvage techniques can result in the saving of large numbers of units of blood. For example, at one institution 7850 U of RBCs were salvaged intraoperatively during 2725 surgical procedures in just 1 year.[15]

Acute normovolemic hemodilution, sometimes termed *perioperative hemodilution,* is another technique for avoiding homologous blood transfusion. The attending anesthesiologist usually performs the procedure by withdrawing blood from the patient after inducing anesthesia. Plasma volume is then expanded with cell-free substitute, to maintain normovolemia. As the patient bleeds during surgery, more of the blood substitute is infused to counteract volume loss; the actual RBC volume lost to perioperative bleeding is much less because the blood lost was diluted. Once hemostasis is restored, the patient's own blood is reinfused. In some cases, perioperative hemodilution can be combined with preoperative autologous blood donation and/or intraoperative blood salvage.

PLATELET TRANSFUSION

More than three-quarters of a century has passed since the discovery that platelet transfusion can arrest thrombocytopenic hemorrhage. During that time, platelet transfusion has been shown to help prolong survival in patients with aplastic anemia and hematologic malignancy. During the early 1960s, platelet transfusions were only available at large hospitals supporting special programs in cancer therapy. All hospitals now have the capacity to provide platelet transfusion therapy, either with platelet concentrates prepared in their own blood banks or with concentrates provided by full-service regional blood centers. In addition, the use of single-donor platelets obtained by plateletpheresis is becoming more widespread. This approach is intended to decrease the number of donors to whom the recipient is exposed, since the number of platelets in one plateletpheresis product is generally equal to the number of platelets in six to eight platelet concentrates.

Indications for Platelet Transfusion

Platelet transfusions are administered to control or prevent bleeding associated with deficiencies in platelet number or function.[16] One unit of platelet concentrate should increase the platelet count in the average adult recipient by at least 5000 platelets/μL (Table 31-1).

Prophylactic platelet transfusion may be indicated to prevent bleeding in patients with severe thrombocytopenia. For the clinically stable patient with an intact vascular system and normal platelet function, prophylactic platelet transfusions may be indicated for platelet counts of less than 10,000–20,000/μL. A patient undergoing an operation or other invasive procedure is unlikely to benefit from prophylactic platelet transfusions if the platelet count is at least 50,000/μL and if thrombocytopenia is the sole abnormality. Platelet transfusions at higher platelet counts may be required for patients with systemic bleeding and for patients at higher risk of bleeding because of additional coagulation defects, sepsis, or platelet dysfunction related to medication or disease.

Platelets should not be transfused to patients with immune thrombocytopenic purpura (unless there is life-threatening bleeding), prophylactically with massive blood transfusion, or prophylactically after cardiopulmonary bypass.[3]

Platelet Dose

An appropriate dose of platelets for transfusion is 1 U/10 kg of body weight. This can be expected to increase the platelet count by at least 5000 platelets/μL (Table 31-1). If platelets are procured by apheresis, the number of platelets obtained is generally equal to those in 6–8 U.

Immune Platelet Disorders

Alloimmune Platelet Disorders

Two clinical syndromes, neonatal alloimmune thrombocytopenic purpura (NAITP) and post-transfusion purpura (PTP) are the direct result of sensitization to platelet-specific alloantigens, usually the P1^{A1} antigen. NAITP is the result of maternal sensitization to paternal alloantigens on fetal platelets. Severe thrombocytopenia may occur in the fetus with resultant bleeding, including in utero intracranial hemorrhage. The disorder frequently occurs during first pregnancies and subsequent pregnancies are managed by treating the mother with intravenous γ globulin or by in utero fetal platelet transfusions. Post-transfusion purpura occurs in previously nontransfused multiparous women who develop severe thrombocytopenia 7–10 days after a transfusion. Intravenous immunoglobulin and plasma exchange appear to be the most effective therapies, although corticosteroids have also been used. Platelet transfusions, even using P1^{A1}-negative platelets, may not be effective.

Refractoriness to Platelet Transfusions

Reaction of a patient's serum in the lymphocytotoxicity test with more than 20% of the lymphocytes in a panel generally indicates that the patient is refractory to platelet transfusions (see below). Platelet-specific antibodies also probably contribute to platelet refractoriness in a minority of instances.

Autoimmune Platelet Disorders

Autoimmune (or idiopathic) thrombocytopenic purpura is probably the most frequent kind of immune thrombocytopenia. Tests for platelet-associated antibody and for serum antibody reactive with platelets are supplementary means of diagnosing this disorder. However, such tests do not have a high degree of sensitivity or specificity.

Drug-Dependent Immune Thrombocytopenia

Immune-mediated thrombocytopenia is a complication of therapy with a variety of drugs. The possible mechanisms by which drug-induced antibodies may result in cytolysis are reviewed under Drug-Induced Immune Hemolytic Anemias.

Platelet Antigens

There are three categories of antigens that have been identified on the platelet surface: platelet-specific antigens, those that are shared with RBCs, and HLA antigens.

Human platelet-specific alloantigens are listed in Table 31-7. A new nomenclature is replacing the more familiar terminology; platelet-specific alloantigens are designated as human platelet antigens (HPA) and are numbered in order of discovery. Allelic antigens are named alphabetically, with the high incidence allele first (=a) and the lower incidence allele second (=b).[17]

Blood group antigens expressed on the platelet surface include ABH, P, Ii, and Le^a. Although some ABH antigen may be absorbed from the plasma, it is clear that some is intrinsic to the platelet membrane.

HLA class I antigens (HLA-A, -B, and -C gene products) are expressed on human platelets, but class II antigens (HLA-DR, -DQ, and -DP) are not. The density of HLA Class I molecules expressed on platelet membranes is highly variable. HLA-C locus molecules are poorly represented on platelets and have not been shown to have relevance in immune platelet disorders.

Also, since clinically important alloimmunization leading to refractoriness to platelet transfusion is usually due to HLA antibodies, platelet alloimmunization is most often defined on the basis of lymphocytotoxicity testing against a panel of lymphocytes.

Laboratory Testing

Neither major nor minor crossmatching is required before transfusion of platelet products. The small volume of unexpected antibodies possibly present in plasma is not considered clinically important.[1] Anti-A or anti-B

Table 31-7. Human Platelet Specific Alloantigens

New Nomenclature	Systems/Antigens	Phenotype Frequency (%) Caucasoids	Orientals	Glycoprotein Assignment
HPA-1a	Zw^a (Pl^{A1})	97.6	100.0	IIIa
-1b	Zw^b (Pl^{A2})	26.2	0	
HPA-2b	Ko^a (Sib^a)	14.3	25.4	Ib
-2a	Ko^b	99.4	?	
HPA-3a	Bak^a	86.7	78.9	IIb
-3b	Bak^b	63.8	?	
HPA-4b	Yuk^a (Pen^b)	0	1.7	IIIa
-4a	Yuk^b (Pen^a)	99.9	99.9	
HPA-5b	Br^a (Zav^a, Hc^a)	20.0	?	Ia
-5a	Br^b (Zav^b)	99.1	?	
—	Nak^a	?	89.6	IV
—	Sr^a	<1.0	?	IIIa

(From Mueller-Eckhardt,[17] with permission.)

in donor plasma may produce a positive direct antiglobulin test and, rarely, shortened RBC survival or frank hemolysis, if the volume of transfused plasma is large relative to the recipient's RBC mass. In this case, it may be desirable to reduce the volume of ABO-incompatible plasma from the platelet product just before it is administered. Laboratory testing regarding platelet transfusions concerns consideration of ABO and Rh blood groups for routine transfusion, as well as HLA typing and platelet crossmatching, for patients who demonstrate refractoriness to platelet transfusions (see below).

Platelet Antigen and Antibody Detection Methods

Platelet typing is done using antisera that have been obtained from normal persons who have been exposed to the alloantigen by pregnancy or transfusion. These antigens have also been identified using immunochemical techniques, monoclonal antibodies and, most recently, molecular biologic technology.

Numerous techniques have been described for the detection of platelet-reactive antibodies.[18] The techniques most commonly used are immunoradiometric assays (using radiolabeled anti-IgG), immunofluorescent assays, flow cytometry, enzyme-linked immunosorbent assays, and solid-phase RBC adherence assays.

ABO and Rh Blood Groups in Platelet Transfusion

Platelet membranes express the antigens of the ABO system, but it is not clear whether these antigens are absorbed from the plasma in which they circulate or are synthesized on the platelet.[16] It may be that the H antigen is intrinsic and that the A and B specificities are passively absorbed. Expression of the A, B, and H antigens is much weaker on the platelet surface than on the RBC surface.

ABO-compatible transfusions give better results than do ABO-incompatible ones, but the differences are usually minor. Also, it is generally impractical to supply ABO-compatible platelets for all platelet transfusions. Therefore, it is inappropriate to delay necessary platelet transfusion if ABO-identical platelets are not available and to wait until ABO-identical platelets become available.

In a small minority of patients, ABO-incompatible platelets are ineffective, whereas ABO-matched platelets give adequate responses.[16] In these unusual cases, it is necessary to provide ABO-compatible platelets for transfusion.

The antigens of the Rh system are probably not on platelet surfaces. However, Rh-negative platelets should be transfused to Rh-negative patients because units of platelets contain small numbers of RBCs, approximately 0.4 mL/U. Thus, RBC alloimmunization caused by contamination of the platelet concentrates by RBCs may occur if Rh-negative patients are transfused with Rh-positive platelet products. If Rh-positive platelets must be given to Rh-negative patients, Rh immunoglobulin may be administered shortly after the platelet transfusion. This is particularly important if the patient is a woman of childbearing age.

Human Leukocyte Antigen Typing

Most patients refractory to random-donor platelets (i.e., patients having a poor post-transfusion platelet count increment) respond to donors selected on the basis of HLA match. Most regional blood centers now have large pools of HLA-typed volunteers who are available to donate platelets by apheresis. With the development of these large pools of donors, HLA-matched platelets are probably available to every refractory patient in the United States.

However, platelets that are perfectly matched at the four A and B HLA loci are only infrequently obtainable, especially if the patient needs repeated platelet transfusions. Thus, platelets that are incompatible at one or more HLA locus may need to be used if an adequate number of perfectly matched donors cannot be found. Also, platelets with cross-reactive antigens are frequently used when perfectly matched platelets are not available. Cross-reactivity, as defined in HLA serology, is based on the in vitro observation that one monospecific serum may react with a single antigen and also may react consistently with additional antigens of the same locus. The original and the additional antigens become known as a cross-reactive group. Experience has shown that some antigens within cross-reactive groups frequently are associated with satisfactory post-transfusion platelet count increments.[16]

Platelet Crossmatch Tests

A significant proportion, perhaps 25–40%, of closely HLA-matched platelet transfusions administered to alloimmunized patients are failures, that is, result in an inadequate post-transfusion platelet count increment. Numerous investigators have reported that platelet crossmatch tests are of value in selecting donors for patients who are alloimmunized and refractory to random or HLA-matched platelets.[19-21]

There is no consensus on the optimal platelet crossmatch test, but numerous methods that measure platelet-associated immunoglobulin have been reported to yield results with a high predictive value. Such methods are used in a manner analogous to the indirect antiglobulin test for RBC crossmatching. That is, the patient's serum is incubated with a sample of the donor platelets. The platelets are then tested for the presence of platelet associated antibody. Methods that have been used include the use of radiolabeled staphylococcal protein A, radiolabeled antiglobulin reagents, enzyme-linked immunosorbent assay (ELISA), or fluorescence. Solid-phase methodology may also be applicable.

The crossmatch test has most often been suggested as an adjunct to HLA matching for the selection of platelets for transfusion to alloimmunized patients, although a number of studies have indicated high predictive values even when the donor and recipient are not HLA matched.[22] Available data suggest that the platelet crossmatch test is underused, and its wider application is to be encouraged.

GRANULOCYTE TRANSFUSION

Indications

Neutropenic patients are at increased risk of infection. The risk increases when the neutrophil count is less than $1000/\mu L$ and becomes severe when the neutrophil level falls below $250/\mu L$. Thus, treatment of infected neutropenic patients with granulocyte replacement therapy is theoretically appealing. However, granulocyte transfusions are not used extensively, in part because the number of granulocytes in the circulation makes it difficult to obtain a large dose for transfusion. Also, the efficacy of granulocyte transfusions is difficult to evaluate. Since the change in the granulocyte count after transfusion is too small to be meaningful, the effectiveness of granulocyte transfusion has been judged on the basis of results of clinical trials that have evaluated large numbers of patients with infections. The survival of patients who were transfused with granulocytes was compared with the survival of those who were not transfused. Such studies have been difficult to perform because potential indications for granulocyte transfusions generally occur in complicated clinical settings, and conflicting conclusions have been reached. Moreover, antibiotics have improved since the trials were performed; thus, controversy remains concerning the indications for granulocyte transfusion.

A commonly used indication in a severely granulocytopenic patient (granulocyte count less than $500/\mu L$ is sepsis, especially when the sepsis is documented by cultures, caused by gram-negative organisms, and is unresponsive to appropriate antibiotic therapy after a period of about 48 hours.[23] Granulocyte transfusions also are used in septic neonates, especially those with depleted granulocyte bone marrow stores and/or those with antibiotic-resistant gram-negative sepsis.[23] Also, granulocyte transfusion may be indicated in patients who have disorders of granulocyte function and who have severe infections. Infections for which the role of granulocyte transfusions is less clear include pneumonia, urinary tract infection, cellulitis, abscesses, fungal infections, and fever of unknown origin.

Laboratory Testing

ABO Typing

Granulocyte concentrates used for transfusion must be ABO compatible with the recipient, even though ABO antigens are not present on granulocytes. This is true because of the RBC content of the concentrates.

Histocompatibility Testing and the Role of the HLA System

For patients who are alloimmunized to HLA antigens, HLA-matched donors should be selected for leukapheresis. Changes in the recipient's granulocyte count after transfusion are small even if the patient is not alloimmunized. Alloimmunization cannot be suspected clinically on the basis of poor post-transfusion granulocyte count increments in a manner analogous to platelet transfusions. Therefore, the only practical approach is to screen the patient's serum for HLA antibodies periodically, especially if the patient has previously received multiple transfusions of cellular blood products.

Granulocyte Dose

The usual granulocyte concentrate contains approximately 1×10^{10} granulocytes. In adults at least 1×10^{10} granulocytes should be transfused per day for at least 4–7 days or until the infection resolves. For neonates, a dose of 1×10^9 granulocytes/kg/d has been recommended.[23] Generally, at least 4 days of transfusion therapy are indicated, unless marked clinical improvement occurs with a sustained elevation of the white blood cell (WBC) count.

Granulocyte Specific Antigen Systems

A number of granulocyte-specific antigen systems have been described and are termed NA, NB, NC, ND, NE, HGA-3, GA, GB, GC, and GR. Antigens at these loci may be detected by granulocyte agglutination, granulocyte cytotoxicity, or immunofluorescence using paraformaldehyde-fixed granulocytes and fluorescein-labelled anti-IgG.

Granulocyte-specific antibodies to these antigens may be responsible for four different clinical syndromes: (1) neonatal alloimmune neutropenia, (2) febrile reactions after transfusion, (3) pulmonary infiltrates after transfusion, and (4) autoimmune neutropenia.

Neonatal alloimmune neutropenia is a rare syndrome analogous to hemolytic disease of the newborn in which severe leukopenia and resultant infections occur as a result of potent IgG antibodies against granulocyte-specific antigens formed by the mother during pregnancy. Febrile transfusion reactions occur during multitransfused patients and their recurrence may be prevented by using leukocyte-depleted blood products. The transfusion of plasma that contains potent leukoagglutinins may cause pulmonary infiltrates, which may be extensive and may be associated with a severe reaction characterized by chills, fever, cough, and dyspnea. Several cases of autoimmune neutropenia associated with severe infections have been described.

TRANSFUSION OF PLASMA AND PLASMA PRODUCTS

Fresh Frozen Plasma

Indications

Fresh frozen plasma (FFP) should be transfused only to increase the level of clotting factors in patients with a demonstrated deficiency.[3] Each unit of FFP transfused will increase the level of any clotting factor by 2–3% in the average adult. Laboratory tests should be used to monitor the patient with a suspected clotting disorder. If prothrombin time (PT) and partial thromboplastin time (PTT) are less than 1.5 times normal, FFP transfusion is rarely indicated.

Patients who have been given the anticoagulant warfarin sodium become deficient in vitamin K-dependent coagulation factors II, VII, IX, and X. If these patients are bleeding or require emergency surgery, they may be candidates for FFP transfusion to achieve immediate hemostasis, when time does not permit warfarin reversal by stopping the drug or administering vitamin K. Patients with rare conditions, such as antithrombin III deficiency and thrombotic thrombocytopenic purpura, may benefit from FFP transfusion.

Fresh frozen plasma should not be transfused for volume expansion, as a nutritional supplement, prophylactically with massive blood transfusion, or prophylactically after cardiopulmonary bypass.[3]

Pretransfusion Testing

Fresh frozen plasma should be ABO compatible with the recipient's RBCs. As a cell-free product, FFP can be given without regard to Rh group. Compatibility testing (minor crossmatch) is not necessary.

Cryoprecipitated Antihemophilic Factor

Cryoprecipitated antihemophilic factor (AHF) is prepared by thawing FFP 1–6°C and recovering the cold precipitate. The cold-insoluble precipitate is refrozen. On the average, each bag of cryoprecipitated AHF contains 80 or more factor VIII (FVIII:C) U and at least 150 mg of fibrinogen in less than 15 mL of plasma. Cryoprecipitated AHF provides a source of coagulation factor VIII, factor XIII, fibrinogen, and von Willebrand factor (AHF-VWF).

Indications

This component is used in the control of bleeding associated with factor VIII deficiency. Its use is also indicated for von Willebrand's disease and for replacement of fibrinogen or factor XIII.

Dosage and Administration

It is preferable but not essential to administer ABO-compatible cryoprecipitate. The volume of each unit is small, but most patients receive many units. With large volumes or with units containing particularly potent ABO antibodies, the isoagglutinins may produce a positive direct antiglobulin test and, rarely, hemolysis.[1] This is more commonly a problem in children, because of their small blood volume, than in adults. Cryoprecipitate can be administered without regard to Rh group, and unexpected antibodies are not usually a problem.

For treatment of bleeding in hemophilia A, rapid infusion (about 10 mL of diluted component per minute) of a loading dose expected to produce the desired level of FVIII:C is usually followed by a smaller maintenance dose every 8–12 hours. To maintain hemostasis after surgery, a regimen of therapy for 10 days or longer may be required. If circulating antibodies to factor VIII are present, larger doses, higher activity concentrates, or other special measures may be indicated.

To calculate dosage, the following formula is helpful:

Number of bags of cryoprecipitate required =
$$\frac{\text{desired FVIII:C level (in \%)} \times \text{patient's plasma volume (in mL)}}{\text{average units of FVIII:C per cryoprecipitate (minimum 80)}}$$

Good patient management requires that the cryoprecipitated AHF treatment responses of factor VIII-deficient recipients be monitored with periodic plasma FVIII:C assays.

For treatment of von Willebrand's disease, smaller amounts of cryoprecipitated AHF will correct the bleeding time. These patients should be monitored by appropriate laboratory studies to determine the frequency of cryoprecipitated AHF administration.

Fibrinogen replacement may be indicated in patients who have severe hypofibrinoginemia as part of the disseminated intravascular coagulation (DIC) syndrome, as a result of massive transfusion or as a rare isolated inherited deficiency. Cryoprecipitate is the only concentrated fibrinogen product available. Fibrinogen preparations formerly available are no longer manufactured because of the high risk of transmitting hepatitis B. Hypofibrinogenemic recipients should be monitored with fibrinogen assays. (For a summary of indications and dosage, see Table 31-1.)

Factor VIII Concentrate

Factor VIII concentrate is prepared by fractionation of pooled human plasma frozen soon after phlebotomy.[24] Several types of factor VIII concentrate are available. A variety of procedures are used to treat factor VIII products to inactivate viruses and reduce the risk of infectious disease transmission. However, no treatment procedure completely eliminates the risk of transmission of viral infections.

Indications

Factor VIII concentrate is indicated for the treatment of hemophilia A patients with moderate to severe congenital factor VIII deficiency and for patients with low titer factor VIII inhibitors (less than 10 Bethesda U/mL).

Dosage and Administration

The quantity of factor VIII coagulant activity (VIII:C) is stated on the bottle in terms of international units. One international unit (IU) is the factor VIII activity present in 1 mL of normal, pooled human plasma less than 1 hour old. The amount of lyophilized factor VIII to be infused is determined by calculating the number of units required to achieve the desired in vivo levels and dividing by the number of units per bottle of concentrate as listed on the label.

Factor IX Concentrate

Two factor IX concentrate products are available.[24] One product has been available for many years and is designated factor IX complex. In addition to factor IX, it contains some quantities of factors II, VII, and X and other proteins. The amount of each factor contained in each bottle is stated on the vial. A newer factor IX product, designated coagulation factor IX, contains trace amounts of factors II, VII, and X. Factor IX concentrates are heat treated to decrease the risk of hepatitis, human immunodeficiency virus type 1 (HIV-1), and other viral diseases.

Indications

Factor IX concentrate products are used for treatment of patients with factor IX deficiency, that is, hemophilia B. Factor IX complex may also be of value for patients with congenital factor VII or X deficiency.

Dosage and Administration

The quantity of factor IX is stated on the bottle in terms of activity units. One unit is the factor IX activity present in 1 mL of normal human plasma. The amount of concentrate to be infused to raise factor IX levels is determined by calculating the number of units required to achieve the desired in vivo levels.

Additional Plasma Derivatives

Additional plasma derivatives include albumin, immune serum globulin, and Rh immunoglobulin. For indications and doses, see Table 31-1.

IMMUNOHEMATOLOGIC TESTS FOR THE DIAGNOSIS OF ACQUIRED IMMUNE HEMOLYTIC ANEMIAS

Special immunohematologic problems are most appropriately resolved in the blood bank, even if transfusion of blood products is unnecessary. Autoimmune hemolytic anemias and drug-induced immune hemolytic anemias require specialized laboratory testing for diagnosis and for selection of blood for transfusion. Frequently, only a few carefully selected serologic tests are required. However, more extensive testing may be necessary when spontaneous agglutination complicates blood typing or when blood transfusion is indicated in a patient who may have RBC alloantibodies in addition to autoantibodies. Table 31-8 summarizes expected findings in patients with autoimmune or drug-induced immune hemolytic anemias.[25]

Collection of Specimens

Both clotted blood for serum and EDTA-anticoagulated blood for RBCs are collected. It is best to perform ABO grouping and Rh phenotyping (using the EDTA-

Table 31-8. Classification and Expected Findings in Autoimmune and Drug-Induced Immune Hemolytic Anemias

Type	Direct Antiglobulin Test	Eluate	Serologic Characteristics	Antibody Specificity
Autoimmune				
Warm antibody AIHA (most common type)	IgG and/or complement (C3)	IgG antibody	IAT positive (57%), agglutinating enzyme premodified cells (90%), hemolyzing enzyme premodified cells (13%)	Usually within Rh system; other specificities include LW, U, I^T, K, Kp^b, K13, Ge, Jk^a, En^a, and Wr^b
Cold agglutinin syndrome	Complement (C3) alone	Negative	Agglutinating activity up to 30°C in albumin; high titer at 4°C (usually >1024)	Usually anti-I; other specificities include i, Pr, Gd, Sd^x
Paroxysmal cold hemoglobinuria	Complement (C3) alone	Negative	Biphasic hemolysin (i.e., sensitizing RBCs in the cold and then hemolyzes them when moved to 37°C);	Anti-P (reacts with all normal RBCs except p or P^k cells)
Drug-induced				
α-methyldopa (Aldomet)	IgG alone	IgG antibody	Similar to warm antibody AIHA	Usually within Rh system
Penicillins	Usually IgG alone but complement (C3) may also be detected	Negative unless penicillin-coated RBCs are tested	Negative unless penicillin-coated RBC are tested	Reacts with penicillin-coated RBCs
Other drugs (i.e., quinidine, phenacetin) —usually reactive due to immune complex formation)	Usually complement (C3) alone, but IgG may also be detected	Negative unless drug + patient's eluate + RBCs tested	Negative unless drug + patient's serum or eluate + RBCs tested	Reacts with RBCs if incubated with drug + patient's serum or eluate

Abbreviations: AIHA, autoimmune hemolytic anemia; RBCs, red blood cells; IAT, indirect antiglobulin test; AIHA, autoimmune hemolytic anemia.
(From Petz and Branch,[25] with permission.)

anticoagulated RBCs) as part of the initial diagnostic studies so that this information is available should transfusion be necessary. Similarly, determination of other RBC antigens also may be important, especially those of the Kidd, Kell, and Duffy blood group systems. Red blood cell typing in the presence of a positive direct antiglobulin test (DAT) necessitates the use of special procedures and reagents as described below.

RBC Antigen Typing in the Presence of Autoagglutination

ABO Red Blood Cell Typing

There is usually no problem in determining the ABO group of patients with autoimmune hemolytic anemia (AIHA). The cells are tested in the usual fashion, with anti-A and anti-B, but a negative control of 6% bovine serum albumin in saline should be used as well. Testing with anti-A,B is indicated only if negative reactions are obtained using anti-A and anti-B. A positive control using 6% bovine serum albumin indicates either nondispersed autoagglutination or spontaneous agglutination of heavily sensitized cells in albumin, and the ABO group results cannot be properly interpreted. When the control is positive in a patient with warm antibody AIHA, washing the patient's cells using saline heated to 45°C, or gently eluting warm antibody by incubating at 45°C in saline for 5–10 minutes, may result in negative controls and allow for reliable typing. Alternatively, the pretreatment of the patient's RBCs using ZZAP reagent can eliminate the spontaneous agglutination and permit reliable ABO grouping.

In patients with cold agglutinins reactive at room temperature, washing the RBCs at 37–45°C may be necessary to prevent cold autoagglutination. Alternatively, the RBCs could be treated with 0.01 M dithiothreitol (DTT) for 30 minutes at 37°C before ABO typing.

ABO Serum Grouping

When the patient's serum is tested against RBCs of group A, B, and O, as well as against the patient's own cells to confirm ABO grouping, it may be necessary to perform these tests using a prewarmed technique at 37°C, if cold autoagglutination occurs.

Rh-Hr Typings

Red blood cells strongly coated with IgG may spontaneously agglutinate when mixed with antisera containing high concentrations of proteins or other potentiators of agglutination. High-protein reagents designated for use by slide or rapid tube tests (sometimes referred to as modified-tube anti-Rh) are most likely to cause problems with IgG-coated RBCs. The inclusion of appropriate controls or the use of chemically modified or saline-reactive reagents may be necessary to avoid erroneous results.[1]

Direct Antiglobulin Test

The DAT should be performed not only with polyspecific antiglobulin serum but also with monospecific anti-IgG and anti-C3 antisera. Such testing provides quite useful, although limited, information.

The results of the DAT may reduce the diagnostic possibilities; for example, the DAT in cold agglutinin syndrome is invariably positive using anti-C3 antiglobulin serum and invariably negative using anti-IgG. Table 31-9 summarizes the expected DAT findings using anti-IgG and anti-C3 in various immune hemolytic anemias.

Characterization of RBC Antibodies in Serum and RBC Eluate

Definitive diagnostic information is provided by characterizing RBC antibodies in the patient's serum and in an eluate from the RBCs. Initially, antibody screening

Table 31-9. Direct Antiglobulin Test Results in Immune Hemolytic Anemias Using Anti-IgG and Anti-C3 Antisera

	IgG	C3[a]
Warm antibody AIHA		
67%	+	+
20%	+	0
13%	0	+
Cold agglutinin syndrome	0	+
Paroxysmal cold hemoglobinuria	0	+
Penicillin or methyldopa induced[b]	+	0
Other drug-induced immune hemolytic anemias[c]	0	+
Warm antibody AIHA associated with SLE	+	+

Abbreviations: AIHA, autoimmune hemolytic anemia; SLE, systemic lupus erythematosus; RBC, red blood cell.

[a] Such cells are primarily sensitized with C3d component of C3.

[b] Weakly positive reactions with anti-C3 may occur; invariably, reactions are strongly positive with anti-IgG.

[c] The most common pattern of RBC sensitization is indicated, but occasionally IgG may be detected with or without C3.

(From Petz and Garratty,[26] with permission.)

tests are performed to detect both warm reactive antibodies and cold agglutinins. When warm antibodies are detected, one must determine whether these are alloantibodies or autoantibodies, or both. This is determined by appropriate, but not exhaustive, specificity testing.

Specificity Tests

When the screening tests are positive, an antibody identification panel is performed as an initial step to determine whether alloantibody(ies) or autoantibody, or both, may be present. A control consisting of the patient's serum and autologous RBCs (autocontrol) must be tested in parallel with the RBC panel.

Positive reactions of the serum with all cells of the panel and with the autocontrol would be expected if warm or cold autoagglutinins are present. Panagglutination may also be caused by serum protein abnormalities, by bacterial contamination of serum or reagents, or by preservatives contained in the reagents being used. When all cells on the panel are agglutinated, but the autocontrol is negative, a mixture of alloantibodies or an alloantibody to a high frequency antigen is likely. Except when autoimmunity is present, autologous RBCs should not react with antibodies in the patient's serum. If the patient has been recently transfused, one must keep in mind that alloantibodies could react with circulating RBCs and produce a positive DAT, which could be misinterpreted.

Characteristic Serologic Findings

The characteristic findings in patients with warm antibody autoimmune hemolytic anemia are as follows: (1) the presence of an acquired hemolytic anemia, (2) a positive DAT, and (3) an "unexpected" autoantibody in the serum and/or eluate that reacts optimally at 37°C. The autoantibody usually reacts similarly with all normal RBCs but, in some cases, may have specificity, usually within the Rh blood group system.

When cold agglutinating antibodies are detected, their clinical significance is related to their thermal amplitude because antibodies that are not reactive up to at least 30°C in albumin do not cause immune hemolytic anemia. The cold agglutinin syndrome may be diagnosed if the following conditions are present: (1) clinical evidence of an acquired hemolytic anemia, (2) a positive direct antiglobulin test caused by sensitization with C3, (3) a negative direct antiglobulin test using anti-IgG antiglobulin serum, and (4) the presence of a cold autoagglutinin with reactivity up to at least 30°C in albumin. Although it is sufficient to determine the pathologic nature of the cold autoantibody by screening tests that include determining the thermal amplitude, it is advisable to perform additional confirmatory tests, to avoid misinterpretation of positive screening results. These should determine the pattern of reactivity at 37, 30, 20, and 4°C and the specificity, if any, within the Ii blood group system.

Paroxysmal cold hemoglobinuria (PCH), the most unusual of the autoimmune hemolytic anemias, should be suspected whenever serologic studies are inconclusive for warm antibody AIHA or the cold agglutinin syndrome. The definitive laboratory test is the biphasic hemolysis test (cold-warm hemolysis), known as the Donath-Landsteiner antibody test. The patient's serum is incubated in the cold (in crushed ice) with normal RBCs for 30 minutes. The RBCs are then incubated in the presence of complement (fresh normal ABO-compatible serum) for 30 minutes. Visible hemolysis constitutes a positive test and is diagnostic of PCH.[26]

Detection of Alloantibodies in the Presence of Warm Autoantibodies

Most warm autoantibodies react with all RBCs of common Rh genotypes. In rare instances, warm autoantibodies demonstrate well-defined specificity for an Rh antigen (e.g., anti-e). Much more commonly, autoantibodies react with all RBCs tested but react to a higher titer (fourfold dilution difference) against RBCs bearing a particular Rh antigen. Such autoantibodies are said to have *relative specificity*. When transfusion is necessary, RBCs that are negative for the antigen to which the patient's serum preferably reacts may survive significantly better than RBCs that are positive for that antigen.[26]

The detection of RBC alloantibodies can be quite difficult in the presence of a warm autoantibody that may react with all RBCs on a panel and thus mask the specific reactivity of alloantibodies. Several serologic techniques are available for detection of alloantibodies in this circumstance.

Comparison of Direct and Indirect Antiglobulin Tests

A comparison of the strength of reactivity of the direct and indirect antiglobulin tests sometimes provides valuable information. In patients with warm antibody

AIHA, the indirect antiglobulin test caused by autoantibody is generally weaker than the direct antiglobulin test. Apparently, most of the antibody is absorbed onto the patient's RBCs in vivo. A coexisting alloantibody may result in a strongly positive indirect antiglobulin test but will not be absorbed by the patient's RBCs. Thus, if the indirect antiglobulin test is significantly stronger than the direct antiglobulin test, the presence of an alloantibody is highly suspect. However, if the direct antiglobulin test is equal or stronger than the indirect antiglobulin test, no conclusion can be reached concerning the presence or absence of alloantibodies.

Testing the Patient's Serum Against a RBC Antibody Identification Panel

If the screening tests for serum antibody demonstrate an antibody reaction at 20°C or 37°C or by means of the indirect antiglobulin technique, the serum should be tested against commercially available panels of phenotyped RBCs. If a strongly reactive RBC alloantibody is present and if the autoantibody results in much weaker reactions, the presence of the alloantibody will be evident, even though reactions are positive against all RBCs on the panel.

Warm Autoabsorption Test for the Detection of Alloantibodies

If the patient has not been transfused within the past 3 months, the best technique currently available for the detection of alloantibodies in the presence of autoantibodies is to absorb the autoantibody from the patient's serum at 37°C using the patient's RBCs after first removing some of the autoantibody from their surface.

The use of ZZAP reagent is the optimal way to remove IgG from the patient's RBCs before absorption. ZZAP consists of 0.1 M DTT and 0.1% cysteine-activated papain.[27] The reagent may be prepared by mixing 2.5 mL of a stock solution of 0.2 M DTT, 0.5 mL of a stock solution of 1% cysteine-activated papain,[27] and 2 mL of phosphate-buffered saline, pH 7.3. The reagent is stable for at least 5 days at 4°C.

IgG is removed from DAT-positive RBCs by incubating 1 volume of packed RBCs with 2 volumes of ZZAP reagent for 30 minutes at 37°C. Usually, two autoabsorptions using two separate aliquots of ZZAP-treated patient's RBCs are sufficient to remove all of the autoantibody. The absorbed serum can then be used for detection and identification of RBC alloantibodies and for crossmatch tests.

Differential Absorption Test for the Detection of Alloantibodies

If the patient has received blood transfusions within the past 3 months, a warm autoabsorption technique for the detection of underlying alloantibodies is not recommended. Conceivably, transfused antigen-positive RBCs may remain and be capable of further absorption of alloantibody in vitro. Thus, false negative results for the presence of significant alloantibody may be obtained.

The differential absorption technique, that is, the absorption of the autoantibody from the patient's serum using allogeneic RBCs of varying phenotypes, should be used instead of the warm autoabsorption method. For example, performing an absorption using R_1R_1 (CDe/CDe) Jk^a-negative RBCs of a serum containing a warm autoantibody plus anti-E and anti-Jk^a alloantibodies will remove the autoantibody, but not the anti-E or the anti-Jk^a. Ideally, sufficient RBCs of varying phenotypes should be obtained from donor centers or laboratory personnel in anticipation of their use for this purpose. These can be aliquoted and stored in a glycerol solution at −20°C until needed. Absorption with aliquots of three carefully selected samples of RBCs is sufficient to permit detection of essentially all the clinically important RBC alloantibodies. Red blood cells having the following phenotypes may be used: R_1R_1 (CDe/CDe), R_2R_2 (cDE/cDE), and rr (cde/cde). In addition, one or all cells must be Kell negative, whereas at least one cell should be Jk^a-negative and one cell Jk^b-negative. All cells should be enzyme premodified before the absorption is performed, thus rendering them all Fy^a-negative.

The differential absorption technique is the most reliable method for the detection of alloantibodies in the presence of autoantibodies in patients who have been recently transfused. Its widespread use in appropriate circumstances should be encouraged.

Performing Compatibility Tests in Patients with Cold Autoantibodies

The optimal way to perform compatibility tests in patients with the cold agglutinin syndrome is to perform the tests strictly at 37°C and to use only normal saline media (i.e., without using albumin or LISS or other potentiators of agglutination). Cold agglutinins from only about 7% of patients with cold agglutinin syndrome react at 37°C in saline, although positive reactions will be obtained about 30% of the time in albumin media. Other more cumbersome approaches are to absorb the cold autoantibody with a series of cold autoabsorptions prior to compatibility testing or to inactivate the cold antibody with DTT, since it is almost always of the IgM class. In those unusual cases in which the cold agglutinin reacts at 37°C, a cold autoabsorption is necessary before compatibility testing.

In patients with PCH, routine compatibility tests will indicate serologic compatibility, because the Donath-Landsteiner antibody will not react, unless incubation in the cold precedes tests at 37°C. However, transfused RBCs will not survive normally. Because the autoantibody in PCH usually has anti-P specificity, there is some logic to transfusing with P-negative RBCs. However, such RBCs are extraordinarily rare and are even difficult to obtain from rare donor files. Patients may require transfusion before such cells are available, and transfusion of RBCs of common P types should not be withheld if transfusion is urgently needed.

DRUG-INDUCED IMMUNE HEMOLYTIC ANEMIAS

In a significant percentage of patients with immune hemolytic anemia, drugs have been incriminated as the etiologic agent.[28,29] Indeed, Petz and Garratty[26] reported that 12.4% of a series of 347 patients with acquired immune hemolytic anemia were caused by drugs. The hemolysis may be acute in onset and of marked severity resulting in severe anemia, hemoglobinemia, hemoglobinuria, renal failure, and even death. Drug-induced immune hemolytic anemia is frequently difficult to diagnose or to exclude with certainty, because (1) a temporal relationship between drug administration and hemolysis is not conclusive, (2) patients are frequently taking multiple drugs, (3) other possible causes of anemia may be present, and (4) in particular because laboratory tests for most drug-related antibodies are not standardized.

Approach to Laboratory Diagnosis

If laboratory findings confirm the diagnosis of an acquired hemolytic anemia and if the patient is taking medications, a diagnosis of drug-induced immune hemolytic anemia must be considered. This is particularly true if the patient is taking drugs that have previously been reported to cause immune hemolysis. It is also true that the list of causative drugs grows each year, so that one must have a high index of suspicion.

The optimal method for laboratory diagnosis generally depends on whether the drug is loosely or tightly bound to RBCs. Also, some drugs cause the development of an antibody that reacts with intrinsic RBC antigens and that has no detectable specificity for the drug. In such cases, diagnosis depends on clinical observations and on the serologic characterization of the RBC autoantibodies.

Drugs Loosely Bound to Red Blood Cells

For most drugs that cause immune hemolytic anemia, the optimal method for detection of the causative antibody is to test the patient's serum and RBC eluate against normal untreated and enzyme-treated RBCs in the presence of the suspected drug. A saturated solution of the drug (or 1 mg/mL of drug, if readily soluble) should be made in appropriately buffered saline. If this concentration of drug causes lysis of normal RBCs, dilutions should be made until the solution no longer causes lysis. An equal volume of this solution is added to the patient's serum, and an equal volume of buffered saline is added to another aliquot of patient's serum as a control. Red blood cells are added, and the mixtures are incubated at 37°C for 1–2 hours. A duplicate set of tubes with the addition of fresh normal serum is also recommended. After incubation at 37°C, the tubes are inspected for hemolysis, agglutination, and agglutination in the indirect antiglobulin test.

A list of drugs that are loosely bound to the erythrocyte is given in Table 31-10. Such drugs frequently cause severe hemolytic anemia with manifestations of acute intravascular hemolysis, such as hemoglobinemia and hemoglobinuria; renal insufficiency is a common consequence.

Drugs Firmly Bound to Red Blood Cells

A number of drugs are firmly bound to the erythrocyte. In this case, the optimal means of detection of the drug-dependent antibody in the laboratory is with drug-coated RBCs. Prototypical drugs are the penicillins; additional drugs are listed in Table 31-11. Clinically, the hemolysis is usually, but not always, less abrupt in onset and less severe without signs of intravascular hemolysis.

Various methods have been described for coupling drugs to erythrocytes. A number of penicillins and cephalosporins are readily bound to RBCs at alkaline pH. Methods for coupling tolbutamide,[30] erythromycin,[31] cisplatin,[32] and tetracycline[33] to RBC membranes vary widely.

Table 31-10. Drugs Reported to Cause Hemolytic Anemia by the Immune Complex Mechanism

Drug	Intravascular Hemolysis[a]	Renal Failure
Acetaminophen	X	
Aminopyrine	X	
p-Aminosalicylic acid (PAS)	X	X
Antazoline	X	X
Butizide	X	X
Carbimazole[b]	X	
Cefotaxime[b]	X	
Ceftriaxone	X	
Chlorpromazine	X	X
Chlorpropamide	X	
Cianidanol	X	X
Dipyrone[b]	X	X
Fluorouracil	X	
Hydralazine		
Hydrochlorothiazide[c]	X	X
9-Hydroxy-methyl-ellipticinium	X	X
Insulin[b]		
Isoniazid[b]	X	
Melphalan		
Methotrexate		
Nalidixic acid	X	X
Nomifensine[d]	X	X
Phenacetin[e]	X	X
Probenecid		
Quinidine[b]		
Quinine	X	
Rifampicin	X	X
Stibophen	X	X
Streptomycin[b,d]		
Sulfonamides	X	X
Teniposide (VM-26)[d]	X	X
Tolmetin[d]	X	X
Triamterene[b]	X	X
Zomax (zomepirac sodium)		

[a] An X in the column indicates that intravascular hemolysis or renal failure have been reported on at least one occasion.
[b] May also bind to red blood cells, and hemolysis may be caused in part by drug adsorption mechanism.
[c] Intravascular hemolysis and renal failure occurred only with an overdose of the drug.
[d] Also caused development of red blood cell autoantibody.
[e] May also cause hemolysis by drug adsorption mechanism and has been associated with the development of autoimmune hemolytic anemia.
(From Petz,[29] with permission.)

Drugs that Cause Autoimmune Hemolytic Anemia

The drugs listed in Table 31-12 lead to the development of autoimmune hemolytic anemia. The antibodies from such patients react directly with normal RBCs in the absence of drug in vitro and, on further characterization, are found to be indistinguishable from those found in patients with idiopathic warm antibody autoimmune hemolytic anemia. Indeed, no serologic proof of a relationship between the antibodies and the drugs has ever been demonstrated; proof that the drugs cause autoimmune hemolytic anemia in such patients has come from clinical observations. Cessation of the drug causes remission of the hemolytic anemia, and the DAT slowly reverts to negative. In some instances, readministration of the drug has caused reappearance of the syndrome, documenting a causal role for the drug.

The applicable diagnostic tests, therefore, consist of characterizing the RBC antibodies as warm autoantibodies and establishing that hemolysis subsides on cessation of the drug. Proof of the etiology of a drug-induced immune hemolytic anemia can only be obtained

Table 31-11. Drugs That Bind Tightly to Red Blood Cell Membrane and Cause Hemolysis by Drug Adsorption Mechanism

Penicillins
Cephalothin
Cephaloridine
Cephalexin
Cefazolin
Cefamandole
Tolbutamide
Erythromycin
Cisplatin
Tetracycline

(From Petz,[29] with permission.)

Table 31-12. Drugs Reported to Cause Autoimmune Hemolytic Anemia

α-Methyldopa
L-Dopa
Mefenamic acid[a]
Procainamide
Phenacetin[b,c]
Chlorpromazine[c]
Streptomycin[c]

[a] Other nonsteroidal anti-inflammatory drugs (ibuprofen, naproxen, tolmetin, feprazone, and fenoprofen) have caused immune hemolysis, but the mechanism is not clear.[38]
[b] Also may cause hemolysis by immune complex or drug adsorption mechanisms.
[c] Only 1 case associated with autoantibodies has been reported.
(From Petz,[29] with permission.)

by restarting the drug, but this is rarely indicated clinically.

Role of Drug Metabolites

In some drug-induced immune hemolytic anemias, the relevant immunogen is not the parent drug but a metabolite.[34,35] Because information about the metabolites of drugs may be incomplete, a number of investigators have used serum and/or urine from patients receiving the drug as a source of metabolites for use in drug-related RBC antibody detection tests. This method has been used for identification of antibodies caused by administration of such drugs as buthiazide and nomifensine,[36] the latter no longer being available in the United States largely because of the frequency with which it caused immune hemolysis.

REFERENCES

1. Walker RH (ed): Technical Manual. 10th Ed. Arlington, VA, American Association of Blood Banks, 1990.
2. Holland PV (ed): Standards for Blood Banks and Transfusion Services. 13th Ed. Arlington, VA, American Association of Blood Banks, 1989.
3. Stehling LC, Cosgrove DM, Moss GS et al: Transfusion Alert. Indications for the Use of Red Blood Cells, Platelets, and Fresh Frozen Plasma. NIH Publication No. 89-2974a. Bethesda, U.S. Department of Health and Human Services, Public Health Service, National Institutes of Health, 1989.
4. Judd WJ: Methods in Immunohematology. Miami, FL, Montgomery Scientific Publications, 1988.
5. Petz LD: Red cell compatibility testing: clinical significance and laboratory methods. pp. 173–211. In Petz LD, Swisher SN (eds): Clinical Practice of Transfusion Medicine. 2nd Ed. New York, Churchill Livingstone, 1989.
6. Low B, Messeter L: Antiglobulin test in low-ionic strength salt solution for rapid antibody screening and cross-matching. Vox Sang 1974;26:53–61.
7. Silvergleid AJ: Autologous, directed, and home transfusion programs. pp. 327–344. In Petz LD, Swisher SN (eds): Clinical Practice of Transfusion Medicine. 2nd Ed. New York, Churchill Livingstone, 1989.
8. Silvergleid AJ: Safety and effectiveness of predeposit autologous transfusions in preteen and adolescent children. JAMA 1987;257:3403–3404.
9. Haugen RK, Hill GE: A large-scale autologous blood program in a community hospital. A contribution to the community's blood supply. JAMA 1987;257:1211–1214.
10. Finch S, Haskins D, Finch CA: Iron metabolism: hematopoiesis following phlebotomy; iron as a limiting factor. J Clin Invest 1950;29:1078–1086.
11. Toy PTCY, Strauss RG, Stehling LC et al: Predeposited autologous blood for elective surgery. A national multicenter study. N Engl J Med. 1987;316:517–520.
12. Silvergleid AJ: Autologous transfusions. Experience in a community blood center. JAMA 1979;241:2724–2725.
13. Thurer RL: Blood conservation in cardiac operations (editorial). Mayo Clin Proc 1988;63:292–293.
14. Novak RW: Autologous blood transfusion in a pediatric population. Safety and efficacy. Clin Pediatr 1987; 27:184–187.
15. Williamson KR, Taswell HF: Intraoperative autologous transfusion (IAT): experience in over 8,000 surgical procedures (abstract). Transfusion 1988;28:11S.
16. Tomasulo PA, Petz LD: Platelet transfusions. pp. 427–467. In Petz LD, Swisher SN (eds): Clinical Practice of Transfusion Medicine. 2nd Ed. New York, Churchill Livingstone, 1989.
17. Mueller-Eckhardt C: Platelet allo- and autoantigens and their clinical implications. pp. 63–93. In Nance ST (ed): Transfusion Medicine in the 1990's. Arlington, VA, American Association of Blood Banks, 1990.
18. Sinor LT, Plapp FV: Platelet antibody detection methods. pp. 55–72. In Smith DM, Summers SH (eds): Platelets. Arlington, VA, American Association of Blood Banks, 1988.
19. Kickler TS, Braine HG, Ness PM et al: A radiolabeled antiglobulin test for crossmatching platelet transfusions. Blood 1983;61:238–242.
20. Yam P, Petz LD, Scott EP, Santos S: Platelet crossmatch tests using radiolabelled staphylococcal protein A or peroxidase anti-peroxidase in alloimmunized patients. Br J Haematol 1984;57:337–347.
21. Rachel JM, Summers TC, Sinor LT, Plapp FV: Use of a solid phase red blood cell adherence method for pretransfusion platelet compatibility testing. Am J Clin Pathol 1988;90:63–68.
22. Petz LD: Platelet Crossmatching (editorial). Am J Clin Pathol 1988;90:114–115.
23. McCullough J: Granulocyte transfusions. pp. 469–484. In Petz LD, Swisher SN (eds): Clinical Practice of Transfusion Medicine. 2nd Ed. New York, Churchill Livingstone, 1989.
24. Pisciotto PT (ed): Blood Transfusion Therapy, A physician's Handbook. 3rd Ed. Arlington, VA, American Association of Blood Banks, 1989.
25. Petz LD, Branch DR: The diagnosis of acquired immune hemolytic anemias. pp. 9–48. In McMillan R (ed): Immune Cytopenias. New York, Churchill Livingstone, 1983.
26. Petz LD, Garratty G: Acquired Immune Hemolytic Anemias. New York, Churchill Livingstone, 1980.
27. Branch DR, Petz LD: A new reagent (ZZAP) having multiple applications in immunohematology. Am J Clin Pathol 1982;78:161–167.
28. Petz LD, Branch DR: Drug-induced immune hemolytic anemia. pp. 47–94. In Chaplin H (ed): Immune Hemolytic Anemias. New York, Churchill Livingstone, 1985.
29. Petz LD: Drug-induced immune hemolytic anemia. pp. 53–75. In Nance ST (ed): Immune Destruction of Red Blood Cells. Arlington, VA, American Association of Blood Banks, 1989.
30. Malacarne P, Castaldi G, Bertusi M, Zavagli G: Tolbutamide-induced hemolytic anemia. Diabetes 1977;26: 156–158.
31. Wong KY, Boose GM, Issitt CH: Erythromycin-induced hemolytic anemia. J Pediatr 1980;98:647–649.
32. Getaz EP, Beckley S, Pitzpatrick J, Dozier A: Cisplatin-induced hemolysis. N Eng J Med 1980;302:334–335.
33. Wenz B, Klein RL, Lalezari P: Tetracycline-induced immune hemolytic anemia. Transfusion 1974;14:265–269.

34. Eisner EV, Shahidi T: Immune thrombocytopenia due to a drug metabolite. N Engl J Med 1972;287:376–381.
35. Salama A, Mueller-Eckhardt C: The role of metabolite-specific antibodies in nomifensine-dependent immune hemolytic anemia. N Engl J Med 1985;313:469–474.
36. Salama A, Mueller-Eckhardt C: Ex vivo antigen preparation for the serological detection of drug-dependent antibodies in immune haemolytic anaemias. Br J Haematol 1984;58:525–531.
37. Calhoun L: Blood product preparation and administration. pp. 239–269. In Petz LD, Swisher SN (eds): Clinical Practice of Transfusion Medicine. 2nd Ed. New York, Churchill Livingstone, 1989.
38. Sanford-Driscoll M, Knodel LC: Induction of hemolytic anemia by nosteroidal antiinflammatory drugs. Drug Intel Clin Pharm 1986;20:925–934.

Index

Page numbers followed by f indicate figures; those followed by t indicate tables.

A

AAT. See α_1-Antitrypsin
AB blood type, 873, 873t
Abetalipoproteinemia, 180
    phospholipids and, 182
    tests for, 185
    vitamin E and, 221
ABG (arterial blood gases) [test], 15–21
abl oncogene, 569
A blood type, 873, 873t
ABO blood group, 873t, 873–874
    and autoagglutination, 890
    compatibility testing, 872–873
    and granulocyte transfusion, 886
    and platelet transfusion, 885
Abscess. *See also specific types*
    aspiration, 689, 692f
    polymicrobic flora infection and, 699, 700f
Absidia, 640, 668, 671t
Absolute eosinophil count [test], 592
Absolute lymphocyte count [test], 838, 840
Abused drugs [tests], 386–389
Acanthamoeba:
    CNS infection, 774, 777t, 778, 782
    cutaneous ulcers, 685
    eye infections, 649, 651, 653
Acanthocytes, 431, 463
Accumulation ratio equation, 336t
ACE. *See* Angiotensin converting enzyme
Acetaminophen:
    and emergency room, 370t
    hemolytic anemia from, 894t
    and hepatic necrosis, 77
    therapeutic range, concentration, and distribution, 334t
    toxicity, 382t, 383f
Acetaminophen [test], 382–383
Acetone, 378
    concentrations from D-Osm, 379t
Acetylcholine receptor, 845t
Acetylcholinesterase, 75
Acetylcholinesterase [test], 403–404, 405t
Acetyl coenzyme A (CoA), 173–174, 222
Acetylsalicylic acid (ASA) [test], 380–382, 381f
AChE. *See* Acetylcholinesterase
Achlorhydria, 99, 100
Acid-base balance, 17–21
Acid-base disorders, 17–21
    mixed, 20, 21f
Acid-base equilibrium equation, 13–14
Acid-base system, 11, 12–15
    amino acids and, 143
    control of blood pH, 14–15, 15f
    function, 12
    open and closed buffering systems, 12–13
    physiologic buffers, 13t, 13–14
Acid buffering power, 12
α_1-Acid glycoprotein, 160
α_1-Acid glycoprotein [test], 165
Acidic phospholipids: in amniotic fluid, 408
Acidified serum lysis test for PNH, 476–477
Acidosis, 18t, 18–19, 19t
    metabolic, 17, 18, 18t, 21
    respiratory, 17, 18t, 18–19, 21
Acid output:
    basal (BAO), 100, 100t
    peak (PAO), 100, 100t
Acid phosphatase [test]:
    stain, 609
    tumor marker, 311–313, 312t
Acid serum test for PNH [test], 476–477
Acid urine, 51–52, 62f
Acinetobacter:
    infections, 624t
    pneumonia, 657, 669t
Acinetobacter calcoaceticus: tissue manifestations, 680t
Acne, 678t
    fulminans, 681t
Acquired immunodeficiency syndrome (AIDS), 860–861. *See also* Human immunodeficiency virus
    adrenal insufficiency and, 259
    Candida and, 641–642, 737, 748
    and CMV, 729, 860
    CNS infections, 769, 785. *See also specific organisms*
    immunology, 860–861
    infectious diarrheas, 751t, 752t, 753t, 754, 755, 756, 860
    infectious esophagitis, 748
    lymphadenopathy, 714
    Mycobacterium avium infections, 620, 626, 728, 754, 755, 756, 860
    opportunistic infections, 860

Acquired immunodeficiency syndrome (AIDS) *(Continued)*
  respiratory disorders and, 657, 658, 661, 662, 672–673
  skin/tissue infections and, 682, 684
  and syphilis, 810
  toxoplasmosis, 704, 714, 777–778, 782, 832
Acrodermatitis enteropathica, 200t, 211–212, 213t, 222
Acromegaloidism, 240
Acromegaly:
  glucose testing and, 128, 133
  and growth hormone, 239–240, 326
  insulin-like growth factor I and, 241
ACTH. *See* Adrenocorticotropic hormone
Actinobacillus, 680t
Actinobacillus actinomycetemcomitans, 624t, 626t
Actinomadura madurae, 681t
Actinomyces:
  CNS abscess, 783
  morphologic characteristics, 671t
  pneumonia, 658, 665, 669t
Actinomyces israelii, 680t
  arthritis, 707
  cultures, 696t
Actinomycetoma, 681t
Activated clotting time (ACT), 524
Activated partial prothrombin time (APTT), 505f, 513, 517f, 518, 518t, 523, 524, 538, 539, 540, 542, 543
Activated partial thromboplastin time [test], 505f, 516t, 518t, 524t, 526–527, 538, 538f
Activation peptide of protein C [test], 509f, 520t, 551
Acute lymphocytic leukemia. *See* Lymphocytic leukemia, acute
Acute myelocytic leukemia. *See* Myelocytic leukemia, acute
Acute phase reaction, 158, 160, 170
  immunoglobulin responses, 157t
Acyl-cholesterol acyltransferase (ACAP), 175
Addison's disease, 259, 273
  autoantibody, 845t
Adenitis, cervical, 714
Adenomas:

  adrenal: idiopathic hyperaldosteronism vs., 274, 274t
  aldosterone-producing, 273
  pituitary
    classification of, 238t
    and growth hormone, 239
Adenopathy: and pneumonia, 660t
Adenosine deaminase deficiency, 858, 859
Adenosine diphosphate (ADP), 25, 61, 501, 505–506, 515f
  measurement, 129
Adenosine triphosphate (ATP), 25, 61, 299, 501
  digoxin and, 357
  measurement, 129
  urinary measurement, 725
Adenosylcobalamin, 471
Adenoviruses:
  blood culture [test], 628t
  CNS infection, 771, 772t, 776
  ear infection, 637
  eye infections, 648, 649t
  gastroenteritis, 751t, 753, 758
  infection frequency, 636t
  lower respiratory infection, 660, 666, 669t
  serology [test], 823
  skin manifestations, 677t
  throat culture, 641, 642
  upper respiratory infections, 636t
  urinary tract infection, 729, 730t
Adenylate cyclase, 501
Adenylate cyclase: and corticotropin (ACTH). *See* Adrenocorticotropic hormone
Adenyl kinase deficiency, 421t
ADH. *See* Antidiuretic hormone
Adipocyte, 443
Adler-Reilly anomaly, 555
Adrenache: DHEA-S levels, 291
Adrenal adenoma, 272, 272t, 290
  idiopathic hyperaldosteronism vs., 274, 274t
  urinary-free cortisol and, 264t
Adrenal autoantibody, 845t
Adrenal carcinoma:
  DHEA-S levels, 291
  hormone markers, 326
  urinary-free cortisol and, 264t
Adrenal cortex, 257–259
  and hyperandrogenism, 288, 288t
  hyperfunction. *See* Adrenal hyperfunction
  hypofunction. *See* Adrenal hypofunction
  zones of, 257

Adrenal hyperfunction, 46, 128, 261–262
  differential diagnosis, 261t, 263t, 266
  laboratory evaluation of, 269f
Adrenal hyperfunction [tests], 262–268
  corticotropin, 264–266, 265f
  corticotropin releasing hormone stimulation, 266
  cortisol, urinary-free, 262–264, 264t
  cortisol (compound F), 262, 263t
  dexamethasone suppression, 266–268
Adrenal hyperplasia, congenital, 259, 271t, 290
  clinical and biocehmical features of, 271t
  DHEA-S levels, 291
Adrenal hyperplasia, congenital [tests], 268–270
  desoxycorticosterone, 270
  11-desoxycortisol, 270
  17-hydroxyprogesterone, 268–270
Adrenal hypofunction, 257–259
Adrenal hypofunction [tests], 259–262
  adrenocorticotropic hormone stimulation, 259–261, 260f
  insulin tolerance, 261
  long ATCH, 261
Adrenal insufficiency, 257–259. *See also* Adrenal hypofunction
  causes of, 259t
  congenital adrenal hyperplasia and, 271t
  DHEA-S levels, 291
  primary vs. secondary causes of, 260
Adrenal insufficiency [tests], 259–262
Adrenal medulla, 277–279
  biochemstry, 277, 278f
  neuroblastoma, 278–279
  pheochromocytoma, 277, 278, 279–281
Adrenal medulla [tests], 279–283
  catecholamines, plasma, 281–282
  catecholamines, urinary (free), 280–281
  3,4 dihydroxyphelalanine, 283
  3,4 dihydroxyphenylglycol, 282–283
  dopamine, 283
  homovanillic acid, 283
  metanephrine, 280

3-methoxy-4-hydroxyphenylglycol, 283
   specimen collection, 277–278
   vanillylmandelic acid, 279–280
Adrenocorticotropic hormone (ACTH), 237, 257, 264–266, 265f
   and aldosterone, 270
   ectopic syndrome, 261t, 265, 266, 269f, 321
   as tumor marker, 321
Adrenocorticotropic hormone (ACTH)-like peptide, 99
Adrenocorticotropic hormone (ACTH) [test], 264–266, 265f
   stimulation, 259–261
   tumor marker, 321
Adrenocorticotropin. See Adrenocorticotropic hormone
Adrenoleukodystrophy: testing for, 419
Adult inclusion conjunctivitis, 648, 652
Adult T-cell leukemia/lymphoma, 441, 576
   immunophenotyping, 602
   T-helper, morphology/manifestations/markers, 575t
Adventitial cell, 443
Aeromonas hydrophila, 680t
   gastroenteritis, 751t, 754, 755, 756
   infections, 624t, 682
Afibrinogenemia, 514t, 516t
AFP. *See* α-Fetoprotein
African eye worm, 649
African histoplasmosis, 677t
African trypanosomiasis (sleeping sickness), 631, 774–775, 779, 782
Agammaglobulinemia, 857
   testing for, 840, 841, 842
Agarose: for high resolution serum protein electrophoresis, 159
Agarose gel inhibitor screening [test], 517f, 542, 542f
Agar overlay method of susceptibility testing, 791t
Agglutination reactions, 805, 809
Agranular platelets, 442
A/G ratio. *See* Albumin-globulin ratio
Ahumada-del Castillo syndrome, 293t
AIDS. *See* Acquired immunodeficiency syndrome
Alanine, 147

biochemistry and reference range, 145t
Alanine aminotransferase, 68–69, 69t, 76, 78
Alanine aminotransferase [test], 67, 67t, 68–69, 69t, 76, 78
   for vitamin B_6, 226
Alanine transaminase: and acetaminophen, 226
Albinism, 150
   enzymatic defect and features of, 146t
Albumin:
   abnormal electrophoretic patterns, 157t
   for alloantibody detection, 877, 878t
   conditions and disorders affecting ranges of, 156t
   and fatty acids, 181
   and fructosamine testing, 138
   functions of, 151
   hypoalbuminemia, 47, 152
   reference range of, 152
   and serum protein electrophoresis, 155, 158
   administration data, 869t
Albumin [test], 67, 76, 151–152
Albumin-globulin ratio [test], 153, 154f, 155f
Albuminuria, 725
Alcohol:
   analytic methods for, 376t
   breath analysis for, 376
   comparative properties, 375t
   drug interactions, 344t, 359, 366, 385, 386
   and emergency room, 370t
   and pseudo-Cushing syndrome, 261, 261t, 264
Alcohol dehydrogenase, 211
   analysis, 375, 376, 376f, 376t
Alcoholic hepatitis, 68t, 69, 70, 74, 77
Alcoholic pancreatitis, 90
Alcoholism:
   and anemia, 451t
   and folate, 473
   GGT and, 79
   and glycohemoglobin, 137
   and hypercholesterolemia, 178
   and hypertriglyceridemia, 180t
   thiamine deficiency and, 229
Alcohols [tests], 374–380
   delta osmolality, 379–380
   ethanol, 375–377
   ethylene glycol, 378–379
   isopropanol, 378
   methanol, 377–378
Aldehyde oxidase, 209

Alder-Reilly anomaly, 436, 558t, 589
Alder-Reilly granules, 436
Aldosterone, 257, 258f, 268, 270
   basal serum test, 273t, 274t
   deficiency, congenital adrenal hyperplasia and, 271t
   and sodium, 46
Aldosterone [test], 272–275, 273t, 274t
Aldosterone glucuronide, 272
Aldosterone-producing adenomas, 273
Aldosterone-producing adrenocorticoid carcinoma, 272, 272t
Aldosterone-renin-angiotensin system, 270–272
Aldosterone-renin-angiotensin system [tests], 272–277
   aldosterone, 272–275, 273t, 274t
   angiotensin converting enzyme, 277
   renin, 275–277, 276t
Aldosteronism, 272t, 272–275
   and hypertension, 276t
   screening tests for primary, 273t
Aliphatic carbon chains, 143
Alkaline phosphatase: zinc and, 211, 213
Alkaline phosphatase [test], 67, 67t, 68t, 70–74, 71f, 71t, 72t, 73t, 74t
   age- and sex-related upper limits, 71f
   and bone disease, 72
   and cardiac disease, 72
   in cholestasis, 72, 77
   diagnostic approach to evaluating, 73t, 73–74, 74t
   elevated, lesions of, 71t
   and gastrointestinal disease, 73
   and hepatic disease, 72, 72t
   increased, with normal bilirubin, 79t
   and ischemic disease, 78
   isoenzymes, 73t, 73–74, 74t, 309–310
   and neoplasia, 73, 74t, 77
   and pulmonary disease, 72–73
   and renal disease, 73
   and splenic disease, 73
   stain, 608–609
   tumor marker, 309t, 309–310
Alkaline urine, 51–52, 62f
Alkalosis, 18t, 19–20, 20t
   metabolic, 17, 18t, 19–20, 20t, 21
   respiratory, 17, 18t, 20, 20t, 21
Alkaptonuria, 148
   enzymatic defect and features of, 146t

ALL. *See* Lymphocytic leukemia, acute
Allen test, 16
Alloantibody detection:
    albumin, 877, 878t
    antiglobulin test, 876, 878t
    autologous control, 875
    clinical significance, 879–880, 880t
    differential absorption test, 892
    enzyme techniques, 876, 878t
    group I–IV, 880, 880t, 881
    interpretation, 877–879, 878t
    low ionic strength solutions (LISS), 876, 877
    reagent RBCs, 875, 875t
    saline test, 876, 878t
    for transfusions, 874–881
    warm autoabsorption test, 892
    and warm autoantibodies, 891
Alloantigens: platelet, 884, 884t
Alloimmune platelet disorders, 883
α_1-Acid glycoprotein, 160
α_1-Acid glycoprotein [test], 165
α-Amino acids, 143
α_2-Antiplasmin, 509, 511f, 512f, 525
    deficiency, 519, 550
α_2-Antiplasmin [test], 512f, 519t, 550
α_1-Antitrypsin, 89
    conditions and disorders affecting ranges of, 156t
α_1-Antitrypsin deficiency, 166
    immunoglobulin responses, 157t
α_1-Antitrypsin [test], 165–166
    genetic disorders, 413–414
α-Fetoprotein:
    CSF, 114
    and serum protein electrophoresis, 158
α-Fetoprotein [test]:
    and liver function, 81
    pleural fluid, 116
    pregnancy, 402–403, 404, 405t
    tumor marker, 314–315, 315t
$\alpha_{1,4}$-Glucosidase deficiency, 421t
α_1-Glycoprotein: conditions and disorders affecting ranges of, 156t
α-Granules, 441
    and plug formation, 501, 503t
α-Heavy chain, 580, 581
α_2-Lipoprotein: conditions and disorders affecting ranges of, 156t, 161
α_2-Macroglobulin, 89, 116
    conditions and disorders affecting ranges of, 156t, 161
    in serum protein electrophoresis test, 155

α_2-Macroglobulin [test], 166
α-Methyldopa: hemolytic anemia from, 889t, 894t
α-Naphthyl acetate esterase [test], 604t, 605–606
α-Naphthyl butyrate esterase [test], 604t, 605–606
α-Thalassemia. *See* Thalassemias
α-Tocopherol, 219, 220, 221t
Alphaviruses: CNS infection, 772t, 774, 777t
Alprazolam:
    and emergency room, 370t
    half-life and therapeutic/toxic concentrations, 384t
ALT. *See* Alanine aminotransferase
Aluminum [test], 60
Alveolar-arterial O_2 concentration, 12
Alveolar dead space, 11
Amebiasis. *See Entamoeba histolytica*
Amenorrhea, 285, 286, 294
    and hypogonadism, 293, 293t
American Association of Blood Banks Standards, 871, 874
American trypanosomiasis serology [test], 832–833
Amides, 143
Amikacin:
    bacterial susceptibility testing, 794
    monitoring [test], 797–798
    reference range, 798t
    therapeutic range, concentration, and distribution, 334t
Amine precursor uptake and decarboxylation (APUD) cells, 101
Amino acids, 143–144
    chromatography, 145, 147
    color tests, 147
    Guthrie test, 147
    hydrophobic and hydrophilic, 143
    metabolism, 144
    nutritionally essential, 144t
    nutritionally nonessential, 145t
    pH, 143
    quantitation, 147
    R group, 143
Amino acid screen [test]: genetic, 414
Amino acid [tests], 144–150
Aminoacidurias, 144–150
    alkaptonuria, 148
    autosomal recessive, 146t
    branched chain ketoaciduria. *See* Maple syrup urine disease
    classification of, 147–148
    cystinuria, 148–149
    homocystinuria, 149

    overflow, 147–148
    phenylalaninemias, 149–150
    renal, 148
    tyrosinuria, 150
γ-Aminobutyric acid (GABA):
    and benzodiazepines, 383
    biochemistry and reference range, 145t
    valproic acid and, 347
3-Amino-9-ethylcarbazole, 604
3-Aminoethylpyrazol (Histalog), 99
Aminoglycosides:
    bacterial susceptibility testing, 794t
    monitoring [test], 797–798
δ-Aminolevulinic acid (ALA), 55, 58t
Aminophylline, 362
Aminopyrine: hemolytic anemia from, 894t
Amino-terminal assay: parathyroid hormone, 300, 301t, 302
Aminotransferase activity assay: for vitamin B_6, 226t
Amiodarone:
    drug interactions, 351
    therapeutic range, concentration, and distribution, 334t
Amitriptyline, 360
    therapeutic range, concentration, and distribution, 334t, 396t
    toxicities, 396t
AML. *See* Myelocytic leukemia, acute
Ammonia:
    glutamine and, 80
    protein, 153
Ammonia [test], 78, 78t
Ammonical silver nitrate test, 147
Ammonium biurate crystals: in urine, 52, 63f
Amniocentesis, 399, 403, 403f, 405t, 413
Amniotic fluid:
    AChE in, 403–404
    bilirubin pigments in, 404–405
    evaluating, 399
    α-fetoprotein in, 402–403, 404, 405t
    phospholipids in, 408–409
Amobarbital [test], 384–386, 385t
Amorphous phosphate crystals: in urine, 52, 63f
Amorphous urate crystals: in urine, 52, 62f
Amoxapine:
    therapeutic range, concentration, and distribution, 334t, 396t
    toxicities, 396t

Amphetamines: testing for, 386–387, 387t, 388t
Ampholytes, 143
Amphotericin B: drug interactions, 364
3′,5′-AMP [test], 58
Amylase:
 activity, 86
 and lung and ovarian cancer, 309
 pleural fluid [test], 116
 serum [test], 86–87, 87f, 90
Amylase/creatinine ratio [test], 87–88
Amylase isoenzymes [test], 87
Amyloidosis: and factor X deficiency, 518
Anaerobes. *See also specific anaerobes*
 blood culture and, 621t
 gastrointestinal, 747
 liver abscess, 701
 myonecrosis, 713
 osteomyelitis, 710
 sinusitis, 640
 susceptibility [test], 792
 urine culture [test], 727
Analbuminemia, 152
Analgesics, non-narcotic [tests], 380–383
 acetaminophen, 382–383
 salicylate (aspirin; ASA), 380–382
Analphalipoproteinemia. *See Tangier's disease*
Analysis, laboratory, 6–7
Analytic variation, 5
Anatomic dead space, 11
Ancylostoma braziliense, 685
Ancylostoma caninum, 685
Ancylostoma duodenale:
 gastrointestinal infection, 761, 763t
 pulmonary infection, 672t
Anderson's disease, 421t
Androgenic tumors, 290
Androgens, 257, 258f
Androstenediol, 292f
Androstenedione, 258f, 268, 287f, 292f
Anemias, 447–448, 448f
 aplastic, 451t, 476
 of chronic disease, 448, 449, 449t, 450t, 450–452, 451t, 452f
 classification, 447–448, 448f
 congenital dyserythropoietic (CDA), type II, 476, 477, 482
 hemolytic. *See hemolytic anemias*
 iron deficiency. *See Iron deficiency anemia*
 macrocytic, 449–450, 451t, 467f, 474t, 610
 macrocytic [tests], 471–476. *See also Macrocytic anemias [tests]*
 megaloblastic. *See Megaloblastic anemia*
 microcytic, 448–449, 449t, 450t
 microcytic [tests], 466–471
 myelophthisic, 451t, 453
 normocytic, 448f, 450–455, 451t, 452f, 454f, 455t
 pernicious, 228, 228t, 447, 469, 472, 475
  autoantibody, 845t
 protein levels and, 156t
 pyridoxine responsive, 227t
 refractory. *See Refractory anemia*
 sickle cell
  testing for, 411, 412
  zinc deficiency and, 211, 212
 sideroblastic, 448, 449t, 566, 567, 567t
 vitamin B_{12} and, 228, 228t
 warm hemolytic, 861
Anencephaly, 402
Aneuploidy, 562
Aneurin. *See Thiamin*
Angioedema, hereditary: complement assay, 849t
Angiostrongylus cantonensis: CNS infection, 775, 777t, 778, 779, 782
Angiotensin I, 59, 275, 277
Angiotensin II, 59, 270, 274t, 277
 and renin secretion, 270
Angiotensin III, 270
Angiotensin converting enzyme (ACE), 270
Angiotensin converting enzyme (ACE) [test], 277
Anileridine: characteristics of, 389t
Animal bite wound specimen [test], 715–716
Anion gap acidosis, increased, 18
Anisocytosis, 431, 457, 461
Ankylosing spondylitis, 707
Anogenital intercourse, 743–744
Anorchia, 290t
Anorexia nervosa: and hypogonadism, 293t
Antacids: drug interactions, 358
Antazoline: hemolytic anemia from, 894t
Anterior pituitary gland, 237
Anterior pituitary gland [tests], 237–243
 arginine infusion, 243
 growth hormone, 237–240
 insulin-like growth factor I, 240–241
 insulin tolerance, 243
 prolactin, 241–243
Anthrax, 659t
 skin manifestations, 677t, 678t, 679t
Antiarrhythmics:
 drug interactions, 344, 353, 355, 356. *See also specific antiarrhythmics*
 oral dose pharmacokinetic formulas, 349t
 pharmacokinetic parameters, 349t
Antiarrhythmics [tests], 348–357
 disopyramide, 348–350
 encainide, 350–351
 flecainide, 351
 lidocaine, 351–352
 mexiletine, 352–353
 procainamide/NAPA, 353–354
 propranolol, 354–355
 quinidine, 355–356
 tocainide, 356–357
Antibiotics: platelet disorders induced by, 516t
Antibiotic therapeutic monitoring [tests], 797–800. *See also Drugs*
Antibodies:
 antigen binding, 838
 auto-, 844–846
 group I–IV, 880, 880t, 881
 incomplete, 876
 as interference, 7
 monoclonal, and antigen cluster designation, 852, 852t
Antibody coated bacteriuria [test], 726–727
Antibody dependent cell-mediated cytotoxicity (ADCC), 438
Antibody detection, 803–805. *See also Serodiagnosis of infectious disease*
 alloantibodies, 874–881
 CSF, 780, 804
 Donath-Landsteiner antibody test, 891
 for transfusions, 874
Anti-CD10, 853t
Anticoagulants, oral:
 drug interactions, 341, 344
 and hemostatic disorders, 518, 549
 therapy monitoring, 523, 524t, 529, 539

Arrhythmias:
  drug-induced, 350, 351, 353, 355, 356, 361
  drugs for, 348–357. *See also* Antiarrhythmics
Arsenic, 199
  monitoring occupational exposure, 392t
  toxic symptoms/concentrations, 391t
Arsenic [test], 390t, 390–392
Arterial blood gases (ABG), 11–12
Arterial blood gases (ABG) [test], 15–21
  reference ranges, 16t
Arthritis:
  differential diagnosis, 708
  gonococcal, 125t
  nonseptic, 125t
  septic, 119–120, 125t
    testing for, 707–709
  synovial fluid examination, 119–120, 125t
  testing for, 850
Arthrocentesis, 708, 710
Ascaris, 705
Ascaris duodenalis, 761
Ascaris lumbricoides, 672, 672t, 673–674, 761, 763t, 765
Ascites, 116
Ascitic fluid tests, 116
Ascorbate, 231
Ascorbate-2-sulfate, 231
Ascorbic acid, 213. *See also* Vitamin C
Ascorbic acid [test], 231–233
ASO test: for *Streptococcus pyogenes*, 808–809
Aspartate aminotransferase [test], 67t, 68t, 69t, 69–70, 70t, 76, 77, 78
  for vitamin B_6, 226
Aspartate transaminase (AST):
  and acetaminophen, 226
  in myocardial infarction, 26f, 31
Aspartic acid: biochemistry and reference range, 145t
Aspergillus:
  antigenemia, 633
  arthritis, 707–708
  and burn wounds, 716, 717
  cultures, 697t
  ear infection, 636
  eye infections, 648
  fungemia, 625
  infections, 624t, 626t
  keratitis, 648
  morphologic characteristics, 671t
  nasal infection, 638–639

osteomyelitis, 710
pericarditis, 711
pulmonary infection, 667–668, 669t
serology [test], 825–827, 826t, 827t
sinusitis, 640
skin manifestations, 679t
upper respiratory infections, 645t
urinary tract infection, 727, 728
Aspirate specimen [test], 700–707
Aspirin:
  drug interactions, 347, 348
  and emergency room, 370t
  platelet disorders induced by, 514, 529–530
  and Reye syndrome, 78
Aspirin [test], 380–382, 381f
Aspirin tolerance [test], 530
Assay precision of a measurement, 5, 6
AST (aspartate aminotransferase) [test], 67t, 68t, 69t, 69–70, 70t, 76, 77, 78
  for vitamin B_6, 226
Asthma: drugs for, 361–363
Astrovirus: gastroenteritis, 751t, 758
Ataxia telangiectasia, 859
Atomic absorption spectrophotometry (AAS): for trace metals, 201, 202, 209, 210
ATP release [test], 514t, 536
Atrial arrhythmias: drugs for, 348, 353, 354
Atrial fibrillation: drugs for, 354, 355
Atrial flutter: drugs for, 355
ATT. *See* α_1-Antitrypsin [test]
Auer bodies (rods), Plate 14B, 436
Autoagglutination: red blood cells, 431
Autoantibodies:
  compatibility testing with cold, 892–893
  essential data on, 845t
Autoantibodies [tests], 844–846, 845t
  thyroid, 254–256, 255f
Autohemolysis [test], 482–483
Autoimmune disorders, 851
  testing for, 840, 841, 844–846, 845t, 850
Autoimmune hemolytic anemia. *See also* Hemolytic anemias
  drug-induced, 894t, 894–895
  testing for, 889–893
Autoimmune platelet disorders, 884
Autologous blood transfusion, 881–882
Automated differential [test], 589–592
Avidin-biotin complex, 222

Avidin-biotin-peroxidase enzyme complex, 601, 601f
Azoospermia, 124, 289, 290t

B

Babesia: blood examination [test], 629t, 630–631
Bacillary angiomatosis, 677t
Bacillus:
  cultures, 697t, 698
  infections, 624t
  respiratory infections, 669t
Bacillus anthracis:
  respiratory infection, 659t, 669t
  skin manifestations, 677t, 678t, 679t
Bacillus cereus:
  cultures, 697t
  gastroenteritis, 751t
Bacteoroides: infections, 624t
Bacteoroides fragilis: infections, 624t
Bacteremia. *See also* Septicemia
  catheter-associated, 633–634
  defined, 620
  gram-negative: complement test and, 168
  infections associated with, 620t
  nosocomial, 633
  testing for, 619–634. *See also* specific bacteria
Bacteria. *See also* specific bacteria
  arthritis, 707–708
  bite wounds, 715–716
  blood cultures [test], 619–627
  bone marrow culture [test], 634
  burn wounds, 716–717
  CNS infections, 770, 775–776, 780, 781
  diarrheas, 751t–753t, 753
  direct blood examination [test], 627
  ear infections, 636–638
  esophageal culture [test], 748
  eye infections, 648–654
  lymphadenitis, 714
  nasal infection, 638–639
  osteomyelitis, 709–711
  pericarditis, 711–712
  peritoneal infection, 700–707
  pneumonia, 657, 657t, 658t, 664–665
  sinusitis, 639–641
  skeletal muscle disease, 712–713
  synovial infection, 707–709

Bacteria *(Continued)*
   throat infections, 641, 642–646
   upper respiratory infections, 635, 641–647, 645t
   in urine, 49–50. *See also* Bacteriuria
   urine culture [test], 721–725
   urine microscopic examination [test], 730–731
Bacterial meningitis. *See* Meningitis, bacterial
Bacterial serology [tests], 806–811
   Borrelia burgdorferi, 807–808
   Brucella, 806
   Francisella tularensis, 811
   Helicobacter pylori, 806
   Legionella, 806
   Leptospira, 807
   Salmonella typhi, 809
   Staphylococcus aureus, 808
   Streptococcus pyogenes, 808–809
   Treponema pallidum, 809–811, 810t
Bacterial tolerance, 790
Bacteriuria, 49–50, 721–729, 730–731. *See also* Urine
   antibody coated [test], 726–727
   count, 723–734
   screening [test], 725
Bacteroides, 640
   CNS abscess, 783
   cultures, 697t
   lymphadenopathy, 714
   peritoneal infection, 701
   respiratory infections, 669t
   traumatic wounds, 718
   vaginosis, 734t
Bacteroides fragilis:
   arthritis, 707
   cultures, 697t, 700f
   liver abscess, 701
   susceptibility testing, 793
Bacteroides melaninogenicus, 644
   osteomyelitis, 710
   susceptibility testing, 793
Baermann funnel technique, 765
BAL. *See* Bronchoalveolar lavage
Balantidium coli: gastroenteritis, 751t, 753, 765–766
Band, 426f, 435
BAO/PAO ratio, 100, 100t
Barbiturates: drug interactions, 344t, 359, 361
Barbiturates [tests], 384–386
Bare-lymphocyte syndrome, 858
Barlow's disease, 231–232
Bartonella bacilliformis:
   direct examination of blood [test], 627

   skin manifestations, 679t, 681t
Basal acid output (BAO), 100, 100t
Base, 11, 12–15. *See also* Acid-base system
   disorders. *See* Acid-base disorders
Basket cell, 440
Basopenia: causes of, 556t, 588
Basophil, 425
   function, 435, 553
   morphology, Plate 8A, 426f, 436
   reference values for cell count and slide differential, 586t–587t
   stain reactions, 604t
Basophilia: causes of, 555t, 588
Basophilic megaloblast, Plate 7, 431
Basophilic normoblast, 427, 429
Basophilic stippling, 431
Bassen-Kanzwez syndrome, 180
Bauer-Kirby method of susceptibility testing, 791t
Bb, 848t, 849t
Bβ 1-42 and Bβ 15-42 [test], 550
B blood type, 873, 873t
B cell. *See* B lymphocytes
B-cell growth factor, 438
B-cell leukemia: testing for, 841
B-cell lymphoma, 580
   EBV and, 859
   immunophenotyping, 603, 856f
B-cell lymphoma, leukemic phase of, 576
   morphology/manifestations/markers, 572t
bcr-abl protein product, 569
bcr gene, 569
Beckman Paragon immunofunction gel, 162f
Bed bug bite, 677t
Beef tapeworm, 761
Bejel, 810
Bence-Jones proteins, 53, 159–160, 162, 163, 164, 165, 169, 580
B endorphin, 321
Benign monoclonal gammopathy (BMG), 581
Bentiromide (tripeptide hydrolysis) [test], 92–93
Benzodiazepines: drug interactions, 344t
Benzodiazepines [tests], 383–384, 384t
Benzoylecgonine, 372, 388
Beriberi, 229t, 229–231
Bernard-Soulier syndrome, 500f, 513, 514t, 515f, 532–533
Beta blockers. *See also specific beta blockers*

   drug interactions, 349, 352, 361
   platelet disorders induced by, 516t
β-Carotene, 216, 217
β-Carotene [test], 97
βδ-Thalassemia. *See* Thalassemias
β-D-Glucose, 129
β-Glucuronidase: as tumor marker, 114
β-hCG. *See* Human chorionic gonadotropin
β-Lactamase test for in vitro susceptibility, 793–794
β-Lipoproteins. *See* Low density lipoproteins
β Lipotrophic hormone, 321
β Melanocyte stimulating hormone, 321
β-Methylcrototonylglycinuria, 223
β_2-Microglobulin:
   conditions and disorders affecting levels of, 157t, 161
   as tumor marker, 114
   urinary measure, 726
β_2-Microglobulin [test], 166–167
β-Thalassemia. *See* Thalassemias
β-Thromboglobulin, 501
β-Thromboglobulin [test], 537
Bethesda assay for factor VIII inhibitors [test], 542–543
Between assay precision of a measurement, 5, 6
BFU. *See* Burst forming unit
Bicarbonate:
   buffer, 13–14
   concentration, 15, 17
   glomerular filtration, 14
   reference ranges for, 48t
Bicarbonate [test], 47–48
Bile acids [test], 81
Bile duct carcinoma: tumor markers, 315
Bile salts: malabsorption and, 91t
Biliary cirrhosis: autoantibody, 845t
Biliary parasites, 702t
Bilirubin:
   alkaline phosphatase and, 72
   α, 75, 75t
   conjugated, 74t, 74–75, 75t, 77
   and erythropoiesis, 427
   unconjugated, 74t, 74–75, 75t, 77
   in urine, 54
   and xanthochromia, 107
Bilirubin [test], 67, 67t, 68t, 74t, 74–75, 75t, 76–77
   differential diagnoses, 75t
Bilirubin pigments in amniotic fluid [test], 404–405
Biologic variation, 5

Bios II (IIB). *See* Biotin [test]
Biotin, 213
   recommended daily intake, 214t
   reference ranges for, 215t
Biotin [test], 222–223
Biotinidase deficiency, 223, 223t
   testing for, 411
Birth defects: testing for, 402–403
Bisalbuminemia, 152
Bite cells, 432, 433, 463
Bites:
   cellulitis, 679t
   wound specimen [test], 715–716
Biuret reaction, 153
Bizarre platelets, Plate 25, 442
BK polyomavirus: urinary, 730, 730t
Black eschar, 679t
Black piedra, 681t
Black widow spider bite, 677t
Bladder bacteriuria, 730. *See also* Bacteriuria
Bladder cancer: tumor marker, 310, 319t, 325
Bladder infection. *See* Cystitis
Bladder washout method, 726
Blastocystis hominis: gastroenteritis, 751t, 760, 760t, 766
Blastomyces dermatitidis:
   arthritis, 707–708
   bites, 716
   eye infections, 648
   morphologic characteristics, 671t
   respiratory infection, 666, 669t
   serology [test], 826t, 827t, 827–828
   skin manifestations, 681t
   urinary tract infection, 727, 728
Blast transformation, 854–855
Bleeding disorders. *See also* Hemostasis
   clinical approach to, 511–519, 513t
   platelet-type vs. fibrin-formation, 513t
   without abnormalities in screening tests, 519, 519t
Bleeding time, 513
Bleeding time [test], 515t, 516t, 529–530
Blepharitis, 635, 648, 650–651
Blind loop syndrome, 475
Blister cells, 432
Blood:
   control of pH, 14–15
   direct examination [test], 627
   intraoperative and postoperative salvage, 882–883
   in urine, 54
   whole, 866t
Blood [tests], 619–634
   antigenemia/endotoxemia, 632–633
   culture, 619–627. *See also* Blood culture [test]
   direct examination, 627
   intravascular catheter culture, 633–634
   for parasites, 629–632
   for transfusion. *See* Transfusions
   viral culture, 627–629
Blood:alcohol concentrations (BAC), 377
Blood bank service, 865–896. *See also* Transfusions
   pretransfusion testing, 865, 871–872
Blood-brain barrier, 107, 112
Blood cell morphology, 425–446
Blood cell profile [test], 457–462, 458f, 459f, 460t, 461t
Blood components: transfusions, 866t–870t
Blood count [test], 457–462, 458f, 459f, 460t, 461t
Blood-CSF barrier, 112
Blood culture [test], 619–627
   brucellosis, 626
   endocarditis, 624
   false positive, 623t
   fungemia, 623, 625
   leptospirosis, 625–626
   and lower respiratory infections, 661
   for *Mycobacterium avium* complex, 626
   for rat bite fever, 626–627
   for rickettsiae, 626
   tularemia, 626
Blood flukes, 706, 762, 762t, 763
   in urine, 53
Blood gases [tests], 15–25
   arterial, 15–21
   oxygen saturation, 23–25
   transcutaneous and continuous arterial blood gas monitoring, 22–23
Blood glucose [test], 132
Blood groups:
   and platelet transfusion, 885
   tests, 873t, 873–874
Blood loss: and anemia, 451t, 453, 464
Blood shunting, 11–12
Blood transfusion. *See* Transfusions
Blood urea nitrogen (BUN) [test], 41–42
Blood viscosity [test], 170–171

B lymphocytes, 438, 837–838, 838f, 839f, 851. *See also* Immunoglobulins
   ALL, 564, 565t, 602, 607
   antigen markers, 599t
   functions, 439, 553
   immunophenotyping by flow cytometry, 600f
   leukemias of differentiated, 571t–573t, 576–581. *See also specific leukemias*
   marker studies, 841t
   monoclonality, 601–602
   morphology, 438
   phenotypes, 856f
   proliferation, 838
B-lymphoma, leukemic phase of: morphology/manifestations/markers, Plates 27B/28A, 573t
Body fluids, 107–126
   ascitic, 116
   cerebrospinal (CSF), 107–114. *See also* Cerebrospinal fluid
   pericardial, 116
   pleural, 114–116
   semen, 122–125
   synovial, 116–122
Body lice, 677t
Body weight, ideal, equation, 336t
Bone:
   alkaline phosphatase: as prostatic tumor marker, 313t
   and calcium regulation, 296t
   γ-carboxyglutamic acid [test], 302–303
   disease
      acid phosphatase and, 312t
      alkaline phosphatase and, 72
      and bone marrow aspiration, 612
      5′-nucleotidase and, 80
   metastases tumor markers, 309, 310
   specimen [test], 709–711
Bone marrow:
   aspirate and biopsy [test], 610–613
   culture [test], 634
   diseases, anemia and, 450, 451t, 453
   examination [test], 610–613
   lymphocytes. *See* B lymphocytes
   transplantation: for leukemia, 559
Bordetella bronchiseptica, 646
Bordetella parapertussis, 646

Bordetella pertussis:
    serology, 805
    upper respiratory infections, 645t, 646–647, 669t
Borrelia: direct examination of blood [test], 627
Borrelia burgdorferi:
    Lyme disease, 677t, 769, 807–808, 810
    serology [test], 807–808, 810
    skin manifestations, 677t
Borrelia recurrentis: skin manifestations, 678t
Boston exanthem, 677t
Botryomycosis, 680t
Botulism. See *Clostridium botulinum*
Bovine papular stomatitis, 681t, 684
Bowel infarction, 90
Boyden chamber technique, 597
Bradycardia syndrome: drugs for, 361–363
Bradykinin, 277
Brain abscess, 639, 769, 781t
    parasitic, 777t, 778, 783
Brain abscess [test], 783–785
Brain biopsy: for viruses, 777, 777t
Branched chain ketoaciduria. See Maple syrup urine disease
Branhamella catarrhalis. See *Moraxella catarrhalis*
Breast cancer:
    CEA elevation in, 319, 319t, 329t
    estrogen receptors and, 326–327, 328
    HER-2/neu and, 327, 328
    metastases, 327
    progesterone receptors and, 327, 328
    tumor markers for, 307, 310, 317, 318, 319, 319t, 326–327, 328–329, 329t
Breath analysis for alcohol, 376
Breath hydrogen test for carbohydrate intolerance [test], 95–96
Brilliant cresyl blue test for hemoglobin H, 488f, 493–494
Broad fish tapeworm, 761
Bromelin: for alloantibody detection, 876
Bromothymol blue, 55
Bromsulphalein (BSP), 82
Bronchiolitis: viral, 660
Bronchitis, 635
Bronchoalveolar lavage, 664, 672–673

Bronchoscopy, 664
Brucella, 620
    arthritis, 707, 708
    bites, 716
    blood culture [test], 622, 626
    bone marrow culture [test], 634
    CNS infections, 770
    and endocarditis, 623, 626t
    environmental exposure, 659t
    infections, 624t
    lymphadenopathy, 715
    serology [test], 804, 805, 806
Brucella abortus, 806
Brucella melitensis, 806
Brucella suis, 806
Brucellosis. See *Brucella*
Brugia malayi, 632, 632t, 681t
BT (bleeding time) [test], 515t, 516t, 529–530
BTG (β-thromboglobulin) [test], 537
B2M. See β_2-Microglobulin
Buboes: and pneumonia, 660t
Buffer acid, 12–13
Buffers:
    open and closed systems, 12–13, 13t
    physiologic, 12, 13t, 13–14
Bulbar poliomyelitis, 771
Bullae: disease, etiology, and tests for, 678t–679t, 687, 688f, 692f
BUN (blood urea nitrogen) [test], 41–42
Bunyaviruses:
    blood culture [test], 628t
    CNS infections, 771, 772t, 776t
    skin manifestations, 677t
Burkitt's leukemia/lymphoma, Plate 21, 445, 564, 579, 603
    c-myc and, 328t
    EBV and, 817t
    phenotyping, 856f
    TdT testing, 607
Burkitt's lymphoma cells, Plate 21A/B, 441
Burns:
    cellulitis, 679t
    wound specimens [test], 716–717
Burr cells, 432
Burrowing ulcer, chronic, 679t
Burst forming unit–erythroid (BFU-E), 426f, 427
Buruli ulcer, 679t
Butabarbital [test], 385t, 385–386
Butalbital [test], 385–386
Butizide: hemolytic anemia from, 894t

Butorphanol: characteristics of, 389t
Bypass surgery: and CK isoform measures, 30

C

C1 inhibitor deficiency: complement assay, 849t
C1q, 846, 848t, 849t
    binding assay, 848, 850, 850t
C2, 848
C3, 846, 848, 848t
C3 proactivator (C3PA), 846
C4, 846, 848, 848t, 849t
C4b binding protein (C4b-BP), 549
C4d, 846, 848, 848t, 849t
C4d/C4 ratio, 846–847, 848, 848t, 849t
C5, 848
CA 15-3 [test], 316, 317, 328–329, 329t
CA 19-9 [test], 316, 319, 329, 329t, 330
CA 50 [test], 317, 329, 330
CA 72 [test], 317, 319–320, 329
CA 125 [test], 317, 329, 329t, 330
CA 195 [test], 318
CA 549 [test], 318, 328–329, 329t
Cabot rings, 432
Cachectin [test]: tumor marker, 325–326
Cacodylic acid [test], 390–392
Cadmium: toxic symptoms/concentrations, 391t
Cadmium [test], 390t, 390–392
Caffeine: therapeutic range, concentration, and distribution, 334t
Caffeine [test], 361
Calabar swellings, 650, 685
Calcitonin: and calcium regulation, 296t
Calcitonin [test], 302
    tumor marker, 307, 320–321
Calcium:
    calcitonin [test], 302
    hormone tests, 300–303
    ionized (free) [test], 297–298
    metabolism disorders, 296, 297t. See also Hypercalcemia; Hypocalcemia
    metabolism tests, 296–303
    osteocalcin [test], 302–303
    parathyroid hormone [test], 300–302, 301t
    and platelet plug formation, 500–501, 502f

regulation, 296t
total [test], 296–297
urine [test], 297–298
vitamin D and, 218
Calcium carbonate crystals: in urine, 52, 63f
Calcium channel blockers:
drug interactions, 355
platelet disorders induced by, 516t
Calcium infusion [test], 141
Calcium oxalate crystals: in urine, 51, 62f
Calcium phosphate crystals: in urine, 52, 62f
Calcium pyrophosphate dehydrate (CPPD) crystals: in synovial fluid, 119t, 123f
Calculi: cystine, 149
Calicivirus: gastroenteritis, 751t
California encephalitis virus, 771, 772t
CALLA. *See* Common acute lymphoblastic leukemia antigen (CD10)
Calymmatobacterium granulomatis:
genital ulcer, 734t, 740, 741
skin manifestations, 679t
cAMP [test], 58
Campylobacter:
gastroenteritis, 751t, 753, 754, 755, 756
rectal discharge, 734t, 744
Campylobacter cinaedi:
anorectal infection, 744, 745t
gastroenteritis, 751t
Campylobacter coli: diarrhea, 753
Campylobacter fennelliae:
anorectal infection, 744, 745t
gastroenteritis, 751t
Campylobacter fetus, 624t
Campylobacter hyointestinalis:
anorectal infection, 744
Campylobacter jejuni:
anorectal infection, 744, 745t
gastroenteritis, 751t, 753, 754, 755, 756
Campylobacter pylori. *See* *Helicobacter pylori*
Cancer. *See* Neoplasia *and specific types*
Cancer antigen. *See* CA
Candida:
and AIDS, 641–642, 860
antigenemia, 633
arthritis, 707–708
bone marrow culture [test], 634
and burns, 679t, 716
catheter infections, 633
CNS infections, 770
cultures, 697t, 698f
ear infection, 636
endocarditis, 623, 626t
esophageal infection, 748
fungemia, 623, 625
infections, 624t
keratitis, 648
morphologic characteristics, 671t
osteomyelitis, 710
pericarditis, 711
peritoneal infection, 701
pulmonary infection, 667–668, 669t
serology [test], 826t, 827t, 828
skin infections, 677t, 678t, 679t, 692, 693, 694, 698f, 699
throat infection, 641–642, 643, 646, 821
upper respiratory infections, 645t
urinary culture, 727–728
urinary tract infections, 722
vaginitis, 734t, 737, 738, 738t, 739
CAPD. *See* Continuous ambulatory peritoneal dialysis
Capillaria philippinensis, 761, 763t
Capillary blood: arterialized, 16
Capillary fragility (tourniquet) [test], 530
Captopril suppression: test for primary aldosteronism, 273t
Carbamazepine, 395
drug interactions, 341, 342, 344t
pharmacokinetic properties, 341t
side effects, 340
therapeutic range, concentration, and distribution, 334t
toxicity monitoring, 342t
Carbamazepine [tests], 340–341
unbound, 341–342
Carbamoyl-phosphate synthase deficiency, 78
Carbimazole: hemolytic anemia from, 894t
Carbohydrates, 127–142
dietary sources, 127
fasting and, 127
intolerance, 95–96, 96t
breath hydrogen test for, 95–96
malabsorption diseases, 96t
metabolism, 127, 128f
Carbohydrate [tests], 128–142
C-peptide, 140
diabetic control, 135–138
fasting glucose, 130–131
fructosamine, 137–138
glucose tolerance, 133–135
glycohemoglobin, 135–137
insulin, 138–140
insulin secretion provocation, 141–142
intravenous glucose tolerance, 135
1-hour postprandial glucose, 135
proinsulin, 140
random glucose, 128–130
routine, 128–132
2-hour postprandial glucose, 131–132
whole blood glucose, 132
Carbon dioxide:
equilibrium, 11
partial pressure of (pCO_2), 11–12, 14, 15, 16t, 16–25
transport, 14, 15f
Carbonic acid (H_2CO_3), 12
Carbonic anhydrase, 211
mechanism, 14–15
Carbon monoxide poisoning, 16
Carbon 14-triolein breath [test], 94
γ-Carboxyglutamic acid (GLA) [test], 302–303
Carboxylic acids: genetic screening, 417
Carboxy-terminal assay: parathyroid hormone, 300, 301t, 302
9-Carboxy THC, 387, 387t, 388
Carcinoembryonic antigen (CEA):
CSF, 114
pleural fluid [test], 116
as tumor marker [test], 315, 318f, 318–319, 319t, 328–329, 329t, 330
Carcinoid syndrome: niacin deficiency and, 224
Carcinoid tumors:
hormone marker, 321
tumor marker, 321
Carcinoplacental (Regan) isoenzyme, 73, 73t
Cardiac disease. *See* Heart disease
Cardiac failure. *See* Congestive heart failure
Cardiac glycosides [tests], 357–359
digitoxin, 358–359
digoxin, 357–358
Cardiac muscle disease, 713
Cardiac serum enzyme [tests], 25–36
creatine kinase, 25–27
creatine kinase isoenzymes, 27–29

Cardiac serum enzyme [tests] *(Continued)*
　　creatine kinase isoforms, 29–31
　　creatine phosphokinase, 25–27
　　creatine phosphokinase isoenzymes, 27–29
　　lactate dehydrogenase, 31–32
　　lactate dehydrogenase isoenzymes, 32–36
Cardiobacterium hominis, 624t, 626t
Cardiogreen, 82
Cardiopulmonary resuscitation, 16
Cardiovascular disorders: malabsorption and, 91t
Cardiovascular drugs:
　　antiarrhythmics, 348–357. *See also* Antiarrhythmics
　　glycosides, 357–359
Carnitine:
　　ascorbic acid and, 231
　　deficiency, 414–415
Carnitine [test]: genetic, 414–415
β-Carotene, 216, 217
β-Carotene [test], 97
Carotenoids [test], 97
Carrion's disease: direct examination of blood [test], 627
Cascade effect, 4
Casein: and breast cancer, 329t
Casoni test, 831
Casts: in urine, 50–51, 62f
Cat bites, 715–716
Catecholamine-producing tumors. *See* Pheochromocytoma
Catecholamines, 277–283
　　fractionation, 281
　　influences of, 279t
　　metabolism, 278f, 279f
　　and renin secretion, 270
　　synthesis, 278f
Catecholamines [tests]:
　　plasma, 281–282
　　urinary (free), 280–281
Catechol O-methyltransferase, 277, 281
Catheters:
　　intravascular culture [test], 633–634
　　urinary indwelling infections, 721, 722, 724, 726
Cat-scratch disease, 678t, 716
　　lymphadenopathy, 714
CBC [test], 457–462, 458f, 459f, 460t, 461t
CD1, 599t, 852t, 853t
CD2, 599t, 855
CD3, 599t, 841t, 852t, 853t, 855
CD4, 599t, 841, 841t, 851, 852t, 853t, 855, 856. *See also* T lymphocytes, helper
　　and AIDS, 860
CD4/CD8 ratio:
　　and AIDS, 860–861
　　therapy-associated changes, 861–862
CD5, 599t, 852t, 853t
CD7, 599t, 841t, 852t, 853t
CD8, 599t, 841, 841t, 851, 852t, 853t, 855, 856. *See also* T lymphocytes, suppressor
　　and AIDS, 860
CD10, 599t, 852t, 853t, 855
CD11, 599t, 852t
CD11b/Cd 18 glycoprotein [test], 597, 599t
CD14, 599t, 852t
CD15, 599t, 852t, 853t
CD16, 599t, 852t, 853t
CD19, 599t, 852t, 853t
CD20, 599t, 841t, 852t, 853t
CD21, 599t, 852t
CD22, 599t, 852t, 853t
CEA. *See* Carcinoembryonic antigen
Cefamandole: hemolytic anemia from, 894t
Cefazolin: hemolytic anemia from, 894t
Cefotaxime:
　　hemolytic anemia from, 894t
Ceftriaxone: hemolytic anemia from, 894t
Celiac disease: and testosterone levels, 289
Cell cluster of differentiation (CD), 599t, 840, 841t. *See also* CD
Cell count:
　　pleural fluid [test], 114–115, 115t
　　synovial fluid [test], 117t, 117–118
Cellophane tape swab, 761, 765
Cells: in cerebrospinal fluid, 108, 108t
Cell surface antigens [test], 598–603
Cell surface markers [test], 598–603
Cellular immunology, 851–862. *See also* T lymphocytes
　　AIDS, 860–861, 861t. *See also* Acquired immunodeficiency syndrome
　　background, 851–852
　　blast transformation, 854–855
　　humoral defects, 857–858
　　immunodeficiency, 856–857
　　immunodeficiency associated with other defects, 859, 859t
　　immunoregulatory abnormalities, 861
　　lymphoproliferative disorders, 855–856, 856f, 857f
　　monoclonal antibodies and antigen cluster designation, 852t
　　primary immunodeficiency states, 857, 858t, 859t
　　reagents, 854
　　specimen requirements, 852–854
　　surface immunoglobulin staining, 854
　　T-cell defects, 858–859, 859t
　　test selection, 852, 853t
　　therapy-associated changes in lymphocyte subpopulations, 861–862
Cellulitis:
　　clostridial, 680t
　　disease, etiology, and tests for, 679t–680t, 688f, 694t
　　facial, 680t
　　orbital, 635, 639–640, 651
　　wound, 687
Cellulose acetate: for high resolution serum protein electrophoresis, 159
Central nervous system, 769–786
　　fluid. *See* Cerebrospinal fluid
　　infections, 769–786
　　　diferential diagnosis, 781t
　　myelin [test], 113t, 113–114
Central nervous system [tests], 769–786
　　brain abscess and other specimens, 783–785
　　cerebrospinal fluid, 108–114, 769–783. *See also* Cerebrospinal fluid
Cephalexin: hemolytic anemia from, 894t
Cephaloridine: hemolytic anemia from, 894t
Cephalosporins: bacterial susceptibility testing, 794t
Cephalosporium: keratitis, 648
Cephalothin, 789
　　bacterial susceptibility testing, 794t
　　hemolytic anemia from, 894t
CER. *See* Ceruloplasmin
c-erb B2 (HER-2/neu) oncogene, 327, 328, 328t
Cercariae, 761
Cerebrospinal fluid (CSF), 107. *See also* Serodiagnosis of infectious disease
　　β_2-microglobulin (B2M), 114
　　causes of increased leukocytes in, 108t

characteristics of normal, 107, 108t
glutamine levels, 80, 111
immunofixation for monoclonal proteins in, 162
isolates, 794t
total volume, 107, 108t
Cerebrospinal fluid (CSF) [tests], 108–114, 769–783
basic, 108
C-reactive protein, 785
culture, 769–783
electrophoresis, 112–113, 113f
glucose, 108–109
glutamine, 111
lactate, 109–111, 110t, 785
lactate dehydrogenase, 111
Limulus lysate, 785
myelin basic protein (MBP), 113t, 113–114
protein, 109
Ceruloplasmin, 202, 203
abnormalities, 200t
and breast cancer, 329t
conditions and disorders affecting ranges of, 156t, 161
and Wilson's disease, 204, 205, 207f, 208, 208t, 209
Ceruloplasmin [test], 169–170
copper and, 205
genetic disorders, 415–416
and liver function, 82
Cervical cancer: tumor marker, 310
Cervical examination [test], 739–740
Cervicitis:
mucopurulent, 740
pathogens, 734t
Cestodes. *See also specific cestodes*
gastrointestinal, 747, 761–762, 763t, 766
pulmonary infections, 672, 672t, 674
Cetromere, 845t
CF. *See* Complement fixation
CF. *See* Cystic fibrosis
CFU. *See* Colony forming unit
CH$_{50}$, 846, 847, 848, 848t, 849t
Chagas disease, 631, 677t, 713. *See also Trypanosoma cruzi*
serology [test], 830t, 832–833
Chancre, syphilitic, 679t, 740–743
Chancroid, 715, 740–743
Charcot-Leyden crystals, 435
Charcot's arthritis, 707
Chédiak-Higashi granules, Plate 12, 436
Chédiak-Higashi syndrome, 436, 514t, 555, 560t, 589, 597

Chelation therapy: for metal toxicity, 392
Chemotaxis, functional assays for [test], 597
Chenodeoxycholic acid, 81
Chest x-ray, 660–661
Chickenpox. *See also* Varicella-zoster virus
lesions and test, 678t, 684
serology [test], 824–825
Chigger bites, 677t
Chilomastix mesnili, 760t
Chlamydia: serology, 814
Chlamydia pneumoniae (TWAR agent):
respiratory infection, 669t
serology, 814
throat infection, 641
Chlamydia psittaci:
pericarditis, 711
respiratory infection, 666, 669t
serology, 814
skin manifestations, 678t
Chlamydia trachomatis:
anorectal infection, 744
cervicitis, 734t, 739–740
ear infection, 637, 638
and endocarditis, 626t
eye infection, 648, 650, 652, 653
pelvic infection, 701
pneumonia, 646–647, 658, 662t, 662–663, 666, 668, 669t
rectal discharge, 734t
serology, 814
skin manifestations, 679t
upper respiratory infections, 645t
urethritis, 734, 734t, 735–737, 736t
urinary tract infections, 722
Chloramphenicol:
drug interactions, 344t, 360, 361, 366
monitoring [test], 799
susceptibility testing, 794t
therapeutic range, concentration, and distribution, 334t
Chloramphenicol hemisuccinate, 333
Chlordiazepoxide: half-life and therapeutic/toxic concentrations, 384t
Chloride: reference ranges for, 47t
Chloride shift, 14
Chloride [test], 47
sweat, 98, 418–419
Chloridorrheas, 47
Chloroacetate esterase [test], 605–606
4-Chloronaphthol, 604
Chlorpromazine:

hemolytic anemia from, 894t
testing for, 394, 394t
Chlorpropamide:
hemolytic anemia from, 894t
toxicity, 138
Chlorzepate: half-life and therapeutic/toxic concentrations, 384t
Cholangiocarcinoma, 762
Cholecalciferol, 217–218. *See also* Vitamin D
Cholecystokinin (CKK), 92, 94
Choledocholithiasis, 72, 77
Cholera. *See also Vibrio cholerae*
pancreatic, 102
Cholestasis, 69, 76, 77, 81
alkaline phosphatase and, 72, 77
and α-bilirubin, 75
classification of, 68t
drug-induced, 77
extrahepatic, 77
GGT and, 79
intrahepatic, 77
Cholesteatoma, 637
Cholesterol, 173–174
and adrenal hormones, 257, 258f
age- and sex-related reference ranges for, 178t
casts in urine, 51
crystals in synovial fluid, 119t, 124f
and estrogen, 292f
and flow chart for evaluation of hyperlipoproteinemias, 186f–187f
and HDLs, 185
and hyperlipoproteinemias, 183t
and hypolipoproteinemias, 184t
and LDLs, 189–190, 191t
Multiple Risk Factor Intervention Trial (MRFIT), 176
National Cholesterol Education Program (NCEP), 176
properties of, 174t
reference ranges for HDL, 188t
structure of, 174f
and testosterone, 287, 287f
total, and low density lipoproteins, 177, 178t
and triglycerides, 177
and VLDLs, 192
Cholesterol [test], 173–178, 174f–176f, 178t, 179t
Cholic: and liver function, 81
Chorioamnionitis: C-reactive protein and, 170
Choriocarcinoma: tumor markers, 315, 315t, 322, 324
Chorionic villus sampling, 412–413

Chorioretinitis, 649, 649t, 653–654
Christmas factor: and vitamin K, 221
Christmas factor. *See* Factor IX
Chromate deficiency, 201
Chromatography:
    for amino acids, 145, 147
    for CK isoenzymes, 27, 29
    gas. *See* Gas chromatography
    high performance liquid (HPLC).
        See High performance
        liquid chromatography
    thin-layer. *See* Thin-layer chromatography
Chromium, 199
    abnormalities, 200t
    body content, 199t
    deficiency, 201
    excretion route, 200t
Chromium [test], 201–202
Chromium 51 RBC survival studies, 484
Chromomycrosis, 681t
Chromosome 14, 579, 580
Chronic burrowing ulcer, 679t
Chronic disease: respiratory disorders and, 657
Chronic obstructive airways disease: drugs for, 361–363
CH50 test, 168
CH100 test, 168
Chylomicrons, 173, 174
    apolipoproteins and, 191
    causes of secondary increases of, 192t
    increased abnormality characteristics, 183t
    properties of, 174t
    and triglycerides, 179
Chylomicrons [test], 191–192
Chymotrypsin, 89, 92, 93
Cianidanol: hemolytic anemia from, 894t
CIE. *See* Counterimmunoelectrophoresis
Cimetidine: drug interactions, 351, 352, 355, 357, 361, 363
Cimetidine [test], 363
Cimex lectularius, 677t
Circulating granulocyte pool (CGP), 435
Circulating immune complexes [test], 848, 850
Circulating monocyte pool (CMP), 437
Circulating platelet aggregates [test], 536
Cirrhosis, 75, 77, 81
    acid phosphatase and, 312t
    alkaline phosphatase and, 72

    aminoaciduria in, 148
    biliary autoantibody, 845t
    cancer antigen (CA) 125 and, 317
    CEA elevation in, 319t
    classification of, 68t
    end-stage, 75, 78
    immunoglobulin responses, 157t
    Indian childhood, 206, 206t, 208t
    leucine crystals and, 52
    and pleural fluid, 115t, 116
    primary biliary, differential diagnosis, 208t
    and protein tests, 155, 158, 165
    and theophylline clearance, 335t
Cisplatin: hemolytic anemia from, 894t
Citrobacter diversus. *See also* Enterobacteriaceae
    CNS infections, 770
Citrobacter freundii. *See* Enterobacteriaceae
Citrulline:
    biochemistry and reference range, 145t
    genetic screening, 414
Citrullinemia: enzymatic defect and features of, 146t
CCK (cholecystokinin), 92, 94
CK (creatine kinase) [test], 25–27
    isoenzymes, 27–29
CK-BB isoenzyme, 26, 27, 27t, 28t, 29
    tumor marker, 310–311
CK-MB isoenzyme, 26, 26f, 27, 27t, 28f, 28t, 28–29, 34f–35f
    isoforms, 28f, 29, 30, 31
    tumor marker, 310–311
CK-MM isoenzyme, 26, 27, 27t, 28, 28f, 28t, 29–31, 30t
    isoforms, 28f, 29–31
c-K-*ras*: and colon cancer, 328t
Clindamycin phosphate, 333
CLL. *See* Lymphocytic leukemia, chronic
Clomiphene testing, 286, 294
Clonazepam:
    half-life and toxic concentrations, 384t
    therapeutic range, concentration, and distribution, 334t, 384t
Clonidine suppression test, 281, 282
Clonorchis sinensis, 702t, 702–703, 762, 762t, 763t
Clostridium:
    infections, 624t
    peritoneal infection, 701
    traumatic wounds, 718

Clostridium botulinum: gastroenteritis, 751t, 753, 756
Clostridium difficile:
    diarrhea, 753, 754, 756–757
    serology, 805
    toxin detection [test], 756–758
Clostridium perfringens:
    cultures, 697t, 700f
    gas gangrene, 713
    gastroenteritis, 751t, 753
    infections, 624t
    pelvic infection, 701
    skin manifestations, 680t, 682
Clostridium septicum: infections, 624t
Clot retraction [test], 536
Clottable fibrinogen [test], 523f, 541
Cluster of differentiation (CD), 840, 841t, 852t, 853t, 854. *See also* CD
CML. *See* Myelocytic leukemia, chronic
CMV. *See* Cytomegalovirus
c-*myc*, 328t
Co. *See* Cobalt
CoA. *See* Acetyl coenzyme A
Coagulation:
    extrinsic pathway, 502
    final common pathway, 504
    intrinsic pathway, 502, 504–505, 505f
Coagulation factors. *See also individual factors*
    functional classification, 505t
    transfusions, 887–888
    and vitamin K, 221
Coagulation factor [tests], 537–542
    clottable fibrinogen, 523f, 541
    factor antigen concentration, 541
    factors II, V, VII, and X, 516t, 523t, 538f, 540
    factor VIII procoagulant, 513t, 517f, 531t, 537–539, 538f
    factor IX procoagulant activity, 539
    factor XI, 540
    factor XII, 540
    factor XIII screen, 507f, 519t, 542
    fibrinogen antigen, 517f, 541–542
    high molecular weight kininogen, 540
    prekallikrein, 540
    prekallikrein activity screen (Fletcher factor assay), 506f, 540
Cobalamin, 227–229. *See also* Vitamin B$_{12}$
    cobalt and, 199, 202
    deficiency, 200t, 471

Cobalamin [test], 471–472, 472t, 473t
Cobalophilins, 227
Cobalt:
    abnormalities, 200t
    body content, 199t
    excretion route, 200t
Cobalt [test], 202
Cocaine:
    and emergency room, 370t
    metabolism, 372
    testing for, 386–387, 387t, 388t
Coccidioides immitis:
    arthritis, 707–708
    bone marrow culture [test], 634
    CNS infections, 770
    environmental exposure, 659t
    eye infections, 648–649
    lymphadenopathy, 714
    morphologic characteristics, 671t
    pericarditis, 712
    pneumonia, 658, 659t
    respiratory infections, 659t, 669t
    serology [test], 826t, 827t, 828
    skin/tissue manifestations, 681t
    urinary tract infection, 727, 728
Codeine:
    characteristics of, 389t
    and emergency room, 370t
Codocytes, 434
Coefficient of variation, 6
Coenzyme R. *See* Biotin
Cold agglutinin syndrome, 889t, 891, 892–893
Cold agglutinin test: for *Mycoplasma*, 814–815
Colipase, 89
Colitis, 744
    antimicrobial-associated (AAC), 744
    pseudomembranous, 754
Collagen vascular disease:
    CEA elevation in, 319t
    and pleural fluid, 115t
Colon cancer:
    and c-K-*ras*, 328t
    tumor markers, 315, 318, 319, 320, 323
Colony forming unit–basophil (CFU-Bas), 426f, 434
Colony forming unit–eosinophil (CFU-Eo), 426f, 434
Colony forming unit–erythroid (CFU-E), 426f, 427
Colony forming unit–granulocyte, erythroid, macrophage, megakaryocyte (CFU-GEMM), 426f, 427, 434, 437, 441
Colony forming unit–granulocyte, monocyte (CFU-GM), 426f, 434, 437
Colony forming unit–lymphoid (CFU-L), 426f, 438
Colony forming unit–megakaryocyte (CFU-Meg), 426f, 441
Colony forming unit–monocyte/-macrophage (CFU-M), 426f, 437
Colony forming unit–neutrophil, monocyte (CFU-NM), 426f, 434, 437
Colony forming unit–neutrophil (CFU-N), 426f, 434
Colony forming unit–spleen (CFU-S), 425, 426f, 427, 434, 437, 438
Colony inhibitory activities (factors) (CIAs; CIFs), 435
Colony stimulating activities (factors) (CSAs; CSFs), 435, 437
Colorado tick fever encephalitis, 772t, 774
Colorectal cancer: tumor markers, 319, 320
Color tests: for amino acids, 147
Combined immunodeficiencies, 858, 859t
    testing for, 840, 841, 857
Common acute lymphoblastic (lymphocytic) leukemia antigen (CALLA) (CD10), 564, 852, 852t, 853t
Common cold, 641
Common variable immunodeficiency (CVID), 858
Complement: total [test], 846–848, 847f, 848t
Complement 3: conditions and disorders affecting ranges of, 156t, 167–168
Complement 4: conditions and disorders affecting ranges of, 156t, 167–168
Complement activation [test], 846–848, 847f, 848t, 849t
Complement by CH$_{50}$, 846
Complement fixation [test], 805. *See also* Serodiagnosis of infectious disease
    for adenovirus, 823
    for blastomycosis, 827, 827t
    for coccidioidomycosis, 828
    for fungi, 825, 825t, 827t
    for histoplasmosis, 827t, 829
    for influenza virus, 823
    for *Mycoplasma*, 814–815
    for paragonimiasis, 830t, 831
    for *Rickettsia*, 811, 812t
    for VZV, 825
Complement pathways:
    alternative, 167, 846–848, 847f, 849t
    classical, 167, 846–848, 847f, 849t
Complement proteins [test], 167–168
Complement split products [test], 846–848, 847f, 848t
Complete blood count (CBC) [test], 457–462, 458f, 459f, 460t, 461t
Compound F [test], 262, 263t
Computed tomography:
    and aldosterone testing, 274t, 275
    and lower respiratory infections, 661
ConA. *See* Concanavalin A
Concanavalin, 315
Concanavalin A (ConA), 853t, 855
Concentration of analyte, 5, 6
Congenital dyserythropoietic anemia (CDA), type II, 476, 477, 482
Congenital erythropoietic porphyria, 57
Congenital erythropoietic protoporphyria, 57
Congenital hemolytic anemia, 477
Congenital photosensitive porphyria, 57
Congestive heart failure:
    and drug distribution volume, 335
    drugs for, 357–359
    LD and, 32, 36, 79f, 79t
    and pleural fluid, 115t, 116
Congo-Crimean hemorrhagic fever, 771, 772t
Conjugate base, 12
Conjunctivitis, 635, 641, 648, 650–651
    adult inclusion, 648, 652
    bilateral follicular, 648, 650
    neonatal, 648
Connective tissue disease, mixed: autoantibody, 845t
Constitutional porphyria, 57
Contact lense infection, 648, 649–650
Container, specimen, 5–6
Contaminants:
    blood culture and, 621t, 623t
    susceptibility testing and, 789
Continuous ambulatory peritoneal dialysis (CAPD): and peritonitis, 701, 703, 705–706

Anticonvulsants:
    benzodiazepine, 384t
    drug interactions, 341t, 352, 356.
        See also specific anticonvulsants
    pharmacokinetic properties, 341t
Anticonvulsants [tests], 340–348
    carbamazepine, 340–342
    ethosuximide, 342–343
    phenobarbital, 343–344
    phenytoin, 344–346
    primadone, 346
    valproic acid, 347–348
Anti-D antigen testing, 873–874
Antidepressants: drug interactions, 341
Antidepressants [tests], 359–361
    desipramine, 359
    imipramine, 359
    lithium, 360
    nortriptyline, 360–361
Antidiuretic hormone (ADH), 237, 257
    and renin secretion, 270
Antidiuretic hormone (ADH) [test], 294–295
    tumor marker, 320
Antidiuretic hormone, syndrome of inappropriate (SIADH), 46, 294–295
    albumin levels and, 152
    disorders associated with, 295t
    water loading test, 295
Anti-DNAse B [test], 808–809
Antifreeze, 378–379
Antigen detection (bacterial):
    CSF test, 775, 780
    urine [test], 725–726
Antigenemia [test], 632–633
Antigen markers: WBC, 599t
Antigens:
    binding, 838
    granulocyte-specific, 887
    HLA, 166–167, 884
    HPA, 166–167, 884
    platelet, 884, 884t
Antigenuria, 726
Antiglobulin test:
    for alloantibody detection, 876, 878t
    direct vs. indirect, 891–892
    for hemolytic anemia, 890, 890t
Antihemolytic factor (AHF), cryoprecipitated, transfusion, 869t, 877–878
Antihemophilic factor, 538. See also Factor VIII
Antihistamines, 363

platelet disorders induced by, 516t
Anti-HLA-Dr, 853t
Anti-hyalurodinase [test], 808–809
Anti-inflammatories: platelet disorders induced by, 514, 516t
Antimicrobial-associated colitis (AAC), 744
Antimicrobial testing [test], 791t, 791–793
Antimicrobial therapy [tests], 787–801. See also Drugs
    therapeutic monitoring, 797–800
    in vitro susceptibility, 789–795
Antimitochondrial antibodies [test], 81
Antineuritic vitamin. See Thiamin
Anti-O agglutinin [test], 809
Anti-oncogenes, 328
α_2-Antiplasmin, 509, 511f, 512f, 525
    deficiency, 519, 550
α_2-Antiplasmin [test], 512f, 519t, 550
Antiscorbutic vitamin. See Vitamin C
Anti-smooth muscle antibodies [test], 81
Anti-streptolysin O (ASO) [test], 808–809
Anti-teichoic acid antibody [test], 808
Antithrombin III, 506–507, 508f, 521, 545
    activity [test], 508f, 520t, 546–548
    antigen [test], 548
    deficiency, 547, 548, 887
Antithymocyte globulin therapy, 862
α_1-Antitrypsin, 89
    conditions and disorders affecting ranges of, 156t
α_1-Antitrypsin deficiency, 166
    immunoglobulin responses, 157t
α_1-Antitrypsin [test], 165–166
    genetic disorders, 413–414
Anti-Vi agglutinin [test], 809
Anxiolytics: benzodiazepine, 384t
AP. See Alkaline phosphatase
APG. See Glomerulonephritis, acute progressive
Aplastic anemia, 451t, 476
    vitamin B_{12} and, 228, 228t
Apnea: drugs for, 361–363
Apoferritin, 466
Apolipoproteins, 151
    A, 174t, 185, 189, 191, 192, 193, 194, 194t, 195t
    B, 189, 191, 193, 194t, 194–195, 195t
    B-48, 174, 174t, 192, 194, 195

B-100, 174t, 175, 192, 194, 195
C, 174t, 185, 191, 192, 193, 194, 194t, 195
and chylomicrons, 191
D, 192, 194t
E, 174, 174t, 185, 192, 193, 194t, 195
G, 195
H, 195
and HDLs, 185
and hyperlipoproteinemias, 183t
and hypolipoproteinemias, 184t
Lp(a), 193
properties of, 174t
reference ranges of, 194t, 195t
V, 193
Apolipoproteins [test], 174t, 183t, 184t, 193–195, 194t, 195t
Apoprotein III, 502
Apoproteins. See Apolipoproteins
APTT. See Activated partial prothrombin time
APUD cells, 101, 321
Apudomas, 101
Arachidonic acid, 181, 182t, 502f
Arachnia propionica, 680t
Arboviruses. See also specific arboviruses
    CNS infection, 776, 776t
    group B, skin manifestations, 677t
    serology [test], 815
    urinary, 730t
Area under the concentration (AUC) time curve for drugs, 337, 338
Arenaviruses:
    CNS infections, 771, 772t
    serology [test], 817
    skin manifestations, 677t
Arginase, 209
Arginine, 143
    biochemistry and reference range, 144t
    and cystinuria, 148
Arginine-asparagine-serine sequence, 506f
Arginine infusion [test], 243
Arginine vasopressin. See Antidiuretic hormone
Argininosuccinate synthetase defect, 146t
Argininosuccinic acid: genetic screening, 414
Argininosuccinic aciduria: enzymatic defect and features of, 146t
Argyll Robertson pupil, 810
Aromatic carbon chains, 143

Continuous scale, 8, 9f
Contraceptives, oral. *See* Oral contraceptives
Control sample, 6
Co-oximeter, 23
Copper, 199
    abnormalities, 200t
    body content, 199t
    ceruloplasmin and, 169
    deficiency, 203t, 203–204, 205
    excess, 203t, 204, 205
    excretion route, 200t
    liver concentrations, 82
    metabolism abnormalities, 203t, 203–204
    toxicity, 204
Copper [tests], 202–209
    ceruloplasmin, 205, 208t
    free (dialysable), 206–209
    genetic disorders, 415–416
    liver, 206, 208t
    radioactive studies, 206, 208, 208t
    serum/urine, 202–205, 208t
    Wilson's disease diagnosis, 206–209, 207f, 208t
Coproporphyria, 58, 418t
Coproporphyrin, 55, 56t, 58, 58t, 418
Coproporphyrinogen oxidase deficiency, 56t
Cori-Forbes disease, 420, 421, 421t, 422
Corneal infections, 635, 648, 651
Corneal scrapings, 651, 652, 653
Coronary heart disease. *See also* Heart disease
    and apolipoproteins, 194–195, 195t
    and cholesterol levels, 175–177, 178t
    HDLs and, 185
    and LDLs, 189–190
    Multiple Risk Factor Intervention Trial, 176
    risk factors for, 178t
Coronavirus:
    gastroenteritis, 751t
    infection frequency, 636t
    throat infection, 641
    upper respiratory infections, 636t
Cor pulmonale: and theophylline clearance, 335t
Corpus luteum, 284f, 285
Corticoids, urinary free [test], 262–264
Corticosteroid-binding globulin (CBG), 262, 263
Corticosteroid crystals: in synovial fluid, 119t

Corticosteroids: drug interactions, 341
Corticosterone, 258f, 269, 270
Corticotropin. *See* Adrenocorticotropic hormone
Corticotropin [test], 264–266, 265f
    tumor marker, 321
Corticotropin releasing factor (CRF) stimulation [test], 264, 266, 269f
Corticotropin releasing hormone (CRH), 257, 326
Corticotropin releasing hormone (CRH) stimulation [test], 264, 266, 269f
Cortisol, 257, 258f, 268, 270
    insulin tolerance test for, 243
Cortisol [test], 262, 263t
    urinary-free, 262–264
Cortrosyn [test], 259–261
Corynebacterium:
    CNS infections, 770
    infections, 624t, 626t
    urinary, 724
Corynebacterium diphtheriae:
    eye infections, 648
    infections, 624t
    skin manifestations, 679t
    throat infection, 642, 644, 645t, 646
    upper respiratory infections, 645t
Corynebacterium haemolyticum:
    skin manifestations, 679t
    throat infection, 641, 642, 644, 645t, 646
    upper respiratory infections, 645t
Corynebacterium jeikeium (JK):
    blood, 624t
    cultures, 696t
    infections, 624t, 699
    skin, 696t
Corynebacterium minutissimum: skin manifestations, 677t
Corynebacterium pyogenes:
    skin manifestations, 679t
    wounds, 680t
Corynebacterium tuberculosis, 680t
Coryneform bacteria: skin manifestations, 678t
Cosyntropin, 259
Coulter S-Plus series, 590, 593, 596f
Counterimmunoelectrophoresis (CIE):
    autoantibody, 845t
    CNS infection, 780
    for fungi, 825, 825t
Cowpox, 684
Coxiella burnetti. *See also* Q fever

    and endocarditis, 623, 626t
    pericarditis, 711
    pneumonia, 658, 669t
    serology [test], 811, 812t
Coxsackie viruses:
    arthritis, 707
    CNS infection, 771, 776, 776t
    eye infection, 648, 649t
    pericarditis, 711
    serology, 816
    skin manifestations, 677t
    stool culture/rectal swab, 759t
    throat infection, 641
    upper respiratory infections, 636t
C-peptide, 138, 139
    clinical indications for measurement of, 140t
C-peptide [test], 140, 140t
C-peptide-glucagon [test], 142
C-peptide suppression [test], 141–142
CPK. *See* Creatine kinase (CK)
CPK (creatine phosphokinase) [test], 25–27
CPK (creatine phosphokinase) isoenzymes [test], 27–29
CPPD (calcium pyrophosphate dehydrate) crystals: in synovial fluid, 119t, 123f
Cr. *See* Chromium
Crab lice, 677t, 745
Crab lice [test], 745
Crack: testing for, 387, 388
Cr3bi receptor complement receptor [test], 597
CR3 deficiency, 560t
C-reactive protein (CRP), 158, 160
C-reactive protein (CRP) [test], 170, 775, 785
Creatine [test], 61
Creatine kinase (CK), 29–31, 61, 70
    BB isoenzyme, 26, 27, 27t, 28t, 29, 310–311
    concentration in tissues, 28t
    isoenzyme time course in myocardial infarction, 33f–35f
    macro, 27, 310–311
    MB isoenzyme, 26, 26f, 27, 27t, 28f, 28t, 28–29, 34f–35f, 310–311
    MM isoenzyme, 26, 27, 27t, 28, 28f, 28t, 29–31, 30t
    as prostatic tumor marker, 313t
Creatine kinase (CK) [test], 25–27
    tumor marker, 310–311, 311f
Creatine kinase isoenzymes (CK isoenzymes) [test], 27–29
Creatine kinase isoforms [test], 29–31

Creatine phosphate, 61
Creatine phosphokinase (CPK) [test], 25–27
Creatine phosphokinase isoenzymes (CPK isoenzymes) [test], 27–29
Creatinine:
　amidohydrolase, 43
　calcium ratio to, 298
　clearance equation, 336t
　clearance of, 43–44, 44t
　deaminase, 43
Creatinine [test], 42–44
Creeping eruptions, 677t, 685
Crenated RBCs, 432
CREST syndrome autoantibody, 845t
Creutzfeldt-Jakob disease, 771t, 772t, 774, 777, 777t, 785
CRH. See Corticotropin releasing hormone
Crigler-Najjar syndrome, 75
Crimean-Congo hemorrhagic fever, 771, 772t
^{51}Cr-Labeled red blood cell volume [test], 496–497
Crohn's disease:
　CEA elevation in, 319t
　protein levels, 170
　zinc deficiency and, 211
Crossed immunoelectrophoresis of VWF [test], 533–534, 534f
Crossmatch:
　for blood transfusion, 874
　for platelet transfusion, 885–886
Croup, 635, 643t, 646
CRP. See C-reactive protein
Crusts: disease, etiology, and tests for, 678t–679t, 686, 687f
Cryoglobulinemia: complement test and, 168
Cryoglobulins [test], 170
Cryoprecipitated antihemolytic factor (AHF): transfusion, 869t, 877–878
Cryptococcosis. See Cryptococcus neoformans
Cryptococcus neoformans:
　antigen testing, 776, 780, 781
　bone marrow aspiration for, 610
　bone marrow culture [test], 634
　CNS infections, 770, 776, 779, 780, 781
　cultures, 697t
　eye infections, 648
　infections, 624t
　morphologic features, 671t
　osteomyelitis, 710
　pulmonary infections, 667, 669t
　serology [test], 826t, 827t, 828–829
　skin manifestations, 680t, 682
　urinary culture, 727, 728
Cryptorchidism, 288, 289, 290t
Cryptosporidiosis. See Cryptosporidium
Cryptosporidium:
　and AIDS, 860
　gastroenteritis, 751t, 753, 759, 760, 760t, 764–765, 766
　pulmonary infection, 672, 672t, 673
Crystals:
　in synovial fluid, 118, 119t, 120f–124f
　in urine, 51–52, 62f–63f
CSF. See Cerebrospinal fluid
CSF lactate [test], 785
CSF Limulus lysate [test], 785
CT. See Calcitonin
^{14}C-triolein breath [test], 94
Cullen's sign, 85, 86t
Cunninghamella, 668, 671t
Curariform drugs: interactions, 353
Curvularia keratitis, 648
Cushing's disease, 261, 261t, 265, 268, 291. See also Cushing syndrome
　DHEA-S levels, 291
Cushing syndrome, 46, 128, 261–262, 290, 326
　and ACTH as tumor marker, 321
　DHEA-S levels, 291
　differential diagnosis, 261t, 263t, 266
　laboratory evaluation of, 269f
Cushing syndrome [tests], 262–268
　corticotropin, 264–266, 265f
　corticotropin releasing hormone stimulation, 266, 326
　cortisol, urinary-free, 262–264, 264t
　cortisol (compound F), 262, 263t
　dexamethasone suppression test, 266–268
　overnight screening, 267
Cutaneous infections. See Skin infections
Cutaneous larva currens, 686
Cutaneous larva migrans, 677t, 686
Cutaneous leishmaniasis: serology, 831
Cutaneous T-cell lymphoma: morphology/manifestations/markers, 574t
Cutoff point, 8, 9

Cyanide-nitroprusside test, 147
　screening, 52
Cyanocobalamin, 471
Cyanocobalamin [test], 227–229. See also Vitamin B$_{12}$
Cyclic adenosine monophosphate (cAMP):
　lithium and, 360
　nephrogenous, 325
　parathyroid hormone-like peptide and, 325
　and platelet plug formation, 501, 502f
Cyclic adenosine monophosphate (cAMP) [test], 58
Cyclic AMP dependent kinase deficiency, 421t
Cyclic AMP [test], 58
Cyclobenzaprine, 395
Cyclo-oxygenase deficiency, 514t
Cyclosporin A. See Cyclosporine
Cyclosporine:
　immunologic effects, 861–862
　therapeutic range, concentration, and distribution, 334t
　toxicity, 364
Cyclosporine [test], 364
Cylindruria, 50
Cystathione β-synthetase deficiency, 149
Cystathioninuria, primary: and vitamin B$_6$, 227t
Cysteine: biochemistry and reference range, 145t
Cysticercosis, 649, 650, 651, 703, 705, 713, 714, 766, 777t, 783, 784. See also Taenia solium
　pulmonary, 673–674
　serology [test], 830, 830t
Cystic fibrosis, 655
　vitamin B$_{12}$ malabsorption and, 96
Cystic fibrosis [tests], 98–99, 411
　restriction fragment length polymorphism, 98–99
　sweat chloride, 98, 418–419
Cystine:
　biochemistry and reference range, 145t
　crystals in urine, 52, 63f
　reductase defect, 146t
Cystinosis: enzymatic defect and features of, 146t
Cystinuria, 148–149, 414
　features of, 146t
Cystitis, 722, 726
　differential diagnosis, 727t
　hemorrhagic, 729
　tests. See Urine [tests]

Cytarabine: drug interactions, 366
Cytochemical tests, 598–610
Cytochrome oxidase, 202
Cytochrome P$_{450}$:
    and acetaminophen, 382
    and alcohol metabolism, 375
Cytokeratins, 602
Cytology:
    ascitic fluid, 116
    pleural fluid [test], 116
Cytomegalovirus, 619
    and AIDS, 729, 860
    blood culture [test], 628, 628t
    chorioretinitis, 649, 649t
    CNS infection, 771, 772t, 773, 776, 776t, 777t
    ear infection, 637
    hepatitis, 702t, 820
    immunology, 861
    mononucleosis, 816
    respiratory infection, 658, 664, 666, 669t
    serology [test], 804, 815–816
    stool culture/rectal swab, 758, 759t
    throat infection, 641, 642
    upper respiratory infections, 636t
    urinary tract infection, 729, 730t, 732
Cytoplasmic granules, 441
Cytoplasmic inclusion disease (CID), 773
Cytotoxic drugs: immunologic effects, 861–862

D

Dacrocytes, 434
DAG (diacylglycerol), 500, 502f
D antigen, 873–874
Dark field microscopy: for syphilis, 741, 742, 743
D-dimer [test], 545–546, 546f–547f
Dead space ventilation, 11
1-Deamino-8-arginine vasopressin (DDAVP), 531
Decision matrix in diagnosis, 3f
Decubitus ulcer, 679t
Degenerative joint disease: synovial fluid examination, 117t
Degranulation, functional assays for [test], 597
Dehydration:
    hyperproteinemia and, 153
    and polycythemia, 456t
    protein levels and, 156t
Dehydration [test], 295–296, 296t
Dehydroascorbic acid (DHAA), 231, 232

Dehydroepiandrosterone (DHEA), 258f, 268, 278f, 292f, 408f
Dehydroepiandrosterone sulfate (DHEA-S) [test], 290, 291t, 291–292
3-Dehydroretinol, 216. *See also* Vitamin A
δ-Granules, 441
Delta OD (optional density) [test], 404–405
Delta osmolality (D-Osm) [test], 376, 376f, 376t, 379t, 379–380
Demoxepam: half-life and therapeutic/toxic concentrations, 384t
Dengue fever virus, 649t, 677t
    hepatitis, 702t
Deoxycholic acid, 81
11-Deoxycortisol, 258f
Deoxyhemoglobin, 12, 14, 23
Deoxyuridilate, 473
Deoxyuridine suppression [test], 476
Depression:
    dexamethasone suppression test for, 267–268
    drugs for, 359–361
    MHPG test for, 283
Dermacentor andersoni, 774
Dermal ulcer, 679t
Dermatomyositis, 861
Dermatophytes:
    cultures, 697t
    skin manifestations, 679t
Desalkylflurazepam: half-life and therapeutic/toxic concentrations, 384t
Desipramine, 360
    therapeutic range, concentration, and distribution, 334t, 396t
    toxicities, 396t
Desipramine [test], 359
Desmethyldiazepam: half-life and therapeutic/toxic concentrations, 384t
20,22-Desmolase:
    deficiency, 270, 271t
    and estrogen, 292
    and testosterone, 287f
Desoxycorticosterone, 257, 258f
    and hypertension, 276t
Desoxycorticosterone [test], 270, 271t
11-Desoxycortisol, 262, 268, 269, 275
11-Desoxycortisol [test], 270, 271t
Dexamethasone suppression [test], 263–264, 264t, 266–268, 269f, 321

    for depression, 267–268
    high dose, 267
    low dose, 267
Dextromethorpan: characteristics of, 389t
DF-2:
    bites, 679t, 715, 716
    infections, 624t
DHEA (dehydroepiandrosterone), 258f, 268, 278f, 292f, 408f
DHEA-S (dehydroepiandrosterone sulfate) [test], 290, 291t, 291–292
DHPG (3,4 dihydroxyphenylglycol), 278, 278f, 282
DHPG (3,4 dihydroxyphenylglycol) [test], 282–283
Diabetes insipidus:
    antidiuretic hormone test for, 295
    cAMP and, 58
    carbamazepine for, 340
    nephrogenic, 295, 295t, 296
    water deprivation test for, 295t, 295–296
Diabetes mellitus:
    autoantibody, 845t
    and fructosamine testing, 137–138
    gestational, 133–134, 135
    and glucose testing, 128, 130, 131, 132, 133–135
    and glucose urine screening, 54
    and hemochromatosis, 98
    and hypercholesterolemia, 178
    and hypertriglyceridemia, 178, 180t
    immunology, 861
    monitoring control of [tests], 135–138
    pregnancy and, 406, 407
    protein levels and, 156t
    zinc deficiency and, 211
Diabetic control monitoring [tests], 135–138
    fructosamine, 137–138
    glycohemoglobin, 135–137
Diacylglycerol (DAG), 500, 502f
Diagnostic immunology, 835–863
    cellular, 851–862. *See also* Cellular immunology
    humoral, 837–850. *See also* Humoral immunology
Diagnostic principles, 1–4
Diagnostic sensitivity, 2, 3f, 4, 5, 6–7, 8
Diagnostic specificity, 2, 3f, 4, 5, 6–7, 8
Dialysis encephalopathy (dementia), 60
Diaminobenzidine, 604

Diarrheas:
  infectious (agents/manifestations), 750–756, 751t–753t
  inflammatory, 751t–753t, 753
  and pneumonia, 660t
  protozoal, 752t, 760
  watery, 751t–753t, 753
Diazepam:
  and emergency room, 370t
  half-life and therapeutic/toxic concentrations, 384t
Diazotized 2,4-dichloroaniline, 54
Dibucaine: and pseudocholinesterase, 76, 76t
DIC. See Disseminated intravascular coagulation
Dicarboxyporphyrin, 55, 56t, 57
2,4-Dichloroaniline, diazotized, 54
Dientamoeba fragilis: gastroenteritis, 752t, 760, 760t, 765
Diet:
  amnino acids, 143, 144t
  carbohydrates in, 127
  and testing, 5
Differential WBC count [test], 583–589
DiGeorge syndrome, 859
Digestion, inadequate: malabsorption and, 91t
Digitoxin [test], 358–359
Digoxin:
  dosing formulas, 358t
  drug interactions, 344, 351, 355, 356, 357
  pharmacokinetic parameters, 349t
  therapeutic range, concentration, and distribution, 334t
  toxicity, 358
Digoxin [test], 357–358
DiGuglielmo syndrome, 565
1,25-Dihydroxy D, 218, 219, 219t, 220t
24,25-Dihydroxy D, 218
3,4 Dihydroxyphelalanine [test], 283
3,4 Dihydroxyphenylglycol (DHPG), 277, 278f, 282
3,4 Dihydroxyphenylglycol (DHPG) [test], 282–283
1,25-Dihydroxyvitamin D:
  and calcium regulation, 296, 296t
  and PTH, 301
2,3-Diketugluconic acid, 231
Dilution methods for in vitro susceptibility, 791–792, 793
Diphenoxylate:
  characteristics of, 389t
  testing for, 388–389, 389t

Diphtheria, 635. See also *Corynebacterium diptheriae*
  ulcer, 679t
Diphtheroids. See also *Corynebacterium*
  cultures, 698
  and ear infections, 636, 638
  prosthetic device infections, 711
Diphyllobothrium latum, 761, 763t
Dipolar ions, 143
Dipropylacetate. See Valproic acid
Dipsticks, 48, 53, 54
Dipstick [test], 725
Dipylidium caninum, 761, 763t
Dipyrone: hemolytic anemia from, 894t
Direct fluorescent antibody (FA) test, 852–854
Direct microscopic examination: of urine, 730–732
Disaccharidase, 95
Disaccharidase deficiency [test], 96
Disaccharides, 95
Disease prevalence, 2
Disk diffusion test for in vitro susceptibility, 792
Disopyramide:
  pharmacokinetic parameters, 349t
  protein binding, 350, 350f
  therapeutic range, concentration, and distribution, 334t
Disopyramide [test], 348–350
Disseminated intravascular coagulation, 518, 521, 522f, 522t, 526, 545, 546, 561, 888
Distribution, test result, 7–8, 8f
Disulfiram: drug interactions, 344t
Dithionite [test], 495–496
Diuretics: drug interactions, 358, 360
Diurnal variations: and testing, 5
Diverticulitis: CEA elevation in, 319t
DNA autoantibody, 845t
DNA hybridization [test], 411–413
Dog bites, 715–716
Döhle bodies, Plate 11B, 436, 589
Donath-Landsteiner antibody test, 453, 891, 893
DOPA (3,4 dihydroxyphelalanine) [test], 283
Dopamine β-hydroxylase, 202
Dopamine [test], 283
Double diffusion, 805
Doumas method, 153
Down syndrome (trisomy 21), 402, 406
  protein levels and, 156t

Doxepin:
  therapeutic range, concentration, and distribution, 334t, 396t
  toxicities, 396t
Doxycycline: drug interactions, 344
D-Penicillamine, 149
2,3 DPG deficiency, 299
Drepanocytes, 433
Driving under the influence (DUI), 375
Driving while intoxicated (DWI), 375
Drug abuse [tests], 386–389. See also Alcohol *and specific drugs*
  opiates and opioids, 388t, 388–389, 389t
  screen, 387–388, 388t
Drug Abuse Warning Network (DAWN), 369
Drug-dependent immune thrombocytopenia, 884
Drug-induced hepatitis, 73, 77
Drug Interference and Effects in Clinical Chemistry, 7
Drug of abuse panel [test], 387–388
Drugs, 333–340, 369–374. See also Drugs [tests] *and specific drugs*
  abuse, 369–398. See also *specific drugs*
  accumulation in body, 336t, 339–340
  and anemia, 451t
  area under the concentration (AUC) time curve, 337, 338
  bioavailability, 333
  concentration monitoring, 340, 340f
  distribution volumes, 334t, 335–336
  elimination half-life, 336–337
  factors affecting choice of, 790
  and G-6-PD deficiency, 477, 478, 480
  and hemolytic anemia, 477, 478–479, 889t, 893–895
  immunologic effects, 861–862
  in vitro susceptibility [tests], 789–795
  Km (affinity of a substrate), 339, 345, 345t, 346f
  minimum bactericidal concentration (MBC), 790, 794–795

Drugs *(Continued)*
  minimum inhibitory concentration (MIC), 789–790
  neutropenia from, 585
  nonlinear pharmacokinetics, 338–339, 339f
  one compartment models, 337
  peak and trough, 337, 338f
  pharmacokinetic equations, 336t
  pharmacokinetic models, 337–339
  pharmacokinetics, 333, 335
  platelet disorders induced by, 514, 516t
  protein binding, 333, 335
  serum concentration monitoring, 340, 340f
  serum concentrations, 333, 334t, 339f, 340, 340f
  steady-state concentration, 333, 336f, 337, 337t, 338f, 340
  sustained release, 340, 341f
  and testing, 5
  therapeutic monitoring [tests], 797–800
  therapeutic ranges, 334t
  total body clearance, 334t, 335–336
  toxicology, 369–398. *See also* Drug toxicology *and specific drugs*
  two compartment models, 337, 339f
  V_{max}, 339, 345, 345t, 346f
Drug screen [test], 387–388
Drugs [tests], 333–368
  aminoglycosides, 797–798
  antiarrhythmics, 348–357
  anticonvulsants, 340–348
  caffeine, 361
  carbamazepine, 340–342
  cardiac glycosides, 357–359
  chloramphenicol, 799
  cimetidine, 363
  cyclosporine, 364
  desipramine, 359
  digitoxin, 358–359
  digoxin, 357–358
  disopyramide, 348–350
  encainide, 350–351
  ethosuximide, 342–343
  flecainide, 351
  flucytosine, 799–800
  gold, 364–365
  imipramine, 359
  and in vitro susceptibility testing, 789–795
  lidocaine, 351–352
  lithium, 360
  methotrexate, 365–366
  mexiletine, 352–353
  NAPA, 353–354
  nortriptyline, 360–361
  phenobarbital, 343–344
  phenytoin, 344–346
  primadone, 346
  procainamide/NAPA, 353–354
  propranolol, 354–355
  psychotropics, 359–361
  quinidine, 355–356
  sulfonamide, 799
  theophylline, 361–363
  therapeutic monitoring, 363
  tocainide, 356–357
  toxicology. *See* Drug toxicology
  valproic acid, 347–348
  vancomycin, 798–799
  xanthines, 361–363
Drug toxicology, 369–398
  analytic methods, 370–374
  comparison of analytic techniques, 374
  drug-specific tests. *See* Drug toxicology [tests]
  gas chromatography, 374, 374f
  high performance liquid chromatography, 373, 373f
  immunoassays, 370–372, 372f
  most frequent drugs encountered, 370t
  panels based on patient presentation, 371t
  pediatric, 369, 370t
  testing availability, 371t
  thin layer chromatography, 372, 373f
Drug toxicology [tests]:
  abused drugs, 386–389
  alcohols, 374–380
  barbiturates, 384–386
  benzodiazepines, 383–384
  metals, 390–392
  non-narcotic analgesics, 380–383
  psychotropics, 392–397
DST. *See* Dexamethasone suppression [test]
Dubin-Johnson syndrome, 58, 74
Duchenne muscular dystrophy: testing for, 411, 413
Duodenal aspirates, 749–750
Duodenal ulcer disease, 100, 100t
  and infections, 749
DU-PAN-2: as tumor marker, 329, 329t
D^u test, 873–874
Dwarfism: zinc deficiency and, 211
D-xylose absorption [test], 95
Dyplastic nucleated red blood cells, Plate 22A, Plate 31B, 431
Dysalbuminemic hyperthyroxinemia, 246, 254, 254f
Dysautonomia, familial, 283
Dysentery, 765. *See also* Diarrheas
  defined, 754
Dyserythropoiesis: in myelodysplasia, 566t
Dysfibrinogenemia, 519, 523t, 528, 541, 545
Dysgerminoma: tumor markers, 315
Dysmegakaryocytosis: in myelodysplasia, 566t
Dysmyelopoietic syndrome, 565
Dysplastic granulocytes, 436
Dysuria, 722, 734
Dysuria-pyuria syndrome, 722

E

E_2. *See* Estradiol
Ear:
  abscess of middle, 638
  external examination [test], 636–637
  infections, 635
  inner cultures [test], 637–638
Eastern equine encephalitis, 772t
Ebola virus, 649t
  serology [test], 817
EBV. *See* Epstein-Barr virus
Ecgonine, 372
Echinococcus granulosus, 674, 702t, 703, 705. *See also* Hydatid disease
  CNS infection, 777t, 778, 782, 783, 784, 785
  serology [test], 830t, 830–831
Echinococcus multiocularis, 702t, 703, 705
Echinocytes, 432
Echinostoma ilocanum, 762t, 763t
Echoviruses:
  CNS infection, 771, 776, 776t
  pericarditis, 711
  skin manifestations, 677t
  stool culture/rectal swab, 759t
  throat infection, 641
  upper respiratory infections, 636t
Ecthyma gangrenosum, 679t
Ecthyma infectiosum, 681t
Eczema, atopic: immunology, 861
EDTA (ethylenediaminetetraacetic acid), 59, 117
Egg white injury preventative factor. *See* Biotin

Ehrlichia canis: serology [test], 811, 813
Ehrlich's reagent, 54, 55
EIA. *See* Enzyme immunoassay
Eikenella corrodens: and endocarditis, 626t
Elastase, 89
Electroimmunodiffusion: for CSF immunoglobulin, 112
Electrolyte exclusion effect, 46
Electrophoresis:
    alkaline phosphatase isoenzymes and, 73t, 73–74, 74t
    for CK isoenzymes, 27, 29, 30t
    CSF [test], 112–113, 113f
    hemoglobin [test], 484–489, 485f, 486t–487t, 488f, 491t
    high resolution serum protein, 158–161, 159f
    serum protein, 154–158, 156t–157t
Electrothermal atomic absorption spectrophotometry: for aluminum, 60
ELISA. *See* Enzyme linked immunosorbent assay
Elliptocytes (ovalocytes), 432
Embden-Meyerhof glycolytic pathway, 483f, 484
Embryonal carcinoma: tumor markers, 315, 315t
Emphysema: protein levels and, 156t
Empyema, 659, 659t, 663, 668
Enanthems, 676
Encainide [test], 350–351
Encephalitis, 769
    CSF lactate and, 111
    granulomatous amebic, 774, 778, 779
    parasitic, 774–775
    viral, 770–774, 771t, 772t, 815
Encephalomyelitis, 773
Endocarditis, infective:
    blood culture, 623
    complement test and, 168
    organisms associated with culture negative, 626t
    skin manifestations, 677t
Endocrine disorders: malabsorption and, 91t
Endocrine function [tests], 58–59
Endocrine neoplasia:
    apudomas, 101
    hormonal assays for, 102
    insulinomas, 102
    MEN syndrome, 101
    VIPomas, 102
Endodermal sinus tumor: tumor markers, 315, 315t

Endolimax nana, 760t
Endometriosis: cancer antigen 125 and, 317
Endomitosis, 441
Endophthalmitis, 635, 648, 651
Endothelial cell, 443
Endothelium cell-derived relaxing factor (EDRF), 506, 507t
Endotoxemia [test], 632–633
Enkephalin, 99
Entamoeba coli, 760t
Entamoeba hartmanni, 760t
Entamoeba histolytica:
    and abscess aspiration, 689
    CNS infection, 777t, 782, 783, 784
    cutaneous ulcers, 685
    direct examination, 693
    gastroenteritis, 752t, 753, 760, 760t, 763, 765
    liver abscess, 702, 704, 706
    proctorectal exudate, 744–745
    pulmonary infection, 672, 672t, 673
    serology [test], 830, 830t
Entamoeba polecki, 760t
Enteric fever, 754
Enterobacter
    traumatic wounds, 718
Enterobacteriaceae, 620
    blood culture, 621t, 623
    CNS infections, 770
    ear infection, 637, 638
    and endocarditis, 623
    infections, 624t
    lower respiratory infection, 657, 669t
    pericarditis, 711
    peritoneal infection, 701
    pylephlebitis, 701
    skin manifestations, 680t
    traumatic wounds, 717
    upper respiratory infections, 645t
    urinary tract infections, 722, 726
Enterobius vermicularis, 761, 763t, 765
    in urine, 53
Enterococcus:
    cultures, 696t
    infections, 624t
    peritoneal infection, 701
    pylephlebitis, 701
    tissue infections, 695, 696t
    traumatic wounds, 718
    urinary tract infections, 722, 726
Enterococcus faecalis:
    cultures, 696t
    trauma/wound infection, 680t, 699
Enterococcus faecium:
    cultures, 696t

infection, 680t
Enteromonas hominis, 760t
Enterotoxins, 750
Enterovirus 68: stool culture/rectal swab, 759t
Enterovirus 70, 771, 771t, 772t
    stool culture/rectal swab, 759t
Enterovirus 71, 771, 771t
    stool culture/rectal swab, 759t
Enteroviruses:
    blood culture [test], 628t
    CNS infection, 771, 771t, 772t, 776, 776t, 777t
    conjunctivitis, 648, 649t
    ear infection, 637
    infection frequency, 636t
    myopericarditis, 713
    pericarditis, 711
    serology [test], 816
    skin manifestations, 677t, 678t, 679t, 684
    stool culture/rectal swab, 759t
Enzymatic alcohol dehydrogenase: in alcohol analysis, 376, 376f, 376t
Enzyme immunoassay (EIA), 805.
    See also Serodiagnosis of infectious disease
    for adenovirus, 823
    for amebiasis, 830, 830t
    for arboviruses, 815
    for *Borrelia*, 808
    for *Brucella*, 806
    for cysticercosis, 830, 830t
    for echinococcosis, 830, 830t
    for HIV, 821–822
    for HTLV-1, 822
    for influenza virus, 823
    for mumps virus, 822
    for *Mycoplasma*, 815
    for rubeola virus, 824
    for schistosomiasis, 830t, 831
    for toxocariasis, 830t, 832
    for toxoplasmosis, 830t, 832
    for trichinosis, 830t, 832
    for VZV, 825
Enzyme linked immunosorbent assay (ELISA), 805
    autoantibody testing, 845t
    for *Borrelia*, 808
    for CSF myelin, 114
    for fungi, 825, 825t
    for *Legionella*, 806
    for paragonimiasis, 830t, 831
    for schistosomiasis, 830t, 831
Enzyme multiplied immunoassay technique (EMIT): in toxicology, 370, 371, 372f, 374t

Enzymes, 150–151. *See also* Proteins
cardiac. *See* Cardiac serum enzyme
Enzyme techniques for alloantibody detection, 876, 878t
Enzyme tumor markers, 308t, 309t, 309–314
    acid phosphatase, 311–313, 312t
    alkaline phosphatase, 309–310
    creatine kinase, 310–311, 311f
    lactate dehydrogenase, 311
    male PAP test, 311–313, 312t
    prostate specific antigen, 313–314
    prostatic acid phosphatase, 311–313, 312t
Eosinopenia: causes of, 556t, 588
Eosinophil(s), 425
    in cerebrospinal fluid, 108, 108t
    function, 435, 553
    morphology, Plate 8B, 426f, 434, 435, 436
    reference values for cell count and slide differential, 586t–587t
    stain reactions, 604t
    in synovial fluid, 118t
    tissue, 443
Eosinophil count [test], 592
Eosinophilia:
    causes of, 555t, 585, 588, 592
    testing for, 592
Ephedrine: drug interactions, 361
Epidemic typhus, 677t
    serology and transmission, 812t
Epidermal autoantibody, 845t
Epidermophyton floccosum: skin manifestations, 678t
Epididymitis, 722
Epidural abscess, 781t, 783
Epiglottitis, 635, 641, 642–643
Epilepsy therapeutic drugs. *See* Anticonvulsants
Epinephrine. *See also* Catecholamines
    and glucogenolysis, 128
    and platelet aggregation, 515f
    synthesis, 277
Epithelial cells:
    renal tubular, 50, 61f
    squamous, 50, 61f
    transitional, 50, 61f
    tubular casts, 51
Epithelial membrane antigen, 602
EPO. *See* Erythropoietin
10,11-Epoxide metabolite, 342
Epstein-Barr virus:
    and B-cell lymphoma, 859
    blood culture [test], 628t
    CNS infection, 771, 772t, 777t

    hepatitis, 702t, 820
    and lymphocytosis, 585
    serology [test], 816–817, 817t
    skin manifestations, 677t
    throat infection, 641, 642
    upper respiratory infections, 636t
Ergocalciferol, 217–218. *See also* Vitamin D
Erysipelas, 677t, 681t
Erysipeloid, 680t, 682
Erysipelothrix fortuitum: skin manifestations, 680t
Erysipelothrix insidiosa: skin manifestations, 681t
Erysipelothrix rhusiopathiae: infections, 624t, 682
Erythema infectiosum, 677t, 822
Erythema marginatum, 677t, 808
Erythrasma, 677t
Erythremic myelosis, chronic, 565
Erythroblasts:
    in bone marrow aspiration, 612t
    stain reactions, 604t
Erythrocuprein, 202
Erythrocyte. *See* Red blood cells
Erythrocyte glutathione reductase activity coefficients (EGRAC), 225, 225t
Erythrocyte hexose monophosphate, 229
Erythrocyte sedimentation rate (ESR) [test], 464–466, 465t
Erythrocytosis, 326
Erythroleukemia, acute, Plate 18, 445, 561, 563t, 608. *See also* Myelocytic leukemia, acute
    vitamin B_{12} and, 228, 228t
Erythromycin: hemolytic anemia from, 894t
Erythropoiesis, 427–434, 430f. *See also* Red blood cells
    abnormal morphology, 431–434
    dysplastic morphology, Plate 1, 431
    megaloblastic morphology, Plate 1, 431
    normoblastic morphology, Plate 1, 427–431
Erythropoietic porphyrias, 56t, 57–58
Erythropoietic protoporphyria, 56t, 57, 418t
Erythropoietic uroporphyria, 57
Erythropoietin:
    conditions and disorders affecting ranges of, 156t

    erythrocytosis, 326
Erythropoietin [test], 497
Escherichia coli:
    0157:57, 752t, 754, 756
    anorectal infection, 744
    antigen detection, 780
    CNS infections, 770, 781, 785
    cultures, 697t, 700f
    enterohemorrhagic, 753
    enteropathogenic, 754
    enterotoxigenic, 747, 754, 756
    gastroenteritis, 752t, 753, 754, 755, 756
    peritoneal infection, 701
    septic arthritis, 707–708
    traumatic wounds, 718
    trauma/wound infection, 680t, 699
    urinary tract infections, 722
Esophageal biopsy, 748
Esophageal cancer: CEA elevation in, 319t
Esophagitis: infectious, 748
Esophagus: bacterial and fungal culture [test], 748
ESR (erythrocyte sedimentation rate) [test], 464–466, 465t
Esterase stain [test], 605–606
Estradiol, 258f, 284f, 285
Estradiol-secreting tumors, 294
Estradiol [test], 292f, 292–294, 293t
Estriol, 292
    unconjugated [test], 405–407, 408f, 409f
Estrogen, 284
    drug interactions, 344t
    synthesis, 292, 292f
Estrogen receptors [test]: tumor marker, 326–327, 328
Estrogen-secreting tumors, 294
Estrone, 292, 292f
ET. *See* Thrombocytopenia, essential
Ethanol:
    concentrations and clinical symtpoms, 377t
    concentrations by D-Osm values, 375f
    properties, 375t
    volatile concentrations from D-Osm, 379t
Ethanol [test], 375–377
Ethosuximide:
    drug interactions, 343, 344t
    therapeutic range, concentration, and distribution, 334t
    toxicity, 343
Ethosuximide [test], 342–343

Ethyl alcohol [test], 375–377
Ethylenediaminetetraacetic acid (EDTA), 59
　for synovial fluid, 117
Ethylene glycol:
　properties, 375t
　　volatile concentrations from D-Osm, 379t, 380
Ethylene glycol [test], 378–379
Euglobulin lysis time [test], 546
Eumycetoma, 680t, 681t
Euthyroid hyperthyroxinemia, 246, 247t
Euthyroid hypothyroxinemia, 246, 247t
Exanthema, 677t
Exanthema subitum, 677t
Exanthems, 676, 677t, 684
Exclusion error, 46
Exocrine function. *See* Pancreatic exocrine function
Exophialia jeanselmi: skin manifestations, 681t
Exophialia werneckii: skin manifestations, 678t, 681t
External quality control, 6
Extrinsic pathway inhibitor, 510, 512f
Extrinsic system, 502, 503f, 512f
Eye, 635
　cultures [test], 648–654

F

FAA. *See* Fumaroylacetoacetate (FAA) hydrolase deficiency
FAB classification system:
　for leukemia, 561, 562, 563t, 564, 564t
　for myelodysplastic syndromes, 566, 567t
Factor antigen concentration [test], 541
Factor B, 848, 848t, 849t
Factor I. *See* Fibrinogen
Factor II. *See* Prothrombin
Factor V, 503, 504, 507
　deficiency, 516t, 539
Factor V [test], 540
Factor Va, 503, 508, 510f, 548
Factor VII, 505
　deficiency, 516t, 518, 888
　and vitamin K, 221
Factor VII [test], 540
Factor VIIa, 502, 503f, 512f
Factor VIII, 504, 507, 518, 526, 530, 537–539
　coagulant antigen, 538
　deficiency, 515–516, 516t, 518, 519, 537–539, 887, 888
　inhibitor assay, quantitative [test], 542–543
　procoagulant protein, 538
　procoagulant [test], 513t, 517f, 531t, 537–539, 538f
　transfusion, 870t, 887, 888
Factor VIIIa, 505f, 508, 510f, 548
Factor IX, 502, 505, 512f, 526
　deficiency, 515–516, 516t, 519, 887, 888
　procoagulant activity [test], 539
　transfusion, 870t, 887, 888
　and vitamin K, 221
Factor X, 502, 503f, 505, 505f, 512f
　deficiency, 516t, 518, 888
Factor X [test], 540
Factor Xa, 501–502, 503, 503f, 504f, 505f, 510, 512f
　inhibition assay [test], 544–545
Factor XI, 504, 505f
　deficiency, 516t, 540
Factor XI [test], 540
Factor XIa, 504, 505f
Factor XII, 499, 505f, 526
　deficiency, 516t, 540
Factor XII [test], 540
Factor XIIa, 505f, 540
Factor XIII, 529
　deficiency, 519, 542
　screen [test], 507f, 519t, 542
Factor XIIIa, 505, 507f
Fallopian tube: ectopic pregnancies in, 400
False negative results, 1–2, 3f
False positive results, 1–2, 3f, 4, 9
Fasciola hepatica, 702t, 702–703, 705, 762, 762t, 763t
Fasciolopsis buski, 761, 762, 762t, 763t
Fast hemoglobin [test], 135–137
Fasting blood sugar [test], 130–131
Fasting glucose [test], 127–128
Fat cell, 443
Fatty acids, 181–182
　common, 182t
　free, 181
　structure of, 181f
Fatty acids [test], 181–182
　very long chain, 419–420
Fatty casts: in urine, 51
Fatty liver, 72
Fatty meal [test], 94–95
Favus, 681t
FBS (fasting blood sugar) [test], 130–131
FDP (fibrin degradation products) [test], 522t, 545, 546f
Fecal fat [test], 93
Fecal flora: polymicrobic tissue infection, 680t, 699, 700f
Fecal-oral transmission, 750, 765
Fentanyl: characteristics of, 389t
Feosol [test], 390–392
Ferrata cell, 443–444
Ferric chloride:
　test, 147
　for urine analysis, 55
Ferritin [test]: for anemia/hemachromatosis, 449, 450t, 466t, 466–468, 467f, 468t, 470
Ferrochelatase, 470
　deficiency, 56t, 57
Ferrous gluconate [test], 390–392
Ferrous sulfate [test], 390–392
Fetal hemoglobin, hereditary persistence of (HPFC), 485, 488, 491t, 492–493, 495, 496
Fetal hemoglobin [tests], 492–493
　Kleihauer-Betke (acid elution), 495
Fetal lung maturity: testing for, 408–410, 410t
Fetal monitoring, 399
α-Fetoprotein:
　CSF, 114
　and serum protein electrophoresis, 158
α-Fetoprotein [test]:
　and liver function, 81
　pleural fluid, 116
　pregnancy, 402–403, 404, 405t
　tumor marker, 314–315, 315t
FFA. *See* Free fatty acids
FFP. *See* Fresh frozen plasma
Fibrin, 151, 505, 507–508, 511f
　D domain, 505, 506f, 507f, 546f–547f
Fibrinase. *See* Factor XIII
Fibrin clot formation, 499, 501–505, 504f, 505f, 505t, 506f, 507f
Fibrin clot formation disorders, 515–519
　acquired, 516–519, 517f, 517t, 518t
　hereditary, 515–516, 516t
Fibrin clot formation [tests], 525–529, 537–551
　acquired inhibitors, 542–544
　activation peptide of protein C, 509f, 520t, 551
　agarose gel inhibitor screening, 517f, 542, 542f

Fibrin clot formation [tests] *(Continued)*
  α_2-antiplasmin, 512f, 519t, 550
  antithrombin III activity, 508f, 520t, 546–548
  antithrombin III antigen, 548
  Bβ 1-42 and Bβ 15-42, 550
  Bethesda assay for factor VIII inhibitors, 542–543
  clottable fibrinogen, 523f, 541
  coagulation factors, 537–542
  D-dimer, 545–546, 546f–547f
  dilute Russell viper venom time, 544
  euglobulin lysis time, 546
  factor antigen concentration, 541
  factors II, V, VII, and X, 516t, 523t, 538f, 540
  factor VIII procoagulant, 513t, 517f, 531t, 537–539, 538f
  factor IX procoagulant activity, 539
  factor Xa inhibition assay, 544–545
  factor XI, 540
  factor XII, 540
  factor XIII screen, 507f, 519t, 542
  fibrin degradation products (FDP), 522t, 545, 546f–547f
  fibrinogen antigen, 517f, 541–542
  fibrinolytic system assessment, 549–550
  fibrinopeptide A, 506f, 551
  heparin cofactor II, 548
  heparin effect measurement, 544–545
  high molecular weight kininogen, 540
  in vivo thrombin activation, 550–551
  intravascular coagulation, 545–546
  plasmin-α_2-antiplasmin complex, 512t, 550
  plasminogen activator inhibition-1, 550
  plasminogen activity, 511f, 512f, 520t, 522f, 523t, 546f–547f, 549–550
  platelet neutralization procedure, 517f, 543–544
  prekallikrein, 540
  prekallikrein activity screen (Fletcher factor assay), 506f, 540
  protamine sulfate and ethanol gelation, 507f, 546
  protein C activity, 509f, 510f, 520t, 548
  protein C antigen, 548–549
  protein C system assessment, 548–549
  protein S antigen, 510f, 520t, 549
  prothrombin fragment 1 + 2, 520t, 534f, 551
  SERPIN family assessment, 546–548
  thrombin-antithrombin III complex, 508f, 520t, 534f, 550–551
  thrombin inhibition, 545
  tissue plasminogen activator, 512f, 519t, 550
  tissue thromboplastin inhibition assay, 517f, 543
Fibrin degradation products (FDP), 521, 522f
Fibrin degradation products (FDP) [test], 522t, 545, 546f–547f
Fibrinogen, 501, 503f, 505, 506f, 507, 527, 546f–547f
  activity [test], 541
  antigen [test], 517f, 541–542
  clottable [test], 523f, 541
Fibrinolytics: therapy monitoring, 525, 545, 550
Fibrinolytic system, 507t, 508–509, 520t
  assessment [tests], 549–550
Fibrinopeptide A, 505, 507f, 521f, 546
Fibrinopeptide A [test], 506f, 551
Fibrinopeptide B, 505, 507f, 521f, 546
Fibrocystic breast disease: CEA elevation in, 319t
Ficin: for alloantibody detection, 876
Ficoll-Hypaque density gradient isolation, 600
Fifth disease, 677t, 822
Filariasis:
  serology [test], 830t, 831
  skin manifestations, 681t, 685
Filoviruses: serology [test], 817
Final common pathway, 504
Fish-eye disease, 189
Fistulae: disease, etiology, and tests for, 680t
5-Hour GTT (glucose tolerance test), 134–135
Flame cell, 440
Flavin adenine dinucleotide (FAD), 224, 225
Flavin mononucleotide (FMN), 224

Flaviviruses: CNS infection, 772t, 774, 776, 777t
Flea bites, 677t, 686
Flecainide:
  drug-induced arrhythmias, 350, 351
  drug interactions, 351
  therapeutic range, concentration, and distribution, 334t
Flecainide [test], 351
Fletcher factor assay [test], 506f, 540
Floating β-lipoprotein [test], 193
Flow cytometry [test], 598–603
Flucytosine monitoring [test], 799–800
Fludrocortisone suppression, 272, 273t, 274
Fluids, body. *See* Body fluids
Fluid specimen [test], 700–707
Flukes, 762–763
Fluorescein isothionate (FITC), 600, 601
Fluorescence polarization immunoassay (FPIA): in drug toxicology, 370, 371, 374t
Fluorescent dye binding systems, 22–23
Fluorescent treponemal test, absorbed (FTA-ABS) [test], 810t, 810–811
Fluoride: and pseudocholinesterase, 76, 76t
Fluoride sensitive esterase [test], 605–606
Fluorouracil: hemolytic anemia from, 894t
Fluphenazine: testing for, 394, 394t
Flurazepam: half-life and therapeutic/toxic concentrations, 384t
Fly maggots, 686
Foam cell, Plate 32B, 443
Folate deficiency, 473–475, 476
  and anemia, 449, 471, 472t
  causes, 474t
  progression, 473–474, 474t
Folate [test]: for anemia, 472t, 473–475, 474t
Folic acid, 213
  ascorbic acid and, 231
Folic acid, serum and red blood cell [test], 472t, 474t, 474–475
Follicle stimulating hormone (FSH), 123, 237, 283–284, 321–322, 400

and menstrual cycle, 284f
  reference intervals, 286t
Follicle stimulating hormone (FSH) [test], 285–286, 286t
Folliculitis: nodular, 681t
Follitropin. *See* Follicle stimulating hormone
Fonsecaea pedrosoi, 681t
Food poisoning, 750
  diarrheas, 753
Formaldehyde, 377
Fournier's disease, 727
F_{1+2} peptide, 504f, 505, 521f, 551
Fragment 1 + 2 assay [test], 520t, 534f, 551
Francisella tularensis:
  bites, 716
  blood culture [test], 622, 626
  environmental exposure, 659t
  eye infections, 648
  pneumonia and, 666–667, 669t
  serology [test], 804, 805, 811
  tissue manifestations, 679t, 681t, 682
Franklin's disease, 164
Free erythrocyte protoporphyrin (FEP) [test], 470–471
Free fatty acids (FFA), 81, 181–182
French-American-British (FAB) classification system:
  for acute leukemia, 562, 564, 564t
  for acute myelocytic leukemia, 561, 563t, 564t
  for myelodysplastic syndromes, 566, 567t
Frequency distribution, 8, 9f
Fresh frozen plasma: transfusion, 868t, 887
Friedwald formula, 190
Fructosamine [test], 137–138
Fructose, 54, 59, 95
  malabsorption, 96t
Fructose 1,6 diphosphate, 128f
  deficiency, 422t
Fructose 6-phosphate, 127
Fructosuria: and glycohemoglobin, 137
FSH. *See* Follicle stimulating hormone
FTA-ABS (fluorescent treponemal test, absorbed) [test], 810t, 810–811
FT_4I (free thyroxine index), 250, 251
Fugitive swellings, 650, 685
Fuller's earth, 43
Fumaroylacetoacetate (FAA) hydrolase deficiency, 150
Fumaryolacetoacetate (FAA) hydrolase deficiency, 146t
Functional assay of adherence and chemotaxis [test], 597
Functional assays of chemotaxis [test], 597
Functional assays of degranulation [test], 597–598
Functional assays of phagocytosis and intracellular killing [test], 597
Fungal serology [tests], 825t, 825–829, 826t, 827t
  aspergillosis, 825–827
  blastomycosis, 827–828
  candidiasis, 828
  coccidioidomycosis, 828
  cryptococcosis, 828–829
  histoplasmosis, 829
  sensitivity/specificity, 825t, 827t
Fungemia:
  agents, 623, 625
  defined, 620
  testing for, 619–634. *See also specific fungi*
Fungi. *See also specific fungi*
  blood culture, 621t, 623, 625
  bone marrow culture [test], 634
  CNS infections, 770, 775–776, 780, 781
  culture of esophagus [test], 748
  direct blood examination [test], 627
  ear infection, 636
  eye infections, 648–649, 651–652
  lymphadenopathy, 714
  nasal infection, 638–639
  pericarditis, 711
  pneumonia, 657, 657t, 658t, 659, 659t, 664–665, 666, 667–668
  serology. *See* Fungal serology
  sinusitis, 640
  skin infections, 699
  throat infections, 641–642, 643, 644, 646
  urine culture [test], 727–728
  urine microscopic examination [test], 730–731
Furosemide:
  drug interactions, 360
  and renin testing, 275
Furuncles: and pneumonia, 660t
Furunculosis, 710
  agent and test, 678t
Fusarium: and burn wounds, 716, 717
Fusobacterium:
  CNS abscess, 783
  infections, 624t
  keratitis, 648
  skin manifestations, 679t
Fusobacterium necrophorum:
  throat infection, 641
  upper respiratory infections, 645t
Fusobacterium nucleatum:
  liver abscess, 701
  respiratory infections, 669t

G

GAE. *See* Granulomatous amebic encephalitis
Gaisböck syndrome (stress erythrocytosis), 456t, 457, 496, 497
Galactokinase assay [test], 416
Galactose, 54
  malabsorption, 96t
Galactosemia: and glycohemoglobin, 137
Galactosemia [test], 411
  genetic, 416
Galactose-1-phosphate uridyl transferase assay [test], 416
Galactosuria, 416
Galactosyltransferase: and ovarian carcinoma, 329t
Gallstones: pancreatitis and, 90
Gambian trypanosomiasis, 631, 774–775
γ-Aminobutyric acid (GABA):
  and benzodiazepines, 383
  biochemistry and reference range, 145t
  valproic acid and, 347
γ-Carboxyglutamic acid, 505, 506f, 518
Gamma globulin. *See* Immunoglobulin G
Gammaglobulin levels, measurement of [test], 842
γ-Glutamyl cysteine synthetase deficiency, 478f, 479
Gamma-glutamyl transpeptidase [test], 77, 79–80
  nonhepatobiliary causes of increases, 80t
γ-Granules, 441
γ-Heavy chain, 580, 581
γ-Melanocyte stimulating hormone (MSH), 265f, 321
Gangliosidoses: GM2, 419
Gangrene, 687, 688f
  gas, 713
  streptococcal, 680t
  synergistic, 680t

Gardnerella vaginalis: vaginosis, 734t, 737, 738, 739
Gas chromatography:
  in alcohol analysis, 376, 376t, 378–379
  in drug toxicology, 374, 374f, 374t
Gas gangrene, 713
Gastric acid secretion [test], 99–100, 100t
Gastric aspirates, 749–750
Gastric biopsy, 749
Gastric carcinoma: tumor markers, 311, 319t, 320
Gastric function, 99
Gastric function [tests], 99–101
  gastric acid secretion, 99–100, 100t
  gastrin, 100–101, 101t
  pepsinogen, 101
Gastric intestinal function [tests], 101–102
  hormonal assays for endocrine neoplasms, 102
  insulin, 102
  vasoactive intestinal peptide, 102
Gastric ulcer disease, 100, 100t
Gastrin, 99
  increased-levels disorders, 101t
  serum concentrations in disease, 101t
Gastrin [test], 100–101, 101t
Gastrinomas, 100
Gastroenteritis:
  defined, 754
  manifestations, 751t–753t, 753–754
  stool culture [test], 750–756
  viral [test], 758–759, 816
Gastrointestinal cancer:
  selenium and, 211
  tumor markers, 316, 317, 318
Gastrointestinal cancer associated antigen (GICA) [test], 316–317
Gastrointestinal tract, 747–767
  alkaline phosphatase and, 73
  and calcium regulation, 296t
  infections, 747–748
  protective mechanisms, 747
  trauma, 706. See also Peritonitis
Gastrointestinal tract [tests], 748–766
  bacterial and fungal culture of esophagus, 748
  Clostridium difficile toxin detection, 756–758
  ova and parasite, 759–766
  serology, 816
  stomach and small intestine culture, 749–750
  stool culture, 750–756, 751t–753t
  viral detection, 758–759, 759t, 816
Gaucher cell, Plate 32A, 443
Gaucher's disease, 311, 312t, 443
Gaussian distribution, 7–8
GC. See Gas chromatography
GD_2 gangliosides, 278
Genetic disorders [tests], 413–420
  amino acid screen, 414
  α_1-antitrypsin, 413–414
  carnitine, 414–415
  copper and ceruloplasmin, 415–416
  galactosemia screening, 416
  mucopolysaccharides, 416–417
  organic acids, 417–418
  prophyrins, 418, 418t
  sweat chloride, 418–419
  Tay-Sachs screening, 419
  very long chain fatty acids, 419–420
Genetic screen [test], 410–411
Genital herpes, 733, 734t, 740, 741, 742, 743
  lymphadenopathy, 715
Genitalia, ambiguous, 259, 288
Genital tract infections, 733–746
Genital tract [tests], 733–746
  cervical examination, 739–740
  lymphadenopathy specimens, 740–743
  proctorectal exudate, 743–745
  pubic lice, 745
  ulcer specimens, 740–743
  urethral exudate, 733–737
  vaginal excretions, 737–739
Genital ulcer, 733, 734t. See also Genital herpes
Genital warts, 733
Gentamicin:
  monitoring [test], 797–798
  reference range, 798t
  therapeutic range, concentration, and distribution, 334t
Geotrichum candidum, 667, 669t
  fungemia, 625
German measles. See Rubella virus
Germ cell tumors:
  α-fetoprotein tumor marker, 314, 315, 315t
  hCG as marker, 322, 324
Gestational trophoblastic disease, 322, 323, 324
GFAAS (graphite furnace atomic absorption spectrometry), 201–202, 210

GGT. See Gamma-glutamyl transpeptidase
GH. See Growth hormone
GHb (glycated hemoglobin:glycosylated hemoglobin) [test], 135–137
Giant platelets, Plate 25, 442
Giardia lamblia:
  gastroenteritis, 752t, 753, 759, 763
  proctorectal exudate, 745
Giardiasis. See *Giardia lamblia*
Gigantism: insulin-like growth factor I and, 241
Gilbert syndrome, 75, 76
Gingivitis:
  and pneumonia, 660t
  ulcerative, 641
Gingivostomatitis, 635, 642, 643t
GLA (γ-carboxyglutamic acid) [test], 302–303
Glanzmann's thrombasthenia, 210, 503f, 513–514, 514t, 536
Glass bead retention time [test], 535
GLC. See Gas chromatography
Globin, 427
Globin chains: composition and genetics, 485, 485f
Globulin content of plasma [test], 842
Glomerular basement membrane (GBM), 845t
Glomerular filtration rate (GFR), 41, 43–44
  inulin clearance and, 59
Glomerular proteinuria, 161
Glomerulonephritis, 51
  acute, and *Streptococcus pyogenes*, 808
  acute progressive autoantibody, 845t
  testing for, 850
Glucagon, 102, 127, 128
Glucocorticoids, 257, 258f
  deficiency, 257, 259
  drug interactions, 358
  and gluconeogenesis, 128
Glucocorticoid-suppressible hyperaldosteronism, 272, 272t, 276t
Glucola, 133
Gluconeogenesis, 127–128
Glucose:
  cerebrospinal fluid [test], 108t, 108–109
  concentrations, 130
  dietary, 127
  and insulin ratios, 139
  malabsorption, 96t

metabolism, 127–129
pleural fluid [test], 116
tolerance. *See* Glucose tolerance
in urine, 54
Glucose dehydrogenase measurement method, 129
Glucose oxidase measurement, 129
Glucose-oxidase-peroxidase system, 54
Glucose 6-phosphatase deficiency, 421t, 422t
Glucose 6-phosphate, 127, 128f
Glucose 6-phosphate dehydrogenase: screen [test] for anemia, 453, 477–479, 478f, 479t
Glucose 6-phosphate dehydrogenase (G-6-PD), 129
Glucose-6 phosphate dehydrogenase (G-6-PD) deficiency: and glycohemoglobin, 137
Glucose 6-phosphate dehydrogenase (G-6-PD) deficiency, 477–479, 478f, 483, 484, 560t, 598
Glucose [tests]:
fasting, 130–131
1-hour postprandial, 135
random, 128–130
2-hour postprandial, 131–132
whole blood, 132
Glucose tolerance:
chromium and, 201
factor (GTF), 201, 223
Glucose tolerance [tests], 5, 96, 128, 129, 132, 133–135
and growth hormone, 239
intravenous, 135
1-hour postprandial, 135
Glucose 6-translocase deficiency, 421t
$\alpha_{1,4}$-Glucosidase deficiency, 421t
β-Glucuronidase, 75, 727
Glutamate oxaloacetate transaminase [test], 69–70
Glutamate pyruvate transaminase [test], 68–69
Glutamic acid: biochemistry and reference range, 145t
Glutamine: biochemistry and reference range, 145t
Glutamine [test], 80, 111
γ-Glutamyl transferase [test], 73, 79–80
nonhepatobiliary causes of increases, 80t
Glutathione, 382, 478f, 484
and hemolytic anemia, 478f
peroxidase, 210
synthetase, 478f

Glycated hemoglobin:glycosylated hemoglobin [test], 135–137
Glycated serum proteins [test], 137–138
Glycerolphosphate, 312t
Glycerophosphatides, 182
Glycine, 55, 144t, 147
biochemistry and reference range, 144t, 145t
Glycinexylidide (GX), 352
Glycocalicin [test], 537
Glycocholates, 81
Glycogen metabolism, 127
Glycogenolysis, 127–128
Glycogen storage diseases, 416, 420
classification and characteristics, 410, 421t
and hypertriglyceridemia, 180t
Glycogen storage diseases [tests], 420–422, 421t
L-lactate, 420–422
Glycohemoglobin [test], 135–137, 136f, 137f
Glycolic acid, 378
Glycolipids: and breast cancer, 329t
α_1-Glycoprotein: conditions and disorders affecting ranges of, 156t
Glycoprotein Ib, 499
Glycoprotein IIb-IIIa complex, 501, 503f, 514, 515f, 522f
deficiency, 536
Glycoprotein tumor markers, 308t, 314–320
α-fetoprotein, 314–315, 315t
cancer antigen 15-3, 316
cancer antigen 19-9, 316–317
cancer antigen 50, 317
cancer antigen 72, 319–320
cancer antigen 125, 317
cancer antigen 195, 318
cancer antigen 549, 318
carcinoembryonic antigen (CEA), 318f, 318–319, 319t
tumor associated glycoprotein, 319–320
Glycosylated serum proteins [test], 137–138
Glycosyl transferases, 209
GM2 gangliosidoses, 419
GnRH. *See* Gonadotropin releasing hormone
Goiter, 244
Gold [test], 364–365
Gonadal dysgenesis, 293t
Gonadotropin cell adenomas, 286
Gonadotropin releasing hormone (GnRH), 239, 284, 292

and menstrual cycle, 284f
Gonadotropin releasing hormone stimulation [test], 286–287
Gonadotropins, 283
Gonadotropins [test], 285–286, 286t
Gonadotropin-secreting tumors, 286
Gonococcal arthritis: synovial fluid lactate examination, 125t
Gonococcal infection. *See Neisseria gonorrhoeae*
Gonococcemia, 677t
Gonorrhea. *See Neisseria gonorrhoeae*
Goof balls: toxicity, 385–386
Gout, 708
and hypercholesterolemia, 178
and hyperuricemia, 45, 52
and synovial fluid examination, 116, 117t
Graft-versus-host disease (GVHD), 858
Grain alcohol [test], 375–377
Granular casts: in urine, 51, 62f
Granules:
α, 441
γ, 441
δ, 441
cytoplasmic, 441
Granulocytes, 425, 426f, 434–437. *See also specific cells*
abnormal, 436–437
Alder-Reilly granules, 436
antigen markers, 599t
Auer bodies (rods), Plate 14B, 436
band, 435
basophil, 436
Chédiak-Higashi granules, Plate 12, 436
circulating pool (CGP), 435
Döhle bodies, Plate 11B, 436
dysplastic, 436
eosinophil, 436
giant metamyelocyte, 436
hypersegmentation (right shift), 436
hyposegmentation (Pelger-Huët cells), Plate 11A, 436, 589
marginal pool (MGP), 435
metamyelocyte, 435
myeloblast, 435
myelocyte, 435
neutrophil, 436
promyelocyte (progranulocyte), 435
stain reactions, 604t
toxic granules, Plate 9A, 437
toxic vacuoles, Plate 9A, 437
transfusion, 868t, 886–887

Granulocyte-specific antigen systems, 887
Granulocytic leukemia, juvenile chronic, 493
Granuloma, swimming pool, 681t
Granuloma inguinale, 734t, 740, 741, 742
Granulomatous amebic encephalitis (GAE), 774, 778, 779
Granulomatous disease, chronic, 560t
Granulomatous lymphadenitis: lymph node biopsy for, 613
Granulopoiesis, 426f, 434–437
  abnormal morphology, 436–437
  morphology, 435–436
Granulopoietins, 435
Granulosa cell, 283, 284
Grape cell, 440
Graphic displays of reports, 7
Graphite furnace atomic absorption spectrometry (GFAAS), 201–202, 210
Graves disease, 244, 252, 255, 256
Gray (agranular) platelets, Plate 25, 442
Gray platelet syndrome, 514t
Grey-Turner's sign, 85, 86t
Gross cystic disease protein: and breast cancer, 329t
Ground itch, 761
Growth factor: and oncogenes, 328
Growth factor releasing factor, 102
Growth hormone:
  arginine infusion for, 243
  and breast cancer, 328
  decreases and increases in, 238t, 238–240
  and glucose testing, 128, 133
  insulin tolerance test for, 243
Growth hormone [test], 237–240
Growth retardation: zinc deficiency and, 211
G-6-P. See Glucose 6-phosphate
Guillain-Barré syndrome, 109, 112, 114, 773, 773t
Gunther's disease, 57
Guthrie bacterial inhibition assay, 411
Guthrie test: for amino acids, 147, 148
Gynecomastia, 294
  hCG levels and, 323–324

H

Haemophilus aprophilus:
  CNS abscess, 783
  infections, 624t, 626t
Haemophilus ducreyi:
  genital ulcer, 734t, 742–743
  lymphadenopathy, 715
Haemophilus influenzae:
  antigen, 671, 726, 775, 780
  antigenemia, 633
  chloramphenicol for, 799
  CNS infections, 770, 775, 779, 780, 781, 785
  ear infection, 637, 638
  eye infections, 648, 650
  infections, 624t, 710
  lower respiratory infection, 657, 665, 666, 670t
  orbital cellulitis and sinusitis, 639–640
  pericarditis, 711
  septic arthritis, 707–708
  and serology testing, 808
  skin manifestations, 677t, 680t
  susceptibility testing, 791, 792
  throat infection, 642, 643
  upper respiratory infections, 645t
Haemophilus parainfluenza:
  culture, 700f
  infections, 624t, 626t
Haemophilus paraprophilus: infections, 624t
Hageman factor. See Factor XII
HAI. See Hemagglutination inhibition test
Hair:
  analysis for trace metals, 201, 212
  direct examination, 694t
Hairy cell, Plate 26A, 440
  stain reactions, 604t
Hairy cell leukemia:
  immunophenotyping, 602, 856f
  morphology/manifestations/markers, Plate 26A, 527t
  TRAP test for, 608
Halazepam: half-life and therapeutic/toxic concentrations, 384t
Half-life, drug, 336–337, 337f, 337t
  equation, 336t
Haloperidol:
  drug interactions, 361
  testing for, 394, 394t
Hamster test, 294
Hamster zona-free ovum test, 294
Ham test, 476–477
Hand, foot, and mouth disease: agent and test, 678t
Hand-Schuller-Christian disease, 581

Hanker-Yeats reagent, 604
Hantzsch reaction, 179, 180
Haptoglobin: conditions and disorders affecting ranges of, 156t, 160, 161
Haptoglobin [test], 166
Hartnup's disease, 414
  features of, 146t
  niacin deficiency and, 223, 224
Hashimoto's thyroiditis, 252, 255, 256
  autoantibody, 845t
HAV. See Hepatitis A virus
HBD (α-hydroxybutyrate), 36
HBV. See Hepatitis B virus
hCG. See Human chorionic gonadotropin
HC II (heparin cofactor II) [test], 548
Hct. See Hematocrit
HCV. See Hepatitis C virus
HDLs. See High density lipoproteins
HDV. See Hepatitis D virus
Head trauma: CSF lactate and, 111
Heart disease:
  alkaline phosphatase and, 72
  coronary. See Coronary heart disease
  muscle, 713
  and polycythemia, 456t
Heart failure. See Congestive heart failure
Heart parasites, 702t, 702–703
Heart tests. See *under* Cardiac
Heat denaturation [test], 484
α-Heavy chain, 580, 581
Heavy chain disease, 581
  immunoelectrophoresis for, 163–165
  immunofixation for, 162
Heavy metals: and renal transport, 41
Heinz bodies, 432, 477
Heinz bodies [test]: for anemia, 453, 478f, 479–480
Helicobacter pylori:
  gastric infection, 749–750
  serology [test], 806
Helmet cells, 432, 433
Helminths. See *also specific species*
  CNS infection, 777t, 778
  extraintestinal infections, 762–763
  gastrointestinal, 759, 761–762, 762t, 766
  infections, 702–703
  lymphadenopathy, 715
  respiratory, direct examination for [test], 671–674
  serology [tests], 830t, 831–832

urine microscopic examination [test], 731–732
Hemagglutination inhibition (HAI) test:
  for adenovirus, 823
  for arboviruses, 815
  for influenza virus, 823
  for rubeola virus, 824
Hemarthrosis: synovial fluid cell count, 117
Hematocrit, 447
  reference values for hemogram, 460t
Hematopoiesis, 425–446
  diagrammatic representation, 426f
Hematopoietic dysplasmia, 565
Hematopoietic sites, 425
Hematopoietic stem cell, 425, 426f, 434
Hematuria, 48, 725
Hemochromatosis, 98
  ferritin and, 466, 468
  testing for, 469, 470
Hemodialysis: aluminum toxicity and, 60
Hemodilution, perioperative, 882–883
Hemoglobin, 447, 453, 455
  abnormalities [tests], 484–496
  in anemia, 461
  buffer, 13t, 13–14
  concentration density (HCD), 459
  dissociation curve, 17, 23f, 23–25, 24f–25f
  distribution width (HDW), 459
  electrophoresis [test], 459f, 484–489, 485f, 486t–487t, 488f, 491t
  fast [test], 135–137
  glycated hemoglobin: glycosylated (GHb) [test], 135–137
  heat stability [test], 484
  in histogram, 458f
  isopropanol denaturation (unstable hemoglobin screen) [test], 494
  mean cell concentration (MCHC), 427, 457, 458f, 459, 460t, 461
  mean cell (MCH), 457, 459, 460t, 461
  in polycythemia, 461
  reference values for hemogram, 460t
  and respiration, 12
  sickle [test], 495–496
  synthesis, 427
  thermolabile [test], 484
  trait vs. disease, 488
  unstable, testing for, 484–496
  unstable screen [test], 484, 494
  in urine, 54
Hemoglobin A, 492
  abnormal proportions, 491t, 492
Hemoglobin A_1 (A_{1a}, A_{1b}, A_{1c}), 136
Hemoglobin A_{1c} [test], 135–137
Hemoglobin A_2 [test], 490–492
Hemoglobin Bart's, 487t, 488, 489, 491t, 494
Hemoglobin C, 488, 491t, 492
  crystals, 432
  disease, 491t, 496
Hemoglobin C-Harlem (Georgetown), 496
Hemoglobin Constant Spring, 449t, 491t
Hemoglobin C-Ziguinchor, 496
Hemoglobin D, 489
Hemoglobin D-Los Angeles (Punjab), 488, 491t
Hemoglobin E, 448, 449t, 488, 491, 491t
  disease, 491t
Hemoglobin F, 137, 492
  abnormal proportions, 491t
  hereditary persistence of (HPFC), 485, 488, 491t, 492–493, 495, 496
Hemoglobin F [tests], 492–493
  Kleihauer-Betke (acid elution), 495
Hemoglobin G-Philadelphia, 488, 489, 491t
Hemoglobin Hasharon, 486t, 495
Hemoglobin H disease, 449t, 491t, 493–494
Hemoglobin H inclusions, 389, 492
Hemoglobin H inclusions [test], 488f, 493–494
Hemoglobin J, 137
Hemoglobin Köln, 491t, 495
Hemoglobin Lepore, 449t, 489, 492, 493
Hemoglobin N, 137
Hemoglobin O, 492
Hemoglobinopathies, 453, 455t
  classification, 485, 486t–487t, 491t
Hemoglobin S, 463, 486, 491t, 492, 495–496
  disease, 491t, 495–496
Hemoglobin S-C disease, 491t
Hemoglobin S-Travis, 496
Hemoglobinuria, 54
  PNH. See Paroxysmal nocturnal hemoglobinuria
Hemoglobin Wayne, 137
Hemoglobin Zurich, 495
Hemogram (CBC) [test], 457–462, 458f, 459f, 460t, 461t
Hemolysis, 453, 454f, 464
Hemolytic activity [test], 846–848, 847f, 848t
Hemolytic anemias, 447, 453–455, 454f, 463
  acquired immune, testing for, 889–893
  autoimmune, 889–893
  bilirubin and, 75
  classification, 455t
  and copper toxicity, 204
  drug-induced, 477, 478–479, 889t, 893–895
  protein ranges in, 156t
  selenium and, 204
  vitamin E and, 220–221
  warm, 861
  warm antibody autoimmune, 889t
Hemolytic anemias [tests], 455t, 476–484
  acidified serum lysis test for PNH, 476–477
  autohemolysis, 482–483
  glucose 6-phosphate dehydrogenase screen, 477–479, 478f, 479t
  Heinz bodies, 478f, 479–480
  immunohematologic, 889–893
  osmotic fragility, 480–481, 481f
  red blood cell enzymes, quantitative, 478f, 483f, 484
  red blood cell half-life, 448f, 455t, 484
  sucrose hemolysis, 481–482
Hemolytic complement, 846
Hemolytic transfusion reactions, 879, 880
Hemolytic uremic syndrome, 521, 522t, 545
Hemopexin: conditions and disorders affecting levels of, 157t
Hemophilia A, 515–516, 516t, 518, 526, 531t, 539, 543, 887, 888
  testing for, 411
  transfusions, 887, 888
Hemophilia B, 515–516, 516t, 526, 539, 887, 888
  transfusions, 887, 888
Hemorrhage: subarachnoid, 107
Hemorrhagic fevers, 677t
  serology [test], 817
Hemorrhagic villonodular synovitis: synovial fluid examination, 117t

Hemosiderosis: ferritin and, 468
Hemostasis, 499–524
    approach to bleeding disorders, 511–519, 513t
    approach to complex disorders, 521–523, 522f, 523f, 523t
    approach to therapeutic monitoring of hemostatic agents, 523–525
    approach to thrombotic disorders, 519–521, 520t, 521f
    fibrin clot formation, 501–505, 504f, 505f, 505t, 506f, 507f
    fibrin clot formation disorders, 515–519
    parameter assessment, 511–525
    platelet disorders, 513–515
    platelet plug formation, 499–501, 500f, 501f, 502f, 503f, 503t
    plug formation, 499–501
    regulation, 500f, 501f, 505–510, 507t, 508f–512f
Hemostasis [tests], 525–530
    activated partial thromboplastin, 505f, 516t, 518t, 524t, 526–527
    fibrin clot formation, 525–529
    prothrombin and proconvertin test, 529
    prothrombin time, 503f, 506f, 516t, 518t, 524t, 525–526
    PTT, APTT, and TT corection (mixing studies), 528–529
    reptilase time, 528
    thrombin time, 517f, 527–528
    thromboelastography, 529
Hemostatic agents, 523–525. *See also specific agents*
    fibrinolytics, 525
    heparin, 524t, 524–525
    monitoring, 523–525
    oral anticoagulants, 523, 524t
HEMPAS, 477
Henderson-Hasselbach equation, 13–14, 17, 20, 48
    modified, 14
Henry's law, 14
Heparan sulfate: and thrombin neutralization, 507, 508f
Heparin:
    APTT and, 524, 524t
    and factor Xa neutralization, 544–545
    therapy monitoring, 524t, 524–525, 526
    and thrombin neutralization, 507, 508f, 516, 524

Heparin cofactor II, 506
Heparin cofactor II [test], 548
Heparin effect measurement [tests], 544–545
Hepatic abscess. *See* Liver abscess
Hepatic coma, 78
Hepatic necrosis:
    acetaminophen and, 382, 382t
    aminoaciduria in, 148
Hepatic porphyrias, 55–57
    acquired, 57
Hepatitis, 702
    alcoholic, 68t, 69, 70, 77
    alkaline phosphatase and, 72
    bilirubin and, 74–75
    CEA elevation in, 319t
    chronic active, 81
        differential diagnosis, 208t
    chronic autoantibody, 845t
    chronic persistent, 68t, 69, 76–77
    classification of, 68t
    α-fetoprotein and, 314
    fulminant, differential diagnosis, 208t
    ischemic, 78
    non-A, non-B (C), 69, 77
    testing for, 704, 705–707
    toxic, 74
    viral, 68, 68t, 69, 70, 74, 75, 77, 702t. *See also specific hepatitis viruses below*
Hepatitis A virus, 702, 702t
    serology [test], 817–818
Hepatitis B virus, 702, 702t
    arthritis, 707
    blood culture [test], 628t
    core antigen, 818, 819t, 820
    e antigen, 819
    serology [test], 818f, 818–820, 819f, 819t
    skin manifestations, 677t
    surface antigen, 818–820, 819t
    urinary, 730t
Hepatitis C virus, 702, 702t
    serology [test], 820
Hepatitis delta virus, 702
    serology [test], 820
Hepatoblastomas: tumor markers, 315
Hepatocellular carcinoma:
    tumor marker, 314, 315, 321, 323, 326
    vitamin B_{12} and, 229
Hepatolenticular degeneration. *See* Wilson's disease
Hepatoma, 702
    α-fetoprotein as marker, 81
    AP isoenzyme, 74t

Hepatotoxicity:
    acetaminophen and, 382, 382t, 383f
    cyclosporine, 364
Heptacarboxyporphyrin, 55, 56t, 57, 58t
Hereditary coproporphyria, 56t, 57
Hereditary persistence of fetal hemoglobin (HPFC), 485, 488, 491t, 492–493, 495, 496
Hermansky-Pudlak syndrome, 210, 514t
HER-2/neu oncogene, 327, 328, 328t
Heroin:
    characteristics of, 389t
    and emergency room, 370t
    testing for, 386, 387t, 388t, 388–389, 389t
Herokinase glucose measurement method, 129
Herpangina: skin manifestations, 679t
Herpes B virus: encephalitis, 772t
Herpes gladitorium, 684
Herpes labialis: and pneumonia, 660t
Herpes simplex virus:
    and AIDS, 860
    blood culture [test], 628t
    cervicitis, 734t, 739–740
    CNS infection, 772t, 773, 776–777
    genital, 715, 733, 734t, 740, 741, 742, 743
    hepatitis, 702t
    keratoconjunctivitis, 648, 649t, 650
    pneumonia, 664, 666, 670t
    rectal discharge, 734t
    serology [test], 804, 820–821
    skin manifestations, 679t, 684, 687f
    throat infection, 641, 642
    upper respiratory infections, 636t
    urethritis, 734, 734t
    urinary tract infection, 729, 730t, 732
Herpesviruses. *See also specific viruses*
    blood culture [test], 627–629
    CNS infections, 772t, 777t
    hepatitis, 702t
    infectious esophagitis, 748
    skin manifestations, 679t
Hers disease, 420, 421, 421t
Heterocyclic imino chains, 143
Heterologous ovum penetration test, 294
Heterophile test: for EBV, 816, 817t

Heterophyes heterophyes, 762, 762t, 763t
Hexacarboxyporphyrin, 55, 56t, 58t
Hexokinase, 127
    measurement, 129
Hexosaminidase A assay [test], 419
Hexose: dietary, 127
Hexose monophosphate shunt, 127, 477, 478f, 484, 556
Hgb. *See* Hemoglobin
Hickman site infection, 680t
High altitude: and polycythemia, 456t
High density lipoproteins, 173, 175, 182
    decreased characteristics, 184t
    factors and diseases associated with abnormal, 189t
    and flow chart for evaluation of hyperlipoproteinemias, 186f–187f
    increased characteristics, 183t
    properties of, 174t, 185
High density lipoproteins [test], 174t, 185–189, 188t, 189t
High molecular weight kininogen deficiency, 516t, 540
High molecular weight kininogen [test], 540
High performance liquid chromatography:
    and α-bilirubin, 75
    for CK isoenzymes, 29, 30t
    in drug toxicology, 373, 373f, 374t
    and porphyrias, 55
    and vitamin tests, 216, 217, 220, 224, 226t, 230
High resolution serum protein electrophoresis [test], 158–161, 159f
Hirsutism, 285, 289–290
    DHEA-S levels, 291
Histalog (3-aminoethylpyrazol), 99
Histamine: ascorbic acid and, 231
Histamine-2 blockers, 363
Histidine, 143, 147
    biochemistry and reference range, 144t
Histidine ammonialyase defect, 146t
Histidinemia: enzymatic defect and features of, 146t
Histiocyte: stain reactions, 604t
Histiocytic malignancies, 559, 581
Histiocytosis, malignant, 581
Histocompatibility antigens (HLA), 851
    and granulocyte transfusion, 886

Histocompatibility Y-chromosome antigen, 167
Histone, 845t
Histones, 151
Histoplasma:
    antigen, 671, 726
    arthritis, 707–708
    bone marrow aspiration for, 610
    bone marrow culture [test], 634
    and endocarditis, 626t
    environmental exposure, 659t
    and fungemia, 625
    lymphadenopathy, 714
    pneumonia, 658, 664, 666, 670t
    serology [test], 826t, 827t, 829
    skin manifestations, 677t, 678t
Histoplasma capsulatum:
    CNS infections, 770
    pericarditis, 712
    urinary test, 712, 727, 728
Histoplasma duboisii: skin manifestations, 677t
Histoplasmosis. *See* *Histoplasma*
HIV. *See* Human immunodeficiency virus
HLA. *See* Human leukocyte antigen
Hodgkin's disease, 577
    Ann Arbor staging system, 578t
    bone marrow aspiration for, 610, 611
    ESR and, 465
    immunophenotyping, 603
    lymph node biopsy for, 613, 615–616
    protein levels and, 156t, 165
    Reed-Sternberg cells and, 443, 577, 603, 615
    Rye histologic classification, 578t
    tumor markers, 310
Hoesch test, 418
Holocarboxylase synthetase deficiency, 223, 223t
Homoarginine: alkaline phosphatase isoenzymes and, 73t, 74, 74t
Homocysteine: elevated, 414
Homocystinuria, 147, 149, 414
    enzymatic defect and features of, 146t
    and vitamin B_6, 227t
Homogentisic acid oxidase deficiency, 146t, 148
Homogentisuria, 55
Homosexuals:
    anal intercourse, 743, 750
    urethritis in, 734
Homovanillic acid, 278f
Homovanillic acid [test], 283

Hookworms, 677t, 761. *See also individual species*
    pulmonary infection, 672, 672t, 673
    skin manifestations, 677t, 685–686
Hormonal assays for endocrine neoplasms, 102
Hormones, 237–306
    adrenal cortex, 257–270. *See also* Adrenal cortex
    adrenal medulla, 277–283. *See also* Adrenal medulla
    aldosterone-renin-angiotensin system, 270–277. *See also* Aldosterone-renin-angiotensin system
    anterior pituitary gland, 237–243. *See also* Anterior pituitary gland
    calcium metabolism, 296–303. *See also* Calcium
    ectopic, 320
    eutopic, 320
    and glucose blood concentration, 128
    hypothalamic-pituitary-adrenal axis, 257–277
    posterior pituitary gland, 294–296
    sex, 283–294. *See also* Sex hormones
    thyroid gland, 243–256. *See also* Thyroid gland
    as tumor markers. *See* Hormone tumor markers
Hormone [tests]:
    adrenocorticotropic hormone stimulation, 259–261
    aldosterone, 272–275
    angiotensin converting enzyme, 277
    antidiuretic hormone, 294–295, 320
    arginine infusion, 243
    calcitonin, 302, 320–321
    calcium metabolism, 296–298
    catecholamines (plasma), 281–282
    catecholamines (urinary), 280–281
    corticotropin, 264–266, 321
    corticotropin releasing hormone, 266
    cortisol, 262
    cortisol, urinary-free, 262–264
    dehydration test, 295–296
    dehydroepiandrosterone sulfate, 291–292
    desoxycorticosterone, 270
    11-desoxycortisol, 270
    dexamethasone suppression, 266–268

Hormone [tests]: *(Continued)*
  3,4 dihydroxyphenyglycol, 282–283
  3,4 dihydroxyphenylalanine, 283
  dopamine, 283
  estradiol, 292–294
  follitropin, 285–286
  free thyroxine, 249–250
  free thyroxine index, 250
  free triiodothyronine, 250–251
  gonadotropin releasing hormone stimulation, 286–287
  gonadotropins, 285–286
  growth hormone, 237–240
  homovanillic acid, 283
  17-hydroxyprogesterone, 268–270
  inhibin, 294
  insulin-like growth factor I, 240–241
  insulin tolerance, 261
  insulin tolerance test, 243
  lutropin, 285–286
  magnesium, 299–300
  metanephrine, 280
  3-methoxy-4-hydroxyphenylglycol, 283
  osteocalcin, 302–303
  parathyroid hormone, 300–302, 324–325
  phosphate (serum), 298–299
  prolactin, 241–243
  protein bound iodine, 251–252
  renin, 275–277
  sperm penetration assay, 294
  testosterone, 287–291
  thyroglobulin, 252
  thyroglobulin antibodies, 255
  thyroid autoantibodies, 254–256
  thyroid microsomal antibodies, 255–256
  thyroid stimulating hormone receptor antibodies, 256
  thyroid stimulating hormone (thyrotropin), 248–249
  thyronine, 252–253
  thyrotropin receptor antibodies, 256
  thyrotropin releasing hormone, 253
  thyroxine, 246–247
  thyroxine, uptake, 250
  thyroxine-binding globulin, 254
  triiodothyronine, 247–248
  triiodothyronine, reverse, 252
  tumor markers. *See* Hormone tumor markers
  vanillylmandelic acid, 279–280
  water deprivation test, 295–296
  water loading test, 295
Hormone tumor markers, 308t, 320t, 320–327
  antidiuretic hormone, 320
  cachectin, 325–326
  calcitonin, 320–321
  corticotropin, 321
  estrogen receptors, 326–327
  human choriogonadotropin, 321–324, 323t, 324t
  parathyroid hormone, 324t, 324–325
  parathyroid hormone-like peptide, 325
  progesterone receptors, 327
  thyrocalcitonin, 320–321
  tumor necrosis factor-α, 325–326
Howell-Jolly bodies, 432, 463
HPA. *See* Hyperphenylalaninemia
HPFC. *See* Hereditary persistence of fetal hemoglobin
HPL. *See* Human placental lactogen
HPLC. *See* High performance liquid chromatography
HSV. *See* Herpes simplex virus
Human bite wounds specimen [test], 715–716
Human bot fly, 681t
Human chorionic gonadotropin (hCG), 283
  comparison of assays, 323t
  CSF, 114
  pregnancy test, 399–401
  serum heterogeneity, 323t
  stimulation test, 289
  as tumor marker, 315, 315t, 321–324, 323t, 324t, 329t
Human chorionic somatomammotropin (HCS) [test], 408
Human herpesvirus 6:
  blood culture [test], 628t
  skin manifestations, 677t
Human immunodeficiency virus (HIV), 733, 860–861. *See also* Acquired immunodeficiency syndrome
  blood culture [test], 627–629, 628t
  and CSF MBP, 114
  encephalopathy, 772t, 774, 776t
  and gastrointestinal infections, 747–748
  immunology, 860–861
  lymphocyte marker studies [test], 840, 841
  serology [test], 821–822
  staging of infection, 861t
  and throat infections, 642
Human leukocyte antigen (HLA), 166–167, 884
  and granulocyte transfusion, 886
  typing, 885
Human menopausal gonadotropin, 294
Human milk fat globule antigen: and ovarian carcinoma, 329t
Human papillomavirus:
  cervicitis, 739, 740
  genital warts, 733
Human placental lactogen: and ovarian carcinoma, 329t
Human placental lactogen [test], 408
Human platelet antigens (HPA), 884, 884t
Human T-cell lymphotropic virus type I (HTLV-I), 771t, 772t, 774
  leukemia and, 856
  serology [test], 822
Human T-cell lymphotropic virus type II (HTLV-II): blood culture [test], 628t
Human T-cell lymphotropic virus type III. *See* Human immunodeficiency virus
Human thyroid/adenylate cyclase stimulator (HTACS), 256
Human thyroid stimulator (HTS), 256
Humoral immunology, 837–850. *See also* B lymphocytes; Immunoglobulins
  autoantibody [test], 844–846, 845t
  basic concepts, 837–838
  cellular events during response, 839f
  complement fixation [test], 846–848, 847f, 848t, 849t
  immune complex [test], 848, 850, 850t
  immunoglobulin quantitation [test], 841–844, 843t
  interrelationship of components, 838f
  lymphocyte marker studies [test], 840–841, 841t
  total lymphocyte count [test], 838, 840
Humster test, 294
Hunter syndrome, 416
Huntington's disease: testing for, 411
Hurler syndrome, 416
HVA (homovanillic acid), 278f
HVA (homovanillic acid) [test], 283
Hyaline casts: in urine, 50, 62f
Hydatid disease, 702, 702t, 705, 777t, 783. *See also Echinococcus granulosus*

alveolar, 702t, 703, 705
pulmonary, 672t, 673–674
serology [test], 830t, 830–831
Hydatidiform moles, 322, 401, 408
Hydralazine: hemolytic anemia from, 894t
Hydrochloric acid, 747
Hydrochlorothiazide: hemolytic anemia from, 894t
Hydrogen peroxide:
and glucose measurement, 129
and vitamin E analysis, 220, 221t
Hydromorphone: characteristics of, 389t
Hydroxy-alprazolam: half-life and therapeutic/toxic concentrations, 384t
Hydroxyapatite crystals: in synovial fluid, 119t
α-Hydroxybutyrate, 36
17-Hydroxycorticosteroid, 264
17-Hydroxycorticosteroid [test], 268, 269f
18-Hydroxycorticosterone, 273, 274t, 275
25-Hydroxy D, 218, 219, 219t, 220t
16α-Hydroxydehydroepiandrosterone sulfate (DHEA-S), 405, 408f
α-Hydroxyketobutyrate, 36
11-Hydroxylase, 258f
deficiency, 262, 270, 271t
17-Hydroxylase, 258f
deficiency, 270, 271t
and testosterone, 287f
18-Hydroxylase, 258f
deficiency, 271t
21-Hydroxylase, 258f
deficiency, 259, 259–261, 260f, 265, 268, 269, 270, 271t, 291
Hydroxylysine: biochemistry and reference range, 145t
9-Hydroxy-methyl-ellipticimium: hemolytic anemia from, 894t
3 Hydroxy-3-methylglutaryl-CoA (HMG-CoA), 174
2-Hydroxy-nortriptyline, 360–361
β-Hydroxy-γ-N-trimethylammonium butyrate. See Carnitine
3-Hydroxy-5-phenylpyrrole-N-tosyl-L-alanine ester, 55
17-Hydroxypregnenolone, 258f
17-Hydroxyprogesterone (17-OHP), 258f, 259, 260f, 268, 269, 270, 291
17-Hydroxyprogesterone (17-OHP) [test], 268-270

Hydroxyproline: biochemistry and reference range, 145t
18-Hydroxysteroid dehydrogenase: deficiency, 271t
3-β Hydroxysteroid dehydrogenase deficiency, 270, 271t
3-β Hydroxysteroid dehydrogenase isomerase: and estrogen, 292f
5-Hydroxytryptophan: ascorbic acid and, 231
25-Hydroxy vitamin D-1-hydroxylase (1-OHase), 218
Hydroxyxylidine, 352
Hymenolepis diminuta, 761, 763t
Hymenolepis nana, 763t
Hyperacidity, 99
Hyperaggregate assay [test], 536
Hyperaldosternoism: primary, and hypertension, 272t
Hyperaldosteronism, 272–275
idiopathic, 272
idiopathic, differentiation from adrenal adenoma, 274, 274t
Hyperalimentation: alkaline phosphatase and, 73
Hyperamylasemia, 86, 87, 90
conditions associated with, 88t
Hyperandrogenism, 288, 288t
Hyperbilirubinemia, 75
Hypercalcemia, 296, 297
causes of, 297t, 298
familial benign (FBH), 297
in malignancy, 324t, 324–325
PTH and, 301
tubular reabsorption of phosphate and, 299
Hypercalciuria, 51, 298, 301
Hypercapnia, 17
Hypercarotenemia: and xanthochromia, 107
Hypercholesterolemia, 178. See also Cholesterol
classification of, 179t
essential familial, 178, 189–191
LDLs and, 189–191
secondary causes of, 178
Hyperchromia, 432
Hyperchylomicronemia, 191–192. See also Chylomicrons
Hypercupremia, 203t, 204
Hypergammaglobulinemia: protein levels and, 157t, 160–161, 169
Hyperglycemia, 54, 128, 130
causes of, 131t
and C-peptide measurement, 140t

and glucose testing, 128
Hypergonadism, 285
Hypergonadotropic hypogonadism, 285–286
Hypergonadotropic syndrome, 290t
Hyperimminoglobulinemia: immunofixation (IFE) test for, 161–163
Hyperkalemia: and renin secretion, 270
Hyperkaluria, 47
Hyperlipidemia, 179. See also Lipids
protein levels and, 156t
Hyperlipoproteinemias, 181, 183t, 185, 186f–187f, 195
flow chart for evaluation of, 186f–187f
Frederickson type, 191
tests for, 185
type II, 192, 193
type IV, 192
type V, 191, 192, 193
Hypermagnesemia, 296, 300
Hypernatremia, 46
Hyperoxaluria, 51
Hyperparathyroidism, 51, 72, 299, 300–302
calcitonin and, 302, 321
familial benign hypercalcemia vs., 297
PTH test, 301–302
Hyperphenylalaninemia (HPA), 147, 149
benign, 149
enzymatic defect and features of, 146t
type I, 146t
type II, 146t
Hyperphosphaturia, 301
Hyperpipecolatemia: testing for, 419
Hyperprolactinemia, 241–242, 242t
and hypogonadism, 293t
Hyperprolinemia (types I and II): enzymatic defect and features of, 146t
Hyperprotinemia, 152–153
Hypersegmentation (right shift) of granulocytes, 436
Hypersensitivity reactions, 851
Hypertension:
catecholamine levels and, 282
congenital adrenal hyperplasia and, 271t
and hypertriglyceridemia, 180t
pheochromocytoma and, 278
plasma renin activity and, 59
primary, 272

Hypertension *(Continued)*
   renin plasma activity test for, 275–277, 276t
   secondary causes of, 272, 272t
Hyperthyroidism, 128, 132, 244, 246, 247–248, 252, 253. *See also specific tests*
   and testosterone levels, 289
Hyperthyroxinemia:
   dysalbuminemic, 246, 254, 254f
   euthyroid, 246, 247t
Hypertriglyceridemia, 178–180. *See also Triglycerides*
   and amylase levels, 88t
   secondary causes of, 180t, 181
   treatment of, 181
Hypertrophic pulmonary osteoarthropathy: synovial fluid examination, 117t
Hyperuricemia, 44t, 45
   and hypertriglyceridemia, 180t
Hyperviscosity syndromes, 171
Hypervitaminosis A, 97, 216
Hypervitaminosis D, 219
Hypnotics, 384t
Hypoalbuminemia, 47, 152
Hypoaldosteronism, 46
Hypoalphalipoproteinemia, familial, 189
Hypocalcemia, 296, 297
   causes of, 297t
Hypocapnia, 17
Hypoceruloplasminemia, 82
Hypochloremia, 47
Hypochloremic acidosis: and maple syrup urine disease, 148
Hypochlorhydria, 100
Hypochromia, 432
Hypocupremia, 203t, 203–204
Hypoestrogenic disorders, 293t, 293–294
Hypofibrinogenemia, 528, 888
Hypogammaglobulinemia:
   and protein tests, 155, 160
   transient of infancy, 858
Hypogeusia: zinc deficiency and, 212
Hypoglycemia:
   causes of, 131t
   and C-peptide measurement, 140t
   and diabetic monitoring tests, 137
   and glucose testing, 128, 130–131
   postprandial, 134–135
   and prolonged (72 hour) fast test, 141
   and provocative tests of insulin secretion, 141
   reactive, 134–135
   symptoms and signs of, 134t
   and tumors, 326
Hypoglycemic index, 134–135
Hypogonadism, 285, 286, 287, 289
   secondary, 289
   in women, 293t
   zinc deficiency and, 211
Hypogonadotropic syndrome, 290t
Hypokalemia: ammonia and, 78
Hypolipoproteinemias, 184t, 185
Hypomagnesemia, 296
   causes of, 300t
Hyponatremia, 47
   renal, 46
Hypoparathyroidism, 58, 299, 300, 301
Hypophosphatasia, 71
Hypophosphatemia, 299, 301
Hypopituitarism, 290t
Hypoprotinemia, 152–153
Hyposegmentation of granulocytes (Pelger-Huët cells), Plate 11A, 436
Hypothalamic-pituitary-adrenal axis, 257–277
   adrenal cortex, 257–259
Hypothalamic-pituitary-gonadal axis, male: laboratory findings, 289, 290t
Hypothalamus: and gonadotropin releasing hormone, 284, 286–287
Hypothyroidism, 71, 244, 248–249, 252, 253, 256. *See also specific tests*
   compensated, 249
   congenital, screening for, 245, 245f
   and hypercholesterolemia, 178
   and hypertriglyceridemia, 180t
   hypothalamic, 249
   neonatal, 256
Hypothyroxinemia: euthyroid, 246, 247t
Hypoxemia, 16–17
Hypoxia, 16–17
   and polycythemia, 456t, 456–457, 496–497

I

iC3b, 846, 848, 848t, 849t
ICG (indocyanine-green excretion) [test], 82
ID. *See* Immunodiffusion
Idiosyncratic porphyria, 57
IDLs. *See* Intermediate density lipoproteins
IFA. *See* Indirect fluorescent antibody test
Ig. *See* Immunoglobulin
IGF I. *See* Insulin-like growth factor I
IGF I/SmC, 240
IHA. *See* Indirect hemagglutination test
Imipramine:
   therapeutic range, concentration, and distribution, 334t, 396t
   toxicities, 396t
Imipramine [test], 359
Immediate spin crossmatch, 874
Immune complexes by C1q binding [test], 848, 850
Immune complex [test], 848, 850, 850t
Immune function, 837–838, 838f, 839f. *See also Cellular immunology; Humoral immunology*
Immune regulatory disorders: testing for, 853t
Immune serum globulin (ISG): transfusion data, 870t
Immunoassays: in drug toxicology, 370–372, 372t
Immunoblast, 440
Immunocompromised patients. *See also Acquired immunodeficiency syndrome*
   chorioretinitis, 649
   CNS infections, 771–772
   and gastrointestinal infections, 747–748, 758
   infectious esophagitis, 748
   nasal infections, 638–639
   sinusitis, 640
Immunodeficiencies, 851. *See also specific disorders*
   associated with other defects, 859, 859t
   combined, 840, 841, 857, 858, 859t
   common variable (CVID), 858
   primary states, 857, 858t, 859t
   testing for, 853t, 856–857
Immunodeficiency with hyper-IgM, 160, 857
Immunodiffusion (ID), 805. *See also Serodiagnosis of infectious disease*
   for aspergillosis, 827t
   autoantibody, 845t
   for blastomycosis, 827t, 827–828
   for candidiasis, 827t, 828
   for coccidioidomycosis, 827t
   for fungi, 825, 825t, 827t
   for histoplasmosis, 827t, 829
Immunoelectrophoresis (IEP) [test]:

protein, 163f, 163–165, 164f, 164t
Immunofixation (IFT) [test]: protein, 161–163, 162f, 164f
Immunogen, 837
Immunoglobulin, 438. *See also* B lymphocytes
  abnormal electrophoretic patterns, 157t, 158
  conditions and disorders affecting levels of, 157t, 168–169
  cryoglobulins and, 170
  deficiencies, 168–169, 857–858
  quantitation [test], 168–169, 841–844, 843t
  Rh, transfusion data, 870t
  surface (SIg) staining, 851, 852, 854
  transfusion data, 870t
Immunoglobulin A:
  conditions and disorders affecting levels of, 157t, 161
  deficiency, 169, 858, 859t
  monoclonal, 162
  myeloma, 164, 171
  quantitation [test], 841–844
  reference range by age, 843t
  in serum protein electrophoresis test, 155
Immunoglobulin D:
  conditions and disorders affecting levels of, 157t, 168
  myeloma, 164
  quantitation [test], 841–844
Immunoglobulin E:
  conditions and disorders affecting levels of, 157t, 168
  quantitation [test], 841–844
  reference range by age, 843t
Immunoglobulin G:
  albumin ratio, 153
  conditions and disorders affecting levels of, 157t, 161, 168
  Fc receptors, 438
  gammopathies, 163f
  index, 112
  myeloma, 159, 164, 171
  NK cells and, 438
  quantitation [test], 841–844
  reference range by age, 843t
  and rubella virus, 824
  synthesis rate, 112
  and thrombocytopenia, 594
  total protein ratio, 112
Immunoglobulin G [test], 111–112
  quantitation, 841–844
Immunoglobulin M:
  conditions and disorders affecting levels of, 157t, 161, 168

gammopathies, 163f, 164, 171
hyper, immunodeficiency with, 160, 857
myeloma, 164, 171
reference range by age, 843t
and rubella virus, 824
and Waldenström's macroglobulinemia, 580, 603
Immunohistochemistry [test], 598–603
Immunologic cell surface studies [test], 598–603
Immunologic tests, 598–610
Immunology, diagnostic. *See* Diagnostic immunology
Immunoperoxidase [test], 598–603
Immunophenotyping [test], 598–603
Immunoproliferative malignancies, 559, 580–581. *See also specific disorders*
Immunoregulatory abnormalities, 861
Impetigo: skin manifestations, 679t
Indian childhood cirrhosis, 206, 206t, 208t
Indirect fluorescent antibody (IFA) test, 852–854
  for hemorrhagic fever viruses, 817
  for *Legionella*, 806
  for malaria, 830t, 831
  for *Mycoplasma*, 814
  for rabies virus, 823
  for schistosomiasis, 830t, 831
  for VZV, 825
Indirect hemagglutination (IHA) test:
  for amebiasis, 830, 830t
  for cysticercosis, 830, 830t
  for echinococcosis, 830t, 830–831
  for filariasis, 830t, 831
  for Rocky Mountain spotted fever, 811
  for strongyloidiasis, 830t, 832
  for trichinosis, 830t, 832
Indirect immunofluorescence (IIF): autoantibody testing, 845t
Indocyanine-green excretion (ICG) [test], 82
β-Indolylacetic acid, 59
Indomethacin: drug interactions, 360
Industrial toxicities, 200t
  chromates, 201
Industrial toxicity [test], 390–392
Infections: C-reactive protein and, 170
Infectious mononucleosis, 677t. *See also* Epstein-Barr virus

and lymphocytosis, 585
serology [test], 816–817, 817t
Infertility:
  gonadotropin levels and, 285
  semen test for, 122–125
  and testosterone levels, 288, 289
Inflammation:
  protein levels and, 156t, 157t, 160, 170
  skin infections and, 683t
Inflammatory bowel disease, 744
Inflammatory diseases:
  and ferritin, 468, 468t
  and iron deficiency, 467f
Influenza virus:
  ear infection, 637
  eye infection, 649t
  infection frequency, 636t
  pneumonia, 657, 658, 660, 664, 666, 668, 670t
  postinfectious syndrome, 773
  serology [test], 823
  throat culture, 641, 642
  upper respiratory infections, 636t
INH. *See* Isoniazid
Inhibin, 284
Inhibin [test], 294
Injection site granuloma, 680t, 681t
Inoculum effect, 789
Inositol triphosphate (IP$_3$), 500, 502f
Insect bites and stings, 686
Insulin, 127, 128
  to glucose ratios, 139
  hemolytic anemia from, 894t
Insulin [test], 102
Insulin-like growth factor I, 238
  increases and decreases in, 241, 241t
Insulin-like growth factor I [test], 240–241
Insulinomas, 102, 138, 140
  testing for, 141
Insulin-producing tumors. *See* Insulinomas, 138, 140
Insulin-secreting pancreatic β-cell tumors, 141–142
Insulin secretion provocation [tests], 141–142
  calcium infusion, 141
  C-peptide-glucagon, 142
  C-peptide suppression, 141–142
  prolonged (72 hour) fast, 141
  tolbutamide tolerance, 141
Insulin stress [test], 261
Insulin [test], 138–140, 139f
Insulin tolerance [test], 243, 261
Interferences, laboratory, 5, 6–7
Interleukin-1, 438, 469

Interleukin-2, 438
    suppression of, 364
Intermediate density lipoproteins, 173, 179, 182
    and flow chart for evaluation of hyperlipoproteinemias, 186f–187f
    increased characteristics, 183t
    properties of, 174t
Intermediate density lipoprotein [test], 193
Internal quality control, 6
International normalized ratio (INR): for prothrombin time, 523, 526, 534t
International sensitivity index (ISI): for thromboplastin, 526
International System (SI) units, 7
Interpretation of test results, 7–10, 8f, 9f
Intestinal infarction, 90
    alkaline phosphatase and, 73
Intestinal perforation, 90
Intestinal wall: parasites, 702t, 702–703
Intra-arterial optode, 22–23
Intracellular killing, functional assays for [test], 597
Intravascular catheter culture [test], 633–634
Intravascular coagulation [tests], 545–546
Intravenous glucose tolerance tests, 135
Intrinsic factor (IF), 96, 845t
    deficiency, 97
    Schilling test and, 475
Intrinsic system, 502, 504–505, 505f
Inulin clearance [test], 44, 59–60
In vitro/in vivo correlation, 789–790, 790t
In vitro susceptibility [tests], 789–795
    anaerobic susceptibility test, 792
    antimicrobial testing, 791–793
    β-lactamase test, 793–794
    dilution methods, 791–792, 793
    disk diffusion test, 792
    indications for, 791t
    interpretative designations defined, 793t
    minimum bactericidal concentration (MBC), 794–795
    serum bactericidal test (SBT), 794–795
Iodamoeba beutschlii, 760t
Iodine, protein bound [test], 251–252
Iodoproteins, 251
Iodotyrosines, 251

Ion-specific electrodes:
    for potassium, 46
    for sodium, 46
Iron, 199
    and hemoglobin, 427
    toxic levels for, 391t
    toxic symptoms/concentrations, 391t
    transferrin and, 468–470
Iron [test]:
    abnormal absorption, 98
    for anemia, 450t, 468–470, 469t
    toxicity, 390t, 390–392
Iron deficiency:
    ferritin test for, 466f, 466–468
    and glycohemoglobin, 137
    inflammatory diseases and, 467f
    PNH and, 482
    protoporphyrin and, 470
    TIBC and, 469
Iron deficiency anemia, 447, 448, 449, 449t, 450t, 451t, 453, 481, 482
    ferritin test for, 466t, 466–468
    immunologic effects, 862
    protein levels and, 156t, 167
    TIBC test for, 469
Iron overload: and scurvy, 233
Iron profile [test]: for anemia, 468–470, 469t
Iron toxicity [test], 390t, 390–392
Islet cells: autoantibody, 845t
Islet cell tumors, 141
Isobutyric acid, 417
Isoelectric focusing: for CK isoenzymes, 29, 30t
Isoelectric point, 143
Isoleucine: biochemistry and reference range, 144t
Isoniazid (INH):
    drug interactions, 341, 344t
    hemolytic anemia from, 894t
    and hepatic necrosis, 77
    vitamin B$_6$ deficiency, 225, 226
Isopropanol:
    properties, 375t
    volatile concentrations from D-Osm, 379t, 380
Isopropanol [test], 378
    denaturation, 494
Isopropyl alcohol [test], 378
Isospora belli:
    and AIDS, 860
    gastroenteritis, 752t, 759, 760, 760t
Isovaleric acid, 414, 417
Isovaleric acidemia, 417
ITT (insulin tolerance test), 243, 261
Ixodes dammini, 807

J

Jaffé reaction, 43
Japanese B encephalitis, 772t
Jaundice:
    differential diagnosis of, 74t
    and pneumonia, 660t
JC polyomavirus, 771t, 777t
    urinary, 730, 730t
Joint disease, degenerative: synovial fluid examination, 117t
Junin virus, 771, 772t
    serology [test], 817
JV virus, 773

K

Kala-azar, 681t, 702, 704, 706
    serology, 831
Kallikrein, 504, 540
Kallman syndrome, 290t
    and hypogonadism, 293t
Kanamycin:
    monitoring [test], 797–798
    reference range, 798t
Kaposi sarcoma, 860
Kasahara isoenzyme, 74t, 310
Katayama fever, 703
Kawasaki disease, 861
Kayser-Fleischer rings, 169, 204, 207f, 208, 415
Keratinin, 151
Keratitis, 635, 648, 651, 652
    ulcerative, 649
Keratoconjunctivitis, 648
Keratocytes, 433
Keratomalacia, 216
Kerion, 681t
    skin manifestations, 679t
Keshan disease, 210
Ketoamines [test], 137–138
α-Ketobutyrate, 36
Ketoconazole: drug interactions, 364
17-Ketogenic steroid, 264
Ketonuria, 54, 55
"Kidney function" factor, 357
Kidneys. *See also* Nephrotic syndrome *and under term* Renal
    and acid-base balance, 12, 14
    and acid-base disturbances, 18t, 18–20
    and calcium regulation, 296t
    LD levels in, 36
    toxicity to. *See* Nephrotoxicity
    tumor markers, 317, 323, 325
Kimmelstiel-Wilson syndrome, 51
Kingella denitrificans, 736

Kinikase II [test], 277
Kininogen, high molecular weight: deficiency, 516t, 540
Kininogen, high molecular weight [test], 540
Kinky hair disease, 200t, 204
Kjeldahl's method, 153
Klebsiella. See also Enterobacteriaceae
    antigenemia, 633
    traumatic wounds, 718
    in urine, 725
Klebsiella ozaenae: nasal infection, 638, 639
Klebsiella pneumoniae:
    and burn wounds, 717
    cultures, 697t
    respiratory infection, 657, 666
Klebsiella rhinoscleromatis:
    nasal infection, 638, 639
    skin/tissue manifestations, 681t
Kleihauer-Betke (acid elution for fetal hemoglobin) [test], 495
Klinefelter syndrome, 290t
"Koagulation" vitamin, 221. *See also* Vitamin K
Koplik spots, 642, 643t, 824
Kupffer cells, 161
Kuru, 774, 777, 777t
Kyasanur Forest disease, 772t

L

LA. *See* Latex agglutination test
Laboratory analysis, 6–7
Laboratory interferences, 5, 6–7
Laboratory tests:
    analysis, 6–7
    criteria for evaluting usefulness, 4t
    decision matrix, 3f
    diagnosis, 1–4
    expenditures on, 1
    interpretation of results, 7–10, 8f, 9f
    patient monitoring, 5
    patient preparation, 5–6, 6t
    principles of, 1–10
    reference ranges, 7t, 7–8
    reports, 7
    screening, 4–5
    selection, 1, 2f
    specimen acquisition, 5–6, 6t
LaCrosse virus, 771, 772t
α-Lactalbumin: and breast cancer, 329t
Lactase deficiency, 96t

Lactate:
    formation of, 128
    pleural fluid [test], 116
    in synovial fluid, 118–120, 125t
Lactate [test], 109–111, 110t, 775, 785
    and bacterial vs. nonbacterial meningitis, 110t
Lactate dehydrogenase (LD):
    and acetaminophen, 226
    activities, 32t, 128
    in cerebrospinal fluid, 108t
    flipped, 35f, 36
    increased, with normal bilirubin, 79t
    isoenzymes
        LD-5, 79, 79f, 727
        LD-6, 78, 79, 79f
        structure and distribution, 32t
        time course in myocardial infarction, 33f–35f
    isoenzymes [test], 32–36
    and myocardial infarction, 26f, 29, 70
    urinary LD-5 isoenzyme, 727
Lactate dehydrogenase (LD) [test], 31–32
    CSF, 111
    and liver function, 78–79, 79f, 79t
    tumor marker, 311
Lactobacillus: urinary, 724
Lactose, 54
    dietary, 127
    malabsorption, 96t
Lactoxylidide (LX), 356
Lamellar bodies: in amniotic fluid, 408–409, 410f
LAP (leukocyte alkaline phosphatase) [test], 608–609
Large cell lymphoma, 856f
Large cell lymphoma cells, 440–441, 856f
Large granular lymphocyte (LGL), 439
Large granular lymphocytic leukemia:
    immunophenotyping, 602
    morphology/manifestations/markers, 574t
Laron dwarfs, 240, 241
Laryngitis, 635, 641
Laryngotracheobronchitis (croup), 635, 643t, 646
Lassa fever virus, 771, 772t
    serology [test], 817
Latex agglutination autoantibody, 845t
Latex agglutination test:
    for coccidioidomycosis, 828

for cryptococcosis, 827t, 828
    for fungi, 825, 825t
    for *Rickettsia*, 811
Latrodectus mactans, 677t
LATS protector, 256
LD. *See* Lactate dehydrogenase
LDH. *See* Lactate dehydrogenase
LDLs. *See* Low density lipoproteins
L-Dopa: hemolytic anemia from, 894t
Lead:
    monitoring occupational exposure, 392t
    toxic symptoms/concentrations, 391t
Lead [test], 390t, 390–392
Lead poisoning, 56t, 58
    and anemia, 448, 449t
    and glycohemoglobin, 137
    protoporphyrin and, 470, 471
LE cells:
    pleural fluid [test], 116
    in synovial fluid, 118t
Lecithin, 182, 185
Lecithin cholesterol acyltransferase, 175
Lecithin-to-sphingomyelin ratio [test], 408–409
Legionella:
    antigens, 671
    and endocarditis, 623, 626t
    environmental exposure, 659t
    pneumonia, 657, 659, 664, 665–666, 668, 670t, 671, 814
    serology [test], 806
Leg ulcers, 679t
Leishmania donovani, 702, 702t
    blood examination [test], 629t, 631–632
    serology [test], 831
    skin/tissue manifestations, 681t, 685
Leishmaniasis. *See also specific species*
    serology [test], 830t, 831
Leishmania tropica: skin/tissue manifestations, 681t, 685
Leprosy:
    lesions, agent, and tests, 678t
    Slavic, 638
Leptocytes, 434
Leptomeningeal metastases: CSF measures, 114
Leptomeningitis, 770
Leptospira, 713
    blood culture [test], 622, 625–626
    lymphadenopathy, 715
    serology [test], 807
    urine culture [test], 728

Leptospira interrogans: environmental exposure, 659t
Lesch-Nyhan syndrome, 45, 52
Letterer-Siwe disease, 581
Leu M3, 853t, 599t
Leu M5, 853t, 599t
Leu 7, 852t, 853t, 599t
Leu 12, 852t, 599t
Leu 14, 852t, 599t
Leu 16, 852t, 599t
Leucine:
    alkaline phosphatase isoenzymes and, 73t, 74, 74t
    biochemistry and reference range, 144t
    crystals in urine, 52, 63f
    and cystinuria, 148
Leucovirin, 365, 366
Leukemia/lymphoma, adult T-cell, 441
    morphology/manifestations/markers, 575t
Leukemias, 556, 559. *See also* Leukemias, acute *and specific leukemias*
    of differentiated B lymphocytes, 571t–573t, 576–581
    of differentiated T lymphocytes, 574t–575t, 576–581
    mast cell, 581
    methotrexate for, 365
    testing for, 841
    tumor markers, 311
    vitamin B_{12} and, 228, 228t
Leukemias, acute, 559–565
    characteristics, 561t
    chromosomal abnormalities in, 562t
    erythro-, Plate 18, 445
    lymphocytic, 564t, 565t. *See also* Lymphocytic leukemia
    megakaryocytic, Plate 19, 561, 563t
    monoblastic, 563t, 564
    monocytic, Plate 17, 445, 561, 562, 563t, 564t
    morphology of, 444t, 444–445
    myelocytic, 561, 563t, 564t. *See also* Myelocytic leukemia
    myelocytic with maturation, Plate 14, 444
    myeloid without maturation, Plate 13, 444
    myelomonocytic, Plate 16, 444, 563t, 564t, 605
    promyelocytic, Plate 15, 444, 561, 563t, 564t
    reaction of leukocyte stains, 604, 604t

Leukemia typing [test], 598–603
Leukemic phase of lymphoma, 576, 579
    B-cell morphology/manifestations/markers, Plates 27B/28A, 572t, 573t
    T-cell morphology/manifestations/markers, 575t
Leukemoid reaction, 567, 569, 569t, 585
    chronic myelocytic leukemia vs., 567, 569t
    differentiation, 569t
        from hematopoietic malignancy, 576t
    disorders associated with, 557t
Leukemoid states: causes of, 557t
Leukocyte. *See* White blood cells
Leukocyte acid phosphatase [test], 609
Leukocyte alkaline phosphatase [test], 608–609
Leukocyte common antigen, 602
Leukocyte count [test], 581–583
Leukocyte differential [test], 583–589
Leukocyte esterase: in urine, 55, 725, 726t
Leukocyte peroxidase [test], 603–605
Leukocyte proteases: α_1-antitrypsin and, 165–166
Leukocytosis, 107
    causes of, 557t
    vitamin B_{12} and, 228, 228t
Leukoerythroblastic reactions: causes of, 588–589, 589t
Leukopenia:
    bone marrow aspiration for, 610
    causes of, 610
Levorphanol: characteristics of, 389t
Lewis A antigen: cancer antigens and, 316, 317
Leydig cell, 122, 283, 285, 289, 293
    testicular failure of, 124
LGV. *See* Lymphogranuloma venereum
LH. *See* Luteinizing hormone
LHRH. *See* Luteinizing releasing hormone
Libermann-Burchard reaction, 177
Lice:
    body, 677t, 745
    pubic, 677t, 745
    pubic [test], 745
Lidocaine:
    continuous infusion, 336f
    drug interactions, 349, 352, 363
    therapeutic range, concentration, and distribution, 334t

Lidocaine [test], 351–352
Light chain disease:
    immunoelectrophoresis for, 163–165
    kappa, 165
    lambda, 165
Light-chain disease, 164
    high resolution serum protein electrophoresis, 159–160, 161
Likelihood ratio, 8–9
Liley chart, 405, 406f
Limulus lysate assay [test], 708
    CSF, 775, 785
Linoleic acid, 181, 182t
Linolenic acid, 181, 182t
Lipase [test], 87f, 88–89, 90
Lipid-lowering drugs: platelet disorders induced by, 516t
Lipid Research Clinics (LRC) programs, 177
Lipids, 173. *See also specific lipids*
    casts in urine, 51
    classification properties of, 174t
Lipids [tests], 173–182
    cholesterol, 173–178, 174f–176f, 178t, 179t
    fatty acids, 181f, 181–182, 182t
    phospholipids, 182
    triglycerides, 178–181, 179f, 180t, 181t
Lipocyte (fat cell), 443
Lipoproteinemias:
    classification of, 182–185, 183t–184t
    hyper-, 183t, 185, 186f–187f
    hypo-, 184t, 185
    primary and secondary, 185
Lipoproteins, 173, 182–185. *See also specific types, e.g.* High density lipoproteins
    α_1, 156t, 161
    α_2, 156t, 161
    β. *See* β-Lipoproteins [tests]
    classification properties of, 174t
    X, 193
Lipoproteins [tests], 185–191, 186f–187f
    apolipoproteins, 174t, 183t, 184t, 193–195, 194t, 195t
    β. *See* low density *below*
    chylomicrons, 191–192
    high density, 174t, 185–189, 188t, 189t
    intermediate density, 193
    low density, 178t, 179f, 189–191, 190f, 191t
    very low density, 192, 192t

β-Lipoproteins [tests], 189–191. *See also* Low density lipoproteins
   floating, 193. *See also* Intermediate density lipoproteins
   pre, 192, 192t. *See also* Very low density lipoproteins
Listeria monocytogenes:
   CNS infections, 770
   infections, 624t
   osteomyelitis, 710
   skin manifestations, 677t, 678t, 679t
Lithic acid [test], 44–45
Lithium:
   therapeutic range, concentration, and distribution, 334t, 393, 393t
   toxicities, 360, 393, 393t
Lithium [test], 360, 392–394
Lithium heparin crystals: in synovial fluid, 119t
Lithocholic acid, 81
Liver abscess, 701, 702–703, 706, 707, 784
   testing for, 704, 705–707
Liver aspiration, 705
Liver biopsy, 705
   copper [test], 206, 206t, 208
   for hemochromatosis, 470
Liver disease:
   and alkaline phosphatase levels, 72, 72t
   aminoaciduria in, 148
   and anemia, 451t
   bilirubin and, 74–75
   CEA elevation in, 319, 319t
   cholestatic, differential diagnosis, 208t
   classification of, 68t
   complement test and, 168
   encephalopathy, 78
   end-stage, 78
   α-fetoprotein tumor marker, 314, 315
   and hemochromatosis, 98
   and hemostatic disorders, 518, 521, 522t, 523, 523t, 526, 527, 540, 549
   hepatitis. *See* Hepatitis
   and hypercholesterolemia, 178
   leucine crystals and, 52
   protein levels and, 156t, 157t, 161
   vitamin B_{12} and, 228, 228t
   zinc deficiency and, 211
Liver flukes, 702–703, 704–705, 706, 762
Liver function, 67–68

   analytes to evaluate, 67t
   information obtained from analytes, 68t
   LD levels and, 32, 36
   metabolic, 67, 67t
Liver function [tests], 68–84
   alanine aminotransferase, 68–69, 69t
   albumin, 76
   and alcoholic hepatitis, 77
   alkaline phosphatase, 70–74, 71f, 71t, 72t, 73t, 74t
   ammonia, 78, 78t
   antimitochondrial antibodies, 81
   anti-smooth muscle antibodies, 81
   aspartate aminotransferase, 69t, 69–70, 70t
   bile acids, 81
   bilirubin, 74t, 74–75, 75t
   ceruloplasmin, 82
   and cholestasis, 77
   and cirrhosis, 77
   and drug-induced hepatitis, 77
   α-fetoprotein, 81
   γ-glutamyl transferase, 79–80, 80t
   glutamine, 80
   indocyanine-green excretion, 82
   interpretation of patterns, 76
   and ischemic disease, 78
   lactate dehydrogenase, 78–79, 79f, 79t
   and neoplasia, 77–78
   5′-nucleotidase, 80
   ornithine carbamoyltransferase, 82
   orthophosphoric monoester phosphohydrolase, 70–74
   pseudocholinesterase, 75–76, 76t
   retinol-binding protein, 83
   serum glutamate oxaloacetate transaminase, 69–70
   serum glutamate pyruvate transaminase, 68–69
   and viral hepatitis, 76–77
Liver infections:
   parasites, 702t, 702–703
   testing for, 702
Liver metastases:
   enzyme activity and, 309, 309t, 310
   tumor markers, 309, 309t, 310, 311, 315
Liver parasites, 702t, 702–703
L-Lactate [test]: glycogen storage diseases, 420–422
L-Lactic acidosis: causes of, 422, 422t
Lloyd's reagent, 43

L-*myc*, 328t
Loa loa, 632, 632t, 649, 650, 651, 685
   lymphadenopathy, 715
Locura manganica, 209
Löffler's syndrome, 673, 761
Long-acting thyroid stimulator (LATS), 256
Lorazepam: half-life and therapeutic/toxic concentrations, 384t
Louping ill, 772t
Low density lipoproteins, 182
   cholesterol and, 189–190, 191t
   conditions and disorders affecting ranges of, 156t
   decreased characteristics, 184t
   and flow chart for evaluation of hyperlipoproteinemias, 186f–187f
   and hypercholesterolemia, 189–191
   increased abnormality characteristics, 183t
   properties of, 174t
   triglycerides and, 179
Low density lipoproteins [test], 178t, 179f, 189–191, 190f, 191t
Low ionic strength solutions (LISS), 876, 877
LRH (luteinizing releasing hormone) stimulation [test], 286–287
LSD (lysurgic acid diethylamide): testing for, 372, 386
L-Tartrate, 313
L-Tyrosine apodecarboxylase assay: for vitamin B_6, 226t
Ludwig's angina, 641
Lumbar puncture, 107, 775. *See also* Cerebrospinal fluid
Lundh [test], 93–94
Lung biopsy, open, 664
Lung cancer:
   amylase production, 309
   and oncogenes, 328t
   tumor markers, 309, 316, 317, 319t, 320–321, 325
Lung fluke, 672t, 674, 762
   serology [test], 831
Lungs. *See also* Respiratory system
   and acid-base disturbances, 18t, 18–20
   disease. *See* Pneumonia; Pulmonary disease.
   fetal maturity testing, 408–410, 410t
   LD levels in, 32, 36

Lupus anticoagulants, 516, 517t, 520, 539, 540, 543, 544
Lupus erythematosus. *See* Systemic lupus erythematosus
Lupus vulgaris, 681t
Luteinizing hormone (LH), 122, 237, 269, 283–284, 284f, 321–322, 400
  and menstrual cycle, 284f
  reference intervals, 286t
Luteinizing hormone (LH) [test], 285–286, 286t
Luteinizing releasing hormone stimulation [test], 286–287
Luteotropic hormone. *See* Luteinizing hormone
Lutropin. *See* Luteinizing hormone
Lyme disease, 677t, 769
  serology, 807–808, 810
Lymphadenitis: causes of, 714–715
Lymphadenopathies:
  architecture of reactive and malignant, 616t
  causes of, 577t, 610, 613–614
  genital tract [test], 740–743
Lymphadenopathy-associated virus. *See* Human immunodeficiency virus
Lymphatic obstruction: malabsorption and, 91t
Lymph node: architecture of, 615f
Lymph node [tests], 714–715
  biopsy, 613–617
Lymphoblast, 439
  stain reactions, 604t
Lymphoblastic lymphoma, 441
Lymphocyte marker studies [test], 840–841, 841t
Lymphocytes, Plate 8A, 425, 439
  absolute count [test], 838, 840
  atypical (reactive), Plate 10A, 440
  B, 438, 837–838. *See also* B lymphocytes
  in bone marrow aspiration, 612t
  in cerebrospinal fluid, 108, 108t
  deficiencies, 553–554
  large granular (LGL), 439
  marker studies [test], 840–841, 841t. *See also* Immunophenotyping [test]
  morphology, 438–439
  in pleural fluid, 115
  production, differentiation, and localization, 553
  reference values for cell count and slide differential, 586t–587t
  specific quantitation [test], 840–841, 841t
  stain reactions, 604t
  subpopulation [test], 840–841, 841t
  T, 438, 837–838. *See also* T lymphocytes
  total count [test], 838, 840
Lymphocytic choriomeningitis virus, 771
  arthritis, 707
Lymphocytic leukemia, acute (ALL), 445, 559, 852
  characteristics, 561t
  chromosomal abnormality, 562t
  classification, 562, 564, 564t, 565t
  immunophenotyping, 602, 856f
  L1, Plate 20, 445, 564, 564t
  L2, 445, 564, 564t
  L3 (Burkitt type), Plate 21, 445, 564, 564t, 579
  TdT testing, 607
  testing for, 855–856
Lymphocytic leukemia, chronic (CLL), 579, 854
  B-cell, 562t
  chromosomal abnormality, 562t
  immunophenotyping, 602, 856f
  morphology/manifestations/markers, 571t
  non-Hodgkin's lymphoma and, 579
  testing for, 855–856
  T-helper, morphology/manifestations/markers, 574t–575t
Lymphocytic leukemia, large granular:
  immunophenotyping, 602
  morphology/manifestations/markers, 574t
Lymphocytic leukocytosis: causes of, 557t
Lymphocytopenia: causes of, 588
Lymphocytopoiesis, 428f, 438–441
Lymphocytosis: causes of, 554t, 585
Lymphogranuloma inguinale: ulcer, 679t, 740, 741, 742
Lymphogranuloma venereum (LGV), 715, 740–743, 814
Lymphoid leukemoid reaction. *See also* Leukemoid reaction
  hematopoietic malignancy vs., 576t, 585
Lymphoid stem cell (LSC), 426f
Lymphokines, 851
Lymphoma, 559, 576–579, 714
  bone marrow aspiration for, 610, 611
  chromosomal abnormalities in, 562t
  immunophenotyping, 603
  leukemic phase of, 572t, 575t, 576, 579
  methotrexate for, 365
  tumor markers, 311
Lymphoma, malignant, 579
  chromosomal abnormality, 562t
Lymphoma, non-Hodgkin's, 577–579
  and AIDS, 860
  classification systems, 615
  immunophenotyping, 603
  lymph node biopsy for, 613
  tissue mast cells and, 443
  Working Formulation, 579t, 615
Lymphoma cells, Plate 21A, Plate 21B, Plate 27B, Plate 28A, 440–441
  stain reactions, 604t
Lymphoma typing [test], 598–603
Lymphopenia: causes of, 556t
Lymphopoiesis: diagrammatic representation, 428f–429f
Lymphoproliferative disorders: testing for, 841, 853t
Lymphoproliferative malignancy: lymphoid leukemoid reaction vs., 576t
Lymphosarcoma cell leukemia, 579
  morphology/manifestations/markers, Plates 27B/28A, 575t
Lysine, 143
  biochemistry and reference range, 144t
  and cystinuria, 148
Lysozyme [test], 606
Lysurgic acid diethylamide (LSD): testing for, 372, 386
Lysyl oxidase, 202

M

Machupo virus, 771, 772t
  serology [test], 817
Macroamylasemia, 88, 90
Macrocytes, 433, 463
Macrocytic anemia, 449–450, 451t, 467f, 474t, 610
Macrocytic anemia [tests], 471–476
  deoxyuridine suppression, 476
  folate, 472t, 473–475, 474t
  methylmalonic acid, 476
  Schilling, 473t, 475–476
  vitamin B_{12} (cobalamin), 471–472, 472t, 473t
Macrocytosis, 462–463
  spurious, 451t
α_2-Macroglobulin, 89, 116
  conditions and disorders affecting ranges of, 156t

in serum protein electrophoresis test, 155
α$_2$-Macroglobulin [test], 166
Macronormoblast, 431
Macro-ovalocyte, 431
Macrophage/histiocyte, Plate 30A, 437–438
Macrophages:
　atypical, 581
　in cerebrospinal fluid, 108t
　malignancies of, 581
　regulatory function, 437
Maculopapules: disease, etiology, and tests for, 677t–678t, 684, 686–687, 688f
Madurella grisea, 681t
Madurella mycetomatis, 681t
Magnesium [test], 299–300
Maintenance dose equation, 336t
Major histocompatibility antigens, 851
Malabsorption, 90–99
　carbohydrate, 95–96, 96t
　classification of, 91t
　pancreatic exocrine function tests, 91–98
　　abnormal iron absorption, 98
　　bentiromide (tripeptide hydrolysis test), 92–93
　　breath hydrogen test, 95–96
　　carbohydrate intolerance, 95–96, 96t
　　β-carotene and carotenoids, 97
　　$_{14}$C-triolein breath, 94
　　disaccharidase deficiency, 96
　　D-xylose absorption, 95
　　fatty meal, 94–95
　　fecal fat, 93
　　Lundh, 93–94
　　Schilling, 96–97
　　secretin, 91–92
　　secretin-cholecystokinin, 92
　　vitamin B$_{12}$ malabsorption, 96–97
　signs and symptoms of, 91t
Malaria, See also *Plasmodium*
　blood examination [test], 629, 629t, 630, 630t
　cerebral, 775, 777t, 778, 782
　serology [test], 830t, 831
Malassezia furfur:
　blood, 624t
　cultures, 697t
　skin manifestations, 678t
Maldigestion, 90. *See also* Malabsorption
Male PAP test: tumor marker, 311–313, 312t

Malignant cells: in synovial fluid, 118t
Malignant histiocytosis, 581
Malignant hypertension: pheochromocytoma and, 278
Malignant lymphoma. *See* Lymphoma, malignant
Malignant pleural effusions, 116
Maltase, 95
　deficiency, 96t
Maltose, 95
　malabsorption, 96t
Maltotriose malabsorption, 96t
Malt-worker's lung, 668
MAM 6: and breast cancer, 329t
Manganese, 199
　abnormalities, 200t
　body content, 199t
　excretion route, 200t
　reference ranges, 209t
Manganese madness, 209
Manganese [test], 209
Manganism, 209
Manic depression: carbamazepine for, 340
Mansonella ozzardi, 632, 632t
Mansonella perstans, 632, 632t
Mansonella streptocerca, 632, 632t
Manual differential [test], 583–589
Maple syrup urine disease, 52, 55, 144t, 147, 148
　enzymatic defect and features of, 146t
　testing for, 411, 414
Maprotiline: therapeutic ranges and toxicities, 396t
Marburg virus, 649t
　serology [test], 817
Marginal granulocyte pool (MGP), 435
Marginal monocyte pool (MMP), 437
Marijuana:
　and emergency room, 370t
　testing for, 386, 387, 387t, 388t
　and theophylline clearance, 335t
Marrow:
　cellularity, 425, 430f
　red, 425
　yellow, 425
Mass spectometry: in drug toxicology, 374, 374t
Mast cell:
　proliferation, 581
　stain reactions, 604t
Mast cell leukemia, 581
Mastocytosis: systemic, 581
Mastoid abscess, 638
Mastoiditis, 637
May-Hegglin anomaly, 555, 558t, 589

MBC. *See* Minimum bactericidal concentration
MBP (myelin basic protein) [test], 113t, 113–114
McArdle's disease, 420, 421, 421t, 422
Mean:
　regression to the, 7
　standard deviation from, 6, 7
Mean cell hemoglobin (MCH), 457, 459, 460t, 461
Mean cell hemoglobin concentration (MCHC), 427, 457, 458f, 459, 460t, 461
Mean cell volume (MCV), 450, 457, 459, 460t, 461, 461t, 462–463
Mean platelet volume [test], 595–596, 596f, 597t
Measles. *See* Rubeola virus
Mechanical ventilation monitoring, 16, 17
Medullary thyroid carcinoma, 302, 307, 321
Mefenamic acid: hemolytic anemia from, 894t
Megakaryoblast, 426f, 441, 442
Megakaryoblastic leukemia, acute, Plate 19, 445
Megakaryocyte, 426f, 441, 442, 609–610
　and bone marrow aspiration, 611–612
　dysplastic, 442
　morphology, 442
　stain reactions, 604t
Megakaryocyte–colony stimulating activity (Meg-CSA), 441
Megakaryocytic leukemia, 561, 563t, 564t, 610
　stains for, 606
Megaloblastic anemia, 449, 451t, 463, 473
　LD levels in, 36
　protein ranges in, 156t
Megaloblastic erythropoiesis, Plate 1, 427, 431
Megaloblastic nucleated red blood cells, Plate 7, 431
Megaloblastoid nucleated red blood cell, 431
Melanocyte stimulating hormone, 265f
Melanogens, 55
Mellidioisis, 659t
Melphalan: hemolytic anemia from, 894t
Membrane glycoprotein expression [test], 537
Menadione, 222

Menaquinones, 221
Mendelian single gene disorders, 411, 412
Meningeal metastases: CSF markers for, 114
Meninges, 768
Meningitis, 769
   acute, 770
   aseptic, 770, 771, 776t, 776–777, 785
   bacterial, 107, 108, 109, 110t, 111, 770, 775–776, 781, 781t, 785
     and lactic acid in CSF, 110t
     protein levels, 170
   chronic, 770
   fungal, 770, 775–776, 781, 781t
   nonbacterial: and lactic acid in CSF, 110t
   pyogenic, 109
   recurrent, 770
   tuberculous, 109, 111
   viral, 770–774, 776t, 776–777, 781t, 781–782
Meningococcemia, 677t
Meningoencephalitis:
   parasitic, 777t, 778, 782
   primary amebic (PAM), 774, 778, 779
   viral, 770–771, 771t, 822
Menkes disease, 200t, 204, 206
   genetic testing, 415–416
Menopause, 285
   and hypogonadism, 293t
Menses, 285
Menstrual cycle, 284, 284f, 285, 292–293
MEN syndrome, 101
Mental retardation, genetic. *See* Genetic disorders
Meperidine:
   characteristics of, 389t
   testing for, 389, 389t
Mephobarbital [test], 384–386, 385t
Mercury:
   monitoring occupational exposure, 392t
   toxic symptoms/concentrations, 391t
Mercury [test], 390t, 390–392
Mesothelial cells: pleural, 115, 116
Metabolic acidosis, 17, 18, 18t, 21
   chloride depletion and, 47
Metabolic alkalosis, 17, 18t, 19–20, 20t, 21
Metabolic bone disease:
   bone marrow aspiration for, 610
   osteocalcin and, 302

Metabolic disorders: malabsorption and, 91t
Metabolic screen [test], 414
Metacercariae, 761
Metagonimus yokogawai, 762, 762t
Metaiodobenzyl-guanidine (MIBG) scintigraphy, 281
Metalloporphyrins, 55
Metals. *See* Trace metals
Metal toxicology [tests], 390–392
Metamyelocyte, 434, 435
   giant, 436
Metamyelocytes: in bone marrow aspiration, 612t
Metanephrines, 277, 278, 279, 280, 281
Metanephrine [test], 280
Metarubricyte, 427
Metastases:
   breast cancer, 327
   enzyme activity in liver, 309, 309t
   lymph node biopsy for, 613, 614
   tumor markers for, 309, 318. *See also* Tumor markers
Methadone:
   characteristics of, 389t
   testing for, 388–389, 389t
Methanol:
   properties, 375t
   volatile concentrations from D-Osm, 379t, 380
Methanol [test], 377–378
Methemoglobin: and xanthochromia, 107
Methemoglobinemia, 456
Methionine, 471
   biochemistry and reference range, 144t
   dietary restriction, 149
   elevated, 414
   metabolism, 471
Methotrexate:
   drug interactions, 366
   hemolytic anemia from, 894t
   therapeutic range, concentration, and distribution, 334t
   toxicity, 365
Methotrexate [test], 365–366
3-Methoxy-4-hydroxymandelic acid, 277, 278f
3-Methoxy-4-hydroxymandelic acid [test], 279–280
3-Methoxy-4-hydroxyphenylglycol, 277, 278f
3-Methoxy-4-hydroxyphenylglycol [test], 283
Methoxymethylenedioxyamphemine (MMDA), 386

Methyl alcohol [test], 377–378
Methylcobalamin, 471
3-Methylcrotonyl-CoA, 222
β-Methylcrototonylglycinuria, 223
α-Methyldopa: hemolytic anemia from, 889t, 894t
Methylenedioxyamphemine (MDA), 386
Methylmalonic acid [test], 476
Methylmalonic acidemia, 78, 417
Methyl malonyl coenzyme A, 471
Methylphenidate: drug interactions, 361
Metoclopramide: drug interactions, 352
Metyrapone test, 268
Mexiletine [test], 352–353
MHA-TP (microhemagglutination antibody, *T. pallidum*) [test], 810t, 810–811
MHPG (3-methoxy-4-hydroxyphenyl-glycol), 277, 278f
MHPG (3-methoxy-4-hydroxyphenyl-glycol) [test], 283
Michaelis-Menten equations, 339, 345t
Microadenomas, 241
Microaerophilic streptococci: skin manifestations, 679t
Micrococcus: cultures, 696t
Microcytes, 433
Microcytic anemias, 448–449, 449t, 450t, 462
Microcytic anemia [tests], 466–471
   ferritin, 466t, 466–468, 467f, 468t
   iron, 468–470, 469t
   protoporphyrin, erythrocyte, 470–471
Microfilariae:
   blood examination [test], 629t, 630, 632
   urinary, 732
β$_2$-Microglobulin (B2M):
   conditions and disorders affecting levels of, 157t, 161
   as tumor marker, 114
   urinary measure, 726
β$_2$-Microglobulin (B2M) [test], 166–167
Microhemagglutination antibody, *T. pallidum* (MHA-TP) [test], 810t, 810–811
Microimmunofluorescence test:
   for aspergillosis, 825–826
   for *Chlamydia*, 814
   for *Rickettsia*, 811, 812t, 813
Microsomal autoantibody, 845t
Microsporum audouinii, 680t

skin manifestations, 678t
Microsporum canis: skin manifestations, 678t
Microsporum tonsurans: skin manifestations, 678t
Midmolecule assay: parathyroid hormone, 300, 301t, 302
MIF. *See* Microimmunofluorescence test
Migraine: carbamazepine for, 340
Milker's nodule, 681t
Millon reaction, 147
Mineralocorticoids, 257, 258f
 deficiency, 257, 259
 and hypertension, 276t
Minimum bactericidal concentration (MBC), 790
Minimum bactericidal concentration (MBC) [test], 794–795
Minimum inhibitory concentration (MIC), 789–790, 792, 793
Mitochondrial autoantibody, 845t
Mitogens, 854–855
Mitogen stimulation test, 853t
Mixed acid-base disorders, 20, 21f
Mixed connective tissue disease autoantibody, 845t
MMM. *See* Myelofibrosis with myeloid metaplasia
Mobiluncus: vaginosis, 734t
Molar disease, 401, 408
Molecular genetic analysis [test], 411–413
Molluscum contagiosum, 681t, 684
 eye infection, 649t
Molybdenum:
 abnormalities, 200t
 body content, 199t
 excretion route, 200t
Molybdenum [test], 209–210
Monoamine oxidase, 277
Monoamine oxidase inhibitors: drug interactions, 341, 359
Monoblast, 426f, 437
 stain reactions, 604t
Monoblastic leukemia, 563t, 564
Monoclonal CEA [test], 318–319
Monoclonal gammopathies, 155, 155f
 benign, 581
 high resolution serum protein electrophoresis, 159–160
 immunoelectrophoresis for, 163f, 163–165, 164t
 immunofixation (IFE) test for, 162, 162f
 secondary, 581
Monoclonal gammopathy of unknown significance (MGUS), 581
Monoclonal proteins: conditions associated with, 164t
Monocytes, 425, 437–438
 antigen markers, 599t
 in bone marrow aspiration, 612t
 circulating pool (CMP), 437
 function, 553
 macrophage/histiocyte, 437–438
 marginal pool (MMP), 437
 monoblast, 437
 morphology, 437
 promonocyte, 437
 reference values for cell count and slide differential, 586t–587t
 in synovial fluid, 118t
Monocytic esterase, 605
Monocytic leukemia, Plate 17, 445, 561, 562, 563t, 564t, 605
 stains for, 606
Monocytopenia: causes of, 556t, 588
Monocytopoiesis, 437–438
 morphology, 437–438
Monocytosis: causes of, 554t, 585
Monoethyl-glycinexylidide (MEGX), 352
Monomyelocytic leukemia, 561
Monophenal monoxygenase, 202
Monosaccharides, 95
Monosodium urate crystals: in synovial fluid, 119t, 120f, 121f, 122f
Montenegro skin test: for leishmaniasis, 831
Moonshine, 377
Moraxella catarrhalis
 conjunctival colonization, 648
 ear infection, 637, 638
 lower respiratory infection, 657, 669t
 sinusitis, 640
 susceptibility testing, 789, 793
 upper respiratory infections, 645t
Moraxella lacunata: eye infections, 648
Moraxella tuberculosis: eye infections, 648
Morphine:
 characteristics of, 389t
 metabolism, 372
 testing for, 387t, 388–389, 389t
Morphine 3-glucuronide, 372
Morquio syndrome, 416
Mott cells, 440
Mouse rosette, 854, 856f
MPD. *See* Myeloproliferative disorders
MPO [test], 603–605
M proteins, 163–165, 166, 169
MPV (mean platelet volume) [test], 595–596, 596f, 597t
MSH, 265f, 321
Mucin, 99
 clot in synovial fluid, 118, 119f
Mucomist, 382
Mucopolysaccharides [test], 416–417
Mucopolysaccharidoses, 589
Mucopurulent cervicitis, 740
Mucopus, 740
Mucor, 640, 668, 671t, 692
 cultures, 697t
Mucus threads: in urine, 53
μ-Heavy chain, 580, 581, 602
Multimetric analysis of VWF [test], 534
Multiple endocrine neoplasia (MEN), 101
 type I, 243
 type II
  calcitonin and, 302
  pheochromocytoma and, 278, 281
Multiple myeloma, 164–165, 580. *See also* Myeloma
 acid phosphatase and, 312t
 high resolution serum protein electrophoresis, 159
 and protein tests, 155, 157t
Multiple sclerosis:
 γ-globulin and, 112, 113f
 immunology, 861
 myelin basic protein and, 113t, 114
Multipotent stem cell, 425, 426f, 434
Mumps virus:
 arthritis, 707
 blood culture [test], 628t
 CNS infection, 772t, 773, 776, 776t
 eye infection, 649t
 serology [test], 822
 urinary infection, 729, 730t
Muramidase [test], 606
Murine typhus: serology and transmission, 812t
Murray Valley encephalitis, 772t
Muscle biopsy [test], 712–714
Muscle disease, 712–713
Mutarotase, 129
My 1, 852t
Myasthenia gravis: autoantibody, 845t
Mycobacterium:
 arthritis, 707
 bone marrow culture [test], 634
 and gastric infections, 749–750
 keratitis, 648
 pneumonia, 658, 662, 664–665, 670t
 urine culture [test], 728

Mycobacterium avium complex, 620
    and AIDS, 620, 626, 728, 754, 755, 756, 860
    blood culture [test], 622, 626
    infections, 624t, 626t
    penumonia, 665, 670t
    and stool culture, 754, 756
    urinary culture, 728
Mycobacterium chelonei:
    skin manifestations, 679t, 680t, 681t
    trauma/wound infection, 680t
Mycobacterium fortuitum: skin manifestations, 680t, 681t, 699
Mycobacterium haemophilum: skin manifestations, 679t
Mycobacterium kansasii: respiratory infection, 670t
Mycobacterium leprae: skin manifestations, 678t
Mycobacterium marinum: skin manifestations, 679t, 681t
Mycobacterium scrofulaceum, 680t
Mycobacterium tuberculosis:
    arthritis, 707–708
    CNS infections, 770, 779, 780, 781
    and ear infection, 637, 638
    eye infections, 648
    myopericarditis, 713
    osteomyelitis, 710
    pericarditis, 711–712
    and peritonitis, 706
    pleural effusion, 668
    pulmonary, 665, 670t
    scrofula, 680t
    skin test, 776
    urinary infection, 721, 728
    verrucosa cutis, 680t
Mycobacterium ulcerans: skin manifestations, 679t
myc oncogene, 328t
Mycoplasma:
    bone marrow aspiration for, 610
    serology [test], 814–815
    upper respiratory infections, 645t
Mycoplasma genitalium: urethritis, 734, 734t
Mycoplasma hominis: vaginosis, 734t, 737
Mycoplasma pneumoniae:
    ear infection, 637
    lower respiratory infection, 657, 659, 660, 661, 662t, 662–663, 666, 670t
    pericarditis, 711
    serology, 814–815
Mycosis fungoides: morphology/manifestations/markers, 574t

Myctalopia, 216
Myelin basic protein (MBP) [test], 113t, 113–114
Myeloblast, 426f, 434, 435
    in bone marrow aspiration, 612t
    stain reactions, 604t
Myeloblastic leukemia. *See* Myelocytic leukemia, acute
Myelocytes, 434, 435
    in bone marrow aspiration, 612t
Myelocytic leukemia, acute (AML), 559, 561, 563t, 564t, 852
    characteristics, 561t
    chromosomal abnormality, 562t
    classification, 561, 563t, 564t
    immunophenotyping, 602
    myelodysplasia transformation to, 566
    stains for, 605, 606
    TdT testing, 607–608
    vitamin B_{12} and, 228, 228t
Myelocytic leukemia, chronic (CML), 559, 561, 567, 568t, 569
    blast crisis, 606–607
    characteristics, 568t
    chromosomal abnormality, 562t
    differential diagnosis, 567, 569
    juvenile, 493
    LAP test for, 607–608
    leukemoid reaction vs., 567, 569t
    testing for, 855
    transformation to ALL, 855
    vitamin B_{12} and, 228, 228t
Myelodysplastic syndromes, 449, 451t, 463, 565–567
    and bone marrow aspiration, 612
    FAB classification, 566, 567t
    LAP test for, 608
    morphologic evidence, 565, 566t
    therapy-related, 567t
Myelofibrosis: vitamin B_{12} and, 228, 228t
Myelofibrosis with myeloid metaplasia, 567, 570, 576
    characteristics, 568t
    chromosomal abnormality, 562t
Myelogeneous leukemia, chronic: immunophenotyping, 602
Myeloid leukemia:
    subacute, 565
    without maturation, Plate 13, 444
Myeloid leukemoid reaction, 569
Myeloma. *See also* Multiple myeloma
    immunoglobulin responses, 157t
    protein ranges in, 156t
    and viscosity ranges, 171
Myelomonocytic leukemia:
    acute, Plate 16, 444, 563t, 564t, 605

    chronic (CMML), 566, 567t
    stains for, 606
Myeloperoxidase, 559
    deficiency, 560t, 603, 605
    stain [test], 603–605, 604t
Myelophthisic anemia, 451t, 453
Myeloproliferative disorders, 567, 569, 570, 576–581, 594–595. *See also specific disorders*
    chronic, 568t
    differential characteristics, 568t
    lysis and, 476
    vitamin B_{12} and, 228, 228t
Myeloproliferative syndrome, acute, 565
Myiasis, 681t, 686
Myocardial autoantibody, 845t
Myocardial infarction:
    alkaline phosphatase and, 72
    AST in, 70
    and drug protein binding, 335
    LD and, 79f, 79t
    protein levels and, 156t, 157t
    serum enzyme tests for, 25–36
Myocarditis, 713–714
Myoglobinuria, 54
Myometritis, 701
Myonecrosis, 713
Myopericarditis, 713
Myosin, 151
Myositis:
    streptococcal, 681t
    testing for, 850
Myristic acid, 182t
Myxedema:
    and anemia, 451t
    thyroid microsomal antibodies and, 256

N

N-Acetylcysteine (NAC), 382, 383
N-Acetyl-imidoquinone, 382
N-Acetyl procainamide (NAPA). *See* Procainamide/NAPA
NADP. *See* Nicotinamide adenine dinucleotide phosphate
Naeglaeria fowleri: CNS infection (PAM), 774, 778, 779, 782
Naegleria fowleri: CNS infection (PAM), 777t
Nagao isoenzyme, 73, 73t, 74t, 310
Nails: direct examination, 694t
Nalidixic acid:
    hemolytic anemia from, 894t
    susceptibility testing, 794t

Naloxone, 389
Nanophyetus salmincola, 762, 762t, 763t
NAPA (N-acetyl procainamide). *See* Procainamide/NAPA
Naphthol AS-D acetate esterase [test], 604t, 605–606
Naphthol AS-D chloroacetate esterase [test], 605–606
α-Naphthyl acetate esterase [test], 604t, 605–606
α-Naphthyl butyrate esterase [test], 604t, 605–606
1-Naphthylphosphate, 312t
2-Naphthylphosphate, 312t
Nasal culture [test], 638–639
Nasal infections, 638–641
Nase: culture [test], 638–639
Nasopharyngeal carcinoma: EBV and, 816–817, 817t
Nasopharyngeal swab, 690f
  for lower respiratory specimen collection, 662–663
Nasopharynx culture [test], 646–647
National Committee for Clinical Laboratory Standards (NCCLS), 7
  for susceptibility testing, 792, 794
National Diabetes Data Group, 131
  glucose tolerance testing criteria, 133t, 134
Natural killer (NK) cells, 438–439
  antigen markers, 599t, 602–603
  immunophenotyping by flow cytometry, 600f
NB 70k: and ovarian carcinoma, 329t
NBT test, 597
N-demethylase, 362
Necator americanus:
  gastrointestinal infection, 761, 763t
  pulmonary infection, 672t
  skin manifestations, 677t
Necrotizing fasciitis, 680t, 717
Negative predictive value, 2, 3f, 4t
Negative results, 1–2
  cutoff point for, 8
  false, 1–2, 3f
  true, 1–2, 3f
Negri bodies, 777
Neisseria:
  blood culture and, 621t
  culture, 700f
  infections, 625t, 626t, 699, 734t
  upper respiratory infections, 645t, 670t

Neisseria gonorrhoeae:
  cervicitis, 734t, 739–740
  eye infections, 648, 650, 652, 653
  gonococcemia, 677t
  infections, 624t, 692, 733
  peritoneal infection, 701, 703, 706
  rectal, 734t, 744
  septic arthritis, 707–708
  susceptibility testing, 791, 792
  throat infection, 641, 642, 644, 645t, 646
  urethritis, 734, 734t, 735, 736, 737
  urine culture [test], 729
Neisseria meningitidis:
  antigen detection, 780
  antigenemia, 633, 726
  arthritis, 707
  CNS infection, 770, 781, 785
  eye infections, 648
  infections, 624t
  meningoccemia, 677t
  pericarditis, 711
  respiratory infection, 657, 670t
  skin manifestations, 678t
Nematodes. *See also specific nematodes*
  eye infections, 649, 650
  gastrointestinal, 747, 761–762, 763t, 765, 766
  pulmonary infections, 672, 672t, 673–674
  tissue infections, 685
Neomycin: monitoring [test], 797–798
Neonatal alloimmune neutropenia, 887
Neonatal alloimmune thrombocytopenic purpura (NAITP), 883
Neonatal hyperviscosity, 171
Neonatal screen [test], 410–411
Neoplasia. *See also specific neoplasias*
  alkaline phosphatase and, 73, 74t
  anemia and, 450
  CK-BB levels and, 29
  and drug protein binding, 335
  endocrine
    apudomas, 101
    hormonal assays for, 102
    insulinomas, 102
    MEN syndrome, 101
    VIPomas, 102
  and ferritin, 468
  α-fetoprotein as marker, 81
  gastrin-secreting (Zollinger-Ellison syndrome), 99, 100, 100t

  humoral syndromes, 308
  insulin-secreting, 102
  liver, 77–78
    and alkaline phosphatase levels, 71–72, 72t
    classification of, 68t
    GGT and, 79
    lactate dehydrogenase and, 78–79
  methotrexate for, 365–366
  neuroendocrine, 101
  pancreatic, 99, 100, 101, 102
  and pleural fluid, 115t
  protein levels and, 156t, 157t
  tumor cells in urine, 52–53
  tumor markers, 307–332. *See also* Tumor markers
  VIP-producing, 102
Nephelometry, 165, 166
Nephrosis: immunoglobulin responses, 157t
Nephrotic syndrome, 51
  aminoaciduria in, 148
  and hypercholesterolemia, 178
  hypoproteinemia and, 153
  protein levels and, 156t, 158
  and serum protein electrophoresis, 158
  vitamin D deficiency and, 219
Nephrotoxicity:
  of aminoglycosides, 798
  cyclosporine, 364
  of vancomycin, 799
Netilmicin:
  monitoring [test], 797–798
  reference range, 798t
Neural tube defects (NTD), 402–403, 404, 404t, 405t
Neuroarthropathy: synovial fluid examination, 117t
Neuroblastoma, 277, 278–279
  homovanillic acid test, 283
  and N-*myc*, 328t
Neuroendocrine neoplasia, 101
Neurophysin, 294, 320
Neurosyphilis, 112, 769, 810, 811
Neutralization test, 805. *See also* Serodiagnosis of infectious disease
  for adenovirus, 823
Neutropenia, 471, 473
  causes of, 555t, 588, 589–590, 596
  neonatal alloimmune, 887
Neutrophil(s):
  causes of disorders, 559t, 596–598
  in cerebrospinal fluid, 108, 108t

Neutrophil(s) *(Continued)*
  function, 435, 553. *See also* Neutrophil function [tests]
  hereditary hypersegmentation of, 556, 558t, 589
  morphology, 426f, 434, 435, 436
  reference values for cell count and slide differential, 586t–587t
  in synovial fluid, 117t
  tissue, 443–444
Neutrophil bands: in bone marrow aspiration, 612t
Neutrophil casts: in urine, 50–51
Neutrophil CR3 [test], 597
Neutrophil dysfunction, 556
  causes of, 556, 559t
  inherited, 556, 560t
Neutrophil function [tests], 596–598
  CR3, 597
  functional assay of adherence and chemotaxis (Rebuck skin window), 597
  functional assays of chemotaxis, 597
  functional assays of degranulation, 597
  functional assays of phagocytosis, 597
  oxidative burst analysis, 598
Neutrophilia: causes of, 554t, 584–585, 589–590
Neutrophilic band, 426f
Neutrophilic leukocytosis: causes of, 557t
Neutrophil myeloperoxidase, 556
Newborn screening [tests], 410–413
  genetic disorders, 413–420. *See also* Genetic disorders
  genetic screen, 410–411
  molecular genetic analysis, 411–413
Newcastle disease virus: eye infection, 649t
N-formidyl tetrahydrofolate, 365
Niacin, 213
  deficiency, 224
  reference ranges for, 215t
  toxicity, 224
Niacinamide. *See* Niacin
Niacin [test], 223–224
Nicotinamide, 223
Nicotinamide adenine dinucleotide (NAD), 129, 223
Nicotinamide adenine dinucleotide phosphate (NADP), 129, 223

  and hemolytic anemia, 477, 478f, 484
  reduced (NADPH), 129, 477, 478f, 484
Nicotinic acid, 213, 223. *See also* Niacin
Niemann-Pick cell (foam cell), Plate 32B, 443
Niemann-Pick disease, 443
  acid phosphatase and, 312t
Night blindness, 216
Nitrates, 54
Nitrite: in urine, 54–55, 725, 726t
Nitroblue tetrazolium test, 597
Nitrofurantoin: susceptibility testing, 794t
Nitrogen: protein, 153
p-Nitrophenyl phosphate, 312t
Nitrosonaphthol test, 147
NK cells. *See* Natural killer cells
N-Methylguanidinoacetic acid [test], 61
N_1-Methylnicotinamide (NMN), 223, 224
N_1-Methyl-2 pyridone-5 carboxamide (2-PYR), 223, 224
N^5-Methyl tetrahydrofolate, 473
N-*myc* oncogene, 278–279, 328t
Nocardia:
  arthritis, 707
  cultures, 696t, 698f
  and endocarditis, 626t
  eye infections, 648
  pneumonia, 658, 662, 665, 666, 667f, 670t
  sulfonamide for, 799
  tissue manifestations, 681t, 692, 694
Nodular folliculitis, 681t
Nodules: disease, etiology, and tests for, 681t, 685–686, 690f
Nomifensine: hemolytic anemia from, 894t
Non-Hodgkin's lymphomas, 577–579
  and AIDS, 860
  classification systems, 615
  immunophenotyping, 603
  lymph node biopsy for, 613
  tissue mast cells and, 443
  Working Formulation, 579t, 615
Nonlinear pharmacokinetics, 338–339
Nonspecific esterase [test], 605–606
Nonsteroidal anti-inflammatory drugs (NSAIDs): drug interactions, 344t, 366
Nonsuppressible insulin-like activity in serum (NSILA-S), 240

Nonurinary tract isolates, 794t
Norepinephrine. *See also* Catecholamines
  ascorbic acid and, 231
  DHPG test and, 282
  synthesis, 277
Normetanephrine, 277, 280
Normoblasts: in bone marrow aspiration, 612t
Normocytic anemias, 448f, 450–455, 451t, 452f, 454f, 455t, 463
  with decreased RBC production, 450–453, 451t
  with increased RBC destruction, 448f, 453–455, 454f, 455t
Nortriptyline:
  therapeutic range, concentration, and distribution, 334t, 396t
  toxicities, 396t
Nortriptyline [test], 360–361
Norwalk agent: gastroenteritis, 747, 752t, 753, 758
Nose: infections, 638–641
NSE [test], 605–606
NT. *See* Neutralization test
5'-Nucleotidase [test], 73, 80

O

Oasthouse syndrome, 52
O blood type, 873, 873t
Octacarboxyporphyrin, 55, 56t, 57, 58t
OCT (ornithine carbamoyltransferase) [test], 82
Odynuria, 722
17-OH corticosteroids (17-OH CS; 17-hydroxycorticosteroid) [test], 268, 269f
OKM1, 852t
OKT1, 852t
OKT3, 852t
OKT4, 852t
OKT5, 852t
OKT6, 852t
OKT8, 852t
OKT11, 852t
Oleic acid, 181, 182t
Oligoclonal banding [test], 112–113, 113f, 161, 162–163
Oligomenorrhea, 286, 293
  DHEA-S levels, 291
Oligonucleotide probes: and genetic disorder testing, 412
Oligospermia, 124, 289, 290t
Omphalocele, 403
Omsk hemorrhagic fever, 772t

Onchocerca volvulus, 632, 632t, 650, 651, 653
  nodules, 685
  urinary infection, 721, 731, 732
Oncogene tumor markers, 308t, 328
One compartment models for drugs, 337
1-Hour postprandial glucose [test], 135
O&P examination. *See* Ova and parasite
Ophthlamic zoster, 648
Opiates:
  addiction: and glycohemoglobin, 137
  characteristics of, 389t
  testing for, 386, 387, 388t, 388–389, 389t
Opiates [test], 388–389, 389t
Opioids: characteristics of, 389t
Opioids [test], 388–389, 389t
Opisthorcis viverrini, 702t, 702–703, 762, 763t
Oral anticoagulants:
  drug interactions, 341, 344
  and hemostatic disorders, 518, 549
  therapy monitoring, 523, 524t, 529, 539
Oral candidiasis, 641–642, 643, 737, 748, 821
Oral contraceptives:
  and cholestasis, 77
  drug interactions, 341
  and hypercholesterolemia, 178
  and hypertriglyceridemia, 180t
  protein levels and, 156t
Oral glucose tolerance test, 133t
Orbital cellulitis, 635, 639–640, 651
Orf, 681t
Organic acidemias, 417–418
Organic acids, 12
Organic acids [test]: for genetic disorders, 417–418
Organic acidurias, 417–418
Oriental sore, 681t
Ornithine:
  biochemistry and reference range, 145t
  and cystinuria, 148
Ornithine carbamoyltransferase (OCT) [test], 82
Ornithine transcarbamoylase, 82
  deficiency, 78
Oropharyngeal flora: polymicrobic tissue infection, 680t, 699, 700f
Oropharynx culture [test], 641–646

Oroya fever: direct examination of blood [test], 627
Orthochromic megaloblast, Plate 7, 431
Orthochromic normoblast, 427, 429
Ortho-dianisidine, 129
Orthophosphoric monoester phosphohydrolase [test], 70–74. *See also* Alkaline phosphatase
Osmol gap [test], 379t, 379–380
Osmometry: in alcohol analysis, 376, 376t
Osmotic fragility [test]: for anemia, 480–481, 481f
Osteoarthropathy, hypertrophic pulmonary: synovial fluid examination, 117t
Osteoblast, 443
Osteocalcin [test], 302–303
Osteochondromatosis: synovial fluid examination, 117t
Osteoclast, 443
Osteogenesis imperfecta: acid phosphatase and, 312t
Osteomalacia:
  alkaline phosphatase and, 72, 73
  vitamin D deficiency and, 218–219
Osteomyelitis: testing for, 709–711
Osteoporosis: acid phosphatase and, 312t
O'Sullivan glucose tolerance testing criteria, 133t, 134
Otitis externa, 635, 636–637
  malignant, 636
Otitis media, 635
  with effusion (OME), 637
o-Tolidine test, 54
Otomycosis, 636
Otorrhea, 637
Ototoxicity: of vancomycin, 799
Ouchterlony method, 805
Outliers, 7
Ova and parasite [test], 759–766
Oval fat bodies: in urine, 52
Ovalocytes, 432
Ovarian carcinoma:
  amylase production, 309
  antigen, 329t
  line (OVCA 433), 317
  progesterone receptors and, 327
  tumor markers for, 309, 310, 316, 317, 318, 320, 323, 325, 329, 329t
Ovarian cysadenocarcinoma antigen, 329t
Ovarian dysfunction: and hyperandrogenism, 288, 288t

Ovarian resistance syndrome, 293t
Ovarian tumors. *See also* Ovarian carcinoma
  androgenic, 290
  DHEA-S levels, 291
  germ cell, 314, 315, 315t
Ovulation, 285
Oxalate, 231
Oxalosis: and vitamin B_6, 227t
Oxazepam: half-life and therapeutic/toxic concentrations, 384t
Oxicillin: bacterial susceptibility testing, 794t
Oxidative burst analysis [test], 597
Oximeter, pulse, 22
Oxycodone: characteristics of, 389t
Oxygen:
  delivery of, 11
  direct transcutaneous monitoring, 22
  dissociation curve, 17, 23f, 23–25, 24f–25f
  equilibrium, 11
  partial pressure of (pO_2), 11–12, 15, 16t, 16–17, 22–25
  saturation, 15, 17, 22, 23–25
Oxygen saturation (measured) [test], 23–25
Oxyhemoglobin, 12, 14, 23
  and xanthochromia, 107
Oxytocin, 237, 294
Ozena, 638

P

PABA (para-amino benzoic acid), 93
Paget's disease:
  alkaline phosphatase and, 72, 312t
  calcitonin levels and, 321
PAI-1 (plasminogen activator inhibitor-1) [test], 550
Palmitic acid, 181, 182t
Palmitoleic acid, 181, 182t
PAM. *See* Primary amebic meningoencephalitis
p-Aminosalicylic acid (PAS): hemolytic anemia from, 894t
Pancreatic carboxypeptidase A, 211
Pancreatic cholera, 102
Pancreatic disease. *See* Pancreatic neoplasia; Pancreatitis
Pancreatic exocrine function [tests], 91–98
  bentiromide (tripeptide hydrolysis), 92–93
  breath hydrogen, for carbohydrate intolerance, 95–96

Pancreatic exocrine function [tests] *(Continued)*
  β-carotene and carotenoids, 97
  ^{14}C-triolein breath, 94
  disaccharidase deficiency, 96
  D-xylose absorption, 95
  fatty meal, 94–95
  fecal fat, 93
  iron absorption, abnormal, 98
  Lundh, 93–94
  secretin, 91–92
  secretin-cholecystokinin, 92
  vitamin B$_{12}$ malabsorption (Schilling), 96–97
Pancreatic function, 85–86
Pancreatic function [tests], 86–90
  amylase/creatinine ratio, 87–88
  amylase isoenzymes, 87
  interpretation of, 89–90
  lipase, 87f, 88–89
  serum amylase, 86–87, 87f
  trypsin (immunoreactive), 87f, 89
Pancreatic neoplasia, 99, 100, 101, 102
  β-cell insulin-secreting tumors, 141–142
  islet cell tumor hormone markers, 321
  tumor markers for, 316, 317, 320, 323, 325, 329t, 329–330
Pancreatic polypeptide, 102
Pancreatic secretory trypsin inhibitor, 89
Pancreatitis, 85–90
  acute, 85, 86
    symptoms and signs, 86t
  alcoholic, 90
  calcitonin levels and, 321
  cancer antigen 125 and, 317
  CEA elevation in, 319t
  chronic, 85–86, 92, 96
  clinical differentiation, 86t, 89
  edematous, 85
  hemorrhagic, 85
  pleural fluid amylase and, 115t, 116
Pancreozymin (PZ), 92
P and P [test], 529
Panel approach, 5
Panencephalitis, 773, 773t
  progressive rubella, 773t
Panmyelopathy, primary acquired, with myeloblastosis, 565
Pantothenic acid, 213
P-AP (plasmin-α$_2$-antiplasmin complex) [test], 512t, 550
PAP. *See* Prostatic acid phosphatase
Papain: for alloantibody detection, 876

Papillomaviruses:
  eye infection, 649t
  warts, 681t, 684, 685t
Papovaviruses: CNS infection, 777t
Pappenheimer bodies, 433, 463
Papular lesions, 677t–678t, 684, 687, 688f
  parasitic, 685–686
Para-amino benzoic acid (PABA), 93
Paracentesis, 705–707
Paracoccidioides brasiliensis: ulcer, 679t
Paragonimiasis. *See Paragonimus*
Paragonimus mexicanus, 762t, 763t
Paragonimus westermanii, 672t, 674, 762, 762t, 763t
  serology [test], 830t, 831
Parainfluenza virus:
  eye infection, 649t
  infection frequency, 636t
  pneumonia, 657, 658, 660, 668, 670t
  serology [test], 823–824
  throat infection, 641, 642, 646
Paralysis, 771t
Paramyxoviruses: CNS infection, 772t, 777t, 782–783
Parapneumonic effusions, 659, 659t, 663, 668
  pleural, 116
Parasites, 702t, 702–703. *See also specific parasites*
  blood [test], 629–632
  CNS infections, 774–775, 777t, 777–778
  eye infections, 649, 650, 651, 653–654
  gastrointestinal tract, 747, 759–766, 762t
  muscle disease, 713–714
  respiratory, direct examination for [test], 671–674
  skin/tissue infections, 676, 685–686, 699
  testing for, 704–705, 706
  in urine, 53
Parasitic eosinophilic meningitis, 775
Parasitic serology [tests], 829–833, 830t
  amebiasis, 830, 830t
  cysticercosis, 830, 830t
  echinococcosis, 830t, 830–831
  filariasis, 830t, 831
  leishmaniasis, 830t, 831
  malaria, 830t, 831
  paragonimiasis, 830t, 831
  schistosomiasis, 830t, 831

  strongyloidiasis, 830t, 831–832
  toxocariasis, 830t, 832
  toxoplasmosis, 830t, 832
  trichinosis, 830t, 832
  trypanosomiasis, 830t, 832–833
Parathion poisoning, 75
Parathyrin. *See* Parathyroid hormone
Parathyroid hormone, 58, 296
  and calcium regulation, 296t
  carboxy-terminal, midmolecule, and amino-terminal, 300, 301t, 302
  and phosphate regulation, 298
Parathyroid hormone [test], 300–302, 301t
  tumor marker, 324t, 324–325
Parathyroid hormone-like peptide [test]: tumor marker, 325
Parietal cells: autoantibody, 845t
Paromomycin monitoring [test], 797–798
Paronychia, 679t
Parotid glands: amylase in, 86, 87, 88t
Paroxysmal cold hemoglobinuria (PCH), 889t, 891, 893
Paroxysmal nocturnal hemoglobinuria [tests]:
  acidified serum lysis, 476–477
  sucrose hemolysis, 481–482
Paroxysmal supraventricular tachycardia: drugs for, 355
Partial pressure of carbon dioxide (pCO_2), 11–12, 14, 15, 16t, 16–25
Partial pressure of oxygen (pO_2), 11–12, 15, 16t, 16–17, 22–25
Partial thromboplastin time (PTT):
  and acetaminophen, 383
  activated [test], 505f, 516t, 518t, 524t, 526–527
  correction [test], 528–529
Particle agglutination assay: for HIV, 821–822
Particle-enhanced immunoassay, 805
Parvovirus:
  arthritis, 707
  serology [test], 822–823
Parvovirus B19: skin manifestations, 677t, 684
PAS (periodic acid-Schiff stain) [test], 608
Pasteurella multocida:
  bites, 679t, 715, 716
  infections, 625t
Patches, 687, 694t
Patient monitoring, 5

Patient preparation, 2f, 5–6, 6t
Paul-Bunnell test, 816
PBG (porphobilinogen), 55, 58t
PBI (protein bound iodine) [test], 251–252
PCH. *See* Paroxysmal cold hemoglobinuria
pCO_2 (partial pressure of carbon dioxide), 11–12, 14, 15, 16t, 16–25
PCP. *See* Phencyclidine
PCR. *See* Polymerase chain reaction
p-Dimethylamino-benzaldehyde, 54
Peak acid output (PAO), 100, 100t
Peak and trough of drugs, 337, 338f
Pediatric poisonings, 369, 370t
Pediculus humanus, 745
  skin manifestations, 677t
Pelger-Huët anomaly, 555, 589
Pelger-Huët cells, Plate 11A, 436
Pellagra, 224
Pellagra preventing factor, 223
Pelvic abscess, 701–702
Pelvic infections, 701–702
Pelvic inflammatory disease (PID), 737
Pemphigus: autoantibody, 845t
Penicillin:
  hemolytic anemia from, 889t, 894t
Penicillium: pulmonary infection, 668, 670t
Pentacarboxyporphyrin, 55, 56t, 57, 58t
Pentagastrin, 99, 302
Pentazocine: characteristics of, 389t
Pentobarbital [test]: toxicity, 384–386, 385t
Pentose: dietary, 127
PEP carboxylase, 128f
Pepsin, 99
Pepsinogen, 99
Pepsinogen [test], 101
Peptic ulcer disease, 99
  CEA elevation in, 319t
  and infections, 749–750
Peptide bonds: protein, 150–151
Peptococcus:
  arthritis, 707
  infections, 625t
Peptococcus magnus: infections, 625t
Peptostreptococcus:
  cultures, 696t, 699
  lymphadenopathy, 714
  respiratory infection, 670t
Percent (%) saturation [test], 468–470
Perfusion, 11
Perianal skin examination, 761

Pericardial effusions, 116, 712
Pericardial fluid [test], 116, 711–712
Pericardial friction rub, 712
Pericardiocentesis, 116, 712
Pericardiotomy, 116
Pericarditis, bacterial, 711–712
Periodic acid-Schiff stain [test], 608
Perioperative hemodilution, 882–883
Peripheral blood smear morphology [test], 462–463
Peristalsis, 747
Peritoneal carcinomatosis, 116
Peritoneal dialysis, continuous ambulatory (CAPD), 701, 703, 705–706
  infectious complications, 705–706
Peritoneal fluid analysis, 706–707
Peritoneal lavage, 705
Peritonitis, 700–701
  cancer antigen 125 and, 317
  testing for, 703, 705–707
Pernicious anemia, 447, 469, 472, 475
  autoantibody, 845t
Pernicious anmeia: vitamin B_{12} and, 228, 228t
Peroxisomes, 441
  defect in, 419–420
Pertussis, 645t, 646, 647
Pesticides [test], 390–392
Petechiae: disease, etiology, and tests for, 677t, 687
PF4 (platelet factor 4) [test], 536–537
pH:
  acid-base disturbances, 17–21
  amino acids, 143
  cerebrospinal fluid, 109, 111
  continuous measurement, 22–23
  control of blood, 14–15
  measures, 15–21
  pericardial fluid, 116
  pleural fluid [test], 116
  of urine, 53
PHA. *See* Phytohemaglutinin
Phaeohyphomycosis, 681t
Phagocytosis, 435
  functional assays for [test], 597
Pharmacokinetic equations, 336t
Pharmacokinetics. *See* Drugs
Pharyngitis, 635, 641–646, 643t
  bacterial, 641
  fungal, 641–642
  and pneumonia, 660t
  viral, 641
Pharyngoconjunctival fever, 648
Phenacetin: hemolytic anemia from, 894t
Phencyclidine (PCP):

  and emergency room, 370t
  testing for, 372, 386, 387, 388, 388t
Phenobarbital, 340, 346
  drug interactions, 344t, 346, 347, 349, 352, 356
  pharmacokinetic properties, 341t
  therapeutic range, concentration, and distribution, 334t
Phenobarbital [test], 343–344
  drug interactions, 344
  toxicity, 384–386, 385t
Phenolic acids: genetic screening, 417
Phenosulfonphthalein (PSP) [test], 60
Phenothiazines:
  and cholestasis, 77
  drug interactions, 361
Phenothiazines [test], 394, 394t
Phenteramine, 388
Phenylacetic acid: elevated, 414
Phenylalanine, 144, 147
  alkaline phosphatase isoenzymes and, 73t, 73–74, 74t
  assay, 411
  biochemistry and reference range, 144t
  elevated, 414
Phenylalanine hydroxylase deficiency, 146t
Phenylalaninemias, 149–150
Phenylamine-phenazone, 129
Phenylbutazone: drug interactions, 344t, 366
Phenylethylmalonamide (PEMA), 346
Phenylketonuria (PKU), 55, 144t
  carrier state, 150
  classic, 149, 150
  Collaborative Study for the Treatment of Children with PKU, 149
  diagnostic parameters, 149–150
  testing for, 411, 414
  variant, 149, 150
Phenytoin, 340, 341, 343, 346
  drug interactions, 344, 344t, 345, 346, 347, 349, 352, 363, 366
  free, 334t
  indications, 345
  nonlinear pharmacokinetics, 339, 339f
  pharmacokinetic properties, 341t
  protein binding, 333, 335
  side effects, 345t
  therapeutic range, concentration, and distribution, 334t
Phenytoin [tests], 344–345
  unbound, 345–346

Pheochromocytoma, 128, 277, 278
  ACTH tumor marker, 321
  calcitonin and, 302
Pheochromocytoma [tests], 279–281
  catecholamines, urinary (free), 280–281
  DHPG, 282–283
  DOPA, 283
  dopamine, 283
  metanephrine, 280
  plasma catecholamines, 281–282
  vanillylmandelic acid, 279–280
Philadelphia (PH) chromosome, 569, 569t, 589
Phlebitis: and pneumonia, 660t
Phosphate, 298–299
  abnormalities, causes of, 299t
  buffer, 13–14
  crystals in urine, 52, 63f
  serum [test], 298–299
  tubular reabsorption, 299
Phosphatidyl choline, 182, 185
Phosphatidyl ethanolamine, 182
Phosphatidyl glycerol, 182
  in amniotic fluid, 408
Phosphatidyl inositol, 182
  pathway, 500, 501f
Phosphatidyl inositol biphosphate (PIP$_2$), 500, 502f
Phosphodiesterase, 501
Phosphofructokinase deficiency, 421t
Phospholipase, 89
Phospholipase C, 500–501, 501f, 502f
Phospholipids:
  in amniotic fluid, 408–409
  and breast cancer, 329t
  and chylomicrons, 191
  and HDLs, 185
Phospholipids [test], 182
Phosphoric acid, 12
Phosphorus, 299
Phosphorylase deficiency, 421t
Phosphorylase kinase deficiency, 421t
Phosphotungstic acid method: for uric acid reference ranges, 45, 45t
Phthirus pubis, 677t, 745
Phycoerythrin (PE), 600, 601
p-Hydroxyphenylpyruvic acid (PHPPA), 147, 150
Phylloquinones, 221
Phytohemaglutinin (PHA), 853t, 855
Pia mater, 768
Pica: zinc and iron deficiencies and, 211
PID (pelvic inflammatory disease), 737

Pili forti, 204, 416
Pink-tooth disease, 57
Pinocytosis: protein, 109
Pinta, 677t, 810
Pinworms, 761, 765
  in urine, 53
Pisano technique, 280
Pituitary function [tests], 237–243
  growth hormone (somatotrophin), 237–240
  insulin-like growth factor I (somatomedin C), 240–241
  prolactin, 241–243
Pituitary sarcoid, 290t
Pituitary tumors:
  prolactin-producing, 241, 242–243
  urinary-free cortisol and, 264t
PKU. *See* Phenylketonuria
Placental alkaline phosphatase (PLAP), 310
  as ovarian tumor marker, 329t
  as prostatic tumor marker, 313t
Plague, 659t. *See also Yersinia pestis*
Plaques: disease, etiology, and tests for, 681t, 688f
Plasma:
  and acid-base balance, 12–15, 13t
  fresh frozen transfusion, 868t, 887
  globulin content of [test], 842
  liquid, transfusion data, 869t
  proteins, 151
Plasmablast, 440
Plasma cells, Plate 29A, 440
  in bone marrow aspiration, 612t
  morphology, 428f, 438–441
  stain reactions, 604t
Plasmacyte. *See* Plasma cells
Plasmacytoid lymphocyte, Plate 10B, 441
Plasmacytoma, 164
Plasma emission spectrometry: for aluminum, 60
Plasma protein fraction: transfusion data, 869t
Plasma renin activity (PRA), 59
Plasma renin activity (PRA) [test], 275–277, 276t
  differentiating adrenal adenomas from hyperaldosteronism, 274t
  screening tests for primary aldosteronism, 273t
Plasma renin concentration [test], 275–277, 276t
Plasmin, 508, 511f, 512f, 546f-547f
Plasmin-α$_2$-antiplasmin complex [test], 512t, 550

Plasminogen, 508, 511f, 525
Plasminogen activator inhibition-1 [test], 550
Plasminogen activity [test], 511f, 512f, 520t, 522f, 523t, 546f–547f, 549–550
Plasmodium. *See also* Malaria
  blood examination [test], 629, 630, 630t
  serology [test], 830t, 831
Plasmodium falciparum, 630, 630t
  cerebral malaria, 775, 777t, 778
Plasmodium malariae, 630, 630t
Plasmodium ovale, 630, 630t
Plasmodium vivax, 630, 630t
Platelet(s), 426f, 442. *See also specific cells*
  α-granule proteins, 503t
  autoantibody, 845t
  bizarre, Plate 25, 442
  causes of increased, 557t, 595
  circulating, 441
  clumping, 594
  giant, Plate 25, 442
  glycolytic action, 129
  gray (agranular), Plate 25, 442
  large, 442
  production and morphology, 426f, 441–442
  transfusion data, 867t–868t. *See also* Platelet transfusion
Platelet [tests], 592–596
  count, 592–595
  mean volume, 595–596
Platelet adhesion, 499–501, 500f
Platelet adhesion [tests], 530–535. *See also* Platelet function [tests]
Platelet aggregation, 499–501, 503f, 515f
Platelet aggregation [test], 513t, 514t, 515f, 515t, 516t, 535
Platelet alloantigens, 884, 884t
Platelet antigens, 884, 884t
  detection, 885
Platelet binding of VWF [test], 500f, 534–535
Platelet count [test], 592–595
Platelet destruction: thrombocytopenia and, 594
Platelet disorders, 513–515. *See also specific disorders*
  acquired qualitative, 501f, 514–515, 515t, 516t
  alloimmune, 883
  autoimmune, 883
  functional, 556, 559t, 560t

hereditary qualitative, 513–514, 514t
immune, 883–884
malignant, 556, 559–565
quantitative and morphologic, 513, 554t–562t, 554–555
Platelet factor III [test], 536
Platelet factor 4 [test], 536–537
Platelet function [tests], 529–537
adhesion, 530–535
aggregation, 513t, 514t, 515f, 515t, 516t, 535
aspirin tolerance, 530
ATP release, 514t, 536
β-thromboglobulin, 537
bleeding time, 515t, 516t, 529–530
capillary fragility (tourniquet test), 530
circulating platelet aggregates, 536
clot retraction, 536
crossed immunoelectrophoresis of VWF, 533–534, 534f
glass bead retention time (Salzman test), 535
glycocalicin, 537
membrane glycoprotein expression, 537
multimetric analysis of VWF, 534
platelet binding of VWF, 500f, 534–535
platelet factor 3, 536
platelet factor 4, 536–537
platelet VWF, 534
ristocetin cofactor activity, 531t, 532
ristocetin-induced aggregation, 500f, 515f, 532–533
serotonin release, 514t, 536
in vivo activation, 536–537
von Willebrand factor antigen, 500f, 515t, 530–532, 531t
Platelet neutralization procedure [test], 517f, 543–544
Platelet peroxidase [test], 609–610
Platelet phospholipid assay [test], 536
Platelet-platelet interaction, 499, 501
Platelet plug formation, 499–501, 500f, 501f, 502f, 503f, 503t
Platelet secretion and aggregation [tests], 535–536. *See also* Platelet function [tests]
Platelet transfusion, 883–886
ABO and RH blood groups in, 885

antigen and antibody detection, 885
crossmatch test, 885–886
data on, 867t–868t
HLA typing, 885
refractoriness, 883–884
Platelet VWF [test], 534
Plesiomonas shigelloides: gastroenteritis, 752t, 754
Pleural biopsy, 663, 663t
Pleural effusions, 114, 668, 671t
exudative, 114, 115t
malignant, 116
parapneumonic, 116
rheumatoid, 116
transudative, 114, 115t
Pleural fluid, 114
CEA measurement in, 319
exudates, 114, 115t
pathologic characteristics, 114, 115t
proteins, 114, 115t
transudates, 114, 115t
Pleural fluid [tests], 114–116
α-fetoprotein, 116
amylase, 116
carcinoembryonic antigen (CEA), 116
cell count, 114–115, 115t
cytology, 116
glucose, 116
LE cells, 116
pH and lactate, 116
protein, 114, 115t
rheumatoid factor, 116
Pluripotent stem cell, 425, 426f, 434
PML (progressive multifocal leukoencephalopathy), 771t, 773, 860
Pneumocystis carinii pneumonia, 658, 661, 662t, 664, 666, 672t, 672–673
and AIDS, 860
Pneumonia, 655. *See also specific pathogens*
aspiration, 749
atypical, 658t, 659–660, 661, 814
bacterial, 657, 657t, 658t, 659, 659t, 664–665
and burns, 716
chlamydial, 646–647, 658, 662t, 662–663, 666, 668
chronic, 658, 658t
community-acquired, 655, 657, 660
diseases asociated with, 656t
extrapulmonary findings, 660t
fungal, 657, 657t, 658t, 659, 659t, 664–665, 666

nosocomial, 657
pathogens, 656t
predisposing factors for infection, 656t
radiography and, 660–661, 661t
specimen collection, 661t, 661–662
typical, 658t, 658–659
viral, 657, 660, 662t, 662–663, 666, 668
PNH. *See* Paroxysmal nocturnal hemoglobinuria
p-Nitrophenyl phosphate, 312t
PNP (platelet neutralization procedure) [test], 517f, 543–544
Poikilocytes, 463
Poikilocytosis, 433, 459, 463
Point mutation: and genetic disorder testing, 412, 413
Poisoning, 369. *See also* Drug toxicity
Pokeweed mitogen (PWM), 853t, 855
Poliomyelitis, 771
Polioviruses, 771, 776, 776t
serology, 816
Polychromasia, 433
Polychromatophilia, 433
Polychromatophilic megaloblast, Plate 7, 431
Polychromatophilic normoblast, 429
Polyclonal gammopathies. *See also* Hypergammaglobulinemia
immunofixation (IFE) test for, 162
Polycystic kidney disease: testing for, 411
Polycystic ovary syndrome, 286, 290, 293
DHEA-S levels, 291
Polycythemias, 455–457, 456t
absolute, 456t, 496–497
erythropoietin and, 326
familial, 456t
relative, 455–456, 456t, 457, 496–497
Polycythemia vera, 456t, 457, 496, 497, 567, 568t, 569–570, 595
characteristics, 568t
chromosomal abnormality, 562t
PVSG diagnosis criteria, 570, 570t
vitamin B_{12} and, 228, 228t
Polycythemia Vera Study Group (PVSG): criteria, 570, 570t
Polydipsia, primary, 295t

Polymerase chain reaction [test], 411–413
  for *Borrelia*, 808
  for HIV, 821
  for parvovirus, 821
Polymicrobic flora:
  fecal infection, 680t, 699, 700f
  oropharyngeal infection, 680t, 699, 700f
Polymyalgia rheumatica: ESR and, 465
Polymyositis, 861
Polyomaviruses: urinary, 730, 730t
Polypeptides, 150–151
Polysaccharides, 95
POMC (pro-opiomelanocortin), 257, 265, 265f, 268, 321
Pompe's disease, 421t
pO_2 (partial pressure of oxygen), 11–12, 15, 16t, 16–17, 22–25
Pork tapeworm. See *Taenia solium*
Porphobilinogen (PBG), 55, 58t, 418
Porphyrias, 55–58, 418, 418t
  acute intermittent, 55, 56t, 57, 418t
  classification of, 56t
  cutanea tarda, 56t, 57, 418t
  erythropoietic, 56t, 57–58, 418t
  hepatic, 55–57
  variegata, 56t, 57, 418t
Porphyrins, 55
  reference ranges, 58t
Porphyrins [test], 56t, 58
Positive predictive value, 2, 3f, 4t
Positive ratio:
  false, 2, 8–9
  true, 2, 8–9
Positive results, 1–2
  cutoff point for, 8
  false, 1–2, 3f, 8
  true, 1–2, 3f
Posterior pituitary [tests], 294–296
  antidiuretic hormone, 294–295
  water deprivation (dehydration), 295–296, 296t
  water loading, 295, 295t
Postinfectious encephalomyelitis, 773t
Postinfectious viral syndrome, 771t, 773t
Postmenopause, 285
Post-test probability, 2, 4
Post-transfusion purpura, 883
Potassium:
  aldosterone and, 270
  reference ranges for, 47t
  test for primary aldosteronism, 273t, 274t

Potassium [test], 46–47
Powassan virus, 772t
Poxvirus: skin manifestations, 681t
p-Phenylenediamine with pyrocatechol, 604
PPO (platelet peroxidase) [test], 609–610
Prazepam: half-life and therapeutic/toxic concentrations, 384t
Prealbumin:
  conditions and disorders affecting ranges of, 156t, 160, 161
  and fatty acids, 181
Prealbumin [test], 165
Preanalytic variation, 5
Pre-B ALL, 564
Pre-β-lipoprotein [test], 192, 192t. *See also* Very low density lipoproteins
Precision of test, 5, 6
Precocious puberty, 290, 290t, 294
Predictive value, 2, 3f, 4t
Pre-employment drug screen [test], 387–388
Pregnancy, 399
  acetylcholinesterase [test], 403–404
  alkaline phosphatase levels in, 71
  α-fetoprotein [test], 402–403
  bilirubin pigments in amniotic fluid [test], 404–405
  cancer antigen 125 and, 317
  cholestasis and, 77
  diabetes in, 133–134
  ectopic, 400, 401
  estriol, unconjugated [test], 405–407
  and gonadotropin tests, 285
  hCG levels and, 322–324, 323t, 324t
  human placental lactogen [test], 408
  lecithin-to-sphingomyelin ratio [test], 408–409
  molar, 323–324
  monitoring tests, 402–410
  multiple, 403
  protein levels and, 156t
  rubella virus and, 824
  testing for, 399–401
  and trophoblastic disease, 322
  urinary infections and, 722
Pregnenolone, 257, 258f, 287f, 292f
Prekallikrein, 504, 505f
  deficiency, 516t, 540
Prekallikrein [test], 540
Prekallikrein activity screen (Fletcher factor assay) [test], 506f, 540
Preleukemia, 565
Premature ventricular contractions: drugs for, 355
Pre-pre-B ALL, 564
Pre-test probability, 2, 4
Pretransfusion testing, 865, 871–872
  age of specimen, 871
  infant specimens, 872
  patient identification, 871
  plasma, 887
  previous records, 872
  retaining and storing specimens, 872
  specimen collection and handling, 871
  specimen labeling, 871
  transfusion request forms, 871
Prevalence of disease, 2
Primadone, 340
  drug interactions, 344t, 347
  pharmacokinetic properties, 341t
  therapeutic range, concentration, and distribution, 334t
Primary amebic meningoencephalitis (PAM), 774, 778, 779
Primidone [test], 385–386
Principles of laboratory medicine, 1–10
Prions, 774
Pro-ACTH, 265
Probability, 2, 4, 5t
  post-test, 2, 4
  pretest, 2, 4
Probenecid:
  drug interactions, 366
  hemolytic anemia from, 894t
Procainamide:
  absorption variance, 354f
  drug interactions, 349, 353
  hemolytic anemia from, 894t
  pharmacokinetic parameters, 349t
  therapeutic range, concentration, and distribution, 334t
Procainamide, n-acetyl: therapeutic range, concentration, and distribution, 334t
Procainamide/NAPA [test], 353–354
Procathepsin D: and breast cancer, 329t
Prochlorperazine: testing for, 394, 394t
Procoagulation factors: and vitamin K, 221
Proconvertin. *See* Factor VII
Proctitis, 744
Proctorectal exudate [test], 743–745

Progesterone, 258f, 284f, 287f
Progesterone challenge test, 286
Progesterone receptors [test]: tumor marker, 327, 328
Progranulocyte, 435
Progressive multifocal leukoencephalopathy (PML), 771t, 773, 860
Progressive rubella panencephalitis, 773t
Proinsulin, 138, 139f, 140, 240
Proinsulin [test], 140
Prolactin, 237
Prolactinomas, 241, 242–243
Prolactin-producing pituitary tumors, 241, 242–243
Prolactin [test], 241–243
Proline: biochemistry and reference range, 145t
Prolonged (72 hour) fast [test], 141
Prolymphocyte, Plate 26B, 439
Prolymphocytic leukemia:
    B-cell, 562t
    chromosomal abnormality, 562t
    immunophenotyping, 602
    morphology/manifestations/markers, Plate 26B, 527t
Promegakaryocyte, 426f, 442
Promegaloblast, Plate 7, 431
Promethazine: testing for, 394, 394t
Promonocyte, 426f, 437
Promyelocytes (progranulocytes), 426f, 435
    in bone marrow aspiration, 612t
Promyelocytic leukemia, Plate 15, 444, 561, 563t, 564t. See also Myelocytic leukemia, acute
Pronormoblast, 426f, 427
Pro-opiomelanocortin (POMC), 257, 265, 265f, 268, 321
Prophyrins [test]: genetic disorders, 418, 418t
Propionibacterium acnes:
    CNS infections, 770
    infections, 625t, 681t
Propionic acid, 417
Propionic acidemia, 78, 223, 417
Propionyl-CoA, 222
Proplasmacyte, Plate 29B, 440
Proporphyrins, 55
Propoxyphene, 388
    characteristics of, 389t
    drug interactions, 344t
    testing for, 388–389, 389t
Propranolol: drug interactions, 349, 351, 352, 355
Propranolol [test], 354–355
Propressophysin, 230, 294

Propronibacterium acnes: prosthetic device infections, 711
Prorubricytes, 427
Prostacyclin, 505, 507t
Prostacyclin synthetase, 505
Prostaglandin pathway, 500
Prostate:
    benign hypertrophy, 311, 314
    biopsy, 311
    infarction, 311
    infection, 726
    tumor markers, 308–314, 313t, 317, 318
Prostatectomy, radical, 314
Prostate specific antigen [test]: tumor marker, 308–309, 312, 313–314
Prostatic acid phosphatase (PAP): reference range, 8
Prostatic acid phosphatase (PAP) [test]: tumor marker, 311–313, 312t
Prostatic carcinoma, 8
    prostate specific antigen as tumor marker, 308–309, 313–314
    prostatic acid phosphatase as tumor marker, 311–313, 312t
    tumor markers, 308–314, 313t
Prostatic hypertrophy, 8
Prostatitis, 314
    bacterial, 722, 726
    differential diagnosis, 727t
    tests. *See* Urine [tests]
Prosthetic devices:
    infections, 711
    and infectious osteomeylitis, 709, 710
Protamine, 517f
Protamine sulfate and ethanol gelation [test], 507f, 546
Protease inhibitor MM (PiMM), 413
Protease inhibitor ZZ (PiZZ), 413
Protective factor X. *See* Biotin
Protein, 150–151
    acute phase reaction, 158
    adsorption of, 151
    ammonia, 153
    Bence-Jones, 53, 159–160, 162, 163, 164, 165, 169, 580
    binding of drugs, 333, 335
    buffer, 13t, 13–14
    C. *See* Protein C
    in cerebrospinal fluid, 108t
    chromatography of, 151
    cobalamin and, 471
    conditions associated with monoclonal, 164t

C-reactive, 158, 160, 170
electrophoresis of, 151
fibrous, 151
globular, 151
immunoprecipitation of, 151
lipo. *See* Lipoproteins
M, 166, 169
nitrogen, 153
pinocytosis, 109
in pleural fluid, 115t
R, 471
refractive index, 153
S. *See* Protein S
separation techniques, 151
structure, 150–151
in synovial fluid, 116
ultracentrifugation of, 151
in urine, 53–54
Z, 166, 413
Protein [tests], 151–171
    α_1-acid glycoprotein (orosomucoid), 165
    α_1-antitrypsin (ATT), 165–166
    albumin, 151–152
    albumin-globulin ratio, 153, 154f, 155f
    α_2-macroglobulin, 166
    β_2-microglobulin, 166–167
    cerebrospinal fluid, 109
    ceruloplasmin (CER), 169–170
    complement proteins, 167–168
    C-reactive protein (CRP), 170
    cryoglobulins, 170
    haptoglobin, 166
    high resolution serum electrophoresis, 158–161, 159f
    immunoelectrophoresis (IEP), 163f, 163–165, 164f, 164t
    immunofixation (IFE), 161–163, 162f
    immunoglobulin (quantitative), 168–169, 841–844, 843t
    myelin basic, 113t, 113–114
    pleural fluid, 114, 115t
    prealbumin, 165
    serum electrophoresis, 154–158, 156t–157t
    total, 152–153
    transferrin, 167
    viscosity (blood and serum), 170–171
Protein bound iodine [test], 251–252
Protein C, 507t, 508, 509f, 510f, 521f, 540, 541
    activation peptide of [test], 509f, 520t, 551
    activity [test], 509f, 510f, 520t, 548
    antigen [test], 548–549

Protein C *(Continued)*
   deficiency, 518, 520t, 548–549
   system assessment [tests], 548–549
   and vitamin K, 221
Protein-calorie malnutrition:
   immunologic effects, 862
   selenium and, 211
   TIBC test and, 469, 470
   zinc deficiency and, 211
Protein kinase C, 500
Protein S, 166, 508, 510f, 540, 541
   antigen [test], 510f, 520t, 549
   deficiency, 518, 549
   and vitamin K, 221
Proteinuria, 50, 54
   glomerular, 161
   mixed, 161
Proteus: osteomyelitis, 710
Proteus mirabilis. *See also* Enterobacteriaceae
   cultures, 697t
Proteus vulgaris. *See also* Enterobacteriaceae
   serology, 805
Prothrombin, 502, 505
   conditions and disorders affecting ranges of, 156t
   deficiency, 516t, 518
   and vitamin K, 221
Prothrombin [test], 516t, 523t, 538f, 540
Prothrombin and proconvertin test, 529
Prothrombinase complex, 504f
Prothrombin complex: transfusion data, 870t
Prothrombin fragment 1 + 2 [test], 520t, 534f, 551
Prothrombin time (PT), 503f, 513, 517f, 518t, 523, 538f
   and acetaminophen, 383
   international normalized ratio (INR), 523, 524t
   and vitamin K, 222
Prothrombin time (PT) [test], 503f, 506f, 516t, 518t, 524t, 525–526, 538f
Protocoproporphyria hereditaria, 57
Proto-oncogenes, 328
Protoporphyria, 57, 418t
Protoporphyrin, 55, 56t, 58, 418, 427
   erythrocyte (free) [test], 470–471
Protoporphyrinogen oxidase deficiency, 56t
Prototheca:
   skin manifestations, 678t
   tissue manifestations, 680t
Protothecosis, 681t

Protozoa. *See also specific species*
   gastrointestinal, 747, 759, 760, 760t, 762t, 765–766
   infections, 702–703
   respiratory, direct examination for [test], 671–674
   serology [tests], 830t, 830–831
   ulcers, 685
   in urine, 53
   urine microscopic examination [test], 731–732
Protriptyline:
   therapeutic range, concentration, and distribution, 334t, 396t
   toxicities, 396t
Providencia. *See also* Enterobacteriaceae
   and burn wounds, 716, 717
   in urine, 725
Provitamin A, 216
PSA. *See* Prostate specific antigen
Pseudoallescharia boydii: sinusitis, 640
Pseudocholinesterase [test], 67, 67t, 68t, 75–76, 76t
Pseudo-Cushing syndrome, 261, 261t, 264
Pseudoephedrine, 388
Pseudogout, 708
   synovial fluid examination, 117t
Pseudohypoparathyroid (PHP), 58, 301
Pseudomembranous colitis, 754
Pseudomonas:
   traumatic wounds, 718
   in urine, 725
Pseudomonas aeruginosa, 620
   burns, 679t, 716, 717
   cultures, 697t
   ear infection, 636, 637, 638
   and endocarditis, 623
   eye infection, 648
   infections, 625t, 655
   osteomyelitis, 710
   peritoneal infection, 701
   pulmonary infection, 657, 670t
   pylephlebitis, 701
   septic arthritis, 707–708
   skin manifestations, 677t, 678t, 679t, 680t, 692, 693
   surgical trauma/wounds, 680t
   susceptibility testing, 794t
   upper respiratory infections, 645t, 670t
   urinary infections, 722, 724, 726
Pseudomonas alcaligenes: tissue manifestations, 680t

Pseudomonas cepacia: infections, 625t
Pseudomonas fluorescens-putida: tissue manifestations, 680t
Pseudomonas mallei: respiratory infection, 659t
Pseudomonas pseudomallei:
   environmental exposure, 659t
   infections, 625t
   pneumonia, 658, 670t
Pseudoneutropenia, 585
Pseudo-Pelger-Huët cells, 436, 558t
Pseudotuberculosis, 680t
Psilocybin, 386
Psittacosis. *See Chlamydia psittaci*
Psoriatic arthritis, 708
PSP (phenosulfonphthalein) [test], 60
Psychotropics [tests], 359–361, 392–397
   desipramine, 359
   imipramine, 359
   lithium, 360
   nortriptyline, 360–361
   poisoning and abuse, 392–397
PTH. *See* Parathyroid hormone
PTT, APTT, and TT correction [tests], 528–529
Puberty, 284, 288–289
   precocious, 290, 290t, 294
Pubic lice, 677t
Pubic lice [test], 745
Pulex irritans: skin manifestations, 677t
Pulmonary abscess, 784
Pulmonary disease. *See also* Pneumonia
   alkaline phosphatase and, 72–73
   CEA elevation in, 319t
   and polycythemia, 456t
   testing for, 655–670
Pulmonary edema: and theophylline clearance, 335t
Pulmonary embolism:
   LD levels in, 32, 36
   and pleural fluid, 115t
Pulmonary function, 11–12
   acid-base system and, 12–15
Pulmonary infarct: alkaline phosphatase and, 72–73
Pulse oximeter, 22
Punctate basophilia, 431
Puncture wound infections, 680t
Purine-nucleoside phosphorylase deficiency, 858, 859
Purpura:
   disease, etiology, and tests for, 677t, 687

neonatal alloimmune thrombocy-
topenic (NAITP), 883
post-transfusion, 883
thrombotic thrombocytopenic
(TTP), 521, 522t, 545,
887
Pustulular lesions: etiology and tests
for, 678t–679t, 684, 687f,
692f, 694t
PV. See Polycythemia vera
PWM. See Pokeweed mitogen
Pyarthrosis, 708
Pyelonephritis, 722, 723
tests. See Urine [tests]
Pylephlebitis, 701
Pyogenic arthritis, acute, 708
Pyomyositis, 713
Pyridine-3-carboxylic acid, 213. See
also Niacin
Pyridoxal-5-phosphate, 225
Pyridoxamine. See Pyridoxine
4-Pyridoxic acid, 225, 226, 226t
Pyridoxine, 213
deficiency, 69, 226, 227t, 448
dependent syndromes, 227t
recommended daily intake, 214t
reference ranges for, 215t, 226,
226t
Pyridoxine [test], 225–227
Pyridoxol. See Pyridoxine
Pyropoikilocytosis, hereditary, 463
Pyrroline-5-carboxylate reductase
defect, 146t
Pyrroloporphyrias, 55, 57
Pyruvate, 222
formation of lactate, 128
Pyruvate carboxylase, 128f
Pyruvate kinase deficiency, 484
Pyuria, 49, 723–724, 730, 731f. See
also Urine
causes of, 724t
screening [test], 725
sterile, 724
PZ (pancreozymin), 92

Q

Q fever, 658, 669t, 713, 814, 820
serology, 811, 812t
Quality control, 6
external, 6
internal, 6
Quantitation of immunoglobulins
(QIgs) [test], 841–844
Quinidine:
continuous infusion, 336f
drug interactions, 341, 349, 357,
359

hemolytic anemia from, 894t
pharmacokinetic parameters,
349t
syncope, 348
therapeutic range, concentration,
and distribution, 334t
Quinidine [test], 355–356
Quinine: hemolytic anemia from,
894t
Quinsy throat, 641

R

Rabies virus:
brain biospy, 785
encephalitis, 772t, 773, 777
serology [test], 823
Radiation therapy: immunologic
effects, 861–862
Radiator fluid, 378–379
Radiography: and lower respiratory
infections, 660–661
Radioimmunoassay (RIA), 813
for fungi, 825, 825t
Raji cell assay [test], 848, 850
Rapid ACTH test, 259–261
Rashes. See Skin
ras oncogene, 328t
Rat bite fever, 716. See also
Spirillum minus
blood culture [test], 626–627
skin lesions, 626–627
Raynaud's phenomenon: cryoglobu-
lins and, 170
RBC. See Red blood cells
RBC compatibility testing, 865,
872–873
RBC distribution width (RDW), 457,
459, 460t, 461, 461t
RBC fragments, 433
RBC mass and plasma volume [test],
496–497
RBC morphology [test], 462–463
RBP (retinol-binding protein) [test]:
and liver function, 83
Rebuck skin window [test], 597
Receiver operating characteristic
(ROC) curve, 9f, 9–10
Recessive oncogenes, 328
Rectal biopsy, 706, 765
Rectal discharge: pathogens, 734t,
744
Rectal exam: for STDs, 743–745
Rectal swabs, 755. See also Stool cul-
ture
Red blood cells (RBC), 431. See also
Erythropoiesis; specific
cells

abnormal morphology, Plate 4,
Plate 5, 431–434
acanthocytes, 431
and acid-base balance, 12–15, 13t
alloantibody detection, 874–881.
See also Alloantibody
detection
anisocytosis, 431
antibodies in serum and eluate,
890–891
antibody detection, 874
antigen typing, 890
autoagglutination, 890
autoagluttination, 431
basophilic normoblast, 429
basophilic stippling, 431
blister cells, 432
blood group tests, 873t, 873–
874
burr cells, 432
Cabot rings, 432
casts in urine, 50, 54, 62f
codocytes, 434
compatibility testing, 865,
872–873
count [test], 457–462
crenated, 432
crossmatch, 874
distribution width (RDW), 457,
459, 460t, 461, 461t
drepanocytes, 433
drugs firmly bound to, 893, 894t
drugs loosely bound to, 893
dyplastic nucleated, Plate 22A,
Plate 31B, 431
elliptocytes (ovalocytes), 432
enzymes, quantitative [test], 478f,
483f, 484
erythropoiesis, 427–434
fragility [test], 480–481, 481f
fragments, 433
frozen-deglycerolized, 867t
glycolytic action, 129
half-life [test], 448f, 455t, 484
Heinz bodies, 432, 477
hemoglobin C crystals, 432
hemolysis, and vitamin E, 220,
221t
Howell-Jolly bodies, 432
hyperchromia, 432
hypochromia, 432
large reticulocyte, 431
LD levels in, 36
leptocytes, 434
macrocytes, 433
macronormoblast, 431
macro-ovalocyte, 431
mass and plasma volume [test],
496–497

Red blood cells (RBC) *(Continued)*
    mean cell volume (MCV), 450, 457, 458f, 459, 460t, 461, 461t, 462–463
    megaloblastic nucleated, Plate 7, 431
    microcytes, 433
    morphology [test], 462–463
    normal morphology, Plate 1, 426f, 427–431
    normochromic, 431
    normocytic, 431
    orthochromic normoblast, 429
    Pappenheimer bodies, 433
    in pleural fluid, 115t
    poikilocytosis, 433
    polychromasia, 433
    polychromatophilic normoblast, 429
    pretransfusion testing, 865, 871–872
    pronormoblast, 427
    reagent, 875, 875t
    reference values for parameters, 459, 460t
    reticulocyte, 429, 431
    rouleaux, 433
    schistocytes, 433
    sickle cells, 433
    sideroblasts, ringed, 433–434
    spherocytes, 434
    spurious parameter results, 459, 460t
    stomatocytes, 434
    target cells, 434
    teardrop cells (dacrocytes), 434
    transfusion, 866t–867t, 872–874. *See also* Transfusions
    in urine, 48–49
    washed, 867t
Red blood cell disorders, 447–498. *See also specific disorders*
    anemia, 447–448, 448f
    macrocytic anemias, 449–450, 451t, 467f, 474t
    microcytic anemias, 448–449, 449t, 450t
    normocytic anemias, 448f, 450–455, 451t, 452f, 454f, 455t
    polycythemias, 455–457, 456t
Red blood cell disorders [tests]:
    for abnormal hemoglobin, 484–496
    acidified serum lysis for PNH, 476–477
    autohemolysis, 482–483
    basic, 457–466
    deoxyuridine suppression, 476
    erythropoietin, 497
    ferritin, 466t, 466–468, 467f, 468t
    folate, 472t, 473–475, 474t
    glucose 6-phosphate dehydrogenase screen, 477–479, 478f, 479t
    heat stability, 484
    Heinz bodies, 453, 478f, 479–480
    hemoglobin A_2, 490–492
    hemoglobin electrophoresis, 484–490, 485f, 486t–487t, 488f, 491t
    hemoglobin F, 492–493
    hemoglobin H, 488f, 493–494
    hemogram (CBC), 457–462, 458f, 459f, 460t, 461t
    for hemolytic anemia, 476–484
    iron, 468–470, 469t
    isopropanol denaturation, 494
    Kleihauer-Betke (acid elution for fetal hemoglobin), 495
    for macrocytic anemia, 471–476
    mass and plasma volume, 496–497
    methylmalonic acid, 476
    for microcytic anemia, 466–471
    osmotic fragility, 480–481, 481f
    protoporphyrin, 470–471
    RBC enzymes, quantitative, 478f, 483f, 484
    RBC half-life, 448f, 455t, 484
    RBC morphology, 462–463
    reticulocyte count, 463–464
    Schilling, 473t, 475–476
    sedimentation rate, 464–466, 465t
    sickle hemoglobin solubility, 495–496
    sucrose hemolysis, 481–482
    vitamin B_{12} (cobalamin), 471–472, 472t, 473t
Reed-Sternberg cell, 443, 577, 603, 615
Reference ranges, 6, 7–8
    influences on, 7t
Refetoff's syndrome, 248
Refractometry: for urine, 55
Refractory anemia (RA), 566, 567, 567t
Refractory anemia with excess of blasts in transformation (RAEB-IT), 566, 567t
Refractory anemia with ringed sideroblasts (RARS), 566, 567t
Refractory megaloblastic leukemia, 565
Refsum's disease: testing for, 419
Regan isoenzyme, 73, 73t, 74t, 310
Regression to the mean, 7
Reiter's cell: in synovial fluid, 118t
Reiter's disease (syndrome), 708
    synovial fluid examination, 117t
Relapsing fever: lesions and tests, 678t
Renal disease:
    alkaline phosphatase and, 73
    categories of, 41
    Mycobacterium tuberculosis, 728–729
    protein ranges in, 156t
    stones, 298
    tumor markers, 317, 323, 325
Renal failure:
    ammonia and, 78
    and anemia, 451t, 452
    CEA elevation in, 319t
    drug half-life equation, 336t
    and hypercholesterolemia, 178
    pancreatitis and, 90
    protein levels and, 157t
    and protein tests, 155, 161
    and PTH test, 302
    zinc deficiency and, 211
Renal function [tests], 41–65
    aluminum, 60
    bicarbonate, 47–48
    chloride, 47
    clearance, 59–60
    creatine, 61
    creatinine, 42–44
    cyclic AMP, 58
    endocrine, 58–59
    inulin clearance, 59–60
    phenosulfonphthalein, 60
    porphyrias, 55–58
    potassium, 46–47
    renin, 58–59
    sodium, 46
    urea nitrogen, 41–42
    uric acid, 44–45
    urinalysis, 48–55
Renal hypertension, 272t
    renin testing and, 276t, 276-277
Renal transplantation:
    α_1-antitrypsin and, 167
    immunologic effects, 862
Renal tubular disorders, 41
Renal tubular epithelial cells: in urine, 50, 61f
Renal vein renin ratios, 276t, 277
Renin, 270
Renin [test], 58–59, 275–277. *See also* Plasmin renin activity
Renin-angiotensin-aldosterone system, 59
Reoviral encephalitis, 772t

Repeating tests, 7
Reports: of laboratory tests, 7
Reptilase time, 516f, 528, 541
Reptilase time [test], 528
Reserpine: drug interactions, 355
Respiration, 11
Respiratory acidosis, 17, 18t, 18–19, 21
Respiratory alkalosis, 17, 18t, 20, 20t, 21
Respiratory function monitoring, 16–17
Respiratory infection serology [test], 823–824
Respiratory syncytial virus:
 bronchiolitis, 647
 ear infection, 637
 infection frequency, 636t
 pneumonia, 657, 658, 660, 668, 670t
 serology [test], 823–824
 throat culture, 641
 upper respiratory infections, 636t, 670t
Respiratory system, 11–12
 and acid-base balance, 12–15
 defenses, 655–656
 lower tract infections, 655–674. *See also* Pneumonia
 predisposing factors for infection, 655, 656t, 657
 seasonal prevalence of infections, 660t
 types of lower tract infection, 657t, 657–658
 upper tract infections, 635, 636, 638–647. *See also* Upper respiratory infections
Respiratory system [tests]:
 direct examination for parasites, 671–674
 lower tract, 655–674
 nasal culture, 638–639
 nasopharynx culture, 646–647
 sputum culture, 655–670
 throat culture, 641–646
Restriction fragment length polymorphism (RFLP) [test], 98–99
Reticulocyte, 427, 429, 431, 463
 count [test], 450, 463–464
 large, 431
 production index, 450, 453, 464
Reticulocytosis, 451t, 453
Reticulum cell, 443, 463
Retinol, 216. *See also* Vitamin A
Retinol-binding protein (RBP) [test]: and liver function, 83
Retortamonas intestinalis, 760t

Retropharyngeal abscess, 635, 642, 643
Retroviruses, 328
Reye syndrome, 78, 773, 773t
RFLP (restriction fragment length polymorphism) [test], 98–99
Rhabdoviruses: CNS infection, 772t, 777t
Rh blood group, 873, 873t
 and autoagglutination, 890
 compatibility testing, 872–873
 and platelet transfusion, 885
Rhesus (Rh) immunoglobulin, 404, 406, 407
Rheumatic fever:
 and *Streptococcus pyogenes*, 808
 synovial fluid examination, 117t
Rheumatoid arthritis, 708
 autoantibody, 845t
 drugs for, 364–365
 ESR and, 465
 hypergammaglobulinemia and, 160
 protein ranges in, 156t
 synovial fluid examination, 117t, 118
 vitamin D deficiency and, 219
Rheumatoid arthritis precipitin (RAP), 845t
Rheumatoid factor, 845t
 pleural fluid [test], 116
Rheumatoid pleural effusions, 116
Rh immunoglobulin transfusion data, 870t
Rhinitis, 635, 641, 643t
Rhinocerebral mucormycosis, 640
Rhinoscleroma, 681t
Rhinoviruses:
 ear infection, 637
 infection frequency, 636t
 throat infection, 641
 upper respiratory infections, 636t
Rhizopus, 640, 671t
 and burn wounds, 717
 cultures, 697t
Rhodesian trypanosomiasis, 631, 774–775
Rhodotorula, 728
 fungemia, 625
RIA. *See* Radioimmunoassay
Riboflavin, 213
 deficiency, 224
 recommended daily intake, 214t
Riboflavin [test], 224–225
Ribonuclease, 89
Rickets:

 alkaline phosphatase and, 72
 vitamin D deficiency and, 218–219, 219t
 X-linked hypophosphatemic, 219
Rickettsia:
 blood culture [test], 622, 626
 lymphadenopathy, 715
 skin manifestations, 677t, 678t, 679t
Rickettsia akari:
 serology and transmission, 812t
 skin manifestations, 679t
Rickettsialpox: serology and transmission, 812t
Rickettsial serology [tests], 811–813, 812t
Rickettsia prowazekii:
 serology and transmission, 812t, 813
 skin manifestations, 677t
Rickettsia quintana: skin manifestations, 678t
Rickettsia rickettsii:
 serology [test], 811, 812t
 skin manifestations, 677t, 678t
Rickettsia tsutsugamushi:
 serology and transmission, 812t, 813
 skin manifestations, 678t, 679t
Rickettsia typhi: serology and transmission, 812t, 813
Rifampicin: hemolytic anemia from, 894t
Rifampin: drug interactions, 349, 356
Rift Valley fever virus, 771, 772t
 chorioretinitis, 649, 649t
Riley-Day syndrome, 283
Ringworm: skin manifestations, 678t
Ristocetin cofactor activity [test], 531t, 532
Ristocetin-induced aggregation [test], 532–533
River blindness, 632
RNP autoantibody, 845t
ROC curve, 9f, 9–10
Rocio virus, 772t
Rocket electrophoresis: for CSF immunoglobulin, 112
Rocky Mountain spotted fever, 677t, 678t
 serology [test], 811, 812t, 813
Rotaviral gastroenteritis, 747, 752t, 758
Rouleaux, 433
R proteins, 471
RPR (rapid plasma reagin) [test], 809–810, 810t
Rubbing alcohol [test], 378

Rubella virus:
  arthritis, 707
  blood culture [test], 628t
  conjunctivitis, 648, 649t
  ear infection, 637
  progressive panencephalitis, 773t
  serology [test], 804, 824
  skin manifestations, 677t, 684
Rubeola virus:
  blood culture [test], 628t
  encephalitis, 773
  eye infections, 648, 649t
  immunology, 861
  oral lesions, 642, 643t
  pneumonia, 670t
  serology [test], 824
  skin manifestations, 677t, 678t
  upper respiratory infections, 636t, 670t
Rubriblast, 427
Rubricytes, 427
Russell bodies, 440
Russell viper venom time, dilute (RVVT) [test], 528, 543, 544
Russian spring-summer encephalitis, 772t

S

Sabin-Feldman dye test, 780
Saccharomyces, 728
Sacrocystis, 766
St. Louis encephalitis, 772t
Salicylate:
  drug interactions, 344t, 366
  and glycohemoglobin, 137
  poisoning, 381, 381f
  therapeutic range, concentration, and distribution, 334t
Salicylate [test], 380–382
Saline:
  suppression test for primary aldosteronism, 273t, 273–274
  test for alloantibody detection, 876, 878t
Salivary amylase, 86, 87, 88t, 90
Salmonella:
  direct examination of blood [test], 627
  infections, 625t
  osteomyelitis, 710
  septic arthritis, 707–708
Salmonella arizona, 716
Salmonella choleraesuis, 754

Salmonella enteritidis: gastroenteritis, 752t, 753, 754, 755, 756
Salmonella paratyphi, 754
Salmonella typhi:
  blood culture, 622
  bone marrow culture [test], 634
  gastroenteritis, 622, 753t, 754
  serology [test], 804, 809
  skin manifestations, 678t
Salpingo-oophoritis, 701–702
Salt retention: hypoproteinemia and, 153
Saltzman test, 535
Sanfilippo syndrome, 416
Saprophytes: gastrointestinal, 747, 755
Sarcocystis hominis: gastroenteritis, 753t, 760, 760t
Sarcocystis lindemanni, 713
Sarcoid:
  ACE test and, 277
  pituitary, 290t
Sarcoptes scabiei: skin manifestations, 678t, 686
SBB [test], 605
Scabies: lesions and tests, 678t, 686
Scalded skin syndrome: lesions, agent, and tests, 678t, 679t
Scales, 681t
Scarlet fever: lesions, agent, and tests, 678t
S-C disease, 463
Schie syndrome, 416
Schilling test, 96–97, 610
  for anemia, 469, 472, 473t, 475–476
Schistocytes, 432, 433, 463
Schistosoma haematobium, 53, 721, 731–732, 762t, 763, 763t, 765
Schistosoma japonicum, 702t, 703, 762t, 763, 763t
Schistosoma mansoni, 702t, 703, 732, 762t, 763, 763t
Schistosoma mekongi, 702t, 703, 762t, 763, 763t
Schistosomiasis, 702t, 703, 704. *See also specific species*
  gastrointestinal, 702t, 703, 704, 763, 765
  serology [test], 830t, 831
  urinary, 731–732
Schlicter test, 795
Scleroderma:
  autoantibody, 845t
  synovial fluid examination, 117t
Scleroma, 638

Screening, 4–5
  criteria for evaluating usefulness of, 4t
Screening differential [test], 589–592
Scrofula, 680t
Scrub typhus:
  lesions, agent, and tests, 678t, 679t
  serology and transmission, 812t
Scurvy, 231–233
Scutulum crust, 681t
Se. *See* Selenium
Sea urchin cells, 432
Secobarbital [test]: toxicity, 384–386, 385t
Secretin, 102
Secretin [test], 91–92
Secretin-cholecystokinin [test], 92, 94
Sedimentation rate [test], 464–466, 465t
Seizure therapeutic drugs. *See* Anticonvulsants
Selenium:
  abnormalities, 200t
  body content, 199t
  excretion route, 200t
  reference ranges for, 211
Selenium [test], 210–211
Semen analysis [test], 122–125
Seminal fluid, 122
Seminoma: tumor markers, 315t
γ-Seminoprotein: as prostatic tumor marker, 313t
Sensitivity, 2, 3f, 4, 5, 6
  ROC curves, 9, 9f
Sepsis: defined, 620
Septic arthritis:
  defined, 798
  synovial fluid examination, 118–119, 125t, 709t
  testing for, 707–709
Septicemia. *See also* Bacteremia
  catheter-associated, 633–634
  defined, 620
Serine, 147
  biochemistry and reference range, 145t
Serine protease inhibitors (SERPINS), 506, 507t, 509, 520t, 550
  assessment [tests], 546–548
Serodiagnosis of infectious disease [tests], 803–833
  agglutination reactions, 805
  analysis, 804–805
  bacterial, 806–811. *See also* Bacterial serology

chlamydial, 814
complement fixation test, 805
enzyme immunoassay, 805
fungal, 825–829. *See also* Fungal serology
immunodiffusion, 805
mycoplasmal, 814–815
overview, 803–805
parasitic, 829–833. *See also* Parasitic serology
particle-enhanced immunoassay, 805
rickettsial, 811–813, 812t
selection, 804
serum neutralization test, 805
specimen collection, 804
viral, 815–825. *See also* Viral serology
Serositis: testing for, 850
Serotonin, 99
Serotonin release [test], 514t, 536
SERPINS (serine protease inhibitors), 506, 507t, 509, 520t, 550
family assessment [tests], 546–548
Serratia. *See also* Enterobacteriaceae
arthritis, 707
septic arthritis, 707–708
Serratia marcescens: and burn wounds, 716, 717
Sertoli cells, 123, 283, 294
Serum amylase [test], 86–87, 87f, 90
Serum and red blood cell folic acid [test], 472t, 474t, 474–475
Serum bactericidal test (SBT) [test], 794–795
Serum glutamate oxaloacetate transaminase (SGOT) [test], 69–70
Serum glutamate pyruvate transaminase (SGPT) [test], 68–69
Serum glycoproteins [test], 137–138
Serum neutralization (NT) test, 805. *See also* Serodiagnosis of infectious disease
Serum protein electrophoresis [test], 154–158, 156t–157t
Serum tumor markers. *See* Tumor markers
Serum viscosity [test], 170–171
Severe combined immunodeficiencies, 858, 859t
testing for, 840, 841
Sex hormone-binding globulin (SHBG), 287–288, 289, 290, 292, 293
Sex hormones, 283–284, 284f
Sex hormones [tests], 283–294
dehydroepiandrosterone sulfate, 291t, 291–292
estradiol, 292f, 292–294, 293t
follitropin, 285–286, 286t
gonadotropin releasing hormone stimulation, 286–287
gonadotropins, 285–286, 286t
inhibin, 294
luteinizing releasing hormone stimulation, 286–287
lutropin, 285–286, 286t
sperm penetration assay, 294
testosterone, 287f, 287–290, 288t, 289t, 290t
bioavailable, 290–291
free, 290
Sexual development anomalous: congenital adrenal hyperplasia and, 271t
Sexually transmitted diseases, 733–746. *See also specific pathogens and diseases*
lymphadenopathy, 714–715
stool cultures, 750
syndromes and pathogens, 734t
testing for, 733–746. *See also* Genital tract [tests]; Urine [tests]
Sézary cell, Plate 27A, 441
Sézary syndrome:
immunophenotyping, 602, 856
morphology/manifestations/markers, 574t
SGOT (serum glutamate oxaloacetate transaminase) [test], 69–70
SGPT (serum glutamate pyruvate transaminase) [test], 68–69
SHBG (sex hormone-binding globulin), 287–288, 289, 290, 292, 293
Sheehan syndrome, 293t
Shiga bacillus, 754
Shigella:
anorectal infection, 744
gastroenteritis, 753t, 754, 755
Shigella dysenteriae: gastroenteritis, 753t, 754
Shingles, 678t, 684, 824. *See also* Varicella-zoster virus
Shock: and lactic acidosis, 422, 422t
Short ACTH test, 259–261
Short tetracosactrin test, 259–261
Shunting:
of blood, 11–12
and hypoxemia, 17
SIADH. *See* Antidiuretic hormone, syndrome of inappropriate
Sialytransferase: and breast cancer, 329t
Sickle cell, 433
Sickle cell anemia:
testing for, 411, 412
zinc deficiency and, 211, 212
Sickle cell disease: and osteomyelitis, 710
Sickle cell preparation [test], 495–496
Sickledex [test], 495–496
Sickle hemoglobin solubility [test], 495–496
Sideroblastic anemias, 448, 449t, 566, 567, 567t
Sideroblasts, ringed, 433–434
Silicon, 199
Silver nitroprusside test, 147
Simulium, 650
Sinus aspirate cultures [test], 639–641
Sinusitis, 639–641, 645t
etiology and tests for, 680t
Sjögren's antigens, 845t
Sjögren's syndrome: autoantibody, 845t
Skeletal muscle autoantibody, 845t
Skeletal muscle disease, 712–713
Skin:
abscess aspiration, 689, 692f
biopsy, 682–683, 694t
cultures, 683, 695, 696t–697t, 698–699
foreign bodies in, 676
infections. *See* Skin infections
normal, 675–676
scrapings, 688–689, 691f, 694t
specimen collection, 688–691
trauma, 676
Skin infections, 675–700
contaminations, 699–700
cultures, 695t, 695–699, 696t–697t
deep infiltrations, 681t
extent of disease, 676, 682
hemorrhage, 677t
history and physical examination, 676
and inflammation, 683t
lesion morphology, 676, 677t–681t
parasitic, 676, 686–686
viral, 676, 683–684, 699
Skin scales, 688, 691f, 694t
Skin tumors: etiology and tests for, 681t

Skin ulcers: etiology and tests for, 679t, 685, 694t
Slavic leprosy, 638
SLE. *See* Systemic lupus erythematosus
Sleep apnea: and polycythemia, 456t
Sleeping pills: toxicity, 385–386
Sleeping sickness, 631, 774–775, 779, 782
Small cell follicular lymphoma:
    cells, Plate 28A, 441, 856f
    immunophenotyping, 603
Small cell lymphocytic lymphoma, 856f
Small cleaved cell lymphoma, 856f
Small intestine culture [test], 749–750
Smallpox: skin manifestations, 678t
Sm antigen, 845t
SmC/IGF I, 240
Smoking:
    CEA elevation in, 319t
    and polycythemia, 456t, 457, 497
    and theophylline clearance, 335t
Smoldering leukemia, 565
Smooth muscle autoantibody, 845t
Smudge cell, 440
Snake bites, 715–716
Sodium [test], 46
    reference ranges for, 46t
Sodium urate crystals: in urine, 52
Soft tissue infections, 675–670
    lesion morphology, 676, 677t–681t
Somatomedin C [test], 240–241
Somatostatin, 99, 102
Somatotrophin [test], 237–240
South African genetic porphyria, 57
Southern blot analysis [test], 411–413, 412f, 602
Specific esterase [test], 605–606
Specificity, 2, 3f, 4, 5, 6
    ROC curves, 9, 9f
Specimen acquisition, 2f, 5–6, 6t
Sperm:
    macrocephalic, 124
    morphology, 124
    motility, 124
Sperm analysis [test], 122–125
Spermatogenesis, 122
Sperm penetration assay [test], 294
Spherocytes, 434, 463, 480–481
Spherocytosis, hereditary, 476, 480, 481, 482–483
Sphingolipids, 182
Sphingomyelin, 182
    in amniotic fluid, 408–409
Spiculated cells, 431
Spina bifida, 402, 405t

Spinal taps, 107. *See also* Cerebrospinal fluid
    traumatic, 107
Spirillum minus (minor):
    blood culture, 622
    and endocarditis, 626t
    rat bite fever, 626–627
    skin manifestations, 678t
Splenic abscess, 701
    testing for, 704, 705–707
Splenic disease: alkaline phosphatase and, 73
Splenic parasites, 702t, 702–703
Spongiform encephalopathy, 771t
Sporothrix schenckii:
    arthritis, 707–708
    eye infections, 649
    skin/tissue manifestations, 679t, 681t
S100 protein, 602
S protein. *See* Protein S
Spur cells, 431
Sputum coloration, 666, 667f
Sputum culture [test], 655–670
    grading quality of sputum, 662t
    for parasites, 672
    specimen collection, 661–662
Squamous epithelial cells: in urine, 50, 61f
Standard deviation (SD), 5, 6
    plus/minus 2 from the mean, 6, 7
    between run, 5
Staphylococcus: blood culture and, 621t
Staphylococcus aureus:
    arthritis, 707
    bites, 679t
    blood culture, 623
    burns, 679t, 716
    catheter infections, 633
    CNS infections, 770
    cultures, 696t, 700f
    ear infection, 636, 638
    eye infections, 648, 650
    gastroenteritis, 753, 753t, 755
    infections, 625t, 655
    lymphadenopathy, 714
    muscle disease, 713
    nasal infection, 639
    orbital cellulitis, 639
    osteomyelitis, 709–710
    pelvic infection, 701
    pericarditis, 711
    puncture wounds, 680t
    respiratory infection, 657, 670t
    serology [test], 808
    skin manifestations, 678t, 679t, 680t, 687f, 692, 693, 699

    susceptibility testing, 792–793, 794t
    throat infection, 641
    traumatic wounds, 718
    upper respiratory infections, 645t
    vancomycin for, 798
Staphylococcus capitis: cultures, 696t
Staphylococcus epidermidis:
    and burn wounds, 716
    conjunctival colonization, 648
    cultures, 696t, 700f
    ear colonization, 636
    endocarditis, 623
    eye infections, 648
    infections, 625t, 699
    oropharyngeal colonization, 670t
    peritoneal infection, 701
    prosthetic device infections, 711
    susceptibility testing, 794t
    traumatic wounds, 718
    urethral contaminant, 736
    urinary, 724, 726
Staphylococcus haemolyticus: cultures, 696t
Staphylococcus saprophyticus: urinary tract infections, 722
Starch:
    dietary, 127
    malabsorption, 96t
Starvation: protein ranges in, 156t
Status epilepticus: phenytoin for, 344–345
STDs. *See* Sexually transmitted diseases
Steady-state concentration, 337, 337t
Steady-state peak formula, 349t
Stearic acid, 181, 182t
Steatorrhea, 93, 94
Stenella arguata: skin manifestations, 678t
Steroid hormones, adrenal, 257
Stibophen: hemolytic anemia from, 894t
Stomach. *See also entries at* Gastric
Stomach biopsy, 749
Stomach culture [test], 749–750
Stomach flu, 754
Stomatitis, vesicular: skin manifestations, 678t
Stomatocytes, 434
Stool culture [test], 750–756, 751t–753t. *See also* Gastroenteritis
    ova and parasite, 759–766
    viral infections, 758, 759t
Stool egg quantitation, 762, 765
Storage of specimen, 6
"Street speed," 361

Streptobacillus moniliformis, 620, 716
   blood culture, 622, 626–627
   infections, 625t, 626t, 626–627
   skin manifestations, 678t, 687f
Streptococcal myositis, 681t
Streptococcus:
   antigenemia, 633, 726
   blood culture and, 621t
   cultures, 696t
   and endocarditis, 626t
   pelvic infection, 701
   pericarditis, 711
   urinary, 724
Streptococcus agalactiae (Group B):
   antigen detection, 780
   CNS infections, 770, 781
   infections, 625t
   pneumonia, 658, 670t
   skin manifestations, 679t
Streptococcus anginosus (milleri):
   infections, 625t
Streptococcus β-hemolytic:
   eye infections, 648
   infections, 625t
   upper respiratory infections, 645t
Streptococcus bovis: infections, 625t
Streptococcus faecalis, 55, 700f
Streptococcus pneumoniae:
   antigen, 671
   CNS infections, 770, 775
   ear infection, 637
   eye infections, 648, 650
   infections, 625t
   lower respiratory infection, 657, 666, 667f, 671t
   orbital cellulitis and sinusitis, 639–640
   skin manifestations, 677t
   and susceptibility testing, 789
   upper respiratory infections, 645t, 671t
Streptococcus pyogenes (Group A):
   bites, 679t, 715
   cultures, 696t
   ear infection, 636–637, 638
   gangrene, 680t
   infections, 625t
   lymphadenopathy, 714
   muscle disease, 713
   peritoneal infection, 701
   pneumonia, 670t
   septic arthritis, 707–708
   serology [test], 808–809
   sinusitis, 640
   skin/tissue manifestations, 677t, 678t, 679t, 680t, 681t, 692, 693, 695, 699
   susceptibility testing, 791
   traumatic wounds, 717–718
   upper respiratory infections, 641, 642, 643–645, 645t, 671t
Streptococcus sanguis, 700f
Streptococcus viridans:
   and endocarditis, 623
   infections, 625t
   skin manifestations, 677t, 699
Streptokinase, 525, 545, 550
Streptomyces somaliensis, 681t
Streptomycin:
   hemolytic anemia from, 894t
   monitoring [test], 797–798
Streptozyme [test], 808–809
Stress erythrocytosis, 456t, 457, 496, 497
Stress reticulocytes, 463
Striational autoantibody, 845t
String test, 760, 764
Strongyloides stercoralis:
   and AIDS, 860
   diarrhea, 753
   gastrointestinal infection, 677t, 686, 763t, 766
   pulmonary infection, 672, 672t
   serology [test], 831–832
   skin manifestations, 677t, 686
Strongyloidiasis. See *Strongyloides stercoralis*
Stuart-Prower factor: and vitamin K, 221
Subacute sclerosing panencephalitis (SSPE), 773, 773t
Subarachnoid hemorrhage:
   CSF lactate and, 111
   traumatic spinal tap vs., 107
Subarachnoid space, 768
Subdural abscess, 781t, 783
Succinylcholine: drug interactions, 360
Succinyl CoA (coenzyme A), 55, 471
Sucrase, 95
Sucrase-isomaltase deficiency, 96t
Sucrose, 127
   malabsorption, 96t
Sucrose hemolysis [test]: for anemia, 481–482
Sudan black B stain [test], 605
Sudanophilia, 605
Sugar metabolism, 95
Sugar water test, 481–482
Suicide: by drugs, 369
Sulfation factor, 240
Sulfisoxasole monitoring [test], 799
Sulfite oxidase, 209, 210
Sulfonamide:
   crystals in urine, 52, 63f
   drug interactions, 366
   hemolytic anemia from, 894t
   monitoring [test], 799
Sulfonylureas: drug interactions, 344t
Sulfuric acid, 12
Superoxide dismutase, 202
Suppressor genes, 328
Suppurative arthritis, 708
Supraventricular tachycardia: drugs for, 354, 355
Surface immunoglobulins (SIg) staining, 851, 852, 854, 856f
Surgical blood salvage, 882–883
Surgical wound infections, 680t, 689, 689f, 693f
Survey programs, 6
Sweat chloride [test], 98, 418–419
Swedish porphyria, 55, 57
Swimming pool granuloma, 681t
Symptomatic cutaneous porphyria, 57
Symptomatic porphyria, 57
Synderman diet, 148
Syndrome of inappropriate antidiuretic hormone (SIADH), 46, 294–295
   albumin levels and, 152
   disorders associated with, 295t
   water loading test, 295
Synovial biopsy, 708
Synovial fluid, 116
   characteristics, 117t, 709t
   eosinophils in, 118t
   LE cells in, 118t
   malignant cells in, 118t
   monocytes in, 118t
   pathologic classification of, 117t
   Reiter's cell in, 118t
Synovial fluid [tests], 116–122
   cell count, 117t, 117–118
   crystals, 118, 119t, 120f–124f
   culture, 707–709, 709t
   lactate, 118–120, 125t
   mucin clot, 118, 119f
Synovitis, hemorrhagic villonodular: synovial fluid examination, 117t
Syphilis. See also *Treponema pallidum*
   chancre, 679t, 740–743
   late, 809–810, 810t
   lymphadenopathy, 715
   neuro-, 112, 769, 810, 811
   primary, 809–810, 810t
   rectal, 744
   secondary, 741, 743, 809–810, 810t
   serology [test], 741, 742, 743, 809–811, 810t
   tertiary, 741, 743

Systemic lupus erythematosus:
   autoantibodies, 844, 845t
   drug-induced, 353, 845t
   hypergammaglobulinemia and, 160
   immunology, 860
   protein levels and, 157t, 168, 169, 170
   synovial fluid examination, 117t

T

T3. See Triiodothyronine
T4. See Thyroxine
T4. See T lymphocytes, helper
T8. See T lymphocytes, suppressor
Tabes dorsalis, 810
Taenia saginata, 761, 763t, 766
Taenia solium, 649, 650, 651, 702t, 703, 713, 714, 763t, 766
   CNS infection, 777t, 782, 783, 784, 785
   eye infections, 649
   gastrontestinal infection, 761
   pulmonary infection, 674
   serology [test], 830
TAG-72 (tumor associated glycoprotein) [test], 317, 319–320, 329
Tamm-Horsfall mucoprotein, 50, 53
Tamoxifen, 327
Tangier's disease:
   HDLs and, 189
   phospholipids and, 182
   protein ranges in, 156t
Tapeworms. *See also specific worms*
   CNS infection, 783–784
   gastrointestinal infection, 761–762, 766
   hepatic infection, 703
   pulmonary infection, 672t, 674
"Tar-baby" effect, 4
Target cells, 434, 463
Tartrate resistant [test], 609
Tartrate resistant acid phosphatase [test], 609
Tartrate resistant isoenzyme 5, 312
Tarul's disease, 421t
T-AT (thrombin-antithrombin III complex) [test], 500f, 550–551
Taurine, 147
   biochemistry and reference range, 145t
Taurocholates, 81
Tay-Sachs screening [test], 419
T cell. *See* T lymphocytes

T-cell CLL: morphology/manifestations/markers, 574t–575t
T-cell leukemia/lymphoma:
   adult, 441, 576, 617, 856
      immunophenotyping, 602, 603
      T-helper, morphology/manifestations/markers, 575t
   HTLV-1 and, 822
T-cell leukemias: testing for, 841, 856
T-cell lymphoma:
   cutaneous: morphology/manifestations/markers, 574t
   leukemic phase of: morphology/manifestations/markers, 575t
T-cell replacement factor, 438
TCT. *See* Thyrocalcitonin
TdT (terminal deoxynucleotidyl transferase) [test], 559, 604t, 606–608, 852, 855–856, 856f
Teardrop cells (dacrocytes), 434, 463
TEG (thromboelastography) [test], 529
Temazepam: half-life and therapeutic/toxic concentrations, 384t
Temporal arteritis: ESR and, 465
Teniposide: hemolytic anemia from, 894t
Teratoma: tumor markers, 315, 315t
Terminal deoxynucleotidyl transferase (TdT) [test], 559, 604t, 606–608, 852, 855–856, 856f
Testes: and testosterone, 288
Testicular damage, 124
Testicular failure, 124, 290t
Testicular tumors, 290
   germ cell, 314, 315t, 322
   hCG as marker, 322, 323, 324
   tumor marker, 310
Testosterone, 122, 258f, 283, 284, 285, 286
   serum reference levels, 289t
   synthesis, 287, 287f
Testosterone [tests], 287f, 287–290, 288t, 289t, 290t
   bioavailable, 290–291
   free, 290
Test probability, 2, 4
Test result distribution, 7–8, 8f
Tests. *See* Laboratory tests
Tetanus skin test, 855
Tetanus toxoid, 855
Tetracarboxyporphyrin, 55, 56f, 57, 58, 58t
Tetracosactrin:
   long [test], 261

short [test], 259–261
Tetracycline:
   drug interactions, 341
   hemolytic anemia from, 894t
   susceptibility testing, 794t
1,2,3,4-Tetrahydrobenzoquinolinol, 55
δ-9-Tetrahydrocannibol (THC), 387, 387t
Tetramethylbenzidine dihydrochloride, 604
Thalassemias, 448, 485
   α, 449t, 450t, 485, 487f, 487t, 491t, 493–494
   β, 449t, 450t, 485, 487t, 489, 491t, 492, 493, 494
   βδ, 485, 487t, 491t, 492, 493
   classification, 485, 486t–487t, 491t
   ferritin and, 467
   homozygous syndromes, 486
   intermedia, 485, 487t
   major, 485, 487t
   minor, 485, 487t
   S/β, 492
   silent trait, 487t
   testing for, 411, 470, 480, 481
   trait, 448–449, 449t, 450t, 455, 461, 485–486
Theophylline:
   adult metabolism, 362
   clearance, factors affecting, 335t
   continuous infusion formulas, 354t
   drug interactions, 360, 363
   infant metabolism, 362
   oral vs. continuous infusion, 362, 363f
   pharmacokinetic parameters, 362t
   therapeutic range, concentration, and distribution, 334t
Theophylline [test], 361–363
Therapeutic drug monitoring, 333–368, 797–800. *See also* Drugs [tests]
Thermolabile hemoglobin [test], 484
Thesaurocyte, 440
Thiamin, 213
   deficiency, 229t, 229–231
   inborn metabolic errors responsive to, 230t
   recommended daily intake, 214t
   reference ranges for, 215t, 230t
Thiamin [test], 229–231
Thiamine. *See* Thiamin
Thiamin load test, 230, 230t
Thiamin pyrophosphate, 229
Thiamin pyrophosphate effect, 230t, 230–231

Thiazide diuretics: drug interactions, 360
Thin-layer chromatography (TLC): in drug toxicology, 370, 372, 373f, 374t
Thiopental [test]: toxicity, 385t, 385–386
Thioridazine, 395
　testing for, 394, 394t
Thoracentesis, 663, 663t
Thormählen's test, 147
Threonine: biochemistry and reference range, 144t
Throat culture [test], 641–646
Throat infections, 635, 641–646
Throat swab: for lower respiratory specimen collection, 662–663
Thrombin, 499, 501, 502f, 503, 503f, 505, 507, 507f, 508, 508f, 509f, 546
　activation, 504–505
　formation, marker proteins and, 521f
Thrombin activation, in vivo [tests], 550–551
Thrombin-antithrombin III complex [test], 508f, 520t, 521f, 534f, 550–551
Thrombin inhibition [test], 545
Thrombin time [test], 517f, 525, 527–528
Thrombocytes. See Platelet(s)
Thrombocythemia, 442, 513
Thrombocytopenia, 442, 513, 521, 523t
　autoantibody, 845t
　bone marrow aspiration for, 610, 611–612
　causes of, 557t, 594, 610
　drug-dependent immune, 884
　essential, 567, 570, 570t
　　characteristics, 568t
　　chromosomal abnormality, 562t
　　PVSG diagnosis criteria, 570, 570t
　heparin-induced, 524t, 524–525
　testing for, 594–596
Thrombocytopenic purpura:
　neonatal alloimmune (NAITP), 883
　thrombotic (TTP), 521, 522t, 545, 887
Thrombocytopoiesis, 426f, 441–442
　morphology, 442
Thrombocytosis, 442, 513
Thromboelastography [test], 529
β-Thromboglobulin [test], 537

Thrombolytic factors: and vitamin K, 221
Thrombolytic therapy: and CK isoform measures, 30–31
Thrombomodulin, 507, 508f
Thrombophlebitis: and burns, 716
Thromboplastin, 526
Thrombotic disorders: approach to, 519–521, 520t, 521f
Thrombotic thrombocytopenic purpura (TTP), 521, 522t, 545, 887
Thromboxane A_2 pathway, 500, 501f
Thromboxane A_2 synthetase deficiency, 514t
Thromboxane synthetase, 505
Thrush, 641–642, 643, 737, 748, 821
Thymidine factor, 240
Thymidine kinase, 211
Thymidylate, 473
Thymolphthaleinmonophosphate, 312t, 313
Thymomas:
　autoantibody, 845t
　tumor markers, 320, 321
Thymosin, 438
Thymus lymphocytes. See T lymphocytes
Thyrocalcitonin [test]: tumor marker, 320–321
Thyroglobulin [test], 252
Thyroglobulin antibodies [test], 255
Thyroid agenesis, 252
Thyroid autoantibodies [tests], 254–256
Thyroid-binding globulin: conditions and disorders affecting ranges of, 156t
Thyroid-binding prealbumin (TBPA), 253, 253f
Thyroid carcinoma, 252
　medullary, 302, 307, 321
Thyroid gland, 243–245
　disease, 244
　and glucogenolysis, 128
Thyroid gland [tests], 243–256
　congenital hypothyroidism screening, 245, 245f
　disease states and, 244
　free hormones, 249–251
　free thyroxine, 249–250
　free thyroxine index, 250
　free triiodothyronine, 250–251
　nonthyroidal illness and, 244–245
　protein bound iodine, 251–252
　screening, 244
　thyroid stimulating hormone (thyrotropin), 244–245, 245f, 248–249, 321–322

　thyroxine, 246–247
　triiodothyronine, 247–248
　T_3 uptake, 250
Thyroid hormone binding ratio (THBR), 250
Thyroiditis, 244, 251–252, 255, 302
　chronic: autoantibody, 845t
　Hashimoto's, 252, 255, 256
Thyroid microsomal antibodies [test], 255–256
Thyroid microsomal thyroglobulin, 845t
Thyroid peroxidase, 255
Thyroid stimulating hormone, 237, 243, 244–245, 283, 400
　thyroxine and, 246
Thyroid stimulating hormone [test], 244–245, 245f, 248–249, 321–322
　antibodies and, 7
　sensitive, 248, 253
　T_4 and, 246
　TRH and, 253, 253f, 254t
Thyroid stimulating hormone receptor antibodies [test], 256
Thyroid stimulating immunoglobulins (TSI), 256
Thyronine [test], 252–253
Thyrotoxicosis, 256
　factitia, 252
　T_3, 246, 248
　T_4, 246, 248
Thyrotropin. See Thyroid stimulating hormone
Thyrotropin receptor antibodies (TRAb) [test], 256
Thyrotropin releasing hormone (TRH), 239, 244, 249, 255f
Thyrotropin releasing hormone (TRH) [test], 244, 253, 253f, 254t
Thyroxine, 243, 244, 244f, 245f
　low T_3 syndrome, 245
　metabolism, 244f
Thyroxine [test], 246–247
　free, 249–250, 251
　free index, 250, 251
　uptake, 250
Thyroxine-binding globulin, 253, 253f
Thyroxine-binding globulin [test], 254
TIBC (total iron binding capacity) [test], 468–470, 469t
Tick bites, 686
Tick-borne encephalitis, 772t, 773
Tick paralysis, 686

Tinea barbae, 678t
Tinea corporis, 678t
Tinea cruris, 678t
Tinea imbricata, 678t
Tinea nigra, 678t
Tinea pedis, 678t
Tinea versicolor, 678t
Tissue biopsies, 610–617
    bone marrow, 610–613
    lymph node, 613–617
Tissue biopsy, 682–683
Tissue cultures, 683
Tissue eosinophil, 443
Tissue factor, 502, 503f, 512f
Tissue infections, 675–670
    lesion morphology, 676, 677t–681t
Tissue mast cell, 443
Tissue neutrophil, 443–444
Tissue plasminogen activator, 509, 511f, 524
Tissue plasminogen activator [test], 512f, 519t, 550
Tissue polypeptide antigen: and breast cancer, 329t
Tissue specimen [test], 700–707
Tissue thromboplastin inhibition assay [test], 517f, 520, 543
T lymphocytes, 438, 837–838, 838f, 839f, 851–862
    ALL and, 564, 565t, 579, 602, 607
    antigen markers, 599t
    CLL and, 574t–575t
    defects, 858–859, 859t
    effector (killer), 838, 851
    functions, 439, 553, 851–852
    helper (CD4), 438, 439, 841t, 851
    CLL morphology/manifestations/markers, 574t–575t
    immunophenotyping by flow cytometry, 600f
    leukemias of differentiated, 574t–575t, 576–581. *See also specific leukemias*
    marker studies, 841t
    morphology, 438–439, 851
    proliferation, 838
    suppressor (CD8), 438, 439, 841t, 851
Tobramycin:
    monitoring [test], 797–798
    reference range, 798t
    therapeutic range, concentration, and distribution, 334t
Tocainide carbamoyl glucuronide (TG), 356
Tocainide [test], 356–357
α-Tocopherol, 219, 220, 221t
Togaviruses:
    encephalitis, 772t, 774, 776t
    hepatitis, 702t
    skin manifestations, 677t
Tolbutamide:
    hemolytic anemia from, 894t
    tolerance [test], 141
o-Tolidine test, 54
Tolmetin: hemolytic anemia from, 894t
Toluidine blue stain [test], 609
Tolypocladium inflatum, 364
Tonsillar abscess, 635, 642, 643
Tonsillitis, 641
Torch agents: serology, 804
Total complement [test], 846–848, 847f, 848t
Total eosinophil count [test], 592
Total iron binding capacity (TIBC) [test]: for anemia, 468–470, 469t
Total lymphocyte count [test], 838, 840
Total protein [test], 152–153
Total ventilation, 11
Touch preparation of biopsy, 610
Tourniquet test, 530
Toxic granules, Plate 9A, 437, 589
Toxicology: of drugs, 369–398. *See also specific drugs*
Toxic shock syndrome: skin manifestations, 678t
Toxic vacuoles, Plate 9A, 437
Toxi-Lab, 372
Toxocara, 703, 705
    eye infections, 649, 650, 651, 654, 703
    serology [test], 830t, 832
Toxocariasis. *See Toxocara*
Toxoplasma gondii, 702, 702t, 713, 714, 820
    and AIDS, 704, 714, 777–778, 782, 832, 860
    CNS infection, 774, 777t, 777–778, 779, 782–783
    eye infections, 649, 650, 653–654
    lymphadenopathy, 715
    pulmonary infection, 672, 672t, 673
    serology [test], 780, 804, 830t, 832
    testing for, 704
Toxoplasmosis. *See Toxoplasma gondii*
Tozer equation, 357
TRAb (thyrotropin receptor antibodies) [test], 256
Trace elements. *See* Trace metals
Trace metals, 199–213
    body content of, 199, 199t
    contamination, 200–201
    excretion routes for, 200t
    laboratory analysis of, 200t, 200–201. *See also* Trace metals [tests]
    toxicity, 200t, 201, 202, 204, 212
    toxicity [tests], 390–392
Trace metals [tests], 201–213
    chromium, 201–202
    cobalt, 202
    copper, 202–205
    copper/ceruloplasmin, 205
    copper (liver), 206
    free (dialysable) copper, 206–209
    manganese, 209
    molybdenum, 209–210
    radiocopper, 206
    selenium, 210–211
    zinc, 211–213
Tracheitis, 635, 641
Trachoma, 648, 652, 814. *See also Chlamydia trachomatis*
Transcobalamin, 227
    I, 471
    II, 471
Transcortin, 262, 263
Transcutaneous and continuous arterial blood gas monitoring [test], 22–23
Transferrin:
    conditions and disorders affecting ranges of, 156t, 160, 161
    and liver function, 67
Transferrin [test], 167
    for anemia, 468–470, 469t
Transfusion reactions, hemolytic, 879, 880
Transfusion request forms, 871
Transfusions, 865–896
    alloantibody detection, 874–881
    antibody detection, 874
    autologous, 881–882
    blood components, 866t–870t
    crossmatch, 874
    cryoprecipitated antihemolytic factor (AHF), 869t, 877–878
    plasma and plasma products, 887–888
    platelet, 883–886
    pretransfusion testing, 865, 871–872
    RBC, 872–874
Transient hypogammaglobulinemia of infancy, 160
Transitional epithelial cells: in urine, 50, 61f
Transketolase test, 230t, 230–231

Transthoracic needle biopsy, 664, 664t
Transtracheal aspiration, 663t, 663–664
TRAP (tartrate resistant acid phosphatase) [test], 609
Traumatic wound specimen [test], 717–718
Trazodone: therapeutic ranges and toxicities, 396t
Trehalose: malabsorption, 96t
Trematodes. *See also specific trematodes*
  extraintestinal infection, 762–763, 763t
  gastrointestinal infection, 761–762, 763t, 766
  pulmonary infections, 672t, 674
  in urine, 53
Trench fever: skin manifestations, 678t
Trench mouth, 641
Trephine biopsy, 610
Treponema carateum: skin manifestations, 677t
Treponema denticola, 743
Treponema pallidum. *See also* Syphilis
  CNS infections, 770
  eye infections, 648
  genital ulcer, 734t, 740–743
  infection, 733
  nontreponemal tests, 809–810, 810t
  serology [test], 809–811, 810t
  skin manifestations, 678t, 679t
  treponemal tests, 810t, 810–811
Treponema pertenue: skin manifestations, 679t
Treponema refringens, 743
TRH (thyrotropin releasing hormone) [test], 253
Triamterene: hemolytic anemia from, 894t
Trichinella spiralis, 713–714
  serology [test], 830t, 832
  skin manifestations, 678t
Trichinosis. *See Trichinella spiralis*
Trichloracetic acid technique: for CSF protein, 109
Trichomonas hominis, 737, 760t, 765
Trichomonas tenax, 737
Trichomonas vaginalis:
  urethritis, 734, 734t
  urinary infection, 721, 731, 732
  in urine, 53
  vaginitis, 734t, 737, 738t, 738–739
Trichophyton concetricum, 678t

Trichophyton mentagrophytes, 678t, 679t, 681t
Trichophyton rubrum, 678t, 681t
Trichophyton schoenleinii, 678t
Trichophyton verrucosum, 678t
Trichophyton violaceum, 678t, 681t
Trichopoliodystrophy. *See* Menkes disease
Trichostrongylus, 761, 763t
Trichuris trichuria, 705, 761, 763t, 765
Tricyclic antidepressants:
  pharmacokinetics, 395
  platelet disorders induced by, 516t
  therapeutic ranges and toxicities, 396t
Tricyclic antidepressants [tests], 395–397
  desipramine, 359
  imipramine, 359
  nortriptyline, 360–361
Trifluoperazine: testing for, 394, 394t
Trigeminal neuralgia: carbamazepine for, 340
Triglycerides:
  casts in urine, 51
  and cholesterol levels, 177
  and chylomicrons, 191
  ^{14}C labeled, 94
  and flow chart for evaluation of hyperlipoproteinemias, 186f–187f
  and HDLs, 185
  and hyperlipoproteinemias, 183t
  and hypolipoproteinemias, 184t
  properties of, 174t
  reference ranges for, 180t
  structure of, 179f
Triglycerides [test], 178–181, 179f, 179t, 180t, 181t
Trihexyphenidyl: drug interactions, 361
Triiodothyronine, 243, 244
  low T_3, low T_4 syndrome, 245
  reverse, 243, 244f, 252
  and thyroxine test, 246–247
Triiodothyronine [test], 247–248
  free, 250–251
  reverse, 252
Trimethoprim/sulfamethoxizole: monitoring, 799
Trimipramine: therapeutic ranges and toxicities, 396t
Trinder's reagent, 129
^{14}C-Triolein breath [test], 94
2,6,8-Trioxypurine [test], 44–45
Tripeptide hydrolysis [test], 92–93

Triple phosphate crystals: in urine, 52, 63f
Trisomy 13, 402
Trisomy 18, 402
Trisomy 21. *See* Down syndrome
Trombicula irritans: skin manifestations, 677t
Trophoblastic disease, gestational: and hCG levels, 322, 323, 324
Tropical phagadenic ulcer, 679t
Tropical spastic paraparesis, 771t, 774, 822
Tropical sprue, 475
True negative ratio, 2, 8–9
True positive ratio, 2, 8–9
Trypanosoma brucei gambiense, 631, 774–775, 777t, 778, 782
Trypanosoma brucei rhodesiense, 631, 774–775, 777t, 778, 782
Trypanosoma cruzi, 631, 702t, 713, 714, 831
  serology [test], 832–833
  skin manifestations, 677t
Trypanosomiasis. *See also specific species*
  African: (sleeping sickness), 631, 774–775, 779, 782
  American, serology [test], 832–833
  blood examination [test], 629t, 631
Trypsin: for alloantibody detection, 876
Trypsin (immunoreactive) [test], 87f, 89, 90
Trypsin inhibitory capacity, 166
Trypsinogen, 89
Tryptophan:
  biochemistry and reference range, 144t
  load test for vitamin B_6, 226t, 226–227
TSH. *See* Thyroid stimulating hormone
TSH assay, 244
TSH-binding inhibitor immunoglobulins (TBII), 256
TSI-block antibodies, 256
TTI (tissue thromboplastin inhibition assay) [test], 517f, 520, 543
TTP. *See* Thrombotic thrombocytopenic purpura
TT (thrombin time) [test], 517f, 525, 527–528
Tube precipitins (TP) test: for coccidioidomycosis, 828

Tuberculin skin test, 776
Tuberculosis:
    and gastric infections, 749
    and pleural fluid, 115t
Tubular acidosis, 46
Tubular epithelial cell casts: in urine, 51
Tularemia, See *Francisella tularensis*
Tumor-associated glycoprotein [test], 317, 319–320, 329
Tumor-associated transplantation antigens, 167
Tumor associated trypsin inhibitor, 329t
Tumor cells: in urine, 52–53
Tumor markers, 307–332
    acid phosphatase, 311–313, 312t
    adrenocorticotropin, 321
    alkaline phosphatase, 309–310
    α-fetoprotein, 314–315, 315t
    antidiuretic hormone, 320
    β_2-microglobulin (B2M), 114
    for breast cancer, 328–329, 329t
    cachectin, 325–326
    calcitonin, 320–321
    cancer antigen 15-3, 316
    cancer antigen 19-9, 316
    cancer antigen 50, 317
    cancer antigen 72, 319–320
    cancer antigen 125, 317
    cancer antigen 195, 318
    cancer antigen 549, 318
    carcinoembryonic antigen, 318f, 318–319, 319t
    characteristics of ideal, 307, 308t
    classification of, 308t, 309
    corticotropin, 321
    creatine kinase, 310–311, 311f
    in CSF, 114
    enzymes, 308t, 309t, 309–314
    estrogen receptors, 326–327
    glycoproteins, 308t, 314–320
    hormones and hormone-like substances, 308t, 320t, 320–327
    human choriogonadotropin, 321–324, 323t, 324t
    lactate dehydrogenase, 311
    male PAP test, 311–313, 312t
    oncogenes and oncogene products, 308t, 328
    for ovarian carcinoma, 329, 329t
    for pancreatic carcinoma, 329t, 329–330
    parathyroid hormone, 324t, 324–325
    parathyroid hormone-like peptide, 325
    production rates, 308
    progesterone receptors, 327
    prostate specific antigen, 313–314
    prostatic acid phosphatase, 311–313, 312t
    thyrocalcitonin, 320–321
    tumor-associated glycoprotein, 319–320
    tumor necrosis factor-α, 325–326
    use of, 307–309, 328–330
Tumor necrosis factor-α [test]: tumor marker, 325–326
Tungsten blue, 45
Turner syndrome, 293t, 403
TWAR agent. See *Chlamydia pneumoniae* (TWAR agent)
Two compartment models for drugs, 337
2-Hour postprandial glucose [test], 131–132
Tympanic membrane rupture, 637
Tympanocentesis, 638
Typhoid fever: skin manifestations, 678t
Typhus:
    epidemic, 677t, 812t
    murine, 812t
    scrub, 678t, 812t
Tyrosinase, 202
Tyrosine:
    ascorbic acid and, 231
    biochemistry and reference range, 145t
    crystals in urine, 52, 63f
    elevated, 414
Tyrosine aminotransferase deficiency, 150
Tyrosinease deficiency, 146t, 150
Tyrosinemia, 55, 147, 149, 414
    enzymatic defect and features of, 146t
    hereditary, 58
Tyrosinosis, 150
Tyrosinuria, 150
Tzanck smear: for genital ulcers, 741–742, 743

U

UFC (urinary-free cortisol) [test], 262–264
Ulcerative colitis: CEA elevation in, 319t
Ulcerative gingivitis, 641
Ulcerative keratitis, 649
Ulceronodules: disease, etiology, and tests for, 681t, 687f
Ulcers, 99, 100, 100t
    chronic burrowing, 679t
    decubitus, 679t
    dermal, 679t, 686
    genital, 733, 734t
    genital tract specimens [test], 740–743
    herpes, 715, 733, 734t, 740, 741, 742, 743
    leg, 679t
    parasitic, 685
    skin: diseases, agents, and tests, 679t, 685, 694t
Ultratrace elements, 199. *See also* Trace metals
"Ulysses" syndrome, 4
Umbrella effect: in immunoelectrophoresis, 163–164
Units of measure, 7
Unstable hemoglobin [test], 484
Upper respiratory infections, 635, 636
    bacterial and fungal pathogens, 645t
    nasopharynx culture [test], 646–647
    testing for, 638–647
    throat culture [test], 641–646
    viruses causing, 636t
Urate crystals:
    amorphous, in urine, 52, 62f
    in synovial fluid, 119t, 120f, 121f, 122f
Urea:
    alkaline phosphatase isoenzymes and, 73t, 74t
    clearance, 42, 43t
    urea nitrogen vs., 42
Urea nitrogen [test], 41–42
    conditions outside reference ranges, 42t
Ureaplasma urealyticum: urethritis, 734, 734t, 737
Urease: gastric, 750
Uremia:
    and glycohemoglobin, 137
    hemodialysis for, 60
    vitamin B_{12} and, 228, 228t
Urethral exudate examination [test], 733–737
Urethral syndrome, acute, 722
Urethritis, 722, 726, 733–737, 734t
    differential diagnosis, 727t
    nongonococcal, 722, 734
    pathogens, 734, 734t
    tests. *See* Urine [tests]
Uric acid [test], 44–45
    conditions with levels outside reference ranges, 44t
    reference ranges for, 45t

Uric acid crystals: in urine, 51–52, 62f
Uricase method: for uric acid reference ranges, 45, 45t
Uridine diphosphate (UDP)-glucose, 416
Urinalysis [test], 48–55. *See also* Urine [tests]
   chemical analysis, 53
Urinary free corticoids [test], 262–264
Urinary indwelling catheter infections, 721, 722, 724, 726
Urinary retention, 314
Urinary tract calculus disease, 149
Urinary tract infection, 721–746. *See also* Urine [tests]
   predisposing factors, 721
   terminology, 722
Urine:
   acid, 51–52, 62f
   alkaline, 51–52, 62f
   AutoMicrobic system, 723
   bacteria in, 49–50
   bacterial count, 723–724
   bilirubin in, 54
   blood in, 54
   casts in, 50–51, 62f
   cells in, 48–50
   color analysis, 48, 49t
   contaminants in, 53, 722–723, 724
   crystals in, 51–52, 62f–63f
   erythrocytes in, 48–49
   glucose in, 54
   ketones in, 54
   leukocyte esterase in, 55
   macroscopic appearance, 48, 49t
   microscopic examination, 48, 61f–63f
   midstream (VB_2), 726, 727t
   mucus threads in, 53
   nitrite in, 54–55
   oval fat bodies in, 52
   parasites in, 53
   pH of, 53
   postmassage prostatic secretions (EPS), 726, 727t
   postmassage (VB_3), 726, 727t
   protein in, 53–54
   specific gravity of, 55
   specimen collection, 722–723
   suprapubic aspiration, 723
   tumor cells in, 52–53
   urobilinogen in, 54
   voided (VB_1), 726, 727t
   yeasts in, 53
Urine [tests], 721–732
   anaerobic culture, 727
   antibody coated bacteriuria, 726–727
   antigen detection, 725–726
   bacterial culture, 721–725
   bacterial microscopic examination, 730–731
   bacteriuria/pyuria screening, 725, 726t
   culture of specially collected specimens, 726, 727t
   direct microscopic examination, 730–732
   fungal culture, 727–728
   fungal microscopic examination, 730–731
   helminthic microscopic examination, 731–732
   Leptospira culture, 728
   to localize infection, 726–727
   Mycobacteria culture, 728
   Neisseria gonorrhoeae culture, 729
   protozoal microscopic examination, 731–732
   reagent strip, 725
   viral culture, 729–730, 730t
   viral microscopic examination, 732
Urine culture [tests]:
   anaerobic, 727
   bacterial, 721–725
   fungal, 727–728
   Leptospira, 728
   Mycobacteria, 728
   Neisseria gonorrhoeae, 729
   for specially collected specimens, 726, 727t
   viral, 729–730
Urine reagent strip [test], 725
Urinometer, 55
Urobilinogen, 418
   in urine, 54
Urokinase, 525, 545, 550
Uroporphyrin, 55, 56t, 58t, 418
Uroporphyrinogen III cosynthetase deficiency, 56t, 57
Urticaria pigmentosa, 581
Uterine cancer: tumor marker, 310, 316

V

Vaccenic acid, 182t
Vaccinia: skin manifestations, 678t, 684
Vaginal excretions [test], 737–739
Vaginitis, 737–739
   pathogens, 734t, 737
Vaginosis: bacterial, 734t, 737, 738t
Valine: biochemistry and reference range, 144t
Valproic acid, 341
   drug interactions, 341, 344, 344t, 347, 348
   pharmacokinetic properties, 341t
   therapeutic range, concentration, and distribution, 334t
Valproic acid [tests], 347
   unbound, 347–348
Vanadium, 199
Vancomycin:
   monitoring [test], 798–799
   therapeutic range, concentration, and distribution, 334t
Vanillylmandelic acid, 277, 278, 278f, 281
   diet, 280
Vanillylmandelic acid [test], 279–280
Variability of test, 5
Variation, coefficient of, 6
Varicella-zoster virus:
   arthritis, 707
   blood culture [test], 628t
   CNS infection, 771, 772t, 773
   ear infection, 637
   eye infection, 648, 649t
   immunology, 861
   pneumonia, 671t
   serology [test], 824–825
   skin manifestations, 678t, 679t, 684
Varicocele, 289, 290t
Vasculitis:
   disseminated, testing for, 850
   skin manifestations, 678t
Vasoactive inhibitory peptide, 99
Vasoactive intestinal peptide (VIP) [test], 102
Vasopressin. *See* Antidiuretic hormone
VDRL (Venereal Disease Research Laboratory) [test], 809–810, 810t
Venereal Disease Research Laboratory (VDRL) [test], 809–810, 810t
Venezuelan equine encephalitis, 772t
Venous admixture, 11
Ventilation, 11
   and respiratory acidosis, 19
Ventilation/perfusion matching, 11
Ventricular arrhythmias: drugs for, 348, 350, 353, 354
Ventricular tachycardia: drugs for, 355
Verapamil: drug interactions, 349, 351, 357

Verminous intoxication, 762
Verner-Morrison syndrome, 102
Verrucosa cutis, 681t
Very long chain fatty acids [test]:
    genetic disorders,
    419–420
Very low density lipoproteins, 175,
    182
    causes of secondary increases of,
        192t
    and flow chart for evaluation of
        hyperlipoproteinemias,
        186f–187f
    increased characteristics, 183t
    properties of, 174t, 174–175
    and triglycerides, 179
Very low density lipoprotein [test],
    192, 192t
Vesicles: disease, etiology, and tests
    for, 678t–679t, 686, 687f,
    692f, 694t
Vesicular lesions, 678t, 679t, 684
Vesicular stomatitis, 678t
Vibrio alginolyticus, 680t
Vibrio cholerae: gastroenteritis, 747,
    753, 753t, 754, 756
Vibrio parahaemolyticus, 680t, 682
    gastroenteritis, 753, 753t, 754,
    756
Vibrio vulnificus, 625t
Vimentin, 602
Vincent's angina, 641
VIP (vasoactive intestinal peptide)
    [test], 102
VIPomas, 102
Viral blood culture [test], 627–629,
    628t
Viral hepatitis, 68, 68t, 69, 70, 74,
    75. *See also* Hepatitis
Viral infections. *See also specific
    viruses*
    arthritis, 707
    blood. *See* Viremia
    brain abscess, 785
    bronchiolitis, 660
    CNS, 770–774, 776t, 776–777,
        780, 781–782
    ear, 637
    eye, 649, 649t, 652
    gastrointestinal tract [test],
        758–759, 759t
    lymphadenitis, 714
    pericarditis, 711–712
    pneumonia, 657, 660, 662t,
        662–663, 666, 668
    serology. *See* Viral serology
    skin, 699
    skin/tissue, 676, 683–684
    throat, 641, 642, 644

upper respiratory, 636t
urine culture [test], 729–730
urine microscopic examination
    [test], 732
Viral serology [tests], 813t, 815–825
    adenovirus, 823
    arbovirus, 815
    cytomegalovirus, 815–816
    EBV, 816–817
    enterovirus, 816
    hemorrhagic fever, 817
    hepatitis, 817–820
    HIV, 821–822
    HSV, 820–821
    HTLV-1, 822
    influenza, 823
    mumps, 822
    parainfluenza, 823–824
    parvovirus, 822–823
    rabies, 823
    respiratory infections, 823–824
    respiratory syncytial virus,
        823–824
    rubella, 824
    rubeola, 824
    VZV, 824–825
Viremia:
    blood culture [test], 627–629
    and burns, 716
    defined, 620
    testing for, 627–629
Viridans streptococci:
    and endocarditis, 623
    infections, 625t
    skin manifestations, 677t, 699
Virilization: congenital adrenal
    hyperplasia and, 271t
Virocyte, Plate 10A, 440
Visceral larva migrans, 703, 705
    eye infections, 649, 650, 651, 654,
        703
    serology [test], 832
Visceral leishmaniasis (kala azar),
    681t, 702, 704, 706
    serology, 831
Viscometer, 171
Vitamin(s), 213–216
    laboratory analysis, 215–216. *See
        also* Vitamin(s) [tests]
    recommended daily intake, 214t
    reference ranges for nutriture,
        215t
Vitamin A, 97, 213
    deficiency, 216
    recommended daily intake, 214t
    reference ranges for, 215t
    relative dose response (RDR), 217
Vitamin A [test], 216–217
Vitamin B_1, 213. *See also* Thiamin

Vitamin B_2, 213
    deficiency, 224
    recommended daily intake, 214t
Vitamin B_2 [test], 224–225
Vitamin B_6, 213
    aspartate aminotransferase [test],
        226
    deficiency, 69, 226, 227t, 448
    dependent syndromes, 227t
    recommended daily intake, 214t
    reference ranges for, 215t, 226,
        226t
    status determination, 226t
Vitamin B_6 [test], 225–227
Vitamin B_{12}, 213
    deficiency, 449, 471–475
    and folate deficiency, 472t,
        473–475, 476
    unsaturated binding capacity
        (UBBC), 227–228,
        228t
Vitamin B_{12} [tests], 227–229
    for anemia, 471–472, 472t, 473t,
        475–476
    Schilling, 96–97, 469, 472, 473t,
        475–476
Vitamin C, 213
    deficiency, 231–232
    factors affecting low levels of,
        231t
    interpretation of serum, blood,
        and leukocyte levels of,
        232t
    loading tests, 233, 233t
    recommended daily intake, 214t
    reference ranges for, 215t
Vitamin C [test], 231–233
Vitamin D, 213
    deficiency, 218, 219t
    metabolites in disease, 220t
    phosphate and, 298
    recommended daily intake, 214t
    reference ranges for, 215t
    toxicity, 219, 299
Vitamin D [test], 217–219
Vitamin D-binding protein (DEP),
    218
Vitamin E, 213
    recommended daily intake, 214t
    reference ranges for, 215t
    and selenium, 210
    toxicity, 221
Vitamin E [test], 219–221
Vitamin F. *See* Thiamin
Vitamin H. *See* Biotin
Vitamin K, 213
    deficiency, 517t, 518–519, 526,
        527, 539, 540
    recommended daily intake, 214t

Vitamin K [test], 221–222
Vitamin K dependent factors, 505, 505t, 506f, 887–888
Vitamin(s) [tests], 216–233. *See also specific vitamins*
  fat-soluble, 216–222
  water-soluble, 222–233
VMA (vanillylmandelic acid), 277, 278, 278f, 280, 281
VMA (vanillylmandelic acid) [test], 279–280
V_{max} (maximum enzymatic biotransformation), 339, 345, 345t, 346f
von Gierke's disease, 420, 421, 421t
von Willebrand factor (VWF), 499, 500f, 515f, 519, 530–531, 532, 887, 888
  antigen [test], 500f, 515t, 530–532, 533, 534
  crossed immunoelectrophoresis (VWF:CIE) [test], 533–534, 534f
  multimetric analysis [test], 534
  platelet binding of [test], 500f, 534
  platelet [test], 534
  ristocetin cofactor activity (VWF:Rcof) [test], 531t, 532, 533
  transfusions, 887, 888
von Willebrand's disease, 500f, 513, 514t, 515f, 516t, 519, 519t, 530–532, 531t, 533
  tranfusions for, 887–888
  types I/II/III, 531t, 531–532, 533, 534
Vulvovaginitis: *Candida*, 734t, 737, 738, 738t, 739
VWF. *See* von Willebrand factor
VWF:Ag [test], 500f, 515t, 530–532, 533, 534
VWF:CIE [test], 533–534, 534f
VWF:Rcof [test], 531t, 532, 533
VZV. *See* Varicella-zoster virus

W

Waldenström's macroglobulinemia, 159, 165, 171, 580, 603, 844, 856f
  protein levels and, 157t
Warfarin: drug interactions, 341, 344, 344t, 347, 349, 356, 363
Warm antibody autoimmune hemolytic anemia, 889t
Warm autoabsorption test, 892

Warm hemolytic anemia, 861
  immunohematologic testing for, 889t, 890t, 891, 892
Warts, 681t, 684, 685t
  genital, 733
Water deprivation (dehydration) [test], 295–296, 296t
Water intoxication: hypoproteinemia and, 153
Water loading [test], 295, 295t
Watson-Schwartz test, 418
Waxy casts: in urine, 51, 62f
WBC. *See* White blood cells
WBC differential, 458
Weil-Felix test, 805, 811
Weil's syndrome, 625
Well differentiated lymphocytic lymphoma (WDLL), 854
Western blot test: for HIV, 821, 822
Western equine encephalitis, 772t
Westergren ESR, 465, 465t
West Nile fever virus, 772t
Wheals: disease, etiology, and tests for, 677t–678t
Whipworm. *See Trichuris trichuria*
White blood cell screening differential [test], 586t–587t, 589–592, 590f, 591f
White blood cell slide differential [test], 583–589, 586t–587t
White blood cells (WBC). *See also specific cells*
  benign morphological abnormalities, 558t
  and bone marrow aspirates, 610611
  casts in urine, 50–51, 61f
  in cerebrospinal fluid, 108t
  count [test], 581–583, 586t–587t, 840
  differential, 458
  glycolytic action, 129
  in pleural fluid, 115, 115t
  in synovial fluid, 117t, 117–118, 119
  in urine, 49–50, 61f
White blood cell disorders, 553–581. *See also specific disorders*
  functional, 556, 559t, 560t
  malignant, 556, 559–565
  quantitative and morphologic, 554t–562t, 554–555
White blood cell [tests], 581–592
  count, 581–583
  screening differential, 586t–587t, 589–592, 590t, 591t
  slide differential, 583–589, 586t–587t

White cell count [test], 581–583, 586t–587t, 840
White piedra, 681t
Whitlow, 684
Whole blood sugar [test], 132
Whooping cough (pertussis), 645t, 646, 647
Widal test, 805, 809
Wilson's disease, 82, 200t, 204, 206, 206t
  diagnosis of, 206–209, 207f, 208t
  differential diagnosis, 208t
  genetic testing, 415–416
  protein ranges in, 156t, 169
Winterbottom sign, 775
Wintrobe ESR, 465
Wiskott-Aldrich syndrome, 442, 514t, 859
Wood alcohol [test], 377–378
World Health Organization (WHO): glucose tolerance testing criteria, 133t, 134
Wound cellulitis, 687
Wounds: disease, etiology, and tests for, 679t–680t, 689, 689f, 693f
Wuchereria bancrofti, 632, 632t, 681t

X

X-amylase deficiency, 96t
Xanthine dehydrogenase, 209
Xanthine oxidase, 209
Xanthines [tests], 361–363
  caffeine, 361
  theophylline, 361–363
Xanthochromia, 107
Xanthomonas maltophilia: tissue manifestations, 680t
Xanthurenic aciduria: and vitamin B_6, 227t
Xerophthalmia, 216
X-glucosidases deficiency, 96t
X-linked hypogammaglobulinemia, 160
X-linked hypophosphatemic rickets, 219
Xylidine, 352
D-Xylose absorption [test], 95

Y

Yaws, 679t, 681t, 810
Yeasts: in urine, 53
Yellow fever virus, 677t
  hepatitis, 702t

Yersinia enterocolitica:
    gastroenteritis, 753, 753t, 754, 755, 756
    infections, 625t
    upper respiratory infections, 645t

Yersinia pestis:
    environmental exposure, 659t
    infections, 625t
    lymphadenopathy, 715
    pneumonia and, 667, 671t
    skin manifestations, 677t

Z

Zellweger syndrome: testing for, 419

Zinc, 199
    abnormalities, 200t
    body content, 199t
    and copper deficiency, 204
    excretion route, 200t
    status in diseases, 213t
    toxicity, 200t, 211

Zinc [test], 211–213

Zinc deficiency, 71, 200t, 211
    and prealbumin, 165

Zinc protoporphyrin (ZnPP) [test], 470–471

Zollinger-Ellison syndrome, 99, 100, 100t, 302, 321, 363

Zomax: hemolytic anemia from, 894t

Z protein, 166

Zwitter ions, 143

Zygomycetes:
    and burn wounds, 716
    cultures, 697t
    and endocarditis, 626t
    fungemia, 625
    morphologic characteristics, 671t
    pulmonary infection, 668, 671t
    sinusitis, 640
    upper respiratory infections, 645t

ZZAP reagent, 892